The GALE
ENCYCLOPEDIA of
ALTERNATIVE
MEDICINE

The GALE ENCYCLOPEDIA of ALTERNATIVE MEDICINE

THIRD EDITION

VOLUME

1

A–C

LAURIE J. FUNDUKIAN, EDITOR

GALE
CENGAGE Learning·

Detroit • New York • San Francisco • New Haven, Conn • Waterville, Maine • London

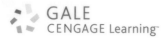
GALE
CENGAGE Learning™

**Gale Encyclopedia of Alternative Medicine,
Third Edition**

Project Editor: Laurie J. Fundukian

Editorial: Donna Batten, Amy Kwolek, Brigham
Narins, Jeffrey Wilson

Product Manager: Kate Hanley

Editorial Support Services: Andrea Lopeman

Indexing Services: Factiva, a Dow Jones Company

Rights Acquisition and Management: Robyn V.
Young

Composition: Evi Abou-El-Seoud, Mary Beth
Trimper

Manufacturing: Wendy Blurton, Dorothy Maki

Imaging: Lezlie Light

Product Design: Pam Galbreath

For product information and technology assistance, contact us at
Gale Customer Support, 1-800-877-4253.
For permission to use material from this text or product,
submit all requests online at **www.cengage.com/permissions.**
Further permissions questions can be emailed to
permissionrequest@cengage.com

While every effort has been made to ensure the reliability of the information presented in this publication, Gale, a part of Cengage Learning, does not guarantee the accuracy of the data contained herein. Gale accepts no payment for listing; and inclusion in the publication of any organization, agency, institution, publication, service, or individual does not imply endorsement of the editors or publisher. Errors brought to the attention of the publisher and verified to the satisfaction of the publisher will be corrected in future editions.

Library of Congress Cataloging-in-Publication Data

The Gale encyclopedia of alternative medicine, 3rd ed. / edited by Laurie J. Fundukian, editor.
    p. cm. --
    Includes bibliographical references and index.
    ISBN 978-1-4144-4872-5 (set) -- ISBN 978-1-4144-4873-2 (vol. 1) --
ISBN 978-1-4144-4874-9 (vol. 2) -- ISBN 978-1-4144-4875-6 (vol. 3) --
ISBN 978-1-4144-4876-3 (vol. 4)
    1. Alternative medicine--Encyclopedias. I. Fundukian, Laurie J. II. Title: Encyclopedia of alternative medicine.
    [DNLM: 1. Complementary Therapies--Encyclopedias--English. 2. Internal Medicine--Encyclopedias--English. WB 13 G1508 2009]

R733.G34 2009
615.5'03--dc22   2008016097

Gale
27500 Drake Rd.
Farmington Hills, MI, 48331-3535

ISBN-13: 978-1-4144-4872-5 (set)   ISBN-10: 1-4144-4872-4 (set)
ISBN-13: 978-1-4144-4873-2 (vol. 1)   ISBN-10: 1-4144-4873-2 (vol. 1)
ISBN-13: 978-1-4144-4874-9 (vol. 2)   ISBN-10: 1-4144-4874-0 (vol. 2)
ISBN-13: 978-1-4144-4875-6 (vol. 3)   ISBN-10: 1-4144-4875-9 (vol. 3)
ISBN-13: 978-1-4144-4876-3 (vol. 4)   ISBN-10: 1-4144-4876-7 (vol. 4)

This title is also available as an e-book.
ISBN-13: 978-1-4144-4877-0 ISBN-10: 1-4144-4877-5
Contact your Gale, a part of Cengage Learning sales representative for ordering information.

Printed in China
1 2 3 4 5 6 7 12 11 10 09 08

CONTENTS

LIST OF ENTRIES

A

Abscess
Acidophilus
Acne
Aconite
Acupressure
Acupuncture
Ademetionine
Adie's pupil
African pygeum
Agastache
Aging
AIDS
Alcoholism
Alexander technique
Alfalfa
Alisma
Allergies
Allium cepa
Aloe
Alpha-hydroxy
Alzheimer's disease
Amenorrhea
Amino acids
Andrographis
Androstenedione
Anemarrhena
Anemia
Angelica root
Angina
Anise
Ankylosing spondylitis
Anorexia nervosa

Anthroposophical medicine
Anti-inflammatory diet
Antioxidants
Anxiety
Apis
Apitherapy
Apple cider vinegar
Applied kinesiology
Apricot seed
Arginine
Arka
Arnica
Aromatherapy
Arrowroot
Arsenicum album
Artichoke
Art therapy
Ashwaganda
Asthma
Astigmatism
Aston-Patterning
Astragalus
Atherosclerosis
Athlete's foot
Atkins diet
Atractylodes (white)
Attention-deficit hyperactivity
  disorder
Aucklandia
Auditory integration training
Aura therapy
Auriculotherapy
Autism
Ayurvedic medicine

B

Bach flower essences
Bad breath
Balm of Gilead
Barberry
Barley grass
Bates method
Bayberry
Bedsores
Bedwetting
Bee pollen
Behavioral therapy
Behavioral optometry
Belladonna
Beta-hydroxy
Beta-methylbutyric acid
Beta carotene
Betaine hydrochloride
Bhakti yoga
Bilberry
Binge eating disorder
Biofeedback
Bioflavonoids
Bioidentical hormone
  therapy
Biota
Biotherapeutic drainage
Biotin
Bipolar disorder
Bird flu
Bites and stings
Bitter melon
Bitters
Black cohosh

Creatine
Crohn's disease
Croup
Crystal healing
Cupping
Curanderismo
Curcumin
Cuscuta
Cuts and scratches
Cymatic therapy
Cyperus

D

Damiana
Dance therapy
Dandelion
Dandruff
Deglycyrrhizanated licorice
Dementia
Depression
Dermatitis
Detoxification
Devil's claw
DHEA
Diabetes mellitus
Diamond diet
Diaper rash
Diarrhea
Diathermy
Diets
Digestive enzymes
Digitalis
Diverticulitis
Dizziness
Dolomite
Dong quai
Dry mouth
Dysbiosis
Dyslexia
Dysmenorrhea

E

Ear infection
Earache

Echinacea
Eczema
Edema
Elder
Electroacupuncture
Elimination diet
Emphysema
Endometriosis
Energy medicine
Environmental therapy
Enzyme therapy
Ephedra
Epididymitis
Epilepsy
Epimedium
Escharotic treatment
Essential fatty acids
Essential oils
Essiac tea
Eucalyptus
Eucommia bark
Eupatorium
Euphrasia
Evening primrose oil
Evodia fruit
Exercise
Eyebright

F

Facial massage
Fasting
Fatigue
Feldenkrais
Feng shui
Fennel
Fenugreek
Ferrum phosphoricum
Fever
Feverfew
Fibrocystic breast disease
Fibromyalgia
Fish oil
5-HTP
Flaxseed
Flower remedies
Fo ti

Folic acid
Food poisoning
Foxglove
Fractures
French green clay
Fritillaria
Frostbite and frostnip
Fructooligosaccharides
Fungal infections

G

Gallstones
Gamma-linoleic acid
Gangrene
Ganoderma
Garcinia
Gardenia
Garlic
Gas
Gastritis
Gastrodia
Gastroenteritis
Gelsemium
Genital herpes
Genital warts
Gentiana
Geriatric massage
Gerson therapy
Ginger
Ginkgo biloba
Ginseng, Siberian
Ginseng, American
Ginseng, Korean
Glaucoma
Glucosamine
Glutamine
Glutathione
Goldenrod
Goldenseal
Gonorrhea
Gotu kola
Gout
Grains-of-paradise fruit
Grape skin
Grape seed extract
Grapefruit seed extract

Leukemia
Lice infestation
Licorice
Light therapy
Linoleic acid
Lipase
Livingston-Wheeler therapy
Lobelia
Lomatium
Lomilomi
Lou Gehrig's disease
Low back pain
Lung cancer
Lutein
Lycium fruit
Lycopene
Lycopodium
Lycopus
Lyme disease
Lymphatic drainage
Lysimachia
Lysine

M

Macrobiotic diet
Macular degeneration
Magnesium
Magnetic therapy
Magnolia
Maitake
Malaria
Malignant lymphoma
Manganese
Mangosteen
Manuka honey
Marijuana
Marsh mallow
Martial arts
Massage therapy
McDougall diet
Measles
Meditation
Mediterranean diet
Medium-chain triglycerides
Melatonin
Memory loss

Méniére's disease
Meningitis
Menopause
Menstruation
Mercurius vivus
Mesoglycan
Metabolic therapies
Methionine
Mexican yam
Migraine headache
Milk thistle
Mind/Body medicine
Mistletoe
Mononucleosis
Morning sickness
Motherwort
Motion sickness
Movement therapy
Moxibustion
MSM
Mugwort leaf
Mullein
Multiple chemical sensitivity
Multiple sclerosis
Mumps
Muscle spasms and cramps
Music therapy
Myopia
Myotherapy
Myrrh

N

Narcolepsy
Native American medicine
Natrum muriaticum
Natural hygiene diet
Natural hormone replacement
  therapy
Naturopathic medicine
Nausea
Neck pain
Neem
Nettle
Neural therapy
Neuralgia
Neurolinguistic programming

Niacin
Night blindness
Noni
Nosebleeds
Notoginseng root
Nutmeg
Nutrition
Nux vomica

O

Oak
Obesity
Obsessive-compulsive disorder
Omega-3 fatty acids
Omega-6 fatty acids
Ophiopogon
Oregano essential oil
Ornish diet
Ortho-bionomy
Orthomolecular medicine
Osha
Osteoarthritis
Osteopathy
Osteoporosis
Ovarian cancer
Ovarian cysts
Oxygen/Ozone therapy

P

Pain
Paleolithic diet
Panchakarma
Pancreatitis
Panic disorder
Pantothenic acid
Parasitic infections
Parkinson's disease
Parsley
Passionflower
Past-life therapy
Pau d'arco
Pelvic inflammatory disease

PLEASE READ—IMPORTANT INFORMATION

INTRODUCTION

The Gale Encyclopedia of Alternative Medicine (GEAM) is a one-stop source for alternative medical information that covers complementary therapies, herbs and remedies, and common medical diseases and conditions. It avoids medical jargon when possible, making it easier for the layperson to use. *The Gale Encyclopedia of Alternative Medicine* presents authoritative, balanced information and is more comprehensive than single-volume family medical guides.

Scope

More than 800 full-length articles are included in *The Gale Encyclopedia of Alternative Medicine*. Many prominent figures are highlighted as sidebar biographies that accompany the therapy entries. Articles follow a standardized format that provides information at a glance. Rubrics include:

Therapies

- Origins
- Benefits
- Description
- Preparations
- Precautions
- Side effects
- Research and general acceptance
- Resources
- Key terms

Herbs/remedies

- General use
- Preparations
- Precautions
- Side effects
- Interactions
- Resources
- Key terms

Diseases/conditions

- Definition
- Description
- Causes and symptoms
- Diagnosis
- Treatment
- Allopathic treatment
- Expected results
- Prevention
- Resources
- Key terms

Inclusion criteria

A preliminary list of therapies, herbs, remedies, diseases, and conditions was compiled from a wide variety of sources, including professional medical guides and textbooks, as well as consumer guides and encyclopedias. The advisory board, made up of three medical and alternative healthcare experts, evaluated the topics and made suggestions for inclusion. Final selection of topics to include was made by the medical advisors in conjunction with Gale editors.

About the Contributors

The essays were compiled by experienced medical writers, including alternative healthcare practitioners and educators, pharmacists, nurses, and other complementary healthcare professionals. *GEAM* medical advisors reviewed more than 95% of the completed essays to insure that they are appropriate, up-to-date, and medically accurate.

How to Use this Book

The Gale Encyclopedia of Alternative Medicine has been designed with ready reference in mind:

• Straight **alphabetical arrangement** allows users to locate information quickly.

• Bold faced terms function as *print hyperlinks* that point the reader to related entries in the encyclopedia.

• A list of **key terms** is provided where appropriate to define unfamiliar words or concepts used within the context of the essay. Additional terms may be found in the **glossary**.

• **Cross-references** placed throughout the encyclopedia direct readers to where information on subjects without their own entries can be found. Synonyms are also cross-referenced.

• A **Resources section** directs users to sources of further complementary medical information.

• An appendix of alternative medical organizations is arranged by type of therapy and includes valuable **contact information**.

• A comprehensive **general index** allows users to easily target detailed aspects of any topic, including Latin names.

Graphics

The Gale Encyclopedia of Alternative Medicine is enhanced with more than 400 images, including photos, tables, and customized line drawings.

ADVISORS

An advisory board made up of prominent individuals from complementary medical communities provided invaluable assistance in the formulation of this encyclopedia. They defined the scope of coverage and reviewed individual entries for accuracy and accessibility. We would therefore like to express our appreciation to them:

Mirka Knaster, PhD
author, editor, consultant in
*   Eastern and Western body-mind*
*   disciplines and spiritual traditions*
Oakland, CA

Diana Quinn, ND
Naturopathic Women's
*   Healthcare, Ann Arbor, MI*
Ann Arbor, MI

Suzanna M. Zick, ND, MPH
University of Michigan
*   Department of Family Medicine*
Ann Arbor, MI

CONTRIBUTORS

Margaret Alic, PhD
Medical Writer
Eastsound, WA

Greg Annussek
Medical Writer
American Society of Journalists
 and Authors
New York, NY

Barbara Boughton
Health and Medical Writer
El Cerrito, CA

Ruth Ann Prag Carter
Freelance Writer
Farmington Hills, MI

Linda Chrisman
*Massage Therapist and
 Educator*
Medical Writer
Oakland, CA

Rhonda Cloos, RN
Medical writer and Nurse
Austin, TX

Gloria Cooksey, CNE
Medical Writer
Sacramento, CA

Amy Cooper, MA, MSI
Medical Writer
Vermillion, SD

Angela Costello
Medical Writer
Northfield, OH

Sharon Crawford
Writer, Editor, Researcher
American Medical Writers
 Association

Periodical Writers Association of
 Canada and the
 Editors' Association of Canada
Toronto, ONT Canada

Sandra Bain Cushman
Massage Therapist
*Alexander Technique Practitioner
 and Educator*
Charlottesville, VA

Helen Davidson
Medical Writer
Portland, OR

Tish Davidson, MA
Medical Writer
Fremont, CA

Lori DeMilto, MJ
Medical Writer
Sicklerville, NJ

Doug Dupler, MA
Medical Writer
Boulder, CO

Paula Ford-Martin, PhD
Medical Writer
Warwick, RI

Rebecca J. Frey, PhD
Medical Writer
New Haven, CT

Lisa Frick
Medical Writer
Columbia, MO

Kathleen Goss
Medical Writer
Darwin, CA

Elliot Greene, MA
*Former President, American
 Massage Therapy Association*

Massage Therapist
Silver Spring, MD

Peter Gregutt
Medical Writer
Asheville, NC

Clare Hanrahan
Medical Writer
Asheville, NC

David Helwig
Medical Writer
London, ONT Canada

Beth A. Kapes
Medical Writer, Editor
Bay Village, OH

Katherine Kim
Medical Writer
Oakland, CA

Erika Lenz
Medical Writer
Lafayette, CO

Lorraine Lica, PhD
Medical Writer
San Diego, CA

Whitney Lowe, LMT
Massage Therapy Educator
Orthopedic Massage
 Education & Research
 Institute
Bend, OR

Mary McNulty
Freelance Writer
St.Charles, IL

Leslie Mertz
Medical Writer, Biologist
Kalkaska, MI

Katherine E. Nelson, ND
Naturopathic Physician
Naples, FL

David E. Newton, Ed.D.
Medical Writer
Ashland, OR

Teresa Odle
Medical Writer
Ute Park, NM

Jodi Ohlsen Read
Medical Writer
Carver, MN

Carole Osborne-Sheets
*Massage Therapist and
    Educator*
Medical Writer
Poway, CA

Lee Ann Paradise
Medical Writer
Lubbock, TX

Patience Paradox
Medical Writer
Bainbridge Island, WA

Belinda Rowland, PhD
Medical Writer
Voorheesville, NY

Joan M. Schonbeck, RN
Medical Writer
Marlborough, MA

Gabriele Schubert, MS
Medical Writer
San Diego, CA

Kim Sharp, M Ln
Medical Writer
Houston, TX

Kathy Shepard Stolley, PhD
Medical Writer
Virginia Beach, VA

Judith Sims, MS
Science Writer
Logan, UT

Patricia Skinner
Medical Writer
Amman, Jordan

Genevieve Slomski, PhD
Medical Writer
New Britain, CT

Jane E. Spear
Medical Writer
Canton, OH

Liz Swain
Medical Writer
San Diego, CA

Judith Turner, DVM
Medical Writer
Sandy, UT

Samuel Uretsky, PharmD
Medical Writer
Wantagh, NY

Ken R. Wells
Science Writer
Laguna Hills, CA

Angela Woodward
Science Writer
Madison, WI

Kathleen Wright, RN
Medical Writer
Delmar, DE

Jennifer L. Wurges
Medical Writer
Rochester Hills, MI

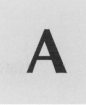

A

Abdominal pain *see* **Stomachaches**

Abscess

Definition

An abscess is a place of accumulation of the creamy white, yellow, or greenish fluid, known as pus, surrounded by reddened tissue. It is the result of the body's inflammatory response to a foreign body or a bacterial, viral, parasitic, or fungal infection. An abscess usually dries out and resolves when it is drained of pus. The most common parts of the body affected by abscesses are the face, armpits, arms and legs, rectum, sebaceous glands (oil glands), and the breast during lactation.

Description

Most abscesses are septic, which means they are the result of an infection. Abscesses occur when white blood cells (WBCs) gather in response to an infection. They produce oxidants (for example, superoxide radical) and enzymes to digest the invading bacteria, viruses, parasites, or fungi. The infective agents are then broken down by the WBCs into small pieces that can be transported through the bloodstream and eliminated from the body. Unfortunately, the enzymes may also digest part of the body's tissues along with the infective agents. The resulting liquid of this digestion is pus, which contains the remains of the infective agents, tissue, white blood cells, and enzymes.

A sterile abscess is one that is not produced by an infection. It is caused by irritants, such as foreign bodies or injected drugs, and medications that have not been totally absorbed. Sterile abscesses quite often heal into hardened scar tissue.

Common types of abscesses

- Boils and carbuncles. Sebaceous glands and superficial skin are the places usually infected.
- Dental abscess. An abscess that develops along the root of a tooth.
- Pilonidal abscess. People who have a birth defect involving a tiny opening in the skin just above the anus may have fecal bacteria enter this opening, causing an infection and a subsequent abscess.
- Retropharyngeal, parapharyngeal, peritonsillar abscess. As a result of throat infections like strep throat and tonsillitis, bacteria invade the deeper tissues of the throat and cause a parapharyngeal or peritonsillar abscess. A retropharyngeal abscess is a result of something usually blood-borne, and not from a direct spread of tonsillitis. These abscesses can compromise swallowing and even breathing.
- Lung abscess. During or after pneumonia, an abscess can develop as a complication.
- Liver abscess. Bacteria, parasites, or amoeba from the intestines can spread through the blood to the liver and cause abscesses.
- Psoas abscess. An abscess can develop in the psoas muscles, when an infection spreads from the appendix, the large intestine, or the fallopian tubes.
- Butin abscess. Any blood-borne organism feeding off bacteria that stimulate pus production (pyogenic organisms). Can cause abscesses in possibly many sites.

Causes and symptoms

Many different agents cause abscesses. The most common are the pyogenic, or pus-forming bacteria, such as *Staphylococcus aureus,* which is nearly always the cause of abscesses directly under the skin. Abscesses are usually caused by organisms that normally inhabit

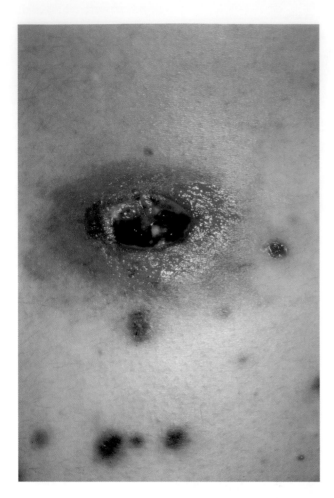

Methicillin resistant *Staphylococcus aureus* skin abscess.
(© Scott Camazine / Alamy)

nearby structures or that infect them. For example, abscesses around the anus may be caused by any of the numerous bacteria found within the large intestine. Brain abscesses and liver abscesses are caused by the bacteria, amoeba, and fungi that are able to travel there through circulation.

Symptoms of an abscess are the general signs of inflammation. Symptoms that identify superficial abscesses include heat, redness, swelling, and **pain** over the affected area. Abscesses in other places may produce only generalized symptoms, such as **fever** and discomfort. A sterile abscess may present as painful lump deep under the site of an injection. A severe infection may bring on fever, **fatigue**, weight loss, and **chills**. Recurrent abscesses may indicate undiscovered **allergies** or decreased immune functioning.

Diagnosis

A general physical examination and a detailed patient history are used to diagnose an abscess. Recent or chronic disease or dysfunction in an organ suggests it may be the site of an abscess. Pain and tenderness on physical examination are common findings. There may also be a leakage of pus from a sinus tract connected to an abscess deep in the body tissue.

Treatment

Bentonite clay packs with a small amount of **goldenseal** powder (*Hydrastis canandensis*) can be placed on the site of a superficial abscess and used to draw out the infection. **Tea tree oil** (*Melaleuca* spp.) and **garlic** (*Allium sativa*) directly applied to abscesses may also help to clear them.

Applications of a hot compress to the skin over the abscess will hasten the draining or the reabsorption of the abscess. Contrast **hydrotherapy**, using alternating hot and cold compresses, can also be used. Additionally, localized warm/hot soaks three to five times daily frequently brings an abscess to heal.

Homeopathic remedies that can be taken to help diminish abscess formation include **belladonna**, **silica**, Hepar sulphuris, and **calendula**. Also, **acupuncture** may be recommended to help treat pain caused by an abscess. In addition, vitamins A and C, beta-carotene, **zinc**, liquid chlorophyll, and garlic are useful as supportive daily nutrients to help clear up abscesses.

Allopathic treatment

Often, the pus of an abscess must be drained by a physician. Ordinarily, the body will handle the remaining infection. Sometimes antibiotics are prescribed. The doctor may often put a piece of cloth or rubber, called a drain, in the cavity of the abscess to prevent it from closing until all the pus has drained.

Expected results

Once the abscess is properly drained, it should clear up in a few days. Any underlying diseases will determine the overall outcome of the condition. Recurrent abscesses, especially those on the skin, return due to either defective/altered immunity, or staph overgrowth, where there is high bacterial colonization on the skin. The patient should consult a physician for treatment with which to wash the skin areas, and treatment to eradicate colonization.

If the abscess ruptures into neighboring areas or if the infectious agent spills into the bloodstream, serious consequences are likely. Abscesses in and around the nasal sinuses, face, ears, and scalp may spread the infection into the brain. Abscesses in the abdominal cavity, such as in the liver, may rupture into that cavity. **Blood poisoning**, or septicemia, is an infection that has spilled into the bloodstream and then spreads throughout the body. These are emergency situations where the patient needs to be seen by a physician as soon as possible.

It is important to take note that abscesses in the hand may be more serious than they might appear. Due to the intricate structure and the overriding importance of the hand, any hand infection must be treated promptly and competently.

Prevention

Infections that are treated early with heat, if superficial, or antibiotics, if deeper, will often resolve without the formation of an abscess. It is even better to avoid infections altogether by promptly cleaning and irrigating open injuries, particularly **bites** and puncture **wounds**.

Resources

BOOKS

Bennett, J. Claude, and Fred Plum, ed. *Cecil Textbook of Medicine*. Philadelphia: W. B. Saunders Co., 1996. (Lee Goldman and Dennis Ausiello, ed. *Cecil Medicine*. [2008]. 23rd ed.)

Duke, James A., et al. *The Green Pharmacy*. Pennsylvania: Rodale, 1997.

Isselbacher, Kurt, et al, ed. *Harrison's Principles of Internal Medicine*. New York: McGraw–Hill, 1997. (Anthony S. Fauci . . . [et al.] [2008]. 17th ed.)

Tierney, Jr., Lawrence M., et al, ed. *Current Medical Diagnosis and Treatment*. Connecticut: Appleton & Lange, 1996.

OTHER

AlternativeMedicine.com. http://www.alternativemedicine. com (December 28, 2000).

Patience Paradox

Absinthe *see* **Wormwood**

Aches and pains *see* **Pain**

Acidophilus

Description

Lactobacillus acidophilus, commonly referred to simply as acidophilus, is a friendly inhabitant of the gastrointestinal (GI) tract. It, as well as some related strains of bacteria, is known as a probiotic. Probiotic organisms secrete enzymes that support healthy digestion. They keep the flora of the intestines and vagina balanced and compete with some pathogenic organisms. When the probiotic population of the body is severely decreased, as can occur with treatment by many antibiotics, yeasts and harmful bacteria may take over and cause illness. Normal and healthy amounts of acidophilus can also be decreased by chronic **diarrhea**, **stress**, **infections**, and poor diet.

The species of *Lactobacilli* that inhabit the GI tract cause an increase of acidity. The bacteria do this by producing lactic acid from milk sugar (lactose). The increased acidity may promote the absorption of **calcium**, as well as of some other minerals. Lowered pH also discourages the growth of many pathogenic species of bacteria and yeasts. The hydrogen peroxide produced by the acidophilus helps to suppress pathogens.

Acidophilus may function in the production of some of the B vitamins, such as **niacin**, **pyridoxine**, **biotin**, and **folic acid**.

General use

Yeast infections

Acidophilus may be used to reduce susceptibility to vaginal yeast infections, which are quite common. Symptoms including **itching**, burning, inflammation, and discharge occur due to an overgrowth of the yeast *Candida albicans*, which is part of the normal vaginal flora. Some women are more prone to yeast infections than others. Antibiotics destroy the normal probiotic flora, and may lead to yeast infections. High sugar levels are another predisposing factor. Diabetics, who tend to have high blood sugar, and persons who consume a processed diet that is high in sugar have more frequent problems with yeast as well. The hormonal states created by **pregnancy** or the use of oral contraceptives also contribute to yeast infections. IUD users can have an increased rate of infection. In rare cases, *Candida* is sexually transmitted and both partners may require treatment in order to control repeated overgrowth. Anyone who has **AIDS** or any other condition causing immunosuppression has increased susceptibility to *Candida* and other types of

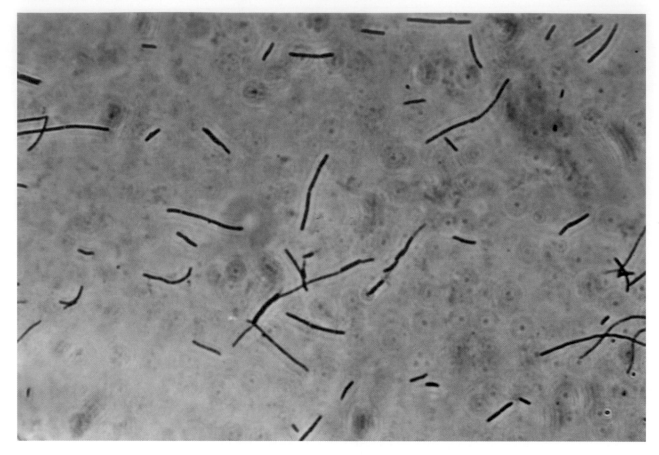

Photomicrograph of *Lactobacillus acidophilus*. This bacterium is considered to be beneficial to health and is part of the normal flora of the gastrointestinal and genitourinary tracts. It is found in yogurt and other dairy products. *(PHOTOTAKE Inc. / Alamy)*

infections. Acidophilus is one of the organisms that competes with *Candida* and decreases its population. Many studies have shown that oral and topical use (by douching) of acidophilus are effective to prevent and treat this condition.

Systemic candidiasis, or yeast hypersensitivity syndrome, is a condition that is not recognized by many allopaths. It is acknowledged by some practitioners of alternative and complementary medicine as a problem with broad-ranging consequences. This theory holds that some people have an allergic reaction to the yeast and/or its toxins, and that they can experience serious symptoms when the organism multiplies in the body to an abnormal degree. **Fatigue**, diarrhea, **constipation**, muscle **pain**, thrush, itching, mood changes, endocrine dysfunction, headaches, and tingling or numbness of the extremities are some of the symptoms that are reportedly associated with systemic candidiasis. A weak immune system may be more prone to allowing yeast to multiply, and large numbers of yeast can act to further suppress the immune function. Acidophilus, in combination with such nutritional supplements as **essential fatty acids**, is often recommended for the prevention and treatment of this syndrome.

Gastrointestinal disorders

Irritable bowel syndrome (IBS) is a functional disturbance of the lower intestine that can cause bloating, cramping, abdominal pain, diarrhea, constipation, and painful bowel movements. This condition is also known as spastic colon. One small study of the use of acidophilus to treat IBS showed more improvement in the treated group than in those who took a placebo. This evidence is not conclusive evidence, but in view of the safety of the treatment and the scarcity of effective alternatives, acidophilus may be worth trying.

Traveler's diarrhea is sometimes suffered by people who consume contaminated food or water in other countries. Some evidence shows that regular use of acidophilus and other **probiotics** may prevent this condition. Two clinical studies published in 2007 reported that probiotics, including acidophilus, can be effective in treating IBS and in preventing and treating mild to moderate ulcerative **colitis** (UC), an inflammation of the walls of the bowel accompanied by the formation of ulcers. The condition can result in permanent bowel damage. One of the studies also showed probiotics appear to be useful in preventing and treating pouchitis, an acute infection in part of the intestines of patients who have undergone an ileostomy (removal of a pouch at the end of the small intestine) and restorative complete colectomy (removal of all four parts of the colon). Both studies concluded there is no evidence to suggest probiotics are effective in treating Crohn's disease, an immune system disorder that effects the small intestine that sometimes spreads to the colon.

High cholesterol levels

Recent evidence suggests that consuming *Lactobacillus acidophilus L1* can be effective in lowering blood **cholesterol**. The February 1999 issue of the *Journal of the American College of Nutrition* reports on two studies done at the University of Kentucky. Subjects who consumed the yogurt containing *L. acidophilus L1* had cholesterol levels drop by 2.4% in one study and 3.2% in the other. Although the percentages are small, the effect on the risk of **heart disease** could be significant.

Immune response

A study published in the December 1998 issue of the *Brazilian Journal of Medical and Biological Research* found that acidophilus induced a nonspecific immune response in experimental mice. Acidophilus is sometimes recommended as an immune booster for people, although as of 2008 the effect has not yet been documented in humans.

Other uses

Acidophilus may possibly be helpful in the treatment of **canker sores**, **feverblisters**, **hives**, and adolescent **acne**. Its use has also been suggested as a preventative for colon **cancer**. Some evidence suggests that acidophilus may reduce the risk of developing an allergic reaction, including **asthma**, **hay fever**, and skin reactions, such as **eczema**. In fact, some early evidence suggests that if mothers who have at least one relative with asthma, or some other allergy-related illness, take this probiotic while pregnant and breastfeeding, their babies may be less likely to develop asthma. Clinical studies also have shown acidophilus can help treat respiratory (lung) infections, including sinusitis, **bronchitis**, and **pneumonia**, according to the University of Maryland Medical Center.

KEY TERMS

Candidiasis—Any of a variety of infections caused by fungi of the genus *Candida*.

Complete colectomy—The surgical removal of all four parts of the colon.

Crohn's disease—An immune system disorder that effects the small intestine that sometimes spreads to the colon.

Ileostomy—The removal of a pouch at the end of the small intestine.

Irritable bowel syndrome—A functional disturbance of the lower intestine that can cause bloating, cramping, abdominal pain, diarrhea, constipation, and painful bowel movements.

Pouchitis—An acute infection in part of the intestines of patients who have undergone an ileostomy and a complete colectomy.

Probiotic—Any strain of bacteria that lives in the human gut and is considered a "friendly" bacterium. Probiotics secrete enzymes that help to keep the digestive system balanced, and compete with some pathogenic organisms. Acidophilus is one of the best-known probiotics.

Traveler's diarrhea—Diarrhea caused by ingesting local bacteria to which one's digestive system has not yet adapted.

Ulcerative colitis—An inflammation of the walls of the bowel accompanied by the formation of ulcers. The condition can result in permanent bowel damage.

Preparations

Acidophilus is taken by mouth. It is available as powder, liquid, tablets, or capsules, and is also present in some types of milk, kefir, yogurt, and some cheeses. Frozen yogurt does not contain live probiotics. Check product labels to see whether live organisms are present. The bacteria are killed by pasteurization. Probiotic products are most potent when kept refrigerated. The potency of a given preparation is usually expressed as the number of organisms per capsule. A usual dose of acidophilus is 1–10 billion organisms, divided into three doses per day.

Precautions

People who are lactose-intolerant may not tolerate acidophilus.

Side effects

The initial use of acidophilus may cause an increase in intestinal **gas**, which decreases with continued use of the product.

Interactions

Taking acidophilus in conjunction with some antibiotics, including ampicillin (Amcill, Ampicin) and amoxicillin (Amoxil, Novamoxin), can prevent the diarrhea that is sometimes caused by their use. One clinical study suggests that acidophilus speeds up the metabolism of sulfasalazine, a medication used to treat ulcerative colitis. The significance of this information is unknown, according to the University of Maryland Medical Center.

Resources

BOOKS

Huffnagle, Gary B., and Sarah Wernick. *The Probiotics Revolution: The Definitive Guide to Safe, Natural Health Solutions Using Probiotic and Prebiotic Foods and Supplements.* New York: Bantam, 2007.

Taylor, John R., and Deborah Mitchell. *The Wonder of Probiotics: A 30-Day Plan to Boost Energy, Enhance Weight Loss, Heal GI Problems, Prevent Disease, and Slow Aging.* New York: St. Martin's Griffin, 2007.

PERIODICALS

Gaby, Alan R. "*Lactobacillus acidophilus* Douche for Bacterial Vaginosis." *Townsend Letter: The Examiner of Alternative Medicine* (October 2007): 50.

Gionchetti, Paolo P., et al. "Antibiotics and Probiotics in Treatment of Inflammatory Bowel Disease." *World Journal of Gastroenterology* (June 2006): 3306–3313.

Hedin, C., et al. "Evidence for the Use of Probiotics and Prebiotics in Inflammatory Bowel Disease: A Review of Clinical Trials." *Proceedings of the Nutrition Society* (August 2007): 307–315.

Moon, Kenneth T. "Does *Lactobacillus acidophilus* Prevent Traveler's Diarrhea?" *American Family Physician* (March 15, 2007): 916.

ORGANIZATIONS

Agriculture and Agri-Foods Canada. Sir John Carling Building, 930 Carling Ave., Ottawa, ON K1A 0C7 Canada. (613) 759-1000. http://www.agr.gc.ca.

Food and Drug Administration. 5600 Fishers Lane, Rockville, MD 20857. (888) 463-6332. http://www.fda.gov.

Nutrition Society. 10 Cambridge Court, 210 Shepherds Bush Road, London W6 7NJ Great Britain. (44) 020-7602-0228. http://www.nutsoc.org.uk.

Judith Turner
Ken R. Wells

Acne

Definition

Acne is a common inflammatory skin disease characterized by pimples on the face, chest, and back. It occurs when the pores of the skin become clogged with oil, dead skin cells, and/or bacteria.

Description

Acne vulgaris, the medical term for common acne, is the most common skin disease. It affects nearly 17 million people in the United States. While acne can occur at any age, it usually begins at puberty and worsens during adolescence. Nearly 85% of people develop acne some time between the ages of 12 and 25 years old. Up to 20% of women develop mild acne. It is also found in some newborns.

The sebaceous glands lie just beneath the skin's surface. They produce sebum, an oily secretion that helps to preserve the flexibility of the hair and moisturizes the skin. These glands and the hair follicles within which they are found are called sebaceous follicles. These follicles open onto the skin through pores that allow the sebum to reach the hair shaft and the skin. In certain situations, the glands excrete excess sebum that cannot be cleared from the pores efficiently. This excess happens, for instance, at puberty when increased levels of the androgen hormones cause overproduction of sebum. In addition, cells lining the follicle are shed too quickly and begin to clump together. The excess sebum combines with the dead cells and forms a plug, or comedo (also called comedones), which is not usually seen, that blocks the pore. When the follicle begins to bulge and show up as a small whitish bump mostly under the skin, it is called a whitehead. If the comedo opens up, the top surface of the plug darkens, and it is referred to as a blackhead.

Infection results when a plugged follicle is invaded by *Propionibacterium acnes,* a bacterium that normally lives on the skin, and possibly other microorganisms. The bacterium produces chemicals and enzymes that bring on inflammation. Pimples are the result of infected blackheads or whiteheads that rupture, releasing sebum, bacteria, dead skin, and white blood cells onto the surrounding tissues. Inflamed pimples near the skin's surface are called papules; they are red and raised and may be quite tender to the touch. The papules may become filled with pus and are then called pustules. If the follicle continues to enlarge rather than rupture, it forms a closed sac, called a cyst, which can be felt as a lump under the skin. Large hard swellings deep within the skin are called nodules. Both nodules and cysts may cause **pain** and scarring.

Causes and symptoms

The exact cause of acne is mostly unknown. One exception is the occurrence of acne in women as a result of excess male hormone production, which is diagnosed by excessive growth of hair, especially in places not usual on a female, called hirsuitism; irregular menstrual cycles; and premenstrual flare-ups of acne. A 2001 study demonstrated that menstrual cycle does affect acne. Surprisingly, the study revealed that 53% of women over age 33 experienced a higher premenstrual acne rate than women under age 20.

Many alternative practitioners assert that acne is often related to a condition of toxicity in the intestines or liver. This condition may be due to the presence of bacteria such as *Clostridia spp.* and *Yersinia enterocolitica,* a result of a low-fiber diet; a lack of friendly gut flora such as *Lactobacillus spp.*; an intestinal overgrowth of *Candida albicans*; and food **allergies**.

The interaction between the body's hormones, skin protein, skin secretions, and bacteria determines the course of acne. Several other factors have also been shown to affect the condition:

- Age. Teenagers are more likely than any other age group to develop acne.
- Gender. Boys have more severe acne and develop it more often than girls.
- Disease. Hormonal disorders can complicate acne in girls.
- Heredity. Individuals with a family history of acne have greater susceptibility to the condition.
- Hormonal changes. Acne can flare up before menstruation, during pregnancy, and menopause.
- Diet. Although they are not the primary cause of acne, certain foods may bring on flare-ups or make the condition worse.
- Drugs. Acne can be a side effect of using antibiotics, oral contraceptives, and anabolic steroids.
- Personal hygiene. Use of abrasive soaps, hard scrubbing of the face, or handling pimples will often make them worse.
- Cosmetics. Oil-based makeup and hair sprays worsen acne.
- Environment. Exposure to oils and greases, polluted air, and sweating in hot weather can all aggravate acne.
- Stress. Emotional stress may contribute to acne.

- Friction. Continual pressure or rubbing on the skin by such objects as bicycle helmets, backpacks, or tight clothing can worsen acne.

The most common sites of acne are the face, chest, shoulders, and back, since these are the parts of the body where the most sebaceous follicles are found. In teenagers, acne is often found on the forehead, nose, and chin. As people age, the condition tends to appear towards the outer part of the face. Adult women may have acne on their chins and around their mouths. The elderly often develop whiteheads and blackheads on the upper cheeks and skin around the eyes. Inflamed lesions may cause redness, pain, tenderness, **itching**, or swelling in affected areas.

Diagnosis

Acne has a characteristic appearance and is, therefore, not difficult to diagnose. A complete medical history should be taken, including questions about skin care, diet, factors that improve or worsen the condition, medication use, and prior treatment. Physical examination includes the face, upper neck, chest, shoulders, back, and other affected areas. Under good lighting, the doctor can determine what types and how many blemishes are present, whether they are inflamed, whether they are deep or superficial, and whether there is scarring or skin discoloration. Blood tests are done when the patient appears to have hormonal or other medical problems. Stool tests can be helpful in determining whether there is a bacterial or yeast overgrowth contributing to the condition. Food allergy testing should also be considered.

Treatment

Alternative treatments for acne focus on proper cleansing to keep the skin oil-free; intermittent **fasting**; eating a good diet; an **elimination diet** in which the individual avoids alcohol, dairy products, **smoking**, **caffeine**, sugar, processed foods, and foods high in **iodine**, a mineral which appears to contribute to acne.

Supplementation with herbs that are blood cleansers or blood purifiers is recommended. These herbs strengthen the action of the liver and the kidneys, helping with **detoxification** and excretion. **Dandelion** root tincture (*Taraxacum officinale*) is recommended. Other recommended products include **burdock root** (*Arctium lappa*), also known as gobo, which can be purchased fresh at health food grocers or in Asian markets. It can be used either raw or cooked in salads, stir-fries, or other vegetable dishes. Burdock root tincture can also be used. **Red clover** (*Trifolium pratense*) makes a pleasant tea that can be consumed throughout the day. **Milk thistle** seed (*Silybum marianum*) can either be taken in tincture form or the seeds can be ground up and eaten in combination with hot cereal, granola, or other foods.

Other herbs useful in the treatment of acne include *Echinacea spp.* and **goldenseal** (*Hydrastis canadensis*). Goldenseal is particularly helpful in clearing up underlying conditions of intestinal toxicity. Herbal remedies used in **traditional Chinese medicine** (TCM) for acne include cnidium seed (*Cnidium monnieri*), and **honeysuckle** flower (*Lonicera japonica*). Supplementation nutrients, such as **essential fatty acids** (EFAs), **vitamin B complex**, **zinc**, **vitamin A** or beta-carotene, and **chromium** are also recommended.

Bowel toxicity may contribute to acne flare-ups and should be addressed. *Lactobacillus acidophilus* and *Lactobacillus bulgaricus* should be taken in yogurt or in capsules to maintain a healthy balance of intestinal flora. Goldenseal can be used to kill toxic bacteria. Allergic foods should be identified and removed from the diet. Dietary fiber, such as oat and wheat bran, beans, fruits and vegetables and their skins, and **psyllium** seed, should be increased in the diet. The fiber absorbs toxins and carries them through the colon to be excreted.

In addition, individuals with acne may want to participate in **movement therapy**, such as **yoga** or **t'ai chi**, or begin an **exercise** regimen. The person may also consider stress reduction or **meditation**.

Allopathic treatment

Acne treatment consists of reducing sebum and keratin production, encouraging the shedding of dead skin cells to help unclog the pores and killing or limiting bacteria. Treatment choice depends upon whether the acne is mild, moderate, or severe. Complicated cases are referred to a dermatologist or an endocrinologist, who treats diseases of the glands and the hormones. Counseling may be necessary to clear up misconceptions about the condition and to offer support regarding the negative effect of acne on the physical appearance.

Topical drugs

Treatment for mild acne consists of reducing the formation of new comedones with over-the-counter acne medications containing benzoyl peroxide (e.g., Clearasil, Fostex), salicylic acid (Stridex), **sulfur** (Therac lotion), or resorcinol (Acnomel cream). Treatment with stronger medications requires a doctor's supervision. Such medications include comedolytics, which are agents that loosen hard plugs and open pores. Adapalene (Differin), the vitamin A acid tretinoin (Retin-A), and concentrated versions of salicylic acid, resorcinol, and sulfur are in this group. Topical antibiotics, such as erythromycin, clindamycin (Cleocin-T), and meclocycline (Meclan), may be added to the treatment regimen. Drugs that act as both comedolytics and antibiotics, such as benzoyl peroxide, azelaic acid (Azelex), or benzoyl peroxide plus erythromycin (Benzamycin), are also used.

After washing with a mild soap, the acne medications are applied alone or in combination, once or twice a day over the entire affected area of skin. It may take many months to years to control the condition with these medications. Possible side effects include mild redness, peeling, irritation, dryness, and an increased sensitivity to sunlight that requires use of a sunscreen.

Oral drugs

When acne is severe and the lesions are deep, oral antibiotics may be taken daily to reduce the spread of bacteria. Tetracycline is the medication most often used. Minocycline, however, may be preferable because it has fewer side effects. Erythromycin and doxycycline are also used, and they also have side effects, including **dizziness**, photosensitivity, gastrointestinal problems, and darkening of the skin. Other possible side effects include allergic reactions, yeast **infections**, dizziness, tooth discoloration, and folliculitis. It is necessary for antibiotics to be used for up to three months to clear up the condition.

Isotretinoin (Accutane) can be used in cases of very severe acne or if antibiotic therapy proves unsuccessful. It may clear up resistant cysts and nodules in up to 90% of people and prevent scarring. Some do require a second course of treatment before this happens, however. Although the medication can be quite helpful, women who might become pregnant should use it with care. Isotretinoin can cause birth defects up to a month after it has stopped being used. Therefore, strict attention is paid to **pregnancy** tests and contraceptive requirements for women of child-bearing age who take this medication.

The course of treatment with isotretinoin lasts about four to five months. If dosage is kept low, a longer course of therapy is needed. Isotretinoin is a strong medication. Side effects are very common, mostly dryness of the eyes, genital mucosa, and lips. Other effects may include increases in **cholesterol**, triglycerides, and abnormal liver enzymes. Blood tests taken each month should be monitored during the course of treatment to ensure that the medication is not causing serious harm.

Anti-androgens, drugs that inhibit androgen production, are used to treat women who are unresponsive to other therapies. Oral contraceptives such as norgestimate/ethinyl estradiol (Ortho-Tri-Cyclen) have been shown to improve acne. In late 2001, a clinical trial demonstrated that ultra low-dose birth control pills (Alesse) prove as effective in treating acne as do pills with higher doses of estrogen. Improvement may take up to four months.

Other drugs, such as spironolactone and corticosteroids, may be used to reduce hormone activity in the adrenal glands, reducing production of sebum. This is the treatment of choice for an extremely severe, but rare type of acne called acne fulminans, found mostly in adolescent males. Acne conglobata, a more common form of severe inflammation, is characterized by numerous, deep, inflammatory nodules that heal with scarring. It is treated with oral isotretinoin and corticosteroids.

Other types of treatment

Several surgical or medical treatments are available to alleviate acne or the resulting scars:

- Comedone extraction. The comedo is removed from the pore with a special tool.
- Chemical peels. Glycolic acid is applied to peel off the top layer of skin to reduce scarring.
- Dermabrasion. The affected skin is frozen with a chemical spray and removed by brushing or planing.
- Punch grafting. Deep scars are excised and the area repaired with small skin grafts.
- Intralesional injection. Corticosteroids are injected directly into inflamed pimples.
- Collagen injection. Shallow scars are elevated by collagen protein injections.
- Laser treatments. Two types of laser treatments are used in treating acne scars. Laser-treated skin heals in three to 10 days, depending on the treatment chosen.

Expected results

Most dermatologists use a combination of therapies to treat acne, depending on the individual. Results of specific treatments vary. Acne is not a serious health threat. The most troubling aspects of this condition are the negative cosmetic effects and potential for permanent scarring. Some people,

---

KEY TERMS

Androgens—Male sex hormones that are linked with the development of acne.

Comedo—A hard plug composed of sebum and dead skin cells.

Follicles—Structures where pimples form. They are found within the skin and house the oil glands and hair.

Isotretinoin—A drug that decreases sebum production and dries up acne pimples.

Sebum—An oily skin moisturizer produced by sebaceous glands.

---

especially teenagers, become emotionally upset about their condition, and this psychological aspect may contribute to social or other emotional problems.

Acne is not considered curable, although it can be controlled by proper treatment, with improvement possibly taking many months. Acne tends to reappear when treatment stops, but it often spontaneously improves over time. Inflammatory acne may leave scars that require further treatment.

Prevention

There are no sure ways to prevent acne, but the following steps may be taken to minimize flare-ups:

- Gentle washing of affected areas once or twice every day.
- Avoidance of abrasive cleansers.
- Limited use of makeup and moisturizers; with avoidance of oil-based brands altogether.
- Frequent shampooing of oily hair which should be worn up, away from the face.
- A healthy, well-balanced diet that emphasizes fresh fruits and vegetables. Foods that seem to trigger flare-ups should be avoided.
- Gentle washing of the face, twice daily, with a soap compounded of sulfur, *Calendula officinalis,* or other substances that are useful against acne.
- Avoidance of handling affected areas excessively. Pimples should not be squeezed or prodded, as this may contribute to scarring, as well as spreading the acne lesions.
- Control over emotional stress.

Resources

BOOKS

Gabriel, Julie. *Clear Skin: Organic Action Plan for Acne.* Lincoln, NE: iUniverse Books, 2007.

Logan, Alan C., and Valori Treloar. *The Clear Skin Diet: A Nutritional Plan for Getting Rid of and Avoiding Acne.* Nashville, TN: Cumberland House, 2007.

Webster, Guy F., and Anthony V. Rawlings, eds. *Acne and Its Therapy.* London: Informa Healthcare, 2007.

PERIODICALS

Ganceviciene, Ruta, and Christos C. Zouboulis. "Isotretinoin: State of the Art Treatment for Acne Vulgaris." *Expert Review of Dermatology* (November 2007): 693–706.

Haedersdal, M., K. Togsverd-Bo, and H. C. Wulf. "Evidence-based Review of Lasers, Light Sources, and Photodynamic Therapy in the Treatment of Acne Vulgaris." *Journal of the European Academy of Dermatology & Venereology* (March 2008): 267–278.

Kumar, Anil, et al. "Treatment of Acne with Special Emphasis on Herbal Remedies." *Expert Review of Dermatology* (February 2008): 111–122.

Simonart, T., M. Dramaix, and V. De Maertelaer. "Efficacy of Tetracyclines in the Treatment of Acne Vulgaris: A Review." *British Journal of Dermatology* (February 2008): 208–216.

OTHER

Harper, Julie C. "Acne Vulgaris." eMedicine. http://www.emedicine.com/DERM/topic2.htm. (February 8, 2008).

Merck Manual. "Acne Vulgaris." http://www.merck.com/mmpe/sec10/ch111/ch111b.html. (February 8, 2008).

Patience Paradox
David Edward Newton, Ed.D.

Acne rosacea *see* **Rosacea**

Aconite

Description

Aconite is the common name for any of 100 or more related species in the *Aconitum* genus. Two of the species, *Aconitum napellus* and *Aconitum carmichaeli* are used medicinally. The more popular remedy, *Aconitum napellus*, is a plant that grows in mountainous regions of Central Asia, Russia, Europe, and Great Britain. This perennial plant from the Ranunculaceae family grows to a height of 3 ft (1 m) and has dark green, glossy leaves and dark blue flowers.

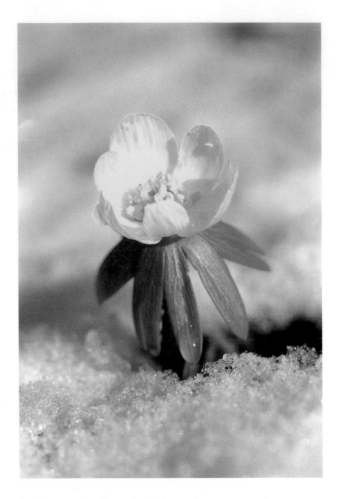

Winter aconite. *(ImageState / Alamy)*

Other names for aconite are wolf's bane, monkshood, blue rocket, and friar's cap. Wolf's bane is a direct translation of the Greek word *Lycotonum*. The Greeks left the plant as poisonous bait for wolves or moistened arrows with the juice of the herb in order to kill wolves. The plant was nicknamed monkshood and friar's cap because of the shape of the flowers.

The plant in its fresh form is highly poisonous. The poison comes from the toxic alkaloid aconitine. Aconitine is found in the whole plant but is concentrated mainly in the root. Symptoms of poisoning include tingling; numbness of the tongue and mouth; **nausea** and **vomiting**; labored breathing; a weak and irregular pulse; and cold, clammy skin. Even the smallest amounts of aconitine inside the mouth cause burning, tingling, and numbness. As little as 2 mg of aconitine can cause death in four hours, which may be one reason why aconite is often chosen by people attempting suicide by poison. The Australian government has declared all species of aconite unfit for human consumption.

General use

Western herbology

Herbalists have used aconite as a medicine for hundreds of years. However, in ancient times the herb was known more for its power to kill rather than heal; it was often used in ancient Rome to commit murders.

The herb acts as a diuretic (a substance that promotes urination) and diaphoretic (a substance that causes sweating). Tinctures are taken internally to slow fevers, **pneumonia**, **laryngitis**, and acute **tonsillitis**. Liniments or ointments made from the herb are applied externally to relieve the **pain** of **neuralgia** and rheumatism.

Traditional Chinese medicine

Aconitum carmichaeli is used in **traditional Chinese medicine**. It is called Fu Zi (sometimes Fu Tzu) in Mandarin; in other parts of China and in Hong Kong, it is known as *chuan wou tou*. This herb is used to treat rheumatism, **bruises**, arthritis, acute hypothermia, **diarrhea**, and **impotence**. The herb has a sweet, spicy taste.

The main function of Fu Zi is to warm the interior of the body. It also works to restore collapsed yang, warm kidney fire, warm the kidney and spleen, drive out the cold, warm the meridians, and relieve pain. Fu Zi is also used by traditional Chinese herbalists in conditions marked by deficient kidney and spleen yang or in conditions with early morning diarrhea or lack of appetite.

Aconitum carmichaeli also contains the toxic alkaloid aconitine. After cooking the herb, the alkaloid is converted to aconine, which is not as toxic.

This herb is poisonous. When it is properly prepared as recommended by a Chinese medicine practitioner, there are rarely any adverse effects. Chinese pharmacies do not sell raw, untreated aconite, as the plant should be dried and then brewed for long periods of time. However, cases of aconite poisoning have been reported in Asian countries, including some that ended in the patient's death from heart arrhythmias. It appears that most of these cases were due either to the herbalist's prescribing a larger dose of aconite than was needed, or to the patient's attempting to prepare the remedy at home.

Homeopathy

Homeopaths prescribe aconite for conditions that come on suddenly as a result of grief, fear, anger, shock, or exposure to cold, dry wind. It is also recommended for people troubled by suicidal thoughts. The remedy is short-acting and is indicated at the onset of acute conditions such as **croup**, colds, **cough**, **bronchitis**, eye and ear **infections**, headaches, and rheumatism. This remedy is one of the best substances for treating **measles**, arthritis, and pneumonia when all of the symptoms are present. Aconite is also useful at the beginning of a **fever**, in early stages of inflammation, and following shock caused by an injury or surgery.

Preparations

Aconite is available as a homeopathic remedy or in dried bulk form, as an ointment or liniment, and as a tincture. Pharmacies, health food stores, and Chinese herbal stores carry the various preparations. They are also available as prescribed by a herbalist, homeopathic doctor, or Chinese medicine practitioner.

The whole plant is used in Western herbal medicine. The leaves and flowers are cut when the flowers are in blossom in June. The roots are collected after the stem has died off, usually in August. The root is dried before use while the leaves, stems, and flowers are used fresh.

The homeopathic preparation of aconite is created in the following manner. When the flowers are in full bloom, the whole plant—but not the root—is collected and pounded to a pulp. The juice from the pulp is pressed and mixed with alcohol. The mixture is then strained and diluted. The final homeopathic remedy is created after the diluted mixture is repeatedly succussed (pounded against a hard surface to break down and mix the substance). The remedy is available at health-food and drug stores in various potencies in the form of tinctures, tablets, and pellets.

In traditional Chinese medicine, the aconite root is generally used in small amounts in combination with other herbs.

Precautions

If symptoms do not improve after the recommended time period, individuals should consult their homeopath or other healthcare practitioner.

Do not exceed the recommended dosage.

Use *Aconitum carmichaeli* only under supervision of a Chinese medical practitioner.

Aconite is poisonous and should not be consumed in its raw state. Persons who gather wild plants to eat should be very careful in identifying what they are gathering. Cases have been reported of aconite poisoning in people who thought they were gathering mountain **chicory**.

KEY TERMS

Aconitine—A toxic alkaloid contained in aconite. As little as 2 mg taken internally may be fatal.

Antidote—A medication or remedy given to counteract the effects of a poison.

Diaphoretic—A substance that causes sweating.

Diuretic—A substance that promotes urination.

Succussion—A process integral to the creation of a homeopathic remedy in which a solution is repeatedly struck against a firm surface. This process is performed to thoroughly mix the substance and magnify its healing properties.

Toxicology—The branch of medical pharmacology dealing with the detection, effects, and antidotes of poisons.

Women who are pregnant, trying to get pregnant, or who are breastfeeding should not use *Aconitum carmichaeli*.

Side effects

Symptoms of poisoning by the fresh aconite plant include tingling, numbness of the tongue and mouth, nausea, vomiting, labored breathing, a weak and irregular pulse, and cold, clammy skin. In cases of severe poisoning, aconite can produce extreme symptoms that include severe pain, convulsions, paralysis, confusion, seizures, and heart failure. The only established treatment for aconite poisoning is supportive; that is, there is no antidote.

Most liniments or lotions made with aconite for external use contain a 1.3% concentration of the herb. Use of these preparations must be limited to unbroken skin, as aconite can be absorbed through the skin and cause toxic symptoms. If a skin reaction occurs, use of the liniment must be discontinued immediately.

Interactions

When taking any homeopathic remedy, individuals should not use **peppermint** products, coffee, or alcohol. These products make the remedy ineffective.

Aconitum carmichaeli should not be used by individuals with a deficiency of yin, or coolness, or with signs of heat such as fever, redness, and agitation.

Resources

BOOKS

Gomella, Leonard G., et al. *Clinician's Pocket Drug Reference*. New York: McGraw Hill, 2008.

PERIODICALS

Fujita, Yuji, et al. "Five Cases of Aconite Poisoning: Toxicokinetics of Aconitines." *Journal of Analytical Toxicology* (April 2007): 132–137.

ORGANIZATIONS

American Academy of Clinical Toxicology, 777 East Park Dr., PO Box 8820, Harrisburg, PA, 17105, (717) 558-7750, http://www.clintox.org/.

National Center for Homeopathy, 801 N. Fairfax St., Suite 306, Alexandria, VA, 22314, (703) 548-7790, http://nationalcenterforhomeopathy.org/.

Jennifer Wurges
Rebecca J. Frey, PhD
David Edward Newton, Ed.D.

Acquired Immunodeficiency syndrome *see* **AIDS**

Acupressure

Definition

Acupressure is a form of touch therapy that uses the principles of **acupuncture** and Chinese medicine. In acupressure, the same points on the body are used as in acupuncture, but they are stimulated with finger pressure instead of with the insertion of needles. Acupressure is used to relieve a variety of symptoms and **pain**.

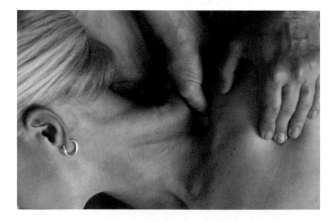

Acupressure massage. *(© Will & Deni McIntyre/Photo Researchers, Inc. Reproduced by permission.)*

Origins

Centuries ago Chinese medicine developed acupuncture, acupressure, herbal remedies, diet, **exercise**, lifestyle changes, and other remedies as part of its healing methods. Many of these historical forms of Oriental medicine are used in the West in the twenty-first century. Acupuncture, acupressure, **shiatsu**, and Chinese herbal medicine have their roots in Chinese medicine. One legend has it that acupuncture and acupressure evolved as early Chinese healers studied the puncture **wounds** of Chinese warriors, noting that certain points on the body created interesting results when stimulated. The oldest known text specifically on acupuncture points, the *Systematic Classic of Acupuncture*, dates to about 282 A.D. Acupressure is the non-invasive form of acupuncture, a result of Chinese physicians having determined that stimulating points on the body with massage and pressure could be effective for treating certain problems.

Outside of Asian American communities, Chinese medicine remained virtually unknown in the United States until the 1970s, when Richard Nixon became the first U.S. president to visit China. On Nixon's trip, journalists were amazed to observe major operations being performed on patients without the use of anesthetics. Instead, fully conscious patients were being operated on, with only acupuncture needles inserted into them to control pain. At that time, a famous columnist for the *New York Times*, James Reston, had to undergo surgery and elected to use acupuncture for anesthesia. Later, he wrote some convincing stories on its effectiveness. Despite being neglected by mainstream medicine and the American Medical Association (AMA), acupuncture and Chinese medicine became an option for alternative medicine practitioners in the United States. In the early 2000s, millions of patients can attest to its effectiveness, and there are nearly 9,000 practitioners dispersed across all 50 states.

Acupressure is used by Chinese medicine practitioners and acupuncturists, as well as by massage therapists. Many massage schools in the United States include acupressure techniques as part of their bodywork programs. Shiatsu massage is very closely related to acupressure, involving the same points on the body and the same general principles, although it was developed over centuries in Japan rather than in China. **Reflexology** is a form of bodywork based on acupressure concepts. Jin Shin Do is a bodywork technique with an increasing number of practitioners in the United States that combines acupressure and shiatsu principles with **qigong**, Reichian theory, and **meditation**.

Benefits

Acupressure massage performed by a therapist can be very effective both as prevention and as a treatment for many health conditions, including headaches, general aches and pains, colds and flu, arthritis, **allergies**, **asthma**, nervous tension, menstrual cramps, sinus problems, **sprains**, **tennis elbow**, and toothaches, among others. Unlike acupuncture, which requires a visit to a professional, acupressure can be performed by a layperson. Acupressure techniques are fairly easy to learn and have been used to provide quick, cost-free, and effective relief from many symptoms. Acupressure points can also be stimulated to increase energy and feelings of well-being, reduce **stress**, stimulate the immune system, and alleviate **sexual dysfunction**.

Description

Acupressure and Chinese medicine

Chinese medicine views the body as a small part of the universe, subject to laws and principles of harmony and balance. Moreover, Chinese medicine does not make as sharp a distinction as Western medicine does between mind and body. The Chinese system asserts that emotions and mental states are every bit as influential on disease as purely physical mechanisms; it considers factors such as work, environment, and relationships as fundamental to health. Chinese medicine also uses very different symbols and ideas to discuss the body and health. While Western medicine typically describes health as mainly physical processes composed of chemical processes, the Chinese use ideas of yin and yang, chi, and the organ system to describe health and the body.

Everything in the universe has properties of yin and yang. Yin is associated with cold, female, passive, downward, inward, dark, wet. Yang can be described as hot, male, active, upward, outward, light, dry, and so on. Nothing is either completely yin or yang. These two principles always interact and affect each other, although the body and its organs can become imbalanced by having either too much or too little of either.

Chi (pronounced *chee*, also spelled *qi* or *ki* in Japanese shiatsu) is the fundamental life energy. It is found in food, air, water, and sunlight, and it travels through the body in channels called *meridians*. There are 12 major meridians in the body that transport chi, corresponding to the 12 main organs categorized by Chinese medicine.

Disease is viewed as an imbalance of the organs and chi in the body. Chinese medicine has developed intricate systems regarding how organs are related to physical and mental symptoms, and it has devised corresponding treatments using the meridian and pressure point networks that are classified and numbered. The goal of acupressure, and acupuncture, is to stimulate and unblock the circulation of chi, by activating very specific points, called pressure points or *acupoints*. Acupressure seeks to stimulate the points on the chi meridians that pass close to the skin, as these are easiest to unblock and manipulate with finger pressure.

Acupressure can be used as part of a Chinese physician's prescription, as a session of **massage therapy**, or as a self-treatment for common aches and illnesses. A Chinese medicine practitioner examines a patient very thoroughly, looking at physical, mental, and emotional activity, taking the pulse usually at the wrists, examining the tongue and complexion, and observing the patient's demeanor and attitude, to get a complete diagnosis of which organs and meridian points are out of balance. When the imbalance is located, the physician recommends specific pressure points for acupuncture or acupressure. If acupressure is recommended, the patient might opt for a series of treatments from a massage therapist.

In massage therapy, acupressurists evaluate a patient's symptoms and overall health, but a massage therapist's diagnostic training is not as extensive as that of a Chinese physician. In a massage therapy treatment, a person usually lies on a table or mat, with thin clothing on. The acupressurist gently feels and palpates the abdomen and other parts of the body to determine energy imbalances. Then, the therapist works with different meridians throughout the body, depending on which organs are imbalanced in the abdomen. The therapist uses different types of finger movements and pressure on different acupoints, depending on whether the chi needs to be increased or dispersed at different points. The therapist observes and guides the energy flow through the patient's body throughout the session. Sometimes, special herbs (*Artemesia vulgaris* or moxa) may be placed on a point to warm it, a process called *moxibustion*. A session of acupressure is generally a very pleasant experience, and some people experience great benefit immediately. For more chronic conditions, several sessions may be necessary to relieve and improve conditions.

As of 2008 the cost of acupressure massage was typically from $30 to $70 per hour session. A visit to a Chinese medicine physician or acupuncturist can be more expensive, comparable to a visit to an allopathic physician if the practitioner is a certified medical doctor (MD). Insurance reimbursement varies widely, and consumers should be inquire as to whether their policies cover alternative treatment, acupuncture, or massage therapy.

Self-treatment

Acupressure is easy to learn, and there are many good books that illustrate the position of acupoints and meridians on the body. The procedure can also be conducted anywhere, and it is a good form of treatment for spouses and partners to give to each other and for parents to perform on children for minor conditions. As effective as acupressure may be, it should not be used to the exclusion of allopathic methods that provide more reliable relief or cure for certain diseases and disorders.

While giving self-treatment or performing acupressure on another, a mental attitude of calmness and attention is important, as one person's energy can be used to help another's. Loose, thin clothing is recommended. There are three general techniques for stimulating a pressure point.

- Tonifying is meant to strengthen weak chi and is done by pressing the thumb or finger into an acupoint with a firm, steady pressure, holding it for up to two minutes.
- Dispersing is meant to move stagnant or blocked chi, and the finger or thumb is moved in a circular motion or slightly in and out of the point for two minutes.
- Calming the chi in a pressure point utilizes the palm to cover the point and gently stroke the area for about two minutes.

There are many pressure points that are easily found and memorized to treat common ailments from headaches to colds.

- For headaches, toothaches, sinus problems, and pain in the upper body, the "LI4" point is recommended. It is located in the web between the thumb and index finger, on the back of the hand. Using the thumb and index finger of the other hand, a person applies a pinching pressure until the point is felt and holds it for two minutes. Pregnant women should never press this point.
- To calm the nerves and stimulate digestion, a person finds the "CV12" point that is four thumb widths above the navel in the center of the abdomen. Calm the point with the palm, using gentle stroking for several minutes.
- To stimulate the immune system, a person finds the "TH5" point on the back of the forearm two thumb widths above the wrist. The dispersing technique, or circular pressure with the thumb or finger, is used for two minutes on each arm.

• For headaches, sinus congestion, and tension, a person locate the "GB20" points at the base of the skull in the back of the head, just behind the bones in back of the ears and then disperses these points for two minutes with the fingers or thumbs. The individual can also find the "yintang" point, which is in the middle of the forehead between the eyebrows and disperse it with gentle pressure for two minutes to clear the mind and to relieve headaches.

Precautions

Acupressure is a safe technique, but it is not meant to replace professional health care. A physician should always be consulted when there are doubts about medical conditions. If a condition is chronic, a professional should be consulted; purely symptomatic treatment can exacerbate chronic conditions. Acupressure should not be applied to open wounds or to places that are swollen or inflamed. Areas of scar tissue, **blisters**, **boils**, **rashes**, or **varicose veins** should be avoided. Finally, certain acupressure points should not be stimulated on people with high or low blood pressure and on pregnant women.

Research and general acceptance

In general, Chinese medicine has been slow to gain acceptance in the West, mainly because it rests on ideas quite unlike the Western scientific model. For instance, Western scientists have trouble with the idea of chi, the invisible energy of the body, and the idea that pressing on certain points can alleviate certain conditions seems incredible.

Western scientists, in trying to account for the action of acupressure, have theorized that chi is actually part of the neuroendocrine system of the body. Celebrated orthopedic surgeon Robert O. Becker, who was twice nominated for the Nobel Prize, wrote a book on the subject called *Cross Currents: The Promise of Electromedicine; The Perils of Electropollution*. By using precise electrical measuring devices, Becker and his colleagues showed that the body has a complex web of electromagnetic energy and that traditional acupressure meridians and points contained amounts of energy that non-acupressure points did not.

The mechanisms of acupuncture and acupressure remain difficult to document in terms of the biochemical processes involved. Numerous testimonials are the primary evidence supporting the effectiveness of acupressure and acupuncture. However, in the 2000s a body of research was growing that verified the effectiveness in acupressure and acupuncture techniques in treating many problems and in controlling pain.

Training and certification

There are two methods for becoming trained in the skill of acupressure. The first is training in traditional acupuncture and Chinese medicine, for which there are many schools and certifying bodies around the United States. The majority of acupressure practitioners are trained as certified massage therapists, either as acupressure or shiatsu specialists.

Resources

BOOKS

Kolster, Bernard C., and Astrid Waskowiak. *The Acupressure Atlas*. Rochester, VT: Healing Arts Press, 2007.

Vora, Devendra. *Health in Your Hands: Acupressure and Other Natural Therapies*, 2nd ed. New Delhi: Navneet, 2007.

Wright, Janet. *Reflexology and Acupressure*. London: Hamlyn Press, 2008.

PERIODICALS

Agarwal, A., et al. "Acupressure for Prevention of Preoperative Anxiety: A Prospective, Randomised, Placebo Controlled Study." *Anaesthesia* (October 2005): 978–981.

Jamigorn, Mattawan, and Vorapong Phupong. "Acupressure and Vitamin B6 to Relieve Nausea and Vomiting in Pregnancy: A Randomized Study." *Archives of Gynecology and Obstetrics* (September 2007): 245–249.

"Non-epidural Pain Relief." *The Informed Choice Initiative (Women's Edition)* (April 2007): 91–98.

Zhou, Wei, and John C. Longhurst. "Review of Trials Examining the Use of Acupuncture to Treat Hypertension." *Future Cardiology* (May 2006): 287–292.

KEY TERMS

Acupoint—A pressure point stimulated in acupressure.

Chi—Basic life energy.

Meridian—A channel through which chi travels in the body.

Moxibustion—An acupuncture technique that involves burning of the herb moxa or mugwort.

Shiatsu—Japanese form of acupressure massage.

Yin/yang—Universal characteristics used to describe aspects of the natural world.

ORGANIZATIONS

Acupressure Institute, 1533 Shattuck Ave., Berkeley, CA, 94709, (800) 442-2232, www.acupressure.com.

American Massage Therapy Association, 500 Davis St., Evanston, IL, 60201, (877) 905-2700, www.amta massage.org.

American Organization for Bodywork Therapies of Asia, 1010 Haddonfield-Berlin Rd., Suite 408, Voorhees, NJ, 08043, (856) 782-1616, http://www.aobta.org/.

Jin Shin Do Foundation for Bodymind Acupressure, PO Box 416, Idyllwild, CA, 92549, (951) 659-5707, http://www.jinshindo.org/.

Douglas Dupler
David Edward Newton, Ed.D.

Acupuncture

Definition

Acupuncture is one of the main forms of treatment in **traditional Chinese medicine**. It involves the use of sharp, thin needles that are inserted in the body at specific points. This process is believed to adjust and alter the body's energy flow into healthier patterns and is used to treat a wide variety of illnesses and health conditions.

Origins

The original text of Chinese medicine is the *Nei Ching, The Yellow Emperor's Classic of Internal Medicine*, which is estimated to be at least 2,500 years old. Thousands of books followed on the subject of Chinese healing, and its basic philosophies spread long ago to other Asian civilizations. Nearly all of the forms of Oriental medicine which are used in the West in the 2000s, including acupuncture, **shiatsu**, **acupressure** massage, and macrobiotics, are part of or have their roots in Chinese medicine. Legend has it that acupuncture developed when early Chinese physicians observed unpredicted effects of puncture **wounds** in Chinese warriors. The oldest known text on acupuncture, the *Systematic Classic of Acupuncture*, dates back to 282 A.D. Although acupuncture is its best known technique, Chinese medicine traditionally uses herbal remedies, dietary therapy, lifestyle changes, and other means to treat patients.

In the early 1900s, only a few Western physicians who had visited China knew about and used acupuncture. But outside of Asian American communities it remained virtually unknown until the 1970s, when Richard Nixon became the first U.S. president to

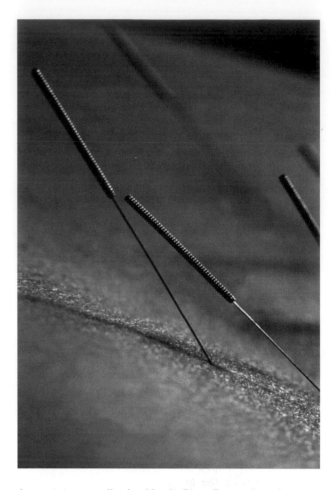

Acupuncture needles in skin. *(© Photo Researchers, Inc. Reproduced by permission.)*

visit China. On Nixon's trip, journalists were amazed to observe major operations being performed on patients without the use of anesthetics. Instead, fully conscious patients were being operated on with only acupuncture needles inserted into them to control **pain**. During that time, a famous columnist for the *New York Times*, James Reston, had to undergo surgery and elected to use acupuncture instead of pain medication, and he wrote some convincing stories on its effectiveness.

As of 2008 acupuncture was practiced in all U.S. 50 states by more than 9,000 practitioners, with about 4,000 medical doctors (MDs) including it in their practices. Acupuncture has shown notable success in treating many conditions, and more than 15 million Americans have used it as a therapy. Acupuncture, however, remains largely unsupported by the medical establishment. The American Medical Association has been resistant to encouraging research, as the practice is based on concepts markedly unlike the Western scientific model.

Several forms of acupuncture are being used as of 2008 in the United States. Japanese acupuncture uses extremely thin needles and does not incorporate herbal medicine in its practice. Auricular acupuncture uses acupuncture points only on the ear, which are believed to stimulate and balance internal organs. In France, where acupuncture is very popular and more widely accepted by the medical establishment, neurologist Paul Nogier developed a system of acupuncture based on neuroendocrine theory rather than on traditional Chinese concepts, which has gained some use in the United States.

Benefits

The World Health Organization (WHO) recommends acupuncture as an effective treatment for over forty medical problems, including **allergies**; respiratory conditions; gastrointestinal disorders; gynecological problems; nervous conditions; and disorders of the eyes, nose and throat; and childhood illnesses; among others. Acupuncture has been used in the treatment of **alcoholism** and **substance abuse**. In 2002, a center in Maine received a unique grant to study acupuncture treatment for substance abuse. Although recognizing that acupuncture had been used before for helping those with abuse problems, this study sought to show that ear acupuncture's effects on **relaxation** response helped those abusing drugs and alcohol better deal with the **anxiety** and life circumstances thought to lead them to substance abuse.

Acupuncture is an effective and low-cost treatment for headaches and chronic pain, associated with problems like back injuries and arthritis. It has also been used to supplement invasive Western treatments such as chemotherapy and surgery. Acupuncture is generally more effective when used as prevention or before a health condition becomes acute, but it has been used to help patients suffering from **cancer** and **AIDS**. In 2002, the National Institutes of Health announced that pain from certain musculoskeletal conditions such as **fibromyalgia** could be helped by acupuncture. Acupuncture has limited value in treating conditions or traumas that require surgery or emergency care (such as for broken bones).

Description

Basic ideas of Chinese medicine

Chinese medicine views the body as a small part of the universe and subject to universal laws and principles of harmony and balance. Chinese medicine does not draw a sharp line, as Western medicine does, between mind and body. The Chinese system believes that emotions and mental states are every bit as influential on disease as purely physical mechanisms and considers factors such as work, environment, lifestyle, and relationships as fundamental to the overall picture of a patient's health. Chinese medicine also uses very different symbols and ideas to discuss the body and health. While Western medicine typically describes health in terms of measurable physical processes made up of chemical reactions, the Chinese use the ideas of yin and yang, chi, the organ system, and the five elements to describe health and the body. To understand the ideas behind acupuncture, it is worthwhile to introduce some of these basic terms.

YIN AND YANG. According to Chinese philosophy, the universe and the body can be described by two separate but complementary principles, that of yin and yang. For example, in temperature, yin is cold and yang is hot. In gender, yin is female and yang is male. In activity, yin is passive and yang is active. In light, yin is dark and yang is bright. In direction yin is inward and downward and yang is outward and up, and so on. Nothing is ever completely yin or yang, but a combination of the two. These two principles are always interacting, opposing, and influencing each other. The goal of Chinese medicine is not to eliminate either yin or yang, but to allow the two to balance each other and exist harmoniously together. For instance, if a person suffers from symptoms of high blood pressure, the Chinese system would say that the heart organ might have too much yang and would recommend methods either to reduce the yang or to increase the yin of the heart, depending on the other symptoms and organs in the body. Thus, acupuncture therapies seek to either increase or reduce yang or increase or reduce yin in particular regions of the body.

CHI. Another fundamental concept of Chinese medicine is that of chi (pronounced *chee*, also spelled *qi*). Chi is the fundamental life energy of the universe. It is invisible and is found in the environment in air, water, food, and sunlight. In the body, it is the invisible vital force that creates and animates life. Humans are all born with inherited amounts of chi, and they also get acquired chi from the food they eat and the air they breathe. The level and quality of a person's chi also depends on the state of physical, mental, and emotional balance. Chi travels through the body along channels called *meridians*.

THE ORGAN SYSTEM. In the Chinese system, there are twelve main organs: the lung, large intestine, stomach, spleen, heart, small intestine, urinary bladder, kidney, liver, gallbladder, pericardium, and the "triple warmer," which represents the entire torso region. Each organ has chi energy associated with it, and each organ interacts with particular emotions on the mental level. As there are twelve organs, there are twelve types of chi that can move through the body, and these move through twelve main channels or meridians. Chinese doctors connect symptoms to organs. That is, symptoms are caused by yin/yang imbalances in one or more organs or by an unhealthy flow of chi to or from one organ to another. Each organ has a different profile of symptoms it can manifest.

THE FIVE ELEMENTS. Another basis of Chinese theory is that the world and body are made up of five main elements: wood, fire, earth, metal, and water. These elements are all interconnected, and each element either generates or controls another element. For instance, water controls fire, and earth generates metal. Each organ is associated with one of the five elements. The Chinese system uses elements and organs to describe and treat conditions. For instance, the kidney is associated with water, and the heart is associated with fire, and the two organs are related as water and fire are related. If the kidney is weak, then there might be a corresponding fire problem in the heart, so treatment might be made by acupuncture or herbs to cool the heart system and/or increase energy in the kidney system.

The Chinese have developed an intricate system that describes how organs and elements are related to physical and mental symptoms, and the above example is a simple one. Although this system sounds suspect to Western scientists, some interesting parallels have been observed. For instance, Western medicine has observed that with severe heart problems, kidney failure often follows, but it still does not know exactly why. In Chinese medicine, this connection between the two organs has long been established.

MEDICAL PROBLEMS AND ACUPUNCTURE. In Chinese medicine, disease as seen as imbalances in the organ system or chi meridians, and the goal of any remedy or treatment is to assist the body in reestablishing its innate harmony. Disease can be caused by internal factors such as emotions, external factors such as the environment and weather, and other factors such as injuries, trauma, diet, and germs. However, infection is seen not as primarily a problem with germs and viruses but as a weakness in the energy of the body that is allowing a sickness to occur. In Chinese medicine, no two illnesses are ever the same, as each body has its own characteristics of symptoms and balance. Acupuncture is used to open or adjust the flow of chi throughout the organ system, which will strengthen the body and prompt it to heal itself.

A VISIT TO THE ACUPUNCTURIST. Typically, an acupuncturist first gets a thorough idea of a patient's medical history and symptoms, both physical and emotional, using a questionnaire and interview. Then the acupuncturist examines the patient to find further symptoms, looking closely at the tongue, the pulse at various points in the body, the complexion, general behavior, and other signs like coughs or pains. From this examination, the practitioner is able to determine patterns of symptoms that indicate which organs and areas are imbalanced. Depending on the problem, the acupuncturist inserts needles to manipulate chi on one or more of the twelve organ meridians. On these twelve meridians, there are nearly 2,000 points that can be used in acupuncture, with around 200 points being most frequently used by traditional acupuncturists. During an individual treatment, one to 20 needles may be used, depending on which meridian points are chosen.

Acupuncture needles are sterilized, and acupuncture is a very safe procedure. The depth of insertion of needles varies, depending on which chi channels are being treated. Some points barely go beyond superficial layers of skin, while some acupuncture points require a depth of 1–3 in (3–8 cm) of needle. The needles generally do not cause pain. Patients sometimes report pinching sensations and often pleasant sensations, as the body experiences healing. Depending on the problem, the acupuncturist might spin or move the needles, or even pass a slight electrical current through some of them. **Moxibustion** may sometimes be used. Moxibustion is a process in which an herbal mixture (moxa or **mugwort**) is either burned like incense on the acupuncture point or on the end of the needle, a process believed to stimulate chi in a particular way. Also, acupuncturists sometimes use *cupping*, during which small suction cups are placed on meridian points to stimulate them.

How long the needles are inserted also varies. Some patients require only a quick in and out insertion to clear problems and provide *tonification* (strengthening of health), while some other conditions might require needles inserted up to an hour or more. The average visit to an acupuncturist takes about 30 minutes. The number of visits to the acupuncturist varies, with some conditions improved in one or two sessions and others requiring a series of six or more visits over the course of weeks or months.

Costs for acupuncture vary, depending on whether the practitioner is a medical physician. Initial visits with non-MD acupuncturists can cost $50–$100, with follow-up visits usually costing less. Insurance reimbursement varies widely, depending on the company and state. Regulations tend to change frequently. Some states authorize Medicaid to cover acupuncture for certain conditions, and some states have mandated that general coverage pay for acupuncture. Consumers should be aware of the provisions for acupuncture in their individual policies.

Precautions

Acupuncture is generally a safe procedure. If individuals are in doubt about a medical condition, more than one physician should be consulted. Also, individuals should feel comfortable and confident that their acupuncturist is knowledgeable and properly trained.

Research and general acceptance

Mainstream medicine has been slow to accept acupuncture. Although more medical doctors are using the technique, the American Medical Association does not recognize it as a specialty. The reason for this position is that the mechanism of acupuncture is difficult to understand or measure scientifically, such as the invisible energy of chi in the body. Western medicine, admitting that acupuncture works in many cases, has theorized that the energy meridians are actually part of the nervous system and that acupuncture relieves pain by releasing endorphins, or natural pain killers, into the bloodstream. Despite the ambiguity in the biochemistry involved, acupuncture continues to show effectiveness in clinical tests, from reducing pain to alleviating the symptoms of chronic illnesses, and in the 2000s research in acupuncture was growing. The Office of Alternative Medicine of the National Institute of Health funded research in the use of acupuncture on a number of conditions, including **depression**, attention-deficit disorder, arthritis, and **post-traumatic stress disorder**.

Training and certification

Medical acupuncture has evolved in the United States in an atmosphere that focuses on traditional Western methods, such as surgical techniques and pain management, and not as part of Chinese medicine overall. Medical acupuncture is performed by an MD or an osteopathic physician (DO). As of 2008, 23 states allowed only this type of acupuncture. Practitioners get their training as part of conventional medical school programs. Since any MD can legally perform acupuncture, the *American Academy of Medical Acupuncture* (AAMA) was chartered in 1987 to support the education and correct practice of physician-trained acupuncturists. Its members must be

| KEY TERMS |

Acupressure—A form of massage using acupuncture points.

Auricular acupuncture—Acupuncture using only points found on the ears.

Chi—Basic life energy.

Meridian—A channel through which chi travels in the body.

Moxibustion—Acupuncture technique that involves burning the herb moxa or mugwort.

Tonification—Acupuncture technique for strengthening the body.

Yin/Yang—Universal characteristics used to describe aspects of the natural world.

either MDs or DOs who have completed proper study of acupuncture techniques.

Resources

BOOKS

Filshie, Jacqueline. *Introduction to Medical Acupuncture.* Oxford, England: Churchill Livingstone, 2008.

Focks, Claudia. *Atlas of Acupuncture.* Oxford, England: Churchill Livingstone, 2008.

Landgren, Kajsa. *Ear Acupuncture: A Practical Guide.* Oxford, England: Churchill Livingstone, 2008.

Maciocia, Giovanni. *The Practice of Chinese Medicine: The Treatment of Diseases with Acupuncture and Chinese Herbs.* Oxford, England: Churchill Livingstone, 2008.

PERIODICALS

Hollifield M., et al. "Acupuncture for Post-traumatic Stress Disorder: A Randomized Controlled Pilot Trial." *Journal of Nervous and Mental Diseases* (June 2007): 504–513.

Mayhew, E., and E. Ernst. "Acupuncture for Fibromyalgia: A Systematic Review of Randomized Clinical Trials." *Rheumatology* (May 2007): 801–804.

Paterson, Charlotte. "Patients' Experiences of Western-style Acupuncture: The Influence of Acupuncture 'Dose', Self-care Strategies and Integration." *Journal of Health Services Research and Policy* (April 2007): 39–45.

Tillisch, Kirsten. "Complementary and Alternative Medicine for Gastrointestinal Disorders." *Clinical Medicine, Journal of the Royal College of Physicians* (June 2007): 224–227.

ORGANIZATIONS

American Academy of Medical Acupuncture, 4929 Wilshire Blvd., Suite 428, Los Angeles, CA, 90010, (323) 937-5514, http://www.medicalacupuncture.org/.

American Association of Acupuncture and Oriental Medicine, PO Box 162340, Sacramento, CA, 95816, (866) 455-7999, http://www.aaom.org/.

National Certification Commission for Acupuncture and Oriental Medicine, 76 South Laura St., Suite 1290, Jacksonville, FL, 32202, (904) 598-1005, http://www.nccaom.org/.

Douglas Dupler
Teresa G. Odle
David Edward Newton, Ed.D.

Acute homeopathic remedies *see* **Homeopathy, acute prescribing**

ADD *see* **Attention-deficit hyperactivity disorder**

Addiction *see* **Alcoholism; Substance abuse and dependence**

Ademetionine

Description

Ademetionine, also known as SAMe (pronounced "sammy"), is a specific form of the amino acid **methionine** (S-adenosyl-methionine). The body manufactures it, and it is found in most tissues of the body. Ademetionine is essential for the formation of **glutathione**, a water-soluble peptide that helps the body fight free radicals. SAMe also helps the liver to process fats (protecting against a fatty liver) and is believed to play a role in protecting the body from **heart disease**.

SAMe is a methyl donor, which means that it provides other molecules with methyl groups that are critical to their metabolism. In general, ademetionine raises the level of functioning of other **amino acids** in the body. Severe deficiencies of SAMe can cause problems with other important body functions, such as secretion of important hormones such as **melatonin**, which plays a key role in regulating sleep and circadian rhythms.

It is believed to increase levels of serotonin and dopamine, and a synthetic version of SAMe may be useful in treating some conditions, including **osteoarthritis** and **depression**.

General use

The synthetic formula of ademetionine was discovered in Italy in 1953 and was researched over the following decades. In the 1970s, Italian researchers investigating its properties as a treatment for **schizophrenia** discovered that it also had antidepressant properties. Ademetionine became a useful treatment during the 1990s, when scientists found a way to stabilize it for research purposes. After that technological development, ademetionine could be sold as a medical supplement.

SAMe has been used to treat depression, osteoarthritis, schizophrenia, liver disease, **peripheral neuropathy**, and other illnesses. As of February 2008, considerable research had been conducted on the use of ademetionine for treating osteoarthritis.

Osteoarthritis

Numerous studies indicated that people diagnosed with osteoarthritis experienced less **pain** while taking ademetionine. SAMe appeared as effective as non-steroidal anti-inflammatory drugs (NSAIDs) and produced fewer side effects, according to organizations, including the Mayo Clinic. However, additional research was needed to verify the findings from those studies. In addition, long-term effects of SAMe use were not known in 2008.

Depression

SAMe has been studied for decades, but research as of 2008 was rated as inconclusive because of factors such as the small number of participants in studies and the absence of a placebo group in some studies. For example, *BMC Psychiatry* in 2004 described an eight-week American study of 20 people diagnosed with HIV/AIDS and major depressive disorder. The people took ademetionine and a "rapid effect" was observed after the first week. "Progressive decreases in depression symptom rating scores" were noted during the subsequent weeks of the study.

Fibromyalgia

Ademetionine may be useful in treating **fibromyalgia**, which is characterized by persistent muscle pain and depression. However, some research involved injections of SAMe. While those studies indicated ademetionine was effective, the body reacts differently to injections than it does to remedies taken orally.

Other conditions

Ademetionine has been suggested for the treatment of conditions, including pain relief, migraine, **Alzheimer's disease**, **Parkinson's disease**, liver function, and peripheral neuropathy. The supplement had not been fully researched as of February 2008 in terms of safety and effectiveness for these and other conditions. Scientifically accepted testing of a large human population should provide answers and clear up inconsistencies in earlier studies. For example, some studies indicated that SAMe would not interfere with the effectiveness of levodopa, the drug most often prescribed for Parkinson's disease. There were no long-term studies on the possible interactions between levodopa and ademetionine.

KEY TERMS

Fibromyalgia—Chronic muscular or nerve pain that has no obvious cause.

Peripheral neuropathy—Damage to the nerve endings of the hands and feet, often as a result of diabetes.

Preparations

Ademetionine is available in preparations for oral, intravenous, and intramuscular administration. The dosage varies with condition, and with the strength and form of the supplement. Treatment with ademetionine should always be monitored by a qualified practitioner. This is particularly important when ademetionine is administered by injection. In February 2008, use of injectable SAMe was more prevalent in Europe than in the United States.

Osteoarthritis patients may be advised to take from 600 mg to 1,200 mg daily. That amount would be divided into three dosages per day. The injected dosage is 400 mg.

For depression, the daily oral dosage ranges from 400 mg to 1,600 mg. The higher strength was used in ademetionine studies. The injected dosage is 200 mg to 400 mg.

People with fibromyalgia could take 200 mg of ademetionine twice daily, increasing to 600 mg doses.

The daily dosages for migraine and liver conditions are 200 mg. For liver function, 200 mg of ademetionine can be taken twice daily, gradually raising the dosage to 400 mg three times daily. Patients with peripheral neuropathy have been given dosages as high as 1,600 mg.

Precautions

The United States Food and Drug Administration does not regulate supplements such as ademetionine, which means that supplements have not proven to be safe or effective. The safety of ademetionine for use by children, pregnant women, and nursing mothers has not been established. In addition, ingredients are not standardized to comply with federal regulations.

SAMe is not suitable for patients with **bipolar disorder**, as it may amplify the manic phase of the condition.

People should consult their doctor or practitioner before taking SAMe. This is especially important for people with pre-existing conditions such as those previously mentioned.

One possible drawback to ademetionine treatment is its cost. One company in 2008 offered a bottle containing 30 200-mg tablets for about $40. Another vendor sold 30 400-mg tablets for that price. Since daily dosages vary by condition, it could cost up to $100 or more for a month's supply of ademetionine. In addition, SAMe is not likely to be covered by medical insurance.

Side effects

Side effects of ademetionine could include gastrointestinal conditions such as **nausea**, **vomiting**, **constipation**, and **diarrhea**. Other side effects include increased thirst, **heartburn**, skin rash, **anxiety**, **dizziness**, headaches, **insomnia**, and sweating.

In patients who are deficient in the B vitamins, notably B_6 and B_{12}, there is a danger that SAMe may break down to form homocysteine, an amino acid that has been linked to heart disease and **stroke**. If the patient's levels of B vitamins are maintained, then, the body will be able to convert the homocysteine back into methionine and glutathione. As a result, use of SAMe will supposedly not increase the risk of heart disease.

Interactions

Ademetionine should not be used in conjunction with prescription medications such as anti-depressants and MAO inhibitors.

Resources

BOOKS

Mayo Clinic Book of Alternative Medicine. New York: Time Inc. Home Entertainment, 2007.

PERIODICALS

Medina, J., and R. Moreno-Otero. "Pathophysiological Basis for Antioxidant Therapy in Chronic Liver Disease." *Medscape Drugs Journal* 65, no. 17 (2005): 2445–2461.

Shippy, R. A., D. Mende, K. Jones, L. Cergnu, and S. E. Karpiak. "S-Adenosylmethionine (SAM-e) for the Treatment of Depression in People Living with HIV/AIDS." *BMC Psychiatry* 4 (2004): 38.

Werneke, U., T. Turner, and S. Priebe. "Complementary Medicines in Psychiatry: Review of Effectiveness and Safety." *British Journal of Psychiatry: The Journal of Mental Science* 188 (June 2006): 587.

ORGANIZATIONS

American Holistic Medicine Association, One Eagle Valley Court, Suite 201, Broadview Heights, OH, 44147, (440) 838-1010, http://www.holisticmedicine.org/index.html.

National Center for Complementary and Alternative Medicine; National Institute of Health (NCCAM), 9000 Rockville Pike, Bethesda, MD, 20892, (888) 644-6226, http://nccam.nih.gov.

Patricia Skinner
Teresa G. Odle
Liz Swain

ADHD *see* **Attention-deficit hyperactivity disorder**

Adie's pupil

Definition

Adie's pupil is a neurological condition that affects the eye and the autonomic nervous system. It is characterized by anisocoria, an inequality in the size of the pupils of the eyes. The pupil of one eye is larger than normal, and it constricts slowly in bright light, a condition known as tonic pupil. The condition may progress to the other eye. Other symptoms of this condition may include the loss of some deep tendon reflexes.

Adie's pupil is also referred to as Holmes-Adie syndrome. Adie's pupil primarily affects young women. It is considered a benign condition with no known cure.

Description

Adie's pupil is thought to be a result of damage to neurons in the ciliary ganglion, the part of the brain that controls eye movement, according to the National Institute of Neurological Disorders and **Stroke** (NINDS). Accommodation, or the adjustment of the eye for distance, is affected. The condition also affects pupillary dilation and contraction, the ability of the eye's iris to open or close in response to ambient light.

The condition also produces damage to the spinal ganglion, the part of the brain related to the autonomic nervous system, which affects deep tendon reflexes such as the knee and ankle jerk reflexes.

Some people may experience tonic pupil along with the loss of deep tendon reflexes and excessive sweating. When these three symptoms are experienced, the condition is generally known as Ross's syndrome, according to NINDS. However, the condition may be diagnosed as a variant of Holmes-Adie syndrome.

Eye function and Adie's pupil

The eyes are a complex anatomical and neurological unit. The outer surface of each eye is protected by a cornea, a normally clear cover that initiates the bending of light rays into the eye. Behind the cornea lies the colorful iris, a membrane containing two muscles capable of contracting and dilating. Behind the iris is the lens. Under the influence of the ciliary body, the lens further bends and directs the incoming light back to the retina. There it is received and transferred through the optic nerve at the back of the eye to the visual center of the brain (the visual cortex) at the back of the head.

The visual cortex sends instruction to the eye based on whether the object of vision is near or far and whether the surrounding light is bright or dim. This instruction goes back to the muscles of the eye—the ciliary body—through the ciliary ganglion. This results in a reshaping of the lens (accommodation) and an opening or closing of the pupil (pupillary reaction) as needed to order to focus more sharply.

Under normal circumstances, brightness and accommodation for near vision result in contracture of the ciliary body and the pupil. Darkness and accommodation for distance normally results in a **relaxation** of the ciliary body and dilation of the pupil. For a person with Adie's pupil, however, nerve signals arriving at the ciliary body of one eye are weaker than to the other eye.

The affected eye muscle is unable to contract, dilate, or focus with the same strength and speed as the unaffected eye. In normal daylight, the pupil of the affected eye is larger than that on the unaffected eye. In a quickly darkened room, the pupil of the affected eye is smaller. Furthermore, the nerve from the ciliary ganglion to the ciliary body has 30 fibers dedicated to changing the shape of the lens and only one fiber dedicated to dilating the iris. As a result, a person with Adie's pupil is even less able to dilate the pupil than to focus. Some research suggests that as the person ages, the ability to dilate gradually lessens to the point that the eye may have a smaller (constricted) pupil almost all the time.

Numerous names

Adie's pupil has been known by many names. These names include: Adie's Tonic Pupil, Tonic Pupil syndrome, Holmes-Adie syndrome and Adie-Holmes syndrome; Psuedotabes, Papillotonic Psuedotabes, and Psuedotabes pupillotonica; Kehrer-Adie syndrome, Markus' syndrome Weill's syndrome, Weill-Reys syndrome, and Weill-Reys-Adie syndrome; Psuedo-Argyll Robertson Pupil, Psuedo-Argyll Robertson syndrome, and Nonluetic Argyll-Robertson Pupil; Myotonic Pupil and Myotonic Pupillary Reaction; and Saenger's syndrome.

These numerous names derive from the lengthy history of the study of this condition. Many designations indicate the name of the person researching the condition. In 1813, London ophthalmologist James Ware described some common symptoms of Adie's pupil. Until 1914, some in the medical community thought the condition was caused by **syphilis**.

William John Adie was among the doctors who studied the condition. His contribution to the research came in 1931 when he maintained the condition was caused by the nervous system. Although Adie was referring to the findings of other doctors during the 1920s, the condition became associated with him. It was first referred to as Adie's syndrome in 1934 by the French neurologist, Jean-Alexandre Barré.

Medical theories

As of February 2008, viral and bacterial **infections** were thought to be the causes of Adie's pupil. Some other theories have been suggested but not proven. One doctor noted that the Adie's pupil affected women between 20 and 40 years of age more than it did men of all ages. The doctor speculated that the condition was related to an autoimmune disorder, especially when the individual lived a stressful lifestyle and other related family members were diagnosed with neurological diseases or disorders.

Heredity is rarely the cause of Adie's pupil, according to the NINDS. NINDS and other institutes of the National Institutes of Health (NIH) conducted research into Holmes-Adie syndrome (HAS) at NIH laboratories. NIH grants also supported research through grants to medical institutions. Research at all locations focused primarily on methods of preventing, treating, and curing conditions such as Adie's pupil.

Causes and symptoms

Adie's pupil is thought to be caused by an infection that damages the neurons in the brain, according to NINDS. A viral or bacterial infection is thought to be the cause of inflammation that damages neurons in the ciliary ganglion and the spinal ganglion.

Symptoms of Adie's pupil

Adie's pupil generally begins gradually in one eye and often progresses to the other eye, according to NINDS. The condition may initially cause the loss of deep tendon reflexes on one side of the body and then progress to the other side. People may sweat excessively, sometimes sweating on just one side of the body.

Adie's pupil has symptoms that may appear in conjunction with other nervous-symptom conditions such as migraine, according to NINDS.

Diagnosis

The diagnosis of Adie's pupil may include a physical examination to rule out other causes. In most cases, a professional in an optometrist's or ophthalmologist's office examines the person. The exam usually includes a test of the eye's reaction to a diluted amount of pilocarpine drops. The drops are an alkaloid substance from the jaborandi tree; they cause the otherwise slow-to-constrict pupil to constrict intensely. In a normal eye, the diluted drops would not cause the pupil to constrict.

In addition, the eyes may be examined with a slit lamp, an intensely bright lamp shielded by a shade with a slit. The diagnosis may be based on observing the pupil's reaction to light and dark conations.

Treatment

Allopathic treatment is necessary for Adie's pupil. Not much is known about this condition so treatments that strengthen or protect the nervous system might be helpful. These include taking the B-complex of vitamins. The complex or group consists of nutrients that are useful to the nervous system and eye health. Stress-reducing activities such as **yoga** or massage may be helpful.

KEY TERMS

Accommodation—The adjustment made through a change in shape of the lens allowing for vision of objects near and far.

Aqueous humor—A clear fluid in the posterior and anterior chambers of the eye that moves from back to front and exits the eye through a small canal into the venous system.

Knee and ankle jerk reflexes—Normal reflexes elicited usually by testing with a reflex hammer and demonstrating, by being present, a healthy and intact nervous system.

Pupillary reaction—The normal change in the size of the pupil due to the amount of ambient light. Under normal circumstances, both pupils respond simultaneously and equally.

Tonic pupil—A pupil that is slow to change.

Allopathic treatment

A doctor may prescribe prescription reading glasses to help correct the vision in the affected eye. In addition, the person may find it helpful to wear sunglasses or tinted indoor glasses.

The doctor may recommend that the patient apply pilocarpine drops to the eye three times a day. These drops constrict the pupil, making it smaller.

Prognosis

Adie's pupil is not a disabling or life-threatening condition, according to NINDS. Although some symptoms in the eyes may worsen, the use of glasses and eyedrops will help correct vision problems. However, the loss of the deep tendon reflexes is permanent.

Prevention

No preventative measures have yet been identified.

Resources

BOOKS

Galloway, Winfried, M. K. Amoaku, Peter H. Galloway, and Andrew C. Browning. *Common Eye Diseases and Their Management*. Berlin: Springer Science + Business Media, 2005.

OTHER

"Adie's syndrome." Who Named It. http://www.whoname dit.com/synd.cfm/1837.html. (February 1, 2008).

"Adie's tonic pupil." *Merck Manuals Online Medical Library Basic and Clinical Science Course Excerpt*. November 2005. http://one.aao.org/CE/Educational Content/snippet.aspx?F = bcsccontent\bcscsec tion5\bcsc2007section5_2007-08-13_050829\thepatient withpupillaryabnormalities\bcsc05100034.xml. (March 1, 2008).

Holistic Online.com. http://holisticonline.com. (March 1, 2008).

"Holmes-Adie's syndrome Information Page." *National Institute of Neurological Disorders and Stroke*. February 13, 2007. http://www.ninds.nih.gov/disorders/holmes_ adie/holmes_adie.htm. (March 1, 2008).

ORGANIZATIONS

American Academy of Ophthalmology, PO Box 7424, San Francisco, CA, 94120-7424, (415) 561-8500, http:// www.aao.org.

American Optometrist Association, 243 N. Lindbergh Blvd., St. Louis, MO, 63141, (800) 365-2219, http:// www.aoa.org.

National Institute of Neurological Disorders and Stroke. NIH Neurological Institute, PO Box 5801, Bethesda, MD, 20824, (800) 352-9424, http://www.ninds.nih.gov.

Katherine E. Nelson, N.D.
Liz Swain

African medicine *see* **Traditional African medicine**

African pygeum

Description

African pygeum (*Prunus africana*), also known as pygeum africanum, pygeum, and African plum tree, is an evergreen tree native to higher elevations of southern Africa. A 150 ft (46 m) tall member of the Rose family (*Rosacea*), pygeum has been found to be useful in treating prostate problems, particularly benign prostatic hypertrophy (BPH), a condition affecting many men.

The tree's bark contains an oil with many active ingredients; waxes, fatty acids, and other less familiar compounds. Pygeum's principal biological activity is traced to a "phytosterol" compound known as beta-sitosterol. Phyto (plant) sterols are structurally similar to, but much less efficiently absorbed from the diet than, **cholesterol**. The biological strength of phytosterols, however, is similar to that of hormones; therefore, a very small amount seems sufficient to initiate a response. Pygeum's phytosterols are anti-inflammatory. Pygeum also reduces **edema** (the swelling caused by an excess of fluids), reduces levels of the hormone prolactin, lowers and inhibits cholesterol activity within the prostate. Prolactin, whose levels are increased by drinking beer, stimulates testosterone uptake by the prostate, reportedly increasing levels of a metabolite responsible for prostatic cell increases, dihydrotestosterone (di-hydro-testosterone), (DHT). Cholesterol is reported to increase the influence of DHT. BPH imlies two prostate changes: increased size and increase tissue density. These changes cause symptoms of frequent urge to urinate small volumes, reduced prostatic secretions, reduced bladder emptying. Incomplete bladder emptying increases risk of bladder **infections**, edema and inflammation, and possibly, prostatic **cancer**. Blood sugar levels and immune function have also been found to improve.

In summary, african pygeum's medicinal actions include:

- anti-inflammation
- reducing edema of the prostate
- inhibit cellular increase
- improving the natural flow of prostatic secretions
- lowering cholesterol
- regulating insulin activity, thereby affecting blood sugar levels
- regulating the immune system

Although pygeum's use is relatively new to the United States, it has been imported from Africa to Europe since the 1700s, and is still used today as a major treatment for BPH. Europeans learned of this plant's usefulness in treating what was then known as "old man's disease". It continues to be *widely popular* in Europe as a remedy for BPH, especially in France where the use of African pygeum for BPH is reported to be about 80%.

General use

Pygeum is primarily used to treat BPH, a condition which affects men as early as their 40s, but increasingly with age: 30% of 50 year olds; 50% of 60 year olds; and nearly 80% of men 70 and older. It has been found to be of use in the related condition of chronic prostatitis, with and without prostate related **sexual dysfunction**, and **infertility** due to reduced prostatic secretions. Due to actions as an immune system "up regulator" and anti-inflammatory, pygeum is also being studied for use with other treatments for **hepatitis** C and HIV.

According to one source, in a double blind placebo controlled study involving 263 men on a dose of 100 mg per day of African pygeum extract for 60 days, the following improvements versus controls were observed:

- 31% decrease in "nocturia," or night-time frequency
- 24.5% decrease in "residual urine," the amount of urine left in the bladder after urination
- 17.2% increase in urine flow
- 50% increase in overall relief and feeling of wellbeing

Two-thirds of the group using Pygeum reported feeling satisfaction. This was twice the improvement reported by the control group on placebo.

In a study on chronic prostatitis, 60% of men with urinary tract infections and nearly 80% of men without infections reported improvements using 100 mg of pygeum extract for five to seven weeks. In the treatment of sexual dysfunction due to chronic prostatitis, a dose of 200 mg for 60 days, with or without an antibiotic, produced improvements in urination and sexual function. The few small and relatively short clinical trials of pygeum in the treatment of hepatitis C and HIV+ infections have been statistically significant; further trials are under way in South Africa.

Preparations

Since the 1960s, in Europe, the most commonly used form is the standardized herbal extract. The process is highly technical and, for pygeum, is designed to target extraction of the active oils using a sequence of laboratory extraction procedures. Standardization is the process whereby the targeted active ingredients are quantified and concentrated to a consistent therapeutic dose. The widely modern use of the extract form of African pygeum instead of the whole plant may derive from the discovery that the plant's activity is primarily due to its alcohol soluble phytosterols. A month's supply in capsules at a daily dosage of 100 mg, standardized to contain approximately 14% of the active beta-sitosterol ingredient, costs between $40 and $50. In some preparations, synergistic ingredients such as **amino acids**, other herbs, and vitamins or minerals, may be included. Studies cited used dosages of 100 mg daily; however, one study compared and found two dosages of 50 mg versus one dose of 100 mg per day had the same therapeutic effect.

Precautions

Precautions include recommendations to seek the guidance of a healthcare professional, and not to self treat. Pygeum may cause a hormonal shift, and is not recommended for children. Pygeum may require several weeks to months to make a noticeable difference; studies noted reported benefits at ranges of five to eight weeks. One source reported pygeum relieves symptoms but does not reduce prostatic size. Another study specifically stated that the active components of pygeum have symptom reversal and prevention characteristics.

Side effects

Pygeum appears to be relatively safe and non-toxic. One report noted rare occurrences of **diarrhea**, **dizziness**, disturbed vision, gastric **pain** and **constipation**. One study reported satisfactory safety profiles after 12 months of using 100 mg daily in 174 subjects. In animal studies it was reported that dogs and rats given amounts equivalent to more than 500 times the therapeutic dose showed no adverse effects, and amounts equivalent to 50 times the therapeutic dose had no effect on fertility. *In vivo* and *in vitro* studies showed no carcinogenic effects, In fact, pygeum's constituents have been found to be anti-carcinogenic. The National Institute of Health (NIH), in 2002, established a grant for a randomized controlled clinical study involving 3,100 men, in order to learn more about the medical potential of this alternative therapy, due to increased BPH diagnoses as the population ages.

Interactions

Synergistic supplements may facilitate benefits. One report advised dietary adjustments to enhance beneficial result. Dietary recommendations to improve prostatic health included avoiding the irritants of coffee and tobacco; eating pumpkin seeds for their **zinc** and Omega 3 anti-inflammatory content; increasing other dietary sources of Omega 3s, including the cold water fishes salmon, sardines, and mackerel; taking **antioxidants** and a good multivitamin; and the synergistic herb **saw palmetto** (*Serenoa repens*), said to be more effective than the pharmaceutical for BPH, Proscar, at inhibiting the conversion of testosterone to its metabolite DHT, implicated in prostatic cell increases. Vitamins E (400 IU) and B$_6$ (50–100 mg) were suggested to synergistically reduce prolactin levels. It was also noted that 200 mcg of **selenium** daily reduce the risk of **prostate cancer**.

No unfavorable interactions were noted. Any lifestyle habit that aggravates prostate health, for example, a high cholesterol, high fat, high red meat, low fiber diet, frequent and high intake of beer, and lack of

---

KEY TERMS

Benign prostatic hypertrophy (BPH)—A condition in many men affecting the prostate, wherein increased number and size of cells produces many urinary related symptoms.

Beta-sitosterol—A plant lipid with considerable biological activity; even in very amounts it is found to be anti-inflammatory and to have positive effects in treating BPH.

Dihydrotestosterone (DHT)—A testosterone metabolite implicated in the increase in size and number of prostatic cells.

Double blind placebo controlled study—A study in which neither the patient nor the drug administrator knows who is receiving the trial drug and who the placebo.

Metabolite—A by-product of the physical and chemical change process known as metabolism.

Prolactin—A hormone found in lactating women, and in men. Levels are increased by drinking beer.

Prostatic secretions—Normal secretions of the prostate gland intended to nourish and protect sperm, improving fertility.

Standardized herbal extract—An herbal product created by using water or alcohol to dissolve and concentrate the active ingredients, which are then quantified for medicinal pharmacological effect.

Synergistic—Describes an association that improves the effectiveness of members of the association.

Testosterone—The primary male reproductive hormone. Uptake into prostatic tissues is stimulated by prolactin; its DHT metabolite stimulates prostatic cell increases.

---

exercise may decrease the effectiveness of pygeum or other medications indicated for prostate health. Because pygeum has been found to upregulate immunity, its use may be contra-indicated where immune system upregulation is undesirable. No unfavorable herb-drug interactions have been noted.

Resources

BOOKS

Chevallier, Andrew. *The Encyclopedia of Medicinal Plants.* D.K. Publishing. 1996. (*Natural health encyclopedia of herbal medicine.* [2000] 2nd Ed.)

PERIODICALS

Brown, Don. "The Male Dilemma: Relief For Prostate Problems." *Total Health* 12 June 1990.

Miller, N.D., Alan L. "Benign Prostatic Hyperplasia, Nutritional and Botanical Therapeutic Options." *Alternative Medicine Review* 1.1. (2001).

Patrick, N.D., Lyn. "Hepatits C: Epidemiology and Review of Complementary/Alternative Medicine Treatments." *Alternative Medicine Review.* (2001).

"Pygeum africanum (*Prunus Africana*) (African plum tree)." *Alternative Medicine Review* 7.1. February 2002.

"The National Institutes of Health is Proceeding on a Study to Determine if the Dietary Supplement Ingredients ... Saw Palmetto and Pygeum." *Food Chemical News* 43.52. February 11, 2002.

OTHER

Iyker, Robert. "Men's Health: Straight Talk On Your Health and Life." *Natural Health* April 1999. http://www.findarticles.com.

Katy Nelson, N.D.

Agastache

Description

Agastache is a genus of plants found almost worldwide. Different species are used in several native cultures for healing. The best known of these is *Agastache rugosa*, also called the giant **hyssop**, wrinkled giant hyssop, Korean mint, or in Chinese *huo xiang*.

Agastache rugosa is a perennial or biennial plant that grows to a height of 4 ft (1.2 m). It is native to China but has spread to Japan, Korea, Laos, and Russia. It grows wild on sunny hillsides and along roads, but it can be cultivated in backyard gardens. The highly aromatic leaves and purple or red flowers are used for healing.

Several other species of agastache found in other parts of the world are used in healing. These include *A. nepetoides* (yellow giant hyssop), *A. foeniculum* (**anise** hyssop), and *A. mexicana*. Leaf and flower color vary considerably among the different species. Many species of agastache also are grown commercially in the United States for landscaping. In southern China and Taiwan, *Pogostemon cablin*, a relative of *Pogostemon*

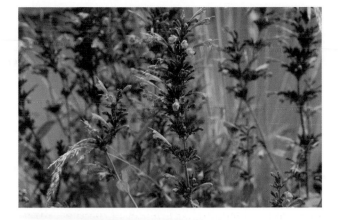

Agastache. *(Plantography / Alamy)*

patchouli, the Indian plant that produces patchouli oil, is used interchangeably with *A. rugosa*.

General use

A. rugosa is used extensively in Chinese herbalism. Its first recorded use dates from about 500 A.D. It is associated with the lungs, spleen, and stomach and is classified as having a warm nature and an acrid and aromatic taste. Traditionally, agastache has been associated the treatment of several different sets of symptoms. It has long been used to treat stomach flu, stomachache, **nausea**, **vomiting**, **diarrhea**, abdominal bloating, and abdominal **pain**. It is combined with *Scutellaria* (**skullcap**) to treat **morning sickness** in pregnant women. It is also a component of formulas that improve digestive balance by aiding the absorption of nutrients and intestinal function.

In Chinese herbalism, *A. rugosa* is also used to treat summer flu or summer colds with accompanying low **fever**, feelings of fullness in the chest, and **headache**. It is also used to treat dark urine and a feeling of heaviness in the arms and legs. A lotion containing *A. rugosa* is applied externally to treat **fungal infections**.

Other cultures independently have discovered similar uses for other species of agastache. *A. mexicana* is grown in Mexico and used to treat gastrointestinal upsets, nervous disorders, and cardiovascular ailments. The leaves of *A. nepetoides* are used by Native Americans to treat skin **rashes** caused by poison ivy. *A. foeniculum* leaves have a strong **licorice** taste (accounting for its English name, anise hyssop). These leaves can be brewed in a tea to treat coughs, fever, and colds.

Rigorous scientific testing of the healing claims made for agastache is scarce. Most of the work that done on this herb involves test-tube studies or animal testing.

Preparations

Agastache can be prepared alone as a tea, incorporated into a lotion, or prepared as a pill. The leaves are strongly aromatic but lose this quality with prolonged boiling (over 15 minutes). Therefore, agastache is added last in formulas that must be boiled.

The best known formulas using agastache are agastache formula and *Huo Xiang Zheng Qi Wan*, or agastache qi-correcting formula. Agastache formula is used to harmonize the stomach. It is given as treatment for gastrointestinal upsets with **chills**, fever, and diarrhea.

Huo Xiang Zheng Qi Wan regulates qi and treats seasonal gastric disorders, especially those occurring during hot, humid weather. This formula is commercially available in both tablet and liquid form. Other cultures prepare agastache either as a tea to be drunk or use the leaves externally.

Precautions

Agastache has a long history of use with no substantial reported problems.

Side effects

No side effects have been reported with the use of agastache.

Interactions

Agastache is often used in conjunction with other herbs with no reported interactions. Since agastache has been used almost exclusively in Chinese medicine, there are no studies of its interactions with Western pharmaceuticals.

Resources

BOOKS

Chevallier, Andrew. *Herbal Remedies.* New York: DK Publishing, 2007.

OTHER

"Agastache rugosa." *Plants for a Future,* June 2004. http://www.pfaf.org/database/plants.php?Agastache + rugosa.

ORGANIZATIONS

Alternative Medicine Foundation, PO Box 60016, Potomac, MD, 20859, (301) 340-1960, http://www.amfoundation.org.

American Association of Oriental Medicine, PO Box 162340, Sacramento, CA, 95816, (866) 455-7999, (914) 443-4770, http://www.aaaomonline.org.

Centre for International Ethnomedicinal Education and Research (CIEER), http://www.cieer.org.

Tish Davidson, A. M.

Aging

Definition

Starting at what is commonly called middle age, operations of the human body become more vulnerable to daily wear and tear. There is a general decline in physical, and possibly mental, functioning. In the Western countries, the length of life often extends into the 70s. However, the upward limit of the life span can be as high as 120 years. During the latter half of life, an individual is more prone to problems with the various functions of the body, and to a number of chronic or fatal diseases. The cardiovascular, digestive, excretory, nervous, reproductive, and urinary systems are particularly affected. The most common diseases of aging include Alzheimer's, arthritis, **cancer**, diabetes, **depression**, and **heart disease**.

Description

Human beings reach a peak of growth and development during their mid 20s. Aging is the normal transition time after that flurry of activity. Although there are quite a few age-related changes that tax the body, disability is not necessarily a part of aging. Health and lifestyle factors, together with the genetic makeup of the individual, determine the response to these changes. Body functions that are most often affected by age include:

- Hearing, which declines especially in relation to the highest pitched tones.
- The proportion of fat to muscle, which may increase by as much as 30%. Typically, the total padding of body fat directly under the skin thins out and accumulates around the stomach. The ability to excrete fats is impaired, and therefore the storage of fats increases, including cholesterol and fat-soluble nutrients.
- The amount of water in the body, which decreases, reducing the body's ability to absorb water-soluble nutrients. Also, there is less saliva and other lubricating fluids.
- Liver and kidney activities, which become less efficient, thus affecting the elimination of wastes.
- The ease of digestion, which is decreased, resulting in a reduction in stomach acid production.
- Muscle strength and coordination, which lessens, with an accompanying loss of mobility, agility, and flexibility.
- Sexual hormones and sexual function, which both decline.
- Sensations of taste and smell, which decrease.
- Cardiovascular and respiratory systems, with changes leading to decreased oxygen and nutrients throughout the body.
- Nervous system, which experiences changes that result in less efficient nerve impulse transmission, reflexes that are not as sharp, and diminished memory and learning.
- Bone strength and density, which decrease.
- Hormone levels, which gradually decline. The thyroid and sexual hormones are particularly affected.
- Visual abilities, which decline. Age-related changes may lead to diseases such as macular degeneration.
- A compromised ability to produce vitamin D from sunlight.
- Protein formation, which is reduced, leading to shrinkage in muscle mass and decreased bone formation, possibly contributing to osteoporosis.

Causes and symptoms

There are several theories on why the aging body loses functioning. It may be that several factors work together or that one particular factor is the culprit in a given individual. These theories include:

- Programmed senescence, or aging clock, theory. The aging of the cells for each individual is programmed into the genes, and there is a preset number of possible rejuvenations in the life of a given cell. When cells die at a rate faster than they are replaced, organs do not function properly, and they become unable to maintain the functions necessary for life.
- Genetic theory. Human cells maintain their own seed of destruction at the chromosome level.
- Connective tissue, or cross-linking theory. Changes in the makeup of the connective tissue alter the stability of body structures, causing a loss of elasticity and functioning, and leading to symptoms of aging.
- Free-radical theory. The most commonly held theory of aging, is based on the fact that ongoing chemical reactions of the cells produce free radicals. In the presence of oxygen, these free radicals cause the cells of the body to break down. As time goes on, more cells die or lose the ability to function, and the body ceases to function as a whole.
- Immunological theory. There are changes in the immune system as it begins to wear out, and the body is more prone to infections and tissue damage, which may ultimately cause death. Also, as the system breaks down, the body is more apt to have autoimmune reactions, in which the body's own cells are mistaken for foreign material and are destroyed or damaged by the immune system.

Diagnosis

Many problems can arise due to age-related changes in the body. Although there is no individual test to measure these changes, a thorough physical exam and a basic blood screening and blood chemistry panel can point to areas in need of further attention. When older people become ill, the first signs of disease are often nonspecific. Further exams should be conducted if any of the following occur:

- diminished, or lack of, desire for food
- increased confusion
- failure to thrive
- urinary incontinence
- dizziness
- weight loss
- falling

Treatment

Nutritional supplements

Consumption of a high-quality multivitamin is recommended. Common nutritional deficiencies connected with aging include B vitamins, **vitamin A** and **vitamin C**, **folic acid**, **calcium**, **magnesium**, **zinc**, **iron**, **chromium**, and trace minerals. Since stomach acids may be decreased, powdered multivitamin formula in gelatin capsules are suggested, as this form is the easiest to digest. Such formulas may also contain enzymes for further help with digestion.

Antioxidants can help neutralize damage caused by free radical actions, which are thought to contribute to problems of aging. They are also helpful in preventing and treating cancer, and in treating **cataracts** and **glaucoma**. Supplements that serve as antioxidants include:

- Vitamin E, 400–1,000 IUs daily. Protects cell membranes against damage. It shows promise in preventing heart disease, and Alzheimer's and Parkinson's diseases.

- Selenium, 50 mg taken twice daily. Research suggests that selenium may play a role in reducing cancer risk.

- Beta-carotene, 25,000–40,000 IUs daily. May help in treating cancer, colds and flu, arthritis, and immune support.

- Vitamin C, 1,000–2,000 mg per day. It may cause diarrhea in large doses. The dosage should be decreased if this occurs.

Other supplements that are helpful in treating age-related problems include:

- B_{12}/B-complex vitamins. Studies show that B_{12} may help reduce mental symptoms, such as confusion, memory loss, and depression.

- Coenzyme Q_{10} may be helpful in treating heart disease. Up to 75% of cardiac patients have been found to lack this heart enzyme.

Hormones

The following hormonc supplements may be taken to prevent or treat various age-related problems. However, caution should be taken before beginning treatment, and the patient should consult his or her health care professional prior to hormone use.

DHEA improves brain functioning and serves as a building block for many other important hormones. It may be helpful in restoring hormone levels that have declined, building muscle mass, strengthening bones, and maintaining a healthy heart.

Melatonin may be helpful for **insomnia**. It has also been used to help fight viruses and bacterial **infections**, reduce the risk of heart disease, improve sexual function, and to protect against cancer.

Human growth hormone (hGH) has been shown to regulate blood sugar levels and to stimulate bone, cartilage, and muscle growth while reducing fat.

Herbs

Garlic (*Allium sativa*) is helpful in preventing heart disease, and improving the tone and texture of skin. Garlic stimulates liver and digestive system functions, and also helps manage heart disease and high blood pressure.

Siberian ginseng (*Eleutherococcus senticosus*) supports the adrenal glands and immune functions. It is believed to be helpful in treating problems related to **stress**. Siberian ginseng also increases mental and physical performance, and may be useful in treating **memory loss**, chronic **fatigue**, and immune dysfunction.

Ginkgo biloba works particularly well on the brain and nervous system. It is effective in reducing the symptoms of such conditions as **Alzheimer's disease**, depression, visual disorders, and problems of blood circulation. It may also help treat heart disease, strokes, **dementia**, Raynaud's disease, head injuries, leg cramps, **macular degeneration**, **tinnitus**, **impotence** due to poor blood flow, and diabetes-related nerve damage.

Proanthocyanidins, or PCO, (brand name Pycnogenol), are derived from grape seeds and skin, as well as pine tree bark. They may help prevent cancer and poor vision.

Green tea has powerful antioxidant qualities, and has been used for centuries as a natural medicine in China, Japan, and other Asian cultures. In alternative medicine, it aids in treating cancer, **rheumatoid arthritis**, high **cholesterol**, heart disease, infection, and impaired immune function. Several scientific studies have shown that antioxidant benefits are obtained by drinking two cups of green tea each day.

In **Ayurvedic medicine**, aging is described as a process of increased vata, in which there is a tendency to become thinner, drier, more nervous, more restless, and more fearful, while experiencing declines in both sleep and appetite. Bananas, almonds, avocados, and coconuts are some of the foods used in correcting such conditions. One of the main herbs used to treat these problems is **gotu kola** (*Centella asiatica*). It is taken to revitalize the nervous system and brain cells, and to fortify the immune system. Gotu kola is also used to treat memory loss, **anxiety**, and insomnia.

In Chinese medicine, most symptoms of aging are regarded as signs of a yin deficiency. Moistening foods are recommended, and include barley soup, tofu, mung beans, **wheat germ**, **spirulina**, potatoes, black sesame seeds, walnuts, and flax seeds. Jing tonics may also be used. These include deer antler, dodder seeds, processed rehmannia, longevity soup, mussels, and chicken.

Allopathic treatment

For the most part, doctors prescribe medications to control the symptoms and diseases of aging. In the United States, about two-thirds of people age 65 and over take medications for various conditions. More women than men use these medications. The most common drugs used by the elderly are painkillers, diuretics or water pills, sedatives, cardiac medications, antibiotics, and mental health remedies.

Estrogen replacement therapy (ERT) is commonly prescribed to alleviate the symptoms of aging in post-menopausal women. It is often used in conjunction with progesterone. These drugs help keep bones strong, reduce the risk of heart disease, restore vaginal lubrication, and improve skin elasticity. Evidence suggests that they may also help maintain mental functions.

Expected results

Aging is unavoidable, but major physical impairment is not. People can lead healthy, disability-free lives throughout their later years. A well-established support system of family, friends, and health care providers, along with a focus on good **nutrition** and lifestyle habits, and effective stress management, can prevent disease and lessen the impact of chronic conditions.

Prevention

Preventive health practices such as healthy diet, daily **exercise**, stress management, and control of lifestyle habits, such as **smoking** and drinking, can lengthen the life span and improve the quality of life as people age. Exercise can improve appetite, bone health, emotional and mental outlook, digestion, and circulation.

Drinking plenty of fluids aids in maintaining healthy skin, good digestion, and proper elimination of wastes. Up to eight glasses of water should be consumed daily, along with plenty of herbal teas, diluted fruit and vegetable juices, and fresh fruits and vegetables that have a high water content.

Because of a decrease in the sense of taste, older people often increase their salt intake, which can contribute to high blood pressure and nutrient loss. Use of sugar is also increased. Seaweeds and small amounts of honey can be used as replacements.

Alcohol, nicotine, and **caffeine** all have potential damaging effects, and consumption should be limited or completely eliminated.

KEY TERMS

Alzheimer's disease—A condition causing a decline in brain function that interferes with the ability to reason and to perform daily activities.

Antioxidants—Substances that counteract the damaging effects of oxidation in the body's tissues.

Senescence—Aging.

Vata—One of the three main constitutional types found under Ayurvedic principles. Keeping one's particular constitution in balance is considered important in maintaining health.

A diet high in fiber and low in fat is recommended. Processed foods should be replaced by such complex carbohydrates as whole grains. If chewing becomes a problem, there should be an increased intake of protein drinks, freshly juiced fruits and vegetables, and creamed cereals.

Resources

BOOKS

Cox, Harold. *Aging*. New York, NY: McGraw Hill College Division, 2004.

Giampapa, Vincent, et al. *The Anti-Aging Solution: 5 Simple Steps to Looking and Feeling Young*. Hoboken, NJ: John Wiley & Sons, 2004.

Landis, Robyn, with Karta Purkh Singh Khalsa. *Herbal Defense: Positioning Yourself to Triumph Over Illness and Aging* New York, NY: Warner Books, 1997.

Panno, Joseph. *Aging: Theories and Potential Therapies* New York, NY: Facts on File, Inc., 2004.

Weil, Andrew M.D. *Healthy Aging* New York, NY: Knopf, 2004.

PERIODICALS

"Chemopreventive Effects of Green Tea Said to Delay Aging of Skin." *Cancer Weekly* (April 13, 2004): 10.

"Discovery Claims to Link DNA Test to Reversing Signs of Aging." *Drug Week* (February 27, 2004): 122.

"Fitness Can Improve Thinking Among Aging." *Obesity, Fitness & Wellness Week* (March 13, 2004): 16.

"Hormonal Activity Plays Role in Body Composition Changes with Aging." *Obesity, Fitness & Wellness Week* (March 20, 2004): 3.

Lofshult, Diane. "Aging Trends for 2004." *IDEA Health & Fitness Source* (March 2004): 14.

"Research Reports on Key Antioxidant to Slow Aging." *Drug Week* (April 2, 2004): 194.

ORGANIZATIONS

The Anti-Aging Institute. 843 William Hilton Parkway, Hilton Head, SC 29928. (912) 238-3383. http://www.anti-aging.org.

The Rosenthal Center for Complementary and Alternative Medicine Research in Aging and Women's Health. Columbia University, College of Physicians and Surgeons, 630 W. 168th St., New York, NY 10032. http://www.rosenthal.hs.columbia.edu.

OTHER

National Institute on Aging Senior Health Web site. http://www.nihseniorhealth.gov.

Patience Paradox
Ken Wells

AIDS

Definition

Acquired immune deficiency syndrome (AIDS) is an infectious disease caused by the human immunodeficiency virus (HIV). It was first recognized in the

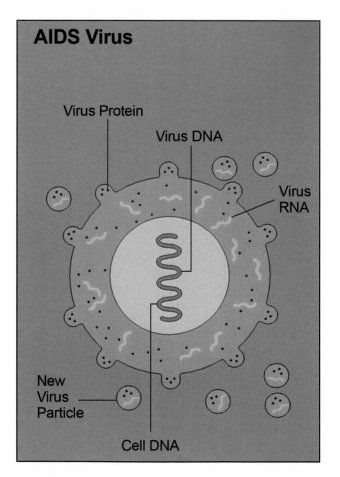

AIDS Virus

Virus Protein
Virus DNA
Virus RNA
New Virus Particle
Cell DNA

The AIDS virus. *(National Institutes of Health, U.S. Department of Health and Human Services)*

Estimated number of adults and children living with AIDS/HIV worldwide as of 2005

Regions	Estimate
Caribbean	330,000
East Asia	680,000
Eastern Europe & Central Asia	1,500,000
Latin America	1,600,000
North Africa & Middle East	440,000
North America	1,300,000
Oceania	78,000
South & Southeast Asia	7,600,000
Sub-Saharan Africa	24,500,000
Western & Central Europe	720,000
Global Total	38,748,000

(Illustration by Corey Light. Cengage Learning, Gale)

United States in 1981. AIDS is the advanced form of infection with the HIV virus, which may not cause disease for a long period after the initial exposure (latency). Infection with HIV weakens the immune system, which makes infected people susceptible to infection and **cancer**.

Description

AIDS is considered one of the most devastating public health problems in recent history. In 2003, the Centers for Disease Control and Prevention (CDC) estimated that one million persons in the United States were HIV-positive, and 223,000 are living with AIDS. Of these patients, 45% are gay or bisexual men, 22% are heterosexual intravenous drug users, and 26% are women. In addition, approximately 100–200 children are born each year with HIV infection. In 2002, the CDC reported 42,136 new AIDS diagnoses in the United States, a 2.2% increase from the previous year. AIDS cases rose among gay and bisexual men (7.1% in 25 states that report regularly). The disease also seems to be rising among older Americans. From

2001 to 2005, the number of cases in Americans age 50 years or older rose from 17% to 24%.

The World Health Organization (WHO) estimates that 18 million adults and 1.5 million children worldwide were infected with HIV as of 1995 with the potential to produce about 4.5 million cases of AIDS. Most of these cases were in the developing countries of Asia and Africa. In 2003, WHO cautioned that if treatment was not delivered soon to nearly 6 million people with AIDS in developing countries, there could be 45 million cases by HIV by 2010.

Risk factors

AIDS can be transmitted in several ways. The risk factors for HIV transmission vary according to category:

- Sexual contact. Persons at greatest risk are those who do not practice safe sex, are not monogamous, participate in anal intercourse, and have sex with a partner with symptoms of advanced HIV infection and/or other sexually transmitted diseases (STDs). In the United States and Europe, most cases of sexually transmitted HIV infection have resulted from homosexual contact, whereas in Africa, the disease is spread primarily through sexual intercourse among heterosexuals.
- Transmission in pregnancy. High-risk mothers include women married to bisexual men or men who have an abnormal blood condition called hemophilia and require blood transfusions, intravenous drug users, and women living in neighborhoods with a high rate of HIV infection among heterosexuals. The chances of transmitting the disease to the child are higher in women in advanced stages of the disease. Breast feeding increases the risk of transmission by 10–20% and is not recommended. The use of zidovudine (ZDV) during pregnancy and delivery can decrease the risk of transmission to the baby.
- Exposure to contaminated blood or blood products. Following the introduction of blood product screening in the mid-1980s, the incidence of HIV transmission in blood transfusions dropped to 1 in 100,000.
- Needle sticks among health care professionals. In the early 2000s, studies indicated that the risk of HIV transmission by a needle stick was about 1 in 250. This rate can be decreased if the injured worker is given AZT or triple therapy (HAART), the standard at the time.

HIV is not transmitted by handshakes or other casual non-sexual contact, coughing or **sneezing**, or by bloodsucking insects such as mosquitoes.

AIDS in women

AIDS in women is a serious public health concern. Women exposed to HIV infection through heterosexual contact are the most rapidly growing risk group in the United States. The percentage of AIDS cases diagnosed in women rose from 7% in 1985 to 18% in 1996. For unknown reasons, women with AIDS do not live as long as men with AIDS.

AIDS in children

Because AIDS can be transmitted from an infected mother to her child during **pregnancy**, during the birth process, or through breast milk, all infants born to HIV-positive mothers are at risk. In 1997, it was estimated that 84% of HIV-positive women are of childbearing age; 41% of them are drug abusers. Between 15–30% of children born to HIV-positive women will be infected with the virus.

AIDS is one of the 10 leading causes of death in children between one and four years of age worldwide. The interval between exposure to HIV and the development of AIDS is shorter in children than in adults. Infants infected with HIV have a 20–30% chance of developing AIDS within a year and dying before age three. In the remainder, AIDS progresses more slowly; the average child patient survives to seven years of age. Some survive into early adolescence.

Causes and symptoms

Because HIV destroys immune system cells, AIDS is a disease that can affect any of the body's major organ systems. HIV attacks the body through three disease processes: immunodeficiency, autoimmunity, and nervous system dysfunction.

Immunodeficiency describes the condition in which the body's immune response is damaged, weakened, or is not functioning properly. In AIDS, immunodeficiency results from the way that the virus binds to a protein called CD4, which is found on certain white blood cells, including helper T cells, macrophages, and monocytes. Once HIV attaches to an immune system cell, it can replicate within the cell and kill the cell. In addition to killing some lymphocytes directly, the AIDS virus disrupts the functioning of other CD4 cells. Because the immune system cells are destroyed, **infections** and cancers that take advantage of a person's weakened immune system (opportunistic) can develop.

Autoimmunity is a condition in which the body's immune system produces antibodies that work against its own cells. Antibodies are specific proteins produced in response to exposure to a specific, usually foreign, protein or particle called an antigen. In this case, the body produces antibodies that bind to blood platelets that are necessary for proper blood clotting and tissue repair. Once bound, the antibodies mark the platelets for removal from the body, and they are filtered out by the spleen. Some AIDS patients develop a disorder, called immune-related thrombocytopenia purpura (ITP), in which the number of blood platelets drops to abnormally low levels.

The course of AIDS generally progresses through three stages, although not all patients follow this progression precisely.

Acute retroviral syndrome

Acute retroviral syndrome is a group of symptoms that can resemble **mononucleosis** and that may be the first sign of HIV infection in 50–70% of all patients and 45–90% of women. The symptoms may include **fever**, **fatigue**, muscle aches, loss of appetite, digestive disturbances, weight loss, skin **rashes**, **headache**, and chronically swollen lymph nodes (lymphadenopathy). Approximately 25–33% of patients experience a form of **meningitis** during this phase, in which the membranes that cover the brain and spinal cord become inflamed. Acute retroviral syndrome develops between one and six weeks after infection and lasts two to four weeks, sometimes up to six weeks. Blood tests during this period indicate the presence of virus (viremia) and the appearance of the viral p24 antigen in the blood.

Latency period

After the HIV virus enters a patient's lymph nodes during the acute retroviral syndrome stage, the disease becomes latent for as many as 10 years or more before symptoms of advanced disease develop. During latency, the virus continues to replicate in the lymph nodes, where it may cause one or more of the following conditions.

PERSISTENT GENERALIZED LYMPHADENOPATHY (PGL). Persistent generalized lymphadenopathy, or PGL, is a condition in which HIV continues to produce chronic painless swellings in the lymph nodes during the latency period. The lymph nodes most frequently affected by PGL are those in the areas of the neck, jaw, groin, and armpits. PGL affects between 50–70% of patients during latency.

CONSTITUTIONAL SYMPTOMS. Many patients develop low-grade fevers, chronic fatigue, and general weakness. HIV also may cause a combination of food malabsorption, loss of appetite, and increased metabolism that contribute to the so-called AIDS wasting or wasting syndrome.

OTHER ORGAN SYSTEMS. At any time during the course of HIV infection, patients may develop a **yeast infection** in the mouth called thrush, open sores or ulcers, or other infections of the mouth; **diarrhea** and other gastrointestinal symptoms that cause malnutrition and weight loss; diseases of the lungs and kidneys; and degeneration of the nerve fibers in the arms and legs. HIV infection of the nervous system leads to general loss of strength, loss of reflexes, and feelings of numbness or burning sensations in the feet or lower legs.

Late-stage AIDS

Late-stage AIDS usually is marked by a sharp decline in the number of CD4+ lymphocytes (a type of white blood cell), followed by a rise in the frequency of opportunistic infections and cancers. Doctors monitor the number and proportion of CD4+ lymphocytes in the patient's blood in order to assess the progression of the disease and the effectiveness of different medications. About 10% of infected individuals never progress to this overt stage of the disease.

OPPORTUNISTIC INFECTIONS. Once the patient's CD4+ lymphocyte count falls below 200 cells/mm^3, he/she is at risk for opportunistic infections. The infectious organisms may include:

- Fungi. Fungal infections include a yeast infection of the mouth (candidiasis or thrush) and cryptococcal meningitis.
- Protozoa. The most common parasitic disease associated with AIDS is *Pneumocystis carinii* pneumonia (PCP). About 70–80% of AIDS patients have at least one episode of PCP prior to death. PCP is the immediate cause of death in 15–20% of AIDS patients. It is an important measure of a patient's prognosis. Toxoplasmosis is another common infection in AIDS patients that is caused by a protozoan. Other diseases in this category include amebiasis and cryptosporidiosis.
- Mycobacteria. AIDS patients may develop tuberculosis or MAC infections. MAC infections are caused by *Mycobacterium avium-intracellulare* and occur in about 40% of AIDS patients.
- Bacteria. AIDS patients are likely to develop bacterial infections of the skin and digestive tract.
- Viruses. AIDS patients are highly vulnerable to cytomegalovirus (CMV), herpes simplex virus (HSV), varicella zoster virus (VZV), and Epstein-Barr virus (EBV) infections. Another virus, JC virus, causes progressive destruction of brain tissue in the brain

stem, cerebrum, and cerebellum (multifocal leukoencephalopathy or PML), which is regarded as an AIDS-defining illness by the CDC.

AIDS DEMENTIA COMPLEX AND NEUROLOGIC COMPLICATIONS. AIDS **dementia** complex is a late complication of the disease. It is unclear whether it is caused by the direct effects of the virus on the brain or by intermediate causes. AIDS dementia complex is marked by loss of reasoning ability, loss of memory, inability to concentrate, apathy and loss of initiative, and unsteadiness or weakness in walking. Some patients also develop seizures.

MUSCULOSKELETAL COMPLICATIONS. Patients in late-stage AIDS may develop inflammations of the muscles, particularly in the hip area, and may have arthritis-like pains in the joints.

ORAL SYMPTOMS. Patients may develop a condition called hairy leukoplakia of the tongue. This condition also is regarded by the CDC as an indicator of AIDS. Hairy leukoplakia is a white area of diseased tissue on the tongue that may be flat or slightly raised. It is caused by the Epstein-Barr virus.

AIDS-RELATED CANCERS. Patients with late-stage AIDS may develop **Kaposi's sarcoma** (KS), a skin tumor that primarily affects homosexual men. KS is the most common AIDS-related malignancy. It is characterized by reddish-purple blotches or patches (brownish in African Americans) on the skin or in the mouth. About 40% of patients with KS develop symptoms in the digestive tract or lungs. KS appears to be caused by a herpes virus.

The second most common form of cancer in AIDS patients is a tumor of the lymphatic system (lymphoma). AIDS-related lymphomas often affect the central nervous system and develop very aggressively.

Invasive cancer of the cervix is an important diagnostic marker of AIDS in women.

Diagnosis

Because HIV infection produces such a wide range of symptoms, the CDC has drawn up a list of 34 conditions regarded as defining AIDS. The physician uses the CDC list to decide whether the patient falls into one of these three groups:

- definitive diagnoses with or without laboratory evidence of HIV infection
- definitive diagnoses with laboratory evidence of HIV infection
- presumptive diagnoses with laboratory evidence of HIV infection

Physical findings

Almost all symptoms of AIDS can occur with other diseases. The general physical examination may range from normal findings to symptoms that are closely associated with AIDS. These symptoms are hairy leukoplakia of the tongue and Kaposi's sarcoma. During the examination, the doctor looks for the overall pattern of symptoms rather than any one finding.

Laboratory tests for HIV infection

BLOOD TESTS (SEROLOGY). The first blood test for AIDS was developed in 1985. Patients who are being tested for HIV infection usually are given an enzyme-linked immunosorbent assay (ELISA) test for the presence of HIV antibody in their blood. Positive ELISA results then are tested with a Western blot or immunofluorescence (IFA) assay for confirmation. The combination of the ELISA and Western blot tests is more than 99.9% accurate in detecting HIV infection within four to eight weeks following exposure. The polymerase chain reaction (PCR) test can be used to detect the presence of viral nucleic acids in the very small number of HIV patients who have false-negative results on the ELISA and Western blot tests. In 2003, a one-step test that was quicker and cheaper was shown to be effective for detecting HIV in the physician office setting. However, further research was ongoing as to its effectiveness in replacing other tests as a first check for HIV.

OTHER LABORATORY TESTS. In addition to diagnostic blood tests, there are other blood tests that are used to track the course of AIDS. These include blood counts, viral load tests, p24 antigen assays, and measurements of β_2-microglobulin (β_2M).

Doctors use a wide variety of tests to diagnose the presence of opportunistic infections, cancers, or other disease conditions in AIDS patients. Tissue biopsies, samples of cerebrospinal fluid, and sophisticated imaging techniques, such as magnetic resonance imaging (MRI) and computed tomography scans (CT) are used to diagnose AIDS-related cancers, some opportunistic infections, damage to the central nervous system, and wasting of the muscles. Urine and stool samples are used to diagnose infections caused by parasites. AIDS patients are also given blood tests for **syphilis** and other sexually transmitted diseases.

Diagnosis in children

Diagnostic blood testing in children older than 18 months is similar to adult testing, with ELISA screening confirmed by Western blot. Younger infants can be diagnosed by direct culture of the HIV virus, PCR testing, and p24 antigen testing.

In terms of symptoms, children are less likely than adults to have an early acute syndrome. They are, however, likely to have delayed growth, a history of frequent illness, recurrent ear infections, a low blood cell count, failure to gain weight, and unexplained fevers. Children with AIDS are more likely to develop bacterial infections, inflammation of the lungs, and AIDS-related brain disorders than are HIV-positive adults.

Treatment

AIDS patients turn to alternative medicine when conventional treatments are ineffective and to supplement conventional treatment, reduce disease symptoms, counteract drug effects, and improve quality of life. Because alternative medicines may interact with conventional medicines, it is important for patients to inform their doctors of all treatments being used.

A report released in 2003 showed trends in increased use of alternative medicine among HIV-positive individuals. The types of therapies they used most were **relaxation** techniques, massage, **chiropractic** care, self-help groups, commercial **diets**, and **acupuncture**.

Supplements

- Lauric oils (coconut oil) are used by the body to make monolaurin, which inactivates HIV.
- Selenium deficiency increases the risk of death due to AIDS-related illness. One study found that 250 micrograms of selenomethionin daily for one year showed no improvement in CD4 cell counts or disease symptoms. Greater than 1,000 micrograms daily is toxic.
- Vitamin C has antioxidant and antiretroviral activities. One study found that treatment caused a trend to decrease viral load.
- DHEA (dehydroepiandrosterone) is commonly used by AIDS patients to counteract wasting. One study found that DHEA had no effect on lymphocytes or p24 antigen levels. However, a 2002 study found that it was associated with a significant increase in measures that indicate mental health improvement.
- Vitamin A deficiency is associated with increased mortality. One study of pregnant women with AIDS found that 5,000 IU of vitamin A daily led to stabilized viral load as compared to a placebo group.

Another study found that 60 mg of vitamin A had no effect on CD4 cells or viral load. Vitamin A has been associated with faster disease progression. Excessive vitamin A during pregnancy can cause birth defects.

- Beta-carotene supplementation for AIDS is controversial as studies have shown both beneficial and detrimental effects. Beta-carotene supplementation has led to elevation in white blood cell counts and changes in the CD4 cell count. Some studies have found that beta-carotene supplementation led to an increase in deaths due to cancer and heart disease.

Naturopathic doctors often recommend the following supplements for AIDS:

- beta-carotene, 150,000 IU daily
- vitamin C, 2000 mg three times daily
- vitamin E, 400 IU twice daily
- cod liver oil, 1 tablespoon daily
- multivitamin, as directed
- coenzyme Q10, 50–60 mg twice daily

Herbals and Chinese medicine

One small study of the effectiveness of Chinese herbal treatment in AIDS showed promise. AIDS patients took a tablet that contained 31 herbs that was based on the formulas Enhance and Clear Heat. Disease symptoms were reduced in the herbal treatment group as compared to the placebo group.

Herbals used in treating AIDS include:

- Maitake mushroom extract. Recommended dose is 10 drops twice daily.
- Licorice (*Glycyrrhiza glabra*) solid extract. Recommended dose is one-quarter to one-half teaspoon twice daily.
- Boxwood extract (SPV-30) has antiviral activity. Recommended dose is one capsule three times daily.
- Garlic concentrate (Allicin) helped reduce bowel movements, stabilized or increased body weight, or cured *Cryptosporidium parvum* infection in affected AIDS patients. However, a 2002 National Institutes of Health study cautioned that garlic supplements could reduce levels of a protease inhibitor that is used to treat AIDS patients, so patients should discuss using garlic supplements with their physicians.
- Tea tree oil (*Malaleuca*) improves or cures infection of the mouth by the yeast *Candida*. Tea tree oil is available as soap, dental floss, toothpick, and mouthwash.
- Marijuana is used to treat wasting. Studies have found that patients who use marijuana had increased food intake and weight gain. The active ingredient

delta-9-tetrahydrocannabinol is licensed for treating AIDS wasting.

Psychotherapy and stress reduction

Many therapies that are directed at improving mental state can have a direct impact on disease severity and quality of life. The effectiveness of many have been proven in clinical studies. These include:

- massage
- laughter/humor
- stress management training
- visualization
- cognitive therapy
- aerobic exercise
- prayer

One study from the New York Institute of Technology claims to have demonstrated that mind power can alter the rate of replication of HIV under laboratory conditions. A more interesting study from the Department of Epidemiology of the University of Washington, published in 2007, reported that people who had engaged in any form of psychological or spiritual treatment for a period of six months to one year had better clinical outcomes, including survival, as compared with other patients.

Other treatments for AIDS include **homeopathy**, naturopathy, acupuncture, and chiropractic.

Allopathic treatment

Treatment for AIDS covers four categories:

Antiretroviral treatment

In the early 2000s researchers developed drugs that suppress HIV replication. The drugs are used in combination with one another and fall into four classes:

- Nucleoside reverse transcriptase inhibitors. These drugs work by interfering with the action of HIV reverse transcriptase, thus ending the virus replication process. These drugs include zidovudine (sometimes called Zidovudine or AZT, trade name Retrovir), didanosine (ddi, Videx), emtricitabine (FTC, Emtriva), zalcitabine (ddC, Hivid), stavudine (d4T, Zerit), abacavir (Ziagen), tenofovir (df, Viread), and lamivudine (3TC, Epivir).
- Protease inhibitors. Protease inhibitors are effective against HIV strains that have developed resistance to nucleoside analogues and often are used in combination with them. These compounds include saquinavir (Fortovase), ritonavir (Norvir), indinavir (Crixivan), amprenavir (Agenerase), lopinavir plus ritonavir (Reyataz), and nelfinavir (Viracept).
- Non-nucleoside reverse transcriptase inhibitors, a newer class of antiretroviral agents. Three are available: nevirapine (Viramune), efavirenz (Sustiva), and delavirdine (Rescriptor).
- Fusion inhibitors. These drugs are less common, expensive, and difficult to use. They block infection early by preventing HIV from fusing with and entering a human cell. This class includes only one compound: Enfuvirtide (Fuzeon).

Treatment guidelines for these agents are in constant change as new medications are developed and introduced. In mid-2003, the U.S. Department of Health and Human Services revised its guidelines for the use of these agents to help clinicians select the best combinations. The new guidelines offer a list of suggested combination regimens classified as either "preferred" or "alternative".

Treatment of opportunistic infections and malignancies

Most AIDS patients require complex long-term treatment with medications for infectious diseases. This treatment often is complicated by the development of resistance in the disease organisms. AIDS-related malignancies in the central nervous system usually are treated with radiation therapy. Cancers elsewhere in the body are treated with chemotherapy.

Prophylactic treatment for opportunistic infections

Prophylactic treatment is treatment that is given to prevent disease. AIDS patients with a history of *Pneumocystis* **pneumonia**; with CD4+ counts below 200 cells/mm^3 or 1% of lymphocytes; weight loss; or thrush are likely to benefit from prophylactic medications. The three drugs given are trimethoprim-sulfamethoxazole, dapsone, or pentamidine in aerosol form.

STIMULATION OF BLOOD CELL PRODUCTION. Because many patients with AIDS have abnormally low levels of both red and white blood cells, they may be given medications to stimulate blood cell production. Epoetin alfa (erythropoietin) may be given to anemic patients. Patients with low white blood cell counts may be given filgrastim or sargramostim.

Treatment in women

Treatment of pregnant women with HIV is particularly important because antiretroviral therapy has been shown to reduce transmission to the infant by 65%

Acute retroviral syndrome—A group of symptoms resembling mononucleosis that often are the first sign of HIV infection.

AIDS dementia complex—A type of brain dysfunction caused by HIV infection that causes difficulty thinking, confusion, and loss of muscular coordination.

Antibody—A specific protein produced by the immune system in response to a specific foreign protein or particle called an antigen.

Antigen—Any substance that stimulates the body to produce antibody.

Autoimmunity—A condition in which the body's immune system produces antibodies in response to its own tissues or blood components instead of to foreign particles or microorganisms.

CD4—A type of protein molecule in human blood. The HIV virus infects cells with CD4 surface proteins and, as a result, depletes the number of T cells, B cells, natural killer cells, and monocytes in the patient's blood.

Hairy leukoplakia of the tongue—A white area of diseased tissue on the tongue that may be flat or slightly raised. Caused by the Epstein-Barr virus, it is an important diagnostic sign of AIDS.

Hemophilia—Hereditary blood clotting disorders occurring almost exclusively in males.

Human immunodeficiency virus (HIV)—A transmissible retrovirus that causes AIDS in humans. Two forms of HIV are recognized: HIV-1, which causes most cases of AIDS in Europe, North and South America, and most parts of Africa; and HIV-2, which is chiefly found in West African patients.

Immunodeficient—A condition in which the body's immune response is damaged, weakened, or is not functioning properly.

Kaposi's sarcoma—A cancer of the connective tissue that produces painless purplish red (in people with light skin) or brown (in people with dark skin) blotches on the skin. It is a major diagnostic marker of AIDS.

Latent period—Also called incubation period, the time between infection with a disease-causing agent and the development of disease.

Lymphocyte—A type of white blood cell that is important in the formation of antibodies and that can be used to monitor the health of AIDS patients.

Lymphoma—A cancerous tumor in the lymphatic system that is associated with a poor prognosis in AIDS patients.

Macrophage—A large white blood cell, found primarily in the bloodstream and connective tissue, that helps the body fight off infections by ingesting the disease-causing organism.

Monocyte—A large white blood cell that is formed in the bone marrow and spleen.

Mycobacterium avium (MAC) infection—A type of opportunistic infection that occurs in about 40% of AIDS patients and is regarded as an AIDS-defining disease.

Opportunistic infection—An infection by organisms that usually do not cause infection in people whose immune systems are working normally.

Persistent generalized lymphadenopathy (PGL)—A condition in which HIV continues to produce chronic painless swellings in the lymph nodes during the latency period.

***Pneumocystis carinii* pneumonia (PCP)**—An opportunistic infection caused by a fungus that is a major cause of death in patients with late-stage AIDS.

Progressive multifocal leukoencephalopathy (PML)—A disease caused by a virus that destroys white matter in localized areas of the brain. It is regarded as an AIDS-defining illness.

Protozoan—A single-celled, usually microscopic organism that has a nucleus and is, therefore, different from bacteria.

Retrovirus—A virus that contains a unique enzyme called reverse transcriptase that allows it to replicate within new host cells.

T cells—Lymphocytes that originate in the thymus gland. CD4 lymphocytes are a subset of T lymphocytes.

Thrush—A yeast infection of the mouth characterized by white patches on the inside of the mouth and cheeks.

Viremia—The measurable presence of virus in the bloodstream that is a characteristic of acute retroviral syndrome.

Wasting syndrome—A progressive loss of weight and muscle tissue caused by the AIDS virus.

Expected results

There is no cure for AIDS. Treatment stresses aggressive combination drug therapy when possible. The use of multi-drug therapies has significantly reduced the number of U.S. deaths resulting from AIDS. The potential exists to prolong life indefinitely using these and other drug therapies to boost the immune system, keep the virus from replicating, and ward off opportunistic infections and malignancies.

Prognosis after the latency period depends on the patient's specific symptoms and the organ systems affected by the disease. Patients with AIDS-related lymphomas of the central nervous system often die within two to three months of diagnosis; those with systemic lymphomas may survive eight to ten months. In the United States, the successful treatment of AIDS patients with highly active anti-retroviral therapy (HAART) has actually led to a growing number of people living with HIV. About 25,000 infected people per year are added to the list of HIV-infected Americans.

HAART and other treatment works to prolong AIDS patients' lives and has led to some improvement in quality of life too. One study shows that HAART therapy substantially reduces risk of AIDS-related pneumonia (PCP), although PCP still remains the most common AIDS-defining illness among opportunistic infections. Other studies show that these protease inhibitors may result in high **cholesterol** and put AIDS patients at eventual risk for **heart disease**. More research must be done, since long-term effects of HAART treatment are still underway. Most clinicians would say the benefits outweigh the risks anyway.

Prevention

As of 2008, there was no vaccine effective against AIDS. Several vaccines to prevent initial HIV infection and disease progression are being tested. In 2002, reports indicated a new "library" vaccine showed potential. The vaccine is composed of up to 32 HIV gene fragments that can induce a number of immune responses. Also in 2002, the British government worked with five African countries in a trial to find an effective gel that would protect women against HIV during sex. The study leaders believed if they could find a lotion that could be applied before intercourse that would help prevent HIV transmission, they would give women the ability to better protect themselves from HIV. In 2003, the first human test of a vaccine against the most common subtype of HIV was undertaken.

Precautions to take to prevent the spread of AIDS include:

- Practicing safe sex and being monogamous. Besides avoiding the risk of HIV infection, condoms are successful in preventing other sexually transmitted diseases and unwanted pregnancies.

- Avoiding needle sharing among intravenous drug users.

- Donating blood before undergoing surgery. Although blood and blood products are carefully monitored, those individuals who are planning to undergo major surgery may wish to donate blood ahead of time to prevent a risk of infection from a blood transfusion.

- Wearing protective gear. Healthcare professionals should wear gloves and masks when handling body fluids and avoid needle-stick injuries.

- Getting tested. Individuals who suspect that they may have become infected should get tested. If treated aggressively and early, the development of AIDS can sometimes be postponed indefinitely. If HIV infection is confirmed, it also is vital to inform sexual partners.

Resources

BOOKS
PERIODICALS

Fitzpatrick, A. L., L. J. Standish, J. Berger, J. G. Kim, C. Calabrese, and N. Polissar. "Survival in HIV-1-positve Adults Practicing Psychological or Spiritual Activities for One Year." *Alternative Therapy Health Medicine* (September/October 2007): 18–20, 22–24.

Xu J; He B. "The Effect of Mind Power on HIV-1: A Pilot Study." *Alternative Therapy Health Medicine* (September/October 2007): 40–42.

ORGANIZATIONS

American Foundation for AIDS Research, 120 Wall St., 13th Fl., New York, NY, 1005–3908, (212) 806-1600., http://www.amfar.org/cgi-bin/iowa/fdoc.html?record = 13.

Gay Men's Health Crisis, 119 W. Twenty-fourth St., New York, NY, 10011-0022, (212) 367-1000, http://www.gmhc.org/donate.html.

National AIDS Hot Line, (800) 342-AIDS (English), (800) 344-SIDA (Spanish), (800) AIDS-TTY (hearing-impaired).

Belinda Rowland
Teresa G. Odle

Alcoholism

Definition

Alcoholism is the layman's term for alcohol dependence and alcohol abuse. According to the *Diagnostic and Statistical Manual of Mental Disorders*, published by the American Psychiatric Association and commonly called DSM–IV, the essential feature of **substance abuse** (in this instance, alcohol abuse) is maladaptive use of the substance with recurrent and significant adverse consequences related to its repeated use. Dependence is a physical addiction with psychological, social, and genetic components. Despite damage to health, finances, reputations, and relationships, the alcohol dependent person continues to drink unless successful intervention occurs. Abuse is distinguished from dependence by the individual's retaining some control over the use of alcohol. Nevertheless both conditions result in many of the same consequences over time, and abuse increases risk of dependence.

Alcohol abuse and alcohol dependence are often associated with abuse of, or dependence on, other substances, including nicotine, **marijuana**, cocaine, heroin, amphetamines, sedatives, and anxiolytics (anti-anxiety drugs). Alcoholism is more common in males than in females, with an estimated male-to-female ratio as high as five-to-one. A U.S. study conducted between 1990 and 1991, using DSM standards, found that 14% of the adult population (ages 15–54) had, at some time, met the criteria for alcohol dependence; and 7% had been alcohol-dependent in the past year. An earlier, similar study showed that about 5% of Americans qualified for a diagnosis of alcohol abuse at some point during their life. In 2006, the Substance Abuse and Mental Health Services Administration reported that 18.2 million Americans over the age of 12 met the criteria for alcohol abuse or dependence in the preceding year. Although it is difficult to develop accurate statistics worldwide, experts know that the incidence of what is called alcoholism has been steadily rising around the globe for several years.

Description

The effects of alcoholism are quite far-reaching. Alcoholism affects every body system, causing a wide range of drinking-related health problems, including lower testosterone, shrinking gonads, erectile dysfunction, interference with reproductive fertility, weak bones, memory disorders, difficulty with balance and walking, liver disease (including **cirrhosis** and **hepatitis**), high blood pressure, weakness of muscles (including the heart), disturbances of heart rhythm, **anemia**, clotting disorders, weak immunity to **infections**, inflammation and irritation of the entire gastrointestinal system, acute and chronic problems with the pancreas, low blood sugar, high blood fat content, and poor **nutrition**.

The mental health implications of alcoholism include marital and other relationship difficulties, **depression**, unemployment, poor performance at

Alcohol concentration and effect relationship

BAC (%)	Effects
0.01-0.029	Mood elevation; slight muscle relaxation; average individual appears normal
0.03-0.06	Relaxation and warmth; increased reaction time; decreased fine muscle coordination; talkativeness; mild euphoria, decreased inhibition
0.06-0.10	Impaired balance, speech, vision, depth perception, hearing, and muscle coordination; euphoria and extroversion
0.11-0.19	Gross impairment of physical and mental control and reaction time; staggering; slurred speech
0.20-0.30	Severly intoxicated; very little control of mind or body, memory blackout
0.40-0.50	Unconscious; deep coma; death from respiratory depression

(Illustration by Corey Light. Cengage Learning, Gale)

school or work, spouse and child abuse, and general family dysfunction. Alcoholism causes or contributes to a variety of severe social problems, such as homelessness, murder, suicide, injury, and violent crime. Alcohol is a contributing factor in half of all deaths from motor vehicle accidents. In fact, 50% of the 100,000 deaths that occur each year due to the effects of alcohol are due to injuries of some sort. By some estimates, alcohol-related problems cost the United States over $150 billion yearly in lost productivity and alcohol-related medical expense.

Causes and symptoms

A physical dependence on alcohol develops insidiously, over time. The body is a magnificent adaptor; therefore, with persistent use, many adaptations occur physically and psychologically, resulting in both a higher tolerance to and increased need for alcohol. The physical adaptation to alcohol involves changing levels and altered balances of neurotransmitters, chemicals in the brain that not only affect physical abilities such as muscle coordination, but also an individual's mood. The abuse of alcohol is associated with a desire to feel better and to avoid feeling poorly. Initially a stimulant, it eventually acts as a central nervous system (CNS) depressant and is used in a majority of societies or cultures in the world as an accepted part of dealing with life events, except where religious opposition bans, discourages, or prohibits its use, as in most Muslim communities. It is included in celebrations and, ironically, its use is perceived as an appropriate response to sadness and loss, such as at wakes.

No single known factor causes some people to be alcohol-dependent and others not. Some genetic studies have demonstrated that close biological relatives of an alcoholic are four times as likely to become alcoholics themselves. Furthermore, this risk holds true even for children who were adopted away from their biological families at birth and raised in non-alcoholic homes, without knowledge of their biological family's difficulties with alcohol. Factors that increase the risk of experiencing problems with alcohol include: being male; being the child of an alcoholic parent or parents; having an extended family history and being of Irish (Celtic), Scandinavian, German, Polish, Russian, or Native American ancestry; beginning drinking as a teenager; and being depressed or highly anxious. Further research may determine if genetic factors are accountable, in part, for differences in alcohol metabolism and increase the risk of an individual's becoming an alcoholic. Other factors contributing to the development of alcoholism include high levels of **stress** and

turmoil or **pain**, and having drinking friends, drinking partners, and enablers—people who facilitate a drinker's habits and denial mechanisms. Ample advertising that makes drinking appear to be sexy or the basis of a good time also contributes. For example, numerous televised sporting events are sponsored heavily by alcohol-related companies.

One of the classic symptoms of alcoholism is denial of a problem with alcohol. An addicted person, under the influence of the addictive substance, is physically and psychologically motivated to perpetuate the addiction. Therefore, intervention often starts when loved ones, recognizing the signs and symptoms, bring attention to the problem and call for help. Occasionally, an intervention requires a whole family unit and outside assistance.

Signs and symptoms of alcohol dependence and abuse may include the following:

- not remembering conversations or commitments
- losing interest in activities that were once pleasurable
- ritualized drinking, before, with, and after dinner and being upset if the pattern is interrupted
- becoming irritable as the so-called happy hour approaches, especially if alcohol is not available
- drinking alone or secretly
- hiding alcohol in unusual places
- ordering doubles, drinking quickly, and drinking to intentionally become drunk
- focusing attention on the source of one's next drink
- unstable relationships, financial, legal, and employment difficulties

Physical symptoms of alcoholism can be divided into two major categories: symptoms of acute alcohol use and symptoms of long-term alcohol use.

Immediate (acute) effects of alcohol use

Although the initial reaction to alcohol may be stimulatory, ultimately alcohol exerts a depressive, uninhibiting effect on the brain. The blood-brain barrier does not prevent alcohol from entering the brain, so the brain alcohol level quickly becomes equivalent to the blood alcohol level. Alcohol's depressive effects result in impaired thinking, feeling, and judgment; short term **memory loss**; muscle weakness; difficulty in walking; poor balance; slurred speech; and generally poor coordination (accounting for the increased likelihood of injury and alcohol-related injury statistics). At higher alcohol levels, a person's breathing and heart rate slows. **Vomiting** may occur, with a high risk of vomitus aspiration (inhaling vomit into the lungs), and may result in further complications, including pneumonia. Still higher alcohol levels may result in coma and death.

Effects of long-term (chronic) alcoholism

Alcohol is considered a lethal poison, requiring continuous **detoxification** by the liver. As drinking continues and alcohol overwhelms the liver's ability to detoxify, long-term consequences to health occur, affecting virtually every organ system of the body.

NERVOUS SYSTEM. Experts estimate that 30–40% of all men in their teens and twenties have experienced alcoholic blackout (loss of consciousness) as a result of drinking a large quantity of alcohol. In an alcoholic blackout, all memory of time and behavior surrounding the episode of drinking is lost. Alcohol causes sleep disturbances, thus affecting overall sleep quality. Numbness and tingling may occur in the arms and legs. Two conditions that may occur either together or separately are Wernicke's and Korsakoff's syndromes. Both are due to the depleted **thiamine** levels found in alcoholics. Wernicke's syndrome results in disordered eye movements, very poor balance, and difficulty walking, whereas Korsakoff's syndrome severely affects one's memory, preventing new learning from taking place.

GASTROINTESTINAL SYSTEM. Alcohol causes a loosening of the muscular ring (the cardiac sphincter) that prevents the stomach's contents from reentering the esophagus. As a result, acid from the stomach flows upward into the esophagus, burning those tissues and causing pain and bleeding, or gastro-esophageal reflux disease (GERD). Inflammation of the stomach can also result in bleeding and pain as well as a decreased desire to eat. A major cause of severe, uncontrollable bleeding (hemorrhage) in an alcoholic is the development in the esophagus of enlarged (dilated) blood vessels, which are called esophageal varices (**varicose veins** of the esophagus). These varices actually develop in response to the toxic effect of alcohol on the liver and are extremely prone to bursting and hemorrhage.

A malnourished state arises from the loss of appetite for food—due to caloric substitution of alcohol and its effects on blood sugar levels—and interference with the absorption of nutrients throughout the intestinal tract. Inflammation of the pancreas (**pancreatitis**) is a serious and painful problem in alcoholics that disrupts carbohydrate and fat digestion and increases the risk of **insulin resistance**, weight gain, hyperlipidemia, diabetes, and pancreatic **cancer**. **Diarrhea** is also a common symptom of chronic alcohol use, due to alcohol's effect on the pancreas.

LIVER. Because alcohol is broken down (metabolized) within the liver, that organ is severely affected by constant levels of alcohol. Alcohol interferes with the large number of important chemical processes that occur in the liver. As alcohol converts to blood sugar, which in turn converts to blood fat, the liver begins to enlarge, filling with fat, a condition called fatty liver. Cirrhosis, a potentially deadly complication, develops when fibrous tissue, while trying to support the extra burden placed on the liver by the accumulation of fat and liver cell weakness, interferes with the liver's normal structure and function. The liver may also become inflamed, a condition called hepatitis, producing **jaundice**, **fatigue**, and elevated liver enzymes indicative of liver cell death and destruction. Because of the liver's important role in digestion, metabolism, and immunity, damage to the liver takes a serious toll throughout the body.

BLOOD. Alcohol can cause changes to any of the types of blood cells. Red blood cells become abnormally large. White blood cells (important for fighting infections) decrease in number, resulting in a weakened immune system. This condition places alcoholics at increased risk for infections and is thought to account in part for an alcoholic's increased risk of cancer (ten times greater than normal). Platelets and blood clotting factors are affected, causing an increased risk of bleeding and hemorrhage, especially when coupled with vascular weaknesses, varices, or aneurism.

HEART AND CIRCULATORY SYSTEM. Small amounts of alcohol cause a drop in blood pressure, but increased use begins to raise blood pressure dangerously. Increased blood pressure negatively affects the kidneys. While some studies demonstrate that one to two alcoholic drinks per night improves **heart disease** risk values, higher amounts and chronic intake produce high levels of circulating fats, which increases the risk of heart disease. Heavy drinking results in an enlarged heart, coronary arterial disease (CAD), peripheral vascular disease, weakening of the heart muscle, abnormal heart rhythms, a risk of **blood clots** forming within the chambers of the heart, and a greatly increased risk of **stroke**. Strokes result when a blood clot from the heart enters the circulatory system, goes to the brain, and blocks a blood vessel. Stroke may also result from a hemorrhage within the brain, as weakened vessel walls give way and platelet deficient blood pours through.

REPRODUCTIVE SYSTEM. Heavy drinking has a negative effect on fertility in both men and women, decreasing testicular and ovarian size, interfering with sperm and egg production and viability, disrupting menstrual cycles, and reducing libido. When **pregnancy**

is achieved reduced quality of sperm and egg may significantly and permanently affect the quality of life, pre-, peri-, and postnatally, of the child. A child born to a woman who abuses alcohol is at risk of being born with fetal alcohol syndrome, which causes distinctive cranial and facial defects, including a smaller head size, shortening of the eyelids, and a lowered IQ. Developmental disabilities, heart defects, and behavioral problems are also more likely.

Diagnosis

The DSM-IV divides substance abuse into specific criteria that can be of aid in diagnosing a substance abuse problem. These criteria are paraphrased here to relate to alcoholism. At least one of the following must have manifested itself within a 12-month period to qualify for a diagnosis of alcohol abuse:

- Recurrent alcohol use that results in failure to fulfill major role obligations at work, school, or home. Specific examples are repeated absences from work or poor work performance related to alcohol use; alcohol-related absences, suspensions, or expulsions from school; and neglect of children or household.
- Recurrent alcohol use in situations in which it is physically hazardous. Specific examples are driving an automobile and operating a machine while impaired by alcohol use.
- Recurrent alcohol-related legal problems, such as arrests for alcohol-related disorderly conduct.
- Continued alcohol use despite having persistent and recurring social or interpersonal problems caused or exacerbated by the effects of the alcohol. Examples include arguments with a spouse about the consequences of intoxication and alcohol-related physical fights.

A diagnosis of alcohol dependence requires habitual, long-term tolerance for and heavy consumption of alcohol as well as the development of symptoms of withdrawal when the amount of alcohol in the system is substantially lowered or completely stopped. Once a pattern of compulsive alcohol use has developed, alcohol-dependent people may devote large portions of their time to the procurement and drinking of alcohol.

A significant number of illnesses categorized in DSM-IV as *alcohol-induced disorders* has come into being as a result of alcohol abuse and dependence, illustrating the negative impacts of alcoholism on physical and mental health. Among the psychiatric diagnoses that are included in alcohol-induced disorders are:

- dementia
- amnestic disorder
- psychotic disorder
- mood disorder
- anxiety disorder
- sexual dysfunction
- sleep disorder

As previously mentioned, due to the strong element of denial and a need, usually, for intervention, diagnosis is often brought about because family members call an alcoholic's difficulties to the attention of a physician. A physician may become suspicious when a patient has repeated injuries or begins to experience medical problems that are related to the use of alcohol. In fact, some estimates suggest that about 20% of a physician's patients are alcoholics, a percentage that is higher than the general population and lower than the increased risk to health posed by alcoholism. In other words, alcohol-related illness may prompt alcoholics to see medical counsel, but their illness may not be recognized as alcohol-related until the disease toll is quite advanced.

Questionnaires that try to determine what aspects of a person's life may be affected by use of alcohol can be an effective diagnostic aid. Determining the exact quantity of alcohol that individuals drink is much less important than determining how their drinking affects health, relationships, jobs, educational goals, and family life. In fact, because the metabolism of alcohol (how the body breaks down and processes alcohol) is so individual, the quantity of alcohol consumed is not part of the criteria list for diagnosing either alcohol dependence or alcohol abuse.

One very simple tool for beginning the diagnosis of alcoholism is called the CAGE questionnaire. It consists of four questions, with the first letter of each key word spelling out the word CAGE:

- Have you ever tried to Cut down on your drinking?
- Have you ever been Annoyed by anyone's comments about your drinking?
- Have you ever felt Guilty about your drinking?
- Do you ever need an Eye-opener (a morning drink of alcohol) to start the day?

Other, longer lists of questions may help determine the severity and effects of a person's alcohol use. A thorough physical examination may reveal the physical signs suggestive of alcoholism, such as an enlarged liver, a visible network of enlarged veins just under the skin around the navel (called *caput medusae* or herniated umbilicus), fluid in the abdomen (ascites), yellowish tone to the skin (jaundice), decreased testicular size or gynecomastia (breast enlargement in men), **osteoporosis**, physical deterioration, loss of teeth, evidence of old injuries, and poor nutritional status. Diagnostic testing may include cardiovascular, CNS, GI, general chemistry, and liver function tests (LFTs) that reveal poor stress test performance, arterial disease, congestive heart failure, palsy, loss of coordination, reflux disease or history of stomach ulcer, **irritable bowel syndrome**, an increased red blood cell size and anemia, abnormal white blood cells (cells responsible for fighting infection) counts or characteristics, abnormal platelets (particles responsible for clotting), and increased liver enzymes. Given the genetic risk factors for alcoholism, determinations of familiar alcoholism related illness and death may be additive.

Treatment

Alternative treatments can be a helpful adjunct for the alcoholic patient once the medical danger of withdrawal has passed. Because many alcoholics have very stressful lives (because of, or leading to, the alcoholism), many of the treatments for alcoholism involve dealing with and relieving stress. These include massage, **meditation**, and **hypnotherapy**. A list from the Mayo Clinic also includes **acupuncture** (may reduce craving, **anxiety**, depression, **tremor**, fatigue, and the symptoms of withdrawal), **biofeedback** (monitoring of internal systems for stress reduction), **behavioral therapy**, motivational enhancement therapy (problem acknowledgment), and aversion therapy (may involve simultaneous use of medications the cause **nausea** or vomiting with relapse).

Nutritionally oriented practitioners may be consulted to address the malnutrition associated with long-term alcohol use. Careful and remedial attention toward a healthier diet and lifestyle, including use of nutritional supplements, such as vitamins A, B complex, and C; certain fatty acids; **amino acids**; **zinc**; **magnesium**; and selenium—supplements that support antioxidant, detoxifying, restorative and corrective deficiencies—may further enhance recovery and lessen the likelihood of relapse.

Herbal treatments include **milk thistle** (*Silybum marianum*), which is thought to protect the liver against damage. Other herbs are thought to be helpful for the patient suffering through withdrawal. Some of these include the antidepressive attributes of **lavender** (*Lavandula officinalis*); the calming and restorative nerve tonifying effects of **skullcap** (*Scutellaria lateriflora*), **chamomile** (*Matricaria recutita*), and **valerian** (*Valeriana officinalis*); the stimulating and GI helpful effects of **peppermint** (*Mentha piperita*); and the bladder aid, **yarrow** (*Achillea millefolium*).

Allopathic treatment

Allopathic treatment of alcoholism has two parts. The first phase is the treatment of acute effects of alcoholism, called detoxification. The second phase involves learning how to live with the disease of alcoholism.

Withdrawal

Detoxification, or withdrawal, involves helping individuals to rid their bodies of alcohol as well as the harmful physical effects of the alcohol. Because their bodies have become accustomed to alcohol, individuals need care and monitoring during withdrawal. Withdrawal is an individual experience, depending on the severity of the alcoholism as measured by the quantity of alcohol ingested daily and the length of time individuals have been drinking (the adaptation factor). Withdrawal symptoms can range from mild to life threatening. Mild withdrawal symptoms include nausea, achiness, diarrhea, difficulty sleeping, excessive sweating, anxiety, and trembling. This phase may last from three to seven days. More severe effects of withdrawal may include hallucinations (in which individuals see, hear, or feel something that is not real), seizures, an unbearable craving for more alcohol, confusion, **fever**, fast heart rate, high blood pressure, and delirium (a fluctuating level of consciousness). Patients at highest risk for the most severe symptoms of withdrawal (referred to as delirium tremens or DTs) are those with other medical problems, such as malnutrition, liver disease, or Wernicke's syndrome. Delirium tremens usually begins about three to five days after the patient's last drink and may last a number of days. Withdrawal usually progresses from the more mild symptoms to the more severe ones.

Patients going through only mild withdrawal, monitored carefully to make sure that more severe symptoms do not develop, may not require medication; however, fluids are encouraged to facilitate detoxifying the person's system. Patients suffering more severe effects of withdrawal may need to be given sedative medications, benzodiazepines such as Valium or Librium, to relieve discomfort and to avoid the potentially life-threatening complications of high blood pressure, fast heart rate, and seizures. Because of the patient's nausea, fluids may need to be given intravenously (through a vein), along with some necessary sugars and salts (electrolyte pushes). It is crucial that thiamine be included in the fluids because it is usually quite low in alcoholic patients, and deficiency of thiamine is responsible for the Wernicke and Korsakoff syndromes. In-patient treatment is usually short-term (three to seven days), though longer reha-bilitation programs lasting weeks or even months are sometimes needed. Any treatment is usually followed by longer-term outpatient treatment.

Recovery

After the physical problems associated with alco-hol withdrawal have been treated, the more difficult task begins: helping individuals recognize the nature and severity of their illness. This is done on both an in-patient and outpatient basis. Alcoholism is a disease of denial; as members of Alcoholics Anonymous (AA) put it, it is "the only disease that keeps telling you that you do not have a disease." Alcoholics can be made aware of their condition through what is called an intervention, a meeting with family and/or significant people who describe for the alcoholic the symptoms of alcoholism that they have witnessed and how these symptoms have affected them. This is important because alcoholics who are actively drinking are often not aware of what they do, nor do they remem-ber later what they have done. (Interventions are sometimes done before the problem becomes serious enough to require detoxification from alcohol.) Essen-tial to recovery is the awareness of powerlessness over the disease, acceptance of having the disease, and abstinence from the substance that perpetuates the disease.

There is no cure for alcoholism. Sessions led by peers, such as AA meetings, are often part of in-patient hospital treatment. AA meetings, in which recovering alcoholics meet regularly and provide sup-port for each other's recovery, are considered among the best methods of preventing a return to drinking (relapse). The AA program is based on a twelve-step program, involving recognizing the destructive power that alcohol has held over the alcoholic's life, looking to a Higher Power for help in overcoming the problem, reflecting on the ways in which the use of alcohol has hurt others, and if possible, making amends to those people. The final step involves carrying the message of hope and recovery to other sick and suffering alco-holics. The Serenity Prayer becomes an ally: "God grant me the strength to accept the things I cannot change, the courage to change the things I can change, and the wisdom to know the difference."

The best programs incorporate the alcoholic's family or loved ones in the therapy because loved ones have undoubtedly been severely affected by the drinking. Many therapists believe that families, in an effort to deal with the alcoholic's drinking problem, develop patterns of behavior that unwittingly support or enable the patient's drinking. This situation is referred to as co-dependency. The twelve-step pro-grams of Al Anon and Adult Children of Alcoholics can be successful in helping the families or loved ones of alcoholics.

There are also medications that may help an alco-holic avoid returning to drinking. These have been used with variable success. Disulfiram (Antabuse) is a drug that, when mixed with alcohol, causes a very unpleasant reaction which includes nausea and vomit-ing, diarrhea, and trembling. Naltrexone (a drug that blocks a narcotic high and may reduce the urge to drink) and acamprosate seem to be helpful in limiting the effects of a relapse. Naltrexone, found to produce liver damaging side effects, may be an option used only as a last resort. None of these medications have been found to be helpful unless individuals are also willing to work hard to change their behavior.

Expected results

There is no cure for alcoholism. Recovery from alcoholism is a lifelong process. In fact, people who have suffered from alcoholism are encouraged to refer to themselves ever after as recovering alcoholics, never as recovered alcoholics. Alcoholism can only be arrested—by abstaining from the drug, alcohol. The potential for relapse (returning to illness) is always there, and it must be acknowledged and respected. Statistics suggest that among middle-class alcoholics in stable financial and family situations who have undergone treatment, 60% or more can successfully stop drinking for at least a year, and many for a lifetime.

Prevention

Prevention is primarily related to education and early intervention. In a culture in which alcohol is so widely accepted and used, education about the dangers of this drug is vitally important, even in early child-hood. Since alcohol is one of the easiest and cheapest drugs to obtain and one commonly used by teens, the first instance of intoxication (drunkenness) with alco-hol usually occurs during the teenage years. It is partic-ularly important that teenagers who are at high risk for alcoholism be made aware of this danger. Those at high risk include those with a family history of alcoholism, an early or frequent use of alcohol, a tendency to drink to drunkenness, alcohol use that interferes with school-work, a poor family environment, or a history of domestic violence. Peers are often the best people to provide this education, and groups such as SADD (Students Against Drunk Driving, a Marlborough, Massachusetts-based organization), appear effective.

KEY TERMS

Blood-brain barrier—A membrane that lines the blood vessels in the brain and prevents many damaging substances from reaching the brain. Certain small molecules are able to cross the barrier, including water, oxygen, carbon dioxide, and alcohol.

Dependence—A state in which a person requires a steady amount of a particular drug in order to avoid experiencing symptoms of withdrawal.

Detoxification—The phase of treatment during which patients stop drinking and are monitored and cared for while they experience withdrawal from alcohol.

Relapse—A return to a disease state after recovery appeared to be occurring. In alcoholism, relapse refers to a patient beginning to drink alcohol again after a period of abstinence.

Tolerance—A phenomenon whereby a drug user becomes physically accustomed to a particular quantity of alcohol (or dosage of a drug) and requires ever-increasing quantities in order to obtain the same effects.

Withdrawal—Those signs and symptoms experienced by individuals who have become physically dependent on a drug, experienced upon decreasing the drug's dosage or discontinuing its use.

Courts and schools sometimes provide education through local substance abuse programs, as well. Setting a good example, developing and practicing communication skills with youngsters, and having frank discussions about the consequences of drinking, are all encouraged as ways to prevent alcoholism-related problems. Developing alternative coping skills to life's problems is also essential, as is encouraging an objective perspective on the pervasive advertising that deceptively promotes alcohol's health-reducing glamour.

Resources

BOOKS

Baye, Douglas R. *New Research on Alcoholism.* Hauppauge, NY: Nova Science, 2007.

Maltzman, Irving M. *Alcoholism: Its Treatments and Mistreatments.* Singapore: World Scientific, 2008.

Prentiss, Chris. *The Alcoholism and Addiction Cure: A Holistic Approach to Total Recovery.* Malibu, CA: Power Press, 2007.

Wyborny, Sheila. *Alcoholism.* Farmington Hills, MI: Lucent Books, 2007.

PERIODICALS

Amodeo, Maryann, et al. "Coping with Stressful Events: Influence of Parental Alcoholism and Race in a Community Sample of Women." *Health and Social Work* (November 2007): 247–257.

Cherpitel, Cheryl. "Alcohol and Injuries: A Review of International Emergency Room Studies Since 1995." *Drug and Alcohol Review* (March 2007): 201–214.

Knop, J., et al. "Paternal Alcoholism Predicts the Occurrence but Not the Remission of Alcoholic Drinking: A 40-year Follow-up." *Acta Psychiatrica Scandinavica* (November 2007): 386–393.

Lawrence, Andrew. "Therapeutics for Alcoholism: What's the Future?" *Drug and Alcohol Review* (January 2007): 3–8.

OTHER

"Alcoholism." *MayoClinic.com.* http://www.mayoclinic.com/print/alcoholism/DS00340/DSECTION = all& METHOD = print (February 9, 2008).

"Alcoholism." *Medline Plus.* National Library of Medicine. http://www.nlm.nih.gov/medlineplus/alcoholism.html (February 9, 2008).

Thompson, Warren. "Alcoholism." *eMedicine.* http://www.emedicine.com/med/topic98.htm (February 9, 2008).

ORGANIZATIONS

Alcoholics Anonymous, AA World Services, Inc, PO Box 459, New York, NY, 10163, (212) 870-3400, http://www.alcoholics–anonymous.org/.

Substance Abuse & Mental Health Services Administration, 1 Choke Cherry Road, Rockville, MD, 20857, http://www.samhsa.gov/.

Katherine E. Nelson, N.D.
David Edward Newton, Ed.D.

Alexander technique

Definition

The Alexander technique is a somatic method for improving physical and mental functioning. Excessive tension, which Frederick Alexander, the originator, recognized as both physical and mental, restricts movement and creates pressure in the joints, the spine, the breathing mechanism, and other organs. The goal of the technique is to restore freedom and expression to the body and clear thinking to the mind.

Origins

Frederick Matthias Alexander was born in 1869 in Tasmania, Australia. He became an actor and Shakespearean reciter, and early in his career he began to suffer from strain on his vocal chords. He sought medical attention for chronic hoarseness, but after treatment with a recommended prescription and extensive periods of rest, his problem persisted.

Alexander realized that his hoarseness began about an hour into a dramatic performance and reasoned that it was something he did in the process of reciting that caused him to lose his voice. Returning to his medical doctor, Alexander told him of his observation. When the doctor admitted that he did not know what Alexander was doing to injure his vocal chords, Alexander decided to try and find out for himself.

Thus began a decade of self-observation and discovery. Using as many as three mirrors to observe himself in the act of reciting, normal speaking, and later standing, walking, and sitting, Alexander managed to improve his coordination and to overcome his vocal problems. One of his most startling discoveries was that in order to change the way he used his body he had to change the way he was thinking, redirecting his thoughts in such a way that he did not produce unnecessary tension when he attempted speech or movement. After making this discovery at the end of the nineteenth century, Alexander became a pioneer in body-mind medicine.

At first, performers and dancers sought guidance from Alexander to overcome physical complaints and to improve the expression and spontaneity of their performances. Soon a great number of people sought help from his teaching for a variety of physical and mental disorders.

Benefits

Because the Alexander technique helps students improve overall functioning, both mental and physical, it offers a wide range of benefits. Nikolaas Tinbergen, in his 1973 Nobel lecture, hailed the "striking improvements in such diverse things as high blood pressure, breathing, depth of sleep, overall cheerfulness and mental alertness, resilience against outside pressures, and the refined skill of playing a musical instrument." He went on to quote a list of other conditions helped by the Alexander technique: "rheumatism, including various forms of arthritis, then respiratory troubles, and even potentially lethal **asthma**; following in their wake, circulation defects, which may lead to high blood pressure and also to some dangerous heart conditions; gastrointestinal disorders of many types, various gynecological conditions, sexual failures, migraines and depressive states."

Literature in the 1980s and 1990s went on to include improvements in back **pain**, chronic pain,

postural problems, repetitive strain injury, benefits during **pregnancy** and **childbirth**, help in applying physical therapy and rehabilitative exercises, improvements in strain caused by computer use, improvements in the posture and performance of school children, and improvements in vocal and dramatic performance among the benefits offered by the technique.

Description

The Alexander technique is primarily taught one-on-one in private lessons. Introductory workshops or workshops for special applications of the technique (e.g., workshops for musicians) are also common. Private lessons range from a half-hour to an hour in length, and are taught in a series. The number of lessons varies according to the severity of the student's difficulties with coordination or to the extent of the student's interest in pursuing the improvements made possible by continued study. The cost of lessons ranges from $40-80 per hour. Insurance coverage is not widely available, but discounts are available for participants in some complementary care insurance plans. Pre-tax Flexible Spending Accounts for health care cover Alexander technique lessons if they are prescribed by a physician.

In lessons, teachers guide students through simple movements (while students are dressed in comfortable clothing) and use their hands to help students identify and stop destructive patterns of tension. Tensing arises from mental processes as well as physical, so discussions of personal reactions or behavior are likely to arise in the course of a lesson.

The technique helps students move with ease and improved coordination. At the beginning of a movement (the lessons are a series of movements), most people pull back their heads, raise their shoulders toward their ears, over-arch their lower backs, tighten their legs, and otherwise produce excessive tension in their bodies. Alexander referred to this as misuse of the body.

At any point in a movement, proper use can be established. If the neck muscles are not over-tensed, the head will carry slightly forward of the spine, simply because it is heavier in the front. When the head is out of balance in the forward direction, it sets off a series of stretch reflexes in the extensor muscles of the back. It is skillful use of these reflexes, along with reflex activity in the feet and legs, the arms and hands, the breathing mechanism, and other parts of the body, that lessons in the technique aim to develop.

Alexander found that optimal functioning of the body was very hard to maintain, even for the short

FREDERICK MATTHIAS ALEXANDER (1869–1955)

Frederick Matthias (F.M.) Alexander was born in Australia where he began a career as a young actor. While leading the theater life, he developed chronic laryngitis. While tragic for a stage career, his lingering ailment would lead to his discovery of the Alexander Technique, which would ultimately help people around the world rid their bodies of tension and stress.

At the age of 19, Alexander became frustrated with a medical practitioner's inability to treat his hoarseness and was determined to find the cause of his malady. Although lacking any medical training, Alexander began to meticulously observe his manner of coordination while speaking and reciting with the use of strategically placed mirrors. After following this method of study for 10 years, Alexander concluded that modern society was causing individuals to severely misuse the human system of locomotion, thus resulting in the dysfunction of other systems of the body. His experiments and technique laid the groundwork in the early 1900s for good habits of coordination and the proper use of the neuromuscular system.

Alexander left Australia for London in 1904. The popularity of the Alexander Technique led him to work with intellectuals such as George Bernard Shaw and Aldous Huxley. Alexander also taught extensively throughout the United States.

The Alexander Technique is taught in 26 countries, and there are nine affiliated societies overseeing a profession of approximately 2,000 teachers of the technique. Alexander's technique continues to have a profound impact on the training of musicians, actors, and dancers from around the world.

period of time it took to complete a single movement. People, especially adults, have very strong tension habits associated with movement. Chronic misuse of the muscles is common. It may be caused by slouching in front of televisions or video monitors, too much sitting or driving and too little walking, or by tension associated with past traumas and injuries. Stiffening the neck after a whiplash injury or favoring a broken or sprained leg long after it has healed are examples of habitual tension caused by injury.

The first thing a teacher of the Alexander technique does is to increase a student's sensory awareness of this excessive habitual tension, particularly that in the neck and spine. Next the student is taught to inhibit the tension. If the student prepares to sit down, for example, he will tense his muscles in his habitual way. If he is asked to put aside the intention to sit and instead to free his neck and allow less constriction in his muscles, he can begin to change his tense habitual response to sitting.

By leaving the head resting on the spine in its natural free balance, by keeping eyes open and focused, not held in a tense stare, by allowing the shoulders to release, the knees to unlock and the back to lengthen and widen, a student greatly reduces strain. In Alexander lessons students learn to direct themselves this way in activity and become skilled in fluid, coordinated movement.

Side effects

The focus of the Alexander technique is educational. Teachers use their hands simply to gently guide students in movement. Therefore, both contraindications and potential physiological side effects are kept to a minimum. No forceful treatment of soft tissue or bony structure is attempted, so damage to tissues, even in the case of errors in teaching, is unlikely.

As students' sensory awareness develops in the course of Alexander lessons, they become more acutely aware of chronic tension patterns. As students learn to release excessive tension in their muscles and to sustain this release in daily activity, they may experience tightness or soreness in the connective tissue. This is caused by the connective tissue adapting to the lengthened and released muscles and the expanded range of movement in the joints.

Occasionally students may get light-headed during a lesson as contracted muscles release and effect the circulatory or respiratory functioning.

Forceful contraction of muscles and rigid postures often indicate suppression of emotion. As muscles release during or after an Alexander lesson, students may experience strong surges of emotion or sudden changes in mood. In some cases, somatic memories surface, bringing to consciousness past injury or trauma. This can cause extreme **anxiety**, and referrals may be made by the teacher for counseling.

Research and general acceptance

Alexander became well known among the intellectual, artistic, and medical communities in London, England during the first half of the twentieth century. Among Alexander's supporters were John Dewey,

Aldous Huxley, Bernard Shaw, and renowned scientists Raymond Dart, G.E. Coghill, Charles Sherrington, and Nikolaas Tinbergen.

Researchers continue to study the effects and applications of the technique in the fields of education, preventive medicine, and rehabilitation. The Alexander technique has proven an effective treatment for reducing **stress**, for improving posture and performance in schoolchildren, for relieving chronic pain, and for improving psychological functioning. The technique has been found to be as effective as beta-blocker medications in controlling stress responses in professional musicians, to enhance respiratory function in normal adults, and to mediate the effects of **scoliosis** in adolescents and adults.

Training and certification

Before his death in 1955, Alexander formed the Society for Teachers of the Alexander Technique (STAT) in London, England. The Society is responsible for upholding the standards for teachers of the technique. In the late 1980s, due to rapid growth of the Alexander teaching profession, STAT authorized replication of its certification body in many countries worldwide.

The American Society for the Alexander Technique (AmSAT) oversees the profession in the United States. Teachers are board certified according to STAT standards. They must receive 1,600 hours of training over three years at an AmSAT approved training program. Alexander Technique International (ATI), a second organization for teachers in the United States, has varied standards for teacher certification.

Resources

BOOKS

Caplan, Deborah. *Back Trouble - A New Approach to Prevention and Recovery Based on the Alexander Technique.* Triad Communications: 1987.

Dimon, Theodore. *THE UNDIVIDED SELF: Alexander Technique and the Control of Stress.* North Atlantic Books: 1999.

Jones, Frank Pierce. *Freedom To Change - The Development and Science of the Alexander Technique.* Mouritz: 1997, imported (First published 1976 as *Body Awareness in Action.*)

PERIODICALS

Stern, Judith C. "The Alexander Technique: An Approach to Pain Control." *Lifeline* (Summer 1992).

Tinbergen, Nikolaas. "Ethology and Stress Diseases." *England Science* 185: (1974) 20-27.

OTHER

Alexander Technique Resource Guide. (includes list of teachers) AmSAT Books, (800) 473-0620 or (413) 584-2359.

Nielsen, Michael. "A Study of Stress Amongst Professional Musicians." *STAT Books* London, 1994.

Reiser, Samuel. "Stress Reduction and Optimal Psychological Functioning." Lecture given at Sixth International Montreaus Congress on Stress, 1994.

ORGANIZATIONS

Alexander Technique International, 1692 Massachusetts Ave., 3rd Floor, Cambridge, MA, 02138, (888) 668-8996, 617-497-2615, ati-usa@ati-net.com, www.ati-net.com.

American Society for the Alexander Technique, P.O. Box 60008, Florence, MA, 01062, (413) 584-2359, (800) 473-0620, 413-584-3097, info@amsat.ws, www.alexandertech.org.

Sandra Bain Cushman

Alfalfa

Description

Alfalfa is the plant *Medicago sativa*. There are many subspecies. It is a perennial plant growing up to 30 in (0.75 m) in height in a wide range of soil conditions. Its small flowers range from yellow to purple. Alfalfa is probably native to the area around the Mediterranean Sea, but it is extensively cultivated as fodder for livestock in all temperate climates.

Alfalfa is a member of the legume family. It has the ability to make nutrients available to other plants both through its very long, deep (6–16 ft [2–5 m]) root

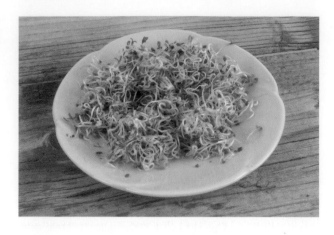

Alfalfa. (© Arco Images / Alamy)

system, and because it hosts beneficial nitrogen-fixing bacteria. For these reasons it is often grown as a soil improver or "green manure." The medicinal parts of alfalfa are the whole plant and the seeds. It is used both in Western and **traditional Chinese medicine**. In Chinese it is called *zi mu*. Other names for alfalfa include buffalo grass, buffalo herb, Chilean clover, purple medick, purple medicle, and lucerne.

General use

Alfalfa has been used for thousands of years in many parts of the world as a source of food for people and livestock and as a medicinal herb. It is probably more useful as a source of easily accessible nutrients than as a medicinal herb. Alfalfa is an excellent source of most vitamins, including vitamins A, D, E, and K. **Vitamin K** is critical in blood clotting, so alfalfa may have some use in improving clotting. It also contains trace minerals such as **calcium**, **magnesium**, **iron**, phosphorous, and **potassium**. Alfalfa is also higher in protein than many other plant foods. This abundance of nutrients has made alfalfa a popular tonic for convalescents when brewed into tea.

In addition to using the seeds and leaves as food, alfalfa has a long history of folk use in Europe as a diuretic or "water pill." It is also said that alfalfa can lower **cholesterol**. Alfalfa is used as to treat arthritis, diabetes, digestive problems, weight loss, ulcers, kidney and bladder problems, prostate conditions, **asthma**, and **hay fever**. Alfalfa is also said to be estrogenic (estrogen-like).

Alfalfa is not native to the United States and did not arrive until around 1850. However, once introduced, it spread rapidly and was adapted by Native Americans as a food source for both humans and animals. The seeds were often ground and used as a flour to make mush. The leaves were eaten as vegetable. The main medical use for alfalfa in the United States was as a nutritious tea or tonic.

In China, alfalfa and a closely related species tooth-bur clover, *Medicago hispida* or *nan mu xu* have been used since the sixth century. Alfalfa is a minor herb in traditional Chinese medicine. It is considered to be bitter in taste and have a neutral nature. Traditional Chinese healers use alfalfa leaves to cleanse the digestive system and to rid the bladder of stones.

The root of alfalfa is used in Chinese medicine to reduce **fever**, improve urine flow, and treat **jaundice**, **kidney stones**, and **night blindness**. Contrary to the Western belief that alfalfa will aid in weight gain, Chinese herbalists believe that extended use of alfalfa will cause weight loss.

Alfalfa contains hundreds of biologically active compounds, making it difficult to analyze and to ascribe healing properties to any particular component. In addition to the nutrients mentioned alfalfa contains two to three percent saponin glycosides. In test tube and animal studies, saponin glycosides have been shown to lower cholesterol, but there is no evidence that this cholesterol-lowering effect occurs in humans. In addition, saponin glycosides are known to cause red blood cells to break open (hemolysis) and to interfere with the body's utilization of **vitamin E**.

No modern scientific evidence exists that alfalfa increases urine output, effectively treats diabetes, aids kidney or bladder disorders, improves arthritis, reduces ulcers, or treats respiratory problems. Similarly, there is no scientific evidence that alfalfa either stimulates the appetite or promotes weight loss. There is no evidence that alfalfa has any estrogenic effect on **menstruation**. There is evidence, however, that although for most people alfalfa is harmless, for some people it can be dangerous to use.

Preparations

Although alfalfa is available as fresh or dried leaf, it is most often taken as a capsule of powdered alfalfa or as a tablet. When dried leaves are used, steeping one ounce of dried leaves in one pint of water for up to 20 minutes makes a tea. Two cups of this tea are drunk daily.

In traditional Chinese medicine, juice squeezed from fresh alfalfa is used to treat kidney and bladder stones. To treat fluid retention, alfalfa leaves are added to a soup along with bean curd and lard.

Precautions

Although alfalfa is harmless to most people when taken in the recommended quantities, people with the autoimmune disease **systemic lupus erythematosus** (SLE) should not take any form of alfalfa. In a well-documented study, people with latent SLE reactivated their symptoms by using alfalfa. In another study, monkeys fed alfalfa sprouts and seeds developed new cases of SLE. People with other autoimmune diseases should stay away from alfalfa as a precautionary measure. In addition, some allergic reactions have been reported to alfalfa tablets contaminated with other substances.

Side effects

No side effects are reported in healthy people using alfalfa in the recommended doses.

Interactions

There are no studies of the interactions of alfalfa and traditional pharmaceuticals.

Resources

BOOKS

Chevallier, Andrew. *Encyclopedia of Medicinal Plants.* London: Dorling Kindersley, 1996. (*Natural health encyclopedia of herbal medicine.* [2000] 2nd Ed.)

Peirce, Andrea. *The American Pharmaceutical Association Practical Guide to Natural Medicines.* New York: William Morrow and Company, 1999.

PDR for Herbal Medicines. Montvale, New Jersey: Medical Economics Company, 1999.

Tish Davidson

Alisma

Description

Alisma, a member of the plant family Alismataceae, is a herb commonly used in **traditional Chinese medicine** (TCM). The medicinal part of the plant is

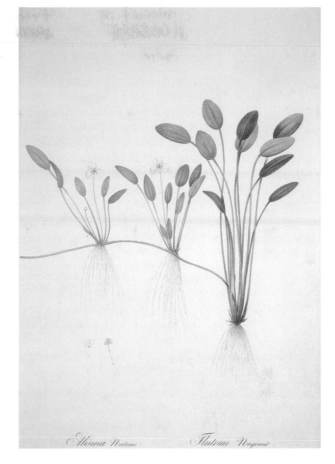

Alisma natans (© The Natural History Museum / Alamy)

the dried root of *Alisma plantago-aquatica*. Alisma is also called mad-dog weed, water **plantain**, American water plantain, or northern water plantain. It belongs to a different species from the edible plantain or cooking banana of the Caribbean or the plantain that produces **psyllium** seed. The Chinese name for alisma is *ze xie*.

Alisma is a perennial plant that grows aggressively in shallow water and boggy spots in parts of Europe, North America, and northern China. Its leaves take different shapes depending on whether the leaves grow above or in the water. The plant rarely reaches a height of more than 30 in (0.9 m). There are several subspecies of *Alisma plantago* found throughout the world, but their medicinal uses are the same.

General use

Alisma has been used for centuries in China. It is also used in North America and Europe. In the categories used by traditional Chinese medicine, which classifies herbs according to energy level (hot, warm, cool, or cold) as well as taste, alisma is said to have a cold nature and a sweet, bland taste. It is used primarily to treat conditions of damp heat associated with the kidney, bladder, and urinary tract.

Alisma is a diuretic and is used to rid the body of excess water. It has mild and safe tonic qualities that especially affect the kidney and bladder. It is often combined with other herbs in general tonic formulas. It is used to treat **kidney stones**, pelvic **infections**, nephritis, and other urinary tract infections, as well as yellowish discharges from the vagina. Alisma is believed to have an antibacterial action that helps control infection. In China, alisma is used to help rid the body of phlegm, to reduce feelings of abdominal bloating, and to treat diabetes. The herb is also widely used in Japan.

Outside of China, alisma leaves are sometimes used medicinally. They can be applied externally to **bruises** and swellings, or taken internally to treat kidney and urinary tract inflammations. The roots are used for kidney and urinary tract disorders, as well as to lower blood pressure and to treat severe **diarrhea**. A minor homeopathic remedy can also be made from the root.

Modern scientific research shows that alisma does act as a mild diuretic. In several studies done in Japan, alisma extracts were shown to reduce artificially induced swelling in the paws of rats. Studies using human subjects have not been done, but test tube and animal studies do seem to indicate that there is a scientific basis for some of the traditional uses of alisma. There is also some indication that alisma does have a mild antibacterial effect, but again, evidence in humans is anecdotal and by observation rather than by controlled trials.

Preparations

Alisma roots are harvested before the plant blooms and is dried for future use. Fresh root is toxic. Heating or drying deactivates the poisonous compounds in the root. If the leaves are used, they must be boiled for a long time before using. Fresh leaves are also poisonous.

Alisma is an ingredient in many common Chinese preparations to improve kidney balance and general health. These include rehmannia eight and rehmannia six combination, lycium chrysanthemum and rehmannia combination, rehmannia and schizandra, rehmannia and **cornus**, rehmannia and magnetitum formula, immortal long life pill, **gentiana**, and hoeln five. An extract of alisma root is commercially available. Some herbalists indicate that a large dose is necessary for

alisma to be completely effective when treating infections, or that it should be combined with other anti-infective herbs.

Precautions

Fresh alisma roots and leaves are poisonous. Dried roots or cooked leaves are safe, even in fairly large doses. However, the **kidney infections** that alisma is used to treat can be serious. Anyone who suspects that they have a kidney infection should see a medical practitioner.

Side effects

Some Chinese herbalists indicate that long-term use of alisma can irritate the intestines.

Interactions

In China and Japan, alisma is often taken together with antibiotics for kidney infections without any negative interactions. Since alisma is primarily an Asian herb, there is no body of information on how it might interact with most Western pharmaceuticals.

Resources

BOOKS

Molony, David. *Complete Guide to Chinese Herbal Medicine*. New York: Berkeley Books, 1998.

PDR for Herbal Medicines. Montvale, New Jersey: Medical Economics Company, 1999.

Teegaurden, Ron. *Radiant Health: The Ancient Wisdom of the Chinese Tonic Herbs*. New York: Warner Books, 1998.

ORGANIZATIONS

American Association of Acupuncture and Oriental Medicine (AAAOM), P.O. Box 162340, Sacramento, CA, 95816, (916) 443-4770, (866) 455-7999, (916) 443-4766, www.aaaomonline.org.

Tish Davidson

Allergic rhinitis *see* **Hay fever**

Allergies

Definition

Allergies are abnormal reactions of the immune system that occur in response to otherwise harmless substances.

Description

Allergies are among the most common medical disorders. The American Academy of Allergy, **Asthma**, and Immunology estimates that more than 50 million Americans, or more than one in every six people, have some form of allergy, with similar proportions throughout much of the rest of the world. Allergy is the single largest reason for school absence and is a major source of lost productivity in the workplace.

An allergy is a type of immune reaction. Normally, the immune system responds to foreign bodies, such as pollen or bacteria, by producing specific proteins called antibodies that are capable of binding to identifying molecules (antigens) on the foreign body. This reaction between antibody and antigen sets off a series of reactions designed to protect the body from infection. Harmless, everyday substances can also trigger this same series of reactions. This condition is known as an allergic response, and the offending substance is called an allergen.

Allergens enter the body through four main routes: the airways, the skin, the gastrointestinal tract, and the circulatory system. The following list describes these pathways and their physiological effects:

- Airborne allergens cause the sneezing, runny nose, and itchy, bloodshot eyes of hay fever (allergic rhinitis). Airborne allergens can also affect the lining of the lungs, causing asthma, or conjunctiva of the eyes, causing conjunctivitis (pink eye).
- Allergens in food can cause itching and swelling of the lips and throat, cramps, and diarrhea. When absorbed into the bloodstream, they may cause hives or more severe reactions, involving recurrent, non-inflammatory swelling of the skin, mucous membranes, organs, and brain (angioedema). Some food allergens may cause anaphylaxis, a potentially life-threatening condition marked by tissue swelling, airway constriction, and drop in blood pressure.
- In contact with the skin, allergens can cause reddening, itching, and blistering, called contact dermatitis. Skin reactions can also occur from allergens introduced through the airways or gastrointestinal tract. This type of reaction is known as atopic dermatitis.
- Injection of allergens, from insect bites and stings or drug administration, can introduce allergens directly into the circulation, where they may cause system-wide responses (including anaphylaxis), as well as the local responses like swelling and irritation at the injection site.

People with allergies are not equally sensitive to all allergens. Allergies may get worse over time. For example, childhood ragweed allergy may progress to year-round dust and pollen allergy. A person may also lose allergic sensitivity. Infant or childhood atopic **dermatitis**, for example, disappears in almost all people. More commonly, what seems to be loss of sensitivity is instead a reduced exposure to allergens or an increased tolerance for the same level of symptoms.

Causes and symptoms

Causes

Immunologists separate allergic reactions into two main types: immediate hypersensitivity reactions, which are mainly mast cell-mediated and occur within minutes of contact with allergen, and delayed hypersensitivity reactions, mediated by T cells (a type of white blood cells) and occurring hours to days after exposure.

In the upper airways and eyes, immediate hypersensitivity reactions cause the runny nose and itchy, bloodshot eyes typical of allergic **rhinitis**. In the gastrointestinal tract, these reactions lead to swelling and irritation of the intestinal lining, which causes the cramping and **diarrhea** typical of food allergy. Allergens that enter the circulation may cause **hives**, angioedema, anaphylaxis, or atopic dermatitis.

Allergens on the skin usually cause delayed hypersensitivity reaction. Roving T cells contact the allergen, setting in motion a more prolonged immune response. This type of allergic response may develop over several days following contact with the allergen, and symptoms may persist for a week or more.

THE ROLE OF INHERITANCE. While allergy to specific allergens is not inherited, the likelihood of developing some type of allergy seems to have a genetic factor, at least for many people. If neither parent has allergies, the chances of a child's developing an allergy is approximately 10–20%; if one parent has allergies, it is 30–50%; and if both have allergies, it is 40–75%.

COMMON ALLERGENS. The most common airborne allergens are the following:

- plant pollens
- animal fur and dander

• body parts from house mites (microscopic creatures found in all houses)

• house dust

• mold spores

• cigarette smoke

• solvents

• cleaners

Common food allergens include the following:

• nuts, especially peanuts, walnuts, and Brazil nuts

• fish, mollusks, and shellfish

• eggs

• wheat

• milk

• food additives and preservatives

Common causes of **contact dermatitis** include the following:

• poison ivy, poison oak, and poison sumac

• nickel or nickel alloys

• latex

Insects and other arthropods whose **bites** or **stings** typically cause allergy include the following:

• bees, wasps, and hornets

• mosquitoes

• fleas

• scabies

Symptoms

Symptoms depend on the specific type of allergic reaction. Allergic rhinitis is characterized by an itchy, runny nose often with a scratchy or irritated throat due to post-nasal drip. Inflammation of the thin membrane covering the eye (allergic **conjunctivitis**) causes redness, irritation, and increased tearing in the eyes. Asthma causes **wheezing**, coughing, and shortness of breath. Symptoms of food allergies depend on the tissues most sensitive to the allergen and whether it is spread systemically by the circulatory system. Gastrointestinal symptoms may include swelling and tingling in the lips, tongue, palate or throat; **nausea**; cramping; diarrhea; and **gas**. Contact dermatitis is marked by reddened, itchy, weepy skin **blisters**.

Whole body or systemic reactions may occur from any type of allergen but are more common following ingestion or injection of an allergen. Skin reactions include the raised, reddened, and itchy patches called hives. A deeper and more extensive skin reaction, involving more extensive fluid collection, is called angioedema. Anaphylaxis, another reaction, is marked by difficulty breathing, blood pressure drop, widespread tissue swelling, heart rhythm abnormalities, lightheadedness, and in some cases, loss of consciousness.

Diagnosis

Allergies can often be diagnosed by a careful medical history, matching the onset of symptoms to the exposure to possible allergens. Allergy tests can be used to identify potential allergens. These tests usually begin with prick tests or patch tests, which expose the skin to small amounts of allergen to observe the response. Reaction will occur on the skin even if the allergen is normally encountered in food or in the airways. Radioallergosorbent testing (RAST) measures the level of reactive antibodies in the blood. Provocation tests, most commonly done with airborne allergens, present the allergen directly through the route normally involved. Food allergen provocation tests require abstinence from the suspect allergen for two weeks or more, followed by ingestion of a measured amount. Provocation tests are not used if anaphylaxis is a concern due to the patient's medical history.

Treatment

Allergic rhinitis

The following treatments can help to relieve the symptoms of airborne allergies:

• Stinging nettle (*Urtica dioica*) has antihistamine and anti-inflammatory properties. The common dose is 300 mg four times daily.

• Grape (*Vitis vinifera*) seed extract has antihistamine and anti-inflammatory properties. The usual dose is 50 mg three times daily.

• Ephedra (*Ephedra sinicia*), also called ma huang, has anti-inflammatory activity and has proven effective in treating allergies. However, ephedra should not be used, as it can raise blood pressure, cause rapid heartbeat, and interfere with adrenal gland function. Because of severe health risks posed by ephedra, the supplement was banned from sale in the United States in April 2004. After a series of lawsuits, the U. S. Court of Appeals for the Tenth District upheld this ban on August 17, 2006. As of July 2007, the supplement can no longer be legally sold in the United States.

• Licorice (*Glycyrrhiza glabra*) has cortisone-like, anti-inflammatory activity, stimulating the adrenals and relieving allergy symptoms. It can be taken as a tea or in 100–300 mg capsules. Long-term use can result in sodium retention or potassium loss.

- Chinese skullcap (*Scutellaria baicalensis*) has bronchodilator activity, is an anti-inflammatory, and prevents allergic reactions. It is taken in combination with other herbs.
- Ginkgo (*Ginkgo biloba*) seeds are used in Chinese medicine for relief from wheezing and coughing.
- Echinacea (*Echinacea* species) may have anti-inflammatory activity and boost the immune system.
- Khellin (*Ammi visnaga*) has bronchodilator activity.
- Cramp (*Viburnum opulus*) bark has bronchodilator activity.
- Traditional Chinese medicine treats allergic rhinitis with various herbs. The patent combination medicines Bu Zhong Yi Qi Wan (Tonify the Middle and Augment the Qi) and Yu Ping Feng San (Jade Windscreen) are used for preventing allergies, and Bi Yan Pian (Rhinitis Infusion) is often prescribed for symptoms affecting the nose.
- The homeopathic remedies *Rhus toxicodendron*, *Apis mellifica*, and *Nux vomica* have decongestant activities. They are taken internally.
- Vitamin C has antihistamine and decongestant activities.
- Vitamins A and E are antioxidants and help to promote normal functioning of the immune system.
- Coenzyme Q10 may help to promote normal functioning of the immune system.
- Zinc may boost the immune system.
- N-acetylcysteine may have decongestant activity.
- Acupuncture has been shown to be as effective as antihistamine drugs in treating allergic rhinitis. It is also used to help prevent allergic reactions by strengthening the immune system.

Skin reactions

A variety of herbal remedies, either applied topically or taken internally, can assist in the treatment of contact dermatitis. A poultice made of jewelweed (*Impatiens* species) or **chickweed** (*Stellaria media*) can soothe the skin. A cream or wash containing **calendula** (*Calendula officinalis*), a natural antiseptic and anti-inflammatory agent, can help heal rash. Chinese herbal remedies have been effective in treating atopic dermatitis. The following are homeopathic remedies to be taken internally:

- Apis (*Apis mellifica*) for hives that feel better with cold application and bee stings
- Poison ivy (*Rhus toxicodendron*) for hives that feel better with hot applications and for poison ivy, oak, or sumac rashes
- Stinging nettle (*Urtica urens*) for hives

- Marsh tea (*Ledum*) for itching insect bites
- Croton (*Croton tiglium*) oil for poison ivy, oak, or sumac rashes

Food allergies

Food allergy may be managed by oral desensitization. Children with allergy to milk, eggs, fish, or apples who follow an oral desensitization procedure may develop resistance to the allergenic food. Oral desensitization exposes the patient to allergens in controlled, but increasing, doses. Control subjects, who had avoided the allergenic food during the study, were still sensitive.

Allopathic treatment

A large number of prescription and over-the-counter drugs are available for treatment of immediate hypersensitivity reactions. Most of these drugs work by decreasing the ability of histamine to provoke symptoms. Other drugs counteract the effects of histamine by stimulating other systems or reducing immune responses in general.

ANTIHISTAMINES. Antihistamines block the histamine receptors on nasal tissue, decreasing the effect of histamine released by mast cells. They may be used after symptoms appear, though they seem to prove more effective when used preventively. A wide variety of antihistamines are available.

DECONGESTANTS. Decongestants constrict blood vessels to counteract the effects of histamine. Nasal sprays and oral systemic preparations are available. Decongestants are stimulants and may cause increased heart rate and blood pressure, headaches, and agitation. Use of nasal sprays for longer than several days can cause loss of effectiveness and produce rebound congestion, in which nasal passages become more severely swollen than before treatment.

TOPICAL CORTICOSTEROIDS. Topical corticosteroids reduce mucous membrane and skin inflammation and are available by prescription. Allergies tend to become worse as the season progresses and topical corticosteroids are especially effective at reducing this seasonal sensitization. As a result, they are best started before allergy season begins. Studies have shown that steroid nasal sprays work better for seasonal allergies on an as-needed basis than do antihistamines. Side effects are usually mild but may include headaches, **nosebleeds**, and unpleasant taste sensations.

MAST CELL STABILIZERS. Cromolyn **sodium** (Nasalcrom) prevents the release of mast cell granules, thereby preventing the release of histamine and other chemicals contained in them. Cromolyn sodium is available as a nasal spray and aerosol (a suspension of particles in gas).

BRONCHODILATORS. Because allergic reactions involving the lungs cause the airways or bronchial tubes to narrow, bronchodilators, which cause the smooth muscle lining the airways to open, can be very effective. Bronchodilators include adrenaline, albuterol, and theophylline. Other drugs, including steroids, are used to prevent and control asthma attacks.

Immunotherapy

Immunotherapy, also known as desensitization or allergy shots, alters the balance of antibody types in the body. Injections involve gradually increasing amounts of allergen, over several weeks or months, with periodic boosters. Full benefits may take up to several years to achieve and are not seen at all in about one in five patients. Individuals receiving all shots will be monitored closely following each shot because of the small risk of anaphylaxis, a condition that can result in difficulty breathing and a sharp drop in blood pressure.

New treatments

Researchers have developed a number of treatments for allergies that employ new approaches to the problem. One class of new medications is the antileukotrienes (also known as leukotriene modifiers). Some members of this class are montelukast (Singulair), zafirlukast (Accolate), and zileuton (Zyflo). These drugs block the action of a group of compounds known as the leukotrienes, which contribute to the development of inflammatory reactions. A second category of new drugs is the IgE modifiers, which interfere with the action of mast cells in producing allergic reactions. The first IgE modifier to be approved for use in the United States by the Food and Drug Administration (FDA) was omalizumab (Xolair), approved in 2003. A third class of antiallergic medications is a group of immunomodulatory medications, topical ointments that interfere with cell mechanisms producing inflammatory responses. Examples of immunomodulatory medications are pimecrolimus (Elidel cream) and tacrolimus (Protopic ointment).

Treatment of contact dermatitis

Calamine lotion applied to affected skin can reduce irritation somewhat. Topical corticosteroid creams are more effective, though overuse may lead to dry and scaly skin.

KEY TERMS

Allergen—A substance that provokes an allergic response.

Allergic rhinitis—Inflammation of the mucous membranes of the nose and eyes in response to an allergen.

Anaphylaxis—Increased sensitivity caused by previous exposure to an allergen that can result in blood vessel dilation and smooth muscle contraction. Anaphylaxis can result in sharp blood pressure drops and difficulty breathing.

Angioedema—Severe non-inflammatory swelling of the skin, organs, and brain that can also be accompanied by fever and muscle pain.

Antibody—A specific protein produced by the immune system in response to a specific foreign particle called an antigen.

Antigen—A foreign particle to which the body reacts by making antibodies.

Asthma—A lung condition in which the airways become narrow due to smooth muscle contraction, causing wheezing, coughing, and shortness of breath.

Atopic dermatitis—Infection of the skin as a result of exposure to airborne or food allergens.

Conjunctivitis—Inflammation of the thin lining of the eye called the conjunctiva.

Contact dermatitis—Inflammation of the skin as a result of contact with a substance.

Histamine—A chemical released by mast cells that activates pain receptors and causes cells to become leaky.

Mast cells—A type of immune system cell that is found in the lining of the nasal passages and eyelids and participates in the allergic response by releasing histamine.

T cells—White blood cells that stimulate cells to create and release antibodies.

Treatment of anaphylaxis

The emergency condition of anaphylaxis is treated with injection of adrenaline, also known as epinephrine. People who are prone to anaphylaxis because of food or insect allergies often carry an Epi-pen containing adrenaline in a hypodermic needle. Prompt injection can prevent a more serious reaction from developing.

Expected results

Allergies can improve over time, although they often worsen. While anaphylaxis and severe asthma are life-threatening, other allergic reactions are not. Learning to recognize and avoid allergy-provoking situations allows most people with allergies to lead normal lives.

Prevention

By determining which allergens are causing the reactions, most people can learn to avoid allergic reactions from food, drugs, and contact allergens. Airborne allergens are more difficult to avoid, although keeping dust and animal dander from collecting in the house may limit exposure. **Vitamin C** may prevent allergy symptoms. Cromolyn sodium can be used for allergy prevention.

Resources

BOOKS

Gensler, Tracy Olgeaty. *Probiotic and Prebiotic Recipes for Health: 100 Recipes that Battle Colitis, Candidiasis, Food Allergies, and Other Digestive Disorders.* Beverly, MA: Fair Winds Press, 2008.

Kay, A. Barry, et al., eds. *Allergy and Allergic Diseases,* 2 vols. New York: Wiley-Blackwell, 2008.

Lockey, Richard F., and Dennis K. Ledford, eds. *Allergens and Allergen Immunotherapy,* 4th ed. London: Informa Healthcare, 2008.

Sutton, Amy L. *Allergies Sourcebook.* Detroit, MI: Omnigraphics, 2007.

PERIODICALS

Björkstén, Bengt, et al. "Worldwide Time Trends for Symptoms of Rhinitis and Conjunctivitis. Phase III of the International Study of Asthma and Allergies in Childhood." *Pediatric Allergy and Immunology* (March 2008): 110–124.

Finegold, Ira. "Immunotherapy: When to Initiate Treatment in Children." *Allergy and Asthma Proceedings* (November/December 2007): 698–705.

Hamelmann, E., et al. "Primary Prevention of Allergy: Avoiding Risk or Providing Protection?" *Clinical & Experimental Allergy* (February 2008): 233–245.

Noimark, Lee, and Helen E. Cox. "Nutritional Problems Related to Food Allergy in Childhood." *Pediatric Allergy and Immunology* (March 2008): 188–195.

Pourpak, Zahra, Mohammad R. Fazlollahi, and Fatemeh Fattahi. "Understanding Adverse Drug Reactions and Drug Allergies: Principles, Diagnosis, and Treatment Aspects." *Recent Patents on Inflammation & Allergy Drug Discovery* (January 2008): 24–46.

OTHER

Gallagher, Patricia E. "American Academy of Allergy, Asthma, and Immunology Patient and Consumer Center." *Journal of Consumer Health on the Internet* June 2007. http://www.aaaai.org/patients.stm (March 1, 2008).

Belinda Rowland
Teresa Norris
David Edward Newton, Ed.D.

Allergy elimination diet *see* **Elimination diet**

Allium cepa

Description

Allium cepa is the common onion. Although it is usually thought of as a vegetable, *A. cepa* also has a long history of medicinal use.

Onions are perennials that are cultivated for food worldwide. There are many varieties. Most onion bulbs are white, yellow, or red. The green stems and leaves are hollow and can reach 3 ft (1 m) in height. The plants bear small flowers that are usually white or purple. The fleshy bulb that grows below the ground is used medicinally as well as for food. Onions are members of the lily family.

General use

Onion has been used as a food source for almost as long as humans have been keeping written records. Their usefulness has been discovered independently by many cultures on several continents. Onions are mentioned in ancient Egyptian writings and were known in

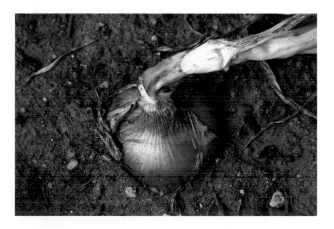

Onion plant. *(©PlantaPhile, Germany. Reproduced by permission.)*

ancient Greece. In medieval Europe, they were used unsuccessfully to ward off plague.

In North America, Native Americans used onion to treat insect **stings** and relieve colds. It is also used in **traditional Chinese medicine**. Homeopaths make a tincture of onion to treat a variety of conditions, including cold, **cough, diarrhea**, facial paralysis, **hay fever**, hernia, **laryngitis, pneumonia**, and trauma.

Over the centuries, onion has been used for healing both internally and externally. Internally, onion has been recommended to treat colds, cough, **bronchitis, whooping cough, asthma**, and other respiratory problems. It is believed to help loosen congestion in the lungs and expand the airways.

Onion is also used internally to relieve excess **gas** and calm an upset stomach. A mixture of rue (*Ruta graveolens*) and onion is used to rid the digestive system of parasites. Onion is also thought to stimulate the appetite.

Onion is believed to have a positive effect on the circulatory system. It has been used as a diuretic to reduce swelling. It is also thought to help reduce arteriosclerosis by lowering blood **cholesterol** levels and preventing the formation of **blood clots**. Onion has been used to treat diabetes and is reputed to lower blood sugar levels.

Externally, fresh onion juice is used to prevent bacterial and **fungal infections**. It can be applied to **wounds** and stings on the skin, used to remove **warts**, used to stimulate hair growth, and even used to reduce unwanted skin blemishes. Warm onion juice dropped in the ear is said to help relieve **earache**. Baked onion is used to draw pus from abscesses.

Modern scientific research supports many of the traditional uses for onion. Onion contains thiosulphinate, a compound that is effective in killing many common bacteria, including *Salmonella typhi, Pseudomonas aeriginosa,* and *Escherichia coli*. This finding supports the folk use of onion to treat wounds and skin **infections** and possibly its use for an upset stomach.

Even more supportive are small clinical studies on humans that show that both fresh onions and commercial onion extracts actually lower blood cholesterol levels, lower blood pressure, and help prevent the formation of blood clots. Although these studies have been done on only a small number of people, they are consistently supported by additional data from animal and test-tube studies. In addition, many of these properties have been found in **garlic** (*A. sativum*) which is a close relative to onion.

In 1990, scientists detected the presence of a compound in onion that partially blocks the development of inflammation. In addition, laboratory animals were protected against induced asthma with fresh onion juice. Humans with asthma have also shown reduced allergy-induced constriction of the airways when given an extract of onion. These findings support the traditional folk administration of onion to treat asthma and respiratory complaints.

Onion has also been shown to contain **antioxidants**, which are compounds that protect the body against free radicals. Free radicals are highly reactive molecules that destabilize other molecules and are associated with a number of degenerative diseases.

The German Federal Health Agency's Commission E, established in 1978 to independently review and evaluate scientific literature and case studies pertaining to herb and plant medications, has approved onion as an antibacterial agent. Although many studies are promising, more information is needed before this endorsement is extended to other uses of onion. In general, however, it appears that onion is a healthful vegetable that may confer many medical benefits.

Cancer

Onion may also be helpful in reducing the risk for a number of cancers, according to a study by Swiss and Italian researchers published in the November 2006 issue of *American Journal of Clinical Nutrition*. The meta-study looked at a number of previous studies of garlic and onion use among approximately 25,000 people in Italy and Switzerland. In people who ate 15–22 portions of onions and garlic per week, the reduced risk of various types of **cancer** was: oral and pharynx, 84%; esophageal, 88%; colorectal, 56%; laryngcal, 83%; breast, 25%; ovarian, 73%; prostate, 71%; and kidney, 38%.

Preparations

A common vegetable, onion can be served cooked or raw. For medicinal purposes, onion is available for internal use as a capsule or tablet containing dehydrated onion or onion extract. One study of the antioxidant activity of onion juice indicates that it is not affected by heating or boiling. For external use, the juice of fresh onion is used. A common dose is 1/4–1 cup of raw onions daily or one teaspoon of juice three times a day. In folk medicine, a cough syrup is made of raw onion liquid and honey.

Precautions

No special precautions are needed when taking onion medicinally.

KEY TERMS

Antioxidant—An enzyme or other organic substance that is capable of counteracting the damaging effects of oxidation in living tissue. Onion has been found to contain antioxidants.

Diuretic—Any substance that increases the production of urine.

Tincture—An alcohol-based extract prepared by soaking plant parts.

Side effects

Although no allergic reactions to the bulb of the onion are reported, some people develop an allergic rash after handling the leaves of the plant. In addition, windblown particles of onion leaves and skin have been shown to irritate the eyes of farm workers employed to harvest onions.

Interactions

There are no studies of the interaction of onion and conventional pharmaceuticals. However, given the long and widespread use of onion as a vegetable, serious interactions appear unlikely.

Resources

BOOKS

Balch, Phyllis A. *Prescription for Nutritional Healing*, 4th ed. New York: Avery Publishing Group, 2007.

ICON Health Publications. *Onions—A Medical Dictionary, Bibliography, and Annotated Research Guide to Internet Resources*. San Diego, CA: ICON Health Publications, 2005.

PERIODICALS

"Compound Found in Onions Linked to Lower Blood Pressure." *Tufts University Health & Nutrition Letter* (January 2008): 6.

Cruz-Correa, Marcia, et al. "Combination Treatment with Curcumin and Quercetin of Adenomas in Familial Adenomatous Polyposis." *Clinical Gastroenterology and Hepatology* (August 2006): 1035–1038.

Galeone, Carlotta, et al. "Onion and Garlic Use and Human Cancer." *American Journal of Clinical Nutrition* (November 2006): 1027–1032.

"Onions and Garlic Could Help Ward Off Cancer." *Tufts University Health & Nutrition Letter* (February 2007): 8.

Wilson, Emily A., and Barbara Demmig-Adams. "Antioxidant, Anti-Inflammatory, and Antimicrobial Properties of Garlic and Onions." *Nutrition & Food Science* (May/June 2007): 178–183.

ORGANIZATIONS

American Association of Acupuncture and Oriental Medicine, PO Box 162340, Sacramento, CA, 95816, (866) 455-7999, http://www.aaaomonline.org.

American Institute of Homeopathy, 801 N. Fairfax St., Suite 306, Alexandria, VA, 22314, (888) 445-9988, http://www.homeopathyusa.org.

Australian Homeopathic Association, 6 Cavan Ave., Renown Park, SA, 5008, Australia, (61) 8-8346-3961, http://www.homeopathyoz.org.

Homeopathic Medical Council of Canada, 3910 Bathurst St., Suite 202, Toronto, ON, M3H 3N8, Canada, (416) 638-4622, http://www.hmcc.ca.

National Center for Alternative and Complementary Medicine, 9000 Rockville Pike, Bethesda, MD, 20892, (888) 644-6226, http://www.nccam.nih.gov.

Tish Davidson
Ken R. Wells

Allium sativa see **Garlic**

Aloe

Definition

Aloe is a genus of flowering succulent plants that includes about four hundred species. Probably the best known and most medically useful member of the genus is *Aloe vera*. The term *aloe* is commonly used to refer to the specific species *Aloe vera*.

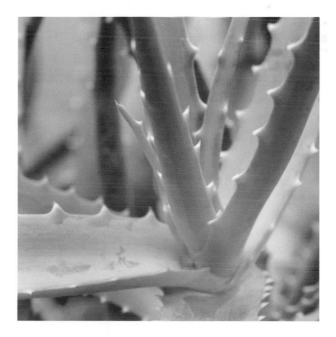

Aloe leaves. (© *blickwinkel / Alamy*)

Description

Appearance

Although it has the appearance of a cactus the aloe is a member of the lily family (Liliaceae). It is indigenous to eastern and southern Africa but has been spread throughout many of the warmer regions of the world and is also popularly grown indoors. The plant has yellow flowers and triangular, fleshy leaves with serrated edges that arise from a central base and may grow to nearly 2 ft (0.6 m) long. Each leaf is composed of three layers. A clear gel, which is the part of the plant used for topical application, is contained within the cells of the generous inner portion. Anthraquinones, which exert a marked laxative effect, are contained in the bitter yellow sap of the middle leaf layer. The fibrous outer part of the leaf serves a protective function.

History

In use for thousands of years, *Aloe vera* is mentioned in records as far back as 1750 B.C. Use of the plant is thought to have originated in Egypt or the Middle East. It was reputedly used in Egyptian embalming procedures, as drawings of *Aloe vera* have been found on burial walls in the region. Legend has it that *Aloe vera* was one of Cleopatra's secrets for keeping her skin soft. Pliny and Dioscorides of ancient Greece wrote of the healing effects of this plant. Additionally, Alexander the Great is said to have acquired Madagascar so that he could use the *Aloe vera* growing there to treat soldiers' **wounds**. The plant has served as a remedy in the Indian practice of **Ayurvedic medicine**.

In the United States, *Aloe vera* was in use by the early 1800s, but primarily as a laxative. A turning point occurred in the mid-1930s, when a woman with chronic and severe **dermatitis** resulting from x-ray treatments was healed by an application of *Aloe vera* leaf gel. Success with this patient encouraged trials with other individuals suffering from radiation **burns**. Evidence of the effectiveness remained anecdotal until 1953, when two American physicians, C. C. Lushbaugh and D. B. Hale, produced a convincing study, using *Aloe vera* to treat beta radiation lesions in rats. Subsequent experimental protocols were carried out using animals, but there was little human research data to describe the degree of effectiveness of *Aloe vera* treatment. Some evidence suggests that it is especially helpful in the elderly and other people with impaired health or failing immune systems.

Biologic components

Aloe vera contains a wealth of substances that are biologically active. The laxative, and in large doses, purgative, effects of *Aloe vera* latex are attributable to a group of chemicals known as the anthraquinones. Aloin, barbaloin, aloe-emodin, and aloectic acid are a few of the anthraquinones contained in the latex layer. Another component was discovered in *Aloe vera*, the biologically active polysaccharide known as acetylated mannose, or acemannan. This substance was shown to be a highly effective immune stimulant, with activity against the viruses causing the flu, **measles**, and early stages of **AIDS**. It has been used effectively against some veterinary cancers, most notably sarcoma, and was investigated as an agent to be used in treating **cancer** in humans. As of 2008, acemannan had been approved for treatment of certain types of cancers in cats and dogs, but it had not yet been approved for use with humans. Acemannan is one of many saccharides contained in *Aloe vera*. Some of the others are arabinose, cellulose, galactose, mannose, and xylose. Prostaglandins, a third important set of compounds, are thought to play a major role in wound healing. *Aloe vera* also contains fatty acids, enzymes, **amino acids**, vitamins, minerals, and other substances. The interaction of all these components produces a favorable environment for wound healing.

General use

Few botanicals are as well known or as highly thought of as the *Aloe vera* plant. Throughout recorded history, it has been used to keep skin beautiful and restore it to health. A frequent moisturizing ingredient in cosmetics and hair care products, it also promotes healing of burns and superficial wounds but should not be used on deep or surgical wounds or punctures. Topical application has been successful in treatment of **sunburn**, **frostbite**, **radiation injuries**, some types of dermatitis, **psoriasis**, **cuts**, insect **stings**, poison ivy, ulcerations, abrasions, and other dermatologic problems. Healing is promoted by the anti-inflammatory components, including several glycoproteins and salicylates, and substances that stimulate growth of skin and connective tissue. *Aloe vera* contains a number of vitamins and minerals that are necessary to healing, including **vitamin C**, **vitamin E**, and **zinc**. It also exerts antifungal and antibacterial effects and thus helps to prevent wound **infections**. One study showed it to have a little more activity than the antiseptic silver sulfadiazine against a number of common bacteria that can infect the skin. It has moisturizing and **pain** relieving properties for the skin lesions, in addition to healing effects.

Aloe vera gel products may also be used internally. They should not contain the laxative chemicals found in the latex layer. There is some evidence that *Aloe vera* juice has a beneficial effect on peptic ulcers, perhaps inhibiting the causative bacteria, *Helicobacter pylori*. It appears to have a soothing effect on the ulcer and interferes with the release of hydrochloric acid by the stomach. **Colitis** and other conditions of the intestinal tract may also respond favorably to the internal use of gel products. *Aloe vera* has been shown to exert a stabilizing effect on blood sugar in studies done on mice, indicating a possible place for it in the treatment of diabetes. One study suggested that giving *Aloe vera* extract orally to patients with **asthma** who are not dependent on steroids could improve symptoms. A healthcare provider should be consulted about these uses. Other suggested, but insufficiently proven, indications for oral *Aloe vera* gel include prevention of **kidney stones** and relief of arthritis pain.

Aloe vera products derived from the latex layer are taken orally for the laxative effect. They can cause painful contractions of the bowel if taken in high doses. Milder measures are recommended first.

The concentration of the immune stimulant acemannan is variable in the natural plant, as well as gel and juice products, but it is also available in a purified, standardized, pharmaceutical grade form. An injectable type is used in veterinary medicine to treat fibrosarcoma and feline **leukemia**, a condition caused by a virus in the same family as AIDS.

Preparations

Commercial products

Choosing effective *Aloe vera* products can be challenging. Once a leaf is cut, enzymes start to break down some of the long chain sugars which make *Aloe vera* gel an effective healing product, so it is important for the plant to have been properly handled and stabilized. Consumers should ask for help in selecting a reputable company as a product source. When shopping for a product to use for topical healing, people should look for *Aloe vera* to be one of the first products listed to ensure that it is not too dilute to be efficacious. Commercial, stabilized gel products may not work as well as the fresh gel, but cold processing is thought to best retain the beneficial properties. The FDA does not regulate labeling of *Aloe vera* products.

Aloe vera juice is most often the form of the gel that is used internally. At least half of the juice should be *Aloe vera* gel. If laxative properties are not desired, users need to be sure that the juice does not contain latex. A product that is made from the whole leaf does not necessarily contain anthraquinones from the latex layer, as those are water-soluble and can be separated out during processing. Capsules and tinctures of the gel are available. Oral forms of the latex extract are generally capsules, as the extract is extremely bitter.

Growing aloe at home

For common topical use, keeping an *Aloe vera* plant at home is one of the easiest ways to get fresh concentrated gel. It is easy to cultivate, requiring only good drainage, mild temperatures, and occasional watering. The plant needs to be brought indoors if outside temperatures are less than 40°F (4°C). It will tolerate either full or partial sunlight but will require more frequent watering in full sun. It should be watered only when the soil is dry. Getting the gel requires breaking off a leaf and cutting it lengthwise to expose the inner layer. The gel can be scooped out and applied generously to the area needing treatment. Leftover gel needs to be discarded because it degenerates quickly. The inner portion of the leaf may also be applied directly to a skin injury and bound to it.

Precautions

Aloe vera gel is generally safe for topical use, but it is best to apply it to a small area first to test for possible allergic reaction. Stinging and generalized dermatitis may result in individuals who are sensitive to it. The vast majority of the warnings apply only to products containing anthraquinones, such as aloin and barbaloin (as well as the numerous others), which are found in the latex layer of the plant. *Aloe vera* latex should not be used internally by children or by women who are pregnant or lactating. This product can cause abortion or stimulate **menstruation**. It may pass into breastmilk. People who have abnormal kidney function, **heart disease**, or gastrointestinal diseases are best advised to avoid any product containing *Aloe vera* latex or anthraquinones. Prolonged, internal use in high doses may produce tolerance so that more is required to obtain the laxative effect. Any *Aloe vera* product intended for internal use is supposed to contain only the gel portion and can become contaminated by the anthraquinones of the latex layer. For this reason, people who have a contraindication for using *Aloe vera* latex should use caution when taking an *Aloe vera* gel product internally.

Side effects

Internal use of *Aloe vera* latex may turn the urine red and abdominal pain or cramps may occur when products containing anthraquinones are consumed.

Interactions

Chronic internal use of products containing *Aloe vera* latex may increase the likelihood of **potassium** loss when used concomitantly with diuretics or corticosteroids. It may possibly compound the risk of toxicity when used with cardiac glycosides (both prescription and herbal types) and antiarrhythmic drugs. Absorption of other oral medications can be decreased. *Aloe vera* latex should not be used with other laxative herbs, which may also lead to excessive potassium loss.

Internal use of *Aloe vera* gel can cause changes in blood sugar, so diabetics should monitor blood glucose levels during use, particularly if insulin or other pharmaceuticals are being used to control hyperglycemia.

Topical *Aloe vera* may enhance the effect of topical corticosteroids and allow for a reduction in the amount of the steroid being used.

Resources

BOOKS

Davis, W. Marvin. *Consumer's Guide to Dietary Supplements and Alternative Medicines: Servings of Hope.* New York: Pharmaceutical Products Press, 2006.

Judith Turner
David Edward Newton, Ed.D.

Alopecia *see* **Hair loss**

Alpha-hydroxy

Description

Alpha-hydroxy is a chemical compound derived from fruit and milk sugars. Alpha-hydroxy acids (AHAs) are used in topical skin care products to exfoliate, or slough away, dead skin cells and promote collagen growth. They may be useful in promoting smoother, even-toned skin and may reduce the appearance of wrinkles and fine lines in some individuals. Products containing AHA may be used to treat **acne**, age spots, and other irregular skin pigmentations.

AHAs are available in a number of different synthetic and natural formulations. Lactic AHA is derived from milk products, while glycolic AHA is derived from sugarcane. Other AHA compounds include citric acid derived from citrus fruit, malic acid derived from apples, and tartaric acid derived from grapes.

General use

AHAs work by removing dead cells at the surface of the skin. In higher concentrations, alpha hydroxy promotes collagen production, which may reduce the appearance of fine lines and wrinkles in the skin. The acids penetrate deep into the skin, where they actually begin to damage skin cells. This skin damage triggers the production of collagen, a fibrous protein and a building block of tissue and skin, as the body attempts to repair the cell damage.

AHA may be an ingredient in over-the-counter products such as creams, lotions, and moisturizers that are marketed for their supposed anti-aging properties. Among the uses of products containing AHA are to smooth fine lines and surface wrinkles, unblock or open pores, improve overall skin appearance and conditions, including acne and oily skin. Over-the-counter products generally have an AHA concentration of 10% or less.

AHA may also be used in chemical peels used to treat skin conditions such as wrinkles, acne, scarring, and oily skin. The concentration of AHA products used by trained cosmetologists may run between 20% and 30%, while those used by doctors may range from 50% to 70%.

Preparations

AHA preparations are available in over-the-counter and prescription products, including gel, lotion, toner, and cream formulations. The United States

Food and Drug Administration (FDA) regulates these products as cosmetics, so the products do not undergo the rigorous testing for safety and effectiveness that is required for drugs. However, the FDA does become involved when it appears that cosmetics may contain ingredients that are harmful to people.

During the 1990s, the FDA received approximately 100 reports from people who said that use of AHA products caused side effects ranging from mild irritation and stinging to blistering and **burns**. These reports led the FDA in 1996 to issue a report, "Effects of Alpha Hydroxy Acid on Skin." The report concluded that additional research was needed.

A report linking AHA usage to increased sensitivity to the sun's ultraviolet (UV) rays was sponsored by the Cosmetic, Toiletry, and Fragrance Association. In December 1996, the association's cosmetic ingredient review panel reported on AHA studies that had started in 1994. The panel stated that over-the-counter products containing AHAs were safe when the alpha-hydroxy concentration was 10% or less. However, the safety depended on the product having a formulation of pH of 3.5 or greater. A lower pH number designates more acidity, which could increase the skin's sensitivity to the sun. On products with a lower pH, the product directions should include daily use of sun protection every day.

Furthermore, the report stated that salon products were safe if the AHA concentrations were less than or equal to 30%. However, safety was based on a pH level of 3.0 or higher.

The FDA's Office of Women's Health sponsored two studies in 2000 that affirmed the connection between AHA and increased sensitivity to the sun. However, that sensitivity diminished soon after a person stopped using products with AHA. In 2002, the FDA required that manufacturers label products containing AHAs with a warning that the acids may increase the risk of **sunburn**.

Selecting AHA products

The manufacturer is not required to list the strength of AHA on the package labeling. However, product ingredients must be listed sequentially in the order of highest concentration, so products that list AHA compounds second or third are usually more beneficial than those who list them in the middle and toward the end of the ingredient list.

Depending on their skin type, certain individuals may find some carrier formulas (i.e., cream, gel, lotion, toner) more effective than others. Those with dry skin may find moisturizing AHA creams and lotions more effective, while individuals with oily skin may prefer a less oily toner or gel.

Individuals who are considering using AHA products for the first time may want to start with a low AHA concentration. It is important to perform a skin-patch test to check for skin sensitivity to the substance. A small, dime-sized drop of the AHA product should be applied to a small patch of skin inside the elbow or wrist. The skin patch should be monitored for 24 hours to ensure no excessive unusual redness, swelling, blistering, or rash occurs. If a reaction does occur, the test may be repeated with an AHA product with a lower alpha-hydroxy acid concentration. Individuals who experience a severe reaction to a skin patch test of AHA are advised not to use the product. A dermatologist or other healthcare professional may be able to recommend a suitable alternative.

Individuals who are prescribed AHA formulations by a healthcare professional should follow their doctor's directions for use of the product.

Precautions

People should carefully read the labels of products containing AHA products that conform to the Cosmetic Ingredient Review guidelines of 10% or less AHA with a 3.5 or higher pH level.

AHA products increase sun sensitivity. Individuals using AHA products should use a sunscreen with an SPF (sun protection factor) of at least 15 to protect against burning. Sunscreen should be applied no less than 15 minutes after the AHA formula is applied to prevent neutralizing the acids. Shading the face with a wide-brimmed hat may also be useful.

Exfoliative products should be used with care, as over-exfoliation can cause damage to the skin. AHA products should not be combined with other exfoliative products such as facial scrubs, buff pads, or loofahs. In addition, individuals should only use one AHA product at a time.

Higher concentration prescription AHA products have a great likelihood of producing side effects, so individuals taking them should contact their healthcare provider immediately if they experience burning, redness, or any other reaction to the product.

Individuals who experience adverse reactions to AHA treatments should report them to both the manufacturer of the product and to the FDA's Office of Consumer Affairs. A patient's dermatologist or healthcare provider may also make this report anonymously for the patient. Although these products do not require FDA approval for market release, the

FDA is responsible for monitoring their safety and may initiate a product recall or removal for a specific brand or formulation if enough adverse effects occur to make these steps necessary.

AHA chemical peels and other high concentration AHA treatments should only be administered by a licensed cosmetologist, licensed dermatologist, or other qualified healthcare professional.

Side effects

The major side effect of using products containing alpha-hydroxy acids is increased sensitivity to the sun's UV rays. This heightened sensitivity may increase the risk of sunburn. People may also experience mild skin irritation. In some cases, products with AHA may cause burning, a rash, or redness. Because of these reactions, it is very important for people to read the directions and warnings on the package before using a product. The person should do a skin-patch test and then use the product sparingly until it is known whether it causes side effects.

Interactions

As of 2008, there were no known interactions between alpha-hydroxy acid products and other medications and substances when these were administered in recommended strengths. However, because over-the-counter AHA products are considered cosmetics and not pharmaceuticals, existing research on possible interactions had thus far been minimal.

Alpha-hydroxy products may enhance the effects of other products or medications with similar therapeutic properties.

Resources

BOOKS

Baumann, Leslie. *The Skin Type Solution*. New York: Bantam Books, 2006.
Day, Doris J., and with Sondra Forsyth. *Forget the Facelift*. New York: Avery (Penguin Group), 2005.

PERIODICALS

Kurtzweil, Paula. "Alpha Hydroxy Acids." FDA Consumer. 32, No. 2 (March/April 1998): 30-6.
Dugas, Barbara. "Choosing the Right Peel for Your Patient." *Plastic Surgical Nursing*. (April/June 2007): 80–84.

OTHER

Mayo Clinic Staff. "Wrinkle Creams: Your Guide To Younger Looking Skin." (October 12, 2006). http://www.mayoclinic.com/health/wrinkle-creams/SN00010 (March 2, 2008).

ORGANIZATIONS

Cosmetic Ingredient Review, 1101 Seventeenth St. N.W., Suite 412, Washington D.C., 20036-4702, (202) 331-0651, http://www.cir-safety.org.
U.S. Food and Drug Administration, 5600 Fishers Lane, Rockville, MD, 20857, (888) 463-6332, http://www.fda.gov.

Paula Ford-Martin
Liz Swain

ALS, Amyotrophic lateral sclerosis *see* **Lou Gehrig's disease**
Alternate nostril breathing *see* **Breath therapy**
Althea occicinal see **Marsh mallow**

Alzheimer's disease

Definition

Alzheimer's disease (AD), the most common form of **dementia**, is a neurologic disease characterized by loss of mental ability severe enough to interfere with normal activities of daily living, lasting at least six months, and not present from birth. AD usually occurs in old age and is marked by a decline in cognitive functions such as remembering, reasoning, and planning.

Description

A person with AD usually has a gradual decline in mental functions, often beginning with slight **memory loss**, followed by losses in the ability to maintain employment, to plan and execute familiar tasks of daily living, and to reason and **exercise** judgment. Communication ability, mood, and personality are also affected. Most people who have AD die within eight years of their diagnosis, although that interval may be as short as one year or as long as 20 years. As of 2008, AD was the eighth leading cause of death in adults in the United States.

In 2007, the Alzheimer's Association estimated that about five million Americans have AD. The National Institute on Aging predicted that that number would grow to as many as 14 million by the middle of the twenty-first century as the population as a whole ages. While a small number of people in their 40s and 50s develop the disease (called early-onset AD), AD affects the elderly predominantly. AD affects about 3% of all people between ages 65 and 74, about 19% of those between 75 and 84, and about 47% of those over 85. Slightly more women than men develop AD, but this may be because women tend to live longer, leaving a higher proportion of women in the most affected age groups.

The cost of caring for a person with AD is considerable and has been estimated at approximately $174,000 per person over the course of the disease. Most people with AD are cared for at home; the cost of extended nursing home care adds substantially to this estimate.

Causes and symptoms

The cause or causes of AD are unknown. Some strong leads have been found through research, and these have also given some theoretical support to several new experimental treatments.

AD affects brain cells, mostly those in brain regions responsible for learning, reasoning, and memory. Autopsies of persons with AD show that these regions of the brain become clogged with two abnormal structures—neurofibrillary tangles and senile plaques. Neurofibrillary tangles are twisted masses of protein fibers inside nerve cells, or neurons. Senile plaques are composed of parts of neurons surrounding a group of brain proteins called beta-amyloid deposits. While it is not clear exactly how these structures cause problems, some researchers believe that their formation is in fact responsible for the mental changes of AD, presumably by interfering with the normal communication between neurons in the brain.

What triggers the formation of plaques and tangles is unknown, although there are several possible candidates. Inflammation of the brain may play a role in their development and use of nonsteroidal anti-inflammatory drugs (NSAIDs) seems to reduce the risk of developing AD. Restriction of blood flow may be part of the problem, perhaps accounting for the beneficial effects of estrogen that increases blood flow in the brain, among its other effects. Highly reactive molecular fragments called free radicals damage cells of all kinds, especially brain cells, which have smaller supplies of protective **antioxidants** thought to protect against free radical damage.

Several genes have been implicated in AD, including the gene for amyloid precursor protein (APP), responsible for producing amyloid. Mutations in this gene are linked to some cases of the relatively uncommon early-onset forms of AD. In 2007, a research team at Harvard University reviewed more than 900 studies on the genetic basis of Alzheimer's. They found ten genes that appear to be implicated in the disease, nine of which they called "minor players." After the study was completed, the Harvard scientists announced that fifteen additional Alzheimer's-related genes had been discovered. Research continued in the 2000s on other genes that may be involved in the development of Alzheimer's, the role they may play, and possible interactions among them.

A potentially important genetic link was discovered in the early 1990s on chromosome 19. A gene on this chromosome, called apoE, codes for a protein involved in transporting lipids into neurons. ApoE occurs in at least three forms—apoE2, apoE3, and apoE4. Each person inherits one apoE from each parent and, therefore, can either have one copy of two different forms, or two copies of one. Compared to those without ApoE4, people with one copy are about three times as likely to develop late-onset AD, and those with two copies are almost four times as likely to do so. Despite this important link, not everyone with apoE4 develops AD, and people without it can still have the disease. Why apoE4 increases the chances of developing AD was not known as of 2008.

Several risk factors increase a person's likelihood of developing AD. The most significant one is age; older people develop AD at much higher rates than younger ones. Another risk factor is having a family history of AD, Down syndrome, or **Parkinson's disease**. People who have had head trauma or **hypothyroidism** may manifest the symptoms of AD more quickly. No other medical conditions have been linked to an increased risk for AD.

Many environmental factors have been suspected of contributing to AD, but population studies had not borne out these links as of 2008. Among these hypothesized factors are pollutants in drinking water, aluminum from commercial products, and metal dental fillings. As of early 2008, none of these factors had been shown to cause AD or increase its likelihood. Further research might yet turn up links to other environmental culprits, although no firm candidates had been identified.

The symptoms of AD begin gradually, usually with short-term memory loss. Occasional memory lapses are common to everyone and do not by themselves signify any change in cognitive function. The person with AD may begin with only the routine sort of memory lapse— forgetting where the car keys are—but progress to more profound or disturbing losses, such as forgetting that one can even drive a car. Becoming lost or disoriented on a walk around the neighborhood becomes more likely as the disease progresses. Individuals with AD may forget the names of family members or forget what was said at the beginning of a sentence by the time they hear the end.

As AD progresses, other symptoms appear, including inability to perform routine tasks, loss of judgment, and personality or behavior changes. Some patients have trouble sleeping and may suffer from confusion or agitation in the evening (called sunsetting). In some cases, people with AD repeat the same ideas, movements, words, or thoughts, a behavior known as perseveration. Some patients may exhibit inappropriate sexual behaviors. In the final stages of the disease, people may have severe problems with eating, communicating, and controlling their bladder and bowel functions.

The Alzheimer's Association developed a list of 10 warning signs of AD. A person with several of these symptoms should see a physician for a thorough evaluation:

- memory loss that affects job skills
- difficulty performing familiar tasks
- problems with language
- disorientation of time and place
- poor or decreased judgment
- problems with abstract thinking
- misplacing belongings
- changes in mood or behavior
- changes in personality
- loss of initiative

Other types of dementia, including some that are reversible, can cause similar symptoms. It is important for the person with these symptoms to be evaluated by a professional who can weigh the possibility that his or her symptoms may have another cause. Approximately 20% of those originally suspected of having AD turn out to have some other disorder; about half of these cases are treatable.

Diagnosis

Diagnosis of AD is complex and may require office visits to several different specialists over several months before a diagnosis can be made. While a confident provisional diagnosis may be made in most cases after thorough testing, AD cannot be definitively diagnosed until autopsy examination of the brain for senile plaques and neurofibrillary tangles.

The diagnosis of AD begins with a thorough physical examination and complete medical history. Except in the disease's earliest stages, accurate history from family members or caregivers is essential. Since there are both prescription and over-the-counter drugs that can cause the same mental changes as AD, a careful review of the patient's drug, medicine, and alcohol use is important. AD-like symptoms can also be provoked by other medical conditions, including tumors, infection, and dementia caused by mild strokes (multi-infarct dementia). These possibilities must be ruled out as well through appropriate blood and urine tests, brain magnetic resonance imaging (MRI) or computed tomography scans (CT), tests of the brain's electrical activity (electroencephalographs or EEGs), or other tests.

Positron emission tomography (PET) scans can also help predict individuals who might develop memory impairment. Although PET scanning is a relatively expensive technology, it has become more readily available. Several types of oral and written tests are used to aid in the AD diagnosis and to follow its progression, including tests of mental status, functional abilities, memory, and concentration. Still, the neurologic exam is normal in most patients in early stages.

One of the most important parts of the diagnostic process is to evaluate the patient for **depression** and delirium, since each of these can be present with AD or may be mistaken for it. (Delirium involves a decreased consciousness or awareness of one's environment.) Depression and memory loss are both common in the elderly, and the combination of the two can often be mistaken for AD. Depression can be treated with drugs, although some antidepressants can worsen dementia if it is present, further complicating both diagnosis and treatment.

A genetic test for the ApoE4 gene is available but it is not used for diagnosis because possessing even two copies does not ensure that a person will develop AD.

Treatment

The mainstay of treatment for individuals with AD continues to be the establishment of daily routines and good nursing care, providing both physical and emotional support for patients. Modifications of the home to increase safety and security are often necessary. Caregivers also need support. Regular medical care by a practitioner with a non-defeatist attitude toward AD is important so that illnesses can be diagnosed and treated properly.

People with AD are also often depressed or anxious and may suffer from sleeplessness, poor **nutrition**, and general poor health. Each of these conditions is treatable to some degree. It is important for persons with AD to eat well and continue to exercise. Professional advice from a nutritionist may be useful to provide healthy, easy-to-prepare meals. Finger foods may be preferable to those requiring utensils to be eaten. Regular exercise (supervised for safety if necessary) promotes overall health. A calm, structured environment with simple tools that support orientation (like calendars and clocks) may reduce **anxiety** and increase safety.

Diet and supplements

DIET. The incidence of AD is lower in countries whose citizens have a diet that is lower in fats and calories. There have been a few reports that a diet rich with fish improves mental function in patients with AD or dementia. AD patients treated with **essential fatty acids** showed greater improvement in mood and mental function than patients on placebo. Because of its disease-preventing properties, red wine in moderation may be beneficial to AD patients.

VITAMIN E. Studies have shown that AD patients have lower blood levels of **vitamin E** than age-matched control subjects. A large, two-year study of moderately affected AD patients found that taking 2,000 IU of vitamin E daily significantly delayed disease progression as compared to patients taking placebo. This delay was equivalent to that seen with patients taking the drug selegiline. Vitamin E is also thought to delay AD onset. High levels of vitamin E put the patient at higher risk for bleeding disorders.

THIAMINE (VITAMIN B₁). Several small studies to determine the effectiveness of **thiamine** (vitamin B_1) on AD have been carried out. Daily doses of 3 g for two to three months have improved mental function and AD assessment scores. Other studies have shown that thiamine had no effect on AD patients. Side effects include **nausea** and **indigestion**.

COBALAMIN (VITAMIN B₁₂). Although results are conflicting, some studies have found that AD patients have lower levels of cobalamin (**vitamin B_{12}**) than others. Some studies have shown that cobalamin

supplementation improves memory and mental function in AD patients whereas other studies have found no effect.

ACETYL L-CARNITINE. Acetyl L-carnitine is similar in structure to the neurotransmitter acetyl-choline. Studies have shown that 2 g or 3 g of acetyl L-carnitine daily slows the progression of AD, especially in patients who developed the disease before age 66. Patients who developed disease after 66 years of age worsened with treatment. Side effects include increased appetite, **body odor**, and rash.

DHEA. DHEA (dehydroepiandrosterone) is a steroid hormone. There may be a link between decreasing levels of DHEA in the elderly and development of AD. Studies on the effect, if any, of DHEA on AD were needed as of 2008. Side effects include **acne**, hair growth, irritability, **insomnia**, **headache**, and menstrual irregularity.

MELATONIN. Melatonin is a hormone that helps to regulate mood and sleep cycles. The effect of melatonin treatment on AD is unknown, but it may be beneficial in regulating sleep cycles. The usual dose is 3 mg taken one to two hours before bedtime. Side effects are drowsiness, confusion, headache, decreased sex drive, and decreased body temperature.

Herbals and Chinese medicine

GINKGO. Ginkgo, the extract from the *Ginkgo biloba* tree is the most commonly used herbal treatment for AD. Several studies have been performed to test the effectiveness of ginkgo for treating AD. The dose range studied were 120–160 mg daily divided into three doses. Although results were mixed, the evidence suggested that ginkgo may be an effective treatment for patients with mild to moderate AD. Side effects are not common but include headache, allergic skin reaction, and gastrointestinal disturbance. Ginkgo also decreases blood coagulation. Individuals with coagulation or platelet disorders should use extreme caution and consult a physician before using ginkgo.

PHYTOESTROGENS. Phytoestrogens may be beneficial in the treatment of AD based on the findings that women with AD who are on hormone replacement therapy have improved mental function and mood. Estrogens may prevent AD, therefore, phytoestrogens may have the same effect. Phytoestrogens are found mainly in soy products.

CLUBMOSS. Huperzine A is a compound isolated from clubmoss (*Huperzia serrata*). Studies have shown that taking 0.1–0.4 mg daily improves mental function in AD patients. Side effects are nausea, **muscle cramps**, **vomiting**, and **diarrhea**.

Therapies

Music therapy has been shown to be effective in treating the depression, agitation, wandering, feelings of isolation, and memory loss associated with AD. AD patients have benefited from listening to favorite music or participating in musical activity. Participation in a music therapy group was more effective at improving memory and decreasing agitation than being part of a verbal (talking) group.

A wide variety of other therapies have been beneficial in the treatment of the psychological symptoms of AD. These include:

- Light therapy in the evening to improve sleep cycle disturbances.
- Supportive therapy through touch, compliments, and displays of affection.
- Sensory stimulation through massage and aromatherapy.
- Socio-environmental therapies using activities fitted to previous interests, favorite foods, and pleasant surroundings.
- Cognitive therapy to reduce negative perceptions and learn coping strategies.
- Insight-oriented psychotherapy to address the patients' awareness of their disease.
- Dance therapy.
- Validation therapy.
- Reminiscence therapy.
- Reality-oriented therapy.

Nursing care and safety

The nursing care required for a person with AD is easy to learn. Caregivers usually need to spend increasing amounts of time grooming patients as the disease progresses. Patients may require assisted feeding early on to make sure that they are taking in enough nutrients. Later on, as movement and swallowing become difficult, a feeding tube may be placed into the stomach through the abdominal wall. A feeding tube requires more attention but is generally easy to care for if patients are not resistant to its use. Incontinence becomes a difficult problem to deal with at home and is a principal reason for pursuing nursing home care. In the early stages, limiting fluid intake and increasing the frequency of toileting can help. Careful attention to hygiene is important to prevent skin irritation and infection from soiled clothing.

In all cases, persons diagnosed with AD should not be allowed to drive because of the increased potential for accidents and the increased likelihood of wandering very far from home while disoriented. In the home, simple measures such as grab bars in the bathroom, bedrails on the bed, and easily negotiable passageways can greatly increase safety. Electrical appliances should be unplugged and put away when not in use. Matches, lighters, knives, or weapons should be stored safely out of reach. The hot water heater temperature may be set lower to prevent accidental scalding. A list of emergency numbers, including the poison control center and the hospital emergency room, should be posted by the phone.

Care for the caregiver

Family members or others caring for a person with AD have an extremely difficult and stressful job that becomes harder as the disease progresses. It is common for caregivers to develop feelings of anger, resentment, guilt, and hopelessness, in addition to the sorrow they feel for their loved one and for themselves. Depression is an extremely common consequence. Becoming a member of an AD caregivers' support group can be one of the most important measures a family member can take, not only for themselves, but for the person with AD as well. The location and contact numbers for AD caregiver support groups are available from the Alzheimer's Association. They may also be available through a local social service agency, the patient's physician, or pharmaceutical companies that manufacture the drugs used to treat AD. Medical treatment for depression may be an important adjunct to group support.

Outside help, nursing homes, and governmental assistance

Most families eventually need outside help to relieve some of the burden of around-the-clock care for individuals with AD. Personal care assistants, either volunteer or paid, may be available through local social service agencies. Adult daycare facilities are increasingly common. Meal delivery, shopping assistance, or respite care may be available as well. Many families consider nursing home care when AD advances to the late-stage.

Several federal government programs may ease the cost of caring for persons with AD, including Social Security Disability, Medicare, and Supplemental Security Income. Each of these programs may provide some assistance for care, medication, or other costs, but none of them pays for nursing home care indefinitely. Medicaid is a state-funded program that may provide for some or all of the cost of nursing home care, although there are important restrictions. Details of the benefits and eligibility requirements of these programs are available through the local Social Security or Medicaid office or from local social service agencies

Allopathic treatment

As of early 2008, the U.S. Food and Drug Administration (FDA) had approved five drugs for use with Alzheimer's disease: memantine (Namenda), galantamine (Razadyne), rivastigmine (Exelon), donepezil (Aricept), and tacrine (Cognex). In most cases, the drugs prevent the breakdown of acetylcholine in the brain, thereby increasing the efficiency with which neurons communicate with each other. These drugs can modestly increase cognition and improve the ability to perform normal activities of daily living. Side effects accompany the use of each drug, the most common of which are diarrhea, nausea, and vomiting. Tacrine has an additional side effect of some concern, promoting an increase in the liver enzyme alanine aminotransferase (ALT). Patients taking tacrine must have a weekly blood test to monitor their ALT levels.

Estrogen, a female sex hormone, has been widely prescribed for post-menopausal women to prevent osteoporosis. Several preliminary studies have shown that women taking estrogen have lower rates of AD, and those who develop AD have a slower progression and less severe symptoms.

Preliminary studies suggested a reduced risk for developing AD in older people who regularly use non-steroidal anti-inflammatory drugs (NSAIDs), including aspirin, ibuprofen (Advil), and naproxen (Aleve), although not acetaminophen. A 2001 study reported that those subjects who used NSAIDs for at least two years were up to 80% less likely to develop Alzheimer's. Later studies have not confirmed this original finding, however, and there was as of 2008 no good reason to recommend the use of NSAIDs in the treatment of AD.

Selegiline, a drug used in the treatment of Parkinson's disease, appears to slow the development of AD. Selegiline is thought to act as an antioxidant, preventing free radical damage. However, it also acts as a stimulant, making it difficult to determine whether the delay in onset of AD symptoms is due to protection from free radicals or to the general elevation of brain activity from the stimulant effect.

Psychiatric symptoms, such as depression, anxiety, hallucinations (seeing or hearing things that aren't there), and delusions (false beliefs) may be treated with drugs if necessary.

KEY TERMS

Acetylcholine—One of the substances in the body that transmits nerve impulses.

Dementia—Impaired intellectual function that interferes with normal social and work activities.

Neurofibrillary tangle—Twisted masses of protein inside nerve cells that develop in the brains of people with AD.

Neuron—A nerve cell.

Senile plaque—Structures composed of parts of neurons surrounding brain proteins called beta-amyloid deposits and found in the brains of people with AD.

Expected results

While Alzheimer's disease may not be the direct cause of death, the generally poorer health of a person with AD increases the risk of life-threatening infection, including **pneumonia**. In addition, other diseases common in old age (**cancer**, **stroke**, and **heart disease**) may lead to more severe consequences in a person with AD. On average, people with AD live eight years past their diagnosis, with a range from 1–20 years.

Prevention

As of 2008, there was no sure way to prevent Alzheimer's disease, although it was hoped that some of the drug treatments discussed may eventually be proven to reduce the risk of developing the disease. The most likely candidates were estrogen, phytoestrogens, NSAIDs, vitamin E, and selegiline. In 2001, researchers found preliminary indications that onset of Alzheimer's might be tied to **cholesterol** levels. Later studies showed, however, that cholesterol-lowering drugs had no effect on the onset or development of Alzheimer's.

Resources

BOOKS

Calo-oy, Starr, and Bob Calo-oy. *Caregiving Tips A-Z, Alzheimer's & Other Dementias.* Fremont, CA: Orchard Publications, 2008.

Chan, A. P. *Alzheimer's Disease Research Trends.* Hauppauge, NY: Nova Science, 2008.

Doraiswamy, P. Murali, Lisa Gwyther, and Tina Adler. *The Alzheimer's Action Plan: The Experts' Guide to the Best Diagnosis and Treatment for Memory Problems.* New York: St. Martin's Press, 2008.

Lerner, Adrienne. *Alzheimer's Disease*. Farmington Hills, MI: Greenhaven Press, 2008.

McCann-Beranger, Judith. *A Caregiver's Guide to Alzheimer's & Related Diseases*. New York: Bunim & Bannigan, 2008.

PERIODICALS

Gruneir, Andrea, et al. "Is Dementia Special Care Really Special? A New Look at an Old Question." *Journal of the American Geriatrics Society* (February 2008): 199–205.

Ji, Hong-fang, and Hong-yu Zhang. "Multipotent Natural Agents to Combat Alzheimer's Disease: Functional Spectrum and Structural Features." *Acta Pharmacologica Sinica* (February 2008): 143–151.

Kontush, Anatol, and Svetlana Schekatolina. "An Update on Using Vitamin E in Alzheimer's Disease." *Expert Opinion on Drug Discovery* (February 2008): 261–271.

Muñoz-Torrero, Diego, and Pelayo Camps. "Huprines for Alzheimer's Disease Drug Development." *Expert Opinion on Drug Discovery* (January 2008): 65–81.

"Statin Use Does Not Prevent the Occurrence of Alzheimer's Disease." *Inpharma* (January 26, 2008): 18.

ORGANIZATIONS

Alzheimer's Association, 225 N. Michigan Ave., 17th Floor, Chicago, IL, 60601-7633, (800) 272-3900, http://www.alz.org/.

National Institute of Aging, Alzheimer's Education and Referral Center, PO Box 8250, Silver Spring, MD, 20907, (800) 438-4380, http://www.nia.nih.gov/alzheimers.

Belinda Rowland
Teresa Norris
David Edward Newton, Ed.D.

Amblyopia *see* **Lazy eye**

Amenorrhea

Definition

Amenorrhea is the absence of menses during the reproductive years.

Description

Amenorrhea is defined as the absence of menses during the childbearing years. It can be physiologic during transitional times such as puberty, **pregnancy** and postpartum, or **menopause**. In other situations the absence of menses in women of childbearing age is considered abnormal and worthy of evaluation. The causes of amenorrhea can be determined by a thorough workup with a licensed heath practitioner, tailoring treatment to the cause of the problem.

Demographics

Amenorrhea is classified as either primary or secondary depending on the time in a woman's life when it occurs. Primary amenorrhea is the absence of menses in a woman who has never menstruated by 16 ½ years of age. This type of amenorrhea is uncommon; the incidence is less than 0.1% of American women. Secondary amenorrhea is defined as an absence of menses for 6–12 months in a woman who has previously menstruated. Approximately 1.8–3% of women in the United States experience amenorrhea at some point in their childbearing years, and it may affect as many as 20% of women seeking treatment for **infertility**.

The age of menarche, or a woman's first menstrual period, occurs on average by 12.3 years. Based on Tanner's stages of puberty for females, menarche typically occurs 2.3 years after breast development begins. When a young woman has not begun menstruating by 16 years of age, but she is progressing through early stages of puberty, it is likely that menarche is simply delayed, but an endocrine evaluation is warranted. If secondary sex characteristics such as breast and pubic hair development have not begun by age 14, primary amenorrhea should be considered and assessed for.

The onset of menses may be delayed for a variety of reasons. Delayed menarche can be caused by low body weight. Girls with the eating disorders **anorexia nervosa** or bulimia often experience delayed menses due to malnutrition. Vigorous **exercise** regimens in the pre–pubertal girl can also cause delayed menarche. These situations can contribute to both primary and secondary amenorrhea.

Causes and symptoms

The most common cause of primary amenorrhea is chromosomal defects that result in normal female external genitalia, but produce alterations in either breast or uterine development. Some examples of these genetic abnormalities are Turner's syndrome, Mullerian anomalies, and Testicular Feminization.

The majority of cases of secondary amenorrhea are due to disorders of the hypothalamus, followed by pituitary disorders and ovarian problems. Least common are cases caused by uterine disorders, which often result from intrauterine adhesions (IUAs) that occur after surgical procedures.

The hypothalamus secretes a hormone that is integral to the normal menstrual cycle, Gonadotropin–releasing hormone (GnRH). This hormone is part of a complex feedback mechanism with estrogen and progesterone. Hypothalamic function may be altered due to a lesion or mass in the hypothalamus or central nervous system, resulting in low circulating levels of GnRH. **Stress**, strenuous exercise and significant weight loss all provoke a drop in GnRH and subsequent decline in estrogen levels resulting in amenorrhea. Amenorrhea due to extreme dieting and exercise is a warning sign for anorexia nervosa. In patients with eating disorders, menses typically resumes with a gain in body weight. Stress–induced amenorrhea is often self–limiting, and is diagnosed by exclusion of a pituitary problem.

The pituitary gland secretes two hormones, leutinizing hormone (LH) and follicle stimulating hormone (FSH). In a healthy menstrual cycle, FSH stimulates maturation of an egg, or ovum, in the ovary. This occurs at the beginning, or follicular phase, of the cycle. During the follicular phase, ovarian production of estrogen rises and peaks, dropping off just before ovulation. Ovulation is the release of the fully mature ovum, and is prompted by a spike in LH, which also rises, peaks and drops off. In the second half of the menstrual cycle, known as the luteal phase, progesterone is secreted by a gland formed from the sac in the ovary that once held the ripening ovum, now called the corpus luteum. Progesterone is the dominant hormone of the luteal phase of the menstrual cycle, accompanied by a gradual rise in estrogen as the cycle prepares to begin again.

Disorders of the pituitary gland leading to amenorrhea include tumors, most commonly benign tumors known as adenomas. These tumors tend to produce hormones that disrupt the menstrual cycle, such as prolactin, adrenocorticotropic hormone (ACTH) or thyroid–stimulating hormone (TSH). Of these, prolactin–secreting tumors are the most common. Prolactin inhibits GnRH and thus disrupts cyclic menses. A common symptom of elevated prolactin is galactorrhea, or milky discharge from the nipples. Because thyroid function closely affects female hormones and the menstrual cycle, thyroid function should be assessed by measuring TSH. Additional abnormalities of the pituitary gland are Sheehan syndrome, which often presents in the postpartum period with an inability to lactate, and Empty Sella Syndrome, an abnormality of the pituitary gland which can be congenital or a result of radiation or surgery.

The ovaries cyclically produce the hormones estrogen and progesterone. Disorders of the ovary can be genetic chromosomal defects resulting in primary amenorrhea, such as Turner's syndrome, Mosaicism and Swyer syndrome. A common cause of secondary amenorrhea is premature ovarian failure, in which women enter menopause under 40 years of age. Premature ovarian failure is also a cause of primary amenorrhea in 10–28% of cases. The cause of premature ovarian failure is usually unknown, although it may have a genetic basis or be due to autoimmune disease. In 10–20% of cases ovarian function resumes. In cases where radiation, chemotherapy or surgical intervention has taken place, ovarian function typically does not resume.

A common ovarian cause of amenorrhea is Polycystic Ovarian Syndrome (PCOS). PCOS, also known as Stein–Leventhal syndrome, is a collection of symptoms which often includes menstrual irregularity, excess growth of facial or chest hair, and **obesity**. Women with PCOS may have irregular, anovulatory cycles and multiple follicular cysts on their ovaries. **Insulin resistance** may also be present, marked by elevated blood glucose and insulin. Masculinization may occur due to elevated testosterone produced by the ovaries.

Diagnosis

Because successful management of amenorrhea requires an accurate diagnosis of the origin of imbalance, a full workup is called for. Amenorrhea, either primary or secondary, is evaluated by the following strategy. First, laboratory analysis of TSH and prolactin are done to rule out **hypothyroidism** or hyperprolactinemia. If prolactin is elevated, an MRI may be indicated to rule out a pituitary adenoma or other pituitary tumor.

If TSH and prolactin levels are normal, the next step in diagnosis is a progesterone challenge. This diagnostic procedure involves the administration of oral or injected progesterone, which should prompt uterine bleeding within two–seven days. This is done to mimic the luteal phase of the menstrual cycle, where a rise and drop in progesterone is followed by **menstruation**. The presence of estrogen in the follicular phase builds the lining of uterus, and the effect of progesterone in the luteal phase is to slough off that lining, prompting menstrual bleeding. If bleeding occurs after a progesterone challenge, a diagnosis can be made of anovulation.

If withdrawal bleeding does not occur, there may be an anatomical abnormality affecting the uterus or vagina, or a low–estrogen state in which the uterus is not building up an endometrial lining. At this point oral estrogen is administered for 21 days, followed by five days of oral progesterone to provoke menstruation. Alternatively, one cycle of oral contraceptive pills may be used. If no withdrawal bleed occurs, an anatomical problem may be the origin of the amenorrhea. If a withdrawal bleed does occur, further workup is still indicated.

Additional tests include FSH and LH levels. Elevated levels suggest premature ovarian failure, as the ovaries are not responding to high levels of stimulating hormones. Normal or low levels of FSH and LH require further assessment of the pituitary gland via imaging techniques.

Treatment

Holistic approaches to treatment of amenorrhea are tailored to address the cause of the imbalance. After appropriate diagnostic measures are taken to identify the cause, a holistic treatment plan will account for the whole person by addressing **nutrition**, exercise, sleep and stress management in addition to therapies to balance the menstrual cycle.

Stress management is an important component to holistic treatment for amenorrhea. Techniques for reducing stress, such as **meditation**, **guided imagery** or deep breathing exercises can be helpful. Gentle stretching exercises like **yoga**, chi gong or tai chi are beneficial for the nervous system. Aerobic exercise for 30 minutes several times per week is essential for cardiovascular and overall health, but vigorous exercise should be avoided in women who are underweight or experiencing exercise–induced amenorrhea. Stress can also be reduced by maintaining a regular sleep routine, as adequate sleep is essential for endocrine health.

Nutrition concerns

Clinical nutrition for amenorrhea is aimed at restoring balance to overall health. For example, for underweight women the goal is to increase calories, dietary protein and high–quality fats. Eating disorders should be evaluated for and treated with appropriate psychiatric intervention. Women experiencing amenorrhea who are overweight with an elevated body mass index may benefit from a diet low in refined carbohydrates and high in fiber and lean proteins to help reduce weight and manage insulin resistance. In all cases, an emphasis on whole foods, complex carbohydrates, legumes, nuts and seeds is ideal. Increasing cold–water fish is beneficial for the essential fatty acid content. Soy foods, which are weakly estrogenic, are helpful in situations where estrogen is low. Optimizing

digestion will benefit overall health, as will incorporating routine in mealtimes.

Therapy

Botanical medicine can be of great help in restoring balance to the menstrual cycle by regulating sex hormones.

- Black Cohosh (*Cimicifuga racemosa*)—Black Cohosh is not a phytoestrogen. It is useful in premature ovarian failure to diminish early symptoms of perimenopause and to reestablish regular menstrual cycles.

- Blue Cohosh (*Caulophyllum thalictroides*)—Blue Cohosh is a uterine stimulant that can stimulate the onset of menses in secondary amenorrhea where there is no underlying pathology. It acts as a progesterone precursor and is helpful in anovulatory cycles with low progesterone in the luteal phase.

- Chastetree Berry (*Vitex agnus cactus*)—Chastetree is indicated for several different causes of amenorrhea. Its action on the hypothalamus and pituitary glands results in an elevation in LH and drop in FSH, causing in an increase in luteal phase progesterone. Chastetree berry can also suppress elevated prolactin levels due to stress. Therefore, Chastetree berry is useful for amenorrhea due to anovulation, such as in PCOS, and in cases of elevated prolactin when no pituitary adenoma is present.

- Dong Quai (*Angelica sinensis*)—Dong Quai is a phytoestrogenic herb that is useful for amenorrhea due to low estrogen or premature ovarian failure.

- Rhodiola (*Rhodiola rosea*)—Rhodiola is an adaptogenic herb that supports the adrenal glands. For this reason it is useful as part of a stress management treatment plan. It also has balancing effects of the nervous system.

- Wild Yam (*Dioscorrhea spp.*)—Wild Yam is a progesterone precursor and is useful for anovulatory cycles with low progesterone in the luteal phase. Wild yam is also the base for many over the counter progesterone creams, as well as being the source material for bioidentical hormone therapy.

Prognosis

Prior to initiating treatment with natural remedies for amenorrhea, a thorough workup to determine the cause is needed. It is advisable to consult with a knowledgeable provider for evaluation and management and treatment.

Prevention

Maintaining a healthy weight and a nutritious diet are important for overall health and can prevent some types of amenorrhea. Stress management, moderate exercise and good sleep habits encourage regular menses.

Resources

BOOKS

Gordon, John David, M.D. and Leon Speroff M.D. *Handbook for Clinical Gynecologic Endocrinology and Infertility*, pp. 211–239. Philadelphia, PA: Lippincott, 2002.

Hudson, Tori, N.D. *Women's Encyclopedia of Natural Medicine: Alternative Therapies and Integrative Medicine*, pp. 15–27. Los Angeles, CA: Keats Publishing, 1999.

Mills, Simon, and Kerry Bone. *Principles and Practice of Phytotherapy: Modern Herbal Medicine*. London, England: Churchill Livingstone, 2000.

Sherman, John A., N.D. *The Complete Botanical Prescriber*. 1993.

Stenchever, Morton, A., M.D., William Droegemueller, M.D., Arthur L. Herbst, M.D., Daniel R. Mishell, Jr., M.D. *Comprehensive Gynecology*, pp. 1099–1119. St. Louis, MO: Elsevier, 2001.

PERIODICALS

Kelly, G. S. "Rhodiola: A Possible Plant Adaptogen." *Alternative Medicine Review* 6, no. 3 (2001): 293–302.

Roemheld–Hamm B. "Chasteberry." *American Family Physician* 78 no. 5 (September 2005): 821–824.

Diana Christoff Quinn, ND

American elm *see* **Slippery elm**

American skullcap *see* **Skullcap**

Amino acids

Description

Amino acids are a group of nitrogen-containing organic compounds composing the structure of proteins. They are essential to human metabolism and to making the human body function properly for good health. All proteins are made of some combination of 20 amino acids. These 20 amino acids are classified into essential and non-essential amino acids. In this context essential means that the human body is unable to synthesize these compounds. It is essential, therefore, that they be included in one's daily diet. Authoritics disagree to some extent as to how amino acids should be classified, at least partly because of the needs of specialized populations (such as those who have deficiency diseases such as phenylketonuria, PKU). The amino acids most commonly listed as essential are histidine, isoleucine, leucine, **lysine**, **methionine**, phenylalanine, threonine, tryptophan, and valine. Five other amino acids are sometimes listed as conditionally essential because they may be essential under special circumstances. For example, **arginine** can be synthesized by adults, but not by children. Other conditionally essential amino acids are cysteine, glycine, **glutamine**, and tyrosine. The non-essential amino acids that can be synthesized by the human body are alanine, asparagine, aspartic acid, glutamic acid, proline, and serine.

The major source for essential amino acids in the human diet is protein from plant and animals sources. Good protein sources include dairy products, meats, fish, poultry, nuts, legumes, and eggs. Those sources are considered more complete than vegetable protein, such as beans, peas, and grains, also considered a good—even if not complete—source of amino acids.

Amino acids became popular as dietary supplements by the end of the twentieth century for various uses, including fitness training, weight loss, and certain chronic diseases. Some proponents of **holistic medicine** believe that amino acid supplements taken in the proper dosage can aid in fighting **depression**, **allergies**, **heart disease**, gastrointestinal problems, high **cholesterol**, muscle weakness, blood sugar problems, arthritis, **insomnia**, bipolar illness, **epilepsy**, **chronic fatigue syndrome**, **autism**, **attention-deficit hyperactivity disorder** (ADHD), and mental exhaustion.

Description

Amino acid therapy as a supplemental aid to a healthy diet joined the fitness craze in the United States by the end of the 1990s. Brenda Adderly in *Better Nutrition,* in September of 1999, stated: "The creation of new protein from amino acids and the breaking down of existing protein into amino acids are ongoing processes." After people **exercise** a lot, amino acides create new protein in order to replace muscle cells. Understanding the balance of amino acids in the body can be often the first clue to understanding why a person has many ailments, ranging from depression to upset stomach to **obesity**. Deficiencies in the proper balance of amino acids is likely to occur in those with poor **diets**. Because **stress**, age, infection, and various other factors, including the amount of exercise a person does, can also affect the levels of amino acids, people with healthy, nutritious diets could also find that they have deficiencies. Unfortunately, amino acid deficiencies are difficult to estimate as there are not recommended daily allowances for them.

Essential amino acids

The amino acids, which are derived only from food and that the body cannot manufacture, perform various functions, as follows:

- Tryptophan is considered a natural relaxant. This amino acid helps alleviate insomnia, helps in the treatment of migraine headaches, helps reduce the risk of artery and heart spasms, and works with lysine to reduce cholesterol levels.
- Lysine aids in proper absorption of calcium; helps form collagen for bone cartilage and connective tissues; and aids in production of antibodies, hormones, and enzymes. Research has indicated it also might be effective against herpes by creating a

balance of nutrients that slows the growth of the herpes virus. A deficiency could result in fatigue, lack of concentration, irritability, bloodshot eyes, retarded growth, hair loss, anemia, and reproductive problems.

- Methionine provides the primary source of sulfur that can prevent disorders of the hair, skin, and nails; lowers cholesterol by increasing the liver's production of lecithin; reduces liver fat; protectes kidneys; and promots hair growth.
- Phenylalanine serves the brain by producing norepinephrine, the chemical responsible for transmitting the signals between the nerve cells and the brain; it maintains alertness, reduces hunger pains, acts as an antidepressant, and improves memory.
- Threonine makes up a substantial portion of the collagen, elastin, and enamel protein; serves the liver by preventing buildup; aids the digestive and intestinal tracts to function better; and acts as a trigger for metabolism.
- Valine promotes mental energy, helps with muscle coordination, and serves as a natural tranquilizer.
- Leucine works with isoleucine to provide for the manufacture of essential biochemical processes in the body that are used for energy, increasing the stimulants to the upper brain for greater mental alertness.

Roles of certain non-essential amino acids

- Glycine facilitates the release of oxygen for the cell-making process and plays a key role in manufacturing of hormones and health of immune system.
- Serine is a source of glucose storage by the liver and muscles, provides antibodies for immune system, and synthesizes fatty acid sheath around nerve fibers.
- Glutamic acid is nature's brain food because it increases mental prowess, helps speed the healing of ulcers, and aids in combating fatigue.

Creatine in the spotlight

One of the most discussed amino acid supplements available on the market is **creatine** monohydrate. Creatine differs from other amino acids discussed in this entry because it is not used in the production of proteins. The body produces small amounts of creatine in the kidneys, liver, and pancreas. Most diets that include red meat or fish also include a few grams of creatine. It is stored in muscle cells and is used in activities, such as weight lifting and sprinting, providing the necessary thrust of energy for such activities. The natural supply of creatine produced by the body is quickly depleted. After approximately 10 seconds, when muscle **fatigue** becomes apparent, the daily production is used.

Timothy Gower, writing for *Esquire* in February of 1998, stated: "Scientists identified creatine 160-odd years ago, but only in the 1980s did they figure out that muscle cells can be 'loaded' with up to 30% more of the compound than they normally carry. Since then, several studies have shown that weight lifters primed on the supplement tire less easily, allowing them to work out longer." Gower also noted that creatine users find that the weight they add on is fat-free, whether that is lean tissue or some is water weight, no one had yet determined, since muscle cells do fill with water during creatine loading. Additionally, while it can add to the burst of the energy a sprinter needs to perform well, creatine does not do anything for the marathon runner going for several hours.

Though creatine has been commercially available since 1993, its long-term effects remain unknown. One 2002 study showed that creatine use improved rehabilitation for injured athletes and another that using the supplement increased risk of injury. It should be noted that some 20–30% of people researched showed no improvement using creatine. One report indicated that creatine could be beneficial for some people in spurring metabolism, burning calories, and helping in weight loss. Those reports were inconclusive as of 2008. In 2008, the National Center for Complementary and Alternative Medicine (NCCAM) reported that initial trials showed that creatine may be effective in treating Huntington's disease. NCCAM reportedly intended to fund further studies on this use of the supplement.

General use

Amino acid supplements to a healthy diet are used for various purposes. The most common uses include: sustaining strength in weight training to build muscles; improving heart and circulatory problems or diseases, particularly in older people; treating chronic fatigue syndrome; treating depression and **anxiety**; treating eating disorders, such as bulimia and/or anorexia, along with overeating; increasing memory; and building up and sustaining the body's immune system in fighting bacteria and viruses. It is important to note that, while the necessity and role of all amino acids was verified in the maintenance of optimum health, research was not extensive enough to provide indisputable verification of the touted benefits of such supplements over the long term.

Nonetheless, some members of the scientific medical community seem to confirm what amino acid proponents have long believed to be true. Rainer Hambrecht and colleagues from the University of Leipzig (Germany) tested the amino acid l-arginine on 38 heart-failure patients. Knowing that the human body converted it into nitric oxide, a chemical that relaxes blood vessels, the researchers gave one group 8 g of it daily for four weeks; another group simply did forearm exercises; and a third group combined the supplement with the exercise. The people who took the supplement alone increased their blood-vessel dilation by a factor of four, as did the exercise group. Those who took both the supplement and performed the exercise increased it by six. Studies on arginine in 2002 found that the supplement may help reduce risk of postoperative **infections**. Further, arginine may enhance women's sexual function. Later studies on the effectiveness of arginine for the treatment of heart disease had variable results. The United States Food and Drug Administration (FDA) prohibited the manufacturers of arginine from claiming that their product is effective in treating heart disease.

Supplements are recommended by alternative medical practitioners particularly for those who are not getting a proper diet, especially vegetarians who might not be getting a balance of complete protein, as well as athletes, anyone under severe stress, and anyone whose alcohol intake level is moderate to high.

Preparations

Supplements of various amino acids are available primarily in capsule, tablet, or powder form. A common way of taking amino acids is in a multiple amino acid gel cap. These contain sources of protein from gelatin, soy, and whey. The market for supplements in wholesale, retail, and Internet sales have been estimated to reach into the millions of dollars, with literally hundreds available. In the 2000s, Internet sales were fast-growing particularly with the use of such supplements as creatine powder publicized by well-known Olympic stars and professional athletes. Daily usage of creatine as evident from research indicated that usage should be leveled at 5 g of powder in a glass of orange juice and could be taken up to four times a day during peak athletic training. Maintenance dosages were recommended at 5 g once a day.

Side effects

Because amino acids are naturally produced substances both in the human body and in the diet protein derived from animal and dairy products, as well as being present in food combinations such as beans and rice, such supplements are not regulated by the United States Food and Drug Administration (FDA), nor are there any specified daily requirements, and they also do not show up in either drug or urine tests. Amino acid supplements might be classified as having no affect at all. Long-term effects had not been identified as of 2008.

Interactions

Interactions of amino acids with drugs has not been sufficiently studied to determine yet if any adverse effects result from using amino acids with medications.

Resources

BOOKS

Cynober, Luc A. *Metabolic and Therapeutic Aspects of Amino Acids in Clinical Nutrition,* 2nd ed. London: Taylor & Francis, 2007.

DiPasquale, Mauro G. *Amino Acids and Proteins for the Athlete: The Anabolic Edge,* 2nd ed. Boca Raton, FL: CRC Press, 2007.

Losso, Jack N., Kenji Sato, and Giuseppe Mazza, eds. *Functional Proteins, Peptides and Amino Acids.* Boca Raton, FL: CRC Press, 2008.

Sahyun, Melville. *Proteins and Amino Acids in Nutrition.* Toronto: Richardson Press, 2007.

PERIODICALS

Brosnan, J. T., and M. E. Brosnan. "The Sulfur-containing Amino Acids: An Overview." *Journal of Nutrition* (June 2006): 1636S–1640S.

Kreider, R. B. "Effects of Creatine Supplementation on Performance and Training Adaptations." *Molecular and Cellular Biochemistry* (February 2003): 89–94.

Maughan, Ron, Doug King, and Trevor Lea. "Dietary Supplements." *Journal of Sports Sciences* (January 2004): 95–113.

Nicolis, Curis E., et al. "Almost All about Citrulline in Mammals." *Amino Acids* (November 2005): 177–205.

Jane Spehar
Teresa G. Odle
David Edward Newton, Ed.D.

Amyotrophic lateral sclerosis *see* **Lou Gehrig's disease**

An-mo *see* **Chinese massage**

Androgaphis

Definition

Androgaphis, a genus of plant belonging to the family Acanthaceae, is native to India and Sri Lanka. Its best known and most widely used exemplar is the species *Androgaphis paniculata.*

Description

Androgaphis paniculata is a flowering perennial that grows wild in thickets throughout south Asia, although it is also cultivated. In summer and autumn, clusters of small white flowers appear. The plant is harvested for commercial and medicinal use when flowers begin to bloom. It is traditionally valued as an herbal remedy in China, where it grows in the Guangdong, Guangxi, Fujian, Yunnan, Sichuan, Jiangsu, and Jianxi provinces.

In Mandarin, androgaphis is called *chuan xin lian, Yi jian xi* and *Lan he lian,* which translate directly as "thread-the-heart lotus." The Cantonese term is *chyun sam ling,* and the Japanese call it *senshinren.* English common names include green chiretta, heart-thread lotus leaf, and kariyat. Its pharmaceutical names, used to distinguish it as a medicine, are *Herba Androgaphitis Paniculatae* or, alternately, *Folium Androgaphis.*

General use

Practitioners of Chinese medicine believe that androgaphis affects the large intestine, lung, stomach, bladder, and liver meridians, or energy pathways in the body. It is thought to dispel heat (such as that associated with **fever** or infection) and is used primarily as a broad-spectrum antibiotic and immunostimulant for a variety of bacterial, viral, and parasitic conditions, including **influenza**, intestinal **infections**, **hepatitis**, **pneumonia**, and infected **wounds**. Androgaphis's medicinal properties are considered very bitter, astringent, cold, dry, and stimulating.

Andrographis is considered most effective for conditions associated with fever, inflammation, and the formation of pus. It clears heat and relieves what is known as fire toxicity manifested as sores and carbuncles on the skin. It is also applied topically for snakebite and **eczema**. Under the supervision of a qualified practitioner, it is used as a uterine stimulant and abortive, to bring on miscarriage or treat prolonged **pregnancy** or retained placenta.

Andrographis can also be used as an inexpensive substitute for another Chinese herb, **coptis** (*huang lian*).

Much research on andrographis has been conducted in China and has focused on pharmacological investigation. Studies there indicate that andrographis cultivated in the plains of Shanghai has significant immune stimulating and anti-infective qualities. In vitro, it inhibits the growth of *Diplococcus pneumoniae* and other bacteria and delays the deterioration of embryonic renal cells caused by a virus. Scientific studies on the safety and efficacy of andrographis in the United States have been inconclusive. A review published in 2008 by Natural Standard, an international collaborative that studies the effectiveness of complementary and alternative medicines, concluded that research on the use of andrographis in the treatment of familial Mediterranean fever, influenza, and upper respiratory tract infection was inadequate to make recommendations on the herb's use.

Major chemical ingredients include andrographan, andrographolide, neoandrographolide, paniculide A, 14-deoxy-11-oxyandrographolide, and beta-sitosterol.

Preparations

Andrographis is not generally available in U.S. health food stores, but it can be found at most Chinese pharmacies and Asian groceries.

The standard dose ranges from 10–15 g as a decoction (strong tea) or 2–5 ml as a tincture. Powder doses range from 0.6 to 1.2 g. Because the herb is extremely bitter, it is recommended that powder be taken in capsule form.

Practitioners of Chinese medicine commonly combine andrographis in patent formulas along with other Chinese herbs. The following are the major herbs with which it is combined and the symptoms for which the combinations are prescribed.

- Pericarpium Citri Reticulatae (*Citrus reticulata, Chen pi*) for cough associated with lung heat.
- Herba et Radix Houttuyniae Cordatae (*Houttuynia cordata, yu xing cao*) and Semen Benincasae Hispidae (*Benincasa hispida, dong gua ren cao*) for lung abscess.
- Flos Lonicerae Japonicae (*Lonicera japonica, jin yin hua*) and Radix Platycodonis Grandiflori (*Platycodon grandiflorum, jie geng*) for early stages of a disease with fever and sore throat.
- Herba Portulacae Oleraceae (*Portulacca oleracea, ma chi xian*) for dysentery.
- Radix et folium Polygoni Cuspidati (*Polygonum cuspidatum, hu zhang*) and Rhizoma Imperatae Cylindricae (*Imperata cylindrical* var. *major, bai mao gen*) for hot, painful urinary dysfunction.

Natural Standard noted that scientific research on the effectiveness of combination treatments was also incomplete and inconclusive.

Precautions

According to tradition, andrographis is never used in cases of deficient, cold intestinal conditions. When used long-term or in large doses, this bitter and cold herb may damage stomach qi, causing gastric distress and loss of appetite.

Andrographis is also capable of producing a miscarriage, and thus should be avoided by pregnant women unless otherwise directed by a knowledgeable practitioner.

Side effects

Gastric distress and loss of appetite have been noted when the herb is taken in large doses. The 2008 Natural Standards review indicated that andrographis is generally safe to use, although a number of unpleasant side effects may occur, including **headache**, **dizziness**, confusion, **nausea**, **diarrhea**, chest and abdominal discomfort, and increased risk of bleeding.

Interactions

Interactions with pharmaceutical drugs and herbs have not been well studied. The 2008 Natural Standards report suggested that interactions may occur with anticoagulant drugs, such as warfarin; antiplatelet drugs, such as clopidogrel; blood pressure medications; some nonsteroidal anti-inflammatory drugs (NSAIDs), such as ibuprofen; and some drugs used for the treatment of diabetes. The report also suggested obtaining professional advice if one is also taking a variety of herbs such as ginkgo, **horse chestnut** seed extract, **black cohosh**, **hawthorn**, or **bitter melon**.

KEY TERMS

Cold—In Chinese pathology, the term defines a condition that has insufficient warmth, either objective (hypothermia) or subjective (feeling cold).

Decoction—A strong tea brewed for 20–30 minutes.

Heat—In Chinese pathology, the term defines a condition that has excessive heat, either objective (fever, infection) or subjective (feeling hot).

Meridians—Energetic pathways inside the body through which *Qi* flows; also called channels.

Patent formulas—Chinese herbal formulas that were patented centuries ago and are believed to be proven over centuries of use and study.

Qi—A Chinese medical term, pronounced *chee,* denoting active physiological energy.

Tincture—A solution of medicinal substance in alcohol, usually more or less diluted; herb tinctures are made by infusing the alcohol with plant material.

Resources

BOOKS

Leung, Ping-Chung, Harry Hong Sang Fong, and Charlie Changli Xue, eds. *Current Review of Chinese Medicine: Quality Control of Herbs And Herbal Material.* Singapore: World Scientific, 2006.

Liu, Chongyun. *Chinese Herbal Medicine: Modern Applications of Traditional Formulas.* London: Taylor & Francis, 2007.

PERIODICALS

Mkrtchyan A., et al. "A Phase I Clinical Study of Andrographis Paniculata Fixed Combination Kan Jang Versus Ginseng and Valerian on the Semen Quality of Healthy Male Subjects." *Phytomedicine* (June 2005): 403–409.

Erika Lenz
David Edward Newton, Ed.D.

Androstenedione

Description

Androstenedione is a hormone that occurs naturally in the body, and is one of those responsible for male characteristics. It is a metabolite of **DHEA**, and as such, a direct precursor to the male hormone testosterone. It is found in some plant matter, notably pollen, and in the gonads of all mammals.

General use

Supplementation with androstenedione increases blood levels of testosterone, which among other things, will lead to an increase in strength and muscle mass. As such, it is mainly of interest to athletes and bodybuilders, for whom it has the added benefits of increasing energy levels, improving levels of nitrogen retention and shortening muscle recovery time. Androstenedione is safer than anabolic steroids because it has a far gentler effect on the body, and potential effects are milder and more transient.

Androstenedione is also taken to improve well being, and to raise levels of mental alertness. In addition, it is thought to have a positive effect on sexual performance. As androstenedione also aids in the conversion of fatty tissue to muscle, it could conceivably be considered an aid to weight loss.

The German patent for androstenedione states that 50 mg administered orally raised testosterone levels from 140%–183% above normal, which although impressive, is considerably less than the increase associated with administration of anabolic steroids. Also, it is a precursor, in that the body retains some control over production of testosterone.

Preparations

When taken orally, androstenedione is metabolized by a single enzyme into testosterone. Athletes generally take between 50 mg–300 mg daily, according to how much time is spent exercising and how much physical improvement is required. Dosage is usually sublingual in the form of a spray or capsules. The spray is felt to be far more effective, due to imperfect absorption through the digestive route.

Levels of testosterone in the blood will begin to rise approximately 15 minutes after administration of androstenedione supplements. They will remain so for about three hours, with testosterone levels peaking roughly 1–1.5 hours after administration.

Precautions

There is no reliable research to prove the claims by supplement companies that androstenedione is useful. Trials that have been conducted are limited in size and scope, and generally do not satisfy the criteria set for medical trials. Some experts warn that as a result of the short time that androstenedione stays in the system, it is unlikely to have any significant bodybuilding effects.

Androstenedione is not suitable for pregnant or lactating women, and should not be taken at all by children. When taken by women, this supplement may cause hirsuitism and virilization. Caution should be exercised when males under the age of 25 years take androstenedione.

Those supplementing with androstenedione on a regular basis are advised to have "cool down" periods when the product is not taken. This can either be a couple of days a week, or one week per month.

Androstenedione is unsuitable for use by men with **prostate cancer** or elevated PSA. It may also stimulate prostate replication, enlarging the prostrate (benign prostate hypertrophy or **cancer**). Many experts are skeptical of the claims made by supplement companies, because they say that natural bodily checks and balances will work against this supplement to ensure that muscle mass and strength do not exceed normal levels for the individual. Taking androstenedione at times other than periods of physical exertion is not recommended, because of the possible effect on mood.

Because of the complex interaction of hormones within the body, it is strongly advised that anyone contemplating supplementing with androstenedione consult a qualified practitioner.

Whereas anabolic steroids are illegal, androstenedione is considered a dietary supplement, and as such is not governed by the same regulations.

As a result of trials conducted by them, the American Medical Association issued a statement to the effect that androstenedione does not raise serum testosterone levels, and in addition, it may have undesirable side effects.

Side effects

Possible effects on the personality of this type of hormone should be considered, as high levels of male hormones have been known to trigger aggressive behavior in some cases, particularly when high doses of the supplement are involved.

It is also possible that long-term use of androstenedione, which is not in accordance with medical recommendations, may eventually have a negative effect on natural levels of testosterone, due to compensation on the part of the pituitary gland. This means that, in the long term, it is possible that supplementation with androstenedione may cause a reduction in levels of testosterone.

The androgen effect of androstenedione may cause males to develop loss of head hair. Other side

---

KEY TERMS

Anabolic steroids—Synthetic male hormones.

DHEA—Dehydroepiandrosterone, which is basically a male hormone.

Hirsuitism—The growth of excess hair on the bodies of women, usually due to a hormone imbalance.

PSA—Prostatic Specific Antigen, elevated levels of which are a precondition to the development of cancer of the prostate gland.

Sublingual—Taken underneath the tongue.

Transient—Of short duration.

Virilization—The development of male characteristics in women.

---

effects that have been associated with androstenedione administration include blurred vision, development of breast-like tissue, and the development of **acne**.

Interactions

This supplement should not be taken in conjunction with other bodybuilding substances, particularly anabolic steroids, unless under the direction of a physician. Lysophosphatidyl **choline**, when taken in conjunction with androstenedione, may enhance absorption.

In addition, manufacturers recommend **saw palmetto** to be taken in conjunction with androstenedione as it can help reduce associated **hair loss**, and is useful in controlling **prostate enlargement**.

Resources

OTHER

Betterbodz (1995-2000). http://www.betterbodz.com/androstenedione.html/ (December 28, 2000).

Nutritionalsupplements.com (1998-2000). http://www.nutritionalsupplements.com/andro5.html/ (December 28, 2000).

Patricia Skinner

Anemarrhena

Description

Anemarrhena (*Anemarrhena asphodeloides* or *Zhi-Mu*) is a rare herb that grows wild in Japan, Korea, and the northern part of China. It has a 2,000-year

---

history of use, and written records of its use date from 200 A.D. It is an attractive-looking plant that belongs to the lily family. At the top of three-foot spikes, it has small, fragrant, white six-petal flowers that bloom at night. The medicinal parts are the rhizomes (roots) and the stems. Rhizomes that are large, hard, and round with pale-yellowish color inside are best for medicinal use.

General use

Traditional Chinese medicine classifies this herb as cold (or yin) and bitter. Yin and yang are the two opposite energies that complement one another. Yin conditions are described as cold, damp, and deficient, while yang is characterized by heat, dry, and excess. Anemarrhena is used to treat heat disorders, which are caused by excessive yang or insufficient yin functions. When there is excessive heat, dryness often follows. For example, fever—an excessive internal heat symptom—is followed by thirst, which is a sign of dryness. Traditional Chinese medicine uses bitter and cold herbs such as anemarrhena to clear the internal heat and provide moisture to the lungs and the kidneys.

Because anemarrhena brings moisture and coolness, it has been said to bring relief to excessive internal heat and dryness symptoms such as **fever**, thirst, irritability, racing pulse, **cough**, bleeding gums, night sweat, **insomnia**, and **hot flashes**. Anemarrhena has been used in herbal combinations such as *Zhi Bai Di Huang Wan* to relieve symptoms such as coughing, ulcers of the mouth, kidney dysfunction, urinary tract infection, insomnia, restlessness, **genital herpes**, and sterility.

Chronic bronchitis

Anemarrhena has been used to eradicate **infections** caused by *Staphylococcus aureus*, the bacterial strain that often causes lung infections. Anemarrhena has also been used to treat **bronchitis** and exacerbating symptoms of chronic bronchitis such as chronic coughing.

Tuberculosis

Anemarrhena is also used to treat **tuberculosis**. However, animal research did not support its use.

Urinary tract infections

Anemarrhena has been used to treat cystitis, an infection of the bladder. It may be effective against *Escherichia coli* (known as *E.coli*), which is a common cause of cystitis in women. If it is proven to be effective, it would be useful against urinary tract infections caused by this bacterial strain.

Other infections

As of 2008 little information was available concerning the use of anemarrhena in other types of infections. However, anemarrhena may have antibacterial activity that is useful against *Salmonella typhi* and *Vibrio cholera*, the bacteria that cause salmonella **food poisoning** and cholera, two common infections of the bowels. Anemarrhena may also be effective against **fungal infections**.

Oliguria

Anemarrhena provides moisture to dry internal organs. Therefore, it is used as a diuretic to improve kidney function.

Ulcers of the mouth and/or bleeding gums

Anemarrhena is thought to restore moisture in these oral conditions that exhibit excessive dryness and inflammation.

Diabetes

Because Chinese herbalists believe that yin deficiency is the underlying cause of diabetes, they often use anemarrhena to treat this disease. Animal studies indicated that anemarrhena contains two pharmacologic agents, mangiferin and mangiferin-7-0-beta glucoside, which appear to increase the effectiveness of insulin and can lower blood glucose levels. In studies, anemarrhena had the greatest effect in mild to moderate diabetic conditions. However, it did not affect glucose levels in nondiabetic conditions. Anemarrhena may be combined with Shi Gao (Gypsum) for additional hypoglycemic effects.

Chemotherapy and radiation side effects

Anemarrhena is thought to be effective in relieving severe adverse reactions associated with conventional chemotherapy and radiation treatments in **cancer** patients. According to traditional Chinese medicine, x rays used in radiation treatment and drugs used in chemotherapy are considered "heat toxins." These agents are very toxic so that they can kill tumor cells. But they are also toxic to the body, causing excessive build-up of heat inside the lungs and damaging the kidneys.

Menopausal symptoms

Another use of anemarrhena is to treat menopausal symptoms such as insomnia, hot flashes, and irregular periods.

High blood pressure

Anemarrhena is often used in combination with phellodendron and rehmannia to treat high blood pressure conditions in patients with symptoms of liver-fire deficiency. These symptoms are **dizziness**, **headache**, ringing in the ears, back **pain**, insomnia, palpitations, dry eyes, and night sweat. Studies of laboratory animals prior to 2000 indicated that this herb was effective in lowering blood pressure.

Preparations

The usual dosage of anamarrhena is 6–12 g per day. It is available as a single ingredient or in combinations in the following forms:

- Powder or pills. These are generally taken with warm water on an empty stomach.
- Decoction. A method often used in traditional Chinese medicine to make an herbal preparation at home. Herbs, usually in combination, are simply boiled down to a concentrated broth or tea to be taken internally.

Precautions

The United States Food and Drug Administration does not regulate herbal remedies such as anemarrhena, which means that the remedies have not been proven to be safe or effective. The safety of anemarrhena has not been established for use by children, pregnant women, and nursing mothers. In addition, ingredients are not standardized to comply with federal regulations.

As of 2008, research claims into the effectiveness of anemarrhena were primarily based on the testing of laboratory animals. The lack of clinical testing on humans raises questions about how anemarrhena would interact with other medications and herbs. In addition, the lack of detailed information about product ingredients drew cautions from organizations, including the American Cancer Society. When the California Department of Health tested Chinese herbal remedies, results showed close to 33% contained prescription drugs or were contaminated with toxic metals such as mercury, arsenic, and lead, according to the society.

Medical precautions

Before beginning any herbal treatment, people should consult a physician or health practitioner. It is especially important for people with conditions such as diabetes to consult with a doctor. Anemarrhena

KEY TERMS

Diuretic—A substance that increases the formation and excretion of urine.

Energy—Includes nonmaterial (such as Qi) as well as material (such as blood) vital forces that create and sustain life.

Fire—An extremely high internal heat condition characterized by severe dehydration, red eyes, red face, constipation, insomnia, and agitation. Fire often affects Lungs, Liver, and Stomach.

Hypoglycemia—Low blood sugar.

Oliguria—A condition in which the kidneys produce small amounts of urine.

should not be regarded as a substitute for other medications, including insulin.

Anemarrhena should not be used when a person has **diarrhea**, chronic loose bowel movements, or hypotension (low blood pressure). Anemarrhena at very high dosages could cause severe drops in blood pressure levels.

Side effects

Taking large dosages of anemarrhena could cause diarrhea, intestinal **colic**, and **gastroenteritis**.

Interactions

Anemarrhena has been known to interact with the following:

- Iron supplements or multivitamin, multimineral supplements containing iron. Patients should take iron supplements at least two hours before or two hours after the herb.
- Iron pots or pans. Patients should not use iron cooking utensils to make decoctions as they may alter the chemistry of the herb.

Resources

BOOKS

Mayo Clinic Book of Alternative Medicine. New York: Time Inc. Home Entertainment, 2007.
PDR for Herbal Medicines, (PDR for Herbal Medicines). Boston: Thomson Healthcare, 2005.

OTHER

"Chinese Herbal Medicine." *American Cancer Society*, June 26, 2007. http://www.cancer.org/docroot/ETO/content/ETO_5_3x_Chinese_Herbal_Medicine.asp. (February 11, 2008).

ORGANIZATIONS

American Association of Acupuncture and Oriental Medicine, PO Box 162340, Sacramento, CA, 95816, (866) 455-7999, http://www.aaom.org.

American Botanical Council, 6200 Manor Rd., Austin, TX, 78723, (512) 926-4900, http://abc.herbalgram.org.

American Diabetes Association, 1701 N. Beauregard St., Alexandria, VA, 22311, (800) 342-2383, http://www.diabetes.org.

American Herbal Products Association, 8484 Georgia Ave., Suite 370, Silver Springs, MD, 20910, (301) 588-1171, http://www.ahpa.org.

Herb Research Foundation, 4140 Fifteenth St., Boulder, CO, 80304, (303) 449-2265, http://www.herbs.org.

National Center for Complementary and Alternative Medicine, National Institute of Health (NCCAM), 9000 Rockville Pike, Bethesda, MD, 20892, (888) 644-6226, http://nccam.nih.gov.

Mai Tran
Liz Swain

Anemia

Definition

Anemia is a condition characterized by abnormally low levels of healthy red blood cells or hemoglobin.

Description

The tissues of the human body need a regular supply of oxygen to stay healthy. Red blood cells, which contain hemoglobin that allows them to deliver oxygen throughout the body, live for only about 120 days. When they die, the **iron** they contain is returned to the bone marrow and used to create new red blood cells. Anemia can develop when heavy bleeding causes significant iron loss. It also occurs when something happens to slow down the production of red blood cells or to increase the rate at which they are destroyed.

Anemia can be mild, moderate, or severe enough to lead to life-threatening complications. Over 400 different types of anemia have been identified. Many of them are rare. More common anemia types include:

- iron deficiency anemia
- folic acid deficiency anemia
- vitamin B_{12} deficiency anemia
- vitamin C deficiency anemia
- autoimmune hemolytic anemia
- hemolytic anemia
- sickle cell anemia
- aplastic anemia
- anemia of chronic disease

Causes and symptoms

Anemia is caused by bleeding, decreased red blood cell production, or increased red blood cell destruction. Poor diet can contribute to vitamin deficiency and iron deficiency anemia, in which an inadequate supply of red blood cells is produced. Hereditary disorders and certain diseases can cause increased blood cell destruction. However, excessive bleeding is the most common cause of anemia, and the speed with which blood loss occurs has a significant effect on the severity of symptoms. Chronic blood loss may be caused by the following conditions:

- heavy menstrual flow
- hemorrhoids
- nosebleeds
- cancer
- gastrointestinal tumors
- diverticulosis
- polyposis
- stomach ulcers
- long-term alcohol abuse

Acute blood loss is usually the result of the following:

- childbirth
- injury
- ruptured blood vessel
- surgery

Iron deficiency anemia

Iron deficiency anemia is the most common form of anemia around the world. In the United States, iron deficiency anemia affects about 240,000 toddlers between one and two years of age and 3.3 million women of childbearing age. This condition is less common in older children and in adults over 50, and it rarely occurs in teenage boys and young men.

Iron deficiency anemia has a gradual onset. The deficiency begins when the body loses more iron than it gains from food and other sources. Because depleted iron stores cannot meet the red blood cells' needs, fewer red blood cells develop. In this early stage of anemia, the red blood cells look normal, but they are reduced in number. Then the body tries to compensate for the iron deficiency by producing more red blood cells, which are characteristically smaller than normal.

Weakness, **fatigue**, and a run-down feeling may be signs of mild anemia. Other signs include skin that is pasty or sallow, or lack of color in the creases of the palm, gums, nail beds, or lining of the eyelids. Someone who is weak, tires easily, is often out of breath, and feels faint or dizzy may be severely anemic. Other symptoms of anemia are:

- angina pectoris (chest pain)
- headache
- inability to concentrate and/or memory loss
- inflammation of the mouth (stomatitis) or tongue (glossitis)
- insomnia
- irregular heartbeat
- loss of appetite
- nails that are dry, brittle, or ridged
- rapid breathing
- sores in the mouth, throat, or rectum
- sweating
- swelling of the hands and feet
- thirst
- tinnitus (ringing in the ears)
- unexplained bleeding or bruising
- pica (a craving to chew ice, paint, or dirt)

Folic acid deficiency anemia

Folic acid deficiency anemia is the most common type of megaloblastic anemia, in which red blood cells are bigger than normal. It is caused by a deficiency of folic acid, a vitamin that the body needs to produce normal cells.

Folic acid anemia is especially common in infants and teenagers. Although this condition usually results from a dietary deficiency, it is sometimes due to an inability to absorb enough folic acid from foods such as the following:

- eggs
- fish
- green vegetables
- meat
- milk and cheese
- mushrooms
- yeast

Smoking raises the risk of developing this condition by interfering with the absorption of **vitamin C**, which the body needs to absorb folic acid. Folic acid anemia can be a complication of **pregnancy**, when a woman's body needs eight times more folic acid than it does otherwise.

Vitamin B₁₂ deficiency anemia

Less common in the United States than folic acid anemia, **vitamin B$_{12}$** deficiency anemia is another type of megaloblastic anemia that develops when the body does not absorb enough of this nutrient. Necessary for the creation of red blood cells, B$_{12}$ is found in meat and vegetables.

Large amounts of B$_{12}$ are stored in the body, so this condition may not become apparent until as long as four years after B$_{12}$ absorption slows down or stops. The resulting drop in red blood cell production can cause the following problems:

- loss of muscle control
- loss of sensation in the legs, hands, and feet
- soreness or burning of the tongue
- weight loss
- yellow-blue color blindness

The most common form of B$_{12}$ deficiency is pernicious anemia. Since most people who eat meat or eggs get enough B$_{12}$ in their **diets**, a deficiency of this vitamin usually means that the body is not absorbing it properly. This condition can occur among people who have had intestinal surgery or those who do not produce adequate amounts of intrinsic factor, a chemical secreted by the stomach lining that combines with B$_{12}$ to help its absorption in the small intestine. Symptoms of pernicious anemia include problems with movement or balance, a slick tongue, tingling in the hands and feet, confusion, **depression**, and **memory loss**. Pernicious anemia can also damage the spinal cord. A doctor should be notified whenever symptoms of this condition occur.

Pernicious anemia usually strikes people 50–60 years of age. Eating disorders or an unbalanced diet increases the risk of developing pernicious anemia. So do **diabetes mellitus**, **gastritis**, stomach **cancer**, stomach surgery, thyroid disease, and family history of pernicious anemia.

Vitamin C deficiency anemia

A rare disorder that causes the bone marrow to manufacture abnormally small red blood cells, vitamin C deficiency anemia results from a severe, long-standing dietary deficiency.

Hemolytic anemia

Some people are born with hemolytic anemia. Some acquire this condition, in which infection or antibodies destroy red blood cells more rapidly than bone marrow can replace them.

Hemolytic anemia can cause enlargement of the spleen and accelerate the destruction of red blood cells (hemolysis). Other complications of hemolytic anemia may include **pain**, shock, **gallstones**, and other serious health problems.

Thalassemias

An inherited form of hemolytic anemia, thalassemia stems from the body's inability to manufacture as much normal hemoglobin as it needs. There are two categories of thalassemia, depending on which of the amino acid chains is affected. (Hemoglobin is composed of four chains of amino acids.) In alpha-thalassemia, there is an imbalance in the production of the alpha chain of **amino acids**; in beta-thalassemia, there is an imbalance in the beta chain. Alpha-thalassemia most commonly affects blacks (25% have at least one gene); beta-thalassemia most commonly affects people of Mediterranean and Southeast Asian ancestry.

Characterized by production of red blood cells that are unusually small and fragile, thalassemia affects only people who inherit the gene for it from each parent (autosomal recessive inheritance).

Autoimmune hemolytic anemia

Warm antibody hemolytic anemia is the most common type of this disorder. This condition occurs when the body produces autoantibodies that coat red blood cells. The coated cells are destroyed by the spleen, liver, or bone marrow.

Warm antibody hemolytic ancmia is more common in women than men. About one-third of patients who have warm antibody hemolytic anemia also have lymphoma, **leukemia**, lupus, or connective tissue disease.

In cold antibody hemolytic anemia, the body attacks red blood cells at or below normal body temperature. The acute form of this condition frequently develops in people who have had **pneumonia**, **mononucleosis**, or other acute **infections**. It tends to be mild and short-lived and disappears without treatment.

Chronic cold antibody hemolytic anemia is most common in women and most often affects those who are over 40 and have arthritis. This condition usually lasts for a lifetime, generally causing few symptoms. However, exposure to cold temperatures can accelerate red blood cell destruction, causing fatigue, joint aches, and discoloration of the arms and hands.

Sickle cell anemia

Sickle cell anemia is a chronic, incurable condition that causes the body to produce defective hemoglobin, which forces red blood cells to assume an abnormal crescent shape. Unlike normal oval cells, fragile sickle cells cannot hold enough hemoglobin to nourish body tissues. The deformed shape makes it hard for sickle cells to pass through narrow blood vessels. When capillaries become obstructed, a life-threatening condition called sickle cell crisis is likely to occur.

Sickle cell anemia is hereditary. It almost always affects people of African or Mediterranean descent. A child who inherits the sickle cell gene from each parent will have the disease, but a child who inherits the gene from only one parent will carry the sickle cell trait but will not have the disease.

Aplastic anemia

Sometimes curable by bone marrow transplant, but potentially fatal, aplastic anemia is characterized by decreased production of red and white blood cells and platelets (disc-shaped cells that allow the blood to clot). This disorder may be inherited or acquired as a result of recent severe illness, long-term exposure to industrial chemicals, or use of anticancer drugs and certain other medications.

Anemia of chronic disease

Cancer, chronic infection or inflammation, and kidney and liver disease often cause mild or moderate anemia. Chronic liver failure generally produces the most severe symptoms.

Diagnosis

Personal and family health history may suggest the presence of certain types of anemia. Laboratory tests that measure the percentage of red blood cells or the amount of hemoglobin in the blood are used to confirm diagnosis and determine which type of anemia is responsible for a patient's symptoms. X rays and examinations of bone marrow may be used to identify the source of bleeding.

Treatment

Individuals who have anemia caused by poor **nutrition** should modify their diet to include more vitamins, minerals, and iron. Foods such as lean red meats, dried beans and fruits, liver, poultry, and enriched breads and cereals are all good sources of iron. In addition, eating foods rich in vitamin C such as citrus fruits and juices can promote the absorption of iron.

Patients diagnosed with iron-deficiency anemia should undergo a thorough physical examination and medical history to determine the cause of the anemia, particularly if chronic or acute blood loss is suspected. The cause of a specific anemia will determine the type of treatment recommended.

Anemia due to nutritional deficiencies can usually be treated at home with iron supplements or self administered injections of vitamin B_{12}. People with folic acid anemia should take oral folic acid replacements. Vitamin C deficiency anemia can be cured by taking daily supplements of vitamin C.

Many therapies for iron-deficiency anemia focus on adding iron-rich foods to the diet or on techniques to improve circulation and digestion. Iron supplementation, especially with iron citrate (less likely to cause **constipation**), can be given in combination with herbs that are rich in iron. Some examples of iron-rich herbs are **dandelion** (*Taraxacum officinale*), **parsley** (*Petroselinum crispum*), and **nettle** (*Urtica dioica*). The homeopathic remedy ferrum phosphoricum (iron sulfate) can also be helpful.

An iron-rich herbal tonic can also be made using the following recipe:

- Soak one-half ounce of yellow dock root and one-half ounce dandelion root in 1 qt of boiled water for 4–8 hours.
- Simmer until the amount of liquid is reduced to 1 cup.
- Remove from heat and add one-half cup black strap molasses, mixing well.
- Store in refrigerator; take one-quarter cup daily.

Other herbal remedies known to promote digestion are prescribed to treat iron-deficiency anemia. Gentian (*Gentiana lutea*) is widely used in Europe to treat anemia and other nutritionally based disorders. The bitter qualities of gentian help stimulate the digestive system, making iron and other nutrients more available for absorption. This bitter herb can be brewed into tea or purchased as an alcoholic extract (tincture).

Other herbs recommended to promote digestion include:

- anise (*Pimpinella anisum*)
- caraway (*Carum carvi*)
- cumin (*Cuminum cyminum*)
- linden (*Tilia* spp.)
- licorice (*Glycyrrhiza glabra*)

Traditional Chinese treatments for anemia include:

- Acupuncture to stimulate a weakened spleen.
- Asian ginseng (*Panax ginseng*) to restore energy.
- Dong quai (*Angelica sinensis*) to control heavy menstrual bleeding.
- A mixture of dong quai and Chinese foxglove (*Rehmannia glutinosa*) to clear a sallow complexion.
- Astragalus (*Astragalus membranaceus*) to treat pallor and dizziness.

Allopathic treatment

Surgery may be necessary to treat anemia caused by excessive loss of blood. Transfusions of red blood cells may be used to accelerate production of red blood cells.

Medication or surgery may also be necessary to control heavy menstrual flow, repair a bleeding ulcer, or remove polyps (growths or nodules) from the bowels.

Patients with thalassemia usually do not require treatment. However, people with a severe form may require periodic hospitalization for blood transfusions and/or bone marrow transplantation.

Sickle cell anemia

Treatment for sickle cell anemia involves regular eye examinations, immunizations for pneumonia and infectious diseases, and prompt treatment for sickle cell crises and infections of any kind. **Psychotherapy** or counseling may help patients deal with the emotional impact of this condition.

Vitamin B_{12} deficiency anemia

A life-long regimen of B_{12} shots is necessary to control symptoms of pernicious anemia. The patient may be advised to limit physical activity until treatment restores strength and balance.

Aplastic anemia

People who have aplastic anemia are especially susceptible to infection. Treatment for aplastic anemia may involve blood transfusions and bone marrow transplant to replace malfunctioning cells with healthy ones.

Anemia of chronic disease

There is no specific treatment for anemia associated with chronic disease, but treating the underlying illness may alleviate this condition. This type of anemia rarely becomes severe. If it does, transfusions or hormone treatments to stimulate red blood cell production may be prescribed.

Hemolytic anemia

There is no specific treatment for cold-antibody hemolytic anemia. About one-third of patients with warm-antibody hemolytic anemia respond well to large doses of intravenous and oral corticosteroids, which are gradually discontinued as the patient's condition improves. Patients with this condition who do not respond to medical therapy must have the spleen surgically removed. This operation controls anemia in about half of the patients on whom it is performed. Immune-system suppressants are prescribed for patients whose surgery is not successful.

Expected results

Folic acid and iron deficiency anemia

It usually takes three to six weeks to correct folic acid or iron deficiency anemia. Patients should continue taking supplements for another six months to replenish iron reserves and should have periodic blood tests to make sure the bleeding has stopped and the anemia has not recurred.

Pernicious anemia

Although pernicious anemia is considered incurable, regular B_{12} shots alleviate symptoms and reverse complications. Some symptoms disappear almost as soon as treatment begins.

Aplastic anemia

Aplastic anemia can sometimes be cured by a bone marrow transplant. If the condition is due to immunosuppressive drugs, symptoms may disappear after the drugs are discontinued.

Sickle cell anemia

Although sickle cell anemia cannot be cured, effective treatments enable patients with this disease to enjoy longer, more productive lives.

Thalassemia

People with mild thalassemia (alpha thalassemia trait or beta thalassemia minor) lead normal lives and do not require treatment. Those with severe thalassemia may require bone marrow transplantation. Genetic therapy is being investigated and is expected to become available.

Hemolytic anemia

Acquired hemolytic anemia can generally be cured when the cause is removed.

KEY TERMS

Aplastic—Exhibiting incomplete or faulty development.

Diabetes mellitus—A disorder of carbohydrate metabolism brought on by a combination of hereditary and environmental factors.

Hemoglobin—An iron-containing pigment of red blood cells composed of four amino acid chains (alpha, beta, delta, gamma) that delivers oxygen from the lungs to the tissues of the body.

Megaloblast—A large erythroblast (a red marrow cell that synthesizes hemoglobin).

Prevention

Inherited anemia cannot be prevented. Genetic counseling can help parents cope with questions and concerns about passing on disease-causing genes to their children.

Avoiding excessive use of alcohol, eating a balanced diet that contains plenty of iron-rich foods, and taking a daily multivitamin can help prevent anemia.

Methods of preventing specific types of anemia include:

- Avoiding lengthy exposure to industrial chemicals and drugs known to cause aplastic anemia.
- Not taking medication that has triggered hemolytic anemia and not eating foods that have caused hemolysis (breakdown of red blood cells).
- Receiving regular B_{12} shots to prevent pernicious anemia resulting from gastritis or stomach surgery.

Resources

BOOKS

Bridges, Kenneth. *Anemias and Other Red Cell Disorders.* New York: McGraw Hill Professional, 2007.

Platt, Allan, and Alan Sacerdote. *Hope and Destiny: A Patient's and Parent's Guide to Sickle Cell Anemia.* Munster, IN: Hilton, 2006.

Weiss, Gunter, Victor R. Gordeuk, and Chaim Hershko, eds. *Anemia of Chronic Disease.* London: Informa Healthcare, 2005.

PERIODICALS

D'Arena, Giovanni, et al. "Rituximab for Warm-type Idiopathic Autoimmune Hemolytic Anemia: A Retrospective Study of 11 Adult Patients." *European Journal of Haematology* (July 2007): 53–58.

Huma, Nuzahat, et al. "Food Fortification Strategy-Preventing Iron Deficiency Anemia: A Review."

Critical Reviews in Food Science and Nutrition (March 2007): 259–265.

Killip, Shersten, John M. Bennett, and Mara D. Chambers. "Iron Deficiency Anemia." *American Family Physician* (March 1, 2007): 671–678.

Paula Ford-Martin
David Edward Newton, Ed.D.

Angelica

Description

Angelica is a genus of plants in the **parsley** family used in both Western healing and **traditional Chinese medicine** (TCM). The most common angelica used in Western healing is the European species, *Angelica archangelica*. Occasionally the North American species, *A. atropurpurea*, is used in the same way as *A. archangelica*. Other names for Western Angelica are European angelica, garden angelica, purple angelica, Alexander's archangel, masterwort, wild angelica, and wild celery.

Western angelica grows to a height of about 4.5 ft (1.5 m) in dappled sun. It has white to yellow flowers and very large three-part leaves. The root is long and fibrous and may be poisonous if used fresh. The plant has a strong, tangy odor and taste.

At least 10 different species of angelica are used in TCM. The most frequently used species is *A. sinensis*, which in Chinese is called *dong quai* (alternate spellings are *dang gui*, *tang kwei*, and *tang gui*). Other Chinese species include *A. pubescens*, called in Chinese *du huo*, and *A. dahurica*, called in Chinese *bai zhi*. The descriptions of the medicinal uses of Chinese angelica in this article refer only to *A. sinensis* or *dong quai*.

Chinese angelica is a perennial that grows to a height of 3 ft (1 m) in moist, fertile soil at high altitudes in China, Korea, and Japan. It has a purple stem and umbrella-like clusters of flowers. The root is used medicinally and as a spice.

The species of angelica used in Western healing have different properties than those used in Eastern medicine. Any properties or benefits ascribed to Western angelica do not necessarily apply to Chinese angelica or vice versa.

General use

Western angelica

Western angelica, or *A. archangelica*, is said to have been named after an angel who revealed the herb to a European monk as a curative. It has a long history of folk use in Europe, Russia, and among Native American tribes.

The leaves of angelica are prepared as a tincture or tea and used to treat coughs, colds, **bronchitis**, and other respiratory complaints. They are considered gentler in action than preparations made from the root. The root is the most medically active part of the plant. It is used as an appetite stimulant and to treat problems of the digestive system and liver. It is said to relieve abdominal bloating and **gas**, **indigestion**, and **heartburn**.

Angelica will induce sweating and is used to treat conditions such as arthritis and rheumatism. In addition, it is used as a diuretic. Externally, angelica is applied as an ointment to treat lice and some skin disorders.

In addition to medicinal use, an essential oil derived from the plant is used in making perfumes and as a food flavoring. Oil from the seeds imparts the distinctive flavor to the Benedictine liqueur. Sometimes candied leaves and stalks are used as sweets.

Despite its widespread folk use, angelica can present some serious health hazards. The root is poisonous when fresh and must be dried thoroughly before use. All members of the genus contain compounds called furocoumarins that can cause a person exposed to the sun or other source of ultraviolet rays to develop severe **sunburn** and/or rash (photodermatitis). In addition, in animal studies furocoumarins have been found to cause **cancer** and cell damage even without exposure to light. The essential oil contains safrole, the cancer-causing substance that caused the United States Food and Drug Administration (FDA) to ban the herb **sassafras**.

Despite these health concerns, the German Federal Health Agency's Commission E, established in 1978 to independently review and evaluate scientific literature and case studies pertaining to herb and plant medications, has approved preparations containing angelica root as a treatment for bloating and as an appetite stimulant.

Chinese angelica

Chinese angelica, or *dong quai*, is considered in TCM to have a warm nature and a sweet, acrid, and bitter taste. The main use of angelica in TCM is to regulate the female reproductive organs and treat irregularities of the menstrual cycle, especially deficient bleeding (amenorhhea). Chinese herbalists also use this herb to treat irregular periods, menstrual cramps, and **infertility**. The root is one component of Four Things Soup, a widely used woman's tonic in China. Because of its use as a tonic for women, *dong quai* is sometimes called "women's ginseng."

Dong quai is one of the most commonly used herbs in China and is one of the traditional Chinese herbs that is increasingly familiar in the West. In addition to treating women's complaints, Chinese angelica is used in general blood tonics to improve conditions such as **anemia**. Because angelica is considered to be a warming herb, it is also used to aid circulation and digestion. Other uses are to treat kidney complaints, **headache**, **constipation**, rheumatism, high blood pressure, and ulcers.

Dong quai contains several active compounds called coumarins. These compounds are well documented as agents that dilate (open up) the blood vessels, stimulate the central nervous system, and help control spasms. It is likely that these compounds do act on the uterus, supporting the use of *dong quai* for some women's problems.

Animal and test-tube studies indicated that *dong quai* may combat **allergies** by altering the immune system response. Other animal studies suggest that the herb is a mild diuretic. Interest in *dong quai* has increased in the twenty-first century and more test tube and animal research is being done on the herb. There are reports that the herb may have estrogen-like properties that would account for its effect on the female reproductive system. As of 2008, laboratory and animal studies of this effect have produced mixed results.

Preparations

Angelica root is harvested in the fall, then dried for future use. The leaves of Western angelica can be made into a tea (1 teaspoon powdered leaves to one cup of boiling water steeped up to 20 minutes), a tincture, or a cream for external use. The root can be made into a tincture or a decoction. The essential oil can be combined with other oils for external use as a massage oil for arthritis.

Dong quai is used in many common Chinese formulas and as a component of many medicinal soups. Because it is most often used with other herbs, dosage varies.

KEY TERMS

Decoction—Decoctions are made by boiling an herb, then straining the solid material out for the resulting liquid.

Diuretic—A diuretic is any substance that increases the production of urine.

Tincture—An alcohol-based extract prepared by soaking plant parts.

Precautions

Pregnant women should not take angelica because of its effects on the reproductive system. It is not known whether angelica passes into breast milk, so breastfeeding women should also avoid the herb. Safe use in children has not been established.

People who are taking blood thinners such as warfarin (Coumadin) should discuss taking any preparations containing angelica with their doctor. The herb appears to have anticlotting effects and may, when taken with other blood-thinning agents, cause excessive bleeding.

Individuals who are allergic to plants in the same family as angelica, including **anise**, caraway, carrot, celery, dill, and parsley, may experience an allergic reaction to *dong quai*.

Women who have or have had estrogen-sensitive cancers should avoid *dong quai* until more research is done on its estrogen-like properties.

Dong quai, like Western angelica, contains compounds that can cause a person exposed to the sun or other source of ultraviolet rays to develop severe sunburn and/or rash. These problems become more severe when using the concentrated essential oil or purified forms of the herb. The essential oil also contains safrole, a known carcinogen.

Side effects

In addition to increasing the risk of photodermatitis, angelica is considered to be a mild laxative and may cause **diarrhea**.

Interactions

Angelica may interact with blood-thinning pharmaceuticals in a way that causes excessive bleeding. Other interactions with Western pharmaceuticals have not been documented. Given the history of its long use in TCM, it appears unlikely that there are any significant interactions with other commonly used Chinese herbs.

Resources

BOOKS

Bensky, Dan, et al. *Chinese Herbal Medicine: Materia Medica,* 3rd ed. Seattle, WA: Eastland Press, 2004.

Blumenthal, Mark, ed. *The Complete German Commission E Monographs: Therapeutic Guide to Herbal Medicines.* Boston: Integrative Medicine Communications, 1998.

Chevallier, Andrew. *Herbal Remedies.* New York: DK Publishing, 2007.

Foster, Steven and Rebecca Johnson. *National Geographic Desk Reference to Nature's Medicine.* Washington, DC: National Geographic Society, 2006.

PDR for Herbal Medicines, 4th ed. Montvale, NJ: Thomson Healthcare, 2007.

OTHER

"*Angelica sinensis.*" *Plants for a Future.* [cited February 19, 2008]. http://www.pfaf.org/database/plants.php? Angelica + sinensis.

"Dong quai (Angelica sinensis [Oliv.] Diels), Chinese angelica." *Mayo Clinic.* September 1, 2006 [cited February 19, 2008]. http://www.mayocli nic.com/health/dong-quai/NS_patient-Dongquai.

"Dong Quai (Angelica sinensis) - Oral." *MedicineNet.com.* March 2, 2005 [cited February 19, 2008]. http://www.medicinenet.com/dong_quai_angelica_sinensis-oral/article.htm.

ORGANIZATIONS

Alternative Medicine Foundation, PO Box 60016, Potomac, MD, 20859, (301) 340-1960, http://www.amfoundation.org.

American Association of Oriental Medicine, PO Box 162340, Sacramento, CA, 95816, (866) 455-7999, (914) 443-4770, http://www.aaaomonline.org.

American Holistic Medical Association, PO Box 2016, Edmonds, WA, 98020, (425) 967-0737, http://www.holisticmedicin.org.

Centre for International Ethnomedicinal Education and Research (CIEER), http://www.cieer.org.

Tish Davidson, A. M.

Angelica archangelica see **Angelica root**
Angelica sinensis see **Dong quai**

Angina

Definition

Angina is **pain**, discomfort, or pressure in the chest that is caused by **ischemia**, an insufficient supply of oxygen-rich blood to the heart muscle. It is sometimes also characterized by a feeling of choking, suffocation, or crushing heaviness. This condition is also called angina pectoris.

Description

Often described as a muscle spasm and choking sensation, angina primarily is chest (thoracic) pain caused by insufficient oxygen to the heart muscle. An episode of angina is not an actual **heart attack**, but rather pain that results when the heart muscle temporarily receives too little blood. This temporary condition may be the result of demanding activities such as **exercise** and does not necessarily indicate that the heart muscle is experiencing permanent damage. In fact, episodes of angina seldom cause permanent damage to heart muscle. An estimated 9.1 million Americans suffer from angina with 500,000 new cases of stable angina diagnosed each year, according to the American Heart Association. In the United Kingdom, about 1.8 million people have angina.

There are five types of angina.

Stable angina

Stable angina is a common disorder caused by the narrowing of the arteries (a condition called **atherosclerosis**) that supply oxygen-rich blood to the heart muscle. In the case of stable angina, the coronary arteries can provide the heart muscle (myocardium) adequate blood during rest but not during periods of exercise, **stress**, or excitement. The resulting pain is relieved by resting or by administering nitroglycerin, a medication that relaxes the heart muscle, opens up the coronary blood vessels, and lowers the blood pressure—all of which reduce the heart's need for oxygen. Patients with stable angina have an increased risk of heart attack (myocardial infarction).

Unstable angina

Unstable angina has symptoms of unexpectant chest pain that occur while the person is at rest. The pain progressively worsens and is more severe than in stable angina. It is an intermediate condition between stable angina and a heart attack. People who experience unstable angina need to seek immediate medical attention.

Variant angina

Variant angina is relatively uncommon and occurs independently of atherosclerosis, which may incidentally be present. Variant angina occurs at rest and is not related to excessive work by the heart muscle. Research indicates that variant angina is caused by coronary artery muscle spasm that does not last long enough and/or is not intense enough to cause an actual heart attack. It is more common in women than men.

Microvascular angina

People with microvascular angina experience chest pain but have no apparent coronary artery blockages. Doctors have found that the pain results from the poor function of tiny blood vessels that nourish the heart as well as the arms and legs. Microvascular angina can be treated with some of the same medications used for stable angina. It is more common in people with diabetes.

Atypical angina

Atypical angina is caused by a sudden narrowing or tightening of an artery that supplies blood to the heart. Symptoms include a vague feeling of discomfort in the chest rather than pain, shortness of breath, **fatigue**, **nausea**, **indigestion**, and back or **neck pain**. It is more common in women than men and in people with diabetes.

Causes and symptoms

Angina is usually caused by an underlying obstruction to the coronary artery due to atherosclerosis. In some cases, it is caused by spasm that occurs naturally or as a result of ingesting cocaine. In rare cases, angina is caused by a coronary embolism or by a disease other than atherosclerosis that places demands on the heart.

Most episodes of angina are brought on by physical exertion, when the heart needs more oxygen than is available from the blood nourishing the heart. Emotional stress, extreme temperatures, heavy meals, cigarette **smoking**, and alcohol can also cause or contribute to an episode of angina.

Angina causes a pressing pain or sensation of heaviness, usually in the chest area under the breast bone (sternum). It is occasionally experienced in the shoulder, arm, neck, or jaw regions. In most cases, the symptoms are relieved within a few minutes by resting or by taking prescribed angina medications.

Diagnosis

Physicians can usually diagnose angina based on the patient's symptoms and the precipitating factors. However, other diagnostic testing is often required to confirm or rule out angina or to determine the severity of the underlying **heart disease**.

Electrocardiogram (ECG)

An electrocardiogram is a test that records electrical impulses from the heart. The resulting graph of electrical activity can show if the heart muscle is not functioning properly as a result of a lack of oxygen. Electrocardiograms are also useful in investigating other possible abnormal features of the heart, such as arrhythmia (irregular heartbeat).

Stress test

For many individuals with angina, the results of an electrocardiogram while at rest will not show any abnormalities. Because the symptoms of angina occur during stress, the heart's function may need to be evaluated under the physical stress of exercise. The stress test records information from the electrocardiogram before, during, and after exercise in search of stress-related abnormalities. Blood pressure is also measured during the stress test and symptoms are noted. In some cases a more involved and complex stress test (for example, thallium scanning) is used to picture the blood flow in the heart muscle during the most intense exercise and after rest.

Angiogram

The angiogram, which is a series of x rays of the coronary artery, has been noted as the most accurate diagnostic test to indicate the presence and extent of coronary disease. In this procedure, a long, thin, flexible tube (catheter) is inserted into an artery located in the forearm or groin. This catheter is passed further through the artery into one of the two major coronary arteries. A dye is injected through the catheter to make the heart, arteries, and blood flow clearer on the x ray. A fluoroscopic film, or series of "moving" x rays, shows the blood flowing through the coronary arteries. This examination reveals any narrowing that can decrease blood flow to the heart muscle and cause symptoms of angina.

Treatment

Controlling existing factors that place the individual at risk is the first step in addressing artery disease that causes angina. These risk factors include cigarette smoking, high blood pressure, high **cholesterol** levels, and **obesity**.

Once the angina has subsided, the cause should be determined and treated. Atherosclerosis, a major associated cause, requires diet and lifestyle adjustments, primarily including regular exercise, reduction of dietary sugar and saturated fats, and increase of dietary fiber.

In the 1990s and 2000s, several specific cholesterol-lowering treatments gained public attention and interest. One popular treatment is ingesting **garlic** (*Allium sativum*). Some studies have shown that garlic can reduce total cholesterol by about 10% and LDL (bad) cholesterol by 15%, and can raise HDL (good) cholesterol by 10%. Other studies have not shown significant benefit. Although its effect on cholesterol is not as great as the effect achieved by medications, garlic may help in relatively mild cases of high cholesterol, without causing the side effects associated with cholesterol-reducing drugs. In 2007, scientists in the United States reported they had discovered why garlic benefits heart health. Researchers found that consuming garlic can boost blood flow by increasing the levels of hydrogen sulphide in the bloodstream, which lowers blood pressure and decreases cholesterol levels, two risk factors for angina.

Several studies have found that red yeast extract can significantly reduce cholesterol when it is taken in conjunction with a low-fat diet. Red yeast extract, available in the United States under the trade name Cholestin, has been used in Chinese medicine to treat heart maladies for hundreds of years. The effectiveness of the extract depends on the patient's cholesterol level and medical history, so individuals should consult with their healthcare professionals before taking the supplement. Additional natural remedies that may help lower cholesterol include oats (*Avena sativa*), **alfalfa** (*Medicago sativa*), **fenugreek** (*Trigonella foenum-graecum*), **Korean ginseng** (*Panax ginseng*), **myrrh** (*Commiphora molmol*), and **turmeric** (*Curcuma longa*).

Yarrow (*Achillea millefolium*), linden (*Tilia europaea*), and **hawthorn** (*Crataegus spp.*) are sometimes recommended for controlling high blood pressure, a risk factor for heart disease. In particular, hawthorn extract appears to benefit the **aging** heart. A 2001 report of a European study reported that patients using hawthorn extract showed improvements in exercise tolerance, fatigue levels, and shortness of breath.

A Chinese herbal medical formula has been used for at least several centuries to treat angina. The formula, called *xue fu zhu yu tang*, contains the following herbs: tao ren (*semen persicae*), hong hua (*flos carthami*), dang gui (*radix angelicae sinensis*), sheng di huang (uncooked *radix rehmanniae*), chuan xiong (*rhizoma chuanxiong*), chi shao (*radix rubra paeoniae*), niu xi (*radix achyranthis bidentatae*), jic geng (*radix platycodi*), chai hu (*radix bupleuri*), zhi ke (*fructus aurantii*), and gan cao (*radix glycyrrhizae*). In a 2006 study, Chinese researchers concluded that the formula was effective in relieving angina pain and had no reported adverse side effects. The formula is sold over the counter in the United States and a one-month supply costs about $40.

Tea (*Camellia sinensis*)—especially green tea—is high in **antioxidants**, and studies have shown that it may help prevent atherosclerosis. Other antioxidants, including **vitamin A (beta carotene)**, **vitamin C**, **vitamin E**, and **selenium**, can also limit the damage to the walls of blood vessels by oxidation, which may be lead to the formation of atherosclerotic plaque.

Vitamin and mineral supplements that reduce, reverse, or protect against coronary artery disease include **chromium**, **calcium**, and **magnesium**, B-complex vitamins, L-carnitine, and **zinc**. **Yoga** and other bodywork, massage, **aromatherapy**, and **music therapy** may also help reduce angina symptoms by promoting **relaxation** and stress reduction.

Traditional Chinese medicine may recommend herbal remedies (such as a ginseng and **aconite** combination), massage, **acupuncture**, and dietary modification. Exercise and a healthy diet, including cold-water fish as a source of **essential fatty acids**, are important components of a regimen to prevent angina and heart disease.

Allopathic treatment

Angina is often controlled by medication, most commonly with nitroglycerin. This drug relieves symptoms of angina by increasing the diameter of the blood vessels that carry blood to the heart muscle. Nitroglycerin is taken whenever discomfort occurs or is expected. It may be taken sublingually, by placing the tablet under the tongue. Or it may be administered transdermally, by placing a medicated patch directly on the skin.

In addition, beta-blockers or calcium channel blockers may be prescribed to decrease the heart's rate and workload. In late 2001, a study reported that the drug Nicorandil had become the first to demonstrate a reduction in risk of angina and to improve symptoms in patients with chronic stable angina. Guidelines released late in 2000 promoted use of clopidogrel to help prevent recurring events. A study group that used clopidogrel and aspirin showed a significant decrease in cardiovascular death, nonfatal heart attack, and **stroke** compared to patients in a control group that received a placebo and aspirin. In 2006, the U.S. Food and Drug Administration (FDA) approved the prescription drug ranolazine (Ranexa) as a second-line treatment of angina. It is recommended for patients with chronic stable angina who do not respond well to other drugs. It was the first new drug in 20 years to be approved by the FDA to treat angina. Further clinical studies of the drug were underway as of late 2007 to determine its effectiveness and safety as a first-line treatment for stable and unstable angina.

When conservative treatments are not effective in reducing angina pain and the risk of heart attack remains high, physicians may recommend angioplasty or surgery. In coronary artery bypass surgery, a blood vessel (often a long vein surgically removed from the leg) is grafted onto the blocked artery to bypass the blocked portion. This newly formed pathway allows blood to flow adequately to the heart muscle.

Another procedure used to improve blood flow to the heart is percutaneous tranluminal coronary angioplasty, usually called coronary or balloon angioplasty. In this procedure, the physician inserts a catheter with a tiny balloon at the end into a forearm or groin artery. The catheter is then threaded up into the coronary arteries, and the balloon is inflated to open the vessel in narrowed sections. Other techniques to open clogged arteries are under development and in limited use, including the use of lasers, stents, and other surgical devices.

A newer but less used treatment for angina is called enhanced external counterpulsation (EECP). The treatment increases blood flow to the heart by wrapping long inflatable cuffs (similar to those used to measure blood pressure) around the calves, thighs, and buttocks of patients. The cuffs inflate and deflate with each heartbeat, pushing blood up the legs towards the heart. EECP is recommended for people with chronic stable angina who are not helped by taking nitrates and who do not qualify for surgery. EECP is a non-surgical procedure that is typically done in an outpatient center. The treatment is given one to two hours a day, five days a week, for seven weeks. A number of studies have reported that EECP treatment is safe, effective, and has no adverse side effects. The treatment costs $8,000 to $10,000 in the United States and is covered by some insurance plans and covered under certain conditions by Medicare.

Expected results

The prognosis for a patient with angina depends on the general health of the individual as well as on the origin, type, and severity of the condition. Individuals can improve their prognosis by seeking prompt medical attention and learning the pattern of their angina, such as what causes the attacks, what they feel like, how long episodes usually last, and whether medication relieves the attacks. Medical help should be sought immediately if patterns of the symptoms change significantly or if symptoms resemble those of a heart attack.

KEY TERMS

Atherosclerosis—Progressive narrowing and hardening of the arteries caused by the buildup of plaque on the artery walls, which results in restricted blood flow.

Enhanced external counterpulsation (EECP)—A noninvasive angina treatment that increases blood flow to the heart.

Ischemia—Decreased blood supply to an organ or body part, often resulting in pain.

Myocardial infarction—A blockage of a coronary artery that cuts off the blood supply to part of the heart. In most cases, the blockage is caused by fatty deposits.

Myocardium—The thick middle layer of the heart that forms the bulk of the heart wall and contracts as the organ beats.

Prevention

In most cases, the best prevention involves changing habits to avoid bringing on attacks of angina. A heart-healthy lifestyle includes eating right, exercising regularly, maintaining an appropriate weight, not smoking, drinking in moderation, controlling **hypertension**, and managing stress. Most healthcare professionals can provide valuable advice on proper diet, weight control, smoking cessation, and maintaining healthy blood cholesterol levels and blood pressure.

Resources

BOOKS

Braverman, Debra. *Heal Your Heart with EECP: The Only Noninvasive Way to Overcome Heart Disease.* San Francisco: Celestial Arts, 2005.

Chermin, Dennis. *The Complete Homeopathic Resource for Common Illnesses.* Berkeley, CA: North Atlantic Books, 2006.

Icon Health Publications. *The Official Patient's Sourcebook on Angina: A Directory for the Internet Age.* San Diego: Icon Health Publications, 2005.

Maciocia, Giovanni. *The Practice of Chinese Medicine: The Treatment of Diseases With Acupuncture and Chinese Herbs.* Burlington, MA: Churchill Livingstone (Elsevier), 2007.

PERIODICALS

Flaws, Bob. "The Chinese Medical Treatment for Coronary Heart Disease Angina." *Townsend Letter: The Examiner of Alternative Medicine* (July 2007): 158–159.

Gupta, Nelly Edmondson, et al. "Stents vs. Medications to Treat Heart Disease: Once Hailed as a Breakthrough in the Care of Angina, Stents Are in the Crosshairs of Skeptics. Two Cardiologists Sort Through the Controversy." *Clinical Advisor* (November 2007): 52(3).

Havranek, Edward. "Enhanced External Counterpulsation (EECP)." *Clinical Reference Systems* (May 31, 2007): N/A.

Koren, Michael J., et al. "Long-Term Safety of a Novel Antianginal Agent in Patients with Severe Chronic Stable Angina." *Journal of the American College of Cardiology* (March 13, 2007): 1027(8).

Moon, Mary Ann. "CABG Relieves Angina Better than PCI." *Family Practice News* (November 1, 2007): 12(2).

Warburton, Louise. "Clinical: How to Diagnose and Treat Angina—The Basics." *GP* (September 14, 2007): 26.

ORGANIZATIONS

American Heart Association, 7320 Greenville Ave., Dallas, TX, 75231, (800) 242-8721, http://www.american heart.org.

American Institute of Homeopathy, 801 N. Fairfax St., Suite 306, Alexandria, VA, 22314, (888) 445-9988, http://www.homeopathyusa.org.

Heart and Stroke Foundation of Canada, 222 Queen St., Suite 1402, Ottawa, ON, K1P 5V9, Canada, (613) 569-4361, http://www.heartandstroke.ca.

Heart Association of Australia, 80 William St., Level 3, Sydney, NSW 2011, Australia, (11) 61-2-300-36-2787, http://www.heartfoundation.org.au.

Homeopathic Medical Council of Canada, 3910 Bathurst St., Suite 202, Toronto, ON , M3H 3N8, Canada, (416) 638-4622, http://www.hmcc.ca.

National Heart, Lung, and Blood Institute, PO Box 30105, Bethesda, MD, 20824-0105, (301) 592-8573, http://www.nhlbi.nih.gov.

Paula Ford-Martin
Ken R. Wells

Animal-assisted therapy *see* **Pet therapy**

Anise

Description

Anise, *Pimpinella anisum*, is a slow-growing annual herb of the **parsley** family (Apiaceae, formerly Umbelliferae). It is related to other plants prized for their aromatic fruits, commonly called seeds, such as dill, cumin, caraway, and **fennel**. It is cultivated chiefly for its licorice-flavored fruits, called aniseed. Although it has a **licorice** flavor, anise is not related to the European plant whose roots are the source of true

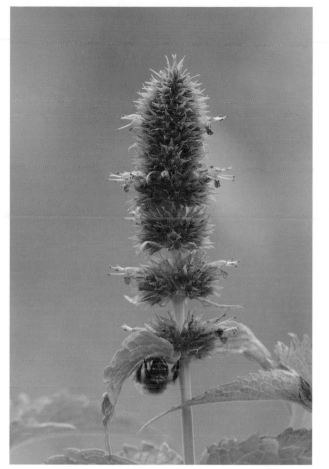

Anise hyssop (*Pimpinella anisum*). (© Arco Images, Inc. / Alamy)

licorice. It has been used as a medicinal and fragrant plant since ancient times.

The plant reaches from 1 to 3 ft (0.3 to 1 m) in height when cultivated, and has finely-divided feather-like bright green leaflets. The name *Pimpinella* (from the Latin *dipinella*) refers to the pinnately divided form of the leaves. The plant bears white to yellowish-white flowers in compound umbels (umbrella-like clusters). When ripe, the fruits are 0.125 in (3 mm) long and oval-shaped with grayish-green coloring.

While the entire plant is fragrant and tastes strongly of anise, it is the aniseed fruit that has been highly valued since antiquity. Seed maturation usually occurs one month after pollination, when the oil content in the dried fruit is about 2.5%. Steam distillation of the crushed aniseed yields from 2.5 to 3.5% of a fragrant, syrupy, essential, or volatile, oil, of which anethole, present at about 90%, is the principal aromatic constituent. Other chemical constituents of the fruit are creosol, alpha-pinene, dianethole, and photoancthole.

In addition to its medicinal properties, anise is widely used for flavoring curries, breads, soups, cakes, candies, desserts, nonalcoholic beverages, and liqueurs such as anisette. The essential oil is valuable in perfumes and soaps and has been used in toothpastes, mouthwashes, and skin creams.

Anise is endemic to the Middle East and Mediterranean regions, including Egypt, Greece, Crete, and Turkey. It was cultivated and used by ancient Egyptians, and used in ancient Greece and Rome, when it was cultivated in Tuscany. Its use and cultivation spread to central Europe in the Middle Ages, and today it is cultivated on a commercial scale in warm areas such as southern Europe, Asia, India, North Africa, Mexico, and Central and South America.

General use

The medicinal properties of anise come from the chemicals that are present in the fruits. The anethole in anise helps to relieve **gas** and settle an upset stomach. The use of anise to season foods, especially meat and vegetable dishes, in many parts of the world may have originated as a digestive aid. The Romans ate aniseed cake at the end of rich meals to prevent **indigestion**. The chemicals creosol and alpha-pinene act as expectorants, loosening mucus and making it easier to cough up. The estrogenic action of anise is from the chemicals dianethole and photoanethole, which act in a way similar to estrogen. The anise fruits and the essential oil of anise contain these chemicals and can be used medicinally. Aniseed can also be used to make an herbal tea which can help relieve physical complaints.

As a medicinal plant, anise has been used as an antibacterial, an antimicrobial, an antiseptic, an antispasmodic, a breath freshener, a carminative, a diaphoretic, a digestive aid, a diuretic, an expectorant, a mild estrogenic, a mild muscle relaxant, a parasiticide, a stimulant, and a stomachic.

Anise may be helpful in the following conditions:

- Anemia. Anise promotes digestion, which may help improve anemia due to inefficient absorption of iron.
- Asthma. Essential oil of anise may be inhaled through the nose to help ease breathing and relieve nasal congestion.
- Bad breath. It can be used in mouthwash or tea to sweeten breath.
- Bronchitis. Aniseed may be used as an expectorant and essential oil of anise may be inhaled through the nose to help ease breathing.
- Catarrh. Drinking aniseed tea soothes mucous membranes.
- Cold. Aniseed can be used as an expectorant and drinking aniseed tea soothes the throat.
- Colic. Drinking anise tea or using essential oil can alleviate gas.
- **Cough**. Can be used as an expectorant, especially for hard, dry coughs where expectoration is difficult.
- Croup. Aniseed can be used to alleviate a persistent cough in a child.
- Emphysema. Essential oil of anise may be inhaled through the nose to help ease breathing and relieve nasal congestion and tea with aniseed will soothe mucous membranes.
- Gas and gas pains. Drinking aniseed tea helps relieve gas, gas pains, and flatulence.
- Menopause. Aniseed tea can help alleviate menopausal symptoms.
- Morning sickness. Tea made from anise can help alleviate morning sickness during pregnancy.
- Nursing. Aniseed tea can help a nursing mother's milk come in.
- Sore throat. Drinking aniseed tea alleviates pain of sore throat.

Preparations

Aniseeds may be added to foods when cooking to flavor and aid digestion, or may be taken whole in doses of 1-3 tsp of dried anise seeds per day.

For tea, one tsp of crushed aniseeds can be steeped in a cup of hot water, then combined with fennel and caraway to help relieve gas and gas pains. To help relieve a cough, **coltsfoot**, **marsh mallow**, **hyssop**, and licorice can be added to the tea. Infants should only receive 1 tsp of boiled, prepared tea.

Preparations of essential oil of anise can be used for inhalation. The essential oil may be taken orally at a dose of 0.01 oz (0.3 g) per day. In addition, the liqueur anisette, which contains anise essential oil, may be administered in hot water to help relieve problems in the bronchial tubes, such as **bronchitis** and spasmodic **asthma**. One to three drops of essential oil administered on sugar may help relieve **colic**.

Precautions

Persons allergic to anise or anethole, its main ingredient, should avoid using aniseed or its essential oil. It is also possible to develop an allergic sensitivity to anise. Care should be taken to monitor the quantity of aniseed oil given to infants. A 2002 report noted an infant brought to the emergency department with seizures as a result of multiple doses of aniseed oil tea.

KEY TERMS

Anemia—Condition in which the blood is deficient in red blood cells, in hemoglobin, or in total volume.

Antiseptic—A substance that checks the growth or action of microorganisms especially in or on living tissue.

Antispasmodic—A substance capable of preventing or relieving spasms or convulsions.

Carminative—A substance that expels gas from the alimentary canal to relieve colic or griping.

Catarrh—Inflammation of a mucous membrane, especially of the nose and air passages.

Diaphoretic—A substance that increases perspiration.

Diuretic—A substance that increases the flow of urine.

Estrogenic—A substance that promotes estrus, the state in which a woman is capable of conceiving.

Expectorant—A substance that promotes the discharge or expulsion of mucus.

Parasiticide—A substance destructive to parasites.

Stomachic—A stimulant or tonic for the stomach.

Side effects

Although anise is generally considered safe, the side effects of its estrogenic property have not been fully studied. Anise oil may induce **nausea**, **vomiting**, seizures, and pulmonary **edema** if it is ingested in sufficient quantities. Also, contact of the skin with the concentrated oil can cause irritation.

It is important to note that Japanese Star Anise is *not* the same herb—it is poisonous.

Interactions

No interactions have been reported.

Resources

BOOKS

Foster, Gertrude B. and Rosemary F. Louden. *Park's Success with Herbs*. Greenwood, SC: G. W. Park Seed Co., 1980.

Grieve, M. *A Modern Herbal: The Medicinal, Culinary, Cosmetic and Economic Properties, Cultivation and Folk-lore of Herbs, Grasses, Fungi, Shrubs, & Trees with All Their Modern Scientific Uses*. New York: Harcourt, Brace and Co., 1931.

Reader's Digest Editors. *Magic and Medicine of Plants*. Pleasantville, NY: Reader's Digest Association, 1986.

Simon, James E., Alena F. Chadwick and Lyle F. Craker. *Herbs: An Indexed Bibliography, 1971-1980: The Scientific Literature on Selected Herbs, and Aromatic and Medicinal Plants of the Temperate Zone*. Hamden, CT.: Archon Books, 1984.

PERIODICALS

Tuckler, V., et al. "Seizure in an Infant from Aniseed Oil Toxicity." *Clinical Toxicology* (August 2002): 689.

OTHER

Herb Society of America. http://www.herbsociety.org/fact sheets/anise.pdf/ (July 12, 2000).

One Planet. http://www.oneplanetnatural.com/anise.htm/ (July 12, 2000).

"*Pimpinella anisum*." http://webmd.lycos.com/content/ article/1677.57580/ (July 12, 2000).

"Herbs." Department of Horticulture, Pennsylvania State University. http://garden.cas.psu.edu/vegcrops/herbs/ Pimpinellaanisum.html/ (July 12, 2000).

Melissa C. McDade
Teresa G. Odle

Ankylosing spondylitis

Definition

Ankylosing spondylitis (AS) is a systemic disorder that involves inflammation of the joints in the spine. AS is the primary disease in a group of conditions known as *seronegative spondylarthropathies*. It is also known as rheumatoid spondylitis or Marie-Strümpell disease (among other names). AS is an autoimmune disease, as are most forms of arthritis. By definition, other joints, in addition to the spine, can be affected, including the shoulders, hips, knees, and feet. Tissues in the eye can also be affected.

Description

A form of arthritis, AS is characterized by chronic inflammation, causing **pain** and stiffness of the back, progressing to the chest and neck. Eventually, the whole back may become curved and inflexible if the bones fuse, which is known as "bamboo spine." Other conditions associated with AS include reactive arthritis, psoriatic arthritis, spondylitis of **inflammatory bowel disease**, and undifferentiated spondyarthropathy. AS may involve multiple organs, such as the following:

- eye (causing an inflammation of the iris, or iritis)
- heart (causing aortic valve disease)

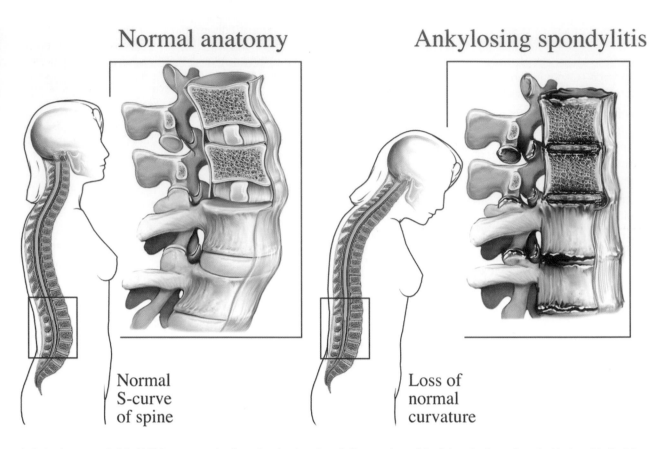

Normal anatomy

Normal
S-curve
of spine

Ankylosing spondylitis

Loss of
normal
curvature

Ankylosing spondylitis (AS) is a systemic disorder that involves inflammation of the joints in the spine. *(© Nucleus Medical Art, Inc. / Alamy)*

- lungs
- skin (causing a scaly skin condition, or psoriasis)
- gastrointestinal tract (causing inflammation within the small intestine, called ileitis, or inflammation of the large intestine, called colitis)

Less than 1% of the population has AS; however, 20% of people with AS have a relative with the disorder.

Causes and symptoms

Genetics, in the form of a gene named HLA-B27, can play an important role in the disease, but the precise cause of AS remains unknown. According to information from the Spondylitis Association of America, HLA-B27 is a perfectly normal gene found in 8% of the general population. Generally speaking, no more than 2% of people born with this gene will eventually get spondylitis. The gene itself does not cause spondylitis, but people with HLA-B27 are more susceptible to getting spondylitis. As of 2008, 31 alleles (subtypes) of HLA-B27 had been identified. They are designated as HLA-B*2701 to HLA-B*2727.

The most common subtypes in the United States are B*2705 and B*2702. The frequency of various HLA-B27 alleles among populations in various parts of the world differs dramatically. For example, the frequency of allele *2704 varies from 80–100% in most of East Asia, but the allele is virtually absent from Europe and Africa. The way in which HLA-B27 interacts with certain other proteins seems to be very important in the genesis of AS, but further research is necessary to determine exactly how this process takes place.

Symptoms of AS include the following:

- low back and hip pain and stiffness
- duration of symptoms longer than three months
- difficulty expanding the chest
- early morning stiffness improved by a warm shower or light exercise
- pain in the neck, shoulders, knees, and ankles
- low-grade fever
- fatigue
- weight loss

AS occurs most often in males between 16 and 35 years of age. Initial symptoms are uncommon after the age of 30, although the diagnosis may not be established until after that age. The incidence of AS in African Americans is about half that among Caucasians.

Some naturopathic healers link the cause of AS to its autoimmune origins in food **allergies** and abnormal bowel function, sometimes referred to as leaky gut syndrome. According to this theory, food allergies combine with the leaky gut and cause increased circulation of gut-derived antigens into other areas of the body. In response to this condition, the body produces antibody-antigen complexes characteristic of **rheumatoid arthritis** to battle these gut-derived foreign antigens, producing the symptoms of AS.

Diagnosis

Doctors usually diagnose ankylosing spondylitis disease simply by observable symptoms of pain and stiffness. Doctors also review spinal and pelvic x rays since involvement of the hip and pelvic joints is common and may be the first abnormality seen on the x ray. Doctors might also order a blood test to determine the presence of HLA-B27 antigen if the x rays have not clearly determined the diagnosis. If the gene is present, it could facilitate the accuracy of the possible AS diagnosis. When a diagnosis is made, patients may be referred to a rheumatologist, a doctor who specializes in treating arthritis. Patients may also be referred to an orthopedic surgeon, a doctor who can surgically correct joint or bone disorders.

Treatment

To reduce inflammation, various herbal remedies, including **white willow** (*Salix alba*), **yarrow** (*Achillea millefolium*), and **lobelia** (*Lobelia inflata*), may be helpful. **Acupuncture**, performed by a trained professional, has helped some patients manage their pain. Homeopathic practitioners may prescribe such remedies as *Bryonia* and *Rhus toxicodendron* for pain relief.

A key alternative treatment for AS is **massage therapy**. Reported benefits include a decrease in pain, increase in circulation, lymph flow improvement, and increase in range of motion. The major benefit of this therapy could be that it provides further motivation for a regular **exercise** program, considered the most beneficial of all treatments for AS.

Diets of various regimens have been offered that include supplements of fatty acids and **antioxidants**, as with other arthritis diets. Naturopaths and some medical doctors have theorized that certain foods should be eliminated from the diet in order to alleviate symptoms. Possible problem foods include wheat, corn, milk and other dairy products, beef, tomatoes, potatoes, and peppers. Tobacco has also been thought to aggravate the condition. Various reports have indicated that a diet high in fiber and fresh fruits and vegetables—minus those listed above—and low in sugar, meat, refined carbohydrates, and animal fats might help in the treatment of the symptoms of AS, particularly with pain or swelling.

Allopathic treatment

Nonsteroidal anti-inflammatory drugs (NSAIDs), such as naproxen (Naprosyn) or indomethacin (Indocin) are used to relieve pain and stiffness. In severe cases, sulfasalazine (Azulfidine), another drug to reduce inflammation, or methotrexate (Rheumatrex), an immune-suppressing drug, are recommended. In cases in which chronic therapy is needed, potential drug side effects must be taken into consideration. Corticosteroid drugs are effective in relieving symptoms but are usually reserved for severe cases that do not improve when NSAIDs are used. To avoid potential side effects, treatment with corticosteroids is usually limited to a short amount of time with a gradual weaning from the drug.

Two other drugs for use with AS work by a somewhat different mechanism than do NSAIDs and corticosteroids. Infliximab (Remicade) is a chimeric (made from both human and mouse components) monoclonal antibody that interferes with the inflammatory response characteristic of the disease. Etanercept (Enbrel) is a recombinant human soluble tumor necrosis factor-alpha (TNFa) receptor fusion protein that functions in a manner similar to that of infliximab, reducing inflammation caused by autoimmune responses in the body. Another TNF blocker, adalimumab (Humira), was approved by the FDA in August 2006 to be used for AS.

Physical therapists prescribe exercises to prevent a stooped posture and breathing problems when the spine starts to fuse and ribs are affected. Back braces may be used to prevent continued deformity of the spine and ribs. Only in severe cases of deformity is surgery performed to straighten and realign the spine or to replace knee, shoulder, or hip joints. Because it is a major and complicated procedure, with a potential for complications, this surgery is recommended cautiously even in severe cases.

Expected results

There is no cure for AS, and the course of the disease is unpredictable. Generally, AS progresses for about 10 years, then levels off. Most patients can lead normal lives with treatment to control symptoms. Claims that homeopathic remedies have cured them had not been verified as of 2008.

Prevention

There is no known way to prevent AS. With advances in gene therapy, the possibility exists for further determination of the factor that HLA-B27 gene plays in its manifestation and what role it could play in preventing it for future generations.

Resources

BOOKS

Parker, Philip M. *Ankylosing Spondylitis: A Bibliography and Dictionary for Physicians, Patients, and Genome Researchers.* San Diego: ICON Group International, 2007.

Van Royen, Barend J., and Ben A. C. Dijkmans, eds. *Ankylosing Spondylitis: Diagnosis and Management.* London: Informa Healthcare, 2006.

Weisman, Michael H., John D. Reveille, and Desiree van der Heijde. *Ankylosing Spondylitis and the Spondyloarthropathies.* St. Louis, MO: Mosby/Elsevier, 2006.

PERIODICALS

Cakar, Engin, et al. "Sexual Problems in Male Ankylosing Spondylitis Patients: Relationship with Functionality, Disease Activity, Quality of Life, and Emotional Status." *Clinical Rheumatology* (October 2007): 1607–1613.

Hoy, Sheridan, and Lesley J. Scott. "Etanercept: A Review of Its Use in the Management of Ankylosing Spondylitis and Psoriatic Arthritis." *Drugs* 67, no. 17 (2007): 2609–2633.

Konttinen, Liisa, et al. "Anti-TNF Therapy in the Treatment of Ankylosing Spondylitis: The Finnish Experience." *Clinical Rheumatology* (October 2007): 1693–1700.

Royen, Barend, et al. "ASKyphoplan: A Program for Deformity Planning in Ankylosing Spondylitis." *European Spine Journal* (September 2007): 1445–1449.

OTHER

"Ankylosing Spondylitis." Merck. http://www.merck.com/mmhe/sec05/ch067/ch067e.html. (February 10, 2008).

Peh, Wilfred C. G. "Ankylosing Spondylitis." *eMedicine.* http://www.emedicine.com/RADIO/topic41.htm. (February 10, 2008).

ORGANIZATIONS

Arthritis Foundation, PO. Box 7669, Atlanta, GA, 30357-0669, (800) 283-7800, http://www.arthritis.org.

National Institute of Arthritis and Musculoskeletal and Skin Diseases, Information Office, Bldg. 31, Room 4C-02, 31 Center Drive, MSC 2350, Bethesda, MD, 20892-2350, (301) 496-8190, www.niams.nih.gov/.

Spondylitis Association of America, PO Box 5872, Sherman Oaks, CA, 91413, (800) 777-8189, http://www.spondylitis.org/.

Jane Spear
Teresa G. Odle
David Edward Newton, Ed.D.

Anorexia nervosa

Definition

Anorexia nervosa is an eating disorder characterized by unrealistic fear of weight gain, self-starvation, and conspicuous distortion of body image. The name comes from two Latin words that together mean "nervous inability to eat." The disorder is sometimes referred to simply as anorexia. In females who have begun to menstruate, anorexia nervosa is usually marked by **amenorrhea**, or missing at least three menstrual periods in a row. The fourth edition of the *Diagnostic and Statistical Manual of Mental Disorders* (*DSM-IV*, 1994) defines two subtypes of anorexia nervosa: a restricting type, characterized by strict dieting and **exercise** without binge eating, and a binge-eating/purging type, marked by episodes of compulsive eating with or without self-induced **vomiting** and the use of laxatives or enemas. *DSM-IV* defines a binge as a time-limited (usually under two hours) episode of compulsive eating in which the individual

Symptoms of anorexia nervosa

Resistance to maintaining body weight at or above a minimally normal weight for age and height

Intense fear of gaining weight or becoming fat, even though underweight

Disturbance in the way in which one's body weight or shape is experienced, undue influence of body weight or shape on self-evaluation, or denial of the seriousness of the current low body weight

Infrequent or absent menstrual periods (in females who have reached puberty)

(Illustration by Corey Light. Cengage Learning, Gale)

consumes a significantly larger amount of food than most people would eat in similar circumstances.

Description

Anorexia nervosa was not officially classified as a psychiatric disorder until the third edition of *DSM* in 1980. It is, however, a growing problem among adolescent females and its incidence in the United States has doubled since 1970. The rise in the number of reported cases reflects a genuine increase in the number of persons affected by the disorder, not simply earlier or more accurate diagnosis. Estimates of the incidence of anorexia range between 0.5–1% of Caucasian female adolescents. Over 90% of patients diagnosed with the disorder as of 1998 were female. It was originally thought that only 5% of anorexics are male, but that estimate was being revised upward as of 2008. The peak age range for onset of the disorder is 14–18 years, although there are patients who develop anorexia as late as their 40s. In the 1970s and 1980s, anorexia was regarded as a disorder of upper- and middle-class women, but that generalization also changed. Subsequent studies indicated that anorexia is increasingly common among women of all races and social classes in the United States.

Anorexia nervosa is a serious public health problem not only because of its rising incidence, but also because it has one of the highest mortality rates of any psychiatric disorder. Moreover, the disorder may cause serious long-term health complications, including congestive heart failure, sudden death, growth retardation, dental problems, **constipation**, stomach rupture, swelling of the salivary glands, loss of kidney function, **osteoporosis**, **anemia**, and other abnormalities of the blood.

Causes and symptoms

Anorexia is a disorder that results from the interaction of cultural and interpersonal as well as biological factors. While the precise cause of the disease is not known, it has been linked to the following factors.

Social influences

The rising incidence of anorexia is thought to reflect the idealization of thinness as a badge of upper-class status as well as of female beauty. In addition, the increase in cases of anorexia includes so-called copycat behavior, with some patients developing the disorder from imitating other girls.

The onset of anorexia in adolescence is attributed to a developmental crisis caused by girls' changing bodies coupled with cultural overemphasis on women's appearance. The increasing influence of the mass media in spreading and reinforcing gender stereotypes has also been noted.

Occupational goals

The risk of developing anorexia is higher among adolescents preparing for careers that require attention to weight and/or appearance. These high-risk groups include dancers, fashion models, professional athletes (including gymnasts, skaters, long-distance runners, and jockeys), and actresses.

Genetic and biological influences

Women whose biological mothers or sisters have the disorder appear to be at increased risk.

Psychological factors

A number of theories have been advanced to explain the psychological aspects of the disorder. No single explanation covers all cases. Anorexia nervosa has been interpreted as connected to the following:

- A rejection of female sexual maturity. This rejection is variously interpreted as a desire to remain a child or as a desire to resemble men as closely as possible.
- A reaction to sexual abuse or assault.
- A desire to appear as fragile and non-threatening as possible. This hypothesis reflects the idea that female passivity and weakness are attractive to men.

- Overemphasis on control, autonomy, and independence. Some anorexics come from achievement-oriented families that stress physical fitness and dieting. Many anorexics are perfectionists and obsessive about schoolwork and other matters in addition to weight control.
- Evidence of family dysfunction. In some families, a daughter's eating disorder serves as a distraction from marital discord or other family tensions.
- Inability to interpret the body's hunger signals accurately due to early experiences of inappropriate feeding.

Male anorexics

Although anorexia nervosa is still considered a disorder that affects women primarily, its incidence in the male population is rising. Less is known about the causes of anorexia in males, but some risk factors are the same as for females. These factors include certain occupational goals and increasing media emphasis on appearance in men.

Diagnosis

Diagnosis of anorexia nervosa is complicated by a number of factors. One is that the disorder varies somewhat in severity from patient to patient. A second factor is denial, which is regarded as an early sign of the disorder. Most anorexics deny that they are ill and are usually brought to treatment by a family member.

Anorexia is usually diagnosed by pediatricians or family practitioners. Anorexics develop emaciated bodies, dry or yellowish skin, and abnormally low blood pressure. There is usually a history of amenorrhea (failure to menstruate) in females and sometimes of abdominal **pain**, constipation, or lack of energy. The patient may feel chilly or have developed lanugo, a growth of downy body hair. If the patient has been vomiting, she may have eroded tooth enamel or Russell's sign (scars on the back of the hand). The second step in diagnosis is measurement of the patient's weight loss. *DSM-IV* specifies a weight loss tending toward a body weight 15% below normal, with some allowance for body build and weight history.

The doctor rules out other physical conditions that can cause weight loss or vomiting after eating, including metabolic disorders, brain tumors (especially hypothalamus and pituitary gland lesions), diseases of the digestive tract, and a condition called superior mesenteric artery syndrome. Persons with this condition sometimes vomit after meals because the blood supply to the intestine is blocked. The doctor usually orders blood tests, an electrocardiogram, urinalysis, and bone densitometry (bone density test) in order to exclude other diseases and to assess the patient's nutritional status.

The doctor also needs to distinguish between anorexia and other psychiatric disorders, including **depression**, **schizophrenia**, social phobia, **obsessive-compulsive disorder**, and body dysmorphic disorder. Two diagnostic tests that are often used are the Eating Attitudes Test (EAT) and the Eating Disorder Inventory (EDI).

Treatment

Alternative treatments should serve as complementary to a conventional treatment program. Alternative therapies for anorexia nervosa include diet and **nutrition**, herbal therapy, **hydrotherapy**, **aromatherapy**, Ayurveda, and **mind/body medicine**.

Nutritional therapy

A naturopath or nutritionist may recommend the following:

- Avoiding sweets or baked goods.
- Following a nutritious and well-balanced diet (when patients resume eating normally).
- Daily multivitamin and mineral supplements.
- Zinc supplements. Zinc is an important mineral needed by the body for normal hormonal activity and enzymatic function.

Herbal therapy

The following herbs may help reduce **anxiety** and depression which are often associated with this disorder:

- chamomile (*Matricaria recutita*)
- lemon balm (*Melissa officinalis*)
- linden (*Tilia* spp.) flowers

Aromatherapy

Essential oils of herbs such as bergamot, basil, **chamomile**, clary **sage**, and **lavender** may help stimulate appetite, relax the body, and fight depression. They can be diffused into the air, inhaled, massaged, or put in bath water.

Relaxation techniques

Relaxation techniques such as **yoga**, **meditation**, and **t'ai chi** can relax the body and release **stress**, anxiety and depression.

Hypnotherapy

Hypnotherapy may help resolve unconscious issues that contribute to anorexic behavior.

Other alternative treatments

Other alternative treatments that may be helpful include hydrotherapy, magnetic field therapy, **acupuncture**, **biofeedback**, Ayurveda and Chinese herbal medicine.

Allopathic treatment

Treatment of anorexia nervosa includes both short-term and long-term measures and requires assessment by dietitians and psychiatrists as well as medical specialists. Therapy is often complicated by the patient's resistance or failure to carry out treatment plan.

Hospital treatment

Hospitalization is recommended for anorexics with any of the following characteristics:

- weight of 40% or more below normal or weight loss over a three-month period of more than 30 pounds
- severely disturbed metabolism
- severe binging and purging
- signs of psychosis
- severe depression or risk of suicide
- family in crisis

Hospital treatment includes individual and group therapy as well as refeeding and monitoring of the patient's physical condition. Treatment usually requires two to four months in the hospital. In extreme cases, hospitalized patients may be force-fed through a tube inserted in the nose (nasogastric tube) or by over-feeding (hyperalimentation techniques).

Outpatient treatment

Anorexics who are not severely malnourished can be treated by outpatient **psychotherapy**. The types of treatment recommended are supportive rather than insight-oriented and include behavioral approaches as well as individual or group therapy. Family therapy is often recommended when the patient's eating disorder is closely tied to family dysfunction. Self-help groups are often useful in helping anorexics find social support and encouragement. Psychotherapy with anorexics is a slow and difficult process; about 50% of patients continue to have serious psychiatric problems after their weight has stabilized.

KEY TERMS

Amenorrhea—Absence of menstruation in a female who has begun to have menstrual periods.

Binge eating—A pattern of eating marked by episodes of rapid consumption of large amounts of food, usually food that is high in calories.

Body dysmorphic disorder—A psychiatric disorder marked by preoccupation with an imagined physical defect.

Hyperalimentation—A method of refeeding anorexics by infusing liquid nutrients and electrolytes directly into central veins through a catheter.

Lanugo—A soft, downy body hair that develops on the chest and arms of anorexic women.

Purging—The use of vomiting, diuretics, or laxatives to clear the stomach and intestines after a binge.

Russell's sign—Scraped or raw areas on the patient's knuckles, caused by self-induced vomiting.

Superior mesenteric artery syndrome—A condition in which a person vomits after meals due to blockage of the blood supply to the intestine.

Medications

Anorexics have been treated with a variety of medications, including antidepressants, anti-anxiety drugs, selective serotonin reuptake inhibitors, and lithium carbonate. The effectiveness of medications in treatment regimens continues to be debated. However, at least one study showed that the antidepressant Prozac helped the patient maintain weight gained while in the hospital.

Expected results

Figures for long-term recovery vary from study to study, but the most reliable estimates are that 40–60% of anorexics make a good physical and social recovery, and 75% gain weight. The long-term mortality rate for anorexia is estimated at around 10%, although some studies give a lower figure of 3–4%. The most frequent causes of death associated with anorexia are starvation, electrolyte imbalance, heart failure, and suicide.

Prevention

Short of major long-term changes in the larger society, the best strategy for prevention of anorexia is the cultivation of healthy attitudes toward food, weight control, and beauty or body image within families.

Resources

BOOKS

Buckroyd, Julia, and Sharon Rother, eds. *Psychological Responses to Eating Disorders and Obesity: Recent and Innovative Work*. New York: Wiley-Interscience, 2008.

Dosil, Joaquin. *Eating Disorders in Athletes*. New York: Wiley-Interscience, 2008.

Lucas, Alexander R. *Demystifying Anorexia Nervosa: An Optimistic Guide to Understanding and Healing*. New York: Oxford University Press, 2008.

Schulherr, Susan. *Eating Disorders for Dummies*. Indianapolis, IN: For Dummies, 2008.

PERIODICALS

Barabasz, Marianne. "Efficacy of Hypnotherapy in the Treatment of Eating Disorders." *International Journal of Clinical and Experimental Hypnosis* (July 2007): 318–335.

Fedyszyn, Izabela Ewa, and Gavin Brent Sullivan. "Ethical Re-evaluation of Contemporary Treatments for Anorexia Nervosa: Is an Aspirational Stance Possible in Practice?" *Australian Psychologist* (September 2007): 198–211.

Maguire, Sarah, et al. "Staging Anorexia Nervosa: Conceptualizing Illness Severity." *Early Intervention in Psychiatry* (February 2008): 3–10.

Nilsson, Karin, et al. "Causes of Adolescent Onset Anorexia Nervosa: Patient Perspectives." *Eating Disorders* (March 2007): 125–133.

OTHER

"Anorexia Nervosa." *MedicineNet.com*. http://www.medicine net.com/anorexia_nervosa/article.htm. (February 10, 2008).

"Anorexia Nervosa." *womenshealth.gov*. http://www.4wo men.gov/faq/easyread/anorexia-etr.htm. (February 10, 2008).

Levey, Robert. "Anorexia Nervosa." *eMedicine*. http://www. emedicine.com/med/topic144.htm. (February 10, 2008).

ORGANIZATIONS

National Association of Anorexia Nervosa and Associated Disorders, PO Box 7, Highland Park, IL, 60035, (847) 433-3996, http://www.anad.org/.

National Eating Disorders Association, 603 Stewart St., Suite 803, Seattle, WA, 98101, (800) 931-2237, http:// www.nationaleatingdisorders.org/.

Mai Tran
David Edward Newton, Ed.D.

Anthroposophical medicine

Definition

Anthroposophical medicine (AM), or anthroposophically extended medicine, is a system of healing based on the spiritual science that was developed by Rudolph Steiner.

Origins

Rudolph Steiner (1861-1925) was an Austrian philosopher and teacher who founded anthroposophy (*anthropos* meaning human and *sophy* meaning wisdom), which is a worldwide spiritual movement that seeks to apply a scientific approach to spiritual perception. Steiner believed that everyone has spiritual powers that can be activated by exercises in mental concentration and **meditation**. During his lifetime, he was an active teacher, attracting many followers to his spiritual ideas. Steiner founded several schools, wrote nearly 30 books, and gave more than 6,000 lectures around the world on subjects including education, medicine, agriculture, social issues, science and art. His ideas have remained influential. The Waldorf school system, which he began, educates thousands of young people each year. Many health food stores carry products produced by Steiner's system of agriculture called biodynamic farming, which considers the health and purity of the soil, water, and air to be of central importance.

Anthroposophical medicine is based on Steiner's concept that spiritual awareness is the foundation of individual health and of the health of society. Steiner believed that many of the oldest systems of healing, such as **traditional Chinese medicine**, **Ayurvedic medicine**, and **Tibetan medicine**, were based on a spiritual perception of the world that modern science has lost. Steiner wanted medicine to get back in touch with **spirituality**, and at the same time keep and use wisely the gains that science and technology have made. Thus, conventional medicine needed to be extended beyond physical science to include a holistic spiritual science.

Steiner formally began application of his philosophy in a series of 20 lectures in the early spring of 1920 to the medical community of a town in Switzerland. It was the first such course for physicians and medical students. He and Dutch medical doctor Ita Wegman co-authored a foundational work for physicians wanting to expand their practice according to anthroposophic principles.

Anthroposophical medicine is still in its early stages. Steiner believed that it would take many years for his medical ideas to be fully applied. There are thousands of anthroposophical doctors and researchers practicing in Europe, where the main school was founded. In America, practitioners can be found in several large cities, but the overall number of anthroposophical physicians is very small.

Benefits

Anthroposophical medicine can be used to treat any health condition. It is particularly recommended for preventive care, **infections**, inflammatory conditions such as arthritis, and the treatment of **cancer** and chronic degenerative diseases associated with **aging**. It is also recommended for pediatric (child) care, with its avoidance of toxic drugs, and is beneficial for children's conditions such as **attention-deficit hyperactivity disorder** (ADHD) and developmental problems.

Description

The anthroposophical concept of the body

Anthroposophical physicians have a different view of the body and health than the conventional scientific model. Human beings are made up of four levels (four-foldness) of being. The first level is the physical body. The second level is the life or *etheric* body, which corresponds to the Chinese idea of *chi* and the Ayurvedic idea of *prana*. The third level is the soul, or astral body, and the fourth level is the spirit. AM doctors believe that all levels of being influence a patient's health.

The physical body is made up of a three-fold system, including the "sense-nerve" system, which comprises the head and nervous system, supporting the mind and the thinking process. Second is the "metabolic-limb" system, which includes the digestive system for elimination, energetic metabolism, and voluntary movement processes, all supporting aspects of human behavior that express the will. Finally, the rhythmic system, which includes the heart and lungs in the chest, is responsible for balancing the head and digestive systems. According to AM, these systems tend to oppose each other in functioning and characteristics, similar to the Chinese concept of yin and yang. For instance, the digestive system is associated with heat and helps to dissolve elements in the body, while the head system is associated with cooling and helps in the formation of elements in the body. Illness is caused when the systems of the body become out of balance. AM involves a broad understanding of the three bodily systems, and the illnesses associated with each system and its imbalance. This model provides practitioners a means for therapeutic insight now recognized as mind-body relationships in health and disease.

In AM, illness is considered a significant event in a person's life, and not just a chance occurrence. One role of the doctor is to understand, and help the patient understand, the significance of the illness on all levels of being. Conventional medicine tends to suppress illness, using drugs to block the symptoms. AM doctors believe that true healing must first bring an illness out in order to heal it, and that healing requires change and development in the patient on several levels.

AM also asserts, as did the early healer Paracelsus, that every illness has a cure that can be found in nature. Paracelsus is the pseudonym for a Swiss-born alchemist and physician who lived from 1493-1541. Nature and the human body are made up of the plant, animal, and mineral kingdoms, and thus AM doctors use medicines that are made from plants, animals (usually in the form of organ extracts), and minerals. AM remedies are usually given in homeopathic doses, which are very diluted, non-toxic solutions.

Treatment by an anthroposophical physician

All anthroposophical physicians are conventionally trained M.D.s, as Steiner believed that conventional training was a necessary first step. However, a visit to an anthroposophical physician may be different than a visit to a regular doctor. Anthroposophical doctors tend to spend much more time with their patients, particularly during the initial visit. Every patient is considered unique, and AM doctors use the first visit to get a broad understanding of patients and their medical histories. To diagnose illnesses, AM doctors may use modern diagnostic tools, but also rely on intuition and an understanding of the patient. Part of training of AM doctors involves improving their powers of perception in order to understand illnesses. Diagnosis is considered a very important process; Steiner believed that if the diagnosis of a problem is done correctly, then the therapeutic (healing) work is much easier. After a problem is thoroughly diagnosed, treatment will be recommended. AM doctors attempt to treat a patient on all four levels of being. For the physical body, remedies will be prescribed. There are hundreds of uniquely formulated medications, similar to homeopathies, as well as botanical medicines. AM doctors try to minimize the use of antibiotics, drugs, and vaccinations.

Anthroposophical medicine also uses allied therapies, which are additional therapies that Steiner recommended to heal patients on other levels than the physical. These include **massage therapy** and a **movement therapy** called *eurythmy*. Eurythmy is a system of movements designed to help patients give expression to inner spiritual movements. **Psychotherapy** may also be recommended to help heal some conditions. AM doctors may apply allied therapies themselves, or refer patients to other healers. The length of treatment with AM depends on the patient and condition. The cost of treatment varies with the practitioner, and is comparable to treatment by conventional M.D.s. AM medications are less expensive than conventional drugs. Because AM practitioners are trained medical doctors, insurance policies often cover their fees, although consumers should be aware of their policy restrictions.

Preparations

AM doctors may give new patients packages of materials before treatment, which include thorough questionnaires and explanations of AM. Anthroposophical physicians encourage patients to prepare for treatment by becoming willing to take responsibility for their condition and health, and to change their behaviors and lifestyles in the interest of healing.

Side effects

AM medications are safe and non-toxic. During treatment, some patients may experience what doctors call "healing crises." During these, patients may temporarily experience a worsening of symptoms as part of the healing process, including **fever**, headaches, **nausea**, weakness, muscle soreness, and other symptoms.

Research and general acceptance

Active research in AM is being regularly conducted in Europe, mainly in Germany, Holland, Switzerland, and France. Several research organizations performing patient-centered research have shown promising results with the AM cure for cancer, which utilizes the herbal remedy **mistletoe** extract, and for other conditions. Other research has shown that AM is less expensive than conventional medical treatment, with 50% fewer illness days than when treated by conventional practitioners. Current research studies appear in the quarterly *Journal of Anthroposophical Medicine*, as well as in European publications.

Training and certification

Currently, there is no course for the certification of AM practitioners, although every AM doctor is required to obtain training as a certified M.D. Afterwards, physicians may specialize in AM by taking a series of courses or by interning with specialists. The Physicians Association for Anthroposophic Medicine (PAAM) is the largest association in North America. The organization for non-M.D. health professionals interested in anthroposophical medicine is *Artemesia, The Association for Anthroposophical Renewal of Healing*.

Resources

BOOKS

Bott, Victor. *Anthroposophical Medicine*. Hudson, New York: Anthroposophic Press, 1985.

Steiner, Rudolph. *Introducing Anthroposophic Medicine*. Hudson, New York: Anthroposophical Press, 1998.

ORGANIZATIONS

Anthroposophic Press (Steiner Books), P.O. Box 749, Great Barrington, MA, 01230, (413) 528-8233, www.steiner books.org.

Artemesia, The Association for Anthroposophical Renewal of Healing, 1923 Geddes Avenue, Ann Arbor, MI, 48104, (734) 930-9462

Gilpin Street Holistic Center. Dr. Philip Incao, M.D, 1624 Gilpin Street, Denver, CO, 80218, (303) 321-2100

Physicians Association for Anthroposophic Medicine (PAAM), 1923 Geddes Avenue, Ann Arbor, MI, 48104, (734) 930-9462

Douglas Dupler

Anti-inflammatory diets

Definition

There is no one anti-inflammatory diet, rather, there are **diets** designed around foods believed to decrease inflammation and that shun foods that aggravate the inflammatory processes. Many anti-inflammatory diets are based around whole grains, legumes, nuts, seeds, fresh vegetables and fruits, wild fish and seafood, grass-fed lean turkey and chicken which are thought to aid in the bodies healing of inflammation. They exclude foods that are thought to trigger inflammation such as refined grains, wheat, corn, full-fat dairy, red meat, **caffeine**, alcohol, peanuts, sugar, saturated and trans-saturated fats.

The common foundation of anti-inflammatory diets is the belief that low grades of inflammation are the precursor and/or antagonizer to many chronic diseases. Once removed, the body can begin healing itself.

Origins

The philosophical genesis of anti-inflammatory diets dates back to the original healers throughout history who have worked with foods, herbs, teas and other natural remedies to assist the body's own healing energy.

Beginning in the 1970s investigators began exploring physiological mechanisms of **fever**, weight loss, and acute phase responses to acute and chronic infection. Research results from these studies began to change the mainstream attitudes about disease pathogenesis. Accumulating evidence linked proteins, produced by macrophages and other immune cells, not pathogens, as formerly believed, to the cause of tissue damage and disease syndromes in experimental animals. Thus, the medical profession began looking into original treatments for chronic diseases. Then in the 1980s, research showed that proteins, newly named cytokines, and hormone-like substances, named prostaglandins and leukotrienes, revealed that they possessed pleiotropic biological activities that were either beneficial or injurious to the bodies' tissues.

From this research emerged the cytokine theory of disease; the concept that cytokines produced by the immune system can cause the signs, symptoms, and damaging after effects of chronic diseases. Change did not occur until the measurement of C-reactive protein (CRP), a marker of inflammation circulating in the blood, was proposed as a method to identify persons at risk of chronic diseases. As pioneering research began to show that higher levels of C-reactive protein was linked to **heart disease**, conventional thought among the medical profession began. Originally discovered by W. S. Tillett and T. Francis Jr. in 1930, C-reactive protein was discovered as a substance in the serum of patients diagnosed with acute inflammation that reacted with the C-polysaccharide of pneumoccocus.

A growing consensus among medical professionals is that inflammation is believed to play a role in the pathogenesis of chronic diseases such as heart disease, **stroke**, diabetes, and colon **cancer** to name a few. Mainstream thinking is beginning to accept that treating the underlying cause may ameliorate

---

KEY TERMS

Anti-oxidant—A chemical compound or substance that inhibits oxidation. A substance, such as vitamin E, vitamin C, or beta-carotene.

Chronic disease—An illness or medical condition that lasts over a long period of time and sometimes causes a long-term change in the body.

C-reactive protein (CRP)— A marker of inflammation circulating in the blood has been proposed as a method to identify persons at risk of these diseases.

Flavonoid—Refers to compounds found in fruits, vegetables, and certain beverages that have diverse beneficial biochemical and antioxidant effects.

Inflammation—Swelling, redness, heat, and pain produced in an area of the body as a reaction to injury or infection.

---

cardiovascular disease, metabolic syndrome, **hypertension**, diabetes, and hyperlipidemia, inflammation caused by visceral adipose tissue.

Description

Inflammation

Inflammation is a localized reaction of tissue to injury, whether caused by bacteria or viral infection, trauma, chemicals, heat or other phenomenon that causes irritation. The irritant causes the tissues within the body to release multiple substances that cause changes within the tissues. This complex response is called inflammation. Inflammation is characterized by such symptoms as (1) vasodilatation of the local blood vessels resulting in excess local blood flow, (2) increases in the permeability of the capillaries with leakage of large quantities of fluid into the interstitial spaces, (3) clotting of the fluid in the interstitial spaces due to excess amounts of fibrinogen and other proteins leaking from the capillaries, (4) relocation of granulocytes and monocytes into the tissue in large quantities, and (5) swelling of the tissue cells.

The common substances released from the tissues that result in inflammation are histamine, bradykinin, serotonin, prostaglandins, multiple hormonal substances called lymphokines that are released by sensitized T-cells and various other reaction products of other systems within the body. Many of these substances activate the macrophage system, which are sent out

---

to dispose of the damaged tissue but also which further injure the still-living tissue and cells.

Conditions with chronic inflammation

Inflammation has been associated as a component of, but not limited to, arthritis, heart disease, diabetes, strokes, **asthma**, **allergies**, irritable bowel disease, **Celiac disease** or other digestive system diseases, **obesity**, chronic **stress**, **sleep disorders** such as **sleep apnea**, Alzheimerís disease, high blood pressure, elevated lipids such as triglycerides and **cholesterol**.

Medical anti-inflammatory treatments

General anti-inflammatory medical treatments include **relaxation**, moderate **exercise** such as walking, weight maintenance or loss, and medications designed to reduce the inflammation and control the **pain** if present.

These medications may include: ibuprofen or aspirin, Non Steroidal Anti-Inflammatory Drugs (NSAIDs), or steroid medications. The NSAIDs are widely used as the initial form of therapy. Unfortunately, long-term use of these medications can irritate the stomach and lead to ulcers. In some cases they can lead to kidney, as well as other medical problems.

Function

Diet and chronic inflammation

Registered dietitians, and naturopathic physicians often prescribe diets to lessen the inflammatory symptoms of diseases. Although these diets have not been compared to other treatments in many formal research settings to date, it is thought that anti-inflammatory diets result in a reduced amount of inflammation and a healthier response by the immune system.

Adding foods that reduce inflammation is thought to improve symptoms of chronic diseases and help decrease risk for chronic diseases. These foods help in supplying the nutrients that are needed to decrease inflammation. One example is **omega-3 fatty acids**. The human body uses these fats to manufacture prostaglandins, chemicals that play an important role in inflammation and a healthy immune response. Another beneficial component of **fish oil** that plays an important role is eicosapentaenoic acid (EPA), an essential fatty acid derived from omega-3 fatty acids. EPA promotes the production of certain forms of prostaglandins having anti-inflammatory properties by reducing inflammation and decreasing the production of inflammatory substances.

Foods that reduce chronic inflammation

Whole grains

Whole grains or foods made from them, whether cracked, crushed, rolled, extruded, and/or cooked, contain the essential parts and nutrients of the entire grain seed. Research has shown that diets high in whole grain products are associated with decreased concentrations of inflammatory markers and increased adiponectin levels. The protective effects of a diet high in whole grains on systemic inflammation may be explained, in part, by reduction in overproduction of oxidative stress that results in inflammation.

A whole grain will include the following parts of the grain kernel–the bran, germ and endosperm. Such whole grains are amaranth, barley, bulgur, wild rice, millet, oats, quinoa, rye, spelt, wheat berries, buckwheat, and whole wheat.

Legumes

Diets high in legumes are inversely related to plasma concentrations of C-reactive protein (CRP). Among the many varieties of legumes are; pinto beans, lentils, kidney beans, borlotti beans, mung beans, soybeans, cannelloni beans, garbanzo or chickpeas, adzuki beans, fava beans, and black beans.

Nuts, seeds

Nuts and seeds are rich in unsaturated fat and other nutrients that may reduce inflammation. Frequent nut consumption is associated with lower levels of inflammatory markers. This may explain why there is a lower risk of cardiovascular disease and type 2 diabetes with frequent nut and seed consumption. With the exception of peanuts, be sure to add in walnuts, flax seeds and pumpkin seeds. Nuts and seeds are best eaten when unsalted and raw.

Fresh vegetables

Green leafy vegetables, and brightly colored vegetables provide beta-carotene; **vitamin C** and other **antioxidants** have been shown to reduce cell damage and to have anti-inflammatory effects. Aim for three or more servings per day.

Fresh fruits

Flavonoids found in fresh fruits among other substances are thought to increase the antioxidant effects of vitamin C. Research has shown that fruits have an anti-inflammatory effect. Aim for two or more servings daily. Be sure to include berries in your weekly choices of fruits such as blueberries, blackberries, and strawberries.

Wild fish and seafood

Oily fish such as herring, mackerel, salmon and trout are an excellent source of omega-3 fatty acids, as are shellfish such as mussels and clams. Including fish or seafood high in omega-3 fatty acids at least three times a week is recommended.

Lean poultry

Protein is used in the body to repair and manufacture cells, make antibodies, enzymes and hormones. Lean protein has been associated with lower levels of inflammatory biomarkers.

When choosing poultry, choose grass-fed animals, which tend to have a higher amount of **essential fatty acids**. Select poultry with limited amounts of, or free of, preservatives, **sodium**, nitrates or coloring. Also, in an ideal diet, only 10-12% of daily calories should come from protein. On average, an adult needs 0.36 grams of protein per pound of body weight.

Soy products

Anti-inflammatory properties of the isoflavones, a micronutrient component of soy, have been reported in several experimental models and disease conditions. Data suggests the possibility of beneficial effects of isoflavone-rich soy foods when added to the diet. Soy products include; soybeans, **edema** me, tofu, tempeh, soymilk, as well as many other products made from soybeans.

Oils

Expeller pressed Canola oil and Extra Virgin Olive oil are types of oils that have been linked to reduced inflammation. Other oils thought to aid in reducing inflammation include rice bran, grape seed, evening primrose and walnut oil. It is suggested to use these oils in moderation when cooking, baking and flavoring of foods. Also, when purchasing oils, make sure they are pure oils rather than blended oils. Blended oil usually contains less healthful oils.

Water in the form of fresh drinking water free of toxic chemicals

Water is an essential substance for every function of the body. It is a medium for chemical processes; a solvent for body wastes and dilutes their toxicity and aids in their excretion. Water aids in ingestion, absorption and transport of vital nutrients that have anti-inflammatory effects. Water is also needed for basic cell functioning, repairing of body tissues and is the base of all blood and fluid secretions.

Herbs and spices

A greater amount of research is emerging on the antioxidant properties of herbs and spices and their use in the management of chronic inflammation. Herbs and spices can be used in recipes to partially or wholly replace less desirable ingredients such as salt, sugar and added saturated fat, know for their inflammatory effects, thus reducing the damaging properties of these foods.

Precautions

Foods that irritate inflammation

Best referred to in research articles as "the western dietary pattern", it credits a diet that is high in refined grains, red meat, butter, processed meats, high-fat dairy, sweets and desserts, pizza, potato, eggs, hydrogenated fats, and soft drinks. This pattern of eating is positively related to an increase in circulating blood CRP levels and higher risks for chronic diseases, obesity and cancers. These foods, termed "pro-inflammatory" may increase inflammation, thus increasing a persons risk for chronic diseases as well as exacerbate symptoms from these chronic conditions.

There is some support for the belief that food sensitivities or allergens to foods may be a trigger for inflammation. Often hard to detect with common blood tests, some people have seen alleviation of symptoms of chronic diseases, such as arthritis, when the aggravating foods are removed from their diet. Common allergic foods are milk and dairy, wheat, corn, eggs, beef, yeast and soy.

Other pro-inflammatory foods have been shown to have substances that activate or support the inflammatory process. Unhealthy trans fats and saturated fats used in preparing and processing certain foods are linked to increased inflammation. Processed meats such as lunchmeats, hot dogs and sausages contain chemicals such as nitrites that are associated with increased inflammation and chronic disease.

Saturated fats naturally found in meats, dairy products and eggs contain fatty acids called arachidonic acid. While some arachidonic acid is essential for health, excess arachidonic acid in the diet has been shown to worsen inflammation.

Research supports that diets high in sugar produce acute oxidative stress within the cells, associating it with inflammation. Elimination of high sugar foods such as sodas, soft drinks, pastries, presweetened cereals and candy has been shown to be beneficial. As well as switching from refined grains to whole grains.

Benefits

The effects of the anti-inflammatory diet are unobtrusive. There is a series of research articles that demonstrate a benefit in reduction of chronic diseases such as cardiovascular disease, neurodegenerative diseases, and cancers when following a dietary pattern associated with the anti-inflammatory diet. But the benefits go beyond disease prevention. Studies have shown an alleviation of symptoms associated with chronic diseases. As well, a person may decrease or discontinue their dosage of medications prescribed to control symptoms related to inflammatory conditions, and reduce the side affects associated with anti-inflammatory agents.

It has also been documented that people who followed the anti-inflammatory diet stated they experienced loss of weight, had an elevation of energy, and reported better mental and emotional health.

Risks

The risks associated with following the anti-inflammatory diet are limited and not supported by research. The general concern associated with following any diet without the consent of a primary physician would apply. Anyone attempting to follow the anti-inflammatory diet should discuss it with their primary care physician and get a referral to see a registered dietitian, educated in the diet for maximal benefit and decreased risk of following a diet that eliminates certain foods from the dietary pattern to ensure proper intake of all macro- and micronutrients.

Research and general acceptance

There is no one anti-inflammatory diet but rather there are foods that are thought to increase the inflammatory process and ones that are beneficial to the inflammatory processed within the body. Because of this, many medical professionals and other health providers may not support the concept of a diet that decreases the anti-inflammatory response within the body.

There is substantial evidence supported through research that shows the beneficial effects on the body in reducing markers of inflammation such as CPH and reduction in chronic disease and its symptoms. Most medical professionals have an easier time accepting the **Mediterranean diet,** which includes many of the foods found in the anti-inflammatory diet, and is the closest termed dietary eating pattern to the anti-inflammatory diet.

Megan C.M. Porter, RD, LD

Antioxidants

Description

Antioxidants are a broad group of compounds that destroy single oxygen molecules, also called free radicals, in the body, thereby protecting against oxidative damage to cells. They are essential to good health and are found naturally in a wide variety of foods and plants, including many fruits and vegetables. Many antioxidants, either singly or in combination, are also available as over-the-counter nutritional supplements in tablet or capsule form. The most commonly used antioxidants are **vitamin C**, **vitamin E**, and **beta carotene**. Others include **grape seed extract**, **vitamin A**, **selenium**, and coenzyme Q10. It is unknown whether supplemental antioxidants provide the same benefits as those occurring naturally in foods.

General use

In brief, antioxidants destroy free radicals in the body. Free radicals are byproducts of oxygen metabolism that can damage cells and are among the causes of many degenerative diseases, especially diseases associated with **aging**. They are also associated with the aging process itself. As a person ages, cell damage accumulates, and supplementing the diet with extra antioxidant-rich foods can help slow the oxidative damage done to cells. Scientific studies validate the role of antioxidants in preventing many diseases. Although studies have shown lower rates of **cancer** and **heart disease** in people who eat a recommended amount of fruits and vegetables, recent clinical studies have shown that supplementation of diet with antioxidant vitamin therapy does not lower risk of cardiovascular disease or certain other diseases.

Many herbs and medicinal plants are good natural sources of antioxidants. These include carrots, tomatoes, yams, leafy greens, blueberries, blackberries, cherries, **ginkgo biloba**, **garlic**, and **green tea**, to name a few. A diet rich in vitamin C, vitamin E, and

Health benefits of antioxidants and their food sources

Antioxidant	Health benefits	Food sources
Selenium	Helps maintain healthy hair and nails, enhances immunity, works with vitamin E to protect cells from damage. Reduces the risk of cancer, particularly lung, prostate, and colorectal.	Garlic, seeds, Brazil nuts, meat, eggs, poultry, seafood, whole grains. The amount in plant sources varies according to the content of the soil.
Beta-carotene	Keeps skin healthy, helps prevent night blindness and infections, promotes growth and bone development.	Red, yellow-orange, and leafy green vegetables and fruits, including carrots, apricots, cantaloupe, peppers, tomatoes, spinach, broccoli, sweet potatoes, and pumpkin.
Vitamin E	Acts as the protector of essential fats in cell membranes and red blood cells. Reduces risk of cancer, heart disease, and other age-associated diseases.	Peanut butter, nuts, seeds, vegetable oils and margarine, wheat germ, avocado, whole grains, salad dressings.
Vitamin C	Destroys free radicals inside and outside cells. Helps in the formation of connective tissue, the healing of wounds, and iron absorption, and also helps to prevent bruising and keep gums healthy. May reduce risk of cataracts, heart disease, and cancer.	Peppers, tomatoes, citrus fruits and juices, berries, broccoli, spinach, cabbage, potatoes, mango, papaya.
Vitamin A	Protects cell membranes and fatty tissue, helps repair damage caused by air pollutants, and boosts the immune system. Helps bones and teeth develop and promotes vision.	Liver, eggs, and fortified dairy products.

(Illustration by GGS Information Services. Cengage Learning, Gale)

beta carotene may help reduce the risk of some cancers, heart disease, **cataracts**, and strokes.

A number of studies were released in 2007 that reported conflicting information on the effectiveness of antioxidants in fighting and preventing disease and their anti-aging properties. In early 2007, the *Journal of the American Medical Association (JAMA)* published an analysis of 68 studies of antioxidant supplements by researchers in Denmark that reported the antioxidants vitamins A, E, and beta carotene did not increase lifespan and, in some cases, shortened it. Some researchers in the United States questioned the accuracy of the study, saying it was flawed because it looked at all causes of death, including murder and auto accidents, even though there clearly is no relationship between taking antioxidant supplements and these types of deaths. Also, U.S. researchers said the studies used in the analysis were not uniform in their length of time or in the dosages taken of the antioxidants. The dosages that were used in the study were extremely high, further tainting the conclusion, some U.S. researchers said.

Two other studies released in 2007 also reported bad news on antioxidants. One of the studies, called the Women's Antioxidant and Cardiovascular Study, reported that taking vitamins C, E, or beta carotene— either alone or in combination—did not protect women from cardiovascular risks, such as **heart attack** and **stroke**. The long-term study of more than 8,000 women was conducted by researchers at Brigham and Women's Hospital in Boston. The second study, conducted by researchers at the University of Paris, reported that taking antioxidant supplements increased the risk of skin cancers in women but not in men. The long-term study of more than 13,000 French men and women involved the antioxidants vitamins C, E, and beta carotene, along with selenium and **zinc**.

Further large-scale clinical studies underway in the United States as of 2007 may shed more light on the antioxidant debate, especially in regards to the anti-cancer benefits of antioxidants. One of these is the Physicians' Health Study-II, which began in 1997 and was scheduled to end in December 2007. As of January 2008, results from the study were still being analyzed and had not been released. The study involved vitamins C, E, and beta carotene, and a multivitamin. It looked at the effects of these antioxidants—together, alone, and in combinations—on preventing cardiovascular disease, cancer in general, **prostate cancer**, colon cancer, aging-related eye disease, and early cognitive decline. Another study is the Selenium and Vitamin E Cancer Prevention Trial (SELECT), a clinical trial to see if either or both of these antioxidants can prevent prostate cancer. More than 35,000 men in the United States, Canada, and Puerto Rico, participated in the study, which began in 2001 and was scheduled to end in 2011. This study was funded by the National Cancer Institute, a branch of the National Institutes of Health.

Vitamin A

A study by the University of Arizona found that vitamin A has a protective affect against many types of cancer, according to Dr. Michael Colgan in his book, *The New Nutrition*. Vitamin A is a fat-soluble antioxidant found in animal products but can be made by the body from its precursor, beta carotene. Foods rich in vitamin A are liver, eggs, and fortified dairy products. Vitamin A helps bones and teeth develop and promotes vision. As an antioxidant, it protects cell membranes and fatty tissue, helps repair damage caused by air pollutants, and boosts the

immune system. A deficiency of this vitamin can result in dry skin, brittle hair, vision problems, blindness, and increased susceptibility to respiratory **infections**.

Vitamin C

Probably the most widely used of all vitamin supplements, vitamin C is a powerful antioxidant that has a myriad of functions and helps strengthen the immune system. It became famous in the 1970s when Nobel Prize-winning scientist Linus Pauling advocated daily mega doses (8–10 grams) of vitamin C to prevent and ease the symptoms of the **common cold**. Many clinical studies show vitamin C is superior to over-the-counter medicines in reducing the symptoms, duration, and severity of colds. As an antioxidant, vitamin C may help fight cardiovascular disease by protecting the linings of arteries from oxidative damage. As of 2007, debate continued on the vitamin's effects on heart disease. One study revealed that Vitamins C and E helped reduce arteriosclerosis (hardening of the arteries) following heart transplants. Yet another study demonstrated that vitamin therapy had no effect on preventing heart disease. There is some evidence and research that vitamin C can help prevent cancer. Studies have shown it is also beneficial in protecting the body against the effects of **smoking** and air pollutants and generally boosts the immune system.

Vitamin E

Vitamin E is a potent antioxidant by itself, but its effectiveness is magnified when taken with other antioxidants, especially vitamin C, selenium, and beta carotene. Some scientific evidence indicates that vitamin E helps promote cardiovascular health. Past studies have demonstrated higher vitamin E intake is associated with decreased incidence of heart disease in both men and women. In fact, the combination of vitamin C and E can slow progression of cardiovascular disease following heart transplant. In 2002, researchers stated that the vitamin combination might also be useful in other organ transplants. In addition, Harvard Medical School reported in the same year that vitamin E might play a role in helping people live longer, citing its role in strengthening the immune system.

Carotenoids

This class of antioxidants, including beta carotene, **lutein**, and **lycopene**, are found in a variety of fruits and vegetables such as carrots, pumpkins, kale, spinach, tomatoes, and pink grapefruit. Research evidence suggests **carotenoids** lower the risk of heart disease and some types of cancer and strengthen the immune system. Lycopene, which is concentrated in the prostate gland, is believed to protect the prostate from cancer. Lutein is thought to prevent **macular degeneration**, a major cause of blindness or stop its progression. Beta carotene increases the lungs' defense system in smokers or those exposed to other air-borne pollutants. It also has been used as an immune system stimulator in people with **AIDS**. In 2002, a report revealed that more than 90% of ophthalmologists and optometrists surveyed believe that lutein helps prevent eye disease.

Bioflavonoids

Bioflavonoids are a group of about 5,000 compounds that act as antioxidants. They occur in fruits, vegetables, green tea, soy products, herbs, and spices. A combination of bioflavonoids has a synergistic effect when taken with vitamin C. They have been shown to be beneficial in treating a variety of conditions, including **allergies**, arthritis, diabetes, **hypertension**, and viral infections. One group of bioflavonoids found to be a powerful antioxidant is oligomeric proanthocyanidins (OPCs), also known generically as pycnogenol. Extremely high concentrations of OPCs are found in maritime pine bark (*Pinus maritima*) extract, grape seed extract, and grape and peanut skins. Due primarily to its much lower cost, grape seed extract is the most commonly used OPC. Procyanidins, a group of compounds found in the extract, are thought to increase the effectiveness of other antioxidants, especially vitamin C and vitamin E, by helping them regenerate after neutralizing free radicals in the blood and tissue.

Other antioxidants

The other widely used antioxidants are selenium, zinc, coenzyme Q10, and certain **amino acids**. Selenium, especially when teamed with vitamin E, may help protect against lung, colon, prostate, and rectum cancers. The antioxidant benefits of coenzyme Q10 may include slowing the aging process, boosting the immune system, and preventing oxidative damage to the brain. Some people suggest its use to treat a variety of cardiovascular diseases. Amino acids that have strong antioxidant effects include alpha lipoic acid, cysteine, **glutathione**, and N-acetyl cysteine (NAC).

Preparations

Bottled antioxidant formulae are available in a single pill or as part of a multivitamin. The usual dosages of antioxidants taken individually can vary widely. The United States Department of Agriculture (USDA) has established recommended daily allowances, but these may be conservative amounts for preventing diseases. For instance, the USDA recommendation for vitamin C is 60 mg a day, but natural health practitioners commonly recommend 500 mg a day or more. The dosage may also depend on whether it is being taken to treat or prevent a specific condition. With that in mind, the common daily dosages for specific antioxidants are: vitamin A, 5,000-15,000 IU; beta carotene, 15,000-25,000 IU; vitamin C, 250-1,500 mg; vitamin E, 30-400 IU; selenium, 50-400 micrograms; bioflavonoids, 100-500 mg; grape seed extract, 150-200 mg; coenzyme Q10, 90-150 mg; alpha lipoic acid, 20-50 mg or 300-600 mg for elevated blood sugar levels; glutathione, 100 mg; N-acetyl cysteine, 600 mg, and zinc, 40–60 mg.

Precautions

Various precautions are available regarding the use of antioxidants:

- Vitamin C: May interfere with some laboratory tests, including urinary sugar spilling for diabetics.
- Vitamin A: Can be toxic in high doses of more than 15,000 IU per day or chronic doses for months and may cause birth defects if taken in high doses during pregnancy. In 2002, one study showed that consistent vitamin A intake could increase the risk of hip fractures in postmenopausal women, but the study was not representative of all women, and more study on the upper limits of safe vitamin A consumption for women in their 40s and 50s is needed.
- Vitamin E: Dangerous in very high doses.
- Carotenoids: No known precautions are indicated for normal doses.
- Bioflavonoids: No known precautions are indicated for normal doses.
- Selenium: No precautions indicated at normal doses, but a physician should be consulted before taking daily doses of more than 200 micrograms.
- Coenzyme Q10: No known precautions are indicated for normal dosage.
- Amino acids: There are no known precautions indicated for alpha lipoic acid, cysteine, glutathione, or NAC.

Side effects

Side effects for consuming antioxidants are as follows:

- Vitamin C: Individual tolerances vary. High doses may cause cramps, diarrhea, ulcer flare-ups, kidney stones, and gout in some people.

- Vitamin A: High doses can lead to headaches, nausea, hair loss, and skin lesions; may cause bone disease in people with chronic kidney failure.

- Vitamin E: Usually no adverse side effects in doses of up to 400 mg a day, high doses may elevate blood pressure and lead to blood-clotting problems.

- Carotenoids: No known side effects occur with normal dosage.

- Bioflavonoids: No known negative side effects in normal doses.

- Selenium: No reported adverse side effects with normal dosage of 200 micrograms, higher doses may cause dizziness and nausea.

- Coenzyme Q10: No adverse side effects have been reported.

- Amino acids: There are no known side effects associated with normal doses of alpha lipoic acid, cysteine, glutathione, or NAC.

Interactions

Information on interactions is available, some of which is as follows:

- Vitamin C: No known common adverse interactions with other drugs.

- Vitamin A: Women taking birth control pills should consult with their doctors before taking extra vitamin A.

- Vitamin E: Should not be used by persons taking anti-coagulation drugs.

- Carotenoids: No known negative interactions with other drugs.

- Bioflavonoids: No known adverse interactions with other drugs.

- Coenzyme Q10: No negative drug interactions yet reported.

- Amino acids: There are no adverse reactions yet reported between alpha lipoic acid, cysteine, glutathione, or NAC and other medications.

KEY TERMS

Atherosclerosis—A buildup of fatty substances in the inside of arteries, resulting in the restriction of blood flow and hardening of the vessels.

Macular degeneration—An eye disease resulting in a loss of central vision in both eyes while peripheral vision is preserved.

Oxidation—The loss of electrons from a molecule by their bonding to an oxygen molecule, rendering the donor molecule positive in charge and the recipient oxygen negative in charge (free radical).

Sinusitis—An inflammation or infection in the sinus cavities in the head.

Resources

BOOKS

Bruning, Nancy Pauling. *The Real Vitamin and Mineral Book: The Definitive Guide to Designing Your Personal Supplement Program,* 4th ed. New York: Avery, 2007.

Jeep, Robin, et al. *The Super Antioxidant Diet and Nutrition Guide: A Health Plan for the Body, Mind, and Spirit.* Charlottesville, VA: Hampton Roads, 2008.

Milbury, Paul E., and Alice C. Richer. *Understanding the Antioxidant Controversy: Scrutinizing the "Fountain of Youth."* Westport, CT: Praeger, 2007.

Panglossi, Harold V., ed. *Antioxidants: New Research.* Haupauge, NY: Nova Science, 2006.

Presman, Alan H., and Sheila Buff. *The Complete Idiot's Guide to Vitamins and Minerals,* 3rd ed. New York: Alpha (Penguin Group), 2007.

PERIODICALS

Antinoro, Linda. "Antioxidant Allies Abound: Where to Look, Surprising Food Sources." *Environmental Nutrition* (March 2006): 1.

"Antioxidant Supplements—Now What? Despite Controversial Analysis Linking Some Antioxidants to Increased Mortality, Experts Still See Possible Preventive Benefits." *Tufts University Health & Nutrition Letter* (June 2007): 4(2).

Brunk, Doug. "Antioxidants Do Not Protect Women Against Heart Risks." *Family Practice News* (September 15, 2007): 17.

Challem, Jack. "Vitamin Basics: To Maintain Optimal Health, It's Often Worthwhile to Venture Beyond What You Get in a Multivitamin. These Are Our Top 10 Picks for Individual Vitamin Supplements." *Better Nutrition* (August 2007): 14(3).

Gable, Christine. "R.O.Y.G.B.I.V.: Eat Your Colors: Color Yourself Healthy with a Rainbow-Inspired Menu that Provides a Balance of Vitamins, Minerals, and Antioxidants." *Better Nutrition* (September 2007): 62–64.

Gottesman, Nancy. "Vitamin Wars—The Latest." *O, The Oprah Magazine* (September 2007): 211–213

Mechcatie, Elizabeth. "Antioxidants May Raise Women's Skin Cancer Risk." *Skin & Allergy News* (October 2007): 4.

ORGANIZATIONS

American Dietetic Association, 120 S. Riverside Plaza, Suite 2000, Chicago, IL, 60606, (800) 877-1600, http://www.eatright.org.

American Institute of Homeopathy, 801 N. Fairfax St., Suite 306, Alexandria, VA, 22314, (888) 445-9988, http://www.homeopathyusa.org.

Canadian Cancer Society, 10 Alcorn Ave., Suite 200, Toronto, ON, M4V 3B1, Canada, (416) 961-7223, http://www.cancer.ca.

Dieticians of Canada, 480 University Ave., Suite 604, Toronto, ON, M5G 1V2, Canada, (416) 596-0857, http://www.dieticians.ca.

National Cancer Institute, 6116 Executive Blvd., Room 3036A, Bethesda, MD, 20892, (800) 422-6237, http://www.cancer.gov.

Office of Dietary Supplements, National Institutes of Health, 6100 Executive Blvd., Room 3B01, MSC 7517, Bethesda, MD, 20892, (301) 435-2920, http://www.ods.od.nih.gov.

Ken R. Wells

Anxiety

Definition

Anxiety is a bodily response to a perceived threat or danger. It is triggered by a combination of biochemical changes in the body, the patient's personal history and memory, and the social situation.

It is important to distinguish between anxiety as a feeling or experience and an anxiety disorder as a psychiatric diagnosis. A person may feel anxious without having an anxiety disorder. Also, a person facing a clear and present danger or experiencing a realistic fear is not usually considered to be in a state of anxiety. In addition, anxiety frequently occurs as a symptom in other categories of psychiatric disturbance.

Description

Anxiety is related to fear, but it is not the same emotion. Fear is a direct, focused response to a specific event or object of which an individual is consciously aware. Most people feel fear if someone points a loaded gun at them or if they see a tornado forming on the horizon. They also recognize that they are afraid. Anxiety, by contrast, is often unfocused, vague, and hard to link to a specific cause.

Sometimes anxiety experienced in the present may stem from an event or person that produced **pain** and fear in the past. In this experience, the anxious individual may not be consciously aware of the original source of the feeling. Anxiety has an aspect of remoteness that makes it hard for people to compare their experiences. Whereas fear is the typical and logical response to physically dangerous situations, anxiety is often triggered by objects or events that are unique and specific to an individual and may seem illogical triggers from other persons' perspectives. An individual may be anxious because of a unique meaning or memory being stimulated by present circumstances rather than because of some immediate danger.

According to the Anxiety Disorders Association of America, anxiety disorders affect 40 million adults in the United States (more than 18% of the population), and are the most common mental illness.

Causes and symptoms

Anxiety is characterized into four categories, each with associated symptoms:

- Somatic. These physical symptoms include headaches, dizziness or lightheadedness, nausea and/or vomiting, diarrhea, tingling, pale complexion, sweating, numbness, difficulty in breathing, and sensations of tightness in the chest, neck, shoulders, or hands. These symptoms are produced by the hormonal, muscular, and cardiovascular reactions involved in the fight-or-flight reaction.

- Behavioral. These symptoms include pacing, trembling, general restlessness, hyperventilation, pressured speech, hand wringing, and finger tapping.

- Cognitive. These symptoms include recurrent or obsessive thoughts, feelings of doom, morbid or fear-inducing thoughts or ideas, and confusion or inability to concentrate.

- Emotional. These symptoms include feelings of tension or nervousness, of being hyper or keyed up, and having a sense of unreality, panic, or terror.

Anxiety can have a number of different causes. It is a multidimensional response to stimuli in the person's environment or a response to an internal stimulus (e.g., a hypochondriac's reaction to stomach rumbling) resulting from a combination of general biological and individual psychological processes.

Physical triggers

In some cases, anxiety is produced by physical responses to **stress** or by certain disease processes or medications.

THE AUTONOMIC NERVOUS SYSTEM (ANS). The nervous system of human beings is hard-wired to respond to dangers or threats. These responses are not subject to conscious control and are the same in humans as in lower animals. They represent an evolutionary adaptation to animal predators and other dangers to which all animals, including primitive humans, had to cope.

The most familiar reaction of this type is the fight-or-flight reaction to a life-threatening situation. When people have fight-or-flight reactions, the level of stress hormones in their blood rises. They become more alert and attentive, their eyes dilate, their heartbeat rate increases, their breathing rate increases, and their digestion slows down, making more energy available to the muscles.

This emergency reaction is regulated by a part of the nervous system called the autonomic nervous system, or ANS. The ANS is regulated by the hypothalamus, a specialized part of the brainstem that is among a group of structures called the limbic system. The limbic system controls human emotions through its connections to glands and muscles; it also connects to the ANS and higher brain centers, such as parts of the cerebral cortex.

One problem with this arrangement is that the limbic system cannot tell the difference between a real physical threat and an anxiety-producing thought or idea. The hypothalamus may trigger the release of stress hormones from the pituitary gland even when there is no external danger.

A second problem is caused by the biochemical side effects of too many false alarms in the ANS. When individuals respond to a real danger, their body relieves itself of the stress hormones by facing up to the danger or fleeing from it. In modern life, however, people often have fight-or-flight reactions in situations in which they can neither run away nor lash out physically. As a result, their bodies have to absorb all the biochemical changes of hyperarousal rather than release them. These biochemical changes can produce anxious feelings as well as muscle tension and other physical symptoms of anxiety.

DISEASES AND DISORDERS. Anxiety can be a symptom of certain medical conditions. For example, anxiety is a symptom of certain endocrine disorders that are characterized by overactivity or underactivity of the thyroid gland. Cushing's syndrome, in which the adrenal cortex overproduces cortisol, is one such disorder. Other medical conditions that can produce anxiety are respiratory distress syndrome, mitral valve prolapse, porphyria, and chest pain caused by inadequate blood supply to the heart (**angina** pectoris).

MEDICATIONS AND SUBSTANCE USE. Numerous medications may cause anxiety-like symptoms as a side effect. They include birth control pills, some thyroid or **asthma** drugs, some psychotropic agents, corticosteroids, antihypertensive drugs, nonsteroidal anti-inflammatory drugs (such as flurbiprofen and ibuprofen), and local anesthetics. **Caffeine** can also cause anxiety-like symptoms when consumed in sufficient quantity.

Withdrawal from certain prescription drugs—primarily beta-blockers and corticosteroids—can cause anxiety. Withdrawal from drugs of abuse, including LSD, cocaine, alcohol, and opiates, can also cause anxiety.

Childhood development and anxiety

Researchers in early childhood development regard anxiety in adult life as a residue of childhood memories of dependency. Humans learn during the first year of life that they are not self-sufficient and that their basic survival depends on others. It is thought that this early experience of helplessness underlies the most common anxieties of adult life, including fear of powerlessness and fear of not being loved. Thus, adults can be made anxious by symbolic threats to their sense of competence or significant relationships, even though they are no longer helpless children.

Symbolization

The psychoanalytic model gives a lot of weight to the symbolic aspect of human anxiety; examples include phobic disorders, obsessions, compulsions, and other forms of anxiety that are highly individualized. Because humans mature slowly, children and adolescents have many opportunities to connect their negative experiences to specific objects or events that can trigger anxious feelings in later life. For example, a person who was frightened as a child by a tall man wearing glasses may feel panicky years later, without consciously knowing why, by something that echoes that person or experience.

Freud thought that anxiety results from a person's internal conflicts. According to his theory, people feel anxious when they feel torn between moral restrictions and desires or urges toward certain actions. In some cases, the person's anxiety may attach itself to an object that represents the inner conflict. For example, someone who feels anxious around money may be pulled between a desire to steal and the belief that stealing is wrong. Money becomes a symbol for the inner conflict between doing what is considered right and doing what one wants.

Phobias

Phobias are a special type of anxiety reaction in which individuals concentrate their anxiety on a specific object or situation and then tries to avoid it. In most cases, the fear is out of proportion to its cause. According to the Anxiety Disorders Association of America, 19 million American adults, representing nearly 9% of the population, have specific phobias. Some phobias—agoraphobia (fear of open spaces), claustrophobia (fear of small or confined spaces), and social phobia, for example—are shared by large numbers of people. Others are less common or are unique to individuals.

Social and environmental stressors

Because humans are social creatures, anxiety often has a social dimension. People frequently report feelings of high anxiety when they anticipate or fear the loss of social approval or love. Social phobia is a specific anxiety disorder that is marked by high levels of anxiety or fear of embarrassment in social situations.

Another social stressor is prejudice. People who belong to groups that are targets of bias have a higher risk of developing anxiety disorders. Some experts think, for example, that the higher rates of phobias and **panic disorder** among women reflects their greater social and economic vulnerability.

Several controversial studies indicate that the increase in violent or upsetting pictures and stories in news reports and entertainment may raise people's anxiety levels. Stress and anxiety management programs often recommend that patients cut down their exposure to upsetting stimuli.

Environmental or occupational factors can also cause anxiety. People who must live or work around sudden or loud noises, bright or flashing lights, chemical vapors, or similar nuisances that they cannot avoid or control may develop heightened anxiety levels.

Diagnosis

Diagnosing anxiety is difficult and complex because of the variety of possible causes and because each person's symptoms arise from highly individualized experiences. When an anxious patient is examined, the healthcare practitioner will first rule out physical conditions and diseases that have anxiety as a symptom. The doctor will then take the patient's history to see if prescription drugs, alcohol or drug abuse, caffeine, work environment, or other external stressors could be triggering the anxiety. In many cases, the most important source of diagnostic information is the patient's psychological and social history. The doctor may administer several brief psychological tests, including the Hamilton Anxiety Scale and the Anxiety Disorders Interview Schedule (ADIS).

Treatment

Meditation and mindfulness training can benefit patients with phobias and panic disorder. **Hydrotherapy**, **massage therapy**, and **aromatherapy** are useful to some anxious patients because these treatments can promote general **relaxation** of the nervous system. **Essential oils** of **lavender**, **chamomile**, neroli, sweet marjoram, and ylang-ylang are commonly recommended by aromatherapists for stress relief and anxiety reduction.

Relaxation training, which is sometimes called anxiety management training, includes breathing exercises and similar techniques intended to help the patient prevent hyperventilation and relieve the muscle tension associated with the fight-or-flight reaction. **Yoga**, aikido, tai chi, and **dance therapy** help patients work with the physical, as well as the emotional, tensions that either promote anxiety or result from the anxiety.

Homeopathy and **traditional Chinese medicine** (TCM) approach anxiety as a symptom of a holistic imbalance. Homeopathic practitioners select a remedy based on other associated symptoms and the patient's general constitution. Homeopathic remedies for anxiety include **ignatia**, **gelsemium**, **aconite**, **pulsatilla**, **arsenicum album**, and coffea cruda. These remedies should be prescribed by a homeopathic healthcare professional.

Chinese medicine regards anxiety as a disruption of *qi*, or energy flow, inside the patient's body. **Acupuncture** and/or herbal therapy are standard remedies for rebalancing the entire system. Reishi (*Ganoderma lucidum* or Ling-Zhi) is a medicinal mushroom prescribed in TCM to reduce anxiety and **insomnia**. However, because reishi can interact with other prescription drugs and is not recommended for patients with certain medical conditions, individuals should consult their healthcare practitioner before taking the remedy. Other TCM herbal remedies for anxiety include the **cordyceps** mushroom (also known as caterpillar fungus) and Chinese **green tea**. In addition, numerous TCM formulas combine multiple herbs for use as an anxiety treatment, depending on the individual problem.

Herbalists or holistic healthcare providers may also prescribe herbs known as *adaptogens* to treat anxiety. These herbs are thought to promote adaptability to stress, and they include Siberian ginseng (*Eleutherococcus senticosus*), ginseng (*Panax ginseng*), wild yam (*Dioscorea villosa*), borage (*Borago officinalis*), **licorice** (*Glycyrrhiza glabra*), chamomile (*Chamaemelum nobile*), **milk thistle** (*Silybum marianum*), and nettles (*Urtica dioica*). Tonics of **skullcap** (*Scutellaria lateriafolia*), and oats (*Avena sativa*) may also be recommended to ease anxiety.

A 2002 preliminary study found that St. John's wort could be an effective treatment for generalized anxiety. Patients taking 900 mg a day and higher doses responded well in early trials. However, further research was needed, particularly at doses higher than 900 mg per day. The Ayurvedic herb **gotu kola**, long used by practitioners of India's holistic medical system to enhance memory and relieve **varicose veins**, may also help patients with anxiety by working against the startle response. In addition, kava extract (also known as kava-kava) has been suggested as a potential treatment for generalized anxiety.

Allopathic treatment

Because anxiety often has more than one cause and patients experience it in highly individual ways, its treatment often requires more than one type of therapy. In some cases, several types of treatment may need to be tried before the best combination is discovered. It usually takes about six to eight weeks to evaluate the effectiveness of a treatment regimen.

Medications

Medications are often prescribed to relieve the physical and psychological symptoms of anxiety. Most medications work by counteracting the biochemical and muscular changes involved in the fight-or-flight reaction. Some work directly on the brain chemicals that are thought to underlie the anxiety.

ANXIOLYTICS. Anxiolytics are sometimes called tranquilizers. Benzodiazepines work by relaxing the skeletal muscles and calming the limbic system. They include such drugs as alprazolam (Xanax) and diazepam (Valium). Barbiturates, once commonly used,

carry a high risk of addiction and abuse and are rarely used in clinical practice. Benzodiazepines are potentially habit-forming and may cause withdrawal symptoms, but they are far less likely than barbiturates to cause physical dependency.

Two other types of anxiolytic medications are meprobamate (Equanil), which is rarely used as of 2008, and buspirone (BuSpar), a later type of anxiolytic that appears to work by increasing the efficiency of the body's own emotion-regulating brain chemicals. Unlike barbiturates and benzodiazepines, buspirone does not cause dependence problems, does not interact with alcohol, and does not affect the patient's ability to drive or operate machinery. It does, however, carry some side effects, and it is not effective against certain types of anxiety, such as panic disorder.

ANTIDEPRESSANTS AND BETA-BLOCKERS. The treatment of choice for **obsessive-compulsive disorder**, panic type anxiety, and other anxiety disorders is a group of antidepressants known as selective serotonin reuptake inhibitors (SSRIs), such as fluoxetine hydrochloride (Prozac) and paroxetine hydrochloride (Paxil). When anxiety occurs in tandem with depressive symptoms, tricyclic antidepressants such as imipramine (Tofranil) or monoamine oxidase inhibitors (MAOIs) such as phenelzine (Nardil) are sometimes prescribed.

Beta-blockers are medications that work by blocking the body's reaction to the stress hormones that are released during the fight-or-flight reaction. They include drugs such as propranolol (Inderal) or atenolol (Tenormin). Beta-blockers are sometimes given to patients with post-traumatic anxiety symptoms or social phobic anxiety.

Psychotherapy

Many patients with anxiety are given some form of **psychotherapy** along with medication. Many patients benefit from insight-oriented therapies, which are designed to help them uncover unconscious conflicts and defense mechanisms in order to understand how their symptoms developed.

Cognitive-behavioral therapy (CBT) also works well with anxious patients. In CBT, individuals are taught to identify thoughts and situations that stimulate their anxiety and to view them more realistically. In the behavioral part of the program, individuals are exposed to the anxiety-provoking object, situation, or internal stimulus (e.g., a rapid heart beat) in gradual stages until they are desensitized to it.

KEY TERMS

Anxiolytic—A type of medication that helps to relieve anxiety.

Aromatherapy—The therapeutic use of plant derived, aromatic essential oils to promote physical and psychological wellbeing.

Autonomic nervous system (ANS)—The part of the nervous system that supplies nerve endings in the blood vessels, heart, intestines, glands, and smooth muscles; it also governs their involuntary functioning. The autonomic nervous system is responsible for the biochemical changes involved in experiences of anxiety.

Endocrine gland—A ductless gland, such as the pituitary, thyroid, or adrenal gland, that secretes its products directly into the blood or lymph.

Hyperarousal—A state or condition of muscular and emotional tension produced by hormones released during the fight-or-flight reaction.

Hypothalamus—A portion of the brain that regulates the autonomic nervous system, the release of hormones from the pituitary gland, sleep cycles, and body temperature.

Limbic system—A group of structures in the brain that includes the hypothalamus, amygdala, and hippocampus. The limbic system plays an important part in regulation of human moods and emotions.

Phobia—In psychoanalytic theory, a psychological defense against anxiety in which the patient displaces anxious feelings onto an external object, activity, or situation.

Expected results

According to the Anxiety Disorders Association of America, nearly half of those people who experience persistent anxiety do not seek treatment. Among those people who do, the prognosis for resolving anxiety depends on the specific disorder and a wide variety of factors, including the patient's age, general health, living situation, belief system, social support network, and responses to different medications and forms of therapy.

Resources

BOOKS

Bourne, Edmund J. *The Anxiety & Phobia Workbook*, 4th ed. Oakland, CA: New Harbinger, 2005.

Challem, Jack, and Melvyn Werbach. *The Food-Mood Solution: All-Natural Ways to Banish Anxiety, Depression, Anger, Stress, Overeating, and Alcohol and Drug Problems—and Feel Good Again*, rep. ed. Hoboken, NJ: Wiley, 2008.

ORGANIZATIONS

American Botanical Council, PO Box 144345, Austin, TX, 78714-4345, (512) 926-4900, http://abc.herbalgram.org/site/PageServer.

Anxiety Disorders Association of America, 8730 Georgia Ave., Suite 600, Silver Spring, MD, 20910, (240) 485-1001, http://www.adaa.org.

Paula Ford-Martin
Leslie Mertz, Ph.D.

Apis

Description

Not all products used in alternative healing come from plants. *Apis mellifica* is the venom of the common honeybee or a tincture made from the whole bee. Various species of honeybees found throughout the world are used for this remedy in homeopathic medicine. The remedy made from them is usually called apis. Other folk medicine traditions use additional bee-related substances in healing such as honey, beeswax, pollen, **royal jelly**, and propolis.

General use

Homeopathic medicine operates on the principle that "like heals like." This means that a disease can be cured by treating it with products that produce the same symptoms as the disease. These products follow

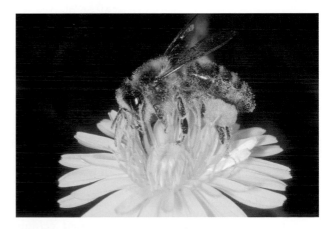

Honey bee, *Apis mellifera*. (© WildPictures / Alamy)

another homeopathic law, the Law of Infinitesimals. In opposition to traditional medicine, the Law of Infinitesimals states that the *lower* a dose of curative, the more effective it is. To make a homeopathic remedy, the curative is diluted many, many times until only a tiny amount remains in a huge amount of the diluting liquid.

In homeopathic terminology, the effectiveness of remedies is "proved" by experimentation and reports by famous homeopathic practitioners. Around 1900, both bee venom and tincture from the entire insect were proved as a remedy by the Central New York State Homeopathic Society.

In homeopathic medicine, apis is used as a remedy for many symptoms similar to those of bee **stings**. These include:

- inflammation with a burning sensation
- stinging pain
- itchy skin
- swollen and sensitive skin
- red, flushed, hot face
- hive-like welts on the skin

Homeopathic practitioners use apis when stinging or burning inflammations appear in all parts of the body, not just on the skin. A homeopath could use apis for sore throats, **mumps**, urinary tract **infections**, and other conditions where there is a stinging or burning sensation.

Symptoms treated by apis usually appear quite rapidly. There is often some swelling (**edema**) along with the stinging sensation. Many people who need apis complain of swollen eyelids, as if they had an eye infection. In keeping with the symptom of edema, often little urine is produced although there may be a strong urge to urinate. Despite this, the patient has little thirst or desire to drink.

Often the patient who will be given apis appears flushed or has a rough rash. The rash may appear, then disappear. The skin will be sensitive to the touch and alternately hot and dry, then sweaty. Patients may also feel nauseated, experience **heartburn**, or have tightness throughout their chest or abdomen that feels as if they will burst if they **cough** or strain.

Certain mental and emotional symptoms also appear in the patient that needs treatment with apis. Sadness, weeping, and **depression** can occur. Apis is often used after a person experiences a strong emotional reaction such as jealousy, fear, rage, or anger.

In homeopathic medicine, the fact that certain symptoms get better or worse under different conditions is used as a diagnostic tool to indicate what remedy will be most effective. Symptoms that benefit from treatment with apis get worse by applying warmth or drinking warm liquids. They also get worse from touch or pressure, or when the person is in a closed, heated room. The symptoms are often worse on the right side, after sleeping and also worsen in the late afternoon. Symptoms improve with the application of cold and exposure to fresh air.

Homeopathy also ascribes certain personality types to certain remedies. The apis personality is said to be fidgety, restless, and unpredictable. People with the apis personality may have wildly inappropriate reactions to emotional situations. They want company, but reject affection, and sometimes insist that they do not need medical attention when they clearly are unwell. People who need apis often have bouts of unprovoked jealousy and unprovoked tears. They may fear ill health and death greatly.

Preparations

There are two homeopathic dilution scales, the decimal (x) scale with a dilution factor of 1:10 and the centesimal (c) scale with a dilution factor of 1:100. Once the mixture is diluted, shaken, strained, then rediluted many times to reach the desired degree of potency, the final mixture is added to lactose (a type of sugar) tablets or pellets. These are then stored away from light. Homeopathic apis venom is available commercially in tablets in many different strengths. Dosage depends on the symptoms being treated. Homeopathic tincture of whole honeybee is also available in a variety of strengths.

Homeopathic and orthodox medical practitioners agree that by the time the initial remedy solution is diluted to strengths used in homeopathic healing, it is likely that very few molecules of the original remedy remain. Homeopaths, however, believe that these remedies continue to work through an effect called "potentization" that has not yet been explained by mainstream scientists.

Precautions

No particular precautions have been noted for using apis. However, people who are allergic or sensitive to bee venom should be cautious. They may react adversely to certain potencies of homeopathic apis.

Side effects

When taken in the recommended dilute form, no side effects from apis have been reported.

Concentrated quantities of the bee venom can cause allergic reactions in susceptible people.

Interactions

Studies on interactions between apis and conventional pharmaceuticals have not been done. No interactions have been reported.

Resources

BOOKS

Chernin, Dennis. *The Complete Homeopathic Resource for Common Illnesses*. Berkeley, CA: North Atlantic Books, 2006.

Cummings, Stephen, and Dana Ullman. *Everybody's Guide to Homeopathic Medicines*. 3rd ed. rev. New York: Tarcher, 2004.

Wolf, C. W. *Apis Mellifica; or, the Poison of the Honeybee, Considered as a Therapeutic Agent*. Originally published Philadelphia: W. Radde, 1858. Reprinted Ann Arbor, MI: Scholarly Publishing Office, University of Michigan Library, 2005.

ORGANIZATIONS

Alternative Medicine Foundation. P. O. Box 60016, Potomac, MD 20859. (301) 340-1960. http://www.amfoundation.org.

American Institute of Homeopathy. 801 N. Fairfax Street, Suite 306, Alexandria, VA 22314. (888) 445-9988. http://homeopathyusa.org.

National Center for Homeopathy. 801 N. Fairfax St., Suite 306, Alexandria, VA 22314. (703) 548-7790. http://www.homeopathic.org/contact.htm.

OTHER

"Apis Mellifica." *ABC Homeopathy*. [cited February 19, 2008]. http://abchomeopathy.com/r.php/Apis.

"British Homeopathic Library." *Hom-Inform*. [cited February 19, 2008]. http://www.hom-inform.org.

Tish Davidson, A. M.

Apitherapy

Definition

Apitherapy involves the therapeutic use of honeybee products, including **bee pollen**, honey, propolis, **royal jelly**, beeswax, and venom, to treat a variety of ailments. The most well-known and well-practiced facet of apitherapy is Bee Venom Therapy (BVT), which involves the medicinal use of bee **stings**. The venom is thought to reduce inflammation and boost the body's immune system. When most people refer to apitherapy, they are referring to BVT.

Origins

The medicinal use of bees goes back to ancient times. Chinese texts dating back 2,000 years mention it, and Hippocrates wrote about it. The Egyptians were said to treat diseases with an ointment made from bees, and Greek physician and writer Galen (129—c. 199), wrote about bee treatments. In 1888, Phillip Terc, an Austrian physician, published a paper on one of the first clinical studies involving bee stings titled *Report About a Peculiar Connection Between the Beestings and Rheumatism*. Thereafter, its use expanded throughout Europe and the United States. It spread as a type of folk remedy popularized by anecdotal accounts, but as the 21st century approached, the medical community began investigating the therapy, studying its use on a pharmacological level. Though clinical studies had begun by 2000, most people using the therapy were either doing it themselves or with the help of lay practitioners. Physicians were beginning to use the therapy but mostly with an injectable form of the venom.

Benefits

The American Apitherapy Society says it has anecdotal evidence showing bee venom is effective in the treatment of:

- immune system problems, such as arthritis and **multiple sclerosis** (MS)
- cardiovascular disease, such as hypertension, arrhythmias, atherosclerosis, and varicose veins
- endocrine disorders, such as premenstrual syndrome, menstrual cramps, irregular periods, and decreased blood glucose levels
- infections, like herpes simplex 1 and 2, warts, mastitis, and laryngitis
- psychological disturbances, such as depression or mood swings

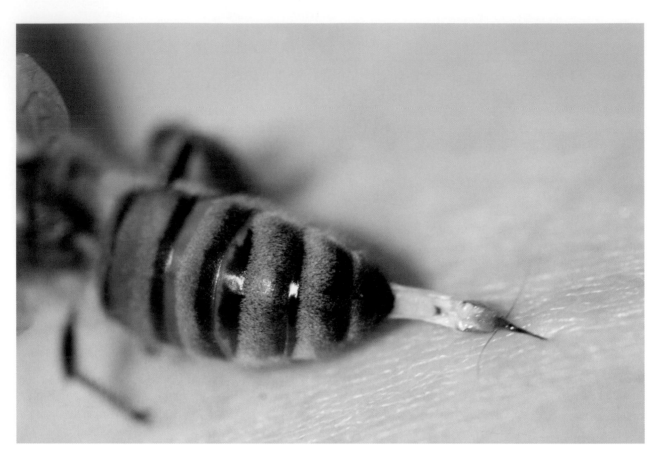

The most well-known facet of apitherapy is Bee Venom Therapy (BVT), which involves the medicinal use of bee stings. The venom is thought to reduce inflammation and boost the body's immune system. *(louise murray / Alamy)*

- rheumatologic disturbances, such as rheumatoid arthritis, osteoarthritis, juvenile rheumatoid arthritis, bursitis and "tennis elbow"
- skin conditions, such as eczema, psoriasis, corns, warts and topical ulcers

Apitherapy is thought of as a last-resort treatment but may be beneficial to those who cannot be helped by traditional therapies and medicines. MS patients have reported increased stability, along with less **fatigue** and muscle spasm, after trying the therapy. Patients with **rheumatoid arthritis** and **osteoarthritis** have said **pain** and swelling have decreased following the stings. It has also been said to shrink the size of rheumatoid nodules. For those who have not achieved relief with other treatments, apitherapy may help.

Description

Honey bee venom contains more than 40 active substances, many of which have physiological effects. The most abundant compound is an anti-inflammatory agent called melittin. This substance causes the body to produce cortisol, which is an agent of the body's own healing process. As an anti-inflammatory, melittin is 100 times more potent than hydrocortisol. It is noted in Paul L. Cerrato's *RN* article that experiments have shown that melittin can slow the body's inflammatory response. That is why the venom may be helpful in treating inflammatory conditions such as rheumatoid arthritis.

Other compounds that may have pharmacological effects include apamin, which works to enhance nerve transmission; adolapin, which is an anti-inflammatory and an analgesic; and other neurotransmitters like norepinephrine and dopamine and seratonin, which figure in **depression**.

The most prevalent use of BVT is for immune system and inflammatory disorders. One of the most promising uses may be relieving the symptoms of treatment-resistant MS. More than 1,300 people with MS have sent testimonials to the American Apitherapy Society in support of the treatment saying the therapy helped relieve fatigue and muscle spasm, as well as to restore stability.

Most people receiving the therapy do it themselves or with the help of a lay practitioner. The cost of learning the therapy and the cost for the bees is generally not covered by insurance. The therapy may be covered, however, if prescribed and administered by a physician who uses an injectable form.

To receive treatment, a bee is taken from a jar or hive with a pair of tweezers and held on the body part to be stung. The stinger should be left in for 10 to 15 minutes. The number of stings delivered in a session and the frequency of the sessions varies, depending on the patient's tolerance and the nature of the problem. To treat tendonitis, a patient might need only two to five therapy sessions involving only two to three stings per session. Treating a more chronic problem like arthritis can take several stings per session two to three times per week for up to three months. Treating MS is a prolonged effort. Those who have used it say the therapy must happen two to three times per week for six months in order to start working.

On average, doctors who use the therapy delivered injections one to two times per week. The number of injections varied widely, from one to 30 per session, depending on the ailment being treated.

Physicians who use the therapy do not use live bees. Instead, they obtain venom in an injectable form and inject it under the skin.

Obviously, the more stings or injections to be administered, the more time the therapy will take per session.

Preparations

Before the therapy is begun, a doctor will inject the patient with a weak form of the venom to test for allergic reaction. The doctor will have a syringe of epinephrine nearby in case a reaction does occur. If the patient is allergic to the venom, the therapy cannot be administered.

Lay practitioners and beekeepers who deliver live stings test patients with an initial sting to the knee or forearm and observe the patient to see if they are allergic. The test sting should only be administered if the practitioner has a bee-sting kit containing epinephrine nearby. If a person is allergic, a reaction will generally occur in 15 to 20 minutes. Up to 2% of the population may be allergic to insect venom.

Ice may be used to numb the area where the stings will occur. It can also be used afterward to soothe the pain.

Precautions

Venom therapy should not be used by those with severe **allergies**, **tuberculosis**, **syphilis**, **gonorrhea**, and transient insulin-dependent diabetes.

Side effects

Pain, **itching**, and swelling are common at the injection or sting site. Patients should also be cautioned that severe anaphylactic allergic reactions can lead to respiratory problems, cardiac collapse, and death. Some may develop nodular masses or ulcers at sting sites.

It seems, however, that major complications are rare. Christopher M. H. Kim, director of the Monmouth Pain Institute in Red Bank, New Jersey, says he has given more than 34,000 injections to 174 patients over the past 15 years and has yet to see any major complications. The venom Kim injects is equivalent to one to ten bee stings. The most common side effect reported by his patients is itching, reported by 80% of his patients after the first session. After 12 sessions, however, only 40% still experienced itching. Of his patients, 29.7% reported swelling; 6.4% reported **headache**; and 5.6% reported flushing.

Research and general acceptance

Due to a growing body of anecdotal evidence to support the use of BVT, formal clinical studies were launched in August 2000. The National Multiple Sclerosis Society funded a study on apitherapy at Georgetown University Medical Center in Washington, D.C. The study evaluated the safety of apitherapy as a treatment for patients with progressive MS. According to the study, although no serious allergic reactions were observed, only two of the nine subjects showed objective improvement and larger studies are necessary to prove effectiveness of the treatment.

During the course of the study, Joseph A. Bellanti, who directed the study, changed his view of the therapy. "In the beginning I thought it was rather strange, but after some investigation, I saw that there are definite immunologic changes after bee venom therapy, and the use of venom began to seem less farfetched."

Over the years, researchers have experimented with the therapy on animals and have found that bee venom can keep arthritis at bay in rodents. A study in which researchers induced a condition similar to rheumatoid arthritis in rats found that

KEY TERMS

Cardiovascular—Refers to the heart and blood vessels as a unified system.

Multiple sclerosis—A chronic, debilitating disease that affects the central nervous system causing a loss of muscular coordination, speech defects, and the like.

Propolis—A brownish, waxy substance that bees collect from the buds of certain trees and use to glue their hives together.

Tendonitis—Refers to an inflammation of the tendons, the fibrous connective tissue that attaches muscle to bone.

daily injections of bee venom suppressed the disease.

Harvard Medical School professor John Mills, who works with arthritis patients, has seen patients achieve short-term relief through the sting therapy, though he does not condone its use. He believes the same response could be achieved through drug therapy without the allergic risk the venom poses to some.

While animal studies, preliminary results of clinical trials, and anecdotal evidence suggest BVT may have therapeutic effects, until clinical trials on humans are completed, there is no way to know if the treatment works. The **placebo effect** may also be responsible for some degree of benefit patients achieve.

Training and certification

Some physicians practice BVT, but the majority of those seeking treatment rely on lay practitioners, bee keepers, themselves, or a partner, who is taught to use the bees.

Those seeking treatment can contact the American Apitherapy Society to find a local practitioner.

Resources

PERIODICALS

Castro, Henry J., et al. "A Phase I Study of the Safety of Honeybee Venom Extract as a Possible Treatment for Patients with Progressive Forms of Multiple Sclerosis." *Allergy and Asthma Proceedings* 26, 6 (November-December 2005): 470-476.

Cerrato, Paul L. "A Therapeutic Bee Sting?" *RN* 61, 8 (August 1998): 57-58.

D'Epiro, Nancy Walsh. "Bee Venom for Multiple Sclerosis." *Patient Care* 33, 14 (September 15, 1999): 27-31.

Granstrom, Chris. "Stinging Away the Pain." *Country Journal* 23, 5 (September/October 1996): 22-25.

Somerfield, Stanley D. "Bee Venom and Arthritis: Magic, Myth or Medicine?" *New Zealand Medical Journal* 99, 800 (April 1986): 281-283.

OTHER

"Bee Venom Therapy." Spectrum Medical Arts. http://www2.shore.net/-spectrum/apitherapy.html (July 13, 2000).

ORGANIZATIONS

American Apitherapy Society, 500 Arthur Street, Centerport, NY, 11721, (631) 470-9446, info@apitherapy.org, http://www.apitherapy.org.

Lisa Frick

Apple cider vinegar

Description

The word vinegar traces back to the French word *vinaigre*, which means sour wine. Apple cider vinegar is created by fermenting cider and other alcoholic liquids. Cider is made by pressing apples into a liquid. Sweet cider is unfermented and nonalcoholic. Hard cider is fermented. When converted into vinegar, the liquid has a strong odor and contains acetic acid. Vinegar is used as a condiment, preservative, and as a folk remedy for numerous conditions.

General use

Vinegar's medicinal uses date back to ancient times. Hippocrates, known as the father of medicine, reportedly used vinegar as an antiseptic.

In the nineteenth century, vinegar became associated with weight loss. The British poet Lord Byron developed a unique diet in 1820. The 194-pound poet scaled down to less than 130 pounds by eating food covered with vinegar. While Byron did not recommend a specific type of vinegar, a twentieth-century American doctor advocated apple cider vinegar as the key to improved health.

Supplement for good health and weight loss

The 1959 bestselling book by DeForest Clinton Jarvis, *Folk Medicine: A Vermont Doctor's Guide to Good Health*, recommended that people consume apple cider vinegar for numerous health conditions. Jarvis based his findings on observing the outcome when cows received vinegar in their food. Jarvis said that adding vinegar to a cow's diet resulted in the birth of a healthy, intelligent, "well-furred" calf.

Jarvis applied his observation to people. He claimed that a pregnant woman who added vinegar and honey to her well-balanced diet would give birth to a baby with thick hair and strong fingernails. Jarvis claimed there was "no limit" to the ailments that could be treated with apple cider vinegar.

While *Time* magazine criticized the remedy as "pseudo science" and "pseudo medicine," the public was not as skeptical. Jarvis's book remained on the bestseller list for months. People paid $2.95 for a 182-page book that advised them to drink vinegar undiluted or with water. However, Jarvis maintained that combining apple cider vinegar with honey produced the best results. A mixture consisting of half vinegar and half honey became known as honegar.

Apple cider vinegar became popular as a weight-loss aid during the 1970s and again in the 1990s. People drank diluted apple cider vinegar before meals because of the liquid's supposed ability to reduce the appetite and burn calories.

By the close of the twentieth century and into the twenty-first, apple cider vinegar in the form of liquid, tablets, and capsules was recommended as a weight-loss aid and a remedy for numerous conditions ranging from arthritis and **asthma** to sore throats and muscles.

Preparation

Apple cider vinegar has long been associated with weight loss, and the condiment may be used as an ingredient for a low-fat salad dressing. Additionally, vinegar was historically a folk remedy for coughs and **sunburn** and a complementary treatment for conditions such as diabetes and high blood pressure. For some conditions, supporters claim that the beneficial effects come from pectin, a water carbohydrate found in ripe fruit.

Some remedies use liquid vinegar; some specify a particular dose. When the dosage is not specified, people should follow the directions on the package or the advice of their physician or health practitioner.

Apple cider vinegar diet

Taking apple cider vinegar before meals is supposed to curb a person's appetite, help the body to burn fat more quickly, and boost metabolism. **Diets**

using vinegar specify dosages ranging from 1 to 3 tsp (5 ml to 15 ml) of apple cider vinegar before meals. Some plans recommend diluting the vinegar in water. The dosage of apple cider vinegar tablets and capsules varies with the strength of the supplement. For some plans, the dosage is 1 to 2 tablets taken before meals.

Many apple cider vinegar weight-loss plans recommend that the dieter **exercise** and eat sensibly. Some diets recommend that people select nutritional food and watch the amount of food consumed. However, people will lose weight without taking apple cider vinegar if they eat sensibly and exercise, according to the American Dietetic Association and other organizations that are skeptical of the benefits of vinegar consumption for weight loss.

Vinegar as a home remedy

Vinegar, in varieties including apple cider, has been recommended for a range of aches and pains. Some treatments are centuries-old home remedies; others are uses recommended by the manufacturers of apple cider vinegar supplement. Conditions and treatments include:

- Sore muscles and cramped legs and feet may be soothed with a compress consisting of a cloth soaked in vinegar. The compress is placed on the aching area for about 15 minutes.
- Headaches may be helped with a compress soaked in a solution that is half vinegar and half water.
- Sunburns can be treated with applications of vinegar compresses.
- Pain from stiff joints may be relieved by ingesting apple cider vinegar in liquid or tablet form. Another remedy is to pour some vinegar in a bath and then soak in it.
- Arthritis pain is said to be helped by a dosage of apple cider vinegar ingested four times daily.
- A sore throat may be soothed by gargling with a solution consisting of 1 tsp apple cider mixed in a glass of water.
- Colds and congestion may be treated by misting a room with 1/4 cup (150 ml) of vinegar in a vaporizer.
- Asthma is supposedly relieved by taking a dosage of apple cider vinegar by mouth or applying a vinegar-soaked cloth to the inside of wrists.

Diabetes and high blood pressure

Apple cider vinegar has also been marketed as a possible remedy for diabetes and high blood pressure. However, research on the effectiveness of this remedy was based on small studies. Lower blood sugar levels were reported in a 2007 study of 11 people diagnosed with Type II diabetes who used 2 T (30 ml) of apple cider vinegar each evening. Furthermore, vinegar reduced the blood pressure in studies involving rats.

As of 2008, larger studies of humans were needed to determine whether apple cider vinegar could help with the treatment of diabetes and high blood pressure.

Precautions

Apple cider vinegar is highly acidic. If not diluted with water or another liquid, vinegar can harm tooth enamel, the mouth, and the esophagus. There is also a risk that it can irritate or burn skin.

Furthermore, apple cider vinegar tablets are classified as supplements and are not evaluated by the U.S. Food and Drug Administration for safety and effectiveness.

In 2005, the University of Arkansas Department of Human Environmental Science tested eight brands of apple cider vinegar tablets after receiving a report that someone taking apple cider vinegar supplements suffered damage to the esophagus. The department's testing covered factors such as pH, which designates acidity and the component acid content. The testing revealed that the supplement size and pH content varied in the eight brands. Furthermore, the researchers noted that doubts remained about whether the brands contained any apple cider vinegar.

People should consult with their doctor or health practitioner before beginning a program that involves regular use of apple cider vinegar. This is especially important for pregnant women, nursing mothers, and people with pre-existing conditions such as diabetes.

Side effects

Possible side effects of apple cider vinegar could result from the acidity in vinegar. The high acid content could cause burning in the mouth and throat, **indigestion**, or **nausea**. Furthermore, a person could experience an allergic reaction. Symptoms of that include difficulty breathing, a rash, and **itching**.

Interactions

When used as a remedy, dosages of apple cider vinegar may potentially react with medications such as insulin and diuretics. The combination could produce complications such as low blood **potassium** levels.

Resources

PERIODICALS

"Bestseller Revisited." *Time* December 18, 1959. http://www.time.com/time/magazine/article/0,9171,811634-1,00.html.

Hill, L., L. H. Woodruff, J. C. Foote, M. Barreto-Alcoba. "Esophageal Injury by Apple Cider Vinegar Tablets and Subsequent Evaluation Of Products." *Journal of the American Dietetic Association* (July 2005): 1141–4.

OTHER

WebMD. "Apple Cider Vinegar." December 4, 2007. http://www.webmd.com/diet/apple-cider-vinegar.

ORGANIZATIONS

American Dietetic Association, 120 S. Riverside Plaza, Suite 2000, Chicago, IL, 60606-6995, (800) 877-1600, http://www.eatright.org.

National Center for Complementary and Alternative Medicine/National Institute of Health (NCCAM), 9000 Rockville Pike, Bethesda, MD, 20892, (888) 644-6226, http://nccam.nih.gov.

Liz Swain

Applied kinesiology

Definition

Applied kinesiology (AK) is the study of muscles and the relationship of muscle strength to health. It incorporates a system of manual muscle testing and therapy. AK is based on the theory that an organ dysfunction is accompanied by a specific muscle weakness. Diseases are diagnosed through muscle-testing procedures and then treated. AK is not the same as kinesiology, or biomechanics, which is the scientific study of movement.

Origins

AK is based on principles of functional neurology, anatomy, physiology, biomechanics, and biochemistry as well as principles from Chinese medicine, **acupuncture**, and massage. It was developed from traditional kinesiology in 1964 by George G. Goodheart, a chiropractor from Detroit, Michigan. He observed that each large muscle relates to a body organ. A weakness in a muscle may mean that there is a problem in the associated organ. Goodheart found that by treating the muscle and making it strong again, he was able to improve the function of the organ as well. For example, if a particular nutritional supplement was given to a patient, and the muscle tested strong, it was the correct supplement for the patient. If the muscle remained weak, it was not. Other methods of treatment can be evaluated in a similar manner. Goodheart also found that painful nodules (small bumps) may be associated with a weak muscle. By deeply massaging the muscle, he was able to improve its strength. Goodheart's findings in 1964 led to the origin and insertion treatment, the first method developed in AK. Other diagnostic and therapeutic procedures were developed for various reflexes described by other chiropractors and doctors. Goodheart incorporated acupuncture meridian therapy into AK after reading the writings of Felix Mann, M.D.

Goodheart considered AK to be a therapeutic tool that incorporates feedback from the body. He said that "applied kinesiology is based on the fact that the body language never lies." He felt that the body's muscles were indicators of disharmony. Once muscle weakness has been ascertained, the problem may be solved in a variety of ways. If a practitioner approaches the problem correctly, he believed, making the proper and adequate diagnosis and treatment, the outcome is satisfactory both to the doctor and to the patient.

Goodheart died March 5, 2008. In addition to pioneering the field of Applied Kinesiology, Goodheart was appointed to the U.S. Olympic Sports Medicine Committee for the 1980 Lake Placid Games.

Benefits

AK is not designed for crisis medicine. For example, an AK practitioner cannot cure **cancer**, arthritis, diabetes, **heart disease**, or **infections**. This therapy is designed to be a part of a holistic approach to preventive medicine. The goals of AK are to (1) restore normal nerve function, (2) achieve normal endocrine, immune, digestive, and other internal organ functions, (3) intervene early in degenerative processes to prevent or delay pathological conditions, and to (4) restore postural balance, correct gait (walking) impairment, and improve range of motion.

Description

According to AK, each muscle in the body relates to a specific meridian or energy pathway (acupuncture lines) in the body. These meridians also relate to organs or glands, allowing the muscles to provide information about organ or gland function and energy. The five areas of diagnosis and therapy for the applied kinesiologist are (1) the nervous system, (2) the lymphatic system, (3) the vascular (blood vessel) system, (4) the cerebrospinal system, and (5) the meridian system.

The first part of AK is muscle testing, which is used to help diagnose what part of the body is functioning abnormally. Muscle testing involves putting the body into a position that requires a certain muscle to remain contracted, and then applying pressure against the muscle. The testing does not measure strength but is meant to reveal stresses and imbalances in the body through the tension in the muscle. The test evaluates the ability of a controlling system (like the nervous system) to adapt the muscle to meet the changing pressure of the examiner's test. AK practitioners also examine structural factors such as posture, gait, and range of motion. Some chiropractors use AK to help them evaluate the success of spinal adjustment. A leg muscle is tested for strength or weakness to determine whether the adjustments made are appropriate.

According to AK, common internal causes of muscle weakness include:

- dysfunction of nerve supply (nerve interference between spine and muscles)
- impairment of lymphatic drainage
- reduction of blood supply
- abnormal pressure in cerebral fluid affecting nerve-to-muscle relationships
- blockage of an acupuncture meridian
- imbalance of chemicals
- dysfunction of organs or glands
- excesses or deficiencies in nutrition

Physiological reactions to chemicals, including those associated with **nutrition** and **allergies**, may also be evaluated using AK. The AK protocol for testing chemical compounds is to place the substance on the patient's tongue so that he tastes the material, and the normal chemical reactions of ingestion begin. In some cases, the substances are inhaled through the nose. The AK practitioner then tests the associated muscle-organ pattern to determine where or if there is a strength or weakness. The patient does not need to swallow the substance for a change in strength or weakness to be identified. David S. Walther, a diplomate of the International College of Applied Kinesiology, has indicated that "it is possible that the central nervous system, recognizing the compound being ingested, relays information to the organs and glands preparing for use of the compound. If the compound is recognized as beneficial, the energy pattern is immediately enhanced, influencing not only the organ or gland, but also the associated muscle."

AK has been used as a diagnostic health tool for a variety of conditions.

Bone health

- neck/low back pain and sciatica
- whiplash
- frozen shoulder

Joint health

- carpal tunnel syndrome
- arthritis (including rheumatoid arthritis)
- sports injuries

Muscle health

- tennis elbow
- heel spurs
- wound healing
- intermittent claudication (pain on walking)
- restless legs
- cramps

Vascular system health

- aching varicose veins
- palpitations
- high blood pressure

Nervous system health

- migraine and other headaches
- trigeminal neuralgia and other face pains
- Bell's palsy
- anxiety
- depression
- fears
- addictions (like smoking)
- claustrophobia
- Meniere's disorder
- neuralgia (severe, throbbing pain)
- travel sickness
- fatigue
- phantom limb pain
- paralysis of leg or arm after a stroke

Respiratory system health

- hay fever
- rhinitis (inflammed nasal passages)
- asthma
- bronchitis
- emphysema (lung disease)

Urinary system health

- cystitis (bladder inflammation), especially in the elderly
- early prostate enlargement
- non-specific urethritis (inflammation of tube from the bladder)
- bedwetting

Reproductive organ health

- menstrual pains
- irregular or excessive menstrual activity
- pelvic pains and endometriosis
- menopausal flushes
- painful, nodular breasts
- preparation for childbirth
- vaginal pain
- post herpetic (shingles) pain
- impotence and infertility

Skin health

- pain after operations
- painful, prominent scars
- wrinkles or bagginess of face
- acne
- psoriasis and eczema (skin diseases)
- boils
- excessive perspiration
- hemorrhoids
- canker sores
- itching

Immune system health

- recurring tonsillitis (inflamed tonsils)
- persisting weakness after a severe illness

Sensory organ health

- tinnitus (ringing ears)
- tired eyes
- retinitis pigmentosa and pterygium retinitis (diseases of the retina)

Digestive system health

- constipation
- colitis or other bowel inflammations
- ulcers
- diarrhea
- obesity

GEORGE GOODHEART (1918–2008)

Dr. George Goodheart was born in Detroit, Michigan, in 1918 and became a second-generation doctor of chiropractic. He graduated from the National College of Chiropractic in 1939 and is recognized as the founder and developer of applied kinesiology. After he joined the U.S. Air Force as an aviation cadet in World War II, he received a promotion to major at the age of 22. He was the youngest ever to attain that rank. He served in active duty from 1941-1946 and continued as a member of the Air Force Reserve until the mid-1950s.

Goodheart held numerous positions of distinction during his career, including director of the National Chiropractic Mutual Insurance Company and director for the International College of Applied Kinesiology-U.S.A. He also lectured and taught throughout the United States, Japan, Europe, and Australia; and he was the official doctor of chiropractic for the Lake Placid Winter Olympic Games in 1980. He contributes to a variety of trade publications on a regular basis.

In 1998 Goodheart received a Lifetime Achievement Award from the International College of Kinesiology. Earlier, in 1987 he was honored with the Leonardo da Vinci Award from the Institute for the Achievement of Human Potential, and he was cited for his research by Logan and Palmer Colleges of Chiropractic. He represented the State of Michigan as a delegate to the American Chiropractic Association and was a fellow at the International College of Chiropractic.

The second part of AK involves the treatment phase. Goodheart and other practitioners of AK have adapted many treatment methods for the problems that are diagnosed with muscle testing. Examples of treatment methods include special **diets**, dietary supplements, **chiropractic** manipulation, osteopathic cranial techniques, acupuncture/meridian therapies, **acupressure**, deep muscle massage, and nervous system coordination procedures. For example, an AK practitioner might treat **asthma** by looking for weaknesses in specific lower back and leg muscles that share a connection with the adrenal glands. The practitioner will strengthen these muscles and help the adrenal gland produce bronchodilators, chemicals that relax or open air passages in the lungs.

The practice of kinesiology requires that it be used in conjunction with other standard diagnostic methods by professionals trained in clinical diagnosis. Most practitioners of AK are chiropractors, but naturopaths, medical doctors, dentists, osteopaths, nutritionists, physical therapists, massage therapists, podiatrists, psychiatrists, and nurse practitioners are also involved. In 2003, 37.6% of 2,574 full-time chiropractors in the United States who responded to a survey by the National Board of Chiropractic Examiners (NBCE) said they used AK in their practice. Previous NBCE surveys indicated that around 31% of chiropractors in Canada, 60% in Australia, and 72% in New Zealand use AK.

Most practitioners of AK utilize a holistic approach and evaluate a person from a triad-based health perspective. Generally, chiropractors approach health and healing from a structural basis, medical doctors generally from a chemical basis, and psychiatrists and psychologists from a mental or emotional basis. Applied kinesiologists attempt to work with all three areas of health, and in some cases, include a spiritual dimension.

The use of AK is often included in insurance coverage if the policy covers chiropractor benefits. The cost of the AK examination is similar to the costs of other chiropractic practices.

Preparations

Since AK is a non-invasive diagnostic tool, there are no preparations required.

Precautions

AK should only by used by trained professionals with the necessary expertise to perform specific and accurate tests. The AK examination should be combined with a standard physical diagnosis, which often includes laboratory tests, x rays, health and dietary history, and other special tests. An AK examination should enhance a standard diagnosis, not replace it. The total diagnostic work-up should be used to determine the final diagnosis.

The use of manual muscle testing to evaluate nutrition is particularly a problem if it is done by a lay nutrition sales person as a tool to sell his/her product. The person should have the educational background to evaluate nutritional needs as well as have a high level of knowledge in the use of proper muscle testing techniques.

Side effects

If AK is performed by a trained practitioner with the appropriate educational background, side effects from the muscle-testing procedures should be minimal.

Research and general acceptance

AK is a tool that is used by many health care professionals, and especially by chiropractors. A literature review published in 1999 by researchers from the School of Medicine at the University of North Carolina at Chapel Hill and the Foundation for Allied Conservative Therapies Research in Chapel Hill stated that, although AK appears to be a promising methodology, there is a lack of research results relevant to clinical practice and outcomes of AK care. They found this lack of results surprising, since cost, satisfaction, utilization, and changes in symptoms are the important results of clinical practice. In addition, they determined that some studies that were supposed to be an evaluation of AK procedures did not actually use clinical practices and principles of AK. However, from studies adhering to AK principles and employing standardized training by well-trained practitioners, they did state there was some evidence that AK is an objectively verifiable phenomenon. They suggested that "future studies of AK should focus on outcomes of care, including symptoms, function, costs, and safety. Only well-designed studies that account for the individual nature of AK diagnosis and treatment and preserve the proper clinical context of AK treatment will be informative. Understanding the individual components of the process of AK treatment remains important. Studies addressing validation of isolated AK procedures need to meet the methodological challenges of studying appropriate subjects that reflects the current recognized practice and understanding of AK. Further evaluation of the basic physiologic phenomena involved and correlation of AK manual muscle test results will also advance understanding of this diagnostic and therapeutic system."

Training and certification

In 1976, a group of doctors who were practicing AK founded the International College of Applied Kinesiology (ICAK). The purpose of the ICAK is to promote teaching and research of AK. The college does not have physical buildings. Instead, it is an organization to bring together those in the health field with common interests and goals and to provide education in the use of AK. The organization has chapters representing Belgium, Luxembourg, and the Netherlands (BeNeLux), Germany, France, Italy, Germany, Scandanavia, United Kingdom, Canada, Australia and Asia (Australasia), and the United States.

AK is performed by a healthcare professional who has basic education in his or her field of practice. To become an applied kinesiologist, the healthcare professional must study the principles in a basic course, which includes 100 hours of classroom study taught by a diplomate of the ICAK. At the end of this course, students take a basic proficiency test. To obtain certification by the board of ICAK, the professional must complete 300 hours of continuing classes, pass a diplomate test (a comprehensive written and practical test), and present two research papers to the general membership of ICAK.

Resources

BOOKS

Holdway, Anne. *Kinesiology: Muscle Testing and Energy Balancing for Health and Well-Being.* Rockport, MA: Element, 1997.

Valentine, Tom, Carol Valentine, and D.P. Hetrick. *Applied Kinesiology.* Rochester, VT: Healing Arts Press, 1989.

ORGANIZATIONS

International College of Applied Kinesiology, 6405 Metcalf Ave., Suite 503, Shawnee Mission, KS, 66202, 913-384-5336, http://www.icakusa.com and http://www.icak.com.

Judith Sims

Apricot seed

Description

Apricot seed is the small kernel enclosed within the wood-like pit at the center of the apricot fruit. The apricot tree carries the botanical name *Prunus armeniaca*. It is a drupe, meaning stone-fruit, and a close relative of the peach. Both are very similar in appearance and qualities. The apricot is also sometimes called apricock or *Armeniaca vulgaris*. Like the plum, both peaches and apricots are distantly related to the rose and are classified as members of the Rosacaeae family.

Apricots grow on small to medium size trees, which are hardy in most temperate areas. White, multi-petaled blossoms with a slight reddish tinge nearer to the base of the flower emerge onto the bare branches in early spring, before the tree's heart-shaped leaves appear. By late July or early August, the apricot fruit ripens. There are more than 20 varieties of apricot known to botanists.

The name *Prunus armeniaca* is actually a misnomer based upon the long-held belief that apricots initially came from Armenia. It is now known that in reality they originated in the Far East, most likely in the Himalayas and Northern China. It is speculated that the apricot had already migrated to the Middle East before the Old Testament and that the apples described in the Garden of Eden in Genesis were actually apricots. During the reign of King Henry VIII in the 1500s, apricots were brought to England from Italy.

Though smaller than the peach, apricots have the same russet-tinted, golden, velvet appearing exterior and deeper golden-orange flesh inside. The innermost layers form the large, woody compressed stone, or pit, that contains at its very center, the kernel, or seed. When pressed, nearly half of this kernel gives forth an oil very chemically similar to the oil found in sweet almond and peach kernels. This oil contains olein, glyceride of **linoleic acid**, and a transparent, crystalline chemical compound, amygdalin, or laetrile. This compound is also known as vitamin B_{17}. The oil is chemically indistinguishable from oil of bitter almond. Although the oil from apricot seeds usually breaks down into a toxic substance capable of causing death within the human body, there are varieties of apricot seed that are reported to be edible.

General use

Because the oil from the apricot seed is far less expensive than oil of almond, confectioners use it in place of bitter almond oil for flavoring sweets and as a culinary seasoning. A liqueur manufactured in France is made from apricot seed and is called *Eau de Noyaux*. Apricot oil is also used extensively in the manufacture of cosmetics, often being fraudulently added to almond oil. It has skin softening properties and is often used in making soaps, hand creams, cold cream, and perfume preparations.

Chinese Medicine practitioners use apricot seed as a treatment in respiratory diseases, including **bronchitis** and **emphysema**. It is believed to act as an **cough** suppressant and expectorant and, because of the oil, also used as a laxative.

There has been considerable controversy regarding apricot seed, and specifically amygdalin, one of its components. Since the 1920s, in many countries around the globe it has been recognized as a possible **cancer** preventative and malignant cell growth inhibitor. In San Francisco biochemist Ernst Krebs's article *The Nitrilosides (Vitamin B_{17})-Their Nature, Occurrence and Metabolic Significance (Antineoplastic Vitamin B_{17})*, theorized that amygdalin, with diet and vitamins, could inhibit cancerous growths. In the years since, it has been used in many countries as a cancer treatment, thought to be especially beneficial in the treatment of smoking-related tumors such as **lung cancer**. Several studies done in the United States throughout the 1970s and early 1980s demonstrated that amygdalin did not kill cancer cells. Review of patients' records where there had been reported cures or remarkable size reduction in tumors did not provide credible evidence of amygdalin ability to treat cancer effectively. There has been significant documentation that amygdalin breaks down into cyanide, a potent poison, in the human body, and when taken in sufficiently high doses, can actually bring on death due to its toxicity.

Preparations

Apricot seed is not sold in American health food stores due to its classification as an unapproved drug by the U.S. Food and Drug Administration (FDA). However, it is available in other countries, including Mexico, and in Chinese pharmacies and Asian markets. It is sold both as the whole kernel or seed, or in decoctions including cough syrups. Chinese practitioners usually combine apricot seed with other herbs, including white mulberry leaf or **ophiopogon**, a tuber grown in Asia. A paste made of apricot seed and sugar has been shown, in some Chinese medical trials, to relieve chronic bronchitis.

Precautions

The amygdalin in apricot seed breaks down within the body into a form of the deadly poison cyanide, or prussic acid. There has been considerable debate concerning its level of toxicity to human beings. Following an Oklahoma judicial decision legalizing the importation of amygdalin in 1986, clinical trials were begun by the FDA and National Cancer Institute in 1987. Amygdalin was used, along with the diet, enzymes, and vitamins suggested by pro-amygdalin factions. The report from this study concludes: "No substantive benefit was observed in terms of cure, improvement, or stabilization of the cancer." They further reported that "the hazards of amygdalin therapy were

PERIODICALS

Krebs, Ernst T., Jr. "The Nitrilosides (Vitamin B-17)-Their Nature, Occurence and Metabolic Significance Antineoplastic Vitamin B-17)." *Journal of Applied Nutrition* 1970.

ORGANIZATIONS

U.S. Food and Drug Administration, HFI-40, Rockville, MD, 2085, 1-888-463-6332, webmail@oc.fda.gov, http://www.fda.gov/bbs/topics/ANSWERS/ANS00309.htm.

Joan Schonbeck

Arbor Vitae *see* **Thuja**

KEY TERMS

Expectorant—An agent that facilitates the removal of the secretions of the bronchopulmonary mucous membrane.

Unapproved drug—The FDA is responsible for ensuring that biological products are safe and effective and in compliance with the law and FDA regulations. Biological products are licensed under the provisions of Section 351 of the Public Health Service Act (42USC)(PHS Act).

---

evidenced in several patients by symptoms of cyanide toxicity or by blood cyanide levels approaching lethal range. Amygdalin is a toxic drug that is not effective as a cancer treatment." It has been reported that ten apricot seeds can kill a child.

Side effects

Chinese practitioners caution using apricot seed if the person being treated has **diarrhea**. **Headache** and **nausea** have been reported following ingestion of small amounts. The most serious side effect of apricot seed is potential cyanide poisoning. When large doses of cyanide are ingested, death is almost instantaneous. Toxicity from smaller doses is manifested by **vomiting**, diarrhea, mental confusion, vertigo, headache, extreme dyspnea, and violent respirations, slow pulse, weakness, glassy or protruding eyes, dilated pupils, and a characteristic (peach blossoms, bitter almond) odor to the breath.

Interactions

Practitioners of Chinese medicine advise that apricot seed should not be given in combination with the herbs **astragalus**, **skullcap**, or **kudzu** root.

Resources

BOOKS

Carper, Jean. *The Food Pharmacy*. Bantam Books, 1988.

Grieve, M. and C. F. Leyel. *A Modern Herbal: The Medical, Culinary, Cosmetic and Economic Properties, Cultivation and Folklore of Herbs, Grasses, Fungi, Shrubs and Trees With All of Their Modern Scientific Uses.* Barnes & Noble Publishing, 1992.

Holvey, David N., MD. *Merck Manual*. Sharp & Dohme Research Laboratories, 1972.

Taber, Clarence Wilbur. *Taber's Cyclopedic Medical Dictionary.* F.A. Davis Co.

Arginine

Description

Arginine is one of the **amino acids** produced in the human body by the digestion, or hydrolysis of proteins. Arginine can also be produced synthetically. Adult humans produce all the arginine they need from the food they eat. For this reason, arginine is usually called a nonessential amino acid. The term nonessential means that it is not necessary to add the amino acid to a person's diet because the body produces all that is needed. Infants, however, are unable to make arginine. Arginine must be added to their diet artificially. For this reason, arginine is also called a semi-essential amino acid. Arginine consists in two forms, called L-arginine and D-arginine. Molecules of the two compounds are mirror images of each other. Although they look very similar, they have different biological properties. The form of arginine most commonly encountered is L-arginine.

General use

Arginine has a number of important functions in the human body. For example, it removes potentially toxic ammonia from the body. Ammonia is formed when proteins are metabolized (broken down). It is then converted to arginine and other compounds for removal from the body by way of the excretory system. Arginine is also involved in cell division, facilitating operation of the immune system, promoting the production of white blood cells, making possible the release of hormones, and taking part in the manufacture of new proteins in the body. Arginine is also a major source of nitric oxide, a compound with a number of important functions in the body. Nitric oxide is a vasodilator, a substance that increases the size of blood vessels, allowing blood to flow more freely through the body. The connection between arginine and nitric oxide was explained by American researchers Robert F. Furchgott, Louis J. Ignarro, and Ferid Murad, who received the 1998 Nobel Prize in physiology or medicine for their studies. This research inspired more than a thousand additional studies on arginine and its relationship to nitric oxide and a variety of biological functions.

Arginine is a popular nutritional supplement because of its many biological properties:

- improves immune response to bacteria, viruses, and tumor cells
- promotes wound healing by repairing tissues
- plays a crucial role in the regeneration of liver
- responsible for release of growth hormones
- promotes muscle growth
- improves cardiovascular functioning

Arginine is used as a supplement in the treatment of heart patients with arterial **heart disease**, as an intravenous supplement to patients with liver dysfunction, and as a supplement for easing exercise-related pains due to the heart muscle not getting enough blood to circulate to the muscles in the calves. A 2000 study by researchers at the University of Leipzig in Germany confirmed the value of arginine in treating patients with chronic heart failure (CHF). The study showed that patients who took arginine had improved blood flow and reduced effects from CHF, whereas those who took arginine and exercised did even better. Supplements that combine arginine with other amino acids, such as ornithine and **lysine**, are purported to assist in muscle-building exercises by minimizing body fat and maximizing muscle tone. Results vary among those who have taken these supplements. Arginine is also present in multi-amino acids capsules that are taken as a dietary supplement.

New information released in 2002 showed that treatment with arginine improved immune function in HIV patients and proved safe for these patients when used short-term on patients. Other research found that arginine supplements worked as an effective anticoagulant, but unlike aspirin and other anticoagulants, could prevent clotting without increasing **stroke** risk. Other research in the 2000s showed arginine's effectiveness in fighting **cancer** and protecting and detoxifying the liver, improving male fertility, and promoting healing.

Preparations

Arginine supplements as an alternative medicine therapy are normally taken in either tablet or capsule form. In naturopathic treatment of liver dysfunction, the supplement is added intravenously as a powder diluted in liquid. Discoveries reported in 2000 indicated that in the treatment of arterial heart disease, the ingestion of arginine tablets or capsules of 6–9 g a day is helpful in dilating blood vessels to ease circulation and prevent the buildup of **cholesterol**.

Precautions

Long-term effects of arginine supplements had not been determined as of 2008. Consultation with a physician regarding individual needs is always advised. Individuals who attempt to treat their own heart ailments or intend to guard against any potential difficulty should seek advice of a physician. Arginine does not show any positive results in treatment of men with damaged valves or enlarged heart tissue.

Arginine has been suspected in the formation of cold sores. Some practitioners suggest that consuming foods high in arginine, such as nuts, grains, and chocolates, can promote cold sores. Reducing intake of foods high in arginine and increasing intake of lysine (another amino acid) can reduce or even eliminate the **cold sore** problem.

Side effects

The use of supplemental arginine should be monitored for use with specific problems. Overdose can result in unforeseen complications, whereas regular use might or might not help ease everyday problems, such as **relaxation** of muscles not due to the specific heart ailment of arterial disease. People who should not take arginine supplements are those predisposed to herpes outbreaks; cancer patients, due to possible increase in cell replication of cancerous cells; those with low blood pressure; and individuals with certain liver or kidney problems. Those taking blood thinners are advised to seek medical advice before taking the supplement. Pregnant women are also cautioned against taking the supplements due to the unknown effect it could have on both mother and fetus.

Interactions

Long-term studies are ongoing. While no adverse reactions of ordinary supplements of 6–9 g a day has been documented, caution is urged. Because amino acids are not drugs, their use is not regulated by the U.S. Food and Drug Administration (FDA). One study in April 1999 in *HealthInform: Essential Information on Alternative Health Care* reported that nutritional supplements of arginine with **omega-3 fatty acids** for outpatients with HIV showed no particular benefits in immunity.

Resources

PERIODICALS

Boeger, Rainer H., and E.S. Ron. "L-Arginine Improves Vascular Function by Overcoming the Deleterious Effects of ADMA, a Novel Cardiovascular Risk Factor." *Alternative Medicine Review* (March 2005): 14–23.

Facchinetti, Fabio, et al. "L-arginine Supplementation in Patients with Gestational Hypertension." *Hypertension in Pregnancy* (January 2007): 121–130.

Schulman, Steven P. "L-Arginine Therapy in Acute Myocardial Infarction." *JAMA* (January 2006): 58–64.

Wilson, Andrew M., et al. "L-Arginine Supplementation in Peripheral Arterial Disease." *Circulation* (July 2007): 188–195.

Jane Spehar
Teresa G. Odle
David Edward Newton, Ed.D.

Arka

Description

Arka is a perennial herb that is in the milkweed family Asclepediaceae (sometimes listed in the subfamily Asclepiadoideae of the family Apocynaceae. It comes in two primary forms—rakta arka (*Calotropis procera*) and sweta arka (*Calotropis gigantea*)—and a number of other less widely used forms. *Calotropis procera* and *Calotropis gigantea* are probably native to India or the Indian subcontinent, although they have spread throughout many areas of Southeast Asia and into Africa. The plants grow in open, often dry areas, including current and past farm fields, and along roadsides. They are often considered weeds and are very widespread. Arka is known by other names, such as yercum, wara, mudar, and mandara, among

many others. It is used in Ayurvedic traditional medicine in India and other folk/traditional remedies.

Plants in the genus *Calotropis* grow in tropical and subtropical Africa and Asia. *Calotropis gigantea* is also known as the crown flower, gigantic swallow wort, giant milkweed, or madar. It is a shrub that grows 8 to 10 ft (2.4–3 m) tall. Its flowers each have five petals of white to light-purple that curl downward from a crown-shaped center. It was introduced to Hawaii and elsewhere. *Calotropis procera* is also known as swallow-wort, apple of Sodom, roostertree, and French cotton. Its flower petals are frequently white toward the center and tipped in shades of pink or lavender. This shrubby plant grows 3 to 6 ft (1 to 2 m) tall. In North America, this plant occurs in California, Hawaii, and Puerto Rico.

Various parts of these two plants, and sometimes the entire plants, have been used in traditional/folk medicine to treat a wide range of ailments, including loss of appetite, respiratory difficulties and disorders, digestive problems, dysentery, **jaundice**, enlarged spleen, leprosy, migraine headaches, poisoning, rheumatism, **syphilis**, eye and ear diseases, **boils**, parasite infestation, chronic **hiccups**, scrofula (a type of **tuberculosis** on the neck) and other skin diseases, snake **bites**, scorpion **stings**, and the bone disorder known as caries. Arka has also been used to promote wound healing.

General use

Alternative medicine practitioners use arka in several ways. They use the dried whole plant as an expectorant to expel mucus and other material from the respiratory system, as a depurative or blood-purification agent, and as an anthelmintic, which combats parasitic **worms**. The dried root bark is used in the same ways as the dried whole plant and also to induce **vomiting**, to reduce **fever**, and as a laxative. Practitioners may prescribe powdered root to treat **asthma**, **bronchitis**, and dyspepsia (**indigestion**). The flowers of the plant are used to aid digestion and as an astringent, and the leaves are used to ease swellings and to reduce fever and also to treat paralysis and joint **pain**. The milky sap is used as an anti-inflammatory to treat various maladies.

Numerous studies of arka have been conducted, much of them since the 1980s. In 1988, for example, researchers examined an extract from the flower of *Calotropis procera* for its anti-inflammatory, fever-reducing (antipyretic), pain-relieving (analgesic), and microbe-fighting activities in rats. They found that it reduced inflammation-caused swelling by 37%, fever by 40%, and significantly decreased the growth of bacteria. Their study found weak analgesic effects, but a later study found that the root yielded a significant pain-relieving response when tested on rats. In 1994, researchers tested the milky sap, or latex, of the plant on rats. They mixed the dried latex in water and found that it significantly reduced inflammation. A study of the pain-relieving properties of latex solution in mice was conducted in 2000, and researchers found that it produced better results than did aspirin. They added, however, that the latex is toxic when taken internally.

Arka has also been shown to assist in wound-healing. Research showed substantial healing in **wounds** to guinea pigs when the animals were treated with a topical application of a solution of *Calotropis procera* latex. When compared with control animals after seven days, the researchers found that the wounds were smaller and the tissue had regenerated faster in the treated guinea pigs. In addition, various studies have shown that arka has antibacterial properties.

A study in 2001 showed that the dry latex of *Calotropis procera* is effective in treating **diarrhea**. In this study, the researchers tested the latex on rats and found that it not only eased existing diarrhea, but also prevented it. In addition, studies have shown that it can fight parasite infection. A study in 2005 demonstrated that powdered flowers of *Calotropis procera* were effective in fighting gastrointestinal nematodes found in sheep.

Studies have also considered arka and diabetes. According to a study published in 2005, dry latex of *Calotropis procera* was effective. The researchers reported, "The efficacy of [dry latex] as an antioxidant and as an anti-diabetic agent was comparable to the standard anti-diabetic drug, glibenclamide."

In addition to its antibacterial, anti-inflammatory, and other properties, arka has been shown to be effective as a sedative, as well as an anticonvulsant and an anti-anxiety agent. An extract made from the roots of *Calotropis gigantea* reduced pain, convulsions, and **anxiety** in rats, and also acted as a sedative.

Arka has an indirect health benefit, too. A study published in 2000 demonstrated that an extract of *Calotropis procera* was effective in killing the larvae of mosquitoes, which transmit numerous illnesses particularly in tropical regions. The researchers tested 16 different plant extracts and found that the extract of *Calotropis procera* latex was one of the most effective. This property, combined with the easy collection of the plant in certain regions of the world that have

mosquito-borne health problems, could make the latex a practical insecticide.

Preparations

Arka is available commercially as tinctures, pills and pellets, liquid solutions, granules, and ointments. In India and many other areas where it is used medicinally, the plants are widespread and sometimes collected by the patient or the herbalist. Dosage recommendations vary greatly depending on the condition and the preparation.

Precautions

Arka is toxic when taken internally. It should be used only under the close supervision of a qualified health-care professional. Anyone using arka products should inform their doctor.

Side effects

Plants in the milkweed family (or subfamily) contain compounds called cardiac glycosides, which are poisonous. In fact, some individuals have orally taken *Calotropis* to commit suicide or to initiate abortion. Extreme care should be taken when using arka, and patients should discuss the use of arka products with their doctor before using them. Topical applications may cause skin irritation.

Interactions

Some people have a reaction to the milky sap of various milkweed plants. In fact, a case study published in 2002 reported that arka appeared to be the cause of **blisters**, lesions, and ulcers at one patient. According to the report, a 79-year-old patient came to the doctor with blisters on his abdomen and back, lesions on his lips, and ulcers in his mouth after taking a regimen of burned *Calotropis procera* leaves to treat joint pain. After developing the symptoms, the patient continued the treatment on the advice of his doctor, but the symptoms worsened and he finally stopped the *Calotropis procera* treatment. After trying several remedies without success, the patient reported to the hospital where he received additional care and finally recovered.

KEY TERMS

Phytoalexin—A compound made by some plants to fight various microbes, such as bacteria, viruses, and fungi.

Phytochemical—A plant chemical.

Resources

BOOKS

Gruenwald, Joerg, Thomas Brendler, and Christof Jaenicke, eds. *PDR for Herbal Medicines,* 4th ed. London: Thomson Healthcare, 2007.

Karalliedde, Lakshman, Rita Fitzpatrick, and Debbie Shaw. *Traditional Herbal Medicines: A Guide to Their Safer Use.* London: Hammersmith Press, 2007.

Mars, Brigitte. *The Desktop Guide to Herbal Medicine: The Ultimate Multidisciplinary Reference to the Amazing Realm of Healing Plants, in a Quick-study, One-stop Guide.* Laguna Beach, CA: Basic Health Publications, 2007.

PERIODICALS

Ahmed, K. K. Mueen, A. C. Rana, and V. K. Dixit. "*Calotropis* Species (Ascelpediaceae)—A Comprehensive Review." *Pharmacognosy Magazine* 1, no. 2 (April/June 2005): 48–52. http://www.phcog.net/phcogmag/review_template.pdf (March 28, 2008).

Argal, Ameeta, and Anupam Kumar Pathak. "CNS activity of *Calotropis gigantea* roots." *Journal of Ethnopharmacology* 106, no. 1 (June 15, 2006): 142–145.

Iqbal, Zafar, Muhammad Lateef, Abdul Jabbar, Ghulam Muhammad, and Muhammad Nisar Khan. "Anthelmintic Activity of *Calotropis procera* (Ait.) Ait. F. Flowers in Sheep." *Journal of Ethnopharmacology* 102, no. 2 (November 14, 2005): 256–261.

Roy, S., R. Sehgal, B. M. Padhy, and V. L. Kumar. "Antioxidant and Protective Effect of Latex of *Calotropis procera* against Alloxan-induced Diabetes in Rats." *Journal of Ethnopharmacology* 102, no. 3 (December 1, 2005): 470–473.

OTHER

"*Calotropis gigantea* (*L.*) R.BR." Medicinal Plants of Conservation Concern. http://envis.frlht.org. [cited March 28, 2008].

"*Calotropis procera* R.BR." Medicinal Plants of Conservation Concern. http://envis.frlht.org. (April 12, 2008).

Leslie Mertz, Ph.D.

Arnica

Description

Arnica (*Arnica montana L.*), known also as leopardsbane, wolfsbane, and European arnica, is a member of the Compositae (Asteraceae) family. This attractive herb is native to the mountains of Siberia

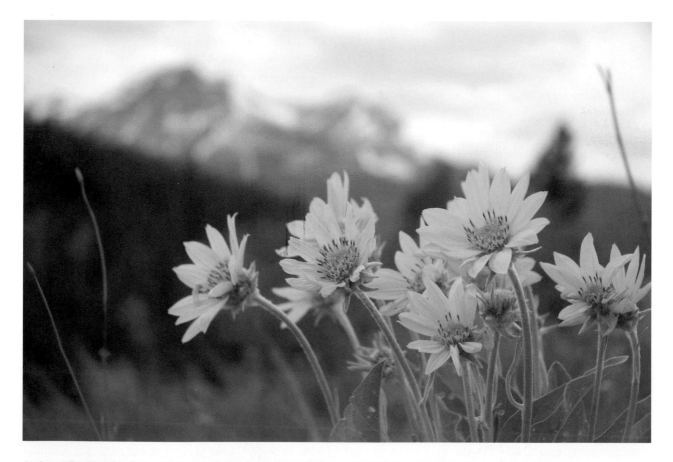

Arnica, a Rocky Mountain wild flower. *(Image copyright Kris Butler, 2008. Used under license from Shutterstock.com.)*

and central Europe, where the leaves were smoked as a substitute for tobacco. This practice led to a common name for the herb: mountain tobacco. There are several North American species of arnica, including *A. fulgens*, *A. sororia*, and *A. cordifolia*. Arnica thrives in the northern mountains of the United States and Canada, in high pastures and woodlands.

Arnica grows from a cylindrical, hairy rhizome with a creeping underground stem. First year leaves are downy and grow in a flat rosette at the base of the stem. In the second year, arnica sends up a round, hairy stem with smaller, sessile leaves growing in one to three opposite pairs. This central stem may branch into three or more stems each with a terminal composite blossom. Arnica's aromatic, daisy-like flowers have 10–14 bright yellow rays, each with three notches at the end. Flower rays are irregularly bent back. The central disk is composed of tubular florets. Arnica blooms from June to August. The flowerheads, when crushed and sniffed, may cause **sneezing**, resulting in another of arnica's common names: sneezewort.

History

Arnica has a history of folk medicine use in many locations, including North America, Germany, and Russian. The herb has been used in folk remedies since the 16th century. A North American indigenous tribe, the Cataulsa, prepared a tea from arnica roots to ease back pains. The German writer Goethe credited arnica with saving his life by bringing down a persistent high **fever**. Arnica preparations are used extensively in Russia. Folk use there includes external treatment of **wounds**, black eye, **sprains**, and contusions. Arnica has been used in Russian folk medicine to treat uterine hemorrhage, myocarditis, arteriosclerosis, **angina** pectoris, cardiac insufficiency, and in numerous other unproven applications.

General use

Arnica flowers, fresh or dried, are used medicinally. Many herbalists consider arnica to be a specific remedy for **bruises**, sprains, and sore muscles. The herb is known by some as "tumbler's cure all," reflecting this common medicinal use. A compress soaked in an arnica infusion may relieve the inflammation of **phlebitis**. A few drops of arnica tincture added to warm water in a foot bath will relieve **fatigue** and soothe sore feet. A hair rinse prepared with arnica extract has been used to treat alopecia neurotica, an **anxiety** condition leading to **hair loss**. The very dilute homeopathic preparation ingested following a shock or muscle/soft tissue trauma is said to be beneficial.

The homeopathic preparation is also used to relieve vertigo, hoarseness, and seasickness. Studies have determined that arnica has properties that act as an immunostimulant. The extract of arnica has been shown to stimulate the action of white blood cells in animal studies, increasing resistance to bacterial **infections**, such as salmonella.

German studies have isolated sesquiterpenoid lactones, including helenalin and dihydrohelenalin, in arnica. These compounds were found to possess the pharmacologic properties responsible for arnica's anti-inflammatory and analgesic effects. Arnica contains sesquiterpene lactones, flavonoid glycosides, alkaloid, volatile oil, tannin, and isomeric alcohol, including arnidio and foradiol.

Arnica is approved for external use as an anti-inflammatory, analgesic, and antiseptic by the German Commission E, an advisory panel on herbal medicines. There are over one hundred medicinal preparations using arnica extracts commercially available in Germany. In the United States, arnica is widely used in topical application for bruises, aches, sprains, and inflammations. Arnica was listed in the *U.S. Pharmacopeia* from the early 1800s until 1960.

Preparations

Arnica is available commercially in the form of liniments and massage oil for external application, and in very dilute homeopathic preparations considered safe for internal use.

Harvest fully open arnica blossoms throughout the flowering season. Pick the flower heads on a sunny day after the morning dew has evaporated. Spread the blossoms on a paper-lined tray to dry in a bright and airy room away from direct sun. Temperature in the drying room should be at least 70°F (21.1°C). When the blossoms are completely dry, store in a dark glass container with an air-tight lid. The dried herb will maintain medicinal potency for 12–18 months. Clearly label the container with the name of the herb and the date and place harvested.

Tincture: Combine four ounces of fresh or dried arnica flowers with one pint of brandy, gin, or vodka in a glass container. The alcohol should be enough to cover the flowers. The ratio should be close to 50/50 alcohol to water. Stir and cover. Place the mixture in a dark cupboard for three to five weeks. Shake the mixture several times each day. Strain and store in a tightly capped, clearly labeled, dark glass bottle. Tinctures, properly prepared and stored, will retain medicinal potency for two years or more. Arnica tincture should not be ingested without supervision of a qualified herbalist or physician.

Ointment: Simmer one ounce of dried and powdered arnica flowers with one ounce of olive oil for several hours on very low heat. Combine this medicinal oil with melted beeswax to desired consistency. Pour into dark glass jars while still warm. Seal with tightly fitting lids when cool and label appropriately.

Infusion: Place two to three teaspoons of chopped, fresh arnica blossoms in a warmed glass container. Bring two cups of fresh, nonchlorinated water to the boiling point, add it to the herbs. Cover. Simmer for about 10 minutes. Strain. The prepared tea will store for about two days in the refrigerator. The infusion may be used to bathe unbroken skin surfaces and to provide relief for rheumatic **pain**, chillbains, bruises, and sprains. Because of the toxicity of arnica, it is best to avoid internal use without qualified medical supervision.

Precautions

Arnica is deadly in large quantities. Do not ingest the herb or the essential oil. Do not use the undiluted essential oil externally. The extremely dilute homeopathic preparation of arnica is considered safe for internal use in proper therapeutic dosages. Overdose of arnica extract has resulted in poisoning, with toxic symptoms such as **vomiting**, **diarrhea**, and hemorrhage, even death. Use externally with caution, and only in dilute preparations. Only the homeopathic tincture can be safely ingested. Discontinue if a skin rash results, and do not use on broken skin. Research has confirmed that alcoholic extracts of arnica have a toxic action on the heart, and can cause an increase in blood pressure.

Side effects

Arnica contains a compound known as helenalin, an allergen that may cause **contact dermatitis** in some persons. If a rash develops discontinue use of the herbal preparation. Prolonged external use of arnica extract in high concentrations can result in blistering, skin ulcers, and surface necroses.

Interactions

None reported.

Resources

BOOKS

Elias, Jason, and Shelagh Ryan Masline. *The A to Z Guide to Healing Herbal Remedies.* Lynn Sonberg Book Associates, 1996.

Hoffmann, David. *The New Holistic Herbal.* 2d ed. Massachusetts: Element, 1986.

Kowalchik, Claire, and William H. Hylton. *Rodale's Illustrated Encyclopedia of Herbs.* Pennsylvania: Rodale Press, 1987.

Lust, John. *The Herb Book.* New York: Bantam Books, 1974.

Magic And Medicine of Plants. The Reader's Digest Association, Inc. 1986.

Meyer, Joseph E. *The Herbalist.* Clarence Meyer, 1973.

Palaise, Jean. *Grandmother's Secrets, Her Green Guide to Health From Plants.* NY: G.P. Putnam's Sons, 1974.

PDR for Herbal Medicines. New Jersey: Medical Economics Company, 1998.

Phillips, Roger, and Nicky Foy. *The Random House Book of Herbs.* New York: Random House, Inc., 1990.

Thomson, M.D., William A. R. *Medicines From The Earth, A Guide to Healing Plants.* San Francisco: Harper & Row, 1978.

Tyler, Varro E., Ph.D. *Herbs Of Choice, The Therapeutic Use of Phytomedicinals.* New York: The Haworth Press, Inc., 1994.

Tyler, Varro E., Ph.D. *The Honest Herbal.* New York: Pharmaceutical Products Press, 1993.

OTHER

Grieve, Mrs. M. "A Modern Herbal, Arnica." http://botanical.com/botanical/mgmh/a/arnic058.html.

Hoffmann, David L. "Herbal Materia Medica, Hyssop." http://www.healthy.net.

Clare Hanrahan

Aromatherapy

Definition

Aromatherapy is the therapeutic use of plant-derived, aromatic **essential oils** to promote physical and psychological well-being. It is sometimes used in combination with massage and other therapeutic techniques as part of a holistic treatment approach.

Origins

Aromatic plants have been employed for their healing, preservative, and pleasurable qualities throughout recorded history in both the East and West. As early as 1500 B.C. the ancient Egyptians used waters, oils, incense, resins, and ointments scented with botanicals for their religious ceremonies.

There is evidence that the Chinese may have recognized the benefits of herbal and aromatic remedies much earlier than this. The oldest known herbal text,

Aromatherapy oils

Name	Description	Conditions treated
Bay laurel	Antiseptic, diuretic, sedative, etc.	Digestive problems, bronchitis, common cold, influenza, and scabies and lice. CAUTION: Don't use if pregnant
Clary sage	Relaxant, anti-convulsive, anti-inflammatory, and antiseptic	Menstrual and menopausal symptoms, burns, eczema, muscle pain and tension, and anxiety. CAUTION: Don't use if pregnant.
Chamomile	Sedative, anti-inflammatory, anti-spasmodic, antiseptic, and pain reliever	Hay fever, burns, acne, arthritis, digestive problems, menstrual and menopausal symptoms, insomnia, and anxiety.
Eucalyptus	Antiseptic, antibacterial, astringent, expectorant, analgesic, and stimulant	Boils, breakouts, cough, common cold, influenza, and sinusitis. CAUTION: Not to be taken orally.
Lavender	Analgesic, antiseptic, calming/soothing, and carminative	Headache, depression, insomnia, stress, sprains, and nausea.
Peppermint	Pain reliever, carminative, anti-inflammatory, anti-spasmodic, analgesic	Indigestion, nausea, headache, motion sickness, muscle pain, ulcerative conditions of the bowels, and tension.
Rosemary	Antiseptic, circulatory and nervine stimulant, diuretic, carminative, anti-spasmodic, and emmenagogue	Indigestion, gas, bronchitis, fluid retention, influenza, and headache. CAUTION: Don't use if pregnant or have epilepsy or hypertension.
Tarragon	Diuretic, laxative, anti-spasmodic, and stimulant	Menstrual and menopausal symptoms, gas, and indigestion. CAUTION: Don't use if pregnant.
Tea tree	Antiseptic and soothing	Common cold, bronchitis, abscesses, acne, vaginitis, and burns.
Thyme	Stimulant, antiseptic, anti-microbial anti-spasmodic, carminative, astringent, expectorant, and anthelmintic	Cough, laryngitis, tonsillitis, coughs, diarrhea, gas, and intestinal worms. CAUTION: Don't use if pregnant or have hypertension.

(Illustration by Corey Light. Cengage Learning, Gale)

Shen Nung's *Pen Ts'ao* (c. 2700-3000 B.C.) catalogs over 200 botanicals. Ayurveda, a practice of traditional Indian medicine that dates back more than 2,500 years, also used aromatic herbs for treatment.

The Romans were well known for their use of fragrances. They bathed with botanicals and integrated them into their state and religious rituals. So did the Greeks, with a growing awareness of the medicinal properties of herbs. Greek physician and surgeon Pedanios Dioscorides, whose renown herbal text *De Materia Medica* (60 A.D.) was the standard textbook for Western medicine for 1,500 years, wrote extensively on the medicinal value of botanical aromatics. The *Medica* contained detailed information on some 500 plants and 4,740 separate medicinal uses for them, including an entire section on aromatics.

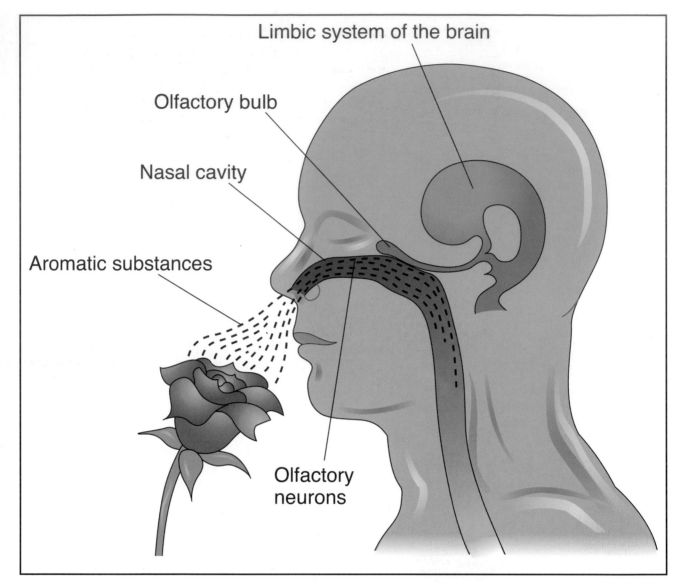

Limbic system of the brain

Olfactory bulb

Nasal cavity

Aromatic substances

Olfactory neurons

As a holistic therapy, aromatherapy is believed to benefit both the mind and body. Here, the aromatic substances from a flower stimulates the olfactory bulb and neurons. The desired emotional response (such as relaxation) is activated from the limbic system of the brain. *(Illustration by GGS Information Services. Cengage Learning, Gale)*

Written records of herbal distillation are found as early as the first century A.D., and around 1000 A.D., the noted Arab physician and naturalist Avicenna described the distillation of rose oil from rose petals, and the medicinal properties of essential oils in his writings. However, it wasn't until 1937, when French chemist René-Maurice Gattefossé published *Aromatherapie: Les Huiles essentielles, hormones végé tales*, that aromatherapie, or aromatherapy, was introduced in Europe as a medical discipline. Gattefossé, who was employed by a French perfumeur, discovered the healing properties of **lavender** oil quite by accident when he suffered a severe burn while working and used the closest available liquid, lavender oil, to soak it.

In the late 20th century, French physician Jean Valnet used botanical aromatics as a front line treatment for wounded soldiers in World War II. He wrote about his use of essential oils and their healing and antiseptic properties, in his 1964 book *Aromatherapie, traitement des maladies par les essences des plantes*, which popularized the use of essential oils for medical and psychiatric treatment throughout France. Later, French biochemist Mauguerite Maury popularized the cosmetic benefits of essential oils, and in 1977 Robert Tisserand wrote the first English language book on the subject, *The Art of Aromatherapy*, which introduced massage as an adjunct treatment to aromatherapy and sparked its popularity in the United Kingdom.

Benefits

Aromatherapy offers diverse physical and psychological benefits, depending on the essential oil or oil combination and method of application used. Some common medicinal properties of essential oils used in aromatherapy include: analgesic, antimicrobial, antiseptic, anti-inflammatory, astringent, sedative, antispasmodic, expectorant, diuretic, and sedative. Essential oils are used to treat a wide range of symptoms and conditions, including, but not limited to, gastrointestinal discomfort, skin conditions, menstrual **pain** and irregularities, stress-related conditions, mood disorders, circulatory problems, respiratory **infections**, and **wounds**.

Description

In aromatherapy, essential oils are carefully selected for their medicinal properties. As essential oils are absorbed into the bloodstream through application to the skin or inhalation, their active components trigger certain pharmalogical effects (e.g., pain relief).

In addition to physical benefits, aromatherapy has strong psychological benefits. The volatility of an oil, or the speed at which it evaporates in open air, is thought to be linked to its specific psychological effect. As a rule of thumb, oils that evaporate quickly are considered emotionally uplifting, while slowly-evaporating oils are thought to have a calming effect.

Essential oils commonly used in aromatherapy treatment include:

- Roman chamomile (*Chamaemelum nobilis*). An anti-inflammatory and analgesic. Useful in treating otitis media (earache), skin conditions, menstrual pains, and depression.
- Clary sage (*Salvia sclarea*). This natural astringent is not only used to treat oily hair and skin, but is also said to be useful in regulating the menstrual cycle, improving mood, and controlling high blood pressure. Clary sage should not be used by pregnant women.
- Lavender (*Lavandula officinalis*). A popular aromatherapy oil that mixes well with most essential oils, lavender has a wide range of medicinal and cosmetic applications, including treatment of insect bites, burns, respiratory infections, intestinal discomfort, nausea, migraine, insomnia, depression, and stress.
- Myrtle (*Myrtus communis*). Myrtle is a fungicide, disinfectant, and antibacterial. It is often used in steam aromatherapy treatments to alleviate the symptoms of whooping cough, bronchitis, and other respiratory infections.
- Neroli (bitter orange), (*Citrus aurantium*). Citrus oil extracted from bitter orange flower and peel and used to treat sore throat, insomnia, and stress and anxiety-related conditions.
- Sweet orange (*Citrus sinensis*). An essential oil used to treat stomach complaints and known for its reported ability to lift the mood while relieving stress.
- Peppermint (*Mentha piperita*). Relaxes and soothes the stomach muscles and gastrointestinal tract. Peppermint's actions as an anti-inflammatory, antiseptic, and antimicrobial also make it an effective skin treatment, and useful in fighting cold and flu symptoms. In addition, research in 2002 found that peppermint scent helped athletes run faster and perform more push-ups than control subjects with odorless strips under their noses.
- Rosemary (*Rosmarinus officinalis*). Stimulating essential oil used to treat muscular and rheumatic complaints, as well as low blood pressure, gastrointestinal problems, and headaches. Recently. Brain scans have shown that fragrance of rosemary increases blood circulation in the brain.
- Tea tree (*Melaleuca alternifolia*). Has bactericidal, virucidal, fungicidal, and anti-inflammatory properties that make it a good choice for fighting infection. Recommended for treating sore throat and respiratory infections, vaginal and bladder infections, wounds, and a variety of skin conditions.
- Ylang ylang (*Cananga odorata*). A sedative essential oil sometimes used to treat hypertension and tachycardia.

Essential oils contain active agents that can have potent physical effects. While some basic aromatherapy home treatments can be self-administered, medical aromatherapy should always be performed under the guidance of an aromatherapist, herbalist, massage therapist, nurse, or physician.

Inhalation

The most basic method of administering aromatherapy is direct or indirect inhalation of essential oils. Several drops of an essential oil can be applied to a tissue or handkerchief and gently inhaled. A small amount of essential oil can also be added to a bowl of hot water and used as a steam treatment. This technique is recommended when aromatherapy is used to treat respiratory and/or skin conditions. Aromatherapy steam devices are also available commercially. A warm bath containing essential oils can have the same effect as steam aromatherapy, with the added benefit of promoting **relaxation**. When used in a bath, water should be lukewarm rather than hot to slow the evaporation of the oil.

Essential oil diffusers, vaporizers, and light bulb rings can be used to disperse essential oils over a large area. These devices can be particularly effective in aromatherapy that uses essential oils to promote a healthier home environment. For example, **eucalyptus** and **tea tree oil** are known for their antiseptic qualities and are frequently used to disinfect sickrooms, and citronella and geranium can be useful in repelling insects.

Direct application

Because of their potency, essential oils are diluted in a carrier oil or lotion before being applied to the skin to prevent an allergic skin reaction. The carrier oil can be a vegetable or olive based one, such as **wheat germ** or avocado. Light oils, such as safflower, sweet almond, grapeseed, hazelnut, **apricot seed**, or peach kernel, may be absorbed more easily by the skin. Standard dilutions of essential oils in carrier oils range from 2–10%. However, some oils can be used at higher concentrations, and others should be diluted further for safe and effective use. The type of carrier oil used and the therapeutic use of the application may also influence how the essential oil is mixed. Individuals should seek guidance from a healthcare professional and/or aromatherapist when diluting essential oils.

Massage is a common therapeutic technique used in conjunction with aromatherapy to both relax the body and thoroughly administer the essential oil treatment. Essential oils can also be used in hot or cold compresses and soaks to treat muscle aches and pains (e.g., lavender and **ginger**). As a **sore throat** remedy, antiseptic and soothing essential oils (e.g., tea tree and **sage**) can be thoroughly mixed with water and used as a gargle or mouthwash.

Internal use

Some essential oils can be administered internally in tincture, infusion, or suppository form to treat certain symptoms or conditions; however, this treatment should never be self-administered. Essential oils should only be taken internally under the supervision of a qualified healthcare professional.

As non-prescription botanical preparations, the essential oils used in aromatherapy are typically not paid for by health insurance. The self-administered nature of the therapy controls costs to some degree. Aromatherapy treatment sessions from a professional aromatherapist are not covered by health insurance in most cases, although aromatherapy performed in conjunction with physical therapy, nursing, therapeutic massage, or other covered medical services may be covered. Individuals should check with their insurance provider to find out about their specific coverage.

The adage "You get what you pay for" usually applies when purchasing essential oils, as bargain oils are often adulterated, diluted, or synthetic. Pure essential oils can be expensive; and the cost of an oil will vary depending on its quality and availability.

Preparations

The method of extracting an essential oil varies by plant type. Common methods include water or steam distillation and cold pressing. Quality essential oils should be unadulterated and extracted from pure botanicals. Many aromatherapy oils on the market are synthetic and/or diluted, contain solvents, or are extracted from botanicals grown with pesticides or herbicides. To ensure best results, essential oils should be made from pure organic botanicals and labeled by their full botanical name. Oils should always be stored in dark bottles out of direct light.

Before using essential oils on the skin, individuals should perform a skin patch test by applying a small amount of the diluted oil behind the wrist and covering it with a bandage or cloth for up to 12 hours. If redness or irritation occurs, the oil should be diluted further and a second skin test performed, or it should be avoided altogether. Individuals should never apply undiluted essential oils to the skin unless advised to do so by a trained healthcare professional.

Precautions

Individuals should only take essential oils internally under the guidance and close supervision of a health care professional. Some oils, such as eucalyptus, **wormwood**, and sage, should never be taken internally. Many essential oils are highly toxic and should not be used at all in aromatherapy. These include (but are not limited to) bitter almond, **pennyroyal**, mustard, **sassafras**, rue, and **mugwort**.

Citrus-based essential oils, including bitter and sweet orange, lime, lemon, grapefruit, and tangerine, are phototoxic, and exposure to direct sunlight should be avoided for at least four hours after their application.

Other essential oils, such as cinnamon leaf, black pepper, **juniper**, lemon, white camphor, eucalyptus blue gum, ginger, **peppermint**, pine needle, and **thyme** can be extremely irritating to the skin if applied in high enough concentration or without a carrier oil or lotion. Caution should always be exercised when applying essential oils topically. Individuals should never apply undiluted essential oils to the skin unless directed to do so by a trained healthcare professional and/or aromatherapist.

Individuals taking homeopathic remedies should avoid black pepper, camphor, eucalyptus, and peppermint essential oils. These oils may act as a remedy antidote to the homeopathic treatment.

Children should only receive aromatherapy treatment under the guidance of a trained aromatherapist or healthcare professional. Some essential oils may not be appropriate for treating children, or may require additional dilution before use on children.

Certain essential oils should not be used by pregnant or nursing women or by people with specific illnesses or physical conditions. Individuals suffering from any chronic or acute health condition should inform their healthcare provider before starting treatment with any essential oil.

Asthmatic individuals should not use steam inhalation for aromatherapy, as it can aggravate their condition.

Essential oils are flammable, and should be kept away from heat sources.

Side effects

Side effects vary by the type of essential oil used. Citrus-based essential oils can cause heightened sensitivity to sunlight. Essential oils may also cause **contact dermatitis**, an allergic reaction characterized by redness and irritation. Anyone experiencing an allergic reaction to an essential oil should discontinue its use and contact their healthcare professional for further guidance. Individuals should do a small skin patch test with new essential oils before using them extensively.

Research and general acceptance

The antiseptic and bactericidal qualities of some essential oils (such as tea tree and peppermint) and their value in fighting infection has been detailed extensively in both ancient and modern medical literature.

Recent research in mainstream medical literature has also shown that aromatherapy has a positive psychological impact on patients. Several clinical studies involving both post-operative and chronically ill subjects showed that massage with essential oils can be helpful in improving emotional well-being, and consequently, promoting the healing process.

Today, the use of holistic aromatherapy is widely accepted in Europe, particularly in Great Britain,

---

KEY TERMS

Antiseptic—Inhibits the growth of microorganisms.

Bactericidal—An agent that destroys bacteria (e.g., *Staphylococci aureus*, *Streptococci pneumoniae*, *Escherichia coli*, *Salmonella enteritidis*).

Carrier oil—An oil used to dilute essential oils for use in massage and other skin care applications.

Contact dermatitis—Skin irritation as a result of contact with a foreign substance.

Essential oil—A volatile oil extracted from the leaves, fruit, flowers, roots, or other components of a plant and used in aromatherapy, perfumes, and foods and beverages.

Holistic—A practice of medicine that focuses on the whole patient, and addresses the social, emotional, and spiritual needs of a patient as well as their physical treatment.

Phototoxic—Causes a harmful skin reaction when exposed to sunlight.

Remedy antidote—Certain foods, beverages, prescription medications, aromatic compounds, and other environmental elements that counteract the efficacy of homeopathic remedies.

Steam distillation—A process of extracting essential oils from plant products through a heating and evaporation process.

Volatile—Something that vaporizes or evaporates quickly when exposed to air.

---

where it is commonly used in conjunction with massage as both a psychological and physiological healing tool. In the United States, where aromatherapy is often misunderstood as solely a cosmetic treatment, the mainstream medical community has been slower to accept its use.

Training and certification

Certification or licensing is currently not required to become an aromatherapist in the United States; however, many states require that healthcare professionals who practice the "hands-on" therapies often used in conjunction with aromatherapy (e.g., massage) to be licensed. There are state-licensed educational institutions that offer certificates and/or diplomas in aromatherapy training. Individuals interested in aromatherapy treatment from a professional aromatherapist may be able to obtain a referral from one of these institutions, or from their current healthcare provider.

Resources

BOOKS

Lawless, Julia. *The Complete Illustrated Guide To Aromatherapy*. Rockport, MA: Element Books Ltd, 1997.

Schnaubelt, Kurt. *Medical Aromatherapy: Healing With Essential Oils*. Berkeley, CA: Frog Ltd, 1999.

PERIODICALS

Claps, Frank. "Training Scents: You May be Able to Sniff Your Way to Better Workouts With Tricks from the Aromatherapist's Bag." *Men's Fitness* (May 2002): 34.

Stanten, Michele, and Selene Yeager. "Smell this for Instant Energy: the Easiest Way to Boost your Workouts. (Fitness News)." *Prevention* (April 2002): 76.

ORGANIZATIONS

National Association of Holistic Aromatherapy, 836 Hanley Industrial Court, St. Louis, MO, 63144, , 888-ASK-NAHA, http://www.naha.org.

Paula Ford-Martin
Teresa G. Odle

Arrowroot

Description

Growing to a height of up to 6 ft (2 m), arrowroot is a tropical perennial with clusters of long, thin stems and small, cream-colored flowers that grow in pairs. Once revered by the ancient Mayans and other inhabitants of Central America as an antidote for poison-tipped arrows, the herb is mainly used today to soothe the stomach and alleviate **diarrhea**. It has also been popular for centuries in the culinary arts and is still used in many American kitchens as a thickening agent. While arrowroot is native to Central America and widely cultivated in the West Indies, it can also be found growing in many tropical regions of the world, including Southeast Asia, South Africa, Australia, and in Florida in the United States. The Latin genus *Maranta* was derived from the name of an Italian doctor, Bartommeo Maranto.

Arrowroot, which belongs to the Marantaceae plant family, is widely considered an easily digested and nutritious starch. The herb is extracted from the fleshy roots, called rhizomes, of the arrowroot plant through an elaborate process of washing, peeling, soaking, and drying in the sun. The end product is a fine, white powder with the same appearance and texture as cornstarch. Arrowroot is valued by herbalists primarily for its demulcent and antidiarrheal properties. Exactly how it produces its therapeutic effects is not known. The chemical composition of the herb has not been thoroughly investigated.

While only *Maranta arundinacea* is considered true arrowroot, the common name for the herb is often applied to a variety of starches. These include other species of *Maranta*, such as *Maranta ramosissima*, *Maranta allouya*, *Maranta nobilis*, as well as Brazilian arrowroot (*Manihot utilissima* or *Manihot palmate*), Tahitian arrowroot (*Tacca oceanica*), and East Indian arrowroot (*Curcuma augustifolia*). While some of these starches may be chemically similar to true arrowroot, it is not clear if they produce the same medicinal effects. Consumers interested in trying arrowroot are advised to choose *Maranta arundinacea*, which is sometimes referred to as West Indian arrowroot or simply Maranta.

Research is still required to determine if arrowroot can produce significant health benefits safely and effectively. The proper dosage of the herb has also yet to be determined.

General use

While not approved by the United States Food and Drug Administration (FDA), arrowroot is thought to have several beneficial effects. However, there is little scientific evidence to support these claims. The herb is primarily used to soothe an uneasy stomach and alleviate diarrhea or **nausea** and **vomiting**. Since it contains **calcium** and carbohydrates as well as other nutrients, arrowroot is also used as an easily digested source of **nutrition** for infants, people recovering from illnesses (especially those with bowel problems), and those on restricted diets. The herb is considered easier on the stomach than other forms of starch.

Because arrowroot has not been studied extensively in people or animals, its effectiveness is based mainly on its reputation as a folk remedy. Despite the lack of scientific evidence, some practitioners of alternative medicine consider it useful for certain conditions. Alternative physicians praise the stomach-soothing powers of arrowroot as well as its nutritional value. Another prominent herbalist recommends arrowroot for preventing athlete's foot. Putting the dried powder inside socks and shoes can help to combat the moisture that contributes to the growth of foot fungus. However, arrowroot is not known to have antifungal properties.

Arrowroot was popular in the past as an antidote for arrow poison. It also had a reputation as a treatment for scorpion and spider **bites** as well as **gangrene**. However, there is no scientific evidence to support these uses. In cases of poisoning, the local poison control center or an emergency care center should be contacted immediately.

Aside from its medicinal uses, arrowroot is still used in cooking. Much like cornstarch, arrowroot is used as a thickener for sauces, soups, and confections.

Preparations

The optimum daily dosage of arrowroot has not been established with any certainty. Consumers should follow the package directions for proper use or consult a doctor experienced in the use of alternative remedies. Arrowroot powder, which is basically flavorless, is often mixed with juice or other beverages before ingestion.

Precautions

Arrowroot is not known to be harmful when taken in recommended dosages. However, it is important to remember that the long-term effects of taking the herb (in any amount) have not been investigated. Due to the lack of sufficient medical research, arrowroot should be used with caution in children, women who are pregnant or breast-feeding, and people with liver or kidney disease.

People who experience vomiting or severe/prolonged diarrhea may be prone to dehydration. They should drink plenty of water (six to eight glasses a day) in order to maintain a proper fluid balance. A doctor should be consulted if the vomiting or diarrhea lasts longer than three days or is accompanied by other symptoms such as **pain** or fever.

Side effects

When taken in recommended dosages, arrowroot is not associated with any significant side effects.

Interactions

Arrowroot is not known to interact adversely with any drug or dietary supplement. It has been combined with milk, lemon and other fruit juices, sugar, and wine without apparent harm.

To avoid **constipation**, consumers should not take arrowroot with other medications or dietary supplements used to alleviate diarrhea.

KEY TERMS

Calcium—A mineral necessary for strong bones and the proper functioning of organs and muscles.

Demulcent—A gelatinous or oily substance that has a protective or soothing influence on irritated mucous membranes.

Gangrene—Localized tissue death caused by lack of blood.

Rhizome—A relatively long and thick plant root that can be distinguished from normal roots by the presence of buds, nodes, or other characteristics.

Resources

BOOKS

Gruenwald, Joerg. *PDR for Herbal Medicines*. New Jersey: Medical Economics, 1998.

PERIODICALS

Rolston D. D., P. Mathew, and V. I. Mathan. "Food-Based Solutions Are a Viable Alternative to Glucose-Electrolyte Solutions for Oral Hydration in Acute Diarrhoea-Studies in a Rat Model of Secretory Diarrhoea." *Transactions of the Royal Society of Tropical Medicine and Hygiene* 84, no. 1 (1990): 156-159.

OTHER

Botanical.com. http://www.botanical.com

ORGANIZATIONS

American Botanical Council, P.O. Box 144345, Austin, TX, 78714-4345.

Greg Annussek

Arsenicum album

Description

Arsenicum album is a homeopathic remedy derived from the metallic element arsenic. Traces of arsenic are found in vegetables and animals. In its crude form, arsenic is poisonous. Gradual accumulations may result in digestive disturbances, **nausea**, **vomiting**, **diarrhea**, dehydration, coma, shock, convulsions, paralysis, and death.

Common names for arsenicum album include arsenic trioxide, white arsenic, white oxide of metallic arsenic, and arsenius acid. Arsenic is indestructible, even by fire, and remains in bone ash after cremation. It has been used to create pigmentation for wallpaper, carpet, and paints. Arsenic has also been used to produce medicines and pesticides.

Arsenic was used as a remedy for certain types of cattle disease as far back as the eighth century. In the seventeenth century, arsenic was applied topically to treat malignant ulcers and skin diseases in humans. Taken internally, it was used to treat fevers. When frequent and repeated doses of arsenic resulted in poisoning and death, arsenic was pronounced unsafe for use. However, housewives and practitioners still used arsenic and were often successful in their treatments. Eventually arsenic use was reinstated. Weak compounds of arsenic were often used to increase strength and endurance, remedy **anemia**, and improve the skin and fur of animals. An ointment made from arsenic was used to treat cancerous growths and tumors.

General use

Arsenicum album is one of the most frequently used homeopathic remedies and is one of the most well-proven remedies. A polychrest with a wide field of action, arsenicum album has the power to affect all parts of the human body.

Arsenicum album is used to treat serious acute ailments, chronic diseases, and acute colds, **bronchitis**, and fevers. Homeopaths prescribe this remedy to treat **asthma**, **anxiety** disorders, panic attacks, skin **infections**, **boils**, **burns** with **blisters**, cystitis, eye inflammations, **chickenpox**, colds, coughs, **indigestion**, **Crohn's disease**, herpes simplex, flu, **insomnia**, **measles**, **mumps**, sore throats, **allergies** and **hay fever**, **food poisoning**, and fevers. Arsenicum album has also been used to treat malarial and septic infections, **alcoholism**, **syphilis**, lupus, and **cancer** (when applied in the early stages of the disease).

Arsenicum album illnesses can be brought about by the use of quinine, tobacco, or alcohol, or from the suppression of skin eruptions, sweat, or mucous membrane discharges.

Common characteristics

People requiring arsenicum album generally fit a particular profile. They are anxious, restless, weak, pale, emaciated, faint, chilled, and catch colds easily. Their eyes are sunken and glassy; their face is yellowish or ashy pale, and mouth, lips, and tongue are parched and dry. They desire liquids in small, frequent amounts. The forehead, face, chest, knees, hands, and feet are often cold, so patients crave warmth. They may suffer from burning, pressing pains throughout the entire body. These pains are aggravated by cold and reduced by heat. Weakness is sudden and is reduced by lying down, although the other symptoms are worsened by it.

Other physical characteristics of this remedy include burning, offensive, and watery discharges; palpitations; profuse, sour sweat; and a red-tipped tongue. There is a tendency to bleed easily and from any place, and vomiting of blood and bleeding from lungs, throat, and mucous membranes are not uncommon.

The mental and emotional symptoms of the patient profile also include anxiety, nervousness, suspicion, impulsiveness, irritability, sadness, hopelessness, and **depression**. People requiring this remedy are often difficult patients. They are critical and argumentative, easily offended, easily startled, insecure, forgetful, sensitive to **pain**, and often suffer from delusions or hallucinations. They think their ailment is more serious than it is and despair of ever getting well, often fearing that they are going to die. They desire company and are afraid of being alone. Patients may be unable to sleep due to their restlessness and anxiety or from physical discomforts such as **fever** or **cough**. When they do sleep, they may have anxious dreams or nightmares. Even though they are extremely weak, arsenicum album patients are clean and tidy, partially to relieve their restlessness.

The symptoms are aggravated by a change in temperature, wet weather, cold food and drink, and by the slightest exertion. They are worse after midnight, upon waking, with alcohol use, and during **menstruation**. Symptoms are improved by heat, hot beverages, the warmth of the bed, fresh air, and lying down.

Arsenicum album is a useful remedy for mental disorders with symptoms of melancholy, irritation, intense anxiety, and restlessness. The patient may be prone to violent fits of anger or rage or have an impulse to commit murder. It also can have a positive effect on alcoholism and can improve diarrhea, weakness, stomach irritation, and emaciation.

Specific indications

Arsenicum album can be used for the following conditions:

- Throbbing, frontal headaches. These are accompanied by a flushed or hot face, heat or burning inside the head, and a feeling that the head will explode. These headaches occur with regularity and are reduced by cool air or cold applications.
- Herpetic or eczematous skin eruptions. These are moist, scabby, pustular, itching, or burning.
- Hot, burning fevers. These sometimes alternate with chills. Fevers are worse at night, particularly after midnight.
- Sore throat. It is accompanied by burning pain that is worse from swallowing or cold drinks and is reduced with hot drinks.
- Hacking coughs. These are frequently dry at night and are relieved by hot drinks. They are worsened by the cold, by fresh air, when lying down, at night (particularly after midnight), and during a fever.
- Chronic nasal congestion. This is often accompanied by bleeding, constant sneezing, chills, fatigue, restlessness, anxiety at night, troublesome dreams, and crusts in the back of the nose.

Preparations

The homeopathic remedy is prepared by separating arsenic from **iron**, cobalt, and nickel when the minerals are baked at high temperatures. The powder is then ground and diluted with milk sugar.

Arsenicum album is available at health food and drug stores in various potencies in the form of tinctures, tablets, and pellets.

Precautions

If symptoms do not improve after the recommended time period, a homeopath or healthcare practitioner should be consulted.

Consumers are advised not to exceed the recommended dose.

Side effects

There are no side effects currently reported.

Interactions

When taking any homeopathic remedy, consumers should not use **peppermint** products, coffee, or alcohol. These products may cause the remedy to be ineffective.

Resources

BOOKS

Cummings, Stephen, M.D., and Ullman, Dana, M.P.H. *Everybody's Guide to Homeopathic Medicines.* New York: Jeremy P. Tarcher/Putnam, 1997.

Kent, James Tyler. *Lectures on Materia Medica.* Delhi, India. B. Jain Publishers, 1996.

Jennifer Wurges

Art therapy

Definition

Art therapy, sometimes called creative arts therapy or expressive arts therapy, encourages people to express and understand emotions through artistic expression and through the creative process.

Origins

Humans have expressed themselves with symbols throughout history. Masks, ritual pottery, costumes, other objects used in rituals, cave drawings, Egyptian hieroglyphics, and Celtic art and symbols are all visual records of self-expression and communication through art. Art has also been associated spiritual power, and artistic forms such as the Hindu and Buddhist mandala and Native American sand painting are considered powerful healing tools.

In the late nineteenth century, French psychiatrists Ambrose Tardieu and Paul-Max Simon both published studies on the similar characteristics of and symbolism in the artwork of the mentally ill. Tardieu and Simon viewed art therapy as an effective diagnostic tool to identify specific types of mental illness or traumatic events. Later, psychologists would use this diagnostic aspect to develop psychological drawing tests (the Draw-A-Man test, the Draw-A-Person Questionnaire [DAP.Q]) and projective personality tests involving visual symbol recognition (e.g., the Rorschach Inkblot Test, the Thematic Apperception Test [TAT], and the Holtzman Inkblot Test [HIT]).

The growing popularity of milieu therapies at psychiatric institutions in the twentieth century was an important factor in the development of art therapy in the United States. Milieu therapies (or **environmental therapy**) focus on putting the patient in a controlled therapeutic social setting that provides the patient with opportunities to gain self-confidence and interact with peers in a positive way. Activities that encourage self-discovery and empowerment such as art, music, dance, and writing are important components of this approach.

Educator and therapist Margaret Naumburg was a follower of both Freud and Jung, and incorporated art into **psychotherapy** as a means for her patients to visualize and recognize the unconscious. She founded the Walden School in 1915, where she used students' artworks in psychological counseling. She published extensively on the subject and taught seminars on the technique at New York University in the 1950s. Today, she is considered the founder of art therapy in the United States.

In the 1930s, Karl, William, and Charles Menninger introduced an art therapy program at their Kansas-based psychiatric hospital, the Menninger Clinic. The Menninger Clinic employed a number of artists in residence in the following years, and the facility was also considered a leader in the art therapy movement through the 1950s and 60s. Other noted art therapy pioneers who emerged in the 50s and 60s include Edith Kramer, Hanna Yaxa Kwiatkowska (National Institute of Mental Health), and Janie Rhyne.

Benefits

Art therapy provides the client-artist with critical insight into emotions, thoughts, and feelings. Key benefits of the art therapy process include:

- Self-discovery. At its most successful, art therapy triggers an emotional catharsis.

- Personal fulfillment. The creation of a tangible reward can build confidence and nurture feelings of self-worth. Personal fulfillment comes from both the creative and the analytical components of the artistic process.

- Empowerment. Art therapy can help people visually express emotions and fears that they cannot express through conventional means, and can give them some sense of control over these feelings.

- Relaxation and stress relief. Chronic stress can be harmful to both mind and body. Stress can weaken and damage the immune system, can cause insomnia and depression, and can trigger circulatory problems (like high blood pressure and irregular heartbeats). When used alone or in combination with other relaxation techniques such as guided imagery, art therapy can effectively relieve stress.

- Symptom relief and physical rehabilitation. Art therapy can also help patients cope with pain. This therapy can promote physiological healing when patients identify and work through anger, resentment, and other emotional stressors. It is often prescribed to accompany pain control therapy for chronically and terminally ill patients.

Description

Art therapy, sometimes called expressive art or art psychology, encourages self-discovery and emotional growth. It is a two part process, involving both the creation of art and the discovery of its meaning. Rooted in Freud and Jung's theories of the subconscious and unconscious, art therapy is based on the assumption that visual symbols and images are the most accessible and natural form of communication to the human experience. Patients are encouraged to visualize, and then create, the thoughts and emotions that they cannot talk about. The resulting artwork is then reviewed and its meaning interpreted by the patient.

The "analysis" of the artwork produced in art therapy typically allows patients to gain some level of insight into their feelings and lets them to work through these issues in a constructive manner. Art therapy is typically practiced with individual, group, or family psychotherapy (talk therapy). While a therapist may provide critical guidance for these activities, a key feature of effective art therapy is that the patient/ artist, not the therapist, directs the interpretation of the artwork.

Art therapy can be a particularly useful treatment tool for children, who frequently have limited language skills. By drawing or using other visual means to express troublesome feelings, younger patients can begin to address these issues, even if they cannot identify or label these emotions with words. Art therapy is also valuable for adolescents and adults who are unable or unwilling to talk about thoughts and feelings.

Beyond its use in mental health treatment, art therapy is also used with traditional medicine to treat organic diseases and conditions. The connection between mental and physical health is well documented, and art therapy can promote healing by relieving **stress** and allowing the patient to develop coping skills.

Art therapy has traditionally centered on visual mediums, like paintings, sculptures, and drawings. Some mental healthcare providers have now broadened the definition to include music, film, dance, writing, and other types of artistic expression.

Art therapy is often one part of a psychiatric inpatient or outpatient treatment program, and can take place in individual or group therapy sessions. Group art therapy sessions often take place in hospital, clinic, shelter, and community program settings. These group therapy sessions can have the added benefits of positive social interaction, empathy, and support from peers. The client-artist can learn that others have similar concerns and issues.

Preparations

Before starting art therapy, the therapist may have an introductory session with the client-artist to discuss art therapy techniques and give the client the opportunity to ask questions about the process. The client-artist's comfort with the artistic process is critical to successful art therapy.

The therapist ensures that appropriate materials and space are available for the client-artist, as well as an adequate amount of time for the session. If the individual artist is exploring art as therapy without the guidance of a trained therapist, adequate materials, space, and time are still important factors in a successful creative experience.

The supplies used in art therapy are limited only by the artist's (and/or therapist's) imagination. Some of the materials often used include paper, canvas, poster board, assorted paints, inks, markers, pencils, charcoals, chalks, fabrics, string, adhesives, clay, wood, glazes, wire, bendable metals, and natural items (like shells, leaves, etc.). Providing artists with a variety of materials in assorted colors and textures can enhance their interest in the process and may result in a richer, more diverse exploration of their emotions in the resulting artwork. Appropriate tools such as scissors, brushes, erasers, easels, supply trays,

glue guns, smocks or aprons, and cleaning materials are also essential.

An appropriate workspace should be available for the creation of art. Ideally, this should be a bright, quiet, comfortable place, with large tables, counters, or other suitable surfaces. The space can be as simple as a kitchen or office table, or as fancy as a specialized artist's studio.

The artist should have adequate time to become comfortable with and explore the creative process. This is especially true for people who do not consider themselves "artists" and may be uncomfortable with the concept. If performed in a therapy group or one-on-one session, the art therapist should be available to answer general questions about materials and/or the creative process. However, the therapist should be careful not to influence the creation or interpretation of the work.

Precautions

Art materials and techniques should match the age and ability of the client. People with impairments, such as traumatic brain injury or an organic neurological condition, may have difficulties with the self-discovery portion of the art therapy process depending on their level of functioning. However, they may still benefit from art therapy through the sensory stimulation it provides and the pleasure they get from artistic creation.

While art is accessible to all (with or without a therapist to guide the process), it may be difficult to tap the full potential of the interpretive part of art therapy without a therapist to guide the process. When art therapy is chosen as a therapeutic tool to cope with a physical condition, it should be treated as a supplemental therapy and not as a substitute for conventional medical treatments.

Research and general acceptance

A wide body of literature supports the use of art therapy in a mental health capacity. And as the mind-body connection between psychological well-being and physical health is further documented by studies in the field, art therapy gains greater acceptance by mainstream medicine as a therapeutic technique for organic illness.

Training and certification

Both undergraduate and graduate art therapy programs are offered at many accredited universities across the United States. Typical art therapy programs combine courses in art and psychology. The majority of these programs meet or exceed standards set by the American Art Therapy Association (AATA).

The Art Therapy Credentials Board (ATCB), a voluntary organization, grants the designation ATR (Art Therapist Registered) to professionals who have completed an approved master's level program of study in art therapy (as described by the AATA) and have accumulated at least 1,000 hours of additional supervised clinical experience. Board certification is also available through the ATCB for art therapists who have met the ATR requirements and have passed a certification exam (ATR-BC). Art therapists with the ATR-BC designation must complete continuing education credits to maintain their certification.

Registration and/or certification is a recognition of professional expertise, not a legal qualification or requirement to practice. Professional licensing requirements for art therapists vary by state. However, if the therapy is intended as a companion treatment to psychological counseling or other mental health treatment, state licensing requirements typically apply. Where licensing is a prerequisite to practice, a combination of education and clinical experience, a written test, and continuing education are required to maintain the license.

Resources

BOOKS

Fausek, Diane. *A Practical Guide to Art Therapy*. Binghamton, New York: Haworth Press, 1997.

Ganim, Barbara. *Art and Healing: Using expressive art to heal your body, mind, and spirit*. New York: Three Rivers Press, 1999.

Malchiodi, Cathy A. *The Art Therapy Sourcebook*. Los Angeles: Lowell House, 1998.

McNiff, Shaun. *Art as Medicine: Creating a Therapy of the Imagination*. Boston: Shambhala, 1992.

ORGANIZATIONS

American Art Therapy Association.1202 Allanson Rd., Mundelein, IL 60060-3808. 888-290-0878 or 847-949-6064. Fax: 847-566-4580. E-mail: arttherapy@ntr.net *www.arttherapy.org*.

Paula Ford-Martin

Arthritis *see* Osteoarthritis; Rheumatoid arthritis

Artichoke

Definition

The artichoke is a perennial plant with purple flowers. Although the artichoke is regarded as a vegetable, the edible portion of the plant is actually the unopened flower bud. Artichoke leaves and roots have been used as remedies to treat conditions ranging from **irritable bowel syndrome** to the prevention of hangovers caused by the consumption of alcohol.

Description

Cynara scolymus is the botanical name for the artichoke, a thistle plant that produces one of the oldest known foods. According to mythology, the Greek god Zeus fell in love with a beautiful woman named Cynara. Zeus transformed her into a goddess and took Cynara to live with him. Cynara did not like her new home and wanted to return to Earth. That angered Zeus. The god sent her home, but Zeus transformed Cynara into the world's first artichoke plant.

The artichoke, a member of the daisy (*Asteraceae*) family, is native to Mediterranean countries in southern Europe, northern Africa, and the Canary Islands. Ancient people recognized the value of the artichoke as both a food and a remedy. Greeks and Romans regarded the artichoke as a delicacy and a treatment for digestive troubles. They also viewed the artichoke as an aphrodisiac, an aid used to enhance romantic feelings and sex drive. Greeks thought that taking artichoke was a remedy for women who wanted to give birth to sons.

There are more than 50 artichoke varieties. These varieties do not include the Jerusalem artichoke, which is a tuber.

The only artichoke grown in the United States is the green globe. Spanish settlers brought the artichoke to the New World during the 1880s, and 80% of green globes are grown in Castroville, California. The town calls itself the "Artichoke Capital of the World." Castroville was among the first to recognize a woman who would become a twentieth century movie goddess. The actress Marilyn Monroe served as the first California Artichoke Queen, a title she received in 1949.

As a food, a medium artichoke contains 25 calories and 3 grams of fiber. It is also a source of **vitamin C**, the B vitamin foliate, and **magnesium**. The leaves contain cynarin, a plant compound that small studies showed may help to lower **cholesterol**.

General use

Considering the legend surrounding the creation of the artichoke, it may not be surprising that the artichoke was considered an aphrodisiac. However, it also served as a folk medicine treatment for a range of other conditions. Over the years, the artichoke was used as a remedy for **anemia**, arthritis and rheumatism, **gallstones**, **gout**, **indigestion**, **itching**, and snakebite.

Contemporary uses of artichoke

Artichoke leaf extract has been used as a remedy for conditions including irritable bowel syndrome, cholesterol management, and hangovers. Other uses include treating indigestion and appetite loss. The artichoke is thought to stimulate bile, the fluid secreted by the liver. By stimulating bile, artichoke leaf extract might provide relief for indigestion.

Artichoke leaf has been approved for some of those conditions in the German Commission E Monographs, a guide to herbal remedies. Those approved uses are the treatment of liver and gallbladder conditions and appetite loss.

In the United States, artichoke leaf is marketed as a dietary supplement because the herbal remedy has not been evaluated by the United States Food and Drug Administration (FDA). The lack of FDA review means that artichoke leaf has not been proven to be safe or effective. Furthermore, ingredients are not standardized to comply with federal regulations.

In 2007, the *American Journal of Health-System Pharmacy* highlighted some of the research into the use of artichoke leaf extract as a remedy for irritable bowel syndrome, cholesterol management, and alcohol-induced hangovers.

IRRITABLE BOWEL SYNDROME. Irritable bowel syndrome is a condition affecting the digestive tract. Symptoms include abdominal bloating, **pain**, and **gas**. In addition, a person may experience **constipation**, **diarrhea**, or both symptoms. Irritable bowel syndrome symptoms may increase during a stressful time or after a person eats.

In a study of 208 people diagnosed with irritable bowel syndrome, the participants were assessed two months before and after treatment with 320 mg or 640 mg of artichoke leaf extract. During the follow-assessment, participants reported a 26.4% decrease in irritable bowel syndrome, according to the *American Journal of Health-System Pharmacy*. The dosage strength did not make a significant difference in the outcome.

The study concluded that artichoke leaf extract may alleviate some symptoms associated with irritable bowel syndrome or dyspepsia (impaired digestion). Furthermore, the *Mayo Clinic Book of Alternative Medicine* noted that a small study "suggests" that artichoke leaf extract could help relieve irritable bowel symptoms.

CHOLESTEROL. Artichoke leaf extract has been marketed as a product that may balance LDL (low-density lipoprotein), which is also known as bad cholesterol. However, studies as of February 2008 had not proven the effectiveness of artichoke on cholesterol management.

HANGOVER. A **hangover** is caused by the body's reaction to alcohol, a substance that is toxic. The amount of alcohol that produces a hangover varies with each person. Hangover symptoms include an intense **headache**, **fatigue**, and dehydration.

Artichoke leaf extract has been marketed as remedy to prevent hangovers. However, the medical community was skeptical about this claim. Small studies showed little proof that artichoke leaf extract was effective at preventing hangovers.

Preparation

Herbal artichoke is available in capsule and extract form. Capsule strength ranges from 170 mg to 320 mg, so people should follow the directions on the product package. The average capsule dosage is 600 mg per day, and the daily artichoke leaf extract dose is about 500 mg per day. People should discuss the dosage with their doctor or health practitioner. This is especially important for women who are pregnant or breastfeeding, and people diagnosed with conditions including diabetes, high blood pressure, liver blockage, and heart or blood vessel disease.

Precautions

Artichoke leaf extract has not been evaluated by the FDA, so its safety and effectiveness have not been established. In addition, ingredients of herbal remedies are not standardized to comply with federal regulations.

Due to the lack of information about the safety of artichoke leaf extract, it should not taken by children under the age of 12, pregnant women, and nursing mothers. In addition, the safety of this remedy has not been determined for people with severe kidney and liver diseases.

Furthermore, people diagnosed with bile-duct obstruction or gallstones should not use artichoke extract as a remedy. The herb could stimulate bile, causing those medical conditions to worsen.

Moreover, artichoke in both herbal form and as a food should be avoided by people who are allergic to daisies, ragweed, chrysanthemums, and marigolds.

Interactions

There are known interactions with artichoke.

Resources

BOOKS

Balch, James, and Mark Stengler. *Prescription for Natural Cures: A Self-care Guide for Treating Health Problems with Natural Remedies, Including Diet and Nutrition, Nutritional Supplements, Bodywork, and More.* John Wiley & Sons, 2004.

Mayo Clinic. *Mayo Clinic Book of Alternative Medicine.* Time Inc. Home Entertainment, 2007.

PERIODICALS

Bundy R., AF Walker, RW Middleton, et al. "Artichoke Leaf Extract Reduces Symptoms Of Irritable Bowel Syndrome And Improves Quality Of Life In Otherwise Healthy Volunteers Suffering From Concomitant Dyspepsia: A Subset Analysis." *The Journal Of Alternative And Complementary Medicine* 10, no. 4 (2004): 667–669.

Joy, Jamie Foster, Stacy L. Haber. "Clinical Uses Of Artichoke Leaf Extract." *American Journal of Health-System Pharmacy.* (September 15, 2007): 1904–1909.

Webb, Denise. "Mysteries of the Artichoke: Fabulous Flavor, Surprising Nutrition." *Environmental Nutrition.* (September 2005): 8.

OTHER

Heubeck, Elizabeth. "Strategies for a Hangover-Free Holiday Season." WebMD Weight Loss Clinic - Feature (December 9, 2004). http://www.medicinenet.com/script/main/art.asp?articlekey=55900 (February 1, 2008).

Holistic Online.com. http://holisticonline.com (Feb. 1, 2008).

ORGANIZATIONS

American Botanical Council, 6200 Manor Rd, Austin, TX, 78723, (512) 926-4900, http://abc.herbalgram.org.

Liz Swain

Ascorbic acid *see* **Vitamin C**

Ashwaganda

Description

Ashwaganda, also spelled ashwagandha, is a member of the pepper family known as *Withania somnifera.* The small evergreen grows in the frost-free drier parts of western India, northern Africa, the Mediterranean, and the Middle East. Ashwaganda grows to a height of 2–3 ft (about 1 m) and has oval leaves, showy yellow flowers, and red, raisin-sized fruits. All parts of the plant, including the root, are used medicinally. Ashwaganda is also called winter cherry, withania, asgandh, and Indian ginseng.

General use

Ashwaganda is a major herb in the Ayurvedic system of health and healing. **Ayurvedic medicine** is a system of individualized healing derived from

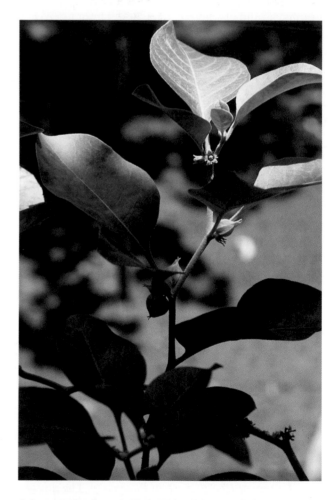

Ashwaganda plant. *(©PlantaPhile, Germany. Reproduced by permission.)*

Hinduism that has been practiced in India for more than 2,000 years. It is a complex system that recognizes different human temperaments and body types. Each of these types has different qualities that affect a person's health and natural balance.

In Ayurvedic medicine, disease can result from any of seven major categories of factors: heredity, congenital, internal, external trauma, seasonal, habits, or supernatural factors. Disease can also be caused by misuse of the five senses: sight, touch, taste, hearing, and smell. Diagnoses are made through questioning, observation, examination, and interpretation. Health is restored by evaluating the exact cause of the imbalance causing the disease or condition and then prescribing herbs, exercises, diet changes and/or **meditation** to help restore the natural balance of body, mind, and spirit. Prescriptions are highly individualized, so that the same symptoms may require different remedies in different people.

Ashwaganda is used to treat a great many different conditions in Ayurvedic medicine. Every part of the plant is used: leaves, fruit, flowers, and root. In addition, the young shoots and seeds are used as food and to thicken plant milks in the making of vegan cheeses. The fruit can be used as a substitute for soap, and the leaves are sometimes used as an insect repellent. Although ashwaganda can be taken alone, it is more often combined with other herbs in tonics to enhance its rejuvenating effects.

Indian ginseng

Ashwaganda is sometimes called the Indian ginseng because its actions and uses are in many ways similar to those of Chinese ginseng, although its cost is much lower. In Hindi, the name of ashwaganda means "horse smell." This unromantic name refers less to the herb's odor than to a horse's strength and health. Ashwaganda is supposed to impart that same horse-like strength to the people who use it.

Ashwaganda is an adaptogen. Adaptogens are substances that non-specifically enhance and regulate the body's ability to withstand **stress** and increase its general performance in ways that help the whole body resist disease. Ashwaganda is celebrated as an adaptogen that will do all of the following:

- boost strength
- increase stamina and relieve fatigue
- enhance sexual energy and rejuvenate the body
- strengthen the immune system
- speed recovery from chronic illness
- strengthen sickly children

- soothe and calm without producing drowsiness
- clarify the mind and improve memory
- slow the aging process

The powdered root of ashwaganda is normally used for whole body tonics that improve general health and well being. For most of these uses, ashwaganda is prepared as part of a *rasayana*, or rejuvenating formula that contains many different herbs. The use of ashwaganda in multi-herb formulas makes it difficult for modern laboratory scientists to assess its specific effects as an adaptogen.

Disease-specific uses

In addition to the whole body effects of ashwaganda, the plant is used for many other specific conditions. Different parts are used for different conditions. Ashwaganda is one of the most frequently used remedies in India. It is taken internally for:

- anemia
- arthritis
- asthma

- bronchitis
- cancer
- chronic fatigue syndrome
- colds
- coughs
- depression
- diarrhea
- fluid retention
- hemorrhoids
- hypertension
- hypoglycemia
- leprosy
- nausea
- rheumatism
- sexually transmitted diseases
- stomach ulcers
- systemic lupus erythematosus
- tuberculosis
- tumors

Ashwaganda can also be made into a poultice for external use, as it is thought to have antibacterial and antifungal properties. It is used to prevent infection in skin **wounds** and to treat skin diseases, including **psoriasis**, ringworm, and **scabies**.

Laboratory studies

University and medical researchers have been studying ashwaganda since at least the early 1960s. Chemical analysis shows that ashwaganda contains compounds thought to have anti-tumor, anti-inflammatory, and anti-fungal properties. Other compounds have been isolated that are associated with ashwaganda's sedative and anti-stress effects.

The most rigorous laboratory tests have been done in test tubes and on rats, mice, and other small laboratory animals. There is no proof that ashwaganda affects humans in the same way that it affects rodents. In animal studies, however, ashwaganda has been shown to have consistent anti-inflammatory, anti-fungal, anti-stress, and sedative effects. In one well-known study, extracts of ashwaganda root were shown to significantly increase the swimming endurance of rats in a test that is considered a classic stress test.

Experimenters have had mixed results in demonstrating anti-tumor and anti-cancer properties of ashwaganda. Many have found that extracts of ashwaganda root slow the growth of tumor cells in test-tube and small-animal experiments, but these results have not yet been reproduced in human subjects. Some researchers report that ashwaganda makes tumors more sensitive to chemotherapy and radiation therapy without increasing side effects caused by these therapies.

Although there is little doubt that ashwaganda contains biologically active compounds that produce some of the healing effects in humans that have been found in test tube and small animal studies, few controlled studies using people have been done. One drawback to arriving at conclusive evidence in humans is that most people take ashwaganda as part of a multiherb tonic, making it difficult for researchers to attribute specific actions to any one particular component of the formula. Scientific interest in ashwaganda is high, and laboratory studies continue to be performed.

Preparations

Ashwaganda is available in many forms, including powders, decoctions, essential oil, tinctures, and teas made from the root, root bark, and the leaves. Commercially ashwaganda is available as capsules. The usual capsule dosage is 300 mg of powdered root, taken once or twice a day. Tincture dosage is often 2–4 ml (0.5–1 tsp) daily. Ashwaganda tea can be made by boiling the roots for about 15 minutes. Three cups a day is recommended. The fruit is often chewed to assist in convalescence from prolonged illness. These are simply representative doses and uses, since Ayurvedic medicine is highly individualized. The dose recommended depends on both the body type of the person and the nature of his or her illness.

Precautions

Ashwaganda is not recommended for use by pregnant women. Thousands of years of use have shown that this plant is quite safe. On the other hand, laboratory tests indicate that rats given high levels of ashwaganda root extract develop kidney lesions. This effect has not been seen in humans, but using the herb in moderation may be prudent.

Ashwaganda has a sedative effect on the central nervous system. It will enhance the effect of any other central nervous system sedatives (e.g., barbiturates or alcohol) that are taken at the same time. People operating heavy equipment or working in situations that require a high level of alertness should keep this in mind when using ashwaganda.

Side effects

No undesirable side effects have been reported with ashwaganda.

Interactions

There are few, if any, studies of how ashwaganda interacts with traditional Western medicines. It has been used for many years in combination with other Ayurvedic herbs without incident. Ayurvedic practitioners believe that when ashwaganda is combined with other herbs in rejuvenation formulas, it enhances the effects of these other herbs.

Resources

BOOKS

Chevallier, Andrew. *Encyclopedia of Medicinal Plants.* London: Dorling Kindersley, 1996.

Peirce, Andrea. *The American Pharmaceutical Association Practical Guide to Natural Medicines.* New York: William Morrow and Company, 1999.

ORGANIZATIONS

American School of Ayurvedic Sciences, 2115 112th Avenue NE, Bellevue, WA 98004, (425) 453-8002.

The Ayurvedic Institute, P. O. Box 23445, Albuquerque, NM 87112, (505) 291-9698.

OTHER

Plants for the Future: Withania somnifera aphrodisiaca. http://www.metalab.unc.edu.

Tish Davidson

Asthma

Definition

Asthma is a chronic inflammatory disease of the airways in the lungs. This inflammation periodically causes the airways to narrow, which produces **wheezing** and breathlessness, sometimes to the point where the patient gasps for air. This obstruction of the air flow either stops spontaneously or responds to a wide range of treatments. Continuing inflammation makes asthmatics hyper-responsive to such stimuli as cold air, **exercise**, dust, pollutants in the air, and even **stress** or **anxiety**.

Description

The American Academy of Allergy Asthma and Immunology (AAAAI) estimates that about 20 million Americans have asthma. That number has been rising since 1980. AAAAI also reports that nine million U.S. children under age 18 have been diagnosed with asthma. African Americans, Hispanics,

---

Inhaled allergens most often triggering asthma attacks

Air pollutants (e.g. tobacco smoke, strong odors, scented products)

Animal dander

Cockroach allergens

Dust mites

Indoor fungi (molds)

Occupational allergens such as chemicals, fumes, particles of industrial materials

Pollen

(Illustration by Corey Light. Cengage Learning, Gale)

Occupations associated with asthma

Animal handling

Bakeries

Cleaning workers

Health care

Jewelry making

Laboratory work

Manufacturing detergents

Nickel plating

Soldering

Snow crab and egg processing

Tanneries

SOURCE: Occupational Safety and Health Administration, U.S. Department of Labor

(Illustration by Corey Light. Cengage Learning, Gale)

American Indians, and Alaskan natives all have higher rates of asthma than whites or Asians in the United States.

The changes that take place in the lungs of asthmatics make their airways (the bronchi and the smaller bronchioles) hyper-reactive to many different types of stimuli that do not affect healthy lungs. In an asthma attack, the muscle tissue in the walls of the bronchi goes into spasm, and the cells that line the airways swell and secrete mucus into the air spaces. Both these actions cause the bronchi to narrow, a change that is called bronchoconstriction. As a result, an asthmatic person has to make a much greater effort to breathe.

Cells in the bronchial walls, called mast cells, release certain substances that cause the bronchial muscle to contract and stimulate mucus formation. These substances, which include histamine and a group of chemicals called leukotrienes, also bring white blood cells into the area. Many patients with asthma are prone to react to substances such as pollen, dust, or animal dander. Substances that produce this reaction are called allergens. Many people with asthma do not realize that allergens are triggering their attacks. However, asthma also affects many patients who are not allergic in this way.

Asthma usually begins in childhood or adolescence, but it also may first appear in adult life. While the symptoms may be similar, certain important aspects of asthma are different in children and adults. When asthma begins in childhood, it often does so in a child who is likely, for genetic reasons, to become sensitized to common allergens in the environment. Such a child is known as an atopic person. In 2004, scientists in Helsinki, Finland, identified two new genes that cause atopic asthma. The discovery may lead to earlier prediction of asthma in children and adults. When these children are exposed to dust, animal proteins, fungi, or other potential allergens, they produce a type of antibody that is intended to engulf and destroy the foreign materials, which has the effect of making the airway cells sensitive to particular materials. Further exposure can lead rapidly to an asthmatic response. This condition of atopy is present in at least one-third and as many as one-half of the general population. When an infant or young child wheezes during viral **infections**, the presence of allergy (in the child or a close relative) is a clue that asthma may well continue throughout childhood. A third asthma gene was discovered in 2007 by a group of scientists from London, France, Germany, and the University of Michigan. The presence of the gene increases a person's chance of contracting asthma by at least 60%.

Allergenic materials may also play a role when adults become asthmatic. Asthma can start at any age and in a wide variety of situations. Many adults who are not allergic have such conditions as sinusitis or nasal polyps, or they may be sensitive to aspirin and related drugs. Another major source of adult asthma is exposure at work to animal products, certain forms of plastic, wood dust, metals, and environmental pollution.

Causes and symptoms

In most cases, asthma is caused by inhaling an allergen that sets off the chain of biochemical and tissue changes leading to airway inflammation, bronchoconstriction, and wheezing. Because avoiding (or at least minimizing) exposure is the most effective way of treating asthma, it is vital to identify the allergen or irritant causing symptoms in a particular patient. Once asthma is present, symptoms can be set off or made worse if the patient also has **rhinitis** (inflammation of the lining of the nose) or sinusitis. The reaction called acid reflux, when stomach acid passes back up the esophagus, can make asthma worse. In addition, a viral infection of the respiratory tract can inflame an asthmatic reaction. Aspirin and drugs called beta-blockers, often used to treat high blood pressure, also can worsen the symptoms of asthma. But the most important inhaled allergens giving rise to attacks of asthma are as follows:

- animal dander
- dust mites
- fungi (molds) that grow indoors
- cockroach allergens
- pollen
- occupational exposure to chemicals, fumes, or particles of industrial materials
- tobacco smoke
- air pollutants

In addition, there are three important factors that regularly produce attacks in certain asthmatic patients, and they may sometimes be the sole cause of symptoms. They are:

- cold air suddenly inhaled (cold-induced asthma)
- exercise-induced asthma (in certain children, asthma attacks are caused simply by exercising)
- stress or a high level of anxiety

Wheezing often is obvious, but mild asthmatic attacks may be confirmed when the physician listens to the patient's chest with a stethoscope. Besides wheezing and being short of breath, the patient may **cough** or report a feeling of tightness in the chest. Children may have **itching** on their back or neck at the start of an attack. Wheezing often is loudest when the patient exhales. Some asthmatics are free of symptoms most of the time but may occasionally be short of breath for a brief time. Others spend much of their days (and nights) coughing and wheezing until properly treated. Crying or even laughing may bring on an attack. Severe episodes often are seen when the patient gets a viral respiratory tract infection or is exposed to a heavy load of an allergen or irritant. Asthmatic attacks may last only a few minutes or can go on for hours or even days. Being short of breath may cause a patient to become very anxious, sit upright, lean forward, and use the muscles of the neck and chest wall to help breathe. The patient may be able to say only a few words at a time before stopping to take a breath. Confusion and a bluish tint to the skin are clues that the oxygen supply is much too low and that emergency treatment is needed. In a severe attack, some of the air sacs in the lung may rupture so that air collects within the chest, which makes it even harder to breathe. The good news is that almost always patients, even with the most severe attacks, recover completely.

Diagnosis

Apart from listening to the patient's chest, the examiner looks for maximum chest expansion during inhalation. Hunched shoulders and contracting neck muscles are other signs of narrowed airways. Nasal polyps or increased amounts of nasal secretions are often noted in asthmatic patients. Skin changes, such as **dermatitis** or **eczema**, are a clue that the patient has allergic problems. Inquiring about a family history of asthma or **allergies** can be a valuable indicator of asthma. A test called spirometry measures how rapidly air is exhaled and how much is retained in the lungs. Repeating the test after the patient inhales a drug that widens the air passages (a bronchodilator) shows whether the narrowing of the airway is reversible, which is a very typical finding in asthma. Often patients use a related instrument, called a peak flow meter, to keep track of asthma severity when at home.

Frequently, it is difficult to determine what is triggering asthma attacks. Allergy skin testing may be used, although an allergic skin response does not always mean that the allergen being tested is causing the asthma. Also, the body's immune system produces an antibody to fight off the allergen, and the amount of antibody can be measured by a blood test. The blood test shows how sensitive the patient is to a particular allergen. If the diagnosis is still in doubt, the patient can inhale a suspect allergen while using a spirometer to detect airway narrowing. Spirometry also can be repeated after a bout of exercise if exercise-induced asthma is a possibility. A chest x-ray helps rule out other disorders.

Treatment

There are many alternative treatments available for asthma that have shown promising results. One strong argument for these treatments is that they try to avoid the drugs that allopathic treatment (combating disease with remedies to produce effects different from those produced by the disease) relies upon, which can be toxic and addictive. Mainstream journals have reported on the toxicity of asthma pharmaceuticals. A 1995 New Zealand study showed that before 1940, death from asthma was very low, but that the death rate promptly increased with the introduction of bronchodilators. The *New England Journal of Medicine* in 1992 reported that albuterol and other asthma drugs cause the lungs to deteriorate when used regularly. A 1989 study in the *Annals of Internal Medicine* showed that respiratory therapists, who are exposed to bronchodilator sprays, develop asthma five times more often than other health professionals, which could imply that the drugs themselves may induce asthma. Theophylline, another popular drug, has been reported to cause personality changes in users. Steroids can also have negative effects on many systems in the body, particularly the hormonal system. Thus, natural and non-toxic methods for treating asthma are the preferred first choice of alternative practitioners, while drugs are used to manage extreme cases and emergencies.

Alternative medicine tends to view asthma as the body's protective reaction to environmental agents and pollutants. As such, the treatment goal is often to restore balance to and strengthen the entire body and provide specific support to the lungs and to the immune and hormonal systems. Asthma sufferers can help by keeping a diary of asthma attacks in order to determine environmental and emotional factors that may be contributing to their condition.

Alternative treatments have minimal side effects, are generally inexpensive, and are convenient forms of self-treatment. They also can be used alongside allopathic treatments to improve their effectiveness and lessen their negative side effects.

Dietary and nutritional therapies

Some alternative practitioners recommend cutting down on or eliminating dairy products from the diet, as these increase mucus secretion in the lungs and are sources of food allergies. Other recommendations include avoiding processed foods, refined starches and sugars, and foods with artificial additives and sulfites. **Diets** should be high in fresh fruits, vegetables, and whole grains, and low in salt. Asthma sufferers should experiment with their diets to determine if food allergies are playing a role in their asthma. Some studies have shown that a sustained vegan (zero animal foods) diet can be effective for asthma, as it does not contain the animal products that frequently cause food allergies and contain chemical additives. A vegan diet also eliminates a fatty acid called arachidonic acid, which is found in animal products and is believed to contribute to allergic reactions. A 1985 Swedish study showed that 92% of patients with asthma improved significantly after one year on a vegan diet. However, some people feel weaker on a vegan diet. In addition, many people are allergic to vegetables rather than to meat.

People with asthma should drink plenty of water, as water helps to keep the passages of the lungs moist. Onions and **garlic** contain **quercetin**, a flavonoid (a chemical compound/biological response modifier) that inhibits the release of histamine, and should be a part of an asthmatic's diet. Quercetin is also available as a supplement and should be taken with the digestive enzyme **bromelain** to increase its absorption.

As nutritional therapy, vitamins A, C, and E have been touted as important treatments for asthma. Also, the B complex vitamins, particularly B_6 and B_{12}, may be helpful for asthma sufferers, as well as **magnesium**, **selenium**, and an omega-3 fatty acid supplement such as **flaxseed** oil. A good multivitamin supplement also is recommended. In 2004, a study of supplements at Cornell University showed that high levels of beta-carotene and **vitamin C** along with selenium lowered risk of asthma. The same study found that **vitamin E** had no effect.

Herbal remedies

Chinese medicine has traditionally used *ma huang* for asthma attacks. Ma huang contains ephedrine, which is a bronchodilator once used in many drugs. However, the U.S. Food and Drug Administration (FDA) issued a ban on the sale of **ephedra** that took effect in April 2004 because it was shown to raise blood pressure and stress the circulatory system, resulting in heart attacks and strokes for some users. Manufacturers of ephedra raised legal challenges to this decision. When the U. S. Supreme Court refused to hear these challenges in 2007, the ban on ephedra became permanent.

Another herbal product, ginkgo, has been shown to reduce the frequency of asthma attacks, and **licorice** is used in Chinese medicine as a natural decongestant and expectorant. There are many formulas used in **traditional Chinese medicine** to prevent or ease asthma attacks, depending on the specific Chinese diagnosis given by the practitioner. For example, ma huang is used to treat so-called wind-cold respiratory ailments.

Other herbs used for asthma include **lobelia**, also called Indian tobacco; **nettle**, which contains a natural antihistamine; **thyme**; elecampane; **mullein**; **feverfew**; **passionflower**; **saw palmetto**; and Asian ginseng. Coffee and tea have been shown to reduce the severity of asthma attacks because **caffeine** works as a bronchodilator. Tea also contains minute amounts of theophylline, a drug commonly used to treat asthma. Ayurvedic (traditional East Indian) medicine recommends the herb *Tylophora asthmatica*.

Mind/body approaches

Mind/body medicine has demonstrated that psychological factors play a complex role in asthma. Emotional stress can trigger asthma attacks. Mind/body techniques strive to reduce stress and help people with asthma manage the psychological component of their condition. A 1992 study by Dr. Erik Peper at the Institute for Holistic Healing Studies in San Francisco used **biofeedback**, a treatment method that uses monitors to reveal physiological information to patients, to teach **relaxation** and deep breathing methods to 21 asthma patients. Eighty percent of them subsequently reported fewer attacks and emergency room visits. A 1993 study by Kaiser Permanente in Northern California worked with 323 adults with moderate to severe asthma. Half the patients got standard care while the other half participated in support groups. The support group patients had cut their asthma-related doctor visits in half after two years. A 2008 study conducted by Anita Kozyrskyj at the University of Manitoba (and her colleagues) found that children whose mothers were chronically stressed experienced a significantly higher rate of asthma that a control group. Some other mind/body techniques used for asthma include relaxation methods, **meditation**, **hypnotherapy**, mental imaging, **psychotherapy**, and visualization.

Yoga and breathing methods

Studies have shown that **yoga** significantly helps asthma sufferers, with exercises specifically designed to expand the lungs, promote deep breathing, and reduce stress. Pranayama is the yogic science of breathing, which includes hundreds of deep breathing techniques. These breathing exercises should be done daily as part of any treatment program for asthma, as they are a very effective and inexpensive measure.

Controlled exercise

Many people believe that people with asthma should not exercise. This belief is especially common among parents of children with asthma. In a 2004 study, researchers reported that 20% of children with asthma do not get enough exercise. Many parents believe it is dangerous for their children with asthma to exercise, but physical activity benefits all children, including those with asthma. Parents should work with their children's healthcare providers and any coach or organized sport leader to carefully monitor the children's activities.

Acupuncture

Acupuncture can be an effective treatment for asthma. It is used in traditional Chinese medicine along with dietary changes. **Acupressure** can also be used as a self-treatment for asthma attacks and prevention. The Lung 1 points, used to stimulate breathing, can be easily found on the chest. These are sensitive, often knotted spots on the muscles that run horizontally about an inch below the collarbone, and about two inches from the center of the chest. The points can be pressed in a circular manner with the thumbs, while the head is allowed to hang forward and the patient takes slow, deep breaths. **Reflexology** also uses particular acupressure points on the hands and feet that are believed to stimulate the lungs.

Other treatments

Aromatherapists recommend **eucalyptus, lavender, rosemary,** and **chamomile** as fragrances that promote free breathing. In Japan, a common treatment for asthma is administering cold baths. This form of **hydrotherapy** has been demonstrated to open constricted air passages. Massage therapies such as **Rolfing** can help asthma sufferers as well, as they strive to open and increase circulation in the chest area. **Homeopathy** uses the remedies *Arsenicum album, Kali carbonicum, Natrum sulphuricum,* and *Aconite.*

Allopathic treatment

Allopaths recommend that asthma patients should be periodically examined and have their lung functions measured by spirometry. The goals are to prevent troublesome symptoms, to maintain lung function as close to normal as possible, and to allow patients to pursue their normal activities, including those requiring exertion. The best drug therapy is that which controls asthmatic symptoms while causing few or no side effects.

Drugs

The chief methylxanthine drug is theophylline. It may exert some anti-inflammatory effect and is especially helpful in controlling nighttime symptoms of asthma. When, for some reason, a patient cannot use an inhaler to maintain long-term control, sustained-release theophylline is a good alternative. The blood levels of the user must be measured periodically, as too high a dose can cause an abnormal heart rhythm or convulsions.

Beta-receptor agonists (drugs that trigger cell response) are bronchodilators. They are the drugs of choice for relieving sudden attacks of asthma and for preventing attacks from being triggered by exercise. Some agonists, such as albuterol, act mainly in lung cells and have little effect on the heart and other organs. These drugs generally start acting within minutes, but their effects last only four to six hours. They may be taken by mouth, inhaled, or injected. In 2004, a new lower concentration of albuterol was approved by the FDA for children ages two to 12.

Steroids are drugs that resemble natural body hormones. They block inflammation and are effective in relieving symptoms of asthma. When steroids are taken by inhalation for a long period, asthma attacks become less frequent as the airways become less sensitive to allergens. Steroids are the strongest medicine for asthma and can control even severe cases over the long term and maintain good lung function. However, steroids can cause numerous side effects, including bleeding from the stomach, loss of **calcium** from bones, **cataracts** in the eye, and a diabetes-like state. Patients using steroids for lengthy periods may also have problems with wound healing, may gain weight, and may suffer mental problems. In children who use steroids, growth may be slowed. Besides being inhaled, steroids may be taken by mouth or injected to rapidly control severe asthma.

Leukotriene modifiers are among a newer type of drug that can be used in place of steroids, for older children or adults who have a mild degree of persistent asthma. They work by counteracting leukotrienes, which are substances released by white blood cells in the lung that cause the air passages to constrict and promote mucus secretion. Other drugs include cromolyn and nedocromil, which are anti-inflammatory drugs that often are used as initial treatments to prevent long-term asthmatic attacks in children. Montelukast **sodium** (Singulair) is a drug taken daily that is used to help prevent asthma attacks rather than to treat an acute attack. In 2004, the FDA approved an oral granule formula of Singulair for young children.

If a patient's asthma is caused by an allergen that cannot be avoided and it has been difficult to control symptoms by drugs, immunotherapy may be worth trying. In a typical course of immunotherapy, a patient is injected with increasing amounts of the allergen over a period of three to five years, so that the body can build up an effective immune response. There is a risk that this treatment may itself cause the airways to become narrowed and bring on an asthmatic attack. Not all experts are enthusiastic about immunotherapy, although some studies have shown that it reduces asthmatic symptoms caused by exposure to dust mites, ragweed pollen, and cats.

Managing asthmatic attacks

A severe asthma attack should be treated as quickly as possible. It is most important for a patient suffering an acute attack to be given extra oxygen. Rarely, it may be necessary to use a mechanical ventilator to help the patient breathe. A beta-receptor agonist is inhaled repeatedly or continuously. If the patient does not respond promptly and completely, a steroid is given. A course of steroid therapy, given after the attack is over, will make a recurrence less likely.

Long-term allopathic treatment for asthma is based on inhaling a beta-receptor agonist using a special inhaler that meters the dose. Patients must be instructed in proper use of an inhaler to be sure that it will deliver the right amount of drug. Once asthma has been controlled for several weeks or months, it is worth trying to cut down on drug treatment, but this tapering must be done gradually. The last drug added should be the first to be reduced. Patients should be seen every one to six months, depending on the frequency of attacks. Starting treatment at home, rather than in a hospital, makes for minimal delay and helps the patient to gain a sense of control over the disease. All patients should be taught how to monitor their symptoms so that they will know when an attack is starting. Those with moderate or severe asthma should know how to use a flow meter. They also should have a written plan to follow if symptoms suddenly become worse, including how to adjust their medication and when to seek medical help. If more intense treatment is necessary, it should be continued for several days. When deciding whether a patient should be hospitalized, the physician must take into account the patient's past history of acute attacks, severity of symptoms, current medication, and the availability of good support at home.

Expected results

Most patients with asthma respond well when the best treatment or combination of treatments is found, and they are able to lead relatively normal lives. Patients who take responsibility for their condition and experiment with various treatments have good chances of keeping symptoms minimal. Having urgent measures to control asthma attacks and ongoing treatment to prevent attacks are important as well. More than one half of affected children stop having attacks by the time they reach 21 years of age. Many others have less frequent and less severe attacks as they grow older. A small minority of patients will have progressively more trouble breathing. Because they run a risk of going into respiratory failure, they must receive intensive treatment.

Prevention

Prevention is extremely important in the treatment of asthma, which includes eliminating all possible allergens from the environment and diet. Homes and work areas should be as dust and pollutant-free as possible. Areas can be tested for allergens and high-quality air filters can be installed to clean the air. If the patient is sensitive to a family pet, removing the animal or at least keeping it out of the bedroom (with the bedroom door closed) is advised. Keeping the pet away from carpets and upholstered furniture, and removing all feathers also helps. To reduce exposure to dust mites, practitioners recommend removal of wall-to-wall carpeting, keeping the humidity low, and using special pillows and mattress covers. Cutting down on stuffed toys and washing them each week in hot water is advised for children with asthma. If cockroach allergen is causing asthma attacks, controlling the roaches (using traps or boric acid) can help.

It is important not to leave food or garbage exposed. Keeping indoor air clean by vacuuming carpets once or twice a week (with the asthmatic person absent) and avoiding use of humidifiers is advised. Those with asthma should avoid exposure to tobacco smoke and should not exercise outside when air pollution levels are high. When asthma is related to exposure at work, taking all precautions, including wearing a mask and, if necessary, arranging to work in a safer area, is recommended. For chronic sufferers who live in heavily polluted areas, moving to less polluted regions may be a viable alternative.

KEY TERMS

Allergen—A foreign substance that causes the airways to narrow and produces symptoms of asthma when inhaled.

Atopy—A state that makes persons more likely to develop allergic reactions of any type, including the inflammation and airway narrowing typical of asthma.

Bronchodilator—A type of medication that acts to open up bronchial tubes that have constricted in an asthmatic attack.

Hypersensitivity—A condition in which very small amounts of allergen can cause the airways to constrict and bring on an asthmatic attack.

Leukotrienes—Substances that are produced by white blood cells in response to antigens and contribute to inflammatory and asthmatic reactions.

Pranayama—Breathing techniques taught in yoga.

Quercetin—A flavonoid (chemical compound/ biological response modifier) found in onions and garlic that may be a useful dietary supplement for asthma patients.

Vegan diet—A vegetarian diet that excludes meat and dairy products.

Resources

BOOKS

Byrne-Ralfs, Christine, and Patrick McKeown. *Stop Asthma Naturally: Incorporating the Buteyko Breathing Method* Vancouver, Canada: Buteyko Books, 2007.

Cutler, Ellen W. *Winning the War against Asthma and Allergies* (Rev. ed.). New York: Delmar, 2007.

Kendall, Kent P. *Allergy and Asthma Control—Naturally.* West Conshohocken, PA: Infinity Press, 2005.

PERIODICALS

"Clinical Applications of Complementary and Alternative Medicine for Asthma." *Alternative & Complementary Therapies* (October 1, 2007): 235–238.

"Complementary and Alternative Medicine Use in Asthma: Who is Using What?" *Respirology* (July 2006): 373–387.

"How Does Exercise Cause Asthma Attacks?" *Current Opinion in Allergy and Clinical Immunology* (February 2006): 37–42.

"New Protein Discovered at Yale May Play a Role in Severe Asthma." *Expert Review of Molecular Diagnostics* (January 2008): 5–7.

ORGANIZATIONS

Allergy and Asthma Magazine, 702 Marshall St., Suite 611, Redwood City, CA, 94063, (605) 780-0546.

Asthma and Allergy Foundation of America, 1125 Fifteenth St. NW, Suite 502, Washington, DC, 20005, (800) 7ASTHMA, http://www.aafa.org.

Center for Complementary and Alternative Medicine Research in Asthma, Allergy, and Immunology. University of California at Davis, 3150B Meyer Hall, Davis, CA, 95616, (916) 752-6575, http://www-camra.ucdavis.edu.

David Newton

Astigmatism

Definition

Astigmatism is visual distortion caused by a misshapen cornea. The cornea acts as a focusing lens for the eye. If the cornea does not have the proper shape, the eye is unable to properly focus an image. Most people have a certain degree of astigmatism. Corrective measures are necessary only in cases in which the distortion is severe.

Description

Light rays entering a normal eye come to a point of focus on the retina through a transparent, dome-shaped layer called the cornea. In astigmatism, an unequal curvature of the cornea causes the light rays to come to focus at more than one point on the retina, and as a result, the person sees a blurred or doubled image. Astigmatism is usually present at birth and may increase during childhood as the eye tissue develops. Usually the degree of astigmatism remains fairly constant throughout adulthood.

Causes and symptoms

It is unknown why some people develop a misshapen cornea. It is possible that astigmatism is an inherited trait. Factors such as **stress**, continual reading in dim lighting, or excessive close-up work may also contribute to the development of astigmatism. It is sometimes caused by pressure from chalazion, a condition that causes the eyelid to swell; from scars on the cornea; or from keratoconus, a condition that involves swelling of the cornea. The main symptom of astigmatism is blurred or distorted vision. Some patients may also experience a history of headaches, eye strain, **fatigue**, and double vision.

Diagnosis

The standard eye examination with a refraction test, given by an optometrist or ophthalmologist, is used to determine the presence of astigmatism. An instrument called a keratometer is used to measure the cornea and calculate the shape of the required corrective lens.

Treatment

The **Bates method** or other type of visual training may be helpful in improving vision and reducing symptoms. Practitioners of alternative medicine may recommend the homeopathic remedies *Ruta graveolens* (from common rue) and *Apis mellifica* (from the honey bee) to relieve eyestrain, one of the main symptoms and possible contributors to astigmatism. They may also suggest **acupuncture** treatment and **traditional Chinese medicine** that have implications for the liver because the liver system is believed to be connected to eye functions. Certain treatments are prescribed to strengthen and correct the skewing of the Liver qi. (*Qi* is the flow of energy in the body. It is sometimes associated with certain organs.)

Allopathic treatment

Astigmatism can be most simply treated with either eyeglasses or contact lenses. The lenses are designed to counteract the shape of the sections of cornea that are causing difficulty. Contact lenses that are used to correct astigmatism are called toric lenses. In the past, only hard contact lenses could treat most cases of astigmatism, but soft contact lenses are now available for all but the most complex prescriptions. The options for keratoconus include soft lenses (for some mild to moderate cases), hard contact lenses, corneal implants, or, in some cases, corneal transplants.

Refractive surgery can be performed to correct the curvature of the cornea. The three most commonly used types are photorefractive keratectomy (PRK), laser-assisted *in situ* keratomileusis (LASIK), and laser-assisted subepithelial keratomileusis (LASEK). In PRK, a laser is used to improve the shape of the cornea by removing micro-thin slices. In LASIK, a flap of the cornea is lifted to reveal the underlying corneal tissue, which is shaved to improve the shape. LASEK is similar to LASIK, but the corneal flap is typically much thinner. LASEK is often recommended for people who are at high risk for eye injury.

KEY TERMS

Chalazion—A condition in which clogging of the meibomiam gland causes a cyst inside the eyelid.

Keratoconus—A progressive condition in which the cornea takes on a cone shape, causing major changes in the eye's refractive power.

Refraction—The turning or bending of light waves as the light passes from one medium or layer to another. In the eye, it means the ability of the eye to bend light so that an image is focused onto the retina.

Refractive surgery—Eye surgery to correct a defect in the eye's ability to focus accurately on an image.

Retina—The substance of the eye, made of nerve tissue. It receives and transmits images to the brain.

These may include individuals who engage in contact sports.

Refractive surgery requires a high level of expertise. Anyone considering it should make sure that the surgeon has a high level of experience in the procedure and should engage in an in-depth discussion of the possible side effects and risks of the procedure. For instance, patients with flatter corneas may experience more light distortion than those with curved corneas.

Expected results

Effects of astigmatism can generally be greatly improved with eyeglasses or contact lenses. Refractive surgery may diminish the need for lenses or make them unnecessary altogether. The major risks of surgery include chronic visual problems, injury to the eye tissue, infection, and over- or under-correction, which would still leave some astigmatism. Complications may require the use of medication or further surgery.

Resources

BOOKS

Gaby, Alan R., and the Healthnotes Medical Team. *The Natural Pharmacy,* 3rd ed. New York: Three Rivers Press, 2006.

Rosenfarb, Andy. *Healing Your Eyes with Chinese Medicine: Acupuncture, Acupressure, & Chinese Herbs.* Berkeley, CA: North Atlantic Books, 2007.

OTHER

"Astigmatism." American Optometric Association. http://www.aoa.org/x4698.xml. (March 25, 2008).

"Astigmatism." Merck Source. August 8, 2006. http://www.mercksource.com/pp/us/cns/cns_hl_adam.jspzQzpgz EzzSzppdocszSzuszSzcnszSzcontentzSzadamzSzen cyzSzarticlezSz001015zPzhtm. (March 25, 2008).

Patience Paradox
Teresa G. Odle
Leslie Mertz, Ph.D.

Aston-Patterning

Definition

Aston-Patterning is an integrated system of movement education, bodywork, ergonomic adjustments, and fitness training that recognizes the relationship between the body and mind for well being. It helps people who seek a remedy from acute or chronic **pain** by teaching them to improve postural and movement patterns.

Origins

Aston-Patterning is a process originated by Judith Aston in 1977. After graduating from college with an advanced degree in dance, Aston began working with athletes, dancers, and actors in movement education programs in California. In 1968, she suffered injuries from two automobile accidents. In seeking relief from pain, she met Dr. Ida Rolf, the developer of **Rolfing**. When Aston recovered from her injuries, Rolf asked her to develop a movement education program that would complement the gains achieved with Rolfing. She worked with Rolf in creating this program from 1971 to 1977.

By 1977, Aston and Rolf's interests and views of bodywork had diverged. Aston left Rolf and established her own techniques, which she called Aston-Patterning. She has also developed a special program for older people called the Aston-Patterning Fitness Program for Seniors. Aston-Patterning is a registered trademark of the Aston Paradigm Corporation, of which Judith Aston is president. Aston Enterprises sells a line of patented products to go along with the Aston-Patterning program.

Benefits

Aston-Patterning assists people in finding more efficient and less stressful ways of performing the simple movements of everyday life in order to dissipate tension in the body. This change is achieved through massage, alteration of the environment, and fitness training.

Description

Seeking to solve movement problems, Aston-Patterning helps make the most of each individual's own body type rather than trying to force everyone to conform to an ideal. Unlike Rolfing, it does not strive for linear symmetry. Rather, it works with asymmetry in the human body to develop patterns of alignment and movement that feel right to the individual. Aston also introduced the idea of working in a three-dimensional spinal pattern.

Aston-Patterning sessions have four general components:

- a personal history that helps the practitioner assess the client's needs
- pre-testing, in which the practitioner and the client explore patterns of movement and potential for improvement
- movement education and bodywork, including massage, myofacial release, and arthrokinetics, to help release tension and make new movement patterns easier
- post-testing, when pre-testing movements are repeated, allowing the client to feel the changes that have taken place and integrate them into daily life

Aston-Patterning requires more participation from the client than many bodywork techniques. The massage aspect of Aston-Patterning is designed around a three-dimensional, non-compressive touch that releases patterns of tension in the body. It is gentler than Rolfing. Myokinetics uses touch to release tension in the face and neck. Arthrokinetics addresses tension at bones and joints. This massage is accompanied by education about the establishment of new movement patterns.

In addition to Aston-Patterning sessions, clients are helped to examine their environment for factors, such as seating or sleeping arrangements, that may limit their body function and introduce tension. Finally, they may choose to participate in the Aston fitness training program that includes loosening techniques based on self-massage, toning, stretching, and cardiovascular fitness.

Preparations

Since clients typically work with an Aston-Patterning practitioner for extended periods, it is important that they feel comfortable with their specific

JUDITH ASTON

Judith Aston was born in Long Beach, California. She graduated from University of California at Los Angeles with a B.A. and a M.F.A. in dance. Her interest in movement arose from working as a dancer. In 1963 Aston established her first movement education program for dancers, actors, and athletes at Long Beach City College.

Five years later, while recovering from injuries sustained during two consecutive automobile accidents, Aston met Ida Rolf, the developer of Rolfing. Aston began working for Rolf, teaching a movement education program called Rolf-Aston Structural Patterning that emphasized using the body with minimum effort and maximum precision.

In time, Rolf and Aston's views on movement diverged, and the partnership was dissolved in 1977. Aston formed her own company called the Aston Paradigm Corporation in Lake Tahoe, California. This company provides training and certification for Aston practitioners. She also began exploring how environmental conditions affect body movement, foreshadowing the ergonomic movement in the workplace that developed in the 1990s. Over time, Aston has expanded her movement work to include a fitness program for older adults. Today, Judith Aston serves as director of Aston Paradigm Corporation.

practitioner. Certified Aston practitioners recommend that prospective clients make a get-acquainted visit before enrolling in a course of treatment.

Precautions

Aston-Patterning can be quite demanding. People with any of the following diseases or disorders should consult a physician before undertaking a course of Aston-Patterning:

- Heart conditions.

- Diabetes. Because diabetes affects blood circulation, diabetics taking Aston-Patterning should ask the practitioner to avoid massage of the legs and feet.

- Carpal tunnel syndrome. Aston-Patterning may worsen the pain associated with this disorder.

- Respiratory disorders, including asthma and emphysema.

- Osteoporosis. The deep tissue massage in Aston-Patterning may cause hairline fractures in brittle bones.

- Bleeding disorders and other disorders requiring treatment with anticoagulant or corticosteroid medications. Drugs in these categories can make the tissues fragile.

- Disorders requiring medications that affect the sense of balance.

- Post-traumatic stress syndromes. People suffering from acute stress disorder, post-traumatic stress disorder (PTSD), or other emotional disorders related to trauma or abuse should consult a psychotherapist as well as a physician before undertaking any form of bodywork. The physical contact involved in Aston-Patterning may cause flashbacks or bring up emotional and psychological issues.

The Aston-Patterning program can be modified to meet the needs of older adults, those in poor health, or persons with special rehabilitation requirements.

Side effects

Most clients of Aston-Patterning report a diminution of tension, improved ease of movement, and an enhanced feeling of well-being. Some clients, however, do report side effects, the most common being pain and exhaustion. To minimize side effects, clients should give the practitioner as much feedback as possible during sessions.

Research and general acceptance

Aston-Patterning is an outgrowth of Rolfing, which has been shown to be of benefit in a limited number of controlled studies. Little controlled research has been done on either the benefits or limitations of Aston-Patterning; as of 2007, no reports had been published in any peer-reviewed medical, alternative medical, or bodywork journals. Its claims have been neither proven nor disproved, although anecdotally many clients report relief from pain and tension as well as improved body movement. Aston-Patterning is a member of the International Alliance of Healthcare Educators (IAHE), and Judith Aston is a frequent speaker at IAHE conferences. In addition, Aston's postural assessment workbook is used by practitioners in other fields of bodywork and physical therapy.

Training and certification

The Aston Training Center in Incline Village, Nevada, offers courses and certification and promotes a code of ethics among its practitioners. Certification

KEY TERMS

Bodywork—Any healing technique involving hands-on massage or manipulation of the body.

Ergonomics—A branch of applied science that coordinates the physical design and arrangement of furniture, machines, and other features of a living or working environment with the needs and requirements of the individuals in that environment.

Rolfing—Developed by Dr. Ida Rolf (1896–1979), rolfing is a systematic approach to relieving stress patterns and dysfunctions in the body's structure through the manipulation of the highly pliant myofacial (connective) tissue. It assists the body in reorganizing its major segments into vertical alignment.

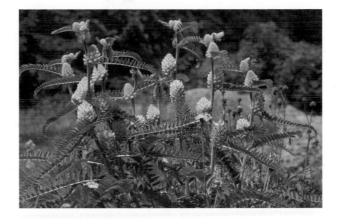

Astragalus is a good source of selenium, an antioxidant and immune system stimulant. (© CuboImages srl / Alamy)

must be renewed frequently. As of 2008, there were certified Aston-Patterning practitioners in fifteen states, with the largest concentrations in California, Washington, and Massachusetts. Certified Aston-Patterning practitioners also were found in Australia, New Zealand, Canada, and the United Kingdom. Some Aston-Patterning practitioners are cross-certified in **Pilates**.

Resources

BOOKS

Aston, Judith. *Aston Postural Assessment Handbook: Skills for Observing and Evaluating Body Patterns.* San Antonio, TX: Therapy Skill Builders, 1998.

ORGANIZATIONS

Aston Training Center, PO Box 3568, Incline Village, NV, 89450, (775) 831-8228, http://www.astonenterprises.com.

International Alliance of Healthcare Educators (IAHE), 11211 Prosperity Farms Road, D-325, Palm Beach Gardens, FL, 34410, (561) 622-4334, www.iahe.com.

Tish Davidson, A. M.

Astragalus

Description

Astragalus, also called milk vetch root, is the root of the *Astragalus membranaceus* plant, which is a member of the pea family. This perennial grows to a height of 2–4 ft. (5–10 cm). It has white or yellow flowers and leaves with 10–18 pairs of leaflets. The large yellow taproots of four- to seven-year-old plants are used for medicinal purposes. Although there are many varieties in the *Astragalus* family, *Astragalus membranaceus* is the sole medicinal type. The plant is found only in the grasslands and mountains of central and western Asia, principally in China, Taiwan, and Korea. Astragalus is a good source of **selenium**, an antioxidant and immune system stimulant.

General use

Astragalus is called *Huang Qi* in **traditional Chinese medicine** (TCM) and is considered to be an important tonic herb. It is used to strengthen what is called the *wei qi*, or the defensive energy of the body against disease. TCM identifies astragalus as being helpful in conditions involving the Spleen, the Lungs, and the Triple Burner. It is a warming tonic, and it improves the functioning of the qi (the flow of energy in the body), the Spleen, the Blood, and the fluids of the body. Astragalus is recommended for Spleen deficiency symptoms, such as **diarrhea**, **fatigue**, sweating, and lack of appetite. It is used as a tonic for the Lungs and is good for shortness of breath, **asthma**, and chronic lung problems. Astragalus is prescribed for arthritis, diarrhea, and nervous symptoms. It is often given to people who are in a state of generally poor or weakened health.

Astragalus is classified as an adaptogen, an herb that increases the body's endurance and resistance to a wide array of physical, chemical, and biological stressors. Adaptogens help normalize the functioning of various body systems by affecting the action of hormones. Adaptogens are usually beneficial in treating chronic conditions. They have been found to enhance the immune response, reduce inflammation, stabilize blood sugar, and support the hormone systems, particularly the adrenal and pituitary glands. Adaptogens should be used for an extended period of time—at least six weeks.

Astragalus helps the body function at its best level. It helps the body deal with **stress** and enhances overall immune function. It has been shown to stimulate production and activation of the white blood cells, which fight infection. It is highly recommended for preventing and alleviating colds and flu. Astragalus can be used to cure chronic weaknesses of the lungs. Because it improves blood circulation and heart function, astragalus is useful in treating **heart disease**. It has also been found to prevent or reduce blood clotting. Astragalus can be taken as a tonic for the kidneys. It has a diuretic (urine-producing) effect and so it flushes out the urinary system. It is thus very effective in treating **kidney infections**, proteinuria (too much protein in the urine), chronic prostate problems, and chronic urinary tract problems.

Astragalus is helpful to those taking chemotherapy and radiation treatments. It reduces toxic side effects and enhances therapeutic effects. **Cancer** patients who take astragalus during or after cancer treatments tend to recover more quickly from the ill effects of the treatment, and they generally have better survival rates. This appears to be connected with the strengthening of the immune system. Astragalus also stimulates the adrenal glands, whose functions are suppressed in cancer. The herb improves poor appetite, diarrhea, weakness, wasting, and night sweats. This makes it helpful for cancer patients as well as **AIDS** patients and those with other debilitating diseases.

Astragalus is recommended as a tonic for the elderly. It protects cells from the **aging** process and may diminish other negative effects of aging. For example, it strengthens digestion, stimulates the appetite, and helps improve mental functioning. Astragalus shows promise in the treatment of Alzheimer's disease. By itself or in combinations, it may be useful in treating viral **infections**, **hypoglycemia**, **diabetes mellitus**, chronic ulcers, **insomnia**, **hyperthyroidism**, **chronic fatigue syndrome**, open **wounds**, liver problems, **sexual dysfunction**, fertility problems, and autoimmune diseases.

Preparations

Astragalus is available as a capsule, a tablet, a tincture, as part of an herbal combination, as a prepared tea, and as a sweet dried root that can be eaten or made into tea. Traditionally, several slices of the

KEY TERMS

Adrenal glands—Glands atop the kidneys that produce hormones.

Blood—In TCM, it is the fluid that transports physical and emotional nourishment.

Heat condition—A disease whose symptoms include fever, rashes, redness, dehydration, and inflammation.

Lungs—In TCM, the parts of the body associated with breathing, such as the lungs and the skin. It also regulates the movement of water and qi through the body channels.

Qi—In the TCM system, the underlying force that controls the body's movement, resistance to disease, use of nourishment, tissue integrity, and temperature. It circulates through channels, or pathways, called meridians.

Spleen—In TCM, the system of organs that includes the pancreas, large muscles, the lips, the eyelids, the lymph system, and the spleen. It also includes the functions that extract nourishment and convert it into qi and Blood.

Triple Burner—The pathways and relationships between the Spleen, the Lungs and the Kidney.

root are often added to soups and stews. A strong tea can be made by boiling three ounces of astragalus root in three cups of water and letting the mixture steep for at least five minutes. Two or three cups of the unheated tea can be taken over the course of a day. In tincture form, 30–60 drops of astragalus can be taken four times per day. Candied roots can be purchased ready-made or prepared in the home. Preparation involves combining four parts of the dried root with one part honey in water, then simmering until the herb is dried and brownish. In TCM, astragalus ointments are used to heal wounds, particularly those that are slow to heal.

Precautions

Since astragalus is a warming herb, its use should be avoided in heat conditions, such as fevers or agitated states. *Astragalus membranaceus* is the only species of its family to have a medicinal use; other species may be toxic. Therefore, local Western varieties should not be used. Use only the root portion of the plant; other parts of the plant may be poisonous.

Side effects

Sometimes individuals experience a slight stomach upset or allergic reaction to astragalus. However, it is generally a very safe herb, even at high doses.

Interactions

Astragalus increases the effectiveness of other herbs when used in combinations. It is often used with **Siberian ginseng**, *Eleutherococcus senticosus; Echinacea spp.;* **dong quai**, *Angelica sinensis;* and *Lingusticum wallichi.* Astragalus may interfere with the actions of diuretics, phenobarbital, beta-blockers, and anticoagulants (substances that prevent blood clotting). Users of these medications should consult a healthcare provider before using the herb.

Resources

BOOKS

Graedon, Joe, and Teresa Graedon. *The People's Pharmacy Guide to Home and Herbal Remedies.* New York: St. Martin's Press, 1999.

Green, James. *The Male Herbal: Health Care for Men and Boys.* Freedom, Calif.: Crossing Press, 1991.

Hart, Carol, and Magnolia Goh. *Traditional Chinese Medicine: The A-Z Guide to Natural Healing from the Orient.* New York: Dell, 1997.

OTHER

"Astragalus." *Go-Symmetry.* http://www.go-symmetry.com/astragalus.htm.

"Astragalus." *The Herbalist.* http://www.theherbalist.com/astragal.htm.

"Astragalus." *HerbsHerbals.com.* http://www.herbsherbals.com/astragalus.html.

"Astragalus." *Pro Health International.* http://www.planet.eon.net/~wiggles/astra1galus.htm.

Patience Paradox

Atherosclerosis

Definition

Atherosclerosis is the build up of plaque on the inside of arteries, the blood vessels that carry blood from the heart to the rest of the body. Atherosclerosis is a specific form of arteriosclerosis, which is a general term for hardening of the arteries. The two terms are sometimes used interchangeably.

Description

Atherosclerosis, a progressive condition responsible for most **heart disease**, is a type of hardening of the arteries. It can be caused by normal **aging** processes, by high blood pressure, and by some diseases such as diabetes. Atherosclerosis can begin in the late teens, but it usually takes decades for the signs and symptoms of the disease to be apparent. Some people experience rapidly progressing atherosclerosis in their 30s or later.

An artery is made up of several layers: an inner lining called the endothelium, an elastic membrane that allows the artery to expand and contract, a layer of smooth muscle, and a layer of connective tissue. Atherosclerosis affects the inner lining of an artery. It is characterized by plaque deposits that reduce or block the flow of blood. Plaque is made of fatty substances, **cholesterol**, waste products from the cells, **calcium**, **iron**, and fibrin, a material that helps blood to clot.

As plaque builds up in and around the cells of the artery walls, they accumulate calcium. The innermost layer thickens, the artery's diameter is reduced, and blood flow and oxygen delivery are decreased. Plaque can rupture or crack open, causing the sudden formation of a blood clot, a process called thrombosis. As a result of thrombosis and/or the buildup of plaque, atherosclerosis can cause a **heart attack** if it completely blocks the blood flow in the coronary arteries. It can cause a **stroke** if it completely blocks the carotid arteries of the brain. Atherosclerosis can also occur in the arteries of the neck, kidneys, thighs, and arms, and may lead to kidney failure, **gangrene**, and even death.

Causes and symptoms

Scientists believe that atherosclerosis is caused by the body's response to damage to the artery wall from cholesterol, high blood pressure, and cigarette **smoking**. A person who has all three of these risk factors is eight times as likely to develop atherosclerosis as is a person who has none of the factors. Physical inactivity, damage by oxidants, diabetes, and **obesity** are also risk factors for atherosclerosis. High levels of the amino acid homocysteine and abnormal levels of fats called lipoproteins also raise the risk. Other risk factors include:

- High triglycerides. Most fat in food and in the body takes the form of triglycerides. Blood triglyceride levels above 400 mg/dL have been linked to atherosclerosis.

- Physical inactivity. Lack of exercise increases the risk of atherosclerosis.
- Diabetes mellitus. The risk of developing atherosclerosis is seriously increased for diabetics and can be lowered by keeping diabetes under control. Many diabetics die from heart attacks caused by atherosclerosis.
- Obesity. Excess weight increases the strain on the heart and increases the risk of developing atherosclerosis, even if no other risk factors are present.
- Heredity. People whose parents have coronary artery disease, atherosclerosis, or stroke at an early age are at increased risk.
- Sex. Before age 60, men are more likely to have heart attacks than women.
- Age. Risk is higher in men who are 45 years of age and older and women who are 55 years of age and older.

The symptoms of atherosclerosis differ depending upon the location. They may involve:

- In the coronary (heart) arteries: chest pain, heart attack, and sudden death.
- In the carotid arteries of the brain: sudden dizziness, weakness, loss of speech, and blindness.
- In the femoral arteries of the legs: cramping and fatigue in the calves of the legs when walking.
- In the renal arteries of the kidneys: high blood pressure resistant to treatment.

Diagnosis

Physicians may be able to make a diagnosis of atherosclerosis during a physical examination by listening to the activity of the arteries and the heart with a stethoscope and probing them with the hands. More definitive tests are usually called for, however. These include an electrocardiogram, which shows the heart's activity; **exercise** electrocardiography, more familiarly known as a **stress** test, conducted while the patient exercises on a treadmill or a stationary bike; echocardiography, a type of ultrasound using sound waves to create an image of the heart's chambers and valves; and ultrasonography to assess arteries of the neck and thighs.

Radionuclide angiography and thallium scanning use radioactive material injected into the bloodstream. These tests enable physicians to see the blood flow through the coronary arteries and the heart chambers and to record pictures of the heart. Coronary angiography is the most accurate diagnostic method for atherosclerosis, and it is also the only invasive procedure. A cardiologist inserts a catheter equipped with a

viewing device into a blood vessel in the leg or arm and guides it into the heart. A contrast dye makes the heart visible to x rays. Motion pictures are taken of the dye flowing though the arteries, and plaques and blockages are well defined.

Treatment

The most common treatments focus on dietary and lifestyle changes to reduce cholesterol and other problems that contribute to atherosclerosis. Dietary modifications usually incorporate eating foods that are low in saturated fats, cholesterol, sugar, and animal proteins. **Diets** should include foods high in fiber, such as fresh fruits and vegetables, and whole grains. By consuming fruits and vegetables, a person also consumes helpful dietary **antioxidants**, such as **carotenoids** found in vegetable pigments, and bioflavenoids in fruit pigments. Nutritionists also recommend liberal use of onions and **garlic**, as well as fish, especially cold–water fish, such as salmon. Smoking, alcohol, and coffee are to be avoided, and exercise is strongly recommended. Several well-known programs are available, such as those created by Nathan and Robert Pritikin and Dean Ornish. These programs may be helpful in setting up and maintaining dietary and lifestyle programs.

Herbal remedies for atherosclerosis include garlic (*Allium sativum*), **ginger** (*Zingiber officinale*), **hawthorn** (*Crataegus oxycantha*), *Ginkgo biloba*, and **Siberian ginseng** root (*Eleutherococcus senticosus*). Gugulipids, or **myrrh** (*Commiphora molmol*) is highly regarded for its ability to lower cholesterol and triglyceride levels. Other herbs with this ability include **alfalfa** (*Medicago sativum*), **turmeric** (*Curcuma longa*), Korean ginseng (*Panax ginseng*), and **fenugreek** (*Trigonella foenum-graecum*). Atherosclerosis is a complex condition. Therefore, a knowledgeable practitioner of herbal healing should be consulted for recommendations on the right combination of herbs and dosages.

Chelation therapy involves injecting a drug called EDTA and drug taken orally called DMSA, together with nutrients into the bloodstream. These drugs work either by binding to the calcium in plaque and transporting it for excretion, or by acting as an antioxidant, or by both methods. Chelation therapy has shown some success, but it remains a controversial method.

Several disciplines can offer helpful long-term treatment strategies for those with atherosclerosis. A knowledgeable practitioner should be consulted. **Ayurvedic medicine** practitioners combine diet, herbal remedies, **relaxation**, and exercises. A homeopath will prescribe a treatment regimen based on a complete assessment of the patient. A **traditional Chinese medicine** practitioner may prescribe a combination of herbs such as siler (*Ledebouriella divaricata*), *Platycodon grandiflorum*, *Polygonum multiflorum*, and *Bupleurum chinense*. **Acupuncture** and massage may be recommended, particularly for the accompanying circulatory problems. A homeopath will prescribe remedies based on an in-depth interview and evaluation.

Stress is known to worsen blood pressure and atherosclerosis, and hasten the progression of the disease. Therapeutic relaxation techniques are, therefore, helpful adjuncts to treatment. Recommended approaches include **yoga**, **meditation**, **guided imagery**, **biofeedback**, and counseling. A 2002 study showed that transcendental meditation, when combined with diet, exercise, and antioxidant food supplements, contributed to nearly a 33% reduction in long-term risk for heart attack and stroke in some patients.

Allopathic treatment

Allopathic treatment includes medications, balloon angioplasty, and coronary artery bypass surgery. Most of the drugs prescribed for atherosclerosis seek to improve conditions that contribute to the disease, such as high cholesterol, **blood clots**, or high blood pressure.

Angioplasty and bypass surgery are invasive procedures that improve blood flow in the coronary arteries. Coronary angioplasty is performed by a cardiologist. It is a procedure in which a catheter tipped with a balloon is threaded from a blood vessel in the thigh into the blocked artery. When the balloon is inflated, it compresses the plaque and enlarges the blood vessel to open the blocked artery. In one–third of patients, the artery narrows again within six months. The procedure may have to be repeated and a wire mesh stent may be placed in the artery to help keep it open. In bypass surgery, a detour is created with grafted or synthetic blood vessels. The blood can then go around the blockage. Other procedures may be used, including catheterization and laser treatments.

Expected results

Atherosclerosis can be successfully treated, but not cured. Studies have shown that atherosclerosis can be delayed, stopped, and even reversed by aggressively lowering cholesterol and changing one's diet.

Prevention

A healthy lifestyle—eating right, regular exercise, maintaining a healthy weight, not smoking, and

---

KEY TERMS

Cardiac catheterization—A treatment using a narrow tube to clear out a blocked blood vessel.

Cholesterol—A fat-like substance that is made by the human body and consumed in animal products. Cholesterol is used to form cell membranes, hormones, and vitamin D. High cholesterol levels contribute to the development of atherosclerosis.

Homocysteine—An amino acid involved with protein use in the body. High levels of homocysteine have been implicated in the development of atherosclerosis.

Triglyceride—A simple fat–like compound derived from food and found in the blood. Elevated triglyceride levels contribute to the development of atherosclerosis.

---

controlling hypertension—can reduce the risk of developing atherosclerosis, help keep the disease from progressing, and sometimes cause it to regress. A 2002 study presented promising news about the impact of simple exercise on modifying the elasticity of one's arteries. A small group of healthy but sedentary postmenopausal women began walking at a moderate pace for 40 to 45 minutes a day five times a week. By the end of 12 weeks, 48% of the women had restored elasticity to their carotid arteries.

Resources

BOOKS

Chilnick, Lawrence D. *Heart Disease: An Essential Guide for the Newly Diagnosed.* Cambridge, Mass.: Da Capo Lifelong Books, 2008.

Kowalski, Robert E. *The Blood Pressure Cure: 8 Weeks to Lower Blood Pressure without Prescription Drugs.* New York: Wiley, 2008.

Sinatra, Stephen T., and James C. Roberts. *Reverse Heart Disease Now: Stop Deadly Cardiovascular Plaque Before It's Too Late.* New York: Wiley, 2008.

PERIODICALS

Expert Panel/Writing Group. "Evidence-Based Guidelines for Cardiovascular Disease Prevention in Women." *Circulation* (January 2004): 672–693.

Falk, Erling. "Pathogenesis of Atherosclerosis." *Journal of the American College of Cardiology* (April 2006): C7–C12.

ORGANIZATIONS

American Heart Association, National Center, 7272 Greenville Avenue, Dallas, TX, 75231-4596, http://www.americanheart.org/.

National Heart, Lung, and Blood Institute, P.O. Box 30105, Bethesda, MD, 20824-0105, http://www.nhlbi.nih.gov/.

Patience Paradox
Teresa G. Odle
David Edward Newton, Ed.D.

Athlete's foot

Definition

Athlete's foot is a common fungus infection in which the skin of the feet, especially on the sole and toes, becomes itchy and sore, cracking and peeling away. Athlete's foot, also known as tinea pedis, can be difficult to clear up completely.

Athlete's foot received its common name because the infection is often found among athletes. The fungi that cause the condition flourish best in and around swimming pools, showers, and locker rooms.

Description

Athlete's foot is very common, so common that most people have at least one episode of this fungal infection in their lives. It is found more often in adult males. Symptoms that appear to be athlete's foot in young children are probably caused by some other skin condition.

Causes and symptoms

Athlete's foot is caused by a fungal infection that most commonly affects the skin between the toes. The fungi that cause athlete's foot include *Trichophyton rubrum, T. mentagrophytes,* and *Epidermophyton floccosum.* These fungi live exclusively on dead body tissue, such as hair, the outer layer of skin, and the nails. The fungus grows best in moist, damp, dark places with poor ventilation. The problem is rare in children and those who customarily go barefoot.

Most people carry fungi on their skin. However, these fungi flourish to the point of causing athlete's foot only if conditions are favorable. The fungi multiply on the skin when it is irritated, weakened, or continuously moist. Sweaty feet, tight shoes, synthetic socks that do not absorb moisture well, a warm climate, and not drying the feet well after swimming or bathing all contribute to overgrowth of the fungi. Symptoms include itchy, sore skin on the toes, with scaling, inflammation, and **blisters**. Blisters that

break, exposing raw patches of tissue, can cause **pain** and swelling. The infected feet also may have an unpleasant smell. As the infection spreads, **itching** and burning may worsen. In severe cases, the skin cracks and seeps fluid. Sometimes a secondary bacterial infection is also present.

If not treated, athlete's foot can spread to the soles of the feet and toenails. Stubborn toenail **infections,** called tinea unguium, may appear at the same time, with crumbling, scaling, and thickened nails, and nail loss. The infection can spread further if patients scratch and then touch themselves elsewhere (especially in the groin or under the arms). The infection may also spread to other parts of the body via contaminated bed sheets, towels, or clothing. Athlete's foot is more severe and more common in people taking antibiotics, corticosteroids, birth control pills, drugs to suppress immune function, and in people are obese or who are living with **AIDS** or **diabetes mellitus**.

Diagnosis

A dermatologist can diagnose the condition by physical examination and by examining a preparation of skin scrapings under a microscope. Not all foot **rashes** are athlete's foot, which is the reason a physician should diagnose the condition before any remedies are used. In order to properly diagnose the infection, the physician may do a fungal culture. Using nonprescription products on a rash that is not athlete's foot can worsen the rash; therefore, proper diagnosis is important.

Treatment

The infected foot should be kept well ventilated. A foot bath containing cinnamon has been shown to slow down the growth of certain molds and fungi and is said to be very effective in clearing up athlete's foot. Eight to ten broken cinnamon sticks are boiled in four cups of water, simmered for five minutes, and then steeped for 45 minutes. The mixture can then be placed in a basin and used daily to soak the feet.

Herbal remedies used externally to treat athlete's foot include **goldenseal** (*Hydrastis canadensis*), **tea tree oil** (*Melaleuca spp.*), **myrrh** (*Commiphora molmol*), **garlic** (*Allium sativa*), oregano oil (though its smell is quite pungent), and **calendula**. The affected area should be swabbed with an herbal mixture twice daily or the feet should be soaked in a herbal footbath. **Pau d'arco**, also called taheebo or lapacho, can be used for athlete's foot as well. The tea bags can be soaked in water for about 10 minutes and then placed on the affected areas, or one can make a tincture that is rubbed directly on the toes.

Aromatherapy may be helpful. Several drops of the **essential oils** of tea tree, **peppermint** (*Mentha piperita*), or **chamomile** (*Matricaria recutita*), can be added to the bath water. Chamomile may be applied directly to the toes.

Allopathic treatment

Simple cases of athlete's foot usually respond to antifungal creams or sprays, such as tolnaftate (Aftate or Tinactin), clotrimazole, miconazole nitrate (Micatin products), or Whitfield's tincture made of salicylic acid and benzoic acid. Athlete's foot may be resistant to topical medication and should not be ignored. If the infection is resistant, the doctor may prescribe an oral antifungal drug such as ketoconozole or griseofulvin. Untreated athlete's foot may lead to a secondary bacterial infection in the skin cracks.

Expected results

Athlete's foot usually responds well to treatment, but it is important to complete the recommended treatment, even if the skin appears to be free of fungus; otherwise, the infection may return. Tinea unguium may accompany athlete's foot. It is typically very hard to treat effectively.

Prevention

A healthy diet should be maintained. Foods with a high sugar content should be avoided, including undiluted fruit juice, honey, and maple syrup.

Good personal hygiene and a few simple precautions can help prevent athlete's foot. These include:

- The feet should be washed daily; care should be taken to avoid contact with other parts of the body.
- The feet should be kept dry, especially between toes.
- Tight shoes and shoes made of synthetic material should not be worn.
- The feet need to be kept well ventilated, especially in the summer; bare feet and sandals are recommended.
- Absorbent polypropylene or white cotton socks are recommended; they should be cleaned and changed often.
- Bathing shoes should be worn in public bathing or showering areas.
- A good quality foot powder should be used to keep the feet dry.

KEY TERMS

Corticosteroids—Synthetic hormones that control nutritional processes in the body as well as the function of several organ systems.

- If anyone in the family has athlete's foot, towels, floors, and shower stalls should be washed with hot water and disinfectant after use.

Resources

BOOKS

Copeland, Glenn, and Stan Solomon. *The Good Foot Book.* Alameda, CA: Hunter House, 2005.
Vonhof, John. *Fixing Your Feet: Prevention and Treatments for Athletes.* Berkeley, CA: Wilderness Press, 2006.

ORGANIZATIONS

American Podiatric Medical Association, 9312 Old Georgetown Rd., Bethesda, MD, 20814, (301) 581-9221, http://www.apma.org/.

Patience Paradox
David Edward Newton, Ed.D.

Atkins diet

Definition

The Atkins diet is a high-protein, high-fat, very low-carbohydrate regimen. It emphasizes meat, cheese, and eggs, while discouraging foods such as bread, pasta, fruit, and sugar. It is a form of ketogenic diet.

Origins

Robert C. Atkins (1930–2003), a cardiologist and internist, developed the diet in the early 1970s. It first came to public attention in 1972 with the publication of *Dr. Atkins' Diet Revolution.* It quickly became a bestseller but, unlike most other fad **diets**, remained popular into the early 2000s. The diet started a "low-carb revolution," leading to development of low carbohydrate choices in grocery stores and restaurants around the world. In addition to his original book, Atkins authored a number of other books on his diet theme before his accidental death (from head injuries incurred from a fall) in 2003.

In 1992, Dr. Atkins updated his *Diet Revolution,* and by 2004 *Dr. Atkins' New Diet Revolution* had sold

ROBERT C. ATKINS (1930–2003)

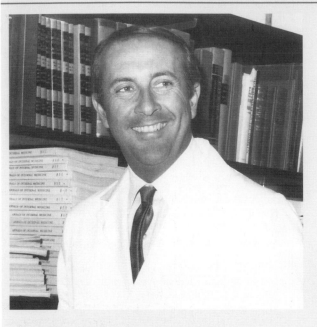

(AP/Wide World Photos. Reproduced by permission.)

Dr. Robert C. Atkins graduated from the University of Michigan in 1951 and received his medical degree from Cornell University Medical School in 1955 with a specialty in cardiology. As an internist and cardiologist he developed the Atkins Diet in the early 1970s. The diet is a ketogenic diet—a high protein, high fat, and very low carbohydrate regimen resulting in ketosis. It emphasizes meat, cheese, and eggs, while discouraging foods such as bread, pasta, fruit, and sugar. It first came to public attention in 1972 with the publication of *Dr. Atkins' Diet Revolution*. The book quickly became a bestseller but unlike most other fad diet books, this one has remained popular. At last count, it had been reprinted 28 times and sold more than 10 million copies worldwide. Since then, Atkins authored a number of other books on his diet theme, including *Dr. Atkins' New Diet Revolution* (1992), *Dr. Atkins' Quick and Easy New Diet Cookbook* (1997), and *The Vita-Nutrient Solution: Nature's Answer to Drugs* (1998).

Atkins saw about 60,000 patients in his more than 30 years of practice. He also appeared on numerous radio and television talk shows, had his own syndicated radio program, *Your Health Choices*, and authored the monthly newsletter *Dr. Atkins' Health Revelations*. Atkins received the World Organization of Alternative Medicine's Recognition of Achievement Award and was named the National Health Federation's Man of the Year. He was director of the Atkins Center for Complementary Medicine, which he founded in the early 1980s. The center is located at 152 E. 55th St., New York, NY 10022.

more than 45 million copies and been translated into 25 languages. The new plan was the same, but the maintenance portion of the diet was made a little more liberal. The diet was extremely popular, as were Atkins Nutritionals products, such as vitamin supplements and numerous food items. A later Web-based version called the Atkins Advantage emphasized the products of Atkins Nutritionals and offered additional books, software, and information on a company Web site to support the program's goals and products.

Benefits

The primary benefit of the diet is rapid and substantial weight loss. By restricting carbohydrate intake, the body **burns** more fat stored in the body. Since there are no limits on the amount of calories or quantities of foods allowed on the diet, there is little hunger between meals. According to Atkins, the diet can alleviate symptoms of conditions such as **fatigue**, irritability, headaches, **depression**, and some types of joint and muscle **pain**.

Some dieters have had at least initial success with the diet and have found the liberal rules regarding protein and fats more tasteful and filling than other diets. Advice from the Atkins plan concerning behavioral changes can be helpful, such as shopping the perimeter of the grocery store, where the unprocessed foods are located. In the 1990s and early 2000s, the program attempted to modify some of its advice to more closely fit traditional advice from registered dieticians. For example, more clearly defining the types of fats to emphasize in the diet may help dieters avoid overeating unhealthy fats and increasing their risk for **heart disease**. However, experts have said that the diet still contradicts mainstream views concerning health promotion and disease prevention.

Description

The regimen is a low-carbohydrate, or ketogenic diet, characterized by initial rapid weight loss, usually due to water loss. Drastically reducing the amount of carbohydrate intake causes liver and muscle glycogen loss, which has a strong but temporary diuretic effect. Long-term weight loss is said to occur because with a low amount of carbohydrate intake, the body burns stored fat for energy.

The four-step diet starts with a two-week induction program designed to rebalance an individual's metabolism. Unlimited amounts of fat and protein are allowed but carbohydrate intake is restricted to 15 to 20 grams per day. Foods allowed include butter, oil, meat, poultry, fish, eggs, cheese, and cream. The daily amount of carbohydrates allowed equals about three cups of salad vegetables, such as lettuce, cucumbers, and celery. High fat condiments such as mayonnaise, sour cream, guacamole, and butter are allowed in virtually unlimited quantities. The Atkins theory is that these high fat foods enhance the flavor of meals, making the Atkins diet easier to maintain. Atkins has reminded dieters that while unlimited quantities of fats and proteins are allowed, the advice is not a license to gorge. Dieters are said to feel hungry for the first 48 hours as their bodies adjust to the abrupt reduction in carbohydrates. Weight loss during the induction phase is said to be significant. The phase is recommended to last at least two weeks.

The second stage of the diet is for ongoing weight loss. It allows 15 to 40 grams of carbohydrates a day. When individuals are about 10 pounds from their desired weight, they begin the pre-maintenance phase. They gradually begin to increase carbohydrate intake by 10 grams per week until weight is gained, then drops back to the previous carbohydrate gram level. Examples of vegetables that contain about 10 grams of carbohydrates are 3/4 c. of carrots, 1/2 c. of acorn squash, 1 c. of beets, and 1/4 c. of white potatoes. Legumes and fruit are the next preferred food groups for adding 10 grams daily. One-half apple contains 10 grams of carbohydrates, as does 1/3 c. of kidney beans.

Once the goal weight is reached the maintenance stage begins. This phase generally allows an adult to consume 90 to 120 grams of carbohydrates a day, depending on age, gender, and activity level, but maintaining goal weight is more likely if carbohydrate intake remains at the level discovered in pre-maintenance. The key, according to Atkins, is never letting weight vary by more than three to five pounds before making corrections.

Like many fad diets, the Atkins plan produces and promotes many food products associated with its diet plan. As of 2007, these products included bars, shakes, and candy. So although the plan argues against processed foods and snacking, the company also heavily promotes use of its nutritional products to support weight loss or maintenance.

Preparations

No advance preparation is needed to go on the diet. However, as with most diets, it is important to consult with a physician and to have a physical evaluation before starting a new nutritional regimen. The evaluation should include blood tests to determine levels of **cholesterol**, triglycerides, glucose, insulin, and uric acid. A glucose tolerance test is also recommended.

Precautions

Adherence to the Atkins diet can result in vitamin and mineral deficiencies. In his books, Atkins recommends a wide range of nutritional supplements, including a multi-vitamin. Among his recommendations, Atkins suggests the following daily dosages: 300-600 micrograms (mcg) of **chromium** picolinate, 100-400 milligrams (mg) of pantetheine, 200 mcg of **selenium**, and 450-675 mcg of **biotin**.

The diet is not recommended for lacto-ovo vegetarians, since it cannot be done as successfully without protein derived from animal products. Also, vegans cannot follow this diet, since a vegan diet is too high in carbohydrates, according to Atkins. Instead, he recommends vegetarians with a serious weight problem give up **vegetarianism**, or at least include fish in their diet. In 2003, a physicians group warned that high-protein diets may cause permanent kidney loss in anyone with reduced kidney function. They also can increase people's risk of colon **cancer** and **osteoporosis**.

Side effects

The average carbohydrate intake recommended by the Atkins diet is well below averages generally recommended by other experts. Studies have shown that even though people may lose weight on the Atkins plan, they do not necessarily keep the weight off long-term because the diet does not teach sustainable lifestyle changes.

Followers of the Atkins diet have reported **muscle cramps**, **diarrhea**, general weakness, and **rashes** more frequently than people on low-fat diets. Others have reported **constipation**, bad breath, **headache**, and fatigue. The American Dietetic Association has warned that any diet that severely limits one food group should raise a red flag to dieters.

Beyond the reported side effects and concerns about the diet's long-term effectiveness, some serious problems may arise for Atkins diet followers. One problem that has been documented is called ketoacidosis, which occurs when there is a buildup of the by-products of fat breakdown because the body does not have enough glucose available. The condition can be dangerous, resulting in cell damage, severe illness, and even death. The low amounts of carbohydrates eaten by those on the diet are below those needed to supply the brain and muscles with sugar. Critics of the diet have also long focused on the risks of unlimited fat intake that the Atkins diet allows. Eating large amounts of saturated fat, even if weight is dropping, can lead to high levels of cholesterol and heart disease. However, this outcome does not inevitably occur. Cholesterol levels tend to decrease in many individuals when they lose weight, even if eating an unbalanced diet. As of 2008, long-term research remained to be done in this area.

People with diabetes who take insulin are at risk of becoming hypoglycemic if they do not eat appropriate carbohydrates. Also, persons who **exercise** regularly may experience low energy levels and muscle fatigue from low carbohydrate intake.

Research and general acceptance

Opinion from the general medical community remains mixed on the Atkins diet but is generally unfavorable. There have been no significant long-term scientific studies on the diet. A number of leading medical and health organizations, including the American Medical Association, American Dietetic Association (ADA), and the American Heart Association oppose it. It is drastically different than the dietary intakes recommended by the U.S. Department of Agriculture and the National Institutes of Health. Much of the opposition comes from the fact that the diet lacks some vitamins and nutrients and is high in fat. In a hearing before the U.S. Congress on February 24, 2000, an ADA representative called the Atkins diet "hazardous" and said it lacked scientific credibility.

In 2004, Jody Gorran, a 53-year-old businessman from Florida, sued the promoters of the Atkins Diet, saying that the plan clogged his arteries and nearly killed him. Gorran claimed that he was seduced by the plan and that by eating the high levels of protein and fats touted by the plan, his cholesterol soared. His lawsuit was backed by the Washington-based advocacy group called Physicians Committee for Responsible Medicine. Gorran sought damages and an injunction preventing the sale of Atkins' books and products without fair and adequate warnings about the dangers of the diet. The lawsuit was dismissed late in 2006 by a judge, but an appeal continued as of 2008.

Atkins' company filed for Chapter 11 bankruptcy protection in July 2005. The company completed its Chapter 11 reorganization by January 2006, having streamlined some operations, and it continued to operate early in 2007, making the Dr. Atkins' diet run more than 35 years long.

Though Dr. Atkins added that numerous studies pointed to the fact that carbohydrates were to blame for weight gain, an explanation for how his diet

---

KEY TERMS

Biotin—The B complex vitamin found naturally in yeast, liver, and egg yolks.

Carbohydrates—Neutral compounds of carbon, hydrogen, and oxygen found in sugar, starches, and cellulose.

Hypertension—Abnormally high arterial blood pressure, which if left untreated can lead to heart disease and stroke.

Ketogenic diet—A diet that supplies an abnormally high amount of fat and small amounts of carbohydrates and protein.

Ketosis—An abnormal increase in ketones in the body, usually found in people with uncontrolled diabetes mellitus.

Pantetheine—A growth factor substance essential in humans and a constituent of coenzyme A.

Triglycerides—A blood fat lipid that increases the risk for heart disease.

---

program worked was never really offered by researchers. Numerous studies continued throughout the 1990s and even after Dr. Atkins' death in 2003. Though some studies showed that people on the Atkins diet often lost weight faster in six months than those on other weight loss programs, the long-term effectiveness and possible harmful effects of the Atkins diet required more study.

Training and certification

There is no formal training or certification required.

Resources

BOOKS

Atkins, Robert C. *Atkins for Life*. New York: St. Martin's, 2003.
Atkins, Robert C. *Dr. Atkins' New Diet Revolution*. New York: St. Martin's Paperbacks, 2004.

PERIODICALS

"Atkins Diet Vindicated But Long-term Success Questionable." *Obesity, Fitness, and Wellness Week* (June 14, 2003): 25.
"Doctor Group Describes Dangers of Atkins Diet." *Obesity, Fitness, and Wellness Week* (August 9, 2003): 33.

OTHER

Atkins Center for Complementary Medicine. 152 E. Fifty-fifth St., New York, NY 10022. (212) 758-2110. http://www.atkinscenter.com.

ORGANIZATIONS

Atkins Nutritionals, 1050 Seventeenth St., Suite 100, Denver, CO, 80265, (800) 6-ATKINS, http://www.atkins.com.

Physicians Committee for Responsible Medicine, 5100 Wisconsin Ave. NW, Suite 400, Washington, DC, 20016, (202) 686-2210, http://www.atkinsdietalert.org.

Ken R. Wells
Teresa G. Odle
Helen Davidson

Atopic dermatitis *see* **Eczema**

Atractylodes

Description

Atractylodes is the dried or steam-dried rhizome (rootstalk) of *Atractylodes macrocephala* or *A. ovata*, perennial north Asian herbs in the Compositae family. It grows in mountain valleys, especially in China's Zhejiang province. It may also be cultivated. In autumn, it presents magenta corolla blooms.

In Mandarin, atractylodes is called *Bai Zhu, Bai Shu, Yu Zhu,* and *Dong Zhu.* The Cantonese term is *Paak Sat,* and the Japanese call it *Byakujutsu.* Common names include large-headed atractylodes, white atractylodes, and white shu. Its pharmaceutical name, used to distinguish it as a medicine, is Rhizoma Atractylodis, and it is one of more than 500 plants recognized as official drugs in **traditional Chinese medicine**. Related species, *A. lancea* and *A. chinensis,* both called black or gray atractylodes, are also used medicinally for similar but distinct purposes.

General use

Practitioners of Chinese medicine believe that atractylodes affects the Spleen and Stomach meridians, or energy pathways in the body. Its medicinal properties are considered warm, mildly bitter, and sweet.

Atractylodes is thought to dry dampness, strengthen the Spleen or digestion, and promote diuresis, the formation and excretion of urine. It is used for **diarrhea**, generalized aching, mental **fatigue, dizziness**, lack of appetite, **vomiting, edema** (accumulation of fluids), and spontaneous sweating. It is also used to prevent miscarriage and to treat restless fetal movement. Other uses include restoring deficient digestion associated with poor absorption, malnutrition, anorexia, metabolic acidosis, hypogylcemia, and rheumatism. It has also been used to treat tumors of the cervix, uterus, breast, and stomach.

KEY TERMS

Cold—In Chinese pathology, the term defines a condition that has insufficient warmth, either objective (hypothermia) or subjective (feeling cold).

Decoction—A strong tea brewed for twenty to thirty minutes.

Heat—In Chinese pathology, the term defines a condition that has excessive heat, either objective (fever, infection) or subjective (feeling hot).

Meridians—Energetic pathways inside the body through which qi flows; also called channels.

Tincture—A solution of medicinal substance in alcohol, usually more or less diluted. Herb tinctures are made by infusing the alcohol with plant material.

Qi—A Chinese medical term denoting active physiological energy.

According to traditional Chinese medicine, both white and black atractylodes may be used for digestive and urinary problems. Black atractylodes is more drying than white. White atractylodes has the additional benefit of being a "Spleen Qi tonic," meaning that it rebuilds metabolic function by increasing **nutrition**, increasing energy, and regulating fluids. White atractylodes is also thought to have restorative, normalizing effects on the digestive system and Liver.

Research on atractylodes has generally been conducted in China and has focused on pharmacological investigation and animal experiments. In-vitro and animal studies show it has significant diuretic, sedative, and hypoglycemic (lowering of blood glucose) effects. Animal studies pinpoint the essential oil as responsible for sedative effects. It also promotes digestion and quells **nausea** and diarrhea.

Major chemical constituents include atractylone, atractylol, butenolide B, acetoxyatractylon, hydroxyatractylon, and **vitamin A**.

Preparations

Atractylodes is not generally available in American health food stores, but it can be found at most Chinese pharmacies and Asian groceries. Good quality atractylodes is large, firm, solid, aromatic, and has a yellowish cross section.

The standard dose is 3–10 g as a decoction (strong tea) or 1–4 ml of tincture. Doses of dried material are 3–12 g.

Atractylodes is commonly prescribed in conjunction with moisture-removing drugs and digestants. Practitioners of Chinese medicine commonly also combine atractylodes with other Chinese herbs. The following are the major herbs with which it is combined and the symptoms for which the combinations are prescribed.

- Radix codonopsis (*Codonopsis pilosula, Dang Shen*) and rhizoma zingiberis (*Zingiber officinalis, Gan Jiang*, dried ginger root) for abdominal pain, distention, vomiting, and diarrhea.

- Fructus Immaturus Citri Aurantii (*Citrus aurantium, Zhi Shi*, unripened bitter orange) for reduced appetite with abdominal distention and fullness due to Spleen deficiency with qi stagnation.

- Gray or black atractylodes (*Atractylodes japonica, Cang Zhu*) for damp-cold painful obstruction or vaginal discharge.

- Sclerotium Poriae Cocos (*Poria cocos; Fu Ling*; tuckahoe, poria, or Indian bread) and Ramulus Cinnamomi Cassiae (*Cinnamomum cassia, Gui Zhi*, cinnamon twig) for congested fluids with distention of the chest and edema due to Spleen deficiency.

- Astragalus (*Astragalus membranaceus, Huang Qi*) and Fructus Tritici (*Triticum aestivum, Fu Xiao Mai*, name wheat grain) for unrelenting spontaneous sweating.

- Ramulus Perillae (*Perilla frutescens, Su Geng*) and Pericarpium Citri Reticulatae (*Citrus reticulata, Chen Pi*, aged tangerine rind) for restless fetus disorder with qi stagnation giving rise to distention and fullness in the chest and abdomen.

Precautions

According to tradition, atractylodes is contraindicated in the presence of deficient heat conditions.

Side effects

None noted.

Interactions

No interactions with pharmaceutical drugs have been noted.

Resources

BOOKS

Bensky, Dan, and Andrew Gamble. *Chinese Herbal Medicine: Materia Medica*. Rev. ed. Seattle: Eastland Press, 1993.

Fan, Warner J-W. *A Manual of Chinese Herbal Medicine: Principles and Practice for Easy Reference*. Boston: Shambhala, 1996.

Holmes, Peter. *Jade Remedies: A Chinese Herbal Reference for the West*. Boulder, CO: Snow Lotus Press, 1996.

Hsu, Hong-yen, et al. *Oriental Materia Medica: A Concise Guide*. Long Beach, CA: Oriental Healing Arts Institute, 1986.

Erika Lenz

Attention-deficit hyperactivity disorder

Definition

Attention-deficit hyperactivity disorder (ADHD) is a developmental disorder characterized by distractibility, hyperactivity, impulsive behaviors, and the inability to remain focused on tasks or activities.

Description

ADHD, also known as hyperkinetic disorder (HKD) outside the United States, is estimated to affect 3–5% of children, or about 2 million children in the United States. It also affects about 4% of adults. The disorder affects boys more often than girls. Although difficult to assess in infancy and toddlerhood, signs of ADHD may begin to appear as early as age two or three, but the symptom picture changes as adolescence approaches. Many symptoms, particularly hyperactivity, diminish in early adulthood. However, impulsivity and inattention problems remain with up to 50% of individuals with ADHD throughout their adult life.

Children with ADHD have short attention spans and are easily bored and/or frustrated with tasks. Although these individuals may be quite intelligent, their lack of focus frequently results in poor grades and difficulties in school. Children with ADHD act impulsively, taking action first and thinking later. They are constantly moving, running, climbing, squirming, and fidgeting, but often have trouble with gross and fine motor skills. As a result, they may be physically clumsy and awkward. Their clumsiness may extend to the social arena, where they are sometimes shunned due to their impulsive and intrusive behavior. Some critics argue that ADHD is a condition created and diagnosed in the Western world, particular to the environment of highly developed countries, since it is not diagnosed in other cultures. These critics of the ADHD diagnosis believe that medicating a child does not address the true underlying problem. They also note that there may not be a problem at all because children are naturally active and impulsive.

Causes and symptoms

The causes of ADHD are not known. However, it appears that heredity plays a major role in the development of ADHD. Children with a parent or sibling with ADHD are more likely to develop the disorder. Before birth, children with ADHD may have been exposed to poor maternal **nutrition**, viral **infections**, or maternal **substance abuse**. In early childhood, exposure to lead or other toxins can cause ADHD-like symptoms. Traumatic brain injury or neurological disorders also may trigger ADHD symptoms. An imbalance of certain neurotransmitters (the chemicals in the brain that send messages between nerve cells) is believed to be the mechanism behind ADHD symptoms.

A widely publicized study conducted by Benjamin Feingold in the early 1970s suggested that **allergies** to certain foods and food additives caused the characteristic hyperactivity of children with ADHD. Although some children may have adverse reactions to certain foods that can affect their behavior (for example, a rash might temporarily cause a child to be distracted from other tasks), carefully controlled follow-up studies uncovered no link between food allergies and ADHD. Another popularly held misconception about food and ADHD is that eating sugar causes hyperactive behavior. Again, studies have shown no link between sugar intake and ADHD. It is important to note that a nutritionally balanced diet is important for normal development in all children.

People with ADHD experience a variety of symptoms, including distraction, not paying attention, inconsistency, forgetfulness of even simple tasks, fidgeting, verbal impulsivity, and many other behaviors. It is interesting to note that everyone experiences these symptoms at times, but an individual with ADHD has more of these symptoms more of the time.

Psychologists and other mental health professionals typically use the criteria listed in the *Diagnostic and Statistical Manual of Mental Disorders, Fourth Edition, Text Revised (DSM-IV-TR)* as a guideline for determining the presence of ADHD. For a diagnosis of ADHD, *DSM-IV-TR* requires the presence of at least six of the following symptoms of inattention or six or more symptoms of hyperactivity and impulsivity combined.

Inattention

- fails to pay close attention to detail or makes careless mistakes in schoolwork or other activities
- has difficulty sustaining attention in tasks or activities
- does not appear to listen when spoken to
- does not follow through on instructions and does not finish tasks
- has difficulty organizing tasks and activities
- avoids or dislikes tasks that require sustained mental effort (such as doing homework)
- is easily distracted
- is forgetful in daily activities

Hyperactivity

- fidgets with hands or feet or squirms in seat
- does not remain seated when expected to do so
- runs or climbs excessively when inappropriate (in adolescents and adults, feelings of restlessness)
- has difficulty playing quietly
- is constantly on the move
- talks excessively

Impulsivity

- blurts out answers before the question has been completed
- has difficulty waiting for his or her turn
- interrupts and/or intrudes on others

DSM-IV-TR also requires that some symptoms develop before age seven and that they significantly impair functioning in two or more settings (e.g., home and school) for at least six months. Children who meet the symptom criteria for inattention, but not for hyperactivity/impulsivity are diagnosed with Attention-Deficit/Hyperactivity Disorder, Predominantly Inattentive Type, commonly called ADD. (Young girls with ADHD may not be diagnosed as frequently because they have mainly this subtype of the disorder.)

Diagnosis

The first step in determining if a child has ADHD is to consult with a pediatrician, a doctor who treats children. The pediatrician can make an initial evaluation of the child's developmental maturity compared to other children in the patient's age group. The doctor also should perform a comprehensive physical examination to rule out any organic causes of ADHD symptoms, such as an overactive thyroid or vision or hearing problems.

If no organic problem can be found, a psychologist, psychiatrist, neurologist, neuropsychologist, or learning specialist typically is consulted to perform a comprehensive ADHD assessment. A complete medical, family, social, psychiatric, and educational history is compiled from existing medical and school records and from interviews with parents and teachers. Interviews also may be conducted with the child, depending on the individual's age. Along with these interviews, several clinical inventories also may be used, such as the Conners Rating Scales (Teacher's Questionnaire and Parent's Questionnaire), Child Behavior Checklist (CBCL), and the Achenbach Child Behavior Rating Scales. These inventories provide valuable information on the child's behavior in different settings and situations. In addition, the Wender Utah Rating Scale has been adapted for use in diagnosing ADHD in adults.

It is important to note that mental disorders such as **depression** and **anxiety** disorder can cause symptoms similar to ADHD. A complete and comprehensive psychiatric assessment is critical to differentiate ADHD from other possible mood and behavioral disorders. **Bipolar disorder**, for example, may be misdiagnosed as ADHD.

Public schools are required by federal law to offer free ADHD testing upon request. A pediatrician also can provide a referral to a psychologist or pediatric specialist for an ADHD assessment. Parents should check with their insurance plans to see if these services are covered.

Treatment

Many treatments are popular for treating children with ADHD. Behavior modification therapy uses a reward system to reinforce good behavior as well as task completion and can be used both in the classroom and at home. A tangible reward such as a sticker may be given to the child every time he completes a task or behaves in an acceptable manner. A chart system may be used to display the stickers and visually illustrate the child's progress. When a certain number of stickers are collected, the child may trade them in for a bigger reward such as a trip to the zoo or a day at the beach. The reward system stays in place until the good behavior becomes ingrained.

A variation of this technique, cognitive-behavioral therapy, works to decrease impulsive behavior by getting the child to recognize the connection between thoughts and behavior and to change behavior by changing negative thinking patterns.

Individual **psychotherapy** can help children with ADHD build self-esteem, give them a place to discuss their worries and anxieties, and help them gain insight into their behavior and feelings. Family therapy also may be beneficial in helping family members develop coping skills and work through feelings of guilt or anger they may be experiencing.

Children with ADHD perform better within a familiar, consistent, and structured routine with positive reinforcements for good behavior and real consequences for bad. Family, friends, and caretakers should be educated on the special needs and behaviors of the child with ADHD. Communication between parents and teachers is especially critical for ensuring that a child with ADHD has an appropriate learning environment.

A number of alternative treatments exist for ADHD. Although there is a lack of controlled studies to prove their efficacy, a 2005 study found more than two out of three families containing a child with ADHD sought complementary or alternative ADHD treatment at some time. Proponents of these treatments report that they are successful in controlling symptoms in some ADHD patients. Some of the more popular alternative treatments are listed.

- Electroencephalograph (EEG) biofeedback. By measuring brain wave activity and teaching the patient with ADHD which type of brain wave is associated with attention, EEG biofeedback attempts to train patients to generate the desired brain wave activity.

- Dietary therapy. Based in part on the Feingold food allergy diet, dietary therapy focuses on a nutritional plan that is high in protein and complex carbohydrates and free of white sugar and salicylate-containing foods such as strawberries, tomatoes, and grapes.

- Herbal therapy. Herbal therapy uses a variety of natural remedies to address the symptoms of ADHD. Ginkgo (*Gingko biloba*) is used for memory and mental sharpness and chamomile (*Matricaria recutita*) extract is used for calming. The safety of herbal remedies has not been demonstrated in controlled studies. For example, it is known that gingko may affect blood coagulation, but controlled studies have not evaluated the risk of the effect.

- Vitamin and mineral supplements. Vitamin and mineral supplements thought to be effective by some alternative practitioners include calcium, zinc, magnesium, iron, inositol, trace minerals, and blue-green algae. Also recommended are the combined amino acids GABA, glycine, taurine, L-glutamine, L phenylalanine, and L-tyrosine.

- Homeopathic medicine. This is probably the most effective alternative therapy for ADD and ADHD because it treats the whole person at a core level. Constitutional homeopathic care is most appropriate and requires consulting with a well-trained homeopath who has experience working with individuals with ADD and ADHD.

- Auricular acupuncture. A small study indicated that this type of acupuncture therapy might be effective in some children, but large well-controlled studies have not been done.

Allopathic treatment

Psychosocial therapy, usually combined with medications, is the treatment approach of choice to alleviate ADHD symptoms. Psychostimulants, such as dextroamphetamine (Dexedrine), pemoline (Cylert), and methylphenidate (Ritalin) commonly are prescribed to control hyperactive and impulsive behavior and increase attention span. They work by stimulating the production of certain neurotransmitters in the brain. Possible side effects of stimulants include nervous tics, irregular heartbeat, loss of appetite, and **insomnia**. The medications usually are well-tolerated and safe in most cases.

In children who do not respond well to stimulant therapy, tricyclic antidepressants such as desipramine (Norpramin, Pertofane) and amitriptyline (Elavil) are frequently recommended. Reported side effects of these drugs include persistent **dry mouth**, sedation, disorientation, and irregular heartbeat (particularly with desipramine). Other medications prescribed for ADHD therapy are buproprion (Wellbutrin), an antidepressant; fluoxetine (Prozac), an antidepressant; and carbamazepine (Tegretol, Atretol), an anticonvulsant drug. Clonidine (Catapres), a medication for high blood pressure, also has been used to control aggression and hyperactivity in some children with ADHD, although it should not be used with Ritalin. A child's response to medication will change with age and maturation, so ADHD symptoms should be monitored closely and prescriptions adjusted accordingly.

In late 2002, the first new drug for treating ADHD released in 30 years was approved by the United States Food and Drug Administration (FDA). The drug atomoxetine (brand name Strattera) was developed by Eli Lilly. Strattera was the first medication for ADHD that was not a stimulant. It was believed that

Strattera would improve ADHD symptoms without many of the negative side effects of stimulants. In 2005 the FDA issued a warning that atomoxetine was linked to increased rates of suicidal thoughts in children and teens who take it. Although the observed rate of children with suicidal thoughts was only 4 in 1,000, and no suicides occurred, the FDA recommended increased vigilance among doctors prescribing atomoxetine and required new warning labels on boxes of Strattera.

Expected results

Untreated, ADHD negatively affects the social and educational performance of children and can seriously damage their sense of self-esteem. Children with ADHD have impaired relationships with their peers and may be seen as social outcasts. They may be seen as slow learners or troublemakers in the classroom. Siblings and even parents may develop resentful feelings toward the child with ADHD.

Some children with ADHD also develop a conduct disorder problem. For those adolescents who have both ADHD and a conduct disorder, up to 25% go on to develop antisocial personality disorder and the criminal behavior, substance abuse, and high rate of suicide attempts that are symptomatic of it. Children diagnosed with ADHD also are more likely to have a learning disorder, a mood disorder such as depression, or an anxiety disorder.

Approximately 70-80% of patients with ADHD who are treated with stimulant medication experience significant relief from symptoms, at least in the short-term. Approximately half of children with ADHD seem to "outgrow" the disorder in adolescence or early adulthood. The other half retain some or all symptoms of ADHD as adults. With early identification and intervention, careful compliance with a treatment program, and a supportive and nurturing home and school environment, children with ADHD can flourish socially and academically.

Resources

BOOKS

Brynie, Faith Hickman. *ADHD: Attention-Deficit Hyper-activity Disorder*. Minneapolis, MN: Twenty-First Century Books, 2008.

Conners, Keith C. *Attention Deficit Hyperactivity Disorder in Children and Adolescents: The Latest Assessment and Treatment Strategies*, 4th ed. Kansas City, MO: Compact Clinicals, 2008.

Diagnostic and Statistical Manual of Mental Disorders, 4th ed. Washington, DC: American Psychiatric Press, 2000.

McBurnett, Keith, and Linda Pfiffner, eds. *Attention Deficit Hyperactivity Disorder: Concepts, Controversies, New Directions*. New York: Informa Healthcare, 2008.

PERIODICAL

Chen, Mandy, Carla M. Seipp, and Charlotte Johnston. "Mothers' and Fathers' Attributions and Beliefs in Families of Girls and Boys with Attention-Deficit/Hyperactivity Disorder." *Child Psychiatry and Human Development* 39, no. 1 (March 2008): 85–100.

Dennis, Tanya, et al. "Attention Deficit Hyperactivity Disorder: Parents' and Professionals' Perceptions." *Community Practitioner* 81, no. 3 (March 2008): 24–29.

ORGANIZATIONS

Attention Deficit Disorder Association, 15000 Commerce Parkway, Suite C, Mount Laurel, NJ, 08054, (856) 439-9099, www.aad.org.

Kim Sharp
Teresa G. Odle

Aucklandia

Description

Aucklandia, also known as costus or *Mu Xiang*, is the root of the plant *Saussurea costus*. Aucklandia has been used for centuries in Chinese and Indian herbal healing. In modern times, it has been used in Western **aromatherapy**.

Aucklandia comes from a perennial plant that grows to about 6 ft (2 m) in height. It is native to northern India and Pakistan. This plant is also cultivated in other parts of India and in southwest China. The long, tapering root is harvested and dried for uses in healing.

In some regions of Asia, several other species of plant are used interchangeably with *Saussurea costus*. These include *Saussurea lappa* and *Saussurea vladimirus*. Locally, aucklandia is also called kuth, kust, kushta, qust-e-shereen, and patchak.

General use

Aucklandia is used in China and India to treat three main categories of complaints concerning the digestive system, the lungs, and **infections**. Aucklandia is used to treat symptoms such as **nausea**, **vomiting**, **diarrhea**, colon spasms, poor digestion, abdominal **gas**, and stomach **pain**. In laboratory studies, aucklandia has been shown to be an antispasmodic, accounting for its effectiveness against such symptoms as nausea and diarrhea. It is also sometimes used to treat **gallstones** and **jaundice**, although no scientific studies have confirmed its effectiveness for these uses.

Aucklandia is used in many places in Asia to treat **asthma**, **bronchitis**, and uncontrolled **cough**. The antispasmodic component of the root extract causes the airways to relax and open more so that breathing becomes easier. This same property causes it to mildly lower blood pressure by relaxing the artery walls. However, it does not lower blood pressure as effectively as some other herbs.

In India, aucklandia is used primarily as an antiseptic, an insecticide, and a fungicide. It is also said to be effective against yeast infections and some parasites. Some research suggests that aucklandia has antibiotic actions and may be effective against infections such as cholera and typhoid. It appears that the use of aucklandia as an antiseptic has some basis in scientific fact.

Other uses of aucklandia that have not been investigated in regulated scientific studies include using it as a treatment for water retention and lung and liver tumors. In addition to its medicinal uses, aucklandia is a fragrance and fixative in perfumes, shampoo, and hair dye. It is used in the Asian food industry to flavor alcoholic beverages, soft drinks, and sweets.

Preparations

Aucklandia can be prepared as either a distilled extract or as an essential oil. The dried roots are chopped fine and softened in warm water, then distilled with steam. The resulting water-based distillate is then subjected to a solvent extraction to remove the active ingredients. The resulting yellow-brown fluid has a long-lasting woody or musty odor. In Chinese medicine, aucklandia is classified as acrid and bitter.

Aucklandia is used in formulas to treat both digestive and respiratory complaints. The best known of these formulas is *Mu Xiang Shun Qi Wan*. It is used to relieve pain and encourage digestion. *Mu Xiang Shun Qi Wan* is also used to treat chronic **hepatitis**, newly

KEY TERMS

Antispasmodic—A substance that relieves spasm or uncontrolled contraction, usually of the smooth or involuntary muscle of the arteries, intestines, or the airways.

Distillate—The material obtained through the process of distilling (vaporized and condensed to separate out different compounds).

Yin aspects—Yin aspects are the opposite of yang aspects and are represented by qualities such as cold, stillness, darkness, and passiveness.

developed **cirrhosis** of the liver, and abdominal pain. This formula is commercially available as pills, with the recommended dose of eight pills twice a day.

Several other common formulas contain aucklandia. Ginseng and longan formula (*Gui Pi Tang*) is used to treat gastrointestinal upsets and various kinds of physical and emotional **stress**. Rhubarb and scutellaria formula (*Li Dan Pian*) is used to treat gallstones. *Tang Gui* and indigo formula (*Chien Chin Chih Tai Wan*) is used to treat vaginal discharge and vaginal infections, as well as lower body pain.

The oil of aucklandia is more commonly used in India than in China, and it is also used in Western aromatherapy. It is applied externally or inhaled. The oil also is used by the cosmetic and perfume industry, where it blends well with other fragrances such as patchouli and floral fragrances.

Precautions

In Chinese medicine, aucklandia should not be used by people with deficient *yin*, which means people who are dehydrated or have a lot of dryness.

Side effects

When used externally, aucklandia causes skin irritation (**contact dermatitis**) in some sensitive individuals.

Interactions

Aucklandia has been used safely in Asia as a medicinal herb and a food and cosmetic additive for centuries. It is often used in conjunction with other herbs with no reported interactions. Since aucklandia has been used almost exclusively in Asian medicine, there are no available studies of its interactions with Western pharmaceuticals.

Resources

BOOKS

Chevallier, Andrew. *Herbal Remedies*. New York: DK Publishing, 2007.

Foster, Steven, and Rebecca Johnson. *National Geographic Desk Reference to Nature's Medicine*. Washington, DC: National Geographic Society, 2006.

PDR for Herbal Medicines, 4th ed. Montvale, NJ: Thompson Healthcare, 2007.

PERIODICALS

Pandey, M. M., S. Rastogi, and A. K. Rasat. "Saussurea costus: Botanical, Chemical, and Pharmacological Review of an Ayurvedic Medicinal Plant." *Journal of Ethnopharmacology* (April 2007): 379–90.

ORGANIZATIONS

Alternative Medicine Foundation, PO Box 60016, Potomac, MD, 20859, (301) 340-1960, www.amfoundation.org.

American Association of Oriental Medicine, PO Box 162340, Sacramento, CA, 95816, (866) 455-7999, (914) 443-4770, http://www.aaaomonline.org.

Centre for International Ethnomedicinal Education and Research (CIEER), www.cieer.org.

Tish Davidson, A. M.

Auditory integration training

Definition

Auditory integration training, or AIT, is one specific type of music/auditory therapy based upon the work of French otolaryngologists Dr. Alfred Tomatis and Dr. Guy Berard.

Origins

The premise upon which most auditory integration programs are based is that distortion in how things are heard contributes to commonly seen behavioral or **learning disorders** in children. Some of these disorders include **attention-deficit hyperactivity disorder** (ADHD), **autism**, **dyslexia**, and central auditory processing disorders (CAPD). Training the patient to listen can stimulate central and cortical organization.

Auditory integration is one facet of what audiologists call central auditory processing. The simplest definition of central auditory processing, or CAP, is University of Buffalo Professor of Audiology Jack Katz's, which is: "What we do with what we hear." Central auditory integration is actually the perception of sound, including the ability to attend to sound, to remember it, retaining it in both the long- and short-term memory, to be able to listen to sound selectively, and to localize it.

Berard developed one of the programs commonly used. Berard's auditory integration training consists of twenty half-hour sessions spent listening to musical sounds via a stereophonic system. The music is random, with filtered frequencies, and the person listens through earphones. These sound waves vibrate and exercise structures in the middle ear. This is normally done in sessions twice a day for 10 days.

Tomatis is also the inventor of the Electronic Ear. This device operates through a series of filters, and reestablishes the dominance of the right ear in hearing. The basis of Tomatis' work is a series of principles that follow:

- The most important purpose of the ear is to adapt sound waves into signals that charge the brain.
- Sound is conducted via both air and bone. It can be considered something that nourishes the nervous system, either stimulating or destimulating it.
- Just as seeing is not the same as looking, hearing is not the same as listening. Hearing is passive. Listening is active.
- A person's ability to listen affects all language development for that person. This process influences every aspect of self-image and social development.
- The capacity to listen can be changed or improved through auditory stimulation using musical and vocal sounds at high frequencies.
- Communication begins in the womb. As early as the beginning of the second trimester, fetuses can hear sounds. These sounds literally cause the brain and nervous system of the baby to develop.

Description

A quartet of CAP defects have been identified that can unfavorably alter how each person processes sound. Among these are:

- Phonetic decoding, a problem that occurs when the brain incorrectly decodes what is being heard. Sounds are unrecognizable, often because the person speaking talks too fast.
- Tolerance-fading memory, a condition with little or poor tolerance for background sounds.
- Auditory integration involves a person's ability to put together things heard with things seen. Characteristically there are long response delays and trouble with phonics, or recognizing the symbols for sounds.
- The fourth problem area, often called auditory organization, overlaps the previous three. It is characterized by disorganization in handling auditory and other information.

Certain audiological tests are carried out to see if the person has a CAP problem, and if so, how severe it is. Other tests give more specific information regarding the nature of the CAP problem. They include:

- Puretone air-conduction threshold testing, which measures peripheral hearing loss. If loss is found, then bone-conduction testing, or evaluation of the vibration of small bones in the inner ear, is also carried out.
- Word discrimination scores (WDS) determines a person's clarity in hearing ideal speech. This is done by presenting 25–50 words at 40 decibels above the person's average sound threshold in each ear. Test scores equal the percentage of words heard correctly.
- Immittance testing is made up of two parts, assessing the status of, and the protective mechanisms of the middle ear.
- Staggered sporadic word (SSW) testing delivers 40 compound words in an overlapping way at 50 decibels above threshold to each ear of the person being tested. This test provides expanded information that makes it possible to break down CAP problems into the four basic types.
- Speech in noise discrimination (SN) testing is similar to Staggered Sporadic Word testing except that other noise is also added and the percentage correct in quiet is compared with that correct when there is added noise.
- Phonemic synthesis (PS) determines serious learning problems. The types of errors made in sounding out written words or associating written letters with the sounds they represent help in determining the type and severity of CAP problems.

Benefits

Upon completion of an auditory integration training program, the person's hearing should be capable of perceiving all frequencies at, or near, the same level. Total improvement from this therapy, in both hearing and behavior, can take up to one year.

Research and general acceptance

Auditory integration training is based upon newly learned information about the brain. Though brain structures and connections are predetermined, probably by heredity, another factor called *plasticity* also comes into play. Learning continues from birth to death. Plasticity is the ability of the brain to actually

ALFRED TOMATIS (1920–2001)

Internationally renowned French otolaryngologist, psychologist, educator and inventor Alfred Tomatis perceived the importance of sound and hearing early in his career. He took his degree as a Doctor of Medicine from the University of Paris and specialized in ear, nose and throat medicine. The son of two opera singers, Tomatis early in his career treated some of his parents' fellow opera singers. From these experiences with the sound of music, he developed the principle that has come to be known as the Tomatis Effect, i.e. that the human voice can only sing what it hears.

Tomatis has been called the Einstein of the ear. It was his research that made the world aware that the ears of an infant in utero are already functioning at four and half months of age. Just as the umbilical cord provides nourishment to the unborn infant's body, Tomatis postulated that the sound of the mother's voice is also a nutrient heard by the fetus. This sound literally charges and stimulates the growth of the brain.

Tomatis took this further, into the realm of language. Tomatis concluded that the need to communicate and to be understood are among our most basic needs. He was a pioneer in perceiving that language problems convert into social problems for people. "Language is what characterizes man and makes him different from other creatures," Tomatis is quoted as saying. The techniques he developed to teach people how to listen effectively are internationally respected tools used in the treatment of autism, attention-deficit disorder, and other learning disabilities.

His listening program, the invention of the Electronic Ear, and his work with the therapeutic use of sound and music for the past fifty years have made Tomatis arguably the best known and most successful ear specialist in the world. There are more than two hundred Tomatis Centers worldwide, treating a vast variety of problems related to the ability to hear.

change its structuring and connections through the process of learning.

Problems with auditory processing are viewed as having a wide–reaching ripple effect in society. It is estimated that 30–40% of children starting school have language-learning skills that can be described as poor. CAP difficulties are a factor in several different learning disabilities. They affect not only academic success, but also nearly every aspect of societal difficulties. One example to illustrate this is a 1989 University of Buffalo study where CAP problems were found to be present in a surprising 97% of youth inmates in an upstate New York corrections facility.

Training and certification

Both Tomatis and Berard have certification programs in their therapies.

Resources

BOOKS

Katz, Jack, Ph.D., Wilma Laufer Gabbay, M.S., Deborah S. Ungerleider, M.A., and Lorin Wilde, M.S. *Handbook of Clinical Audiology.* Waverly Press, Inc., 1985.

PERIODICALS

Katz, Jack, Ph.D. "Central Auditory Processing Evaluation." (1996).
Masters, M. Gay. "Speech and Language Management of CAPD." (1996).

Musiek, Frank, Ph.D. "Auditory Training: An Eclectic Approach." *American Journal of Audiology* (1995).

OTHER

Cooper, Rachel. "What is Auditory Integration Training?" http://www.vision3d.com/adhd/ (December 2000).
Dejean, Valerie. *About the Tomatis Method, 1997.* Tomatis Auditory Training Spectrum Center, Bethseda, MD.
Masters, M. Gay, and Jack Stecker Katz, N.A. *Central Auditory Processing Disorders: Characteristic Difficulties.* Miniseminar, 1994.
The Spectrum Center. "Auditory Integration and Alfred Tomatis." http://listeningtraining.com/ (December 2000).

Joan Schonbeck

Aura therapy

Definition

Aura therapy is a healing technique based on reading a person's aura, or vital energy field, and then treating diseases revealed by the aura color or colors. Aura therapy is generally considered a subtype of biofield therapy, which is a form of energy therapy that utilizes energies thought to reside in or emanate from the human body (as distinct from electromagnetic energy therapies). There are several variations of treatment,

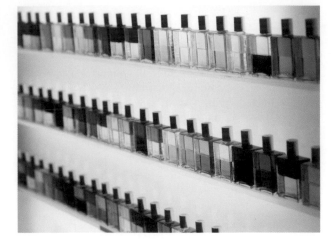

Colored bottles used for aura therapy. *(© Anneke Doorenbosch/ Alamy)*

but in general aura therapy emphasizes manipulating the aura energy back into a positive balance.

Origins

The exact origin of aura therapy is unknown, but historical references to it date back about 5,000 years. East Indian, Chinese, Jewish, and Christian faiths all have references to auras as energies that vibrate through physical matter. The energies are seen as colors and represent such states of being emotional, mental, astral, and celestial. Halos have also been considered a kind of aura. Historically, it was believed that the special powers of a psychic, mystic, or clairvoyant were needed to see auras. Today, there are many New Age centers that teach the art of aura reading and therapy.

In the late 1890s, the scientist and inventor Nicola Tesla (1856–1943) became the first person to photograph an aura. Auric photography took a big leap forward in the late 1930s when Semyon and Valentina Kirlian introduced a high-voltage imaging process that became known as **Kirlian photography**. Although there have been challenges to the use of Kirlian photography, the process was designed to photograph aura energy emitted by life forms, including plants, animals, and humans. A newer variation is aura imaging photography, which uses a special camera to take instant photos of a person's aura. The size, shape, and color of the aura can then be analyzed to reveal specific physical, emotional, and mental problems.

Types of aura therapy

Since the early 1970s, several different forms of aura therapy have emerged within the alternative medicine field.

Aura color therapy

Aura **color therapy** is more closely related to **light therapy** than to such other forms of aura therapy as **therapeutic touch**. In aura color therapy, the proportions of the colors in a person's aura as well as their clarity or intensity are analyzed and treated. Aura color therapists maintain that the aura of a healthy person will have an undistorted oval shape around the body, with clear lines of light energy and a perfect balance of the seven colors of the rainbow. Muddy colors, bulges or swirls in the energy lines, or an absence of any of the major colors signal energy imbalances. For example, a depressed person will have large amounts of blue and green in the aura with no orange or yellow. A chronically angry person will have too much red and little or no blue.

Color therapy treatment consists of adding extra colors to a dull or depleted aura or using complementary colors to correct a color imbalance in the aura. For example, orange, which is the complementary color of blue, would be used to treat the aura of a depressed person. Several different techniques may be used to add or balance the colors, the most common being the use of colored lights to irradiate the client's body, or the placement of colored gemstones on the client's body while he or she lies on the floor or on a massage table. In another variation of aura color therapy, the client is advised to wear clothing in colors intended to balance or correct the aura.

Therapeutic touch (TT)

Therapeutic touch, or TT, is a form of energy therapy that was developed in the United States in 1972 by Dora Kunz, a psychic healer, and Dolores Krieger, a professor of nursing at New York University. In TT, the practitioner alters the patient's energy field through a transfer of energy from his or her hands to the patient. When illness occurs, it creates a disturbance or blockage in the aura or vital energy field. The TT practitioner uses her/his hands to discern the blockage or disturbance. Although the technique is called "therapeutic touch," there is generally no touching of the client's physical body, only his or her energetic body or biofield. TT is usually performed on fully clothed patients who are either lying down on a flat surface or sitting up in a chair.

A therapeutic touch session consists of five steps or phases. The first step is a period of **meditation** on the practitioner's part, to become spiritually centered and energized for the task of healing. The second step is assessment or discernment of the energy imbalances in the patient's aura. In this step, the TT practitioner holds his or her hands about 2–3 inches above the patient's body and moves them in long, sweeping strokes from the patient's head downward to the feet. The practitioner may feel a sense of warmth, heaviness, tingling, or similar cues, as they are known in TT. The cues are thought to reveal the location of the energy disturbances or imbalances. In the third step, known as the unruffling process, the practitioner removes the energy disturbances with downward sweeping movements. In the fourth step, the practitioner serves as a channel for the transfer of universal energy to the patient. The fifth step consists of smoothing the patient's energy field and restoring a symmetrical pattern of energy flow. After the treatment, the patient rests for 10–15 minutes.

Tellington touch (Ttouch)

Tellington touch, which is also known as Ttouch, is an interesting instance of an alternative therapy that began in veterinary practice and was later extended to humans. Ttouch was developed in England by Linda Tellington-Jones, a graduate of **Feldenkrais** training.

The Feldenkrais method, which is usually considered a bodywork therapy, originated with Dr. Moshe Feldenkrais (1904-1984), a scientist and engineer who was also a judo instructor. The Feldenkrais method is based on redirecting the client's habitual patterns of body movement, but it is unusual among bodywork therapies in its emphasis on new patterns of thinking and imagination as byproducts of the body's reeducation. Tellington-Jones, who was employed as a horse trainer, began using Feldenkrais techniques on horses in 1975. In 1983 she developed the pattern of circular touching motions known as Tellington touch.

In the 1980s, Ttouch expanded from treating behavioral problems in horses to treating cats, dogs, and other household pets. In the 1990s, Ttouch was introduced into nursing school curricula for the treatment of humans. It has been used to treat patients suffering from such chronic conditions as **pain** syndromes, **Alzheimer's disease**, arthritis, and **multiple sclerosis** as well as patients recovering from traumatic injuries or **stroke**. Ttouch is growing in popularity among hospice nurses as an alternative treatment for patients facing death.

In Ttouch, the practitioner touches the client's skin but does not manipulate the underlying muscles or bones. The practitioner imagines the face of a clock on the client's body and places a lightly curved finger at the 6-o'clock position. He or she then pushes the skin clockwise around the face of the clock for one and one-quarter circles, maintaining a constant pressure. The client's body is gently supported with the practitioner's free hand, which is placed opposite the hand making the circle. After each circular touch, the practitioner gently slides the hand down the body and repeats the circle.

Benefits

Aura therapy is generally designed to bring imbalances in the aura back into physical, mental, emotional, and spiritual balance. The benefits can be subtle (like a general feeling of peace and well-being) or dramatic (like experiencing a spiritual transformation or feelings of ecstasy). Changes may be immediate or can occur over several days. Repeated therapy sessions can maintain and deepen the aura energy balance.

Persons who have received therapeutic touch or Tellington touch from nurses frequently mention "comfort" or "humanizing of health care" as important benefits.

Therapeutic touch and Tellington touch appear to benefit patients in intensive care units (ICUs), who frequently develop mild psychiatric disturbances from being isolated and from the fact that ICU equipment interferes with normal human sensory perception. It is thought that TT and Ttouch help to break down the patient's feelings of isolation and disconnection from other people.

Description

Traditionally, an aura is a protective psychic and spiritual energy field that surrounds the physical body. Energy from an aura is usually not static. It is constantly flowing, flashing, vibrating, expanding, and decreasing. The colors detected usually indicate emotions, such as:

- lavender and purple for spirituality
- red/orange for sexual passion
- white for truth
- rose or pink for love
- red for anger
- yellow for intellect

Slow, deep breaths expand the aura while fast, shallow breaths decrease it. Spaces or gaps in the aura usually signify disease. These gaps often appear near the affected area, such as around the heart to signify **heart disease**. In general, auras have seven levels. Physical and ethereal auras extend up to a foot from the body, imagination and emotional auras extend about two feet, while the mental, archetypal (destiny), and spiritual auras extend about three feet.

There seems to be a general consensus among aura therapists that more than one session is required for optimal balancing. Many suggest three sessions within two or three weeks. The first session focuses on the physical aura, the next on the emotional, and the third on the spiritual. Once the aura levels are in balance, follow-up sessions are encouraged every six months to a year. Aura therapy is not covered by medical insurance. The cost can range from $50 to $100 or more per session.

Preparations

No advance preparation is required. Many aura readers and therapists say the patient should have a genuine desire for better health and happiness. Also, many therapists suggest patients abstain from recreational drugs, alcohol, and sex for several days before the therapy for a better sense of clarity and focus.

Precautions

There are no known precautions associated with aura therapy.

Side effects

No negative side effects associated with aura therapy have been reported, although a small minority of patients treated with TT or Ttouch report feeling uncomfortable with being touched by strangers.

Research and general acceptance

Aura color therapy is considered a New Age treatment and is not generally accepted as valid by the conventional medical community. Skeptics argue that there are no scientific studies documenting the benefits of aura therapy or the existence of a human biofield. Most reports of the benefits of aura color therapy are anecdotal and appear in New Age journals and magazines.

Although therapeutic touch has become a popular alternative/complementary approach in some schools of nursing in the United States and Canada, acceptance by the mainstream medical community varies. Many hospitals permit nurses and staff to perform TT on patients at no extra charge. On the other hand, therapeutic touch became national news in April 1998 when an elementary-school student carried out research for a science project that questioned its claims. Twenty-one TT practitioners with experience ranging from one to 27 years were blindfolded and asked to identify whether the investigator's hand was closer to their right hand or their left. Placement of the investigator's hand was determined by flipping a coin. The TT practitioners were able to identify the correct hand in only 123 (44%) of 280 trials, a figure that could result from random chance alone. Debate about the merits of TT filled the editorial pages of the *Journal of the American Medical Association* for nearly a year after the news reports.

Tellington touch training is offered by some schools of veterinary medicine in the United States, and is also offered in continuing education programs in schools of nursing. It appears to be gaining wider support from the mainstream medical community as a useful technique in calming patients facing unpleasant or painful procedures. One study found that patients awaiting venipuncture who received Ttouch were more relaxed before the procedure and had significantly less discomfort afterward.

Training and certification

No formal training or certification is required to practice aura reading, aura color therapy, TT, or Ttouch. However, a number of alternative medicine and New Age healing schools offer formal training and certification. Therapeutic touch and Tellington touch have their own training and certification programs.

Resources

BOOKS

Bain, Gabriel Hudson. *Auras 101: A Basic Study of Human Auras and the Techniques to See Them.* Flagstaff, AZ: Light Technology Publications, 1998.

Bartlett, Sarah. *Auras and How to See Them.* London, UK: Collins & Brown, 2000.

Chiazzari, Suzy. *The Complete Book of Color: Using Color for Lifestyle, Health, and Well-Being,* Part Six: Healing Through the Aura. Boston, MA: Element, 1998.

Krieger, Dolores, Ph.D., R.N. *Accepting Your Power to Heal: The Personal Practice of Therapeutic Touch.* New York: Bear & Company, 1993.

MacFarlane, Muriel. *Heal Your Aura: Finding True Love by Generating A Positive Personal Energy Field.* Secaucus, NJ: Citadel Press, 1999.

Oslie, Pamela. *Life Colors: What the Colors in Your Aura Reveal.* Novato, CA: New World Library, 2000.

Snellgrove, Brian. *The Magic in Your Hands: How to See Auras and Use Them for Diagnosis and Healing.* Essex, UK: C. W. Daniel, 1998.

Tellington-Jones, Linda, and Sybil Taylor. *The Tellington Touch: A Breakthrough Technique to Train and Care for Your Favorite Animal.* New York and London, UK: Penguin Books, 1995.

PERIODICALS

Demmer, C., and J. Sauer. "Assessing Complementary Therapy Services in a Hospice Program." *American Journal of Hospice and Palliative Care* 19 (September-October 2002): 306-314.

Hewitt, J. "Psychoaffective Disorder in Intensive Care Units: A Review." *Journal of Clinical Nursing* 11 (September 2002): 575-584.

Rosa, Linda, MSN; Emily Rosa; Larry Sarner; and Stephen Barrett, MD. "A Close Look at Therapeutic Touch." *Journal of the American Medical Association* 279 (April 1, 1998): 1005-11.

"Somesthetic Aura: The Experience of Alice in Wonderland." *The Lancet* (June 27, 1998): 1934.

Wendler, M. Cecilia. "Tellington Touch Before Venipuncture: An Exploratory Descriptive Study." *Holistic Nursing Practice* 16 (July 2002): 51-64.

ORGANIZATIONS

Feldenkrais Guild of North America. 3611 S.W. Hood Avenue, Suite 100, Portland, OR 97201. (800) 775-2118 or (503) 221-6612. Fax: (503) 221-6616. www.feldenkrais.com.

International Society for the Study of Subtle Energies and Energy Medicine (ISSSEEM). 356 Goldco Circle. Golden, CO 80401. (303) 278-2228. www.vitalenergy.com/ISSSEEM.

National Center for Complementary and Alternative Medicine (NCCAM) Clearinghouse. P.O. Box 7923, Gaithersburg, MD 20898. (888) 644-6226. TTY: (866) 464-3615. Fax: (866) 464-3616. www.nccam.nih.gov.

The Nurse Healers Professional Associates International (NH-PAI), the Official Organization of Therapeutic Touch. 3760 S. Highland Drive, Salt Lake City, UT 84106. (801) 273-3399. nhpai@therapeutic-touch.org. www.therapeutic-touch.org.

TTEAM/Ttouch in USA. P. O. Box 3793, Santa Fe, NM 87506. (800) 854-8326. www.tellingtontouch.com.

TTEAM/Ttouch in Canada. Rochdell Road, Vernon, BC V1B 3E8. (250) 545-2336. www.tellingtontouch.com.

OTHER

Auras website. The Healing Channel. http://www.healingchannel. org/aura.html.

Ken R. Wells
Rebecca J. Frey, PhD

Auriculotherapy

Definition

Auriculotherapy, also called ear **acupuncture**, applies the principles of acupuncture to specific points on the ear. Auriculotherapists believe that healing processes can be promoted by working with these points on the ear, because the ear contains many blood vessels and nerve endings that, when stimulated, influence the organs and bodily functions.

Origins

Acupuncture is one of the world's oldest therapeutic techniques, having its roots in ancient China. Some of the oldest texts of Chinese medicine mention acupuncture points and massage techniques specifically for the ear. For eye problems, silver or gold earrings were sometimes prescribed in ancient times to provide constant healing stimulation at points on the ear, a practice that is still performed in some areas of the world, including parts of Europe. The ancient Egyptians and Greeks believed that working with the ears could influence health. Hippocrates, the Greek father of medicine, mentioned a point on the ear that could be operated on as a birth control measure in men. In Europe in the Middle Ages, doctors

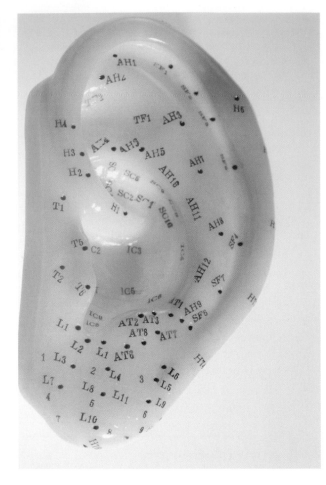

Image of a dummy ear to be used for auriculotherapy. *(© Image Source Limited / Phototake. Reproduced by permission.)*

scientific experiments in auriculotherapy, and showed some significant and surprising results in both treatment and diagnosis of conditions. In 2002, a center in Maine received a unique grant to study auriculotherapy for **substance abuse**. Although recognizing that acupuncture had been used before for helping those with abuse, this study sought to show that auriculotherapy's effects on **relaxation** response helped those abusing drugs and alcohol better deal with the **anxiety** and life circumstances thought to lead them to substance abuse.

Benefits

Auriculotherapy is a quick, inexpensive, and noninvasive method of pain control. Ear acupuncture is also used as anesthesia during medical procedures. It is used frequently to help people overcome drug, tobacco, and alcohol addictions, and is used to treat chronic health conditions and diseases.

Description

After an initial exam and interview, auriculotherapists begin treatment by checking the patient's ears closely. Practitioners may palpate (feel) the ears with their hands, and check for any irregularities or painful spots. They may check for spots that are insensitive or numb by using cold or hot needles on the ear. They may also rely on electrical devices that measure skin resistance at points on the ear.

Several techniques may be used during auriculotherapy. Acupuncture needles are typically extremely thin. More than one needle may be used at one time, inserted deeply, or just pricked slightly along the contours of the ear. On some points, needles may be twisted or slanted to create more healing effects. Needles may be left in from a few minutes to half an hour or more.

Auriculotherapists may use *permanent press needles*. These small, tack-shaped needles may be attached to the ear with a narrow band of tape for several days or weeks. They are used for conditions that may require constant stimulation to acupuncture

prescribed surgery on a particular spot on the ear for a condition called **sciatica**, which causes nerve **pain** in the hips and thighs.

In modern times, auriculotherapy has been advanced by Paul Nogier of France. Beginning his work and experiments in the 1950s, Nogier laid out an intricate map of points on the ear that correspond to the organs and processes in the body. Nogier believed that the ear is shaped like an upside down human fetus, and the acupuncture points on the ear correspond to the body parts of the fetus shape, with the earlobe representing the head. Nogier theorized that by stimulating these points on the ear, the corresponding organs and bodily processes would be stimulated by nerve impulses. Nogier also theorized that by measuring electrical impulses on the skin of the ear, problems could be detected in the internal organs, and therefore auriculotherapy could be used to diagnose illnesses. Nogier and many followers, including ear acupuncturists in America and China, conducted points on the ear, such as addictions, chronic (long-lasting) **infections**, and other health problems.

Auriculotherapists also practice **electroacupuncture**, which utilizes electrical devices to send small electrical currents into the ear or through the body. Electroacupuncture is used for conditions such as paralysis or nerve damage in the body, drug and alcohol addictions, and chronic pain. Auriculotherapists may also employ *bleeding*, which removes one or two drops of blood at certain points on the ear. Bleeding is used for health problems such as high blood pressure, high **cholesterol**, or **heart disease**.

Auriculotherapy is generally performed once per week on patients for a sequence of several months, although the frequency of treatment depends on the patient and condition. Treatment may last for several months. The initial visit to an acupuncturist is typically the most expensive, costing from $80 to $200. Follow-up visits are less expensive, from $50 to $100 on average. Auriculotherapists may also prescribe herbal and nutritional remedies. Insurance coverage of acupuncture fees varies, depending on individual policies.

Preparations

Before treatment, an auriculotherapist may perform a thorough examination and interview the patient to determine health conditions and any precautions or adjustments that must be made. Acupuncturists often rely on **pulse diagnosis** and other diagnostic techniques before and during treatment.

For treatment, the patient should lie in a horizontal position on a comfortable surface in a calm, stress-free environment. After treatment, the patient should be permitted to lie down until feeling capable of leaving the practitioner's office.

Acupuncture needles should be sterilized before use. The ears should be disinfected before acupuncture as well, which is usually done with a cotton ball dipped in rubbing alcohol.

Precautions

Auriculotherapy, like all acupuncture, should not be performed on weak or exhausted patients, nor on those who are very hungry or have just eaten a meal or drunk alcohol. Auriculotherapy should not be performed on pregnant women during the first two trimesters (six months) of **pregnancy**, and afterwards only on very particular points on the ear for pain control. Auriculotherapy is not recommended for children under seven years old, and should be performed with care on the elderly. Ear acupuncture is to be avoided by those with **anemia** (low red blood cell quantity in the blood). Patients with nervous conditions should be thoroughly relaxed and prepared before treatment. For people that find acupuncture disagreeable, ear massage and **acupressure** may be preferable to treatment with needles.

Side effects

Some patients may experience uncomfortable side effects during or after acupuncture. Side effects that may occur after treatment include fainting, **dizziness**, **nausea**, numbness, headaches, sweating, or sharp pains throughout the body. These reactions may be due to anxiety or because acupuncture needles have been inserted too deeply or in the wrong area. Side effects can be alleviated by removing the needles and allowing the patient to lie down under supervision. Some side effects that occur during treatment, such as **hot flashes**, increased pulse, and temporarily increased symptoms, are considered normal and usually disappear quickly.

Training and certification

The American Academy of Medical Acupuncture (AAMA) was chartered in 1987 to support the education and correct practice of physician-trained acupuncturists. Its members must be either MDs or DOs who have completed proper study of acupuncture techniques.

The National Commission for Certification of Acupuncturists (NCCA) conducts certification exams, promotes national standards, and registers members. Most states that license acupuncturists use the NCCA standards as certification.

The American Association of Acupuncture and Oriental Medicine (AAAOM) is the largest organization for practitioners, with more than 1,600 members.

Resources

BOOKS

Fleischman, Dr. Gary. *Acupuncture: Everything You Ever Wanted to Know*. Barrytown, NY: Station Hill, 1998.

Hicks, Angela. *Thorson's Principles of Acupuncture*. New York: HarperCollins, 1997.

Requena, Yves, MD. *Terrains and Pathology in Acupuncture*. Massachusetts: Paradigm, 1986.

PERIODICALS

American Journal of Acupuncture. 1840 41st Ave., Suite 102, P.O. Box 610, Capitola, CA 95010.

Savage, Lorraine. "Grant to Study Acupuncture's Effectiveness on Patients Suffering from Substance Abuse."*Healthcare Review*. (March 19, 2002): 16.

ORGANIZATIONS
American Academy of Medical Acupuncture. 5820 Wilshire Blvd., Suite 500, Los Angeles, CA 90036, (213) 937-5514.
American Association of Acupuncture and Oriental Medicine. 433 Front St., Catasaugua, PA 18032, (610) 266-1433.
National Commission for Certification of Acupuncturists. 1424 16th St. NW, Suite 501, Washington, D.C. 20036, (202) 232-1404.

Douglas Dupler
Teresa G. Odle

Autism

Definition

Autism is a chronic and often severe disorder of brain functioning that begins during childhood. It is marked by problems with social contact, intelligence, and language, coupled with ritualistic or compulsive behavior, sensory integration and processing problems, and abnormal environmental responses.

Description

Autism is a lifelong disorder that interferes with a person's ability to understand what is seen, heard, and touched. This condition can cause profound problems in personal behavior and in a person's ability to relate to others. A person with autism must learn how to communicate normally and how to relate to people, objects, and events. Not all patients have the same degree of impairment. The severity of the condition varies among individuals, ranging from extremely unusual and aggressive behavior to a mild personality disorder or a learning disability.

Autism occurs in as many as one in 1,000 children, and incidence is rapidly increasing. It is found three to four times as often in boys as in girls. The condition occurs around the world in all races and all social backgrounds. Autism usually is evident in the first three years of life, although in some children it is difficult to pinpoint when the problem actually takes hold. Often, the condition may not be diagnosed until

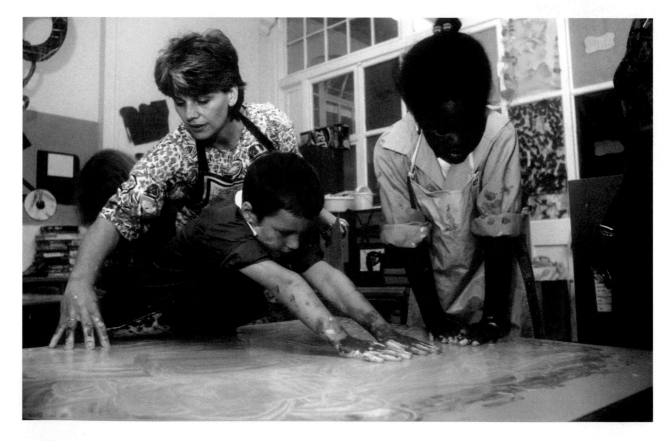

Working with autistic children. *(© Janine Wiedel Photolibrary / Alamy)*

the child enters school. A person with autism can have symptoms ranging from mild to severe.

Two subgroups of autism have been explained by clinicians. Those with essential autism, as defined by diagnostic tests, appear to have higher IQ scores and fewer seizures than those with complex autism, which offers a poorer outcome.

Causes and symptoms

Although the exact causes of autism are unknown, many possibilities have been proposed. Most experts believe that several independent factors contribute to development of autism. The number and combinations of these factors probably differ from person to person. Research points to such precipitating conditions as fetal alcohol syndrome, genetic connections (as with identical twins), brain stem defects, **lead poisoning**, a nervous system defect, **infections**, food and inhalant **allergies**, infant vaccination reactions, and digestive system deficiencies.

Further studies point to major disturbances in the body chemistry of children with autism. Disruption is most often found in fatty acid metabolism, electrolyte balances, problems with digestive functioning, production of red and white blood cells, and the body's balance of minerals. Diseases that may trigger autistic behavior include **rubella** in the pregnant mother; tuberous sclerosis; candiasis infection's fragile X syndrome; encephalitis; cytomegalovirus (CMV), a severe form of a herpes simplex infection; and untreated phenylketonuria.

There also appears to be a strong genetic basis for autism. In October 2001, the National Institutes of Health (NIH) reported that two regions of chromosomes contain genes involved with autism and that two other chromosomes had a weaker relation to autism-related genes. Genetically identical twins are much more likely than fraternal twins to both have autism if one is affected. In a family with one autistic child, the chance of having another child with autism is about one in 20, much higher than in the normal population. Sometimes, relatives of an autistic child have mild behaviors that look very much like autism, such as repetitive behaviors and social or communication problems. Research also has found that some emotional disorders, such as manic **depression**, occur more often in families of a child with autism. At least one group of researchers has also found a link between an abnormal gene and autism. The gene may be just one of at least three to five genes that interact in some way to cause the condition. Scientists suspect that a faulty gene or genes might make a person vulnerable to develop autism in the presence of other factors, such as chemical imbalance, infection, or a lack of oxygen at birth. In general, the genetic basis for autism appears fundamentally important, although still unclear. In a review of research in the area reported in 2007, scientists at Trinity College, in Dublin, Ireland, noted that seven chromosomal regions appear to contain genes that are involved in the development of autism in some way or another. They recommended that future research be focused on these seven areas.

Autism affects the way in which the brain uses or transmits information. Studies have found abnormalities in several parts of the brains of individuals with autism that almost certainly occurred during fetal development. The problem may be centered in the parts of the brain responsible for processing language and information from the senses. Profound problems with social interactions are the most common symptoms of autism. Infants with the disorder will not cuddle, tend to avoid eye contact, and in general do not seem to like or require physical contact or affection. Often, the child will not form attachments to parents or the rest of the family. The child may not speak at all, or will speak very little and may show bizarre patterns of speech, such as endlessly repeating words or phrases. About 10% of those with autism have an exceptional ability in particular areas, such as mathematics, memory, art, or music. Such individuals are known as autistic savants.

Most autistic children appear to be mentally retarded to at least some degree. Bizarre behavior patterns are very common and may include repeated mimicking of the actions of others, complex rituals, screaming fits, rhythmic rocking, arm flapping, finger twiddling, and crying without tears. Many of these children may react to sounds by banging their head or flapping fingers. Some less affected autistic adults who have written books about their childhood experiences report that sounds were often excruciatingly painful to them, forcing them to withdraw from the environment or to try to cope by withdrawing into their own invented world. A common characteristic of individuals with autism is an insistence on routine. There may be strong reactions to changes in food, clothing, and objects or events.

Diagnosis

Autism is diagnosed by obtaining a developmental history of the child and observing and evaluating the child's behavior, communication skills, and social interactions. Because the symptoms of autism are so varied, the condition may go undiagnosed for some time. There is no medical test for autism. The condition is often missed, especially in mild cases or when additional handicaps are present. Special screening tools help physicians diagnose the condition. Medical tests are sometimes used to rule out other possible causes of autistic symptoms.

Treatment

Early intervention proves critical in managing autism. The American Academy of Pediatrics (AAP) states that many parents have chosen alternative therapies when more traditional therapies do not produce desired results. Among therapies mentioned in the group's report are nutritional supplements, elimination **diets**, immune globulin therapy, and secretin (a hormone) therapy.

There is often a strong nutritional dysfunction involved in autism. A major overhaul of the child's diet should be done, but very gradually. A healthy diet of whole foods with no preservatives or additives, including food dyes, is recommended. Autistic children may have particular difficulty handling certain artificial ingredients, such as the sweetener aspartame, and monosodium glutamate (MSG), as these chemicals may further interfere with already disrupted nerve impulses. Processed foods such as white flour, white sugar, margarine, and hydrogenated fats should be avoided because they may interfere with the stability of blood chemistry.

Many autistic children may be unable to effectively break down the protein in grains such as wheat, barley, and oats called gluten, and the protein in milk called casein. Overgrowths of *Candida albicans* may be present and should be tested for and treated. Testing should also be done for food, chemical, and inhalant allergies. Digestive functioning should be tested and monitored. Extensive testing should be done for blood levels of chemicals in the body, as well. Allergens should be subsequently removed from the diet and environment; further dietary changes should be made to correct chemical imbalances. Possible gut and immune system dysfunction should also be addressed.

Studies have shown that supplementation with megadoses of vitamin B_6 together with **magnesium** improves eye contact, speech, and behavior problems. Vitamin B_6 causes fewer side effects than other medications, but megadoses should be given only under the supervision of a healthcare provider. A B-complex vitamin is probably the best way to give B_6, due to the interdependent functioning of the B vitamins. **Zinc** and **vitamin C** supplementation is also recommended. In addition, dimethylglycine (DMG) has been reported to improve speech in some children with autism in as little as a week's time. Other therapeutic methods that have been shown to be helpful include special **auditory integration training** (AIT) based on the Berard method or the Tomatis method. **Craniosacral therapy** may also improve symptoms of autism by relieving compressions of the skull bones and membranes. Autism is a complex condition. A practitioner who has already worked with cases of autism successfully will be able to offer a comprehensive treatment plan.

Allopathic treatment

Many experts recommend a complex treatment regimen for autism that begins early in life and continues through the teenage years. Behavioral therapies are used in conjunction with medications and special diets. Because the symptoms vary so widely from one person to the next, there is no single approach that works best for every person. Interventions include special training in music, listening, vision, and speech and language. Sensory integration training may be used to normalize sensory functions. Training to change aberrant behaviors should be started as early in the autistic child's life as possible, since early intervention appears to have the most influence on brain development and functioning. A child with autism is able to learn best in a specialized, structured program that emphasizes individualized instruction.

As of 2008, no single medication had proved highly effective for the major features of autism. However, a variety of drugs can control self-injurious, aggressive, and other behaviors. Drugs also can control **epilepsy**, which afflicts up to 20% of people with autism. Types of recommended medication may include stimulants, such as methylphenidate (Ritalin); antidepressants, such as fluroxamine (Luvox); opiate blockers, such as naltrexone (ReVia); antipsychotics; and tranquilizers.

Expected results

Studies show that people with autism can improve significantly with proper treatment. While there is no cure, the negative behaviors of autism can be modified. Earlier generations placed autistic children in institutions; in the 2000s, even severely disabled children can be helped to eventually become more responsive to others. Children with autism usually can learn to better understand and deal with the world around them. Some can even lead nearly mainstream lives.

Hall, Laura J. *Autism Spectrum Disorders: From Theory to Practice.* Upper Saddle River, NJ: Prentice Hall, 2008.

Jepson, Bryan. *Changing the Course of Autism: A Scientific Approach for Parents and Physicians.* Boulder, CO: Sentient, 2007.

Mackenzie, Heather. *Reaching and Teaching the Child with Autism Spectrum Disorder: Using Learning Preferences and Strengths.* London: Jessica Kingsley, 2008.

PERIODICALS

Knott, Fiona, Aline-Wendy Dunlop, and Tommy Mackay. "Living with ASD: How Do Children and Their Parents Assess Their Difficulties with Social Interaction and Understanding?" *Autism* (November 1, 2006): 609–617.

Schmitz, C., and P. Rezaie. "The Neuropathology of Autism: Where Do We Stand?" *Neuropathology & Applied Neurobiology* (February 2008): 4–11.

Wendling, Patricia. "CAM Use High among Autism Patients." *Family Practice News* (February 15, 2005): 43.

Patience Paradox
Teresa Norris
David Edward Newton, Ed.D.

Autoimmune arthritis *see* **Ankylosing spondylitis**

KEY TERMS

Antidepressant—A type of medication that is used to treat depression; also sometimes used to treat autism.

Asperger syndrome—A condition in which individuals have autistic behavior but normal language skills.

Encephalitis—A rare inflammation of the brain caused by a viral infection, linked to the development of autism.

Fragile X syndrome—A genetic condition related to the X chromosome that affects mental, physical, and sensory development.

Phenylketonuria (PKU)—An enzyme deficiency present at birth that disrupts metabolism and causes brain damage; this rare inherited defect may be linked to the development of autism.

Rubella—Also known as German measles. When a woman contracts rubella during pregnancy, her developing fetus may be damaged. One of the problems that may result is autism.

Tuberous sclerosis—A genetic disease that causes skin problems, seizures, and mental retardation; it may be confused with autism.

Prevention

The mechanisms of autism are poorly understood. As of 2008 there was no known method of prevention for the condition. However, there was much debate as to what part the **measles**, **mumps**, and rubella (MMR) vaccination and the diphtheria, pertussis, and **tetanus** (DPT) vaccination may play in the onset of autism. Some people believe strongly that vaccines may be responsible for a significant number of autism cases. As of 2008, however, virtually no scientific evidence was available to support that hypothesis. Public health authorities were virtually unanimous in their recommendation that all young children have the traditional series of vaccinations for dangerous and potentially fatal diseases.

Resources

BOOKS

Boucher, Jill M. *Autism: Characteristics, Causes, and Basic Issues.* Thousand Oaks, CA: Sage Publications, 2008.

Exkorn, Karen Siff. *The Autism Sourcebook: Everything You Need to Know About Diagnosis, Treatment, Coping, and Healing.* Doughcloyne, Wilton, Cork, Ireland: Collins Press, 2005.

Ayurvedic medicine

Definition

Ayurvedic medicine is a system of healing that originated in ancient India. In Sanskrit, *ayur* means life or living, and *veda* means knowledge, so Ayurveda has been defined as the "knowledge of living" or the "science of longevity." Ayurvedic medicine utilizes diet, **detoxification** and purification techniques, herbal and mineral remedies, **yoga**, breathing exercises, **meditation**, and **massage therapy** as holistic healing methods. Ayurvedic medicine is widely practiced in modern India and has been steadily gaining followers in the West. In this form of medicine, the physician treats the whole person, rather than only focusing on the medical issues that an individual experiences.

Origins

Ayurvedic medicine originated in the early civilizations of India some 3,000–5,000 years ago. It is mentioned in the *Vedas*, the ancient religious and philosophical texts that are the oldest surviving literature in the world, which makes Ayurvedic medicine

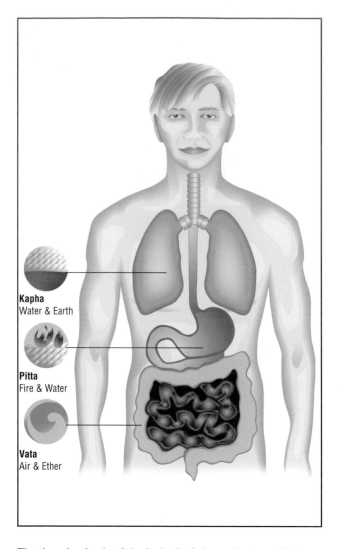

Kapha
Water & Earth

Pitta
Fire & Water

Vata
Air & Ether

The three basic physiological principles or doshas. *(Illustration by GGS Information Services, Inc. Cengage Learning, Gale)*

the oldest surviving healing system. According to the texts, Ayurveda was conceived by enlightened wise men as a system of living harmoniously and maintaining the body so that mental and spiritual awareness could be possible. Medical historians believe that Ayurvedic ideas were transported from ancient India to China and were instrumental in the development of Chinese medicine.

Ayurvedic medicine is used by 80% of the population in India. Aided by the efforts of Deepak Chopra and the Maharishi Mahesh Yogi (1918–2008, founder of Transcendental Meditation), it became an increasingly accepted alternative medical treatment in the United States during the 1980s and 1990s. Chopra, who has an MD, has written several bestsellers based on Ayurvedic ideas. He also helped develop the Center

for **Mind/Body Medicine** in La Jolla, California, a major Ayurvedic center that trains physicians in Ayurvedic principles, produces herbal remedies, and conducts research and documentation of its healing techniques.

Benefits

According to the original texts, the goal of Ayurveda is prevention as well as promotion of the body's own capacity for maintenance and balance. Ayurvedic treatment is non-invasive and non-toxic, so it can be used safely as an alternative therapy or alongside conventional therapies. Ayurvedic physicians claim that their methods can also help stress-related, metabolic, and chronic conditions. Ayurveda has been used to treat various physical problems, including **acne**, **allergies**, **asthma**, **anxiety**, arthritis, **chronic fatigue syndrome**, colds, **colitis**, **constipation**, **depression**, diabetes, flu, **heart disease**, **hypertension**, immune problems, inflammation, **insomnia**, nervous disorders, **obesity**, skin problems, and ulcers.

Ayurvedic physicians seek to discover the roots of a disease before it gets so advanced that more radical treatments are necessary. Thus, Ayurveda seems to be of limited usefulness in treating severely advanced conditions, traumatic injuries, acute **pain**, and conditions and injuries requiring invasive surgery. Ayurvedic techniques have also been used alongside chemotherapy and surgery to assist patients in recovery and healing.

Description

To understand Ayurvedic treatment, it is necessary to have an idea how the Ayurvedic system views the body. The basic life force in the body is *prana*, which is also found in the elements and is similar to the Chinese notion of *chi*. As Swami Vishnudevananda, a yogi and expert, put it, "Prana is in the air, but is not the oxygen, nor any of its chemical constituents. It is in food, water, and in the sunlight, yet it is not vitamin, heat, or light-rays. Food, water, air, etc., are only the media through which the prana is carried."

In Ayurveda, there are five basic elements that contain prana: earth, water, fire, air, and ether. These elements interact and are further organized in the human body as three main categories or basic physiological principles that govern all bodily functions known as the *doshas*. The three doshas are *vata, pitta,* and *kapha.* Each person has a unique blend of the three doshas, known as the person's *prakriti*, which is why Ayurvedic treatment is always individualized. In Ayurveda, disease is viewed as a state of imbalance

Ayurvedic body types (DOSHAS)

	Vata	Pitta	Kapha
Physical characteristics	Thin	Average build	Large build
	Prominent features	Fair, thin hair	Wavy, thick hair
	Cool, dry skin	Warm, moist skin	Pale, cool, oily skin
	Susceptible to constipation, and skin, neurological and mental diseases	Ulcers, heartburn, hemmorrhoids, heart disease, and arthritis	Obesity, allergies, and sinus problems/asthma, gallbladder problems, and diabetes
	Cramps	Acne	High cholesterol
Emotional characteristics	Moody	Intense	Relaxed
	Vivacious	Quick tempered	Not easily angered
	Imaginative	Intelligent	Affectionate
	Enthusiastic	Loving	Tolerant
	Intuitive	Articulate	Compassionate
Behavioral characteristics	Unscheduled sleep and meal times	Orderly	Slow, graceful
	Nervous disorders	Structured sleep and meal times	Long sleeper and slow eater
	Anxiety	Perfectionist	Procrastination
Dominant Elements	Space and air	Fire and water	Earth and water

(*Illustration by Corey Light. Cengage Learning, Gale*)

in one or more of a person's doshas, and an Ayurvedic physician strives to adjust and balance the doshas, using a variety of techniques.

The vata dosha is associated with air and ether, and in the body it promotes movement and lightness. Vata people are generally thin and light physically, dry-skinned, and very energetic and mentally restless. When vata is out of balance, there are often nervous problems, hyperactivity, sleeplessness, lower back pains, and headaches.

Pitta is associated with fire and water. In the body, it is responsible for metabolism and digestion. Pitta characteristics are medium-built bodies, fair skin, strong digestion, and good mental concentration. Pitta imbalances show up as anger and aggression and stress-related conditions such as **gastritis**, ulcers, liver problems, and hypertension.

The kapha dosha is associated with water and earth. People characterized as kapha are generally large or heavy with more oily complexions. They tend to be slow, calm, and peaceful. Kapha disorders manifest emotionally as greed and possessiveness, and physically as obesity, **fatigue**, **bronchitis**, and sinus problems.

Diagnosis

In Ayurvedic medicine, disease is always seen as an imbalance in the dosha system, so the diagnostic process strives to determine which doshas are underactive or overactive in a body. Diagnosis is often taken over a course of days in order for the Ayurvedic physician to accurately determine what parts of the body are being affected. To diagnose problems, Ayurvedic physicians often use long questionnaires and interviews to determine a person's dosha patterns and physical and psychological histories. Ayurvedic physicians also intricately observe the pulse, tongue, face, lips, eyes, and fingernails for abnormalities or patterns that they believe can indicate deeper problems in the internal

DEEPAK CHOPRA (1946–)

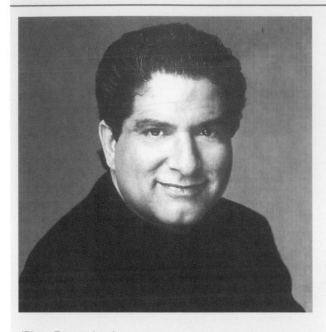

(Photo Researchers)

Deepak Chopra was born in India and studied medicine at the All India Institute of Medical Science. He left his home for the United States in 1970 and completed residencies in internal medicine and endocrinology. He went on to teaching posts at major medical institutions—Tufts

University and Boston University schools of medicine—while establishing a very successful private practice. By the time he was thirty-five, Chopra had become chief of staff at New England Memorial Hospital.

Disturbed by Western medicine's reliance on medication, he began a search for alternatives and discovered one in the teachings of the Maharishi Mahesh Yogi, an Indian spiritualist who had gained a cult following in the late sixties teaching Transcendental Meditation (TM). Chopra began practicing TM fervently and eventually met the Maharishi. In 1985 Chopra established the Ayurvedic Health Center for Stress Management and Behavioral Medicine in Lancaster, Massachusetts, where he began his practice of integrating the best aspects of Eastern and Western medicine.

In 1993, he published *Creating Affluence: Wealth Consciousness in the Field of All Possibilities*, and the enormously successful best seller, *Ageless Body, Timeless Mind*. In the latter he presents his most radical thesis: that aging is not the inevitable deterioration of organs and mind that we have been traditionally taught to think of it as. It is a process that can be influenced, slowed down, and even reversed with the correct kinds of therapies, almost all of which are self-administered or self-taught. He teaches that applying a regimen of nutritional balance, meditation, and emotional clarity characterized by such factors as learning to easily and quickly express anger, for instance, can lead to increased lifespans of up to 120 years.

systems. Some Ayurvedic physicians also use laboratory tests to assist in diagnosis.

Treatment

Ayurvedic treatment seeks to re-establish balance and harmony in the body's systems. Usually the first method of treatment involves some sort of detoxification and cleansing of the body, in the belief that accumulated toxins must be removed before any other methods of treatment will be effective. Methods of detoxification include therapeutic **vomiting**, laxatives, medicated enemas, **fasting**, and cleansing of the sinuses. Many Ayurvedic clinics combine all of these cleansing methods into intensive sessions known as *panchakarma*. **Panchakarma** methods can take several days or even weeks, and they are more than elimination therapies. They also include herbalized oil massage and herbalized heat treatments. After individuals undergo purification, Ayurvedic physicians use herbal and mineral remedies to balance the body. Ayurvedic

medicine contains a vast knowledge of herbs and their uses for specific health problems.

Ayurvedic medicine also emphasizes how people live their lives from day to day, asserting that proper lifestyles and routines accentuate balance, rest, diet, and prevention. Ayurveda recommends yoga as a form of **exercise** to build strength and health, and it also advises massage therapy and self-massage as ways of increasing circulation and reducing **stress**. Yogic breathing techniques and meditation are also part of a healthy Ayurvedic regimen for reducing stress and improving mental energy.

Of all treatments, though, diet is one of the most basic and widely used therapies in the Ayurvedic system. An Ayurvedic diet is a very well planned and individualized regimen. According to Ayurveda, there are six basic tastes: sweet, sour, salty, pungent, bitter, and astringent. Certain tastes and foods can either calm or aggravate a particular dosha. For instance, sweet, sour, and salty decrease vata problems and increase kapha. Sour, salty, and pungent can increase pitta. After an Ayurvedic physician determines a person's dosha profile, he or she will recommend a specific diet to correct imbalances and increase health. The Ayurvedic diet emphasizes primarily vegetarian foods of high quality and freshness, tailored to the season and time of day. Cooling foods are eaten in the summer and heating ones in the winter, always within a person's dosha requirements. In daily routine, the heaviest meal of the day is lunch, and dinner is eaten well before bedtime to allow for complete digestion. Also, eating meals in a calm manner with proper chewing and state of mind is important, as is combining foods properly and avoiding overeating.

Cost

Costs of Ayurvedic treatments vary, with initial consultations running from $40 to over $100, with follow-up visits costing less. In the United States, a half-hour consultation may range from to $25 to $50. Herbal treatments may cost from $10 to $50 per month and are often available from health food or bulk herb stores. Some clinics offer panchakarma, the intensive Ayurvedic detoxification treatment, which can include overnight stays for up to several weeks. The prices for these programs vary significantly, depending on the services and length of stay. Insurance reimbursement may depend on whether the primary physician is a licensed medical doctor.

Preparations

Ayurveda is a mind/body system of health that contains some ideas foreign to the Western scientific model. Those people considering Ayurveda should approach it with an open mind and willingness to experiment. Also, because Ayurveda is a whole-body system of healing and health, patience and discipline are helpful, as some conditions and diseases are believed to be brought on by years of bad health habits and require time and effort to correct. Finally, the Ayurvedic philosophy affirms that all individuals have the ability to heal themselves, so those considering Ayurveda should be prepared to bring responsibility and participation into the treatment.

Precautions

An Ayurvedic practitioner should be consulted by individuals who want to use herbal preparations. Care should be taken to ensure that a trained practitioner prepares individualized remedies. In 2002, a New York City hospital emergency department cautioned other hospitals when they encountered a case of a patient who came in with severe abdominal pain, occasional vomiting, and eventually seizures. The patient had suffered severe lead toxicity from an ayurvedic compound. In 2004, the Centers for Disease Control and Prevention received 12 reports of **lead poisoning**, which were associated with the use of Ayurvedic treatments. The reports came from consumers in California, Massachusetts, New Hampshire, New York, and Texas.

Side effects

During Ayurvedic detoxification programs, some people report fatigue, muscle soreness, and general sickness. As Ayurveda seeks to release mental stresses and psychological problems from the patient, some people can experience mental disturbances and depression during treatment, and psychological counseling may be part of a sound program.

Research and general acceptance

Because Ayurveda had been outside the Western scientific system for years, research in the United States dates only from the last part of the twentieth century. Another difficulty in documentation arises because Ayurvedic treatment is strictly individualized; two people with the same disease but different dosha patterns are likely to be treated differently. Much more scientific research was conducted in India during the last third of the twentieth century.

Outside India, many groups tried to market the Ayurvedic remedies by duplicating processes and formulas and calling them their own. The Indian government appointed a task force in January 2000 to develop traditional medicines and to prevent piracy of traditional Indian medical knowledge. The task force developed a digital library with international and Indian languages describing about 35,000 Ayurvedic herbal processes and formulas. The library became available in early 2003 on the Internet.

Some Ayurvedic herbal mixtures have been proven to have high antioxidant properties, much stronger than vitamins A, C, and E, and some have also been shown in laboratory tests to reduce or eliminate tumors in mice and to inhibit **cancer** growth in human lung tumor cells. In a 1987 study at MIT, an Ayurvedic herbal remedy was shown to significantly reduce colon cancer in rats. Another study was performed in the Netherlands with Maharishi Ayur-Ved products. A group of patients with chronic illnesses, including asthma, chronic bronchitis, hypertension, **eczema**, **psoriasis**, constipation, **rheumatoid arthritis**, headaches, and non-insulin dependent **diabetes mellitus**, were given Ayurvedic treatment. Strong results were

KEY TERMS

Dosha—One of three constitutional types (vata, pitta, or kapha) identified in Ayurvedic medicine.

Meditation—Technique focusing and concentration in order to calm the mind and body.

Panchakarma—Intensive Ayurvedic cleansing and detoxification program.

Prakriti—An individual's unique dosha pattern.

Prana—Basic life energy found in the elements.

Yoga—System of body and breathing exercises.

observed, with nearly 80% of the patients improving and some chronic conditions being completely cured.

Other studies have shown that Ayurvedic therapies can significantly lower **cholesterol** and blood pressure in stress-related problems. Diabetes, acne, and allergies have also been successfully treated with Ayurvedic remedies. Ayurvedic products have been shown to increase short-term memory and reduce headaches. Also, Ayurvedic remedies have been used successfully to support the healing process of patients undergoing chemotherapy, as these remedies have been demonstrated to increase immune system activity. The herb **gotu kola** has been reported to relieve anxiety and enhance memory.

Training and certification

In the United States, as of 2008, there was no standardized program for the certification of Ayurvedic practitioners. Many practitioners have primary degrees, either as medical doctors, homeopaths, or naturopathic physicians, with additional training in Ayurveda. Others train at an Ayurvedic medical school or college in India. A number of Ayurvedic organizations have worked toward developing licensing standards. Those seeking Ayurvedic treatment should inquire about the Ayurvedic training that a practitioner has completed.

Resources

PERIODICALS

"A Closer Look at Ayurvedic Medicine." *Focus on Complementary and Alternative Medicine* 12, no. 4 (Fall 2005/ Winter 2006).

ORGANIZATIONS

American Institute of Vedic Studies. PO Box 8357, Santa Fe, NM 87504. (505) 983-9385. http://www.vedanet.com/.

Ayurvedic and Naturopathic Medical Clinic. 10025 NE Fourth St., Bellevue, WA 98004. (206) 453-8022. http://www.ayurvedicscience.com/.

Ayurveda Holistic Center. Bayville, Long Island, NY. (516) 759-7731. http://www.Ayurvedahc.com.

Ayurvedic Institute. 11311 Menaul, NE Albuquerque, NM 87112. (505) 291-9698. http://www.Ayurveda.com.

Bastyr University of Natural Health Sciences. 144 NE Fifty-fourth St., Seattle, WA 98105. (206) 523-9585. http://www.bastyr.edu/.

Center for Mind/Body Medicine. PO Box 1048, La Jolla, CA 92038. (619) 794-2425. http://www.cmbm.org/.

Centers for Disease Control and Prevention. 1600 Clifton Rd., Atlanta, GA 30333. (404) 498-1515; (800) 311-3435. http://www.cdc.gov.

National Institute of Ayurvedic Medicine. 375 Fifth Ave., New York, NY 10016. (212) 685-8600. http://www.niam.com.

Rocky Mountain Institute of Yoga and Ayurveda. PO Box 1091, Boulder, CO 80306. (303) 443-6923. http://www.rmiya.org/index.php/.

OTHER

"Inside Ayurveda: An Independent Journal of Ayurvedic Health Care." PO Box 3021, Quincy, CA 95971. http://www.insideayurveda.com.

Douglas Dupler
Rhonda Cloos, RN

B

Bach flower essences

Description

Bach Flower Essences are specially prepared flower concentrates, containing the healing energy of plants. They are prescribed according to a patient's emotional disposition, as determined by the health practitioner or patients themselves. Bach Flower Essences are more homeopathic than herbal in the way they work, effecting energy levels rather than chemical balances in human and animal bodies. The theory is that they capture the flowers' healing energy, and they are said to overcome negative emotions and so relieve blockages in the flow of human energy that can cause illness. This theory also applies to pets.

The theory behind Bach Flower Essences was originated in the 1920s by British physician and bacteriologist, Edward Bach (1886–1936). Bach noticed that patients with physical complaints often suffered from **anxiety** or some kind of negative emotion. He concluded that determining a patient's emotional disposition and then prescribing an appropriate flower essence could treat the physical illness. Bach was a licensed medical doctor, but he also practiced **homeopathy**.

Following his own serious illness in 1917, Bach began a search for a new and simple system of medicine that would treat the whole person. In 1930, he gave up his medical practice in London and went to Wales and the English countryside to devote his life to his research. At this point, he stopped dispensing the mixtures of homeopathy and allopathic medicine that he had been using. Instead, he began investigating the healing properties of plant essences and discovered that he possessed an intuition for judging the properties of each flower. Through this research, including experimenting with each essence on himself, he developed the system of treatment that bears his name and is also the foundation for all other flower-remedy systems. In 1932 he discovered the first of his flower essences. In the years before his death in 1936, he discovered the remaining 37 essences that came to make up his system of remedies.

The system consists of 38 flower essences, each for a different emotional disposition. The basic theory is that if the remedy for the correct emotion is chosen, the physical illness resulting from that emotional state can then be treated. Bach also developed a combination formula, called **Rescue Remedy**, that contains five of the essences—cherry plum, clematis, impatiens, rock rose, and star of Bethlehem—and is recommended for treating any kind of physical or emotional shock.

Bach Flower Essences cost about $15 per 20 ml vial. There is no set time limit for treatment, which may take days, weeks, or in some cases months. The essences are not generally covered by medical insurance, including Medicare Part D drug plans.

General use

The 38 Bach Flower Essences are divided into seven emotional groups: fear, uncertainty, insufficient interest in present circumstances, despondency and despair, over-sensitivity to the influences or ideas of others, over-care for the welfare of others, and loneliness. The flower essences associated with each group and the specific emotion they are used to treat are as follows:

Fear

- Red rose: Used to treat terror or fright and in situations in which a person feels frozen and unable to move or to think clearly.
- Mimulus: Helps to treat identifiable fears and phobias, such as the fear of spiders or snakes, the fear of being alone, losing a job, or becoming sick. It also alleviates the anxiety of speaking about a fear to others and helps relieve shyness.
- Cherry plum: A remedy for people who fear losing control of their thoughts or actions, and of enacting

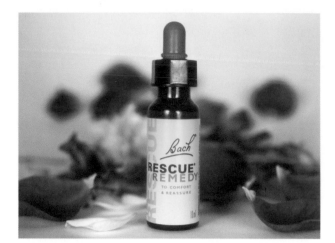

Bach Flower Essences are specially prepared flower concentrates, containing the healing energy of plants. *(Cordelia Molloy / Photo Researchers, Inc.)*

choices that are bad for them or that they believe are wrong. It also helps people to trust in themselves and to take actions that they believe are best for them.
- Aspen: Helps alleviate undefined, vague, or unexplainable fears.
- Red chestnut: Helps a person not feel anxious for others, especially loved ones.

Uncertainty

- Cerato: Helps individuals trust their own judgment when making a decision.
- Scleranthus: Helps a person to make a choice when faced with several different options.
- Gentian: Relieves feelings of discouragement and depression when something goes wrong or when one is faced with delays or difficulties.
- Gorse: Alleviates feelings of hopelessness and a sense that nothing more can be done about a situation.
- Hornbeam: Helps indiviudals believe they have the mental or physical strength to deal with the problems of everyday life.
- Wild oat: Helps individuals choose a direction when they reach a crossroad in their lives.

Insufficient interest in current circumstances

- Clematis: A relief for people who feel absorbed, impractical, indifferent, or withdrawn into fantasies, and helps to foster clarity and creativity.
- Honeysuckle: Offers help to people who are homesick, living in the past, or nostalgic.
- Wild rose: Alleviates apathy and resignation, and helps people take a more active interest in their lives.

- Olive: A remedy for exhaustion, which also helps users regain energy, vitality, and an interest in life.
- White chestnut: A help for people who are worried, preoccupied, or who want to get rid of unwanted thoughts.
- Mustard: A relief for sadness and depression caused by unknown reasons.
- Chestnut bud: An aid for people who repeatedly make the same mistake.

Loneliness

- Water violet: Helps people attain a warmer relationship with others and relieves feelings of aloofness.
- Impatiens: A remedy for impatience, irritability, and impulsiveness, and lowers stress and allows people to have empathy and understanding.
- Heather: An aid for people who feel self-centered, egotistical, or self-absorbed, which helps users find companionship and talk about their problems with others.

Over-sensitivity to influences and ideas

- Agrimony: Helps people to communicate their true feelings, and helps people who are normally cheerful but who get upset by arguments.
- Centaury: Helps people who are submissive and weak-willed and makes it easier to say no to others.
- Walnut: Helps to free people from old ties, during times of major life changes, and helps people who have difficulty accepting change.
- Holly: A relief for people who feel anger, jealousy, envy, hatred, and suspicion.

Despondency or despair

- Larch: Helps people regain self-esteem and confidence.
- Pine: Helps relieve feelings of guilt and self-blame. Also helps people who are never satisfied with their efforts and results.
- Elm: Offers relief to people who feel overwhelmed or inadequate and those who are depressed and exhausted.
- Sweet chestnut: Helps people when they feel anguish, despair, or hopelessness.
- Star of Bethlehem: A remedy for grief and distress, such as getting bad news, losing a loved one, or coping with a serious accident.
- Willow: Helps relieve feelings of self-pity and bitterness.
- Oak: A relief for people who are obstinate, inflexible, and overachievers.

- Crab apple: Helps people who feel ashamed and dislike themselves without cause, also known as the cleansing essence.

Over-care for the welfare of others

- Chicory: Helps people to be less critical, opinionated, controlling, or argumentative.
- Vervain: A remedy for people who are overbearing, fanatical, or have an overactive mind.
- Vine: An aid for those who are arrogant, ruthless, and inflexible.
- Beech: Helps people who are critical, intolerant, and negative.
- Rock water: Helps when a person is obsessive, repressive, or perfectionistic.

Preparations

The Bach Flower Essences are made from spring water infused with wild flowers, either by steeping in the sun for two to four hours or by boiling. They are produced by hand at a facility in England and contain 27% grape brandy as a preservative.

The 38 Bach Flower Essences can be taken individually or in any combination. The most common form of the essences is liquid concentrates although there is a combination in cream form, called Rescue Remedy. The liquid essences come in 20 ml (two-third of an ounce) dropper bottles. The recommended dosage is four drops four times a day until relief from the ailment is achieved. The drops can be taken directly into the mouth, placed in a glass of water, or applied on the skin behind the ears or on the inside of the wrists. To use a combination of essences, a small treatment bottle, usually one ounce or 30 ml, is filled with fresh spring water, leaving enough room for the appropriate number of drops. Dr. Bach recommended using two drops of each desired essence, with a maximum of six or seven essences in a single treatment bottle. One teaspoon of brandy, **apple cider vinegar**, or vegetable glycerin can be added as a preservative, if desired.

Precautions

Bach Flower Essences are highly diluted and have not been shown to be addictive, toxic, or cause adverse health effects when taken in normal dosages. Recovering alcoholics and people who avoid alcohol should not take Bach Flower Essences as they contain brandy.

The American **Cancer** Society (ACS) is one of several organizations that maintains there is no available scientific evidence to support claims that flower essences are effective in treating cancer or any other disease. The ACS cites a 2005 Israeli study that reported flower essences were ineffective in treating children with attention deficit hyperactivity disorder. The ACS also points to a 2001 German study that states both flower essences and a placebo were effective in reducing **stress** anxiety in children. This showed that a treatment can be effective if people simply think or are told it will be effective, something called the **placebo effect**, according to the ACS.

Side effects

Few, if any, adverse side effects have been reported by people using Bach Flower Essences.

Interactions

People taking the antibiotic metronidazole (Flagyl) or antialcoholic medications such as disulfiram (Antabuse) should avoid taking Bach Flower Essences since the essences contain brandy and can cause **nausea** and **vomiting**. Bach Flower Essences have not been tested to determine if they interact with medicines, foods, herbs, spices, and dietary supplements.

Resources

BOOKS

Bach, Edward. *The Essential Writings of Dr. Edward Bach: The Twelve Healers and Heal Thyself.* London: Random House UK, 2005.

Bradford, Nikki. *Heal Yourself with Flowers and Other Essences.* London: Quadrille, 2007.

Pallasdowney, Rhonda. *The Healing Power of Flowers: Bridging Herbalism, Homeopathy, Flower Essences, and the Human Energy System.* Orem, UT: Woodland, 2007.

KEY TERMS

Allopathic—Conventional medical treatment of disease symptoms that uses substances or techniques to oppose or suppress the symptoms.

Essence—The basic constituent of a plant that determines its characteristics.

Homeopathic—An alternative or complementary disease treatment system in which a patient is given minute doses of natural substances that in larger doses would produce symptoms of the disease itself.

Placebo—Something prescribed for patients that contains no medicine, but is given for the positive psychological effect it may have because the patients believe that they are receiving treatment.

Salmon, Philip, and Anna Jeoffroy. *Dr. Bach's Flower Remedies: Tapping into the Positive Emotional Qualities of the Chakras.* Berkeley, CA: North Atlantic Books, 2007.

PERIODICALS

"Independent Nurse: Clinical-Complementary Medicine—Flower Remedies." *GP* (October 21, 2005): 20.

Howard, Judy. "Do Bach Flower Remedies Have a Role to Play in Pain Control?" *Complementary Therapies in Clinical Practice* (August 2007): 174(10).

Pintov, S., et al. "Bach Flower Remedies Used for Attention Deficit Hyperactivity Disorder in Children—A Prospective Double-Blind Controlled Study." *European Journal of Paediatric Neurology* (October 27, 2005): 395–398.

Wedam, Norene F. "Biological Liquid Crystals: A Scientific Explanation of Bach Flower Essences." *Townsend Letter: The Examiner of Alternative Medicine* (July 2006): 91(3).

ORGANIZATIONS

American Institute of Homeopathy, 801 N. Fairfax St., Suite 306, Alexandria, VA, 22314, (888) 445-9988, http://www.homeopathyusa.org.

Dr. Edward Bach Centre, Mount Vernon, Bakers Lane, Brightwell-cum-SotwellOxon, OX10 0PZ , U.K, (44) 01491-834678, http://www.bachcentre.com.

Flower Essence Society, PO Box 459, Nevada City, CA, 95959, (800) 736-9222, http://www.flowersociety. org.

Homeopathic Medical Council of Canada, 3910 Bathurst St., Suite 202, Toronto, ON, M3H 3N8, Canada, (416) 638-4622, http://www.hmcc.ca.

National Center for Alternative and Complementary Medicine, 9000 Rockville Pike, Bethesda, MD, 20892, (888) 644-6226, http://www.nccam.nih.gov.

Ken R. Wells

Bach flower remedies *see* **Flower remedies**

Back pain *see* **Low back pain**

Bad breath *see* **Halitosis**

Bai gou *see* **Ginkgo biloba**

Bai thu *see* **Atractylodes (white)**

Balding *see* **Hair loss**

Balm of Gilead

Description

Balm of Gilead (*Cammiphora opobalsamum*, known as *Populus candicans* in the United States) is a substance used in perfumes that is derived from the resinous juices of the balsam poplar tree. The tree is a member of the Bursera family. The variety that is native to the continents of Africa and Asia is a small tree of 10–12 ft

---

(3-3.6 m)in height. The cultivated North American variety can grow to heights of 100 ft (30 m).

The herb's name derives from the ancient region of Gilead in Palestine, known for the great healing powers of its balm. Balm of Gilead is mentioned several times in the Bible (e.g., Jeremiah 8:22). The writings of Pliny the Elder indicate that the tree was brought to Rome in the first century A.D. The historian Josephus recorded that the Queen of Sheba made a gift of balm of Gilead to King Solomon.

General use

In addition to being used in the composition of perfumes, balm of Gilead is used to soothe ailments of the mucous membranes. It is taken internally to ease coughs and respiratory **infections**. The balm is also said to relieve **laryngitis** and sore throats. It can also be combined with **coltsfoot** to make a **cough** suppressant.

Preparations

The resin of the balsam poplar tree is collected when it seeps out of the tree during the summer months. Seepage increases when humidity levels are high. Slits may be made in the tree's bark to collect the resin more rapidly. The bark and leaf buds are also collected.

For the internal treatment of chest congestion, balm of Gilead is made into a tincture or a syrup. To make a syrup, the balm is combined with equal parts of elecampane, wild **cherry bark** and one-half part of **licorice** mixed with honey. The syrup can be taken by tablespoons as needed.

For external treatment of **bruises**, swellings and minor skin irritations, the balm is combined with lard or oil and applied as needed. The bark, which contains traces of salicylic acid, can be combined with willow and **rosemary** and used as a analgesic to relieve fevers, muscle aches and arthritic **pain**.

Precautions

The sale and use of herbs as medicines, including balm of Gilead, are not regulated by government agencies. Therefore, consumers should **exercise** caution in purchasing and using herbs in this manner. Consultation with a physician or pharmacist is always recommended.

Side effects

In general, balm of Gilead is safe to use in small amounts for coughs and other minor health problems. Some people, however, may have allergic reactions to the resin. In addition, patients with kidney and liver disease, as well as pregnant and nursing women, should avoid the internal use of balm of Gilead.

Interactions

Balm of Gilead has no known interactions with standard pharmaceutical preparations.

Resources

BOOKS

Elias, Jason, and Shelagh Ryan Masline. *Healing Herbal Remedies.* New York: Dell, 1995.

Tierra, Michael. *The Way of Herbs.* New York: Pocket Books, 1990.

OTHER

Grieve, M. "Balsam of Gilead." http://www.botanical.com/ (December 2000).

Mary McNulty

Balneology *see* **Hydrotherapy**
Ban xia *see* **Pinellia**

Barberry

Description

Barberry, Latin name *Berberis vulgaris*, is native to Europe, where it is commonly used as an ornamental shrub. It is also commonly grown in North America. Its close relative, *Berberis aquifolium*, is a native of North America, and is also known as Oregon grape. Native Americans originally taught settlers its value as a medicinal herb. Two other species of the plant,

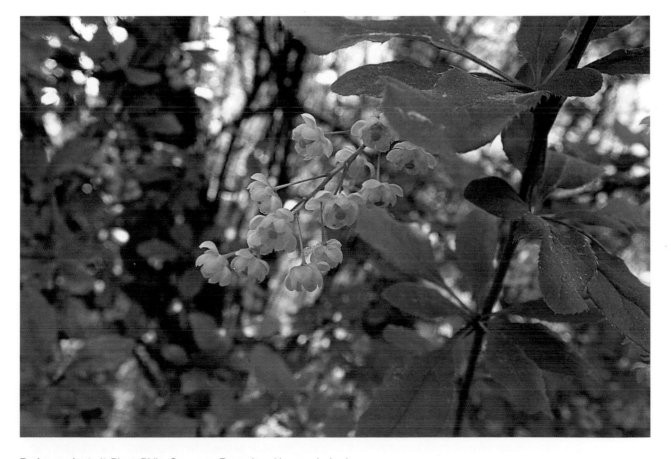

Barberry plant. *(©PlantaPhile, Germany. Reproduced by permission.)*

Nepalese and Indian barberry, are native to those areas and possess similar qualities.

Barberry is a perennial herb that is usually around 8 ft (2.4 m) tall, but can grow up to 10 ft (3 m) high. It bears yellow flowers, red or black berries, and small rounded fleshy leaves. It flourishes in dry sandy soil, and prefers a sunny location. Research has established that the active alkaloids in barberry belong to the isoquinoline family. They are berberine, berbamine, oxyacanthine, bervulcine, columbamine, isotetrandrine, jatrorrhizine, magnoflorine, and vulvracine. Other components include resin, tannin, and chelidonic acid, among others.

General use

Barberry and other berberine-containing plants have been used throughout history for their medicinal properties. Chinese medicine has records of such use dating back over 3,000 years. In addition to the fact that these plants have been tried and tested over time, recent research has indeed confirmed what herbalists have been teaching for millennia—berberine has remarkable properties.

The berries of the barberry plant are traditionally used to make jams and jellies, and the plant is used to make a dye. However, its culinary use is only minor compared to its importance as a member of the herbal *Materia Medica*.

The medicinal actions of barberry are traditionally classified as being cholagogue, hepatic, antiemetic, bitter and laxative. Its main active constituent, berberine, has recently been the subject of much research (it is the active constituent of a number of valuable herbs, barberry and **goldenseal** being two important examples), and has been proven effective against a variety of ailments.

Barberry is chiefly valued as an efficient liver cleanser, due to its ability to correct liver function and promote the flow of bile. It is good for **heartburn**, stomach upsets, including **gastritis**, ulcers and ulcerative bowel conditions, and is an effective appetite stimulant. It has also been recommended for renal **colic** and the treatment of renal calculi, where it is claimed to allay burning and soreness.

The herb has significant antibacterial, antiviral and antifungal properties, and has even demonstrated antiprotozoal properties, so it is an extremely valuable weapon against infection and **fever**. It is recommended for use against **diarrhea**, whether of non-specific type, such as **gastroenteritis**, or from an identified source such as cholera. It is also capable of inhibiting the growth of *Giardia lamblia, Trichomonas vaginalis* and *Entamoeba*

histolytica. In fact, barberry is capable of similar action to Metronidazole, a common antiprotozoal medication, but has the advantage of no side effects.

Berberine, the active constituent of barberry, inhibits *Candida* and other fungal growth, but does not affect beneficial bacteria such as *Acidophilus* and *Bifidus*. Barberry is particularly useful for skin **infections**, for which it is often taken internally, and has even been found effective against **psoriasis**.

It is often used against bronchial infections, as it is capable of breaking down and dispersing mucous accumulations, and controlling further secretions. It is an effective sedative, is capable of lowering blood pressure, and is an effective uterine stimulant. Barberry is also taken for **gallstones** and inflammation of the gallbladder. It has the ability to correct an enlarged spleen.

Barberry is useful for correcting menstrual irregularities, correcting **anemia**, as a treatment for **vaginitis**, and even as a tonic for a **hangover**. It is a suitable medication for gouty constitutions. It is recommended for strengthening the patient during convalescence, as it acts as an immune stimulant.

Barberry can be used to treat **malaria** and even Leishmaniasis, which is a protozoal infection. Nicholas Culpeper praised the barberry plant highly, and stated that the berries are just as useful as the bark. He recommended their use for the cure of ringworm, in addition to the ailments already mentioned.

Because it is capable of increasing blood supply, barberry may be of use to those suffering from ventricular heart defects. Berberine is used in China to treat white blood cell **depression** caused by chemotherapy or radiation treatments.

Preparations

The bark of the roots or stems are the parts used medicinally.

The dried herb may be taken in a decoction, for which place one teaspoonful of the herb in a cup of water and bring to the boil. Leave for about fifteen minutes and drink. This may be taken three time daily. The decoction may also be used as a gargle in cases of **sore throat**.

If a tincture is being used, 1–2 ml may be taken three times daily.

Herbalists recommend that in cases of gallbladder disease, barberry combined with fringe tree bark and black root are an effective treatment.

For an effective liver cleanse, herbalists recommend a combination of one part barberry, one part wild yam, one part **dandelion**, and one half part **licorice** root, simmered in one pint of water for ten minutes, then strained through a coffee filter.

The bark is sometimes made into a poultice for the treatment of skin lesions, and a compress is useful for swollen eye lids and **conjunctivitis**.

Precautions

Barberry root should not be taken by pregnant women because of its stimulant effect on the uterus. Those with **heart disease** or chronic respiratory problems should only take barberry after consultation with a herbalist, naturopath, or medical specialist.

The cultivation of barberry is restricted in some areas, as it hosts and promotes stem rust, a scourge to cereal crops.

If in any doubt, it is always best to consult an herbal practitioner regarding dosage of herbs.

Side effects

Berberine (an active ingredient of barberry), has been found to affect normal bilirubin in infants, so in theory, it may have an adverse effect on **jaundice**.

Strong extracts may cause stomach upsets, so use of barberry for a period of more than two consecutive weeks is not recommended.

Barberry, if taken to excess may cause nose bleeds, lethargy, kidney irritation, skin and eye inflammation, in addition to headaches and low blood sugar.

Interactions

Barberry, or any herb containing berberine, has been found to interact with Sumycin, Helidac (Tetrecycline), Vibramycin, Helidac (Tetracycline), Doxycycline, and Achromycin, causing them to be less effective, and to affect their absorption.

Resources

BOOKS

Culpeper, Nicholas. *Culpeper's Complete Herbal*. London: Bloomsbury Books, 1992.

Duke, James A. *The Green Pharmacy*. New York: St. Martin's Paperbacks, 1998.

Grieve, M. *A Modern Herbal*. London: Tiger Books International, 1992.

OTHER

Hoffman, David L. "Barberry." Health World Online. http://www.healthy.net/asp.

Birdsall, Timothy and Gregory Kelly. "Berberine: Theraputic Potential of an Alkaloid found in several Medicinal plants." In *Alternative Medicine Review* [online database] Vol. 2, no. 2 (March 1997) http://www.thorne.com/altmedrev/fulltext/berb.html.

Patricia Skinner

Barley grass

Description

Barley grass is the leaf portion of the barley plant (*Hordeum vulgare*), which remains after the seeds have been removed. As a grass, it is also known as a *distichon*, meaning that it grows in two separate ranks, or rows. The rows of barley grass are parallel to the central axis, forming a loose sheath over the stem, which is sometimes called the *culm*. This stem is hollow and jointed, and the seeds are elliptical and furrowed. The barley plant, an annual that requires reseeding each year, reaches a height of up to 3 ft (about 1 m). The plant has an extensive history in human and animal **nutrition**. As a nutritional supplement, it is preferable to use young barley plants that have not yet developed seeds.

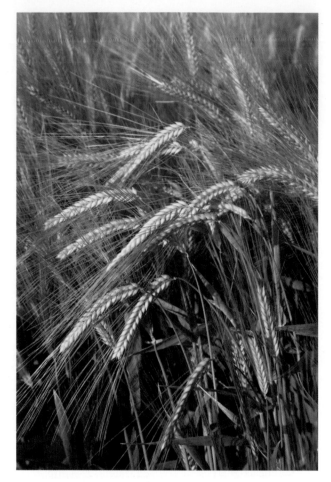

Barley growing in a field in California. *(© inga spence / Alamy)*

General use

The barley plant appears to have been used by the ancient Egyptians, Romans, and Vikings. It is believed that Columbus brought it to the Americas in 1493. Barley seeds have been used in both human nutrition and medicine. When the seeds are boiled, they release a thick substance that soothes sore throats. Barley seeds are used for the preparation of malt extract, which has a high sugar content that makes it suitable as a flavoring agent in pharmaceutical preparations.

Marketers make a number of claims regarding barley grass, including:

- It is the only vegetation on earth that can supply sole nutritional support from birth to old age.
- Barley grass juice contains nutrients such as vitamins C and E, which are much more potent together than when taken separately.
- Barley grass is high in calcium, iron, all essential amino acids, vitamin C, the flavonoids, vitamin B$_{12}$, and a number of enzymes and minerals.

- Barley grass can be used to treat disorders of the stomach and duodenum; pancreatitis; and as an anti-inflammatory agent.
- Barley grass contains superoxide dismutase (SOD), a powerful antioxidant enzyme that protects the cells against toxic free radicals.

Although not substantiated, one source has claimed that barley grass is good for the following conditions:

- skin diseases
- hepatitis
- asthma
- anemia
- diabetes
- arthritis
- obesity

Barley grass contains vitamins, particularly B vitamins, as well minerals such as **potassium**, **calcium**, **iron**, **phosphorus**, and **magnesium**. Enzymes contained in the plant include SOD and nitrogen reductase. The latter reduces nitrogen—an element commonly found in protein—in a biological process. Although barley grass contains enzymes, the health benefits of these substances remain unclear. Enzymes are proteins, which are normally broken down into their component chemicals during digestion. However, the enzymes found in raw foods remain technologically unprotected from normal digestive processes. The medical literature is not consistent on whether any SOD is actually absorbed intact through the digestive tract. In fact, the percentage absorbed may be very small. Techniques are being developed to encapsulate enzymes into other molecules. This will allow the enzymes to be absorbed intact, so that they will remain active following digestion.

Barley grass and other cereal grasses may or may not be useful sources of natural vitamins and minerals. Evidence may be insufficient to justify claims that these products improve physical health or cure disease. Barley grass has not been reviewed by the United States Food and Drug Administration (FDA) or the German Commission E. Nutrient concentration in barley grass products varies with the conditions under which the plant is grown. Like other natural supplements, commercial barley grass is not standardized; therefore, different crops contain varying amounts of nutrients. Young barley grass plants appear to contain higher concentrations of nutrients than older plants.

One well-publicized Chinese study reported that barley grass was beneficial in lowering **cholesterol**

KEY TERMS

Amino acid—An organic compound containing an amino group (NH_2), a carboxylic acid group (COOH), and various side groups. Amino acids are bound together to form proteins.

Diabetes type 2—A form of diabetes mellitus that usually occurs in adults. The pancreas produces insulin, but the muscle cells are resistant to the effects of the insulin. This was formerly called maturity (or adult) onset diabetes.

Enzyme—A protein, produced by a living organism, that functions as an organic catalyst (a chemical that increases the speed of a reaction without being involved in the reaction itself).

Vitamin—Any of various organic carbon-containing substances that are essential in minute amounts for normal growth and activity of the body, and are obtained naturally from plant and animal foods.

levels in patients with type 2 diabetes. This may be due to the plant's antioxidant abilities. Similar results were achieved by other researchers who studied the antioxidant effects of red wine and tomato juice.

Other health claims made for barley grass remain unconfirmed. For example, chlorophyll, the pigment found in barley grass and all green plants, may have some antibacterial effects. Chlorophyll reportedly inhibits the growth of **cancer** cells under laboratory conditions, but its value in human health is unknown.

Similarly, the claim that barley grass can provide full nutrition is subject to dispute. One researcher found that people on a vegan diet that included barley grass were likely to show reduced levels of **vitamin B$_{12}$**, and to require supplementation with this essential nutrient.

Preparations

Barley grass is available in capsule, powder, and tablet formulations. Capsules are sold in strengths of 470 mg, 475 mg, and 500 mg. Tablets are available in 350 mg and 500 mg strengths.

Precautions

Barley grass may sometimes be rich in **vitamin K**, which interferes with the action of anticoagulants such as Coumadin (the brand name for warfarin, a drug used to treat and prevent **blood clots**). Other than an allergic reaction, there are no known adverse effects attributed to barley grass.

Side effects

There are no known side effects attributed to barley grass.

Interactions

No drug interactions have been associated with barley grass, with the exception of samples that are high in vitamin K (interferes with Coumidin).

Resources

BOOKS

Lust J *The Herb Book*. New York, NY: Bantam Books, 1984.

Reynolds J., ed. *Martindale The Extra Pharmacopoeia*. 30th ed. London: The Pharmaceutical Press, 1993.

Seibold, R. *Cereal Grass, Nature's Greatest Health Gift*. New Canaan, CT: Keats Publishing Inc., 1991.

PERIODICALS

Donaldson, M.S. "Metabolic Vitamin B$_{12}$ Status on a Mostly Raw Vegan Diet with Follow-up Using Tablets, Nutritional Yeast, or Probiotic Supplements." *Annals of Nutrition and Metabolism* 44 (2000): 229–34.

Gowri, J. W., M. S. Turner, J. Nichols, et al. "Lipoprotein Oxidation for Individuals with Type 2 Diabetes Mellitus." *Journal of the American College of Nutrition* 18 (October 1999): 451–61.

Yu, Y. M., Chang, W. C., Chang, C. T., et al. "Effects of Young Barley Leaf Extract and Antioxidative Vitamins on LDL Oxidation and Free Radical Scavenging Activities in Type 2 Diabetes." *Diabetes Metab*. (April 28, 2002): 107–14.

OTHER

Alberta Barley Commission. #200, 3601A - 21 Street N.E. Calgary, Alberta T2E 6T5 CANADA. (403) 291-9111. (800) 265-9111. Fax: (403) 291-0190. http://www.albertabarley.com/kids/about.shtml.

Green Green Grass.com. 7925-A N Oracle Rd #281 Tucson, AZ 85704. (888) 773-9808. info@greengreengrass.com. http://www.greengreengrass.com/barleygreen_premium.html.

Herbal Information Center. 3507 Marsala Ct. Punta Gorda, FL 33950 http://www.kcweb.com/herb/barley.htm.

Samuel Uretsky, Pharm.D.

Bates method

Definition

The Bates method, popularized in the early twentieth century by ophthalmologist William Horatio Bates, involves the use of therapeutic eye exercises.

Bates claims these exercises will correct vision problems, thus alleviating the need for glasses or contact lenses. Patients practice eye exercises aimed at strengthening and training their eye muscles in an effort to overcome such problems as farsightedness (**hyperopia**), nearsightedness (**myopia**), and **astigmatism**.

Origins

The method was devised by Bates, who was born in 1860 in Newark, New Jersey. In 1885, he received his medical degree and began practicing in New York City. Over the years, he began to notice that eye conditions like myopia, which is caused by a refractive error, could become better or worse for no apparent reason. Based on this observation, he began to question a basic tenet of traditional ophthalmology, which held that once a person had a refractive error like myopia, the only way to correct it was by wearing glasses.

While traditional ophthalmologists believed that the lens was responsible for the eye's focus, Bates maintained that it was the muscles around the eye that caused the eye to focus. Thus, traditional ophthalmologists blamed problems like nearsightedness on a failure of the lens to properly focus, while Bates believed it was due to a dysfunction of the muscles surrounding the eyeball. Bates had come to this conclusion after performing eye surgery on cataract patients and finding that some of them could still see distance without glasses even though he had removed the lens from their eyes; therefore, he determined that the lens did not play a role in refractive errors such as myopia.

At this point, Bates broke from his counterparts and began focusing his attention on the muscles surrounding the eye. He came to view eye problems as a result of poor evolution, believing that the eye had not kept up with human progress and had not evolved to allow reading. He also blamed problems on artificial light, which kept the eyes working longer hours each day than they were intended to. Bates developed a series of eye exercises to retrain the optic muscles to solve this evolutionary glitch.

Bates believed that eye strain caused vision to deteriorate, and his treatment was simple: like any other muscles, the eye muscles need periods of rest and **exercise** in order to achieve optimal performance. He focused on the functioning of the six small muscles that control the eye's shape. When they become tense, they gradually grow weak and result in nearsightedness, farsightedness, astigmatism, or "lazy eye."

The Bates method received acclaim several years after Bates's death (1931), when author Aldous

---

KEY TERMS

Astigmatism—An eye condition that causes a person to see distorted images due to an abnormality in the curvature of the eye's lens.

Farsightedness—Being able to see more clearly those objects far away as opposed to those that are near. Also called hyperopic.

Nearsightedness—Being able to see more clearly those objects that are near as opposed to those in the distance. Also called myopia.

Huxley boasted that after two months on the Bates program, he went from being almost blind to being able to read without wearing glasses.

Benefits

An advantage of the Bates method is that the treatment is relaxing. Also, if patients stick to the routine and eye improvement is gained, they may benefit by being able to discard their corrective lenses, escaping a lifetime of costs for glasses, lenses, and contact solutions. The treatment is also much less invasive than refractive surgery, which is costly and has risks, just like any other operation.

Description

The Bates method maintains that vision problems are caused by physiological and psychological **strains** and therefore cannot be corrected by wearing glasses. He believed that a combination of rest and exercise would mend the eyes and devised several exercises aimed at strengthening and retraining the eye muscles.

The exercises themselves are simple, but Bates stressed that it takes discipline and attention to detail in order to achieve improvement. Some of the principal exercises of the Bates method are described below.

Palming

Palming is aimed at calming the visual system. In this exercise, patients close their eyes and cover them with the palms of their hands, allowing the fingers to cross on the forehead. The hands should be cupped so that no pressure is put on the eyeballs. Next, the patient should open his or her eyes and see if any light is getting in. If so, the hands should be moved so that no light enters and then close the eyes again. The warmth of a person's hands, combined with blocking out all light, will relax a pair of tense eyeballs.

Sitting at a table is a good palming position. A person can place a cushion on the table on which to rest their arms, and should check the height to be sure their hands are not too high or too low. Lying on the back, with knees raised and feet flat on the floor, is also a good position. While palming, patients should imagine a relaxing scene, such as a sunrise or ocean.

A description of the exercise posted on the Bates Association for Vision Education website suggests palming in 5–10 minute sessions, at least once a day. If this is found unpleasant, a person can try mini-sessions, palming for a period of 15 breaths, up to 20 times a day. Palming may also help when the eyes become tired and bleary.

Swinging

Swinging is meant to train the eyes not to stare. Bates maintained that the rigidity of staring was bad for the eyes. To do this exercise, the patient should focus on a fixed object, then swing the head or the entire body from side to side while keeping the object in view by moving the head instead of the eyes.

Test-card practice

Based on the idea that practice makes perfect, this exercise involves practicing eye charts. Patients are asked to focus on a letter, then close their eyes and visualize the black letter for several seconds. After several sessions, Bates maintains, the letters will appear blacker and clearer.

Sunning

Sunning is aimed at reducing light sensitivity. Bates believed the sun has a therapeutic effect, so patients are asked to close their eyes and face the sun. It is advised to sun only in the morning or evening and only for short periods of time.

Centralization

Centralization, or central fixation, is aimed at training the eye not to overstrain itself by taking in too much at once. This exercise involves training the eyes to focus on a single point, rather than an entire picture. The eye has a point in the middle of the vision field where vision is sharpest. This exercise is aimed at training people to look only at that point. Patients are asked to look at an object piece by piece instead of trying to look at it in its entirety, which Bates maintains is beyond the physical capabilities of the eye. Bates believed that looking at an entire picture created strain, causing bad eyesight. This is not an exercise per se, but rather something patients are asked to do all day long.

Color days

This involves spending the day focused on looking for a specific color. When looking at a color, patients are asked to focus on the color, not the form. Colors change every day.

People interested in the Bates method can pay a professional trained in the method to teach them the exercises or they can simply read about them in books or on the internet for no cost. Bates believed that improvement would vary, depending on the degree of problem and a person's devotion to doing the exercises.

Preparations

There are no pre-therapy procedures.

Precautions

People should be aware that the theory remains untested and they may be wasting their time on the exercises. This method should not be a substitute for appropriate medical treatment in the case of **cataracts**, **glaucoma**, and other eye diseases.

Side effects

There are no side effects, but patients should be cautious when using the sunning exercise, which may cause solar retinitis, or inflammation of the retina, causing permanent damage.

Research and general acceptance

Though the Bates method was devised a century ago, it has never been tested in a clinical setting. At best, anecdotal evidence is all there is to substantiate its use.

The orthodox ophthalmologists of Bates's time, as well as those of today, have largely dismissed his theories as based on flawed science. Traditional ophthalmologists hold that the lens—not the eye muscles—is responsible for focus and therefore cannot be fixed through a series of exercises. Traditional ophthalmologists believe that problems like nearsightedness are anatomic conditions that cannot be fixed by strengthening the eye muscles.

As Philip Pollack noted in his book *The Truth About Eye Exercises*, Bates used testimonials and case histories depicting successful treatment as scientific proof his theory was sound. Pollack also lambasted Bates for describing rare cases as the norm, using them as justification for his methods.

The Bates method has not found widespread use and is generally not accepted by the medical establishment. In his book *Health Education Authority Guide to Complementary Medicine and Therapies*, A. Woodham cautions that the medical consensus is that "eye exercises can improve the sight in some cases, but these need a lot of dedication and perseverance. Do not expect miracles."

Training and certification

Natural vision improvement techniques, such as the Bates method, are generally taught by behavioral optometrists or vision therapists. Vision therapists may not necessarily be trained in optometry. It is possible, however, to find practicing optometrists trained by the Bates Association for Vision Education, which offers courses on the method.

Resources

BOOKS

Bates, W. *The Bates Method for Better Eyesight without Glasses*. New York: Henry Holt & Co., 1987.

Cheney, E. *The Eyes Have It: A Self-Help Manual for Better Vision*. York Beach, Maine: Samuel Weiser, Inc., 1987.

PERIODICALS

Booth, Brian. "Nature Cures: Hydrotherapy, Bates Method." *Nursing Times* 91 no. 20 (May 1995): 42–43.

Karatz, May Annexton. "William Horatio Bates, M.D., and the Bates Method of Eye Exercises." *New York State Journal of Medicine* 75 no. 7 (June 1975): 1105–1110.

ORGANIZATIONS

College of Optometrics in Vision Development. P.O. Box 285, Chula Vista, CA 91912. (619) 425-6191. Fax: (619) 425-0733.

OTHER

"Bates Method." *The Vision Improvement Site.* http://lightning.prohosting.com/-hanwen/vision/bates.htm. 16 July 2000.

"Fallacies of the Bates System." *Quackwatch.com.* http://www.quackwatch.com. 14 July 2000.

"Who Was Dr. Bates?" *Bates Association for Vision Education.* http://www.seeing.org/intro/faq/faq01.htm. 14 July 2000.

Lisa Frick

Bayberry

Description

Bayberry, also known as wax myrtle, waxberry, or candelberry, is both a shrub and a tree. All members of the bayberry family are classified botanically as *Myricaceae*, and many varieties are found all over the world, including Japan, South America, the West Indies, the United Kingdom, and in the United States.

American bayberry (*Myrica cerifera*) is a shrub that grows 3–8 ft (1–2.4 m) high. It is found in eastern North America, in marshes and bogs near sandy Atlantic coastal areas, as well as in similar areas along the shores of the Great Lakes. American bayberry is the variety most often mentioned by herbalists.

American bayberry and its British Isles cousin, English bog myrtle, are very alike in appearance, and grow to a similar height. Foliage is evergreen and consists of knife-blade shaped shiny leaves that have small spots on them. When crumpled in one's hand, bayberry leaves and its bark produce a pleasant, balsamic aroma. However, they have a very bitter, astringent taste. The small berries are in globular clusters at stem junctions, crusted with a greenish-white waxy substance sprinkled with small black flecks. The exterior of bayberry root bark is mottled, with smooth reddish-brown cork underneath.

General use

Both American bayberry and English bog myrtle, besides sharing a similar appearance, have similar medicinal qualities. Like all bayberry varieties, they are classified as astringent herbs. Some evidence suggests that these herbs have antimicrobial capabilities, in that they are able to prevent the development of pathogenic activity from microbes, and are useful in regulating mucus in the body.

Both varieties' bark and roots contain starch, lignin, gum, albumen, tannic and gallic acids, astringent resin, a red coloring substance, a vaporous oil, and an acid similar to saponin. Powdered bayberry root is useful as a bowel astringent in the treatment of **diarrhea** and **colitis**, a soothing and helpful gargle for the **common cold** or a **sore throat**, and as a douche in the treatment of leukorrhea, an abnormal white or yellow mucoid discharge from the vagina or cervix. In the *Herbal Materia Medica*, bayberry root bark is classified as an astringent, a circulatory stimulant, as well as a diaphoretic, a remedy which dilates superficial capillaries and induces perspiration, sometimes used to reduce fevers.

The berries of both American bayberry and English bog myrtle, when boiled in water, produce myrtle wax, which is composed of stearic, palmitic, myristic, and oleaic acids. This is used in making bayberry-scented soaps and bayberry candles, which are fragrant, more brittle than bees' wax candles, and are virtually smokeless. Four pounds of berries produce approximately one pound of wax. A briskly stimulating shaving cream was also made from this bayberry wax.

The wax's modern medicinal uses were first discovered and came into use in 1722, and included the making of surgeon's soap plasters. The water that the berries were boiled in during wax-extraction, when boiled down to an extract, has been used in the North Country of England and Scotland for centuries as a treatment for dysentery. Narcotic properties are also attributed to bayberry wax.

In *A Modern Herbal*, it was written that the leaves of English bog myrtle were commonly used in France to induce both **menstruation** and abortion.

In China, bayberry leaves are infused to make a tea which is used both to relieve stomach problems, and as a cordial, which is a stimulating medicine or drink.

A mouthwash particularly useful in inhibiting halitosis can be made from either the powdered root or leaves.

Bayberry bark has traditionally been used to tan leather and dye wool.

Bayberry branches have been used in lieu of **hops** in the fermentation of *gale beer*, popular in northern England, and reported to have more than the usual "thirst-quenching" ability.

Bayberries can be ground to use as spice, or added to broths.

In the West Indies, *Pimenta acris*, commonly called wild cinnamon or bayberry, is used in making both bay rum and oil of bayberry.

M. pennsylvanica's root can be used to induce **vomiting**.

The Brazilian species, *Tabocas combicurdo*, is described in *A Modern Herbal* as a "pick-me-up."

Preparations

Bayberry preparations are made by collecting root bark in late fall or early winter, drying thoroughly, and either pulvarizing into a powder or chopping the bark. It should be stored in a tightly sealed container, away from light.

A decoction or tea is prepared by adding a teaspoonful of powdered bayberry bark to a cup of cold water and bringing this to a boil. If using chopped, not powdered, bark, the decoction is simmered. This *tea* is then left to steep for 15–20 minutes before drinking. It may be taken up to three times a day for a limited period of time, as chronic use at this dosage could damage a person's kidneys and liver. The same preparation can be used as a gargle for sore throat.

Tincture of bayberry preparations are also available in some locales. Usual dosage is one-half teaspoonful in water.

Precautions

As noted previously, English bog myrtle has historically been shown as having characteristics capable of inducing abortion. Its leaves, in nature, also have a poisonous, volatile oil present, which can be removed by boiling. Though no studies were found indicating the same capabilities for American bayberry, because of their many similarities, it should be assumed that neither English bog myrtle nor American bayberry leaves should be ingested in their natural, unprepared state. Additionally, aforementioned dosages of a bayberry decoction or tea should not be taken on a chronic basis, as damage to the kidneys and liver could occur.

Side effects

Powdered bayberry root, if inhaled, can cause convulsive episodes of both **sneezing** and coughing.

Several varieties of the bayberry family are used as emetics, which are agents used to induce vomiting, and can also cause **nausea**.

Interactions

To date, no reported interactions with either food, drug, or other herbal preparations have been found.

Resources

BOOKS

Grieve, M. and C.F. Leyel Barnes. *A Modern Herbal: The Medical, Culinary, Cosmetic and Economic Properties, Cultivation and Folklore of Herbs, Grasses, Fungi, Shrubs and Trees With All of Their Modern Scientific Uses.* Barnes and Noble Publishing, 1992.

Hoffman, David and Linda Quayle. *The Complete Illustrated Herbal: A Safe and Practical Guide to Making and Using Herbal Remedies.* Barnes and Noble Publishing, 1999.

Thayer, Henry. *Fluid and Solid Extracts.* Geo.C.Rand & Avery, 1866.

Joan Schonbeck

Bearberry *see* **Uva ursi**

Beard moss *see* **Usnea**

Bedsores

Definition

Bedsores are the result of inflammation and damage caused by irritation to the skin and inhibited blood flow. The condition occurs when skin is rubbed against a bed, chair, cast, or other hard object for an extended period of time. Bedsores can range from mild inflammation to deep **wounds** that involve muscle and bone. **Infections** can be a serious complication to the condition.

Description

Bedsores are also called decubitus ulcers, pressure ulcers, or pressure sores. They often start out with shiny red skin that becomes itchy or painful, then quickly **blisters** and deteriorates into open sores. Once there is a break in the skin, there is a strong possibility of the sore becoming infected, causing further medical problems. Bedsores are most apt to develop over the bony prominences of the ankles, the hip bones, the lower back, the shoulders, the spinal column, the buttocks, and the heels of the feet. Bedsores are most likely to occur in people who must use wheelchairs or who are confined to bed.

Bedsores are medically categorized by stages:

- Stage I: The skin reddens, but it remains unbroken.
- Stage II: Redness, swelling, and blisters develop. There is possibly peeling of the outer layer of the skin.
- Stage III: A shallow open wound develops on the skin.
- Stage IV: The sore deepens, spreading through layers of skin and fat down to muscle tissue.
- Stage V: Muscle tissue is broken down.
- Stage VI: The underlying bone is exposed, and there is danger of severe damage and infection.

Causes and symptoms

Bedsores most often happen when the most superficial blood vessels are pressed against the skin and squeezed shut, closing off the flow of blood. If the supply of blood to an area of skin is cut off for more than an hour, the tissue will began to die due to lack of oxygen and nutrients. Ordinarily, the layer of fat under the bony areas of the skin helps keep the blood vessels from being compressed in this way. Also, people have a normal impulse to change positions frequently when they are sitting or lying down, so the blood supply is usually not kept from any area of the skin for very long. Bedsores are most likely to occur in people who have lost the protective fat layer or whose movement impulse is hindered.

Friction or rubbing from poorly fitted shoes or clothing and wrinkled bedding often cause a sore to develop. Constant exposure to the moisture of urine, feces, and perspiration may also cause the skin to deteriorate. In such cases there is an increased the risk of skin infection as well as sores.

Risk factors for bedsores:

- older than 60 years of age
- heart disease
- diabetes
- diminished tactile sensation
- incontinence
- malnutrition
- obesity
- paralysis or immobility
- poor circulation
- prolonged bed rest
- spinal cord injury
- anemia
- disuse atrophy

KEY TERMS

Disuse atrophy—Condition of muscles that have lost size, strength, and function due to lack of mobility.

Gangrene—A serious condition where there is decay or death of an organ, tissue, or bone caused by a lack of oxygen and nutrients and by bacterial infections.

Incontinence—Inability to control bladder or bowel movements.

Inflammation—An immune reaction to tissue injury or damage, usually characterized by pain, swelling and redness.

Poultice—Moistened herbs applied directly to a site of injury or infection.

Tactile sense—Receiving information about the body and the environment via contact with the skin. When this is lost through illness, a person may receive injuries without being aware of it.

Diagnosis

Physical examination of the skin, medical history, and patient and caregiver observations are the basis of diagnosis. Any sign of reddening of the skin will be closely monitored.

Treatment

Contrasting hot and cold local applications can increase circulation to problem areas and help flush out waste products, speeding the healing process. Hot compresses should be applied for three minutes, followed by 30 seconds of cold compress application, repeating the cycle three times. The cycle should always end with the cold compress. In addition, **zinc** and vitamins A, C, E, and B-complex should be taken to help maintain healthy skin and repair injuries.

Herbal remedies

A poultice can be made of equal parts of powdered **slippery elm**, *Ulmus fulva*; **marsh mallow** root, *Althaea officinalis*; and *Echinacea spp.* The herbs should be blended together with a small amount of hot water and applied to the skin three or four times per day to relieve inflammation. Poultices used on broken skin or infected areas should never be reused.

An infection-fighting rinse can be made by diluting two drops of essential **tea tree oil**, *Melaleuca spp.*, in eight ounces of water. This should be used to bathe the wound when bandages are changed.

An herbal tea made from *Calendula officinalis* can be used as an antiseptic wash and a wound healing agent. **Calendula** cream can also be applied to the affected area.

A poultice made from **goldenseal**, *Hydrastis canadensis,* and water or goldenseal ointment can be applied to areas of inflammation several times per day to heal the skin and prevent infection.

Allopathic treatment

A healthcare provider should be consulted whenever a person develops bedsores. An emergency situation may be indicated if sores become tender, swollen, or warm to the touch, if the patient develops a **fever**, or if the sore has pus or a foul-smelling discharge.

For mild bedsores, treatment basically involves relieving pressure on the area and keeping the skin clean and dry. When the skin is broken, a non-stick covering may be used. A saline solution is often used to clean the wound site whenever a fresh bandage is applied. Disinfectants are applied if the site is infected.

The doctor may also prescribe antibiotics, special dressings or drying agents, and ointments to be applied to the wound. Heat lamps are used quite successfully to dry out and heal the sores. Warm whirlpool treatments are sometimes also recommended for sores on the arm, hand, foot, or leg.

In a procedure called debridement, a scalpel may be used to remove dead tissue or other debris from the wound. Deep sores that don't respond to other therapy may require skin grafts or plastic surgery. If there is a major infection, oral antibiotics may be given. If a bone infection, called osteomyelitis, develops or infection spreads through the bloodstream, aggressive treatment with antibiotics over the course of several weeks may be required.

Expected results

With proper treatment, bedsores should begin to heal two to four weeks after treatment begins. Left untreated, however, **gangrene**, osteomyelitis, or a systemic infection may develop. In the United States, about 60,000 deaths a year are attributable to complications caused by bedsores.

Prevention

Prompt medical attention can prevent pressure sores from deepening into more serious infections. People whose movement or sense of touch is limited by disability and disease should be monitored to insure that the skin remains clean, dry, and healthy. A bed-ridden patient should be repositioned at least once every two hours while awake. A person who uses a wheelchair should remember to shift the body's position often or they should be helped to reposition the body at least once an hour. To avoid injury, it is important to lift, rather than drag, a person being repositioned. Wheelchair users should sit up as straight as possible, with pillows behind the head and between the legs if needed. Donut-shaped seat cushions should not be used because they may restrict blood flow.

Even slight friction can remove the top layer of skin and damage the blood vessels beneath it. Pillows or foam wedges can be used to keep the ankles from rubbing together and irritating each other; pillows placed under the lower legs can raise the heels off the bed. To minimize pressure sores, there should be adequate padding in beds, chairs, and wheelchairs. Those who are bed-ridden can be protected by using sheepskin pads, specialized cushions, and mattresses filled with air or water. In addition, a 1997 study indicates that topical use of **essential fatty acids** can help the skin stay healthy.

Resources

BOOKS

Berkow, MD, Robert, editor in-chief, et al. *The Merck Manual of Medical Information, Home Edition.* New York: Pocket Books, 1997.

The Editors of Time-Life Books. *The Medical Advisor: The Complete Guide to Alternative and Conventional Treatments.* Virginia: Time-Life, Inc., 1996.

PERIODICALS

Declair, V. *Ostomy Wound Management* 43, no. 5 (1997): 48-52.

ORGANIZATIONS

International Association of Enterstomal Therapy, 27241 La Paz Road, Suite 121, Laguna Niguel, CA 92656

National Pressure Ulcer Advisory Panel, SUNY at Buffalo, Beck Hall, 3435 Main Street, Buffalo, NY 14214 Website: http://www.npuap.org.

Patience Paradox

Bedwetting

Definition

Bedwetting, or enuresis, is a childhood condition of urinating in bed while asleep at night. It is a chronic condition that often resolves by itself before the teenage years.

Description

One of the major tasks of toddlerhood is to learn how to achieve conscious control over the timing of urination. Most children do not become fully toilet trained until they are about two to four years old. Before then, the parts of the nervous system in charge of bladder control are not fully developed and functional. In general, boys take longer to learn to control their bladders than girls, and daytime bladder control is easier for a child than overnight bladder control. There is a genetic aspect to bedwetting, so that parents who once had the condition often have children who wet the bed at night.

Causes and symptoms

Bedwetting is often due to the normal immaturity of the nervous system and the urinary system. For instance, up to age six, bedwetting is often due to nothing more than the bladder having a small capacity. In addition, the muscles that control the opening and closing of the urethra may not be sufficiently developed.

Often it takes a while for a child to learn recognition of bladder fullness, waking up, and going to the toilet. In most cases, urinary capacity and control increase over time, and the bedwetting problem will eventually be outgrown.

Surprisingly, a major cause of bedwetting is lack of sleep. If a child is not sleeping enough hours, then there will be less of the light, rapid eye movement (REM) sleep, and more periods of heavy, deep sleep. During the periods of deep sleep some children will have difficulty becoming aware of the urge to urinate and awakening to go to the toilet.

Bedwetting may be a sign of allergic reactions, which end up irritating sphincter muscles around the urethra. This contributes to a loss of bladder control during sleep. Heavy **snoring**, mouth breathing, and night sweats may all be indications of the presence of **allergies**.

Bedwetting can sometimes be due to emotional and psychological **stress**, including major life changes such as moving or a divorce. This usually leads to the type of bedwetting called secondary enuresis, in which a previous level of accomplishment with bladder control is lost. In other words, a child who has been dry at night will suddenly start wetting the bed again. This may indicate an underlying problem such as **constipation**, diabetes, physical defects in the urinary tract, sacral nerve disorders, a pelvic growth, urinary stasis, infection, **kidney stones**, or kidney damage. Secondary enuresis also frequently occurs in children who are being physically or sexually abused. A pediatrician should be consulted if the condition persists.

Only about 1% of bedwetting is caused by a serious underlying problem. If the following symptoms are present, a pediatrician or a pediatric urologist should be consulted:

- straining during urination
- a burning feeling or other discomfort during urination
- constant or recurrent dribbling of urine
- cloudy or pink urine
- bloodstains or other discharge on underpants or nightclothes
- an unpleasant urine odor
- onset of abdominal pain, backache or fever
- constant thirst, especially at night
- sudden loss of bladder control previously mastered
- a child over the age of two who still shows no signs of being ready to learn bladder control

Diagnosis

When bedwetting is resistant to home treatments or when more serious symptoms are present, a visit should be made to a healthcare provider. This is especially warranted if the child is older than six. A thorough history and physical exam should be taken along with a urine sample. Analysis and culture tests can be done on the urine to determine if an infection is present. Further evaluations may be made using ultrasound, an x ray of the kidney, or a consultation with a urologist. If the bedwetting appears to be connected with issues of stress or family problems, a mental health consultation may be recommended.

Treatment

Sitting in a cool sitz bath (pelvic area only immersed) for about five minutes daily can tone up the urethral sphincter. This can be done using a bathtub filled with about two or three inches of water, having the child sit in a large basin of water or using a sitz basin (available from larger drugstores and medical supply stores).

"Hands-on" treatments such as **acupressure**, **reflexology**, and **shiatsu** can be used to relax the child, counteract stress, and improve the actions of the nervous system. **Hypnotherapy** can also be helpful in improving bedwetting. Among other things, the child will be given positive goal affirmations to say before going to bed. This should help make the urge to urinate during the night more conscious, and therefore encourage the child to awaken and go to the toilet.

The best way to use **homeopathy** is to see a homeopath for individual prescribing. *Equisetum* 6c, may be useful, especially if there are dreams or nightmares connected with the bedwetting. For bedwetting in very excitable, outgoing children, which occurs soon after falling asleep, *Causticum* 6c may be recommended. The remedies should be given once per day at bedtime for up to two weeks. A practitioner should be consulted for more specific remedies.

Herbal medicine

A strong tea can also be made using equal parts of **horsetail**, *Equisetum arvense;* **St. John's wort**; **cornsilk**, *Zea mays;* and **lemon balm**, *Melissa offinalis.* Two to three handfuls of the mixture should be placed in a quart or liter jar and then covered with boiling water. The tea should be allowed to steep overnight. The child should be given half a cup of the tea three times per day, with the last dose being given at least two hours before bedtime.

Nettles, *Urtica dioica,* can be made into a pleasant tea and consumed throughout the day as a tonic for the kidneys. The tea can be mixed with equal parts of fruit juice as a pleasant drink for the child.

Aromatherapy uses the essential oil of cypress, *Cupressus sempervirens* to treat chronic bedwetting. Several drops of cypress oil should be put in olive oil for massage. The oil should be rubbed onto the child's stomach right before bedtime.

Behavior modification programs may be suggested. In one type, alarms that are triggered by body moisture are worn overnight, waking the child at the first sign of bedwetting. The child can then go use the toilet to finish emptying the bladder. This will eventually train the child to awaken and use the toilet upon experiencing the sensation of a full bladder. Nighttime toilet training using the alarm may take up to four or five months to be effective, however. Another program focuses on the child's effort with urinating before going to bed, recording wet and dry nights, changing wet clothing and bedding, and discussing progress. Positive reinforcements, such as gold stars on a chart and other rewards, are given for nights that the child does not urinate in bed.

Allopathic treatment

If other treatments fail to work, treatment with medication may be suggested. With the use of the drug imipramine, improvement will usually occur in the first week of treatment if it is going to be helpful. The drug can be discontinued if it does not work within a week or after a month has gone by with no bedwetting. Unfortunately, relapses are very common with this treatment. Also, since imipramine is a strong drug, the blood needs to be tested every other week for abnormal side effects. A nasal spray containing Demopressin, an antidiuretic drug, has been shown to be effective in diminishing bedwetting. It is necessary to use the spray at least four to six weeks for maximum effectiveness. Demopressin also has negative side effects and is, therefore, only recommended for short-term use.

Expected results

Bedwetting is usually outgrown at some point. However, underlying disease conditions may have to be assessed and treated.

Prevention

Caffeine has a diuretic effect, and should be avoided. It is found in coffee, chocolate, tea, and many sodas. Food labels should be examined to determine caffeine content.

Resources

BOOKS

The Editors of Time-Life Books. *The Medical Advisor: The Complete Guide to Alternative and Conventional Treatments.* Virginia: Time-Life, Inc., 1996.

Kirchheimer, Sid and the editors of Prevention Magazine Health Books. *The Doctors Book of Home Remedies II: Over 1,200 New Doctor-Tested Tips and Techniques Anyone Can Use to Heal Hundreds of Everyday Health Problems.* Pennsylvania: Rodale Press, 1993.

Lockie, Dr. Andrew and Dr. Nicola Geddes. *The Complete Guide to homeopathy: The principles and Practice of Treatment with a Comprehensive Range of Self-Help Remedies for Common Ailments.* London: Dorling Kindersley, Ltd., 1995.

OTHER

AlternativeMedicine.com. http://www.alternative medicine.com

American Academy of Pediatrics. http://www.aap.org/ family/bedwet.htm.

Medicinal Herbs Online. http://www.egregore.com/ diseases/ bedwetting.html.

Patience Paradox

Bee pollen
Description

Bee pollen is the dust-size male seed found on the stamen of any flower blossom. The pollen collects on the legs of honeybees as they move from flower to flower. The bees secrete a number of enzymes into the pollen. Pollen is usually collected commercially by placing a special device at the entrance of beehives that brushes the substance from their hind legs into a collection receptacle.

General use

Bee pollen is among the oldest known dietary supplements. Its use as a rejuvenator and medicine date back to the early Egyptians and ancient Chinese. It has been called many things, from a fountain of youth to an "ambrosia of the gods." The Greek physician Hippocrates, sometimes called the father of modern medicine, used it as a healing substance 2,500 years ago. It is rich in vitamins, especially B vitamins, and contains trace amounts of minerals, elements, **amino acids**, and enzymes.

The pollen is composed of 55% carbohydrates, 35% protein, 3% minerals and vitamins, 2% fatty acids, and 5% other substances. It contains very small amounts of many substances considered to be **antioxidants**, including betacarotene, vitamins C and E, **lycopene**, **selenium**, and flavonoids.

Proponents of bee pollen offer a wide range of claims regarding its nutritional and healing properties. These include enhancing the immune system, controlling weight, relieving allergy symptoms, increasing strength, improving sexual function, enhancing vitality and stamina, slowing the **aging** process, and prolonging life. None of these claims have been substantiated by scientific studies.

Bee pollen is said to strengthen the immune system through its antioxidant properties. Antioxidants are used to deactivate free radicals in the body. Free radicals are byproducts of oxygen that can damage cells and are linked to many degenerative diseases, especially those associated with aging. They are also associated with the aging process itself. Antioxidants may block further damage and even reverse much of the cell oxidation already done. Bee pollen is suggested to help counteract the effects of radiation and environmental pollutants that weaken the immune system, supporters say.

In the January 2000 issue of *Bee Online*, an Internet publication of the American **Apitherapy** Society,

KEY TERMS

Antioxidant—A substance that opposes oxidation damage anywhere in the body caused by free oxygen radicals.

Flavonoids—A group of about 5,000 substances, mostly derived from food, that have super antioxidant qualities

Free oxygen radicals—Also called free radicals, these are by-products of oxygen that cause oxidative damage to the body's cells.

Gout—A disease causing inflammation of the joints, especially the knees, toes, and fingers due to the deposit of crystallized uric acid in the joints.

Stamen—The male fertilizing organ of flowering plants, bearing pollen.

Uric acid—A compound that can form deposits in joints and tissues. This disease is known as gout or hyperuricemia.

Steve Schecter, naturopathic doctor, said bee pollen is beneficial in reducing the effects of radiation treatment in women with **cancer**. A group of 25 women undergoing treatment for **uterine cancer** also took 20 g (about two teaspoons) of bee pollen three times a day. The women reported improvements in their appetites and sense of well being, and less severe **nausea** associated with radiation therapy. Their serum protein levels increased and red and white blood cell counts also improved.

Although many plant pollens can cause or exacerbate **allergies** and **hay fever**, bee pollen can actually help reduce the symptoms of these conditions. Local bee pollen therapy is recommended to start before the allergy season begins and it may take a few weeks for the pollen to work. According to an article in the February 1998 issue of *Better Nutrition*, an Oklahoma allergist successfully used bee pollen to treat 22,000 patients with allergies. However, those allergic to bee **stings** may experience severe (anaphylactic) reactions to the pollen.

Bee pollen is often used by athletes to improve strength, endurance, energy, and speed. It is said to help muscles recover more quickly from **exercise** and to increase mental stamina. "Bee pollen is used by almost every Olympic athlete in the world," said James Higgins, treasurer of the American Apitherapy Society, in an interview in the August 1999 issue of *Better Nutrition*. "It gives them more energy and better performance for events like marathons, and they aren't as exhausted the next day."

Preparations

It takes about two hours for bee pollen to be absorbed into the bloodstream. It is available in health food stores in gelatin capsules, tablets, and granules. Capsules and tablets generally contain 500-1000 mg of bee pollen. A 100-count bottle costs $5-8 on average. Granules are sold by the ounce or pound. A one-pound bag costs about $20. The recommended dosages for preventative purposes are an eighth to a quarter teaspoon of granules once a day to start, gradually increasing over a month to one to two teaspoons, one to three times a day. The dosage for short-term therapeutic use is 3/8-3/4 teaspoon to start, increasing to three to six teaspoons, one to three times a day. The recommended preventative dosage for capsules is two 450-580 mg capsules, three to four times a day, and three times that dosage for therapeutic purposes. Bee pollen is also available in liquid, cream, salve, and tincture form, mainly for use on skin conditions, sores, pounds, and **bruises**. Bee pollen should not be heated, since it will lose its potency.

Precautions

Persons who are allergic to bee stings or products should not use bee pollen since it may cause a serious allergic reaction, including death. Anyone uncertain if they are allergic to bee pollen should sample only a few granules first to see if there is any type of reaction, or have an allergy test. Those using bee pollen to reduce hay **fever** should be sure to consume local bee pollen to obtain the best results.

Side effects

There are rare cases of minor side effects, such as gastrointestinal irritation and **diarrhea**, associated with ingesting bee pollen.

Interactions

Bee pollen has no known negative interactions with other drugs, vitamins, or supplements.

Resources

BOOKS

Balch, James F. *Prescription for Nutritional Healing.* Avery Publishing Group, 1997.

Elkins, Rita. *Bee Pollen, Royal Jelly, Propolis, and Honey: An Extraordinary Energy and Health-Promoting Ensemble.* Woodland Publishing, 1999.

Geelhoed, Glenn W. and Jean Barilla. *Natural Health Secrets From Around the World*. Keats Publishing, 1997.

Jensen, Bernard *Bee Well, Bee Wise*. Bernard Jensen Publisher, 1994.

Wade, Carlson. *Carlson Wade's New Fact Book on Bee Pollen and Your Health*. Keats Publishing, 1994.

PERIODICALS

Adderly, Brenda. "The Latest Buzz on Products of the Hive." *Better Nutrition* (August 1999): 42.

Hovey, Sue. "One Pill Makes You Larger." *Women's Sports and Fitness* (April 1997): 79-80.

Satel, Sally and James Taranto. "Bogus Bee Pollen." *The New Republic* (January 8, 1996): 24-26.

Scheer, James. "Products of the Hive: Sticky, Sweet and Healthful." *Better Nutrition* (February 1998): 60-63.

Somer, Elizabeth. "Tasty Relief: The Benefits of Using Food as Nutrition." *Men's Fitness* (July 1998): 44-46.

ORGANIZATIONS

American Apitherapy Society. 5390 Grande Road, Hillsboro, OH 45133. (937) 364-1108. aasoffice@in-touch.net. http://www.apitherapy.org.

Ken R. Wells

Bee sting therapy *see* **Apitherapy**

Bee stings *see* **Bites and stings**

Behavioral medicine *see* **Mind/Body medicine**

Behavioral optometry

Definition

Behavioral optometry is a system of eye care that emphasizes visual training as a way to improve the way a patient uses his or her eyes. Rather than simply prescribe lenses to compensate for eyesight weaknesses, behavioral optometrists attempt to train the patient to see better across a range of different circumstances.

Origins

Behavioral optometry traces its roots to the writings of Dr. William H. Bates, a New York City ophthalmologist. Bates began writing in the 1920s about alternatives to the use of corrective lenses. He believed that many physical and emotional stresses caused vision problems, and that alleviating these stresses could improve vision. He noted that modern humans spend an inordinate amount of time doing close work such as reading, while the human eye may have been originally adapted for distance vision. Bates devised a program of eye training that allowed patients to gradually improve their vision without glasses. The English novelist Aldous Huxley recovered from near-blindness using Bates's system, and wrote a book about his experience. Other optometrists built on Bates's insights, supplementing his research and ideas. Some researchers focused on the fact that the need for corrective lenses rises in proportion to a person's level of education. They concluded that the **stress** of reading was probably responsible for poor eyesight. Others noted that vision problems increase as cultures become increasingly industrialized and developed. Practitioners of behavioral optometry who built on and extended Bates's ideas include Dr. Raymond L. Gottlieb and Dr. Jacob Liberman, both influential authors and teachers. Behavioral optometrists are distinctly a minority in the field of optometry, but they can be found across the United States and worldwide.

Benefits

Behavioral optometrists promise many benefits from this way of treating vision problems. Perhaps the foremost is that people can learn to live without the discomfort and bother of wearing eyeglasses or contact lenses. Behavioral optometry also focuses on children, particularly those with learning difficulties. These children can benefit from learning to train their eyes and so overcome reading problems due to inability to concentrate or inability to keep the eyes in place on the page. Behavioral optometry also tries to help patients deal with stress, so that vision training can lead to a more relaxed and healthy lifestyle. In addition, behavioral optometry has been used to develop the special visual acuity that is needed for sports; and some practitioners are trained to treat patients who have suffered vision trauma such as **stroke**, or to work with autistic or disabled children.

Description

Behavioral optometry aims to treat the whole patient, not just correct his or her vision. The first step in an examination may be a wide-ranging series of tests and questions, geared to determine the patient's overall visual abilities. This term means not just how well the eyes read letters on a chart, but such broader areas of visual perception as hand-eye coordination and color perception. Behavioral optometrists will prescribe corrective lenses, but these are usually somewhat different from traditional glasses. The lenses are designed to relieve the stress caused by such close-focus work as reading or working at a

KEY TERMS

Ophthalmologist—A physician who specializes in treating diseases and disorders of the eye.

Optometrist—A professional who examines the eyes for vision defects in order to fit the patient with corrective lenses or prescribe other appropriate treatment.

computer. But for distance seeing, the lenses may not be as accurate as traditional lenses, since the behavioral optometrist seeks to teach the eyes to relearn distance vision skills that have atrophied. Many behavioral optometrists prescribe lenses that include a series of small prisms, which are supposed to help the eyes develop better vision patterns. Behavioral optometrists also practice vision therapy, in which the optometrist works closely with the patient in step-by-step exercises to help the eyes relax and relearn lost skills. These are not merely eye exercises, because exercising the muscles around the eye can **fatigue** them instead of strengthen them. The therapy might involve learning new skills such as juggling, drawing, dancing, or ball games, as well as **relaxation** techniques. The optometrist may also work with the patient to alter diet, sleep patterns, and lifestyle stress.

Research and general acceptance

Though behavioral optometrists are definitely a minority within the field of optometry, a body of research supports their methods. This can be found in professional journals such as *Journal of Behavioral Optometry* and *Journal of Optometric Vision Development*. Bates's method has been in use since the 1920s, and much anecdotal evidence attests to its efficacy, including the dramatic case of writer Aldous Huxley. Other patients and practitioners have written of their ability to function without glasses and overcome learning disabilities through behavioral optometry. And one of the major contentions of behavioral optometry is that conventional optometry does not cure the eye conditions it treats. Myopic patients are given glasses, and then a stronger pair of glasses, and then a stronger, as vision gradually worsens. Behavioral optometrists use this development as evidence that conventional optometry fails its patients.

Training and certification

In the United States, there are three major training institutions for behavioral optometry. The College of Optometrists and Vision Development offers courses and examinations leading to an international certificate in behavioral optometry. Clinical education workshops are offered by the Optometric Extension Program Foundation in Santa Ana, California. The Baltimore Academy of Behavioral Optometry offers in-depth coursework in behavioral optometry to qualified optometrists. Only people who already have a degree in optometry can take these courses. Technicians also work with behavioral optometrists. These technicians need have no specific educational background, but to become certified, they must work for 2,000 hours under a certified behavioral optometrist and pass a written and oral examination.

Resources

BOOKS

Bates, William. *The Bates Method for Better Eyesight Without Glasses*. New York: Henry Holt & Co., 1981.

Liberman, Jacob. *Take Off Your Glasses and See*. New York: Crown Publishers, 1995.

ORGANIZATIONS

Baltimore Academy of Behavioral Optometry. 16 Greenmeadow Drive, Suite 103. Timonium, MD 21093. (800) 447-0370.

College of Optometrists in Vision Development. 353 H. Street, Suite C. Chula Vista, CA 91910. (888) 268-3770.

Optometric Extension Program Foundation. 2912 South Daimler Street, Suite 100. Santa Ana, CA 92705. (949) 250-8070.

Angela Woodward

Behavioral therapy

Definition

Behavioral therapy, or behavioral modification, is a psychological technique based on the premise that specific, observable, maladaptive, badly adjusted, or self-destructing behaviors can be modified by learning new, more appropriate behaviors to replace them.

Origins

Reward and punishment systems have been used historically in an attempt to influence behavior, from child rearing to the criminal justice system. Modern behavioral therapy began in the 1950s with the work of B. F. Skinner (1904–1990) and Joseph Wolpe (1915–1997). Wolpe treated his patients who suffered from **phobias** with a technique he developed called systematic desensitization. Systematic desensitization involved gradually exposing a patient to an anxiety-provoking stimuli until the **anxiety** response was extinguished, or eliminated.

Skinner introduced a behavioral technique he called operant conditioning. Operant conditioning is based on the idea that individuals will choose their behavior based on past experiences of consequences of that behavior. If a behavior was associated with positive reinforcements or rewards in the past, individuals will choose it over behavior associated with punishments.

By the 1970s, behavior therapy enjoyed widespread popularity as a treatment approach. After that, the attention of behavioral therapists focused increasingly on their clients' cognitive processes, and many therapists began to use cognitive behavior therapy to change clients' unhealthy behavior by replacing negative or self-defeating thought patterns with more positive ones.

Benefits

Behavioral therapy can be a useful treatment tool in an array of mental illnesses and symptoms of mental illness that involve maladaptive behavior, such as **substance abuse**, aggressive behavior, anger management, eating disorders, phobias, and anxiety disorders. It is also sometimes used to treat organic disorders such as incontinence and **insomnia** by changing the behaviors that might be contributing to these disorders.

Cognitive-behavioral therapy is an offshoot of behavioral therapy that focuses on changing maladaptive behaviors by changing the faulty thinking patterns behind them. It is a recommended treatment option for a number of mental disorders, including affective (mood) disorders, personality disorders, social phobia, **schizophrenia**, obsessive compulsive disorder (OCD), agoraphobia, **post-traumatic stress disorder** (PTSD), and **attention-deficit hyperactivity disorder** (ADHD). It is also frequently used as a tool to deal with chronic **pain** for patients with illnesses such as **rheumatoid arthritis**, back problems, and **cancer**.

Behavioral therapy techniques are sometimes combined with other interventions such as medication. Treatment depends on the individual patient and the severity of symptoms surrounding the behavioral problem.

Description

Behavioral therapy, or behavior modification, is based on the assumption that emotional problems, like any behavior, are learned responses to the environment and can be unlearned. Unlike psychodynamic therapies, it does not focus on uncovering or understanding the unconscious motivations that may be behind the maladaptive behavior. In other words, behavioral therapists do not try to find out why their patients behave the way they do; they just help them learn to change the behavior.

Initial treatment sessions are typically spent explaining the basic tenets of behavioral therapy to the patient and establishing a positive working relationship between therapist and patient. Behavioral therapy is a collaborative, action-oriented therapy, and as such, it empowers patients by giving them an active role in the treatment process. It also discourages overdependence on the therapist, a situation that may occur in other therapeutic relationships. Treatment is typically administered in an outpatient setting in either group or individual sessions. Treatment is relatively short compared to other forms of **psychotherapy**, usually lasting no longer than 16 weeks or sessions.

There are a number of different techniques used in behavioral therapy to help patients change their behaviors. These include:

- Behavioral homework assignments. The therapist often requests that the patient complete homework assignments between therapy sessions. These may consist of real-life behavioral experiments in which patients are encouraged to try new responses to situations discussed in therapy sessions.
- Contingency contracting. In conjunction with the patient, the therapist outlines a written or verbal contract of desired behaviors for the patient. The contract may have certain positive reinforcements (rewards) associated with appropriate behaviors and negative reinforcements (punishments) associated with maladaptive behavior.
- Modeling. The patient learns a new behavior through observation.
- Rehearsed behavior. The therapist and patient engage in role-playing exercises in which the therapist acts out appropriate behaviors or responses to situations.
- Skills training techniques. The patient undergoes an education program to learn social, parenting, or other relevant life skills.
- Conditioning. The therapist uses reinforcement to encourage a particular behavior. For example, a child with ADHD may get a gold star every time he stays focused on tasks and accomplishes certain daily chores. The gold star reinforces and increases the desired behavior by identifying it with something

positive. Reinforcement can also be used to extinguish unwanted behaviors by imposing negative consequences (also called punishment and response).

- Systematic desensitization. Patients are gradually exposed to a situation they fear, either in a role-playing situation or in reality. The therapist employs relaxation techniques to help them cope with their fear reaction and eventually eliminate the anxiety altogether. For example, patients in treatment for agoraphobia, a fear of open or public places, relax and then picture themselves on the sidewalk outside of their house. In the next session, patients may relax themselves and then imagine a visit to a crowded shopping mall. The imagery gets progressively more intense until eventually, therapist and patient approach the anxiety-producing situation in real life by visiting a mall. By repeatedly pairing a desired response (relaxation) with a fear-producing situation (open, public spaces), the patient gradually becomes desensitized to the old response of fear and learns to react with feelings of relaxation.

- Flooding. Flooding is an accelerated version of systematic desensitization, in which patients are exposed directly to the anxiety-provoking situation that they fear most (either through mental visualization or real life contact) in an effort to extinguish the fear response.

- Progressive relaxation. As the name implies, progressive relaxation involves complete relaxation of the muscle groups of the body and smooth, even breathing until the body is completely tension free. It is used by behavioral therapists both as a relaxation exercise to relieve anxiety and stress and as a method of preparing the patient for systematic desensitization. Progressive relaxation is performed by first tensing and then relaxing the muscles of the body, one group at a time. The therapist may suggest that the patient use one of many available instructional relaxation recordings for practicing this technique at home.

Cognitive-behavioral therapy (CBT) integrates features of behavioral modification into the traditional cognitive restructuring approach. In this approach, the therapist works with the patient to identify the thoughts that are causing distress and employs behavioral therapy techniques to alter the resulting behavior. Patients may have certain fundamental core beliefs, known as schemas, which are flawed and are having a negative impact on the patients' behavior and functioning. For example, patients suffering from **depression** may develop a social phobia because they are convinced they are uninteresting and unlikable. A cognitive-behavioral therapist would test this assumption, or schema, by asking patients to name family and

friends that care for them and enjoy their company. By showing patients that others value them, the therapist exposes the irrationality of the assumption. The therapist thus provides a new model of thought for patients to use in changing their previous behavior pattern (i.e., an affirmation, such as "I am an interesting and likeable person; therefore, I make new social acquaintances with ease"). Additional behavioral techniques such as conditioning and systematic desensitization may then be used to gradually reintroduce patients to social situations.

Additional treatment techniques that may be employed with cognitive-behavioral therapy include:

- Cognitive rehearsal. Patients imagine a difficult situation, and the therapist guides them through the step-by-step process of facing and successfully dealing with it. Patients then work on practicing, or rehearsing, these steps mentally. Ideally, when the actual situation arises in real life, patients draw on the rehearsed behavior to address it.

- Journal therapy. Patients keep a detailed diary recounting their thoughts, feelings, and actions when specific situations arise. The journal helps to make patients aware of their maladaptive thoughts and their consequences on behavior. In later stages of therapy, the journal may serve to demonstrate and reinforce positive behavior.

- Validity testing. Patients are asked to test the validity of the automatic thoughts and schemas they encounter. The therapist may ask patients to defend or produce evidence that a schema is true. If patients are unable to meet the challenge, the faulty nature of that schema is exposed.

Biofeedback, a patient-guided treatment also associated with behavioral therapy, teaches individuals to control muscle tension, pain, body temperature, brain waves, and other bodily functions and processes through **relaxation**, visualization, and other techniques. In some cases, positive reinforcements are used to reward patients who generate the correct biofeedback response during treatment. The term biofeedback refers to the biological signals that are fed back to the patient in order for the patient to develop techniques of controlling them.

Preparations

Patients may seek therapy independently or be referred for treatment by a primary physician, psychologist, psychiatrist, or other healthcare professional. Because patients and therapists work closely together to achieve specific therapeutic objectives, it is important that their working relationship be comfortable and that their treatment goals are compatible. Prior to beginning treatment, the patient and therapist have a consultation session, or mutual interview. The consultation gives the therapist the opportunity to make an initial assessment (a detailed behavioral analysis of the particular incidents which lead up to and ensue after a specific unwanted behavior) of the patient and recommend a course of treatment and goals for therapy. It also gives the patient an opportunity to find out important details about the therapist's approach to treatment, professional credentials, and any other relevant, important issues.

In some managed-care clinical settings, an intake interview or evaluation is required before a patient begins therapy. The intake interview is used to evaluate the patient and assign the person to a therapist. It may be conducted by a psychiatric nurse, counselor, or social worker.

Precautions

Behavioral therapy may not be suitable for some patients. Those who do not have a specific behavioral issue they wish to address and whose goals for therapy are to gain insight into the past may be better served by psychodynamic therapy. Patients must also be willing to take a very active role in the treatment process.

Behavioral therapy may also be inappropriate for cognitively impaired individuals (e.g., patients with organic brain disease or a traumatic brain injury) depending on their level of functioning.

Because of the brief nature of behavioral therapy, relapse is reported in some patient populations. However, follow-up sessions can frequently put patients back on track to recovery.

Research and general acceptance

The use of behavioral modification techniques to treat an array of mental health problems has been extensively described and studied in medical literature. Much research by the medical community on behavioral therapy focuses on exploring its effectiveness as a treatment for various types of problems. Behavioral therapy is a well accepted form of treatment for some problems, such as phobias. As of 2008, using behavioral therapy to treat other problems, such as chronic pain, is newer and less widely accepted application.

Types of problems that have been documented as successfully treated by behavioral therapy or a combination of behavioral therapy and other interventions include binge-eating, management of chronic lower

---

KEY TERMS

Cognitive-behavioral therapy—An offshoot of behavioral therapy that focuses on changing maladaptive behaviors by changing the faulty thinking patterns behind them.

Cognitive restructuring—A technique used in cognitive-behavioral therapy. The process of replacing maladaptive thought patterns with constructive thoughts and beliefs.

Maladaptive—Unsuitable; maladaptive behavior is behavior that is inappropriate to a given situation.

Psychodynamic therapy—A therapeutic approach that assumes improper or unwanted behavior is caused by unconscious, internal conflicts and focuses on gaining insight into these motivations.

Relapse—A return of behaviors or symptoms after initial treatment.

Schemas—Fundamental core beliefs or assumptions that are part of the perceptual filter through which people view the world. Cognitive-behavioral therapy seeks to change maladaptive schemas.

---

back pain, depression, and **obsessive-compulsive disorder**.

Training and certification

Behavioral therapists are typically psychologists (PhD, PsyD, EdD, or MA), clinical social workers (MSW, DSW, or LSW), counselors (MA or MS), or psychiatrists (MD with specialization in psychiatry). Other healthcare providers may suggest brief behavioral interventions, but more extensive treatment should be done by individuals who are specifically trained in behavioral therapy techniques.

Resources

BOOKS

Edelman, Sarah. *Change Your Thinking: Overcome Stress, Combat Anxiety and Depression, and Improve Your Life with CBT.* New York: Marlowe, 2007.

Keegan, Mary Eamon. *Empowering Vulnerable Populations: Cognitive-Behavioral Interventions.* Chicago: Lyceum Books, 2008.

Lam, Danny C. K. *Cognitive Behavioral Therapy: A Practical Guide to Helping People Take Control.* New York: Routledge, 2008.

Ramsay, J. Russell, and Anthony L. Rostain. *Cognitive Behavioral Therapy for Adult ADHD: An Integrative Psychosocial and Medical Approach.* New York: Routledge, 2007.

PERIODICALS

Bland, Phillip. "Internet-Based CBT Not Effective as Intervention for Depression." *The Practitioner* (September 25, 2007): 20.

Diefenbach, Gretchen J., et al. "Changes in Quality of Life Following Cognitive-Behavioral Therapy for Obsessive-Compulsive Disorder." *Behavior Research and Therapy* 45, no. 12 (December 2007): 3060–3069.

Jancin, Bruce. "CBT Eases Psychiatric Aspects of Irritable Bowel Syndrome." *Family Practice News* 38, no. 1 (January 1, 2008): 32.

ORGANIZATIONS

National Association of Cognitive-Behavioral Therapists, PO Box 2195, Weirton, WV, 26062, (800) 853-1135, http://www.nacbt.org/.

Paula Ford-Martin
Helen Davidson

Belladonna

Description

Belladonna (*Atropa belladonna*), also known as as deadly nightshade, devil's cherries, devil's herb, divale, dwale, dwayberry, great morel, naughty man's cherries, and poison black cherry, is a perennial herb that has been valued for its medicinal properties for over five centuries. Belladonna is a member of the Solanaceae (nightshade) family and can be identified by its bell-shaped, purple flowers and cherry-sized green berries that mature to a dark purple or black color. The tall, branching plant can grow to a height of at least 5 ft (1.5 m) and is native to Europe, North Africa, and Asia and is cultivated in North America and the United Kingdom. Introduced to a number of places, including the United States and Ireland, belladonna grows wild there.

Belladonna leaves are large (up to 10 in [25 cm] in length) and grow in pairs on either side of the plant stem. Near the flowers or blossoms, one of each leaf pair is noticeably smaller in size. Both the leaves and root have a sharp, unpleasant odor and bitter taste. As the name deadly nightshade suggests, the herb is highly toxic even when taken in extremely low concentrations.

One of the first widespread uses of the herb was purely for cosmetic purposes. Sixteenth-century Italian women reportedly applied belladonna solutions to their eyes to dilate the pupils and achieve a dreamy and supposedly more desirable appearance (hence the name belladonna, which is Italian for beautiful lady).

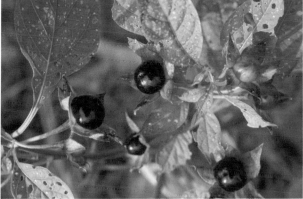

Deadly nightshade Atropa belladonna fruits. *(© blickwinkel / Alamy)*

Atropine, an alkaloid of belladonna that blocks certain nerve impulses, is still used in modern times by some ophthalmologists to dilate the pupils for eye examinations.

General use

Belladonna has a long history of medicinal applications in healthcare. Belladonna alkaloids are anticholinergic, which means that they block certain nerve impulses involved in the parasympathetic nervous system that regulates certain involuntary bodily functions or reflexes, including pupil dilation, heart rate, secretion of glands and organs, and the constriction of the bronchioles in the lungs and the alimentary canal (digestive tract). Belladonna relaxes the smooth muscles of the internal organs and inhibits or dries up secretions (e.g., perspiration, mucous, breast milk, and saliva).

Belladonna alkaloids, the active ingredients of the plant, include atropine and scopolamine. These alkaloids are extracted from the leaves and root of the plant and administered either alone or in combination with other herbal remedies or prescription medications. However, even tiny doses are toxic and should be taken only by prescription.

Belladonna alkaloids are used to treat a variety of symptoms and conditions, including the following:

- Gastrointestinal disorders. Because the alkaloids relax the smooth muscles of the gastrointestinal tract and reduce stomach acid secretions, they are useful in treating colitis, diverticulitis, irritable bowel syndrome, colic, diarrhea, and peptic ulcer.
- Asthma. By relaxing the bronchioles, belladonna alleviates the wheezing symptoms of an asthma attack.

- Excessive sweating. Belladonna slows gland and organ secretion, which makes it useful in controlling conditions that cause excessive sweating.
- Nighttime incontinence. Belladonna acts as a diuretic and can be helpful in treating excessive nighttime urination and incontinence.
- Headaches and migraines. The pain-relieving properties of atropine, a belladonna alkaloid, are useful in treating headaches.
- Muscle pains and spasms. Belladonna is frequently prescribed to ease severe menstrual cramps.
- Motion sickness. Scopolamine, an alkaloid of belladonna, is helpful in treating motion sickness and vertigo.
- Parkinson's disease. Belladonna can alleviate the excessive sweating and salivation associated with the disease, as well as controlling tremors and muscle rigidity.
- Biliary colic. Muscle spasm, or colic, of the gallbladder and liver can be relieved through the muscle relaxing properties of belladonna.

Homeopathic use

Belladonna is a frequently prescribed homeopathic remedy used to treat illnesses that manifest symptoms similar to those that belladonna poisoning triggers (i.e., high **fever**, **nausea**, delirium, **muscle spasms**, flushed skin, dilated pupils). These include the **common cold**, otitis media (**earache**), fever, arthritis, menstrual cramps, **diverticulitis**, muscle **pain**, sunstroke, **toothache** and teething discomfort, **conjunctivitis**, headaches, **sore throat**, and **boils** and abscesses. As with all homeopathic remedies, the prescription of belladonna depends on the individual's overall symptom picture, mood, and temperament. When used as a homeopathic remedy, belladonna is administered in a highly diluted form to trigger the body's natural healing response without risk of belladonna poisoning or death.

Results of a clinical trial performed at the National **Cancer** Institute of Milan, Italy, indicated that homeopathic remedies of belladonna can be useful in relieving the discomfort, warmth, and swelling of the skin associated with radiotherapy for **breast cancer** (i.e., radiodermatitis).

Preparations

Belladonna leaf is harvested between May and July and dried at temperatures no greater than 140°F (60° C). The roots of *Atropa belladonna* plants that are two to four years old are also harvested for herbal preparations in early fall between mid-October and mid-

November. The roots are then cleaned and dried at temperatures no greater than 122°F (50°C). After drying, the leaves and roots are crushed for use in a number of forms, including decoctions, tinctures, infusions, plasters, pills, suppositories, liquid solutions or suspensions, and powders. They can be used both alone and in combination with other herbs and medications.

It is extremely dangerous to self-prescribe belladonna, and it should always be taken under the direction of a doctor or other qualified healthcare professional. The frequency and quantity of dosage will depend on both the patient and the illness for which the herb is prescribed, but the doses are always extremely small. For example the *Physicians Desk Reference (PDR) for Herbal Medicines* recommends an average single dose of 0.05–0.10 g. Each patient's illness is different and some patients experience toxicity at unusually low doses.

For homeopathic remedies, the plant is broken apart and juice is extracted through a pressing process. The extract is then mixed with a water/alcohol solution by a ratio of either 1:10 or 1:100, and this process is repeated up to 30 times to form an extremely diluted dose of the extract. Homeopathic belladonna remedy is generally added to pellets of sugar for easier administration. The dilution and dosage frequency depend on the symptoms being treated, but homeopathic remedies are typically administered only until the patient starts to show signs of improvement so that the body's natural healing response can take over.

Belladonna is available by prescription both alone (in high concentration strength) and in combination with other drugs. As of 2008 available prescription combinations included belladonna with opium (for uterine pain), kaolin and pectin (for **diarrhea**), phenobarbital (for menopausal symptoms and migraine prophylactic), other barbiturates (for **insomnia** and for cramping and muscle spasms in the digestive tract), or belladonna and opium suppositories (for severe intestinal cramping).

Belladonna preparations should be stored in airtight containers away from direct light. Under these conditions, most preparations will remain potent for up to three years.

Precautions

Ingestion of high concentrations of atropine, a potent alkaloid found in belladonna, can cause severe illness and death. Atropine is fatal in doses as small as 100 mg, which is equivalent to 5–50 g of belladonna herb, depending on the potency of the particular plant. For children, a fatal dose is significantly less. For this reason, belladonna should never be used unless prescribed by a trained practitioner.

Individuals suffering from kidney disease, intestinal blockage, **glaucoma**, enlarged prostate, urinary blockage, severe ulcerative **colitis**, or myasthenia gravis are advised not to take belladonna, as are those patients with a known allergy to belladonna. Patients with chronic health conditions should never take belladonna without a doctor's prescription.

Pregnant or breastfeeding women should avoid all but homeopathic belladonna, unless prescribed by a doctor.

Because of the sedative qualities of belladonna, individuals taking the herb should use caution when driving or operating machinery. Alcohol and other central nervous system (CNS) depressants should also be avoided, as they may increase drowsiness and **dizziness** in the patient taking belladonna.

If individuals taking homeopathic dilutions of belladonna experience worsening of their symptoms (known as a homeopathic aggravation), they should contact their healthcare professional. A homeopathic aggravation can be an early indication that a remedy is working properly, but it can also be a sign that a different remedy is called for.

Side effects

Toxic signs of belladonna include **dry mouth**, drowsiness, dizziness, **constipation**, and nausea. Some side effects, including pupil dilation, blurred vision, fever (due to the inability to perspire), inability to urinate, arrhythmia, and excessive dry mouth and eyes, can also be early indications of belladonna overdose. Individuals experiencing these side effects should inform their healthcare practitioner immediately.

Belladonna overdose is also indicated by a burning throat, delirium, restlessness and mania, hallucinations, difficulty breathing, and flushed skin that is hot and dry. Without proper treatment, constriction of the airway can cause suffocation. If any of these symptoms occur, individuals should seek emergency medical attention immediately. Treatment of belladonna overdose is typically gastric lavage, which involves the insertion of a tube down the patient's throat and washing out the stomach with a solution of **activated charcoal** or tannic acid to neutralize the atropine. Oxygen may also be required until breathing is stabilized, and barbiturates may be administered to counteract mania and/or excitation.

KEY TERMS

Alkaloids—A family of chemical compounds whose members contain nitrogen.

Allopathic—Healthcare practice that uses remedies and treatments that cause different effects than the symptoms they are intended to treat; conventional medicine is usually considered allopathic in nature.

Anticholinergic—A medication or other substance that blocks certain parasympathetic nerve impulses.

Decoction—An herbal extract produced by mixing an herb in cold water, bringing the mixture to a boil, and letting it simmer to extract water. The decoction is then strained and drunk hot or cold. Decoctions are usually chosen over infusion when the botanical in question is a root or bark.

Homeopathic—Remedies and treatments that cause similar effects to the symptoms they are intended to treat in an effort to stimulate the body's natural immune response system.

Infusion—An herbal preparation made by pouring boiling water over an herb and letting the brew steep for 20 minutes, then straining. Tea is made by infusion.

Mania—Hyperelevated, or excessively excited mood.

Naturalized—Plants that are introduced in the wild.

Prophylactic—A preventative treatment.

Radiodermatitis—Red, irritated, and inflamed skin caused by x rays, radiation treatment, or other radiation exposure.

Tinctures—An alcohol liquid extract of an herb.

USP—The *U.S. Pharmacopoeia* contains nationally and internationally recognized drug standards published by the United States Pharmacopeia Convention and used as a standard by FDA and other federal regulatory agencies.

Interactions

Certain medications may increase the effects of belladonna. These medications include central nervous system (CNS) depressants, monoamine oxidase (MAO) inhibitors, tricyclic antidepressants, quinidine, amantadine, antihistamines, and other anticholinergics. Other medications, including anticoagulants (blood thinners) and corticotropin (ACTH), become less effective when used with belladonna, while some drugs, such as diarrhea medicines containing kaolin and attapulgite, may decrease the therapeutic response to belladonna when they are taken with the herb. Patients taking these or any other medications or herbal remedies should inform their healthcare professional.

Alcohol, a CNS depressant, can also enhance the sedative effect of belladonna and should be avoided during belladonna treatment.

Individuals considering treatment with homeopathic dilutions of belladonna should consult their healthcare professional about possible interactions with certain foods, beverages, prescription medications, aromatic compounds, and other environmental elements that could counteract the efficacy of belladonna treatment.

Resources

BOOKS

Gruenwald, Joerg, Thomas Brendler, and Christof Jaenicke, eds. *PDR for Herbal Medicines.*, 4th ed. London: Thomson Healthcare, 2007.

Ratsch, Christian. *The Encyclopedia of Psychoactive Plants: Ethnopharmacology and Its Applications.* South Paris, ME: Park Street Press, 2005.

PERIODICALS

Piccillo, G., et al. "Anticholinergic Syndrome Due to 'Devil's Herb': When Risks Come from the Ancient Time." *International Journal of Clinical Practice* (April 2006): 492–494.

Ulbricht, Catherine, et al. "An Evidence-Based Systematic Review of Belladonna by the Natural Standard Research Collaboration." *Journal of Herbal Pharmacotherapy* (May 2005): 61–90.

ORGANIZATIONS

American Botanical Council, PO Box 144345, Austin, TX, 78714-4345, (512) 926-4900, http://www.herbalgram.org.

Office of Dietary Supplements. National Institutes of Health, Building 31, Room 1B25, 31 Center Dr., MSC 2086, Bethesda, MD, 20892-2086, (301) 435-2920, http://odp.od.nih.gov/ods/.

Paula Ford-Martin
David Edward Newton, Ed.D.

Benign prostatic hypertrophy *see* **Prostate enlargement**

Bernard training *see* **Auditory integration training**

Beta-methylbutyric acid

Description

Beta-methylbutyric acid, technically known as "beta-hydroxy beta-methylbutyric acid," or more commonly known as "HMB," is a metabolite of the amino acid leucine. The dietary supplement HMB is used by athletes to build muscles. It has also been used to treat the muscle deterioration in cases of **AIDS** (acquired immunodeficiency syndrome), and by people seeking to lose weight or manage their **cholesterol**.

General use

Human muscles have a particularly high concentration of leucine, so this amino acid is often broken down and utilized during strenuous **exercise**. HMB is found in citrus fruit, catfish, and **alfalfa**. It was first found to be of use in agriculture as an additive to help pigs, chickens, and other farm animals gain muscle and lose fat. After a research trial conducted by the University of Iowa at Iowa City showed positive results, HMB caught attention as promising for human use.

A four-week double-blind study in 1995 involved 17 exercise-trained and 23 untrained males, divided into two groups. One group took daily capsules containing 3 g of HMB, and the other took placebos. Everyone observed an identical weight-training regimen three times a week. Upon the trial's completion, the group that took the HMB demonstrated an average 3.1% increase in lean muscle mass, as compared with 1.9% for those who took the placebos. Also, the HMB group lost an average of 7.3% initial body fat, against 2.2% for the placebo group. The men who took HMB were able to average 22 pounds more with the bench press than they did at the beginning of the study. The men who did not, averaged a 14-pound increase. The results indicated that when taken as a supplement of up to 3 g a day, HMB could increase lean muscle mass and strength in athletes who use it during weight training. Theories suggested that HMB possibly suppresses protein breakdown that follows exercise that is rigorous and of long-term duration.

By the Summer Olympics in Atlanta in 1996, the publicity of the possible benefits of HMB had spread among athletes. Because it was not a banned substance, demand was heavy, and it continued to remain popular among athletes as a nutritional supplement. Its popularity was particularly evident among weight trainers, but it was also reported as useful for any athlete undergoing resistance training.

In the years that followed, HMB research focused on use of the supplement by athletes, AIDS patients, and people seeking to manage their cholesterol. A study described in the May/June 2000 issue of *Journal of Parenteral and Enteral Nutrition* described research into the effect of HMB on the lean tissue loss in people living with AIDS. In the double-blind study, 68 people received a placebo or a combination of three nutrients. The combination mixture consisted of 3 g HMB, 14 g L-glutamine (Gln), and 14 g L-arginine (Arg). Participants took this dosage daily for eight weeks. The study ended with 43 participants, and the conclusion that the combination "can markedly alter" lean tissue loss.

Sports Nutrition Review Journal, 2004 evaluated HMB and concluded that there was "fairly good evidence" that the supplement enhanced training adaptations for people who initiated training. The journal maintained more research was needed to determine if it would enhance "training adaptations in athletes."

Studies of HMB and exercise during the 1990s and 2000s involved small numbers of participants and produced varied results. In some cases, improvement was reported; in others, the outcome indicated little or no benefit. In addition, cholesterol was studied in research into the effect of HMB in activities such as weight training. As of February 2008, some in the medical community maintained that larger clinical studies were needed to determine the effectiveness of HMB. In addition, research into the longtime use of HMB was needed.

Preparations

HMB is available in powder, capsule, and tablet form. In addition, combination products containing HMB include capsules, fruit-flavored mixes, protein bars, and meal-replacement shakes. HMB is frequently combined with **creatine** monohydrate, an amino acid found in muscles. That combination is thought by some to increase the effect of each supplement and could be helpful for people who plan to do intense training.

According to some studies, a person taking HMB could see "measurable increases" in strength and lean body mass within several weeks. That information was posted on the Web site of Metabolic Technologies, Inc. (MTI), a research-based company in Iowa that developed HMB.

The usual dosage of HMB is 3 g per day. However, the amount will vary based on the reason the person is taking the supplement. According to MTI, a person may customize the daily dosage by calculating an amount based on the formula of 38 mg multiplied by body weight that is expressed in kilograms.

Another consideration is that product strengths vary, so it is important to follow package directions or consult with a health-care professional. Seeing a physician before taking any dietary supplement is particularly important for adolescents and people with a pre-existing condition such as high blood pressure, heart valve or blood valve diseases, and severe liver and kidney diseases.

Pregnant women and nursing mothers should not take HMB because safety studies have not been performed for those population groups, according to the MTI Web site in February 2008.

Precautions

The U.S. Food and Drug Administration does not regulate dietary supplements such as HMB, so these products do not have to undergo the rigorous testing that is required for the approval of drugs. Thus, supplements have not proven to be safe or effective. Furthermore, ingredients are not standardized to comply with federal regulations.

Side effects

People who take HMB may find they are allergic to it and experience symptoms such as breathing problems, chest **pain**, and skin **hives**, according to *Physicians' Desktop Reference*. Other symptoms include tightness in the chest or throat, a rash, and itchy or swollen skin. People experiencing those symptoms should immediately stop taking the supplement and contact their doctor.

Interactions

As of February 2008, there were no known adverse reactions when HMB was taken with other drugs or food supplements.

Resources

OTHER

"HMB." *Physician's Desktop Reference*. http://www.pdrhealth.com/drugs/altmed/altmed-mono.aspx?contentFileName=amc0435.xml&contentName=HMB&contentId=591 (February 24, 2008).

Iowa State University Extension. "Eat to Compete," January 12, 2006. http://www.extension.iastate.edu/nutrition/sport/supplements.html (February 14, 2008).

Mississippi Baptist Health Systems EBSCO Content. "Hydroxymethyl Butyrate (HMB)." http://www.mbmc.org/healthgate/GetHGContent.aspx?token=9c315661-83b7-472d-a7ab-bc8582171f86&chunkiid=21551 (February 14, 2008).

Sports Nutrition Society. *Sports Nutrition Review Journal,* 2004. http://www.sportsnutritionsociety.org/site/pdf/Kreider-SNRJ-1-1-1-44-2004.pdf (February 14, 2008).

ORGANIZATIONS

Metabolic Technologies, Inc, 2711 S. Loop Dr., Suite 4400, Ames, Iowa, 50010-8656, http://www.hmb.org.

National Center for Complementary and Alternative Medicine, National Institute of Health (NCCAM), 9000 Rockville Pike, Bethesda, MD, 20892, (888) 644-6226, http://nccam.nih.gov.

Jane Spehar
Liz Swain

Beta carotene

Description

Beta carotene is one of the most important naturally occurring **antioxidants**. It is a fat-soluble pigment found in plants (notably carrots and many colorful vegetables and fruits) and in the sea alga *Dunaleilla salina* and *D. bardawil*. Natural beta carotene supplements are derived primarily from *D. salina*. Beta carotene is one of the major dietary **carotenoids** and one of the most biologically active of approximately 800 carotenes and more than 1,000 carotenoids present in food. It is responsible for the orange or yellow colors of many fruits and vegetables. In the human body, beta carotene is found in lipids and in fat tissues. Sometimes beta carotene is called provitamin A because it is more easily converted to **vitamin A** (retinol) in the liver than other carotenoids. Beta carotene is considered to be a conditionally essential

Beta carotene content of some common foods

Vegetable	Serving	International Units (IU)	Daily Allowance (DA)
Carrot	1 whole raw, 7.5 in (19 cm)	20,250	410%
Carrot	Sliced and boiled, 0.5 cup (118 ml)	19,150	380%
Carrot juice	Canned, 0.5 cup (118 ml)	12,915	260%
Spinach	Frozen and boiled, 0.5 cup (118 ml)	7,395	150%
Sweet potatoes	Canned and drained, 0.5 cup (118 ml)	7,015	140%
Mango	Sliced raw, 0.5 cup (118 ml)	6,425	130%
Vegetable soup	Canned, ready to serve, 1 cup (237 ml)	5,880	115%
Cantaloupe	Raw, 1 cup (237 ml)	5,160	100%
Kale	Frozen and boiled, 0.5 cup (118 ml)	4,130	80%
Pumpkin	1 cup cooked, boiled, drained, without salt	2,650	50%
Spinach	Raw, 1 cup (237 ml)	2,015	40%
Apricot nectar	Canned, 0.5 cup (118 ml)	1,650	35%
Oatmeal	1 packet instant plain	1,510	30%
Tomato juice	Canned, 6 oz. (177 ml)	1,010	20%
Apricots	2 halves with skin packed in juice	610	10%
Red pepper	1 raw ring, 3 in (7.8 cm); 0.25 in (0.64 cm) thick	570	10%
Peas	Frozen and boiled, 0.5 cup (118 ml)	535	10%
Peaches	1 medium raw fruit	525	10%
Peaches	Canned halves or slices in water, 1 cup (237 ml)	470	10%
Papaya	Raw cubes, 1 cup (237 ml)	400	8%

(Illustration by Corey Light. Cengage Learning, Gale)

nutrient because it becomes essential when vitamin A intake is low.

Beta carotene consists of a chain of 40 carbon atoms, with conjugated double bonds and a ring structure at each end of the chain. Depending on the positions of the molecular groups attached to the carbon chain, naturally occurring beta carotene may be any of the following:

- All-*trans* beta-carotene
- 9-*cis* beta-carotene
- 13-*cis* beta-carotene, in smaller amounts. Synthetic beta carotene is primarily all-*trans*.

In plants and alga, beta carotene and other carotenoids attract light for photosynthesis and provide protection from toxic forms of oxygen. Beta carotene is a powerful antioxidant because it destroys toxic free radicals, including singlet oxygen —an oxygen atom that is missing an electron and is very damaging to human tissue if not taken up quickly and deactivated.

General use

Vitamin A precursor

Vitamin A is obtained in the diet from animal products or is made in the liver from beta carotene and other carotenoids. Vitamin A is essential for the following:

- vision and eye health
- normal cell division
- growth
- reproduction and fertility
- immune system function
- skin and mucous membrane health

In sub-Saharan Africa about three million children under the age of five suffer from an eye disorder caused by vitamin-A deficiency that can lead to blindness and death. Although red palm oil, a traditional African food, contains high provitamin A, its substitution by imported cooking oils has reduced this dietary source in many homes. Many vegetables and fruits also contain provitamin A but are not always consumed in adequate amounts. Vitamin A deficiency is the leading cause of blindness worldwide.

In the 1920s vitamin-A deficiency was linked to stomach **cancer** and to precancerous conditions in the epithelial (lining) cells of the throat and lungs. In 1977 vitamin A supplementation was shown to inhibit certain cancers and to reduce the growth of certain tumors in at-risk animals.

Dietary beta carotene

Carotenoids, including beta carotene, that are obtained from food may have the following:

- antioxidant activity
- immune-system-enhancing activity
- activity against some cancers and precancerous conditions
- a role in preventing coronary heart disease, including heart attack and stroke

Epidemiological studies that looked at cancer rates and diet found that at least five daily servings of green, orange, red, and yellow vegetables and fruits appeared to significantly reduce the risk of stomach, lung, prostate, breast, head, and neck cancer, and possibly slow the progression of others. In 1971 a large study of humans linked cancer death rates to low levels of beta carotene in the blood. Subsequent studies linked high blood levels of dietary beta carotene to lower cancer risks. However, subsequent evidence linked these results to a combination of antioxidants found in fruits and vegetables, rather then to beta carotene alone. High beta carotene levels in the blood may be associated with a reduced risk of **asthma**.

Supplemental beta carotene

Supplemental beta carotene has been claimed to do the following:

- inhibit precancerous lesions in those at risk of oral cancer
- protect against gastric and esophageal cancers
- reduce the risk of prostate cancer
- lower the overall cancer risk
- protect against sunburn

However, as of 2008 there was very little evidence that supplemental beta carotene is an effective cancer-preventing substance, except perhaps in those with poor **nutrition** or low baseline levels of beta carotene in the blood. Additional studies showed that beta carotene supplements do not reduce the risk of cancer, **heart disease**, or **cataracts**. Two studies of beta carotene and cancer produced mixed results. A Swedish study of 82,000 men and women reported in 2007 that people who had high intakes of beta carotene, alpha carotene, and vitamin A, were 40% to 60% less likely to develop stomach cancer than people with low intakes of the three supplements. However, in smokers, the supplements offered no protection against stomach cancer. A long-term French study of nearly 60,000 women reported in 2006 that those with high intakes of beta carotene who were non-smokers had a significantly decreased risk for developing tobacco-related cancers whereas smokers who had a high intake of beta carotene significantly increased their risk of getting tobacco-related cancers. Lung, head, neck, urinary tract, digestive tract, cervix, thyroid, and ovarian cancers are associated with **smoking**. Previous studies had found no such increases in **lung cancer** in those taking beta carotene. Since there is conflicting research, it is probably best for smokers and people being treated for asbestos exposure to avoid taking beta carotene supplements.

A long-term study of 16,548 men in the United States reported in 2006 that taking a high dose of beta carotene had no effect on the risk of developing **prostate cancer**.

Yet supplemental beta carotene does appear to increase the amounts of some types of immune-system cells. Studies have shown that women with low dietary intake or low blood levels of beta carotene are at increased risk for **cervical dysplasia** (abnormal cell growth) and cervical cancer.

The Age-Related Eye Disease Study found that a combined supplement of beta carotene, **vitamin C**, **vitamin E**, **zinc**, and **copper** reduced the risk of disease progression and vision loss in people with advanced **macular degeneration**. The supplement did not slow disease progression in those with early-stage macular degeneration. However, a controlled study of 22,000 males aged 40–84 years reported in 2007 that long-term beta-carotene supplementation neither decreased nor increased the risk of the eye condition age-related maculopathy, also called macular **retinopathy**, that is, any condition or disease of the macula, the small spot in the retina where vision is keenest.

One study found that supplementation with a mixture of antioxidants—beta carotene, alpha-tocopherol, and plant sterols—lowered **cholesterol** levels in the blood.

Beta carotene at 25,000 international units (IU) daily may be useful for treating **psoriasis**, a skin condition. Beta carotene supplements also are used to treat **acne**. Two 25,000-IU supplements daily, in combination with other supplements, sometimes are used to treat stomach ulcers.

Studies reported in 2006 and 2007 that antioxidants, including beta carotene, did not protect women from developing heart disease; that beta carotene supplementation did not improve cognitive performance in older men who took it for less than 15 years but improved it in men who took it for 15 years or longer, including reducing the risk of developing **dementia**;

and that people who had a diet high in beta carotene slowed age-related loss of lung power by 32%.

Preparations

Measuring beta carotene

As of the late 2000s, a recommended dietary allowance (RDA) for beta carotene had not been established and most foods were not labeled as to vitamin A content. There are two incompatible systems for quantifying beta carotene. IUs are used most often for nutritional labeling:

- 1 IU equals 0.6 µg of all-*trans* beta carotene
- 3.33 IU of all-*trans* beta carotene, 2 µg is equal to 1 µg of all-*trans* retinol (vitamin A)
- 5,000 IU equals 3 mg of beta carotene, the RDA for vitamin A
- 1 IU equals 1.2 µg of other provitamin A carotenoids

The second system uses retinol equivalents (RE):

- 1 RE equals 1 µg of all-*trans* retinol
- 1 RE equals 6 µg of all-*trans* beta carotene
- 1 RE equals 12 µg of other provitamin A carotenoids

Dietary beta carotene

Daily values (DVs) are determined from the RDA. They are based on a 2,000-calorie diet and usually are expressed as a percentage of an RDA. The IUs and DVs for beta carotene, per serving, in common foods are listed in table 1.

Carrots and sweet potatoes that are more orange contain more beta carotene. New carrot cultivars that contain more beta carotene have been developed and high-beta-carotene sweet potatoes have been introduced into sub-Saharan Africa to treat vitamin-A deficiency.

Other foods that contain beta carotene include:

- avocados
- broccoli
- chard
- coffee
- collard greens
- palm oil and other food colorants
- squash
- string beans
- watermelon
- yams

According to the Institute of Medicine, a daily intake of 3–6 mg of beta carotene keeps the blood level within the range associated with a lower risk for chronic diseases. The recommended daily diet of five or more servings of fruits and vegetables provides 3–6 mg of beta carotene (if carrots, sweet potatoes, papaya, apricots, or other very high carotenoid food is used, the RDA can be met in a single serving). In contrast, the average American diet contains 1.3–2.9 mg daily. Vegetarians may have twice as much beta carotene in their blood as compared to non-vegetarians because they generally consume more greens and fruits.

Beta carotene in food is found within an oil or a matrix of sugars and proteins; therefore, the absorption of beta carotene by the body varies greatly. The elderly and those with poor digestion and liver trouble may be at risk for insufficient absorption from an adequate beta carotene diet.

Animal sources of vitamin A are more easily absorbed than plant sources of beta carotene, particularly if the vegetables and fruits are eaten raw or whole. Although beta carotene can be converted to vitamin A in the body, it has its own unique physiological functions. Beta carotene and vitamin A are not totally identical in the health benefits they deliver, so it is good to eat sources of both. While supplementation is helpful to those who have trouble absorbing adequate beta carotene, getting all or some beta carotene through food sources rather than supplements alone is by far the best. This is substantiated by research showing there are many beneficial carotenoids in foods and that they may also work together synergistically to optimize health.

Supplemental beta carotene

Beta carotene supplements are inexpensive and readily available over-the-counter. They are available as pills, powders, and oils, and they vary greatly in potency. Some supplements contain a mixture of carotenoids. There is a major problem with shelf life stability for beta carotene, as it "oxidizes" quickly when in pure form. When buying a supplement of it, shelf life stability or the presence of such stabilizers as vitamin E can guarantee biological activity of the capsule.

Supplemental intake of beta carotene probably should not exceed 3–15 mg per day. Common preparation of supplemental beta carotene include:

- 30- or 60-mg capsules
- 5,000-, 10,000-, or 25,000-IU capsules
- 10,000- or 25,000-IU tablets A typical dosage of beta carotene for treating cancer is 75,000–150,000 IU

daily. Absorption of beta carotene in nutritional supplements can be 70% or more. There is no established maximum daily intake for beta carotene.

Some common beta carotene nutritional supplements are:

- A-Caro-25
- B-Caro-T
- Biotene
- Caroguard
- Caro-Plete
- Dry Beta Carotene
- Lumitene
- Marine Carotene
- Mega Carotene
- Oceanic Beta Carotene
- Superbeta Carotene
- Ultra Beta Carotene

Manufacturers often supplement food with beta carotene. One study showed that bakery products enriched with beta carotene increased beta carotene levels in the blood.

Precautions

Antioxidants such as beta carotene often work together with other antioxidants and an excess or deficiency of one can inhibit the other. The Food and Nutrition Board of the Institute of Medicine does not recommend beta carotene supplementation except in cases of vitamin A deficiency.

Pregnant and nursing mothers should limit their intake of supplemental beta carotene to 6 mg per day or less.

Side effects

Even long-term high-dosage use of supplemental beta carotene appears to be non-toxic. Daily doses of 30 mg or more over a long period may cause carotenosis (carotenodermia), a yellowing of the skin, which is harmless and reversible. In contrast, very high daily doses of vitamin A are dangerous and damage the liver and other organs, as well as provoke **hair loss**).

Interactions

Drugs and other substances that may interfere with beta-carotene absorption include:

- Cholestyramine
- Colestipol

KEY TERMS

Alpha-tocopherol—An antioxidant derivative of vitamin E that stabilizes cell membranes.

Antioxidant—A substance that prevents oxidation, such as cellular damage caused by free radicals.

Carotenoid—A large class of red and yellow pigments found in some plants and in animal fat.

Carotenosis (carotenodermia, carotenemia)—A yellowish pigmentation of the skin caused by high levels of carotene in the blood.

Cholesterol—An important sterol that is deposited on blood vessel walls in arteriolosclerosis.

Daily value (DV)—The percentage of the RDA of a nutrient that is present in a food or supplement.

Epithelium—Layers of cells covering internal and external body surfaces.

Free radical—An atom or compound with an unpaired electron; oxygen free radicals can damage cells and cell constituents.

Immune system—The body system that protects against foreign pathogens and abnormal cells.

International unit (IU)—A widely accepted definition that is used to quantify a given substance.

Macular degeneration—Progressive deterioration of the macula—the light-sensitive cells of the central retina of the eye.

Provitamin A—A carotenoid, such as beta carotene, that can be converted into vitamin A in the liver.

Recommended dietary allowance (RDA)—The average daily dietary intake of a nutrient that is sufficient to meet the nutritional requirements of 97–98% of healthy individuals of a given age and gender.

Retinol equivalent (RE)—1 μg of all-*trans* retinol (vitamin A), 6 μg of all-*trans* beta carotene.

Vitamin A (retinol).—An essential nutrient for vision that is obtained from animal products or made in the liver from carotenoids such as beta carotene.

- mineral oil
- Olestra
- Orlistat
- pectin

The absorption of luteine, another carotenoid antioxidant, may be reduced if taken in conjunction with beta carotene.

Resources

BOOKS

Bruning, Nancy Pauling. *The Real Vitamin and Mineral Book: The Definitive Guide to Designing Your Personal Supplement Program,* 4th ed. New York: Avery, 2007.

Jeep, Robin, et al. *The Super Antioxidant Diet and Nutrition Guide: A Health Plan for the Body, Mind, and Spirit.* Charlottesville, VA: Hampton Roads, 2008.

Milbury, Paul E., and Alice C. Richer. *Understanding the Antioxidant Controversy: Scrutinizing the "Fountain of Youth."* Westport, CT: Praeger, 2007.

Panglossi, Harold V., ed. *Antioxidants: New Research.* Haupauge, NY: Nova Science, 2006.

Presman, Alan H., and Sheila Buff. *The Complete Idiot's Guide to Vitamins and Minerals,* 3rd ed. New York: Alpha (Penguin Group), 2007.

PERIODICALS

Brunk, Doug. "Antioxidants Do Not Protect Women Against Heart Risks." *Family Practice News* (September 15, 2007): 17.

Challem, Jack. "Are Antioxidant Supplements Still Safe? Were Important Details Omitted from a Recent Study on Antioxidants? A Closer Look Reveals the Real Story." *Better Nutrition* (May 2007): 16.

Gaby, Alan R. "Beta-Carotene and Cancer: Good for Non-Smokers, Bad for Smokers?" *Townsend Letter: The Examiner of Alternative Medicine* (August/September 2006): 51(2).

MacDougall, David S. "Benefits of Antioxidants Are Limited: Vitamin E, Vitamin C, or Beta-Carotene Supplements Do Not Cut Population's Risk for Prostate Cancer." *Renal & Urology News* (April 2006): 38.

Medley, Jennifer. "Beta-Carotene: With Most Food-Based Nutrients, We Simply Have to Trust that They Are There, but If You're on the Lookout for Beta-Carotene-Rich Foods, Just Turn to the Rainbow." *Kiwi Magazine* (November/December 2007): 26.

Moon, Mary Ann. "Antioxidant Doesn't Benefit Cognitive Performance Short Term." *Family Practice News* (December 15, 2007): 27.

ORGANIZATIONS

American Dietetic Association, 120 S. Riverside Plaza, Suite 2000, Chicago, IL, 60606, (800) 877-1600, http://www.eatright.org.

American Institute of Homeopathy, 801 N. Fairfax St., Suite 306, Alexandria, VA, 22314, (888) 445-9988, http://www.homeopathyusa.org.

Dieticians of Canada, 480 University Ave., Suite 604, Toronto, ON, M5G 1V2, Canada, (416) 596-0857, http://www.dieticians.ca.

Office of Dietary Supplements, National Institutes of Health, 6100 Executive Blvd., Room 3B01, MSC 7517, Bethesda, MD, 20892, (301) 435-2920, http://www.ods.od.nih.gov.

Margaret Alic
Ken R. Wells

Beta hydroxy

Description

Beta hydroxy acids (BHAs) are a group of acids once used primarily for the treatment of dry skin, **acne**, and **warts**. During the 1990s, beta hydroxy acids "increasingly appeared" in anti-aging cosmetics, according to the U.S. Food and Drug Administration (FDA). The cosmetics were promoted for the supposed ability of the skin-care products to reduce the appearance of fine lines and wrinkles. Manufacturers claimed that products containing BHAs improved skin quality.

Common beta hydroxy acids include salicylic acid, benzoic acid and beta hydroxybutanoic acid. Salicylic acid is the most widely used BHA in skin care products, and it is widely regarded by the public, medical community and skin care product manufacturers as a BHA. However, according to the FDA, salicylic acid is not considered to be a true BHA. Salicylic acid may be listed by that name or as related substances such as salicylate, **sodium** salicylate, and willow extract, according to the FDA.

BHAs are exfoliants, which means that they cause the top layers of the skin to exfoliate or peel. Exfoliation leaves behind fresh skin that is also smoother and softer than before. Beta hydroxys are said to work by speeding up the turnover of skin cells. They dissolve the glue that holds dead skin cells in the top layers, allowing the fresh cells beneath to emerge. Chemical exfoliation with beta hydroxys is said to peel away a variety of such age-related skin problems as wrinkles, acne, age spots, blemishes, and skin unevenness. Used on a regular basis at a low concentration in cleansers or acne treatments, BHAs refresh the skin and clear away the dirt and oils that often cause acne eruptions. In addition to cosmetic applications, these chemicals also are used as treatments for a variety of skin disorders including **psoriasis**, seborrhea, **dandruff**, and warts.

BHAs are found in many skin care products. They are also found naturally in fresh fruit (berries, pineapple, papaya, etc.), milk and yogurt, **wintergreen** leaves, sweet birch, and some other plants.

Structurally, BHAs appear to be very similar to another group of chemicals used in skin care products, the alpha hydroxy acids or AHAs. These two groups of chemicals have similar activities as well; both are skin exfoliants. BHAs, however, are believed to be less irritating to the skin than AHAs. They are also more effective in preventing acne eruptions and smoothing the skin.

General use

Skin cleansing

Many skin cleansers contain BHAs because they help remove excess oil from the face. They can, however, remove oil only on the surface and cannot affect oil production under the skin. To help maintain healthy skin, these cleansers should be used once or twice a week to improve skin tone and texture. BHA-containing preparations should be left on the face for a short time only and rinsed off with generous amounts of water. Because the skin is more sensitive to sunlight after the use of products containing BHAs, users should apply sunscreens and avoid prolonged sun exposure.

Wrinkles and age spots

Wrinkles are signs of the normal **aging** process. Over the years, the skin becomes thinner, drier and less elastic as its collagen and elastin fibers gradually lose their elasticity. To improve the appearance of the skin and to correct minor blemishes and unevenness, some people have chemical peels with hydroxy acids. Chemical peels have become one of the most popular methods for removing wrinkles. This process uses concentrated preparations of BHAs, alpha hydroxy acids, or combinations of both to remove the top layer of skin. The chemical peel allows a newer layer of skin to replace the older layer. Some fine lines and wrinkles may also be removed.

Because of potential scarring and other severe adverse reactions, chemical peels should be performed by a professional, usually a board-certified dermatologist or a licensed estheticist (skin care specialist).

For best results, chemical peels are often used in combination with such other anti-wrinkle treatments as collagen, fat implants or laser surgery. For relatively young people, a chemical peel with BHA often provides satisfactory results. Those above the age of 40 sometimes choose to have collagen or fat implants together with the peel. Some older patients may have both a chemical peel and a special kind of laser surgery called laser resurfacing. While chemical peels can remove some fine wrinkle lines, laser resurfacing is a more powerful tool. It can remove deeper wrinkles and skin imperfections.

Acne therapy

Acne is a skin disorder caused by excessive production of oil under the uppermost layers of skin. When the oil cannot pass through the hair follicles, the pores under the skin are plugged up, trapping the oil and dead skin cells underneath the skin. These plugged pores become fertile breeding grounds for a type of bacterium called *Propionibacterium acnes*, sometimes called the acne bacillus, to grow inside the pore, causing irritation, inflammation, and in due time, pimples.

Because it is an effective cleanser, a 1% solution of salicylic acid can enter the pores and help to remove excess oil, dirt, and dead skin cells. It reduces skin breakouts by preventing the buildup of dead skin cells associated with acne formation. Beta hydroxy acids, including salicylic acid, are good treatments for acne because they are relatively mild. Because they are applied topically, they do not cause systemic side effects as oral antibiotics sometimes do. In addition, they are especially appropriate for the treatment of acne because they have anti-inflammatory properties. BHAs, however, do not have the antimicrobial properties of such topical medications as benzoyl peroxide.

Psoriasis

Psoriasis is a chronic skin condition requiring lifelong treatment with topical lotions and creams, phototherapy (using radiation or ultraviolet light), or medications taken by mouth. Salicylic acid can be used to treat psoriasis. Salicylic acid facilitates the removal of scaly skin. In so doing, it helps moisturizers and other topical medications for psoriasis work more effectively.

Warts

Salicylic acid is also an effective and mild treatment for warts and plantar warts. Patients should wash and dry the area around the wart thoroughly before applying the product. Then they should apply a thin film of salicylic acid over each wart and allow it to dry. The product should be applied once or twice a day. Salicylic acid acts slowly and may take as long as 12 weeks before one can see results.

Other uses

The anti-inflammatory properties of BHAs are useful in treating such other skin conditions as dandruff or seborrheic **dermatitis**, a condition characterized by oily skin.

Preparations

Salicylic acid is often found in many over-the-counter skin care products such as soaps, cleansers, acne medications, and anti-wrinkle creams. These products, however, contain only 2% of salicylic acid. This concentration is strong enough for exfoliation but not for chemical peel treatment.

Chemical peel preparations contain very high concentrations (up to 30%) of beta hydroxy acids in combination with alpha hydroxy acids. Because of the potential for scarring and other severe adverse reactions, these prescription-strength products are not sold to the general public. They are available only to licensed dermatologists or estheticians.

Individuals who are prescribed AHA formulations by a healthcare professional should follow their doctor's directions for use of the product.

BHAs can also be found in certain fruits and vegetables. For example, thin layers of papaya can be applied on the face and allowed to remain for a while. Papaya pulp helps soften the skin and decrease its unevenness. It is most beneficial to dry, sun-damaged skin, although it may also cause allergic reactions in some sensitive people. Pineapple is another natural product that contains beta hydroxy acid. Pineapple can be put into a blender or juicer to obtain fresh juice. The juice can be applied to the skin; again, however, it may cause allergic reactions.

Skin test

Before using a new product containing BHA, it is important to test the substance on a small portion of the skin. A small, dime-sized drop of the BHA product should be applied to a small patch of skin inside the elbow or wrist. The skin patch should be monitored for 24 hours for reactions such as irritation or stinging. If the person experiences those reactions, a doctor should be consulted.

Precautions

The FDA regulates skin care products as if they were cosmetics, so products containing BHA don't undergo the rigorous testing for safety and effectiveness that is required for drugs. However, the FDA does become involved when it appears that cosmetics may contain ingredients that are harmful to people.

People who use skin care products containing BHAs should be aware of the following considerations and side effects:

- Increased sensitivity to sunlight. Exfoliated skin is very tender and sensitive to sunlight. Studies have shown that skin treated with these exfoliants has twice the sun damage compared to untreated skin. Therefore, it is important to use suncreen with an SPF (sun protection factor) of at least 15. People should avoid direct exposure to the sun when using products containing BHAs.

KEY TERMS

Cystinuria—Excess cystine, lysine, arginine, and ornithine in urine due to defective transport system of these acids in kidney and intestines.

Gastric acid—Also, stomach acid; helps break up fats and proteins for further digestion, aids in the absorption of nutrients through the walls of the intestines into the blood, and helps protect the gastrointestinal tract from harmful bacteria.

Homocysteine—An amino acid in the blood, too much of which is related to a higher risk of vascular disease.

Lipotropic—Substances that help prevent or correct excessive fat deposits in liver.

the lining of the stomach. If a burning sensation is experienced, betaine hydrochloride should be immediately discontinued.

Side effects

Side effects are seldom seen, but as of 2008 betaine hydrochloride had not been through rigorous safety studies. Its safety, especially for young children, pregnant or nursing women, or those with severe liver or kidney disease, is not known.

In very high doses, betaine hydrochlorine has been associated with heartburn.

Interactions

People taking nonsteroidal anti-inflammatory drugs (NSAIDs), cortisone-like drugs, or other medications that could cause peptic ulcers should not take betaine hydrochloride.

Resources

PERIODICALS

Challem, Jack. "Navigating the labyrinth: 30 things you need to know about nutritional supplements." *Vegetarian Times* (January 1998), no. 245: 66-67.
Gormley, James J. "Healthful weight loss includes L-carnitine, chromium, and lipotropics." *Better Nutrition* (May 1996) 58, no. 5: 40-41.

OTHER

PharmaSave Library. http://www.pharmasave.com/health-library.php/.

Melissa C. McDade
Rhonda Cloos, RN

Bhakti yoga

Definition

Bhakti **yoga** is one of six major branches of yoga, representing the path of self-transcending love or complete devotion to God or the divine. A practitioner of bhakti yoga regards God as present in every person or sentient being. Although bhakti yoga developed within a Hindu culture, it can be practiced by members of Western religions, as it focuses the believer's mind and heart on God as a supreme Person rather than an impersonal Absolute. Unlike **hatha yoga**, which is the form of yoga most familiar to Americans, bhakti yoga does not place great emphasis on breathing patterns or asanas (physical postures), but rather on acts of worship, devotion, and service.

Origins

Bhakti yoga is thought by some to be the oldest form of yoga, with its roots in the Vedas, or ancient scriptures of India. Some of the hymns in the Vedas are thought to be four thousand years old. Bhakti yoga did not emerge as a distinctive form of yoga, however, until about 500 B.C., the time of the composition of the *Bhagavad-Gita*, a Sanskrit work containing the teachings of Krishna, one of the most beloved of Hindu deities.

Bhakti yoga eventually became the focus of a popular devotional movement in India known as the bhakti-marga or "road of devotion." This movement flourished between 800 and 1100 A.D.. Around 900, devotees of Krishna who belonged to the bhakti-marga produced a scripture known as the *Bhagavad-Purana*, which contains Krishna's instructions to his worshipers. In one passage from the *Bhagavad-Purana*, Krishna praises bhakti above all other paths to bliss. He is represented as saying, "The wise person should abandon bad company and associate with the virtuous, for the virtuous ones sever the mind's attachments [to worldly concerns] by their utterances.... O greatly blessed devotee, these blessed ones constantly tell my story, by listening to which people are released from sin. Those who respectfully listen to, esteem, and recite my story become dedicated to me and attain faith and devotion to me."

Benefits

The chief benefit of bhakti yoga, from the perspective of its practitioners, is greater love for and closeness to God, and to other people (and all beings) as reflections of God. Although bhakti yoga is also beneficial to mental and physical well-being, improved health is not the primary reason most adherents choose this form of yoga.

Description

The Hindu sacred texts list nine forms of bhakti yoga:

- Sravana. Sravana is the Sanskrit term for listening to poems or stories about God's virtues and mighty deeds. Sravana bhakti cannot be practiced in isolation, however; the devotee must hear the stories from a wise teacher, and seek the companionship of holy people.

- Kirtana. Kirtana refers to singing or chanting God's praises. Ram Dass has said of this form of bhakti "When you are in love with God, the very sound of the Name brings great joy."

- Smarana. Smarana is remembrance of God at all times, or keeping God in the forefront of one's consciousness. In Christian terms, smarana is what the French monk Brother Lawrence (1605–1691) meant by "the practice of the presence of God."

- Padasevana. This form of bhakti yoga expresses love toward God through service to others, especially the sick.

- Archana. Archana refers to worship of God through such external images as icons or religious pictures, or through internal visualizations. The purpose of archana is to purify the heart through love of God.

- Vandana. Vandana refers to prayer and prostration (lying face downward on the ground with arms outstretched). This form of bhakti yoga is intended to curb self-absorption and self-centeredness.

- Dasya. In dasya bhakti, the devotee regards him- or herself as God's slave or servant, carrying out God's commandments, meditating on the words of God, caring for the sick and the poor, and helping to clean or repair sacred buildings or places.

- Sakha-bhava. This form of bhakti yoga is a cultivation of friendship-love toward God—to love God as a member of one's family or dearest friend, and delight in companionship with God.

- Atma-nivedana. Atma-nivedana is complete self-offering or self-surrender to God. Unlike some other forms of yoga, however, bhakti yoga does not teach that the devotee completely loses his or her personal identity through absorption into the divine. God is regarded as infinitely greater than the human worshiper, even one at the highest levels of spiritual attainment.

The nine types of bhakti yoga are not considered a hierarchy in the sense that some are regarded as superior

to others in guiding people toward God. An Indian teacher of bhakti yoga has said, "A devotee can take up any of these paths and reach the highest state. The path of bhakti is the easiest of all [types of yoga] and is not very much against the nature of human inclinations. It slowly and gradually takes the individual to the Supreme without frustrating his [sic] human instincts."

Preparations

The practice of bhakti yoga does not require any special physical or emotional preparation. It is a good idea, however, for Western readers to gather more information about a specific form of bhakti yoga that may interest or attract them. This preparation is particularly important because the tendency of Western culture to separate intellect from feeling leads many people to think of bhakti as sheer emotional fervor that does not engage the mind, whereas many of the great teachers of bhakti yoga were known for their wisdom and mindfulness as well as intensity of devotion. Useful resources for learning more about bhakti yoga include such periodicals as *Yoga Journal* and the various organizations listed below.

Precautions

Bhakti yoga tends to attract persons of a strongly emotional nature. There is some risk, however, of such individuals remaining spiritually immature or joining cult-like groups. The Hare Krishna movement, for example, is an offshoot of one school of bhakti yoga, the Gaudiya vaishnava tradition. Although some members of the movement consider their participation meaningful, others have left because they experienced it as repressive and intolerant of other faiths.

Side effects

There are no known side effects associated with the practice of bhakti yoga.

Research and general acceptance

A number of research studies have shown that such spiritual and devotional practices as those associated with bhakti yoga have positive effects on physical as well as emotional health. The positive physical effects include strengthening of the immune system, lowered blood pressure, and improved ability to cope with chronic **pain**. Chanting or hymn singing (kirtana) has been shown to be particularly effective in pain management.

Several research studies published in early 2004 report that all forms of yoga are becoming increasingly popular among Americans over 40—particularly women and people living in urban areas—for general wellness as well as back pain or other specific health problems. At least 15 million adults in the United States have participated in yoga programs, according to a study conducted at Harvard Medical School. Ninety percent of those contacted by telephone in a research sample said that they found yoga very or somewhat helpful. A survey of **cancer** patients in a supportive care program at Stanford University found that yoga and **massage therapy** were the activities that drew the largest number of participants.

Training and certification

There are no international or nationwide licensing or credentialing procedures for spiritual guides or teachers of bhakti yoga. The web site of the American Yoga Association (AYA) does, however, include an article on "How to Choose a Qualified Teacher."

Resources

BOOKS

Dass, Ram. *Journey of Awakening: A Meditator's Guidebook*. New York: Bantam Books, 1978. Contains some prayers, hymns, chants, and other suggestions for devotion drawn from Christian and Jewish sources that can be used in the practice of bhakti yoga.

Dossey, Larry, MD. *Healing Beyond the Body: Medicine and the Infinite Reach of the Mind*. Boston: Shambhala Publications, Inc., 2001.

Feuerstein, Georg, and Stephan Bodian, eds. *Living Yoga: A Comprehensive Guide for Daily Life*, Part III, "Cultivating Love: Bhakti Yoga." New York: Jeremy P. Tarcher/Perigee Books, 1993.

Pelletier, Kenneth, MD. *The Best Alternative Medicine*, Chapter 2, "Sound Mind, Sound Body." New York: Simon & Schuster, 2002.

Sivananda, Swami, and the Staff of the Sivananda Vedanta Yoga Center. *Yoga Mind and Body*. New York: DK Publishing, 1998.

PERIODICALS

Rosenbaum, E., H. Gautier, P. Fobair, et al. "Cancer Supportive Care, Improving the Quality of Life for Cancer Patients. A Program Evaluation Report." *Supportive Care in Cancer* 12 (May 2004): 293–301.

Saper, R. B., D. M. Eisenberg, R. B. Davis, et al. "Prevalence and Patterns of Adult Yoga Use in the United States: Results of a National Survey." *Alternative Therapies in Health and Medicine* 10 (March-April 2004): 44–49.

Wolsko, P. M., D. M. Eisenberg, R. B. Davis, and R. S. Phillips. "Use of Mind-Body Medical Therapies." *Journal of General Internal Medicine* 19 (January 2004): 43–50.

OTHER

Yoga.com Staff. "History of Bhakti Yoga." [cited May 23, 2004]. http://www.yoga.com/ydc/enlighten/enlighten_document.asp.

ORGANIZATIONS

American Yoga Association (AYA), P.O. Box 19986,, Sarasota,, FL, 34276, (941) 927-4977, Fax: (941) 921-9844, http://www.americanyogaassociation.org.

Yoga Alliance, 122 West Lancaster Avenue, Suite 204,, Reading,, PA, 19607-1874, (610) 777-7793, Fax:(610) 777-0556, http://www.yogaalliance.org.

Yoga Research and Education Center (YREC), P. O. Box 426,, Manton,, CA, 96059, (530) 474-5700, http://www.yrec.org.

Rebecca Frey

Bilberry

Description

Bilberry, *Vaccinium myrtillus*, is a European berry shrub that is related to the blueberry, huckleberry, and bearberry plants that grow in the United States. Bilberry is a small, wild, perennial shrub that grows throughout Europe and is now cultivated from the Far East to the United States. The shrub yields large amounts of small, darkish blue berries. Besides their medicinal use, they are often eaten fresh or made into jams and preserves. The leaves of the plant are used medicinally as well, but to a lesser extent than the berries. The qualities of the herb are sour, astringent, cold, and drying.

Bilberry has been used by European herbalists for centuries. In Elizabethan times, bilberries were mixed with honey and made into a syrup called *rob* that was prescribed for **diarrhea** and stomach problems. The berries were also used for **infections**, scurvy, and **kidney stones**. The leaves of the plant were used as a folk remedy for diabetes. Bilberry is most famous, though, for its long use as a medicine for eye and vision

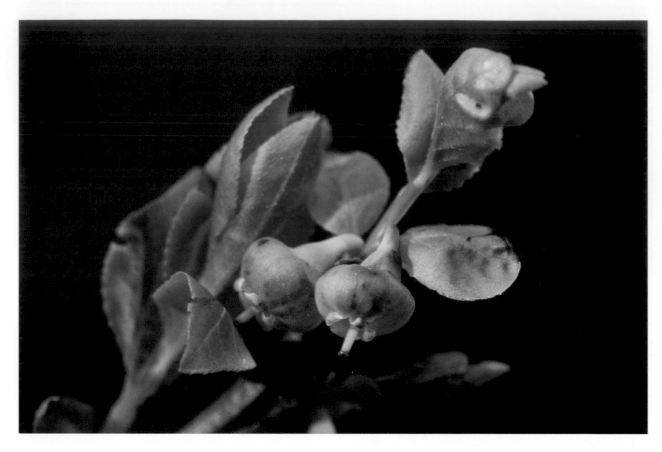

Northern Bilberry. (© Arco Images / Alamy)

problems. Legend has it that during World War II, British and American pilots discovered that eating bilberry jam before night missions greatly improved their night vision. Bilberries then became a staple for Air Force pilots. Since then, extensive research in Europe has shown that bilberries contain specific compounds that have beneficial effects on the eyes and circulatory system. In France, bilberries have been prescribed since 1945 for diabetic **retinopathy**, a major cause of blindness in diabetics.

Bilberries are high in substances called *flavonoids*, which are found in many fruits, vegetables, grains, beans, peas, and are particularly abundant in citrus fruits and berries. Flavonoids are chemicals technically known as polyphenols. Flavonoids have antioxidant and disease-fighting properties. **Antioxidants** are substances that help cells in the body resist and repair damage. The flavonoids found in bilberry provide the blue color of the berry. The bilberry flavonoids are called *anthocyanosides*, which were found to be the main active ingredients.

Bilberry flavonoids can increase certain enzymes and substances in the eyes that are crucial to good vision and eye function. Furthermore, anthocyanosides can increase circulation in the blood vessels in the eyes, and help these blood vessels repair and protect themselves. Specifically, research has shown that anthocyanosides help stabilize and protect a protein called collagen, which is a basic building block of veins, arteries, capillaries, and connective tissue. Particularly, anthocyanosides seem to work favorably in the tissues found in the retina, the back of the eye where major functions of vision take place. The retina is composed of millions of tiny nerve cells and blood vessels, which anthocyanosides can help support. Bilberry is a common treatment for many varieties of retinopathy, a disorder in which the intricate blood and nerve vessels in the retina are damaged. Retinopathy particularly affects people with diabetes, high blood pressure, and **sickle cell anemia**.

Many studies have documented bilberry's usefulness as a medicinal herb. One study demonstrated that bilberry extract used with **Vitamin E** prevented the progression of **cataracts** in 48 of 50 patients with cataract formations. In animal studies, bilberry reduced and stabilized blood sugar levels. In an Italian

KEY TERMS

Atherosclerosis—Disease in which the arteries and circulation are impaired from hardening and clogging, often from high cholesterol levels.

Cataracts—Eye condition in which the lenses harden and lose their clarity.

Glaucoma—Eye disease that can cause blindness; characterized by excess fluid between the iris and cornea of the eye.

Macular degeneration—Disease in which the macula, the part of the retina responsible for precise vision, deteriorates.

study, bilberry's flavonoids lowered **cholesterol** levels in the blood and improved circulation.

General use

Bilberry is most commonly used as a component of treatment for various vision and eye disorders, including **glaucoma**, cataracts, and **macular degeneration**. However, people with glaucoma should be monitored by an eye doctor regularly, and those with acute glaucoma should not depend on bilberry alone to protect their vision. They can use bilberry along with other emergency medical treatments. Bilberry is included in the treatments for many types of retinopathy and is also used for eye **fatigue**, poor night vision, and nearsightedness. It can be used as a preventative measure for glaucoma and cataracts, and to help those who require precise night vision like cab drivers and pilots. Bilberry's circulation improving and cholesterol lowering qualities make it useful in the treatment of **varicose veins** and **atherosclerosis**. It is also occasionally prescribed for arthritis.

Preparations

Fresh bilberries can be eaten like blueberries, although they are difficult to find outside of Europe. Two to four ounce servings of the fresh fruit can be eaten three times a day. One to two cups each day is a good dose. Dried bilberries are sometimes available in herb or organic health food stores, and two or three small handfuls can be eaten per day. However, dried berries are likely to contain only a small amount of the flavonoids.

Bilberry supplements are widely available in health food stores. They can be purchased as capsules and liquid extracts. A high-quality supplement may contain a standardized formula of up to 25% anthocyanocides. The dosage recommended with this percentage of active ingredients is 80-160 mg taken three times daily. Bilberry supplements may be taken with food or on an empty stomach. Bilberry jam and syrup may also be used.

For eye and circulatory problems, bilberry can be taken with ginkgo to increase its beneficial effects. Vitamins A, C and E may also enhance bilberry's healing effects in the eye. Some suggestions have been made that other flavonoid-containing supplements, such as **pine bark extract** and **grape seed extract**, can possibly enhance bilberry's healing properties.

Precautions

Bilberry may be used as prevention and herbal support for eye conditions, but should not replace medical care. People with vision problems should be thoroughly and immediately examined by an ophthalmologist (eye specialist) before any treatment or remedy is used.

Side effects

Bilberries can be taken in large doses without any side effects. However, bilberry leaves shouldn't be taken in large doses or over long periods of time because they are toxic.

Resources

BOOKS

Keville, Kathi. *Herbs: An Illustrated Encyclopedia.* New York: Friedman/Fairfax, 1994.

Mayell, Mark. *Off-the-Shelf Natural Health.* New York: Bantam, 1995.

PERIODICALS

HerbalGram (a quarterly journal of the American Botanical Council and Herb Research Foundation) P.O. Box 144345, Austin, TX 78714-4345, (800) 373-7105, http://www.herbalgram.org.

ORGANIZATIONS

Herb Research Foundation. 1007 Pearl Street, Boulder, CO 80302.

OTHER

Dietary Supplement Quality Initiative. http://www.dsqi.org.

Douglas Dupler

Binge eating disorder

Definition

Binge eating disorder (BED) is characterized by a loss of control over eating behaviors. The binge eater consumes unnaturally large amounts of food in a short time period, but unlike a bulimic, doesn't regularly engage in any inappropriate weight-reducing behaviors (like excessive **exercise**, **vomiting**, taking laxatives) after the binge episodes.

Description

About three percent of women and one-tenth as many men have duffered from either bulimia or binge eating disorder at some time in their lives. BED typically strikes individuals between their adolescent years and their early 20s. Because of the nature of the

disorder, most BED patients are overweight or obese. Studies of weight loss programs have shown that an average of 30% of individuals enrolling in these programs report binge eating behavior. Binge eating in milder forms is even more common, as are attempts to compensate for the binges.

Causes and symptoms

Binge eating episodes may act as a psychological release for excessive emotional **stress**. Other circumstances that may predispose an individual to BED include heredity and mood disorders, such as major **depression**. BED patients are also more likely to have an additional diagnosis of impulsive behaviors (for example, compulsive shopping), **post-traumatic stress disorder** (PTSD), **panic disorder**, or personality disorders. More than half also have a history of major depression. In 2002, the American Psychiatric Association was considering including BED as a psychiatric diagnosis.

Individuals who develop BED often come from families who put an unnatural emphasis on the importance of food. For example, these families may use food as a source of comfort in times of emotional distress. As children, BED patients may have been taught to clean their plates regardless of their appetite, or to be a good girl or boy and finish all of the meal. Cultural attitudes towards beauty and thinness may also be a factor in BED.

During binge episodes, BED patients experience a definite sense of lost control over their eating. They eat quickly and to the point of discomfort, even if they aren't hungry. They typically binge alone two or more times a week, and often feel depressed and guilty when the episode is over.

Diagnosis

BED is usually diagnosed and treated by a psychiatrist and/or a psychologist. In addition to an

---

Symptoms of binge-eating disorder

Recurrent episodes of binge eating, characterized by eating an excessive amount of food within a discrete period of time and by a sense of lack of control over eating during the episode

The binge-eating episodes are associated with at least 3 of the following: eating much more rapidly than normal; eating until feeling uncomfortably full; eating large amounts of food when not feeling physically hungry; eating alone because of being embarrassed by how much one is eating; feeling disgusted with oneself, depressed, or very guilty after overeating

Marked distress about the binge-eating behavior

The binge eating occurs, on average, at least 2 days a week for 6 months

The binge eating is not associated with the regular use of inappropriate compensatory behaviors (e.g., purging, fasting, excessive exercise)

(Illustration by Corey Light. Cengage Learning, Gale)

interview with the patient, personality and behavioral inventories, such as the Minnesota Multiphasic Personality Inventory (MMPI), may be administered as part of the assessment process. One of several clinical inventories, or scales, may also be used to assess depressive symptoms, including the Hamilton Depression Scale (HAM-D) or Beck Depression Inventory (BDI). These tests may be administered in an outpatient or hospital setting.

Treatment

Many BED individuals binge after long periods of excessive dieting; therapy helps normalize this pattern. The initial goal of BED treatment is to teach the patient to gain control over his or her eating behavior by focusing on eating regular meals and avoiding snacking. Cognitive **behavioral therapy**, group therapy, or interpersonal **psychotherapy** may be used to uncover the emotional motives, distorted thinking, and behavioral patterns behind the binge eating. The overweight BED patient may be placed on a moderate exercise program and a nutritionist may be consulted to educate the patient on healthy food choices and strategies for weight loss.

Initial treatment may focus on curbing the depression that is a characteristic feature of BED. Recommended herbal remedies to ease the symptoms of depression may include **damiana** (*Turnera diffusa*), ginseng (*Panax ginseng*), kola (*Cola nitida*), lady's slipper (*Cypripedium calceolus*), **lavender** (*Lavandula angustifolia*), lime blossom (*Tilia x vulgaris*), oats (*Avena sativa*), **rosemary** (*Rosmarinus officinalis*), **skullcap** (*Scutellaria laterifolia*), **St. John's wort** (*Hypericum perforatum*), **valerian** (*Valeriana officinalis*), and vervain (*Verbena officinalis*).

Binge-eating episodes that appear to be triggered by stress may be curbed by educating the patient in **relaxation** exercises and techniques, including **aromatherapy**, breathing exercises, **biofeedback**, **music therapy**, **yoga**, and massage. Herbs known as adaptogens may also be prescribed by an herbalist or holistic healthcare professional. These herbs are thought to promote adaptability to stress, and include **Siberian ginseng** (*Eleutherococcus senticosus*), ginseng (*Panax ginseng*), wild yam (*Dioscorea villosa*), borage (*Borago officinalis*), **licorice** (*Glycyrrhiza glabra*), **chamomile** (*Chamaemelum nobile*), and nettles (*Urtica dioica*). Tonics of skullcap (*Scutellaria lateriafolia*), and oats (*Avena sativa*), may also be recommended to ease **anxiety**.

Allopathic treatment

Treatment with antidepressants may be prescribed for BED patients. Selective serotonin reuptake inhibitors (such as Prozac) are usually preferred because they offer fewer side effects. However, clinical studies don't show much effectiveness for use of antidepressants in treating BED. Psychotherapy shows better results. Once the binge eating behavior is curbed and depressive symptoms are controlled, the physical symptoms of the disorder can be addressed.

Expected results

The poor dietary habits and **obesity** that are symptomatic of BED can lead to serious health problems, such as high blood pressure, heart attacks, and diabetes, if left unchecked. BED is a chronic condition that requires ongoing medical and psychological management. To bring long-term relief to the BED patient, it is critical to address the underlying psychological causes behind binge eating behaviors. It appears that up to 50% of BED patients will stop bingeing with cognitive behavioral therapy.

Resources

BOOKS

Abraham, Suzanne and Derek Llewellyn-Jones. *Eating Disorders: The Facts.* 4th ed. Oxford: Oxford University Press, 1997.

American Psychiatric Association. *Diagnostic and Statistical Manual of Mental Disorders,* 4th ed. Washington, DC: American Psychiatric Press, Inc., 1994.

Siegel, Michele, Judith Brisman, and Margot Weinshel. *Surviving an Eating Disorder: Strategies for Family and Friends,* 2nd ed. New York: Harper Perennial, 1997.

PERIODICALS

Brewerton, Timothy D. "Binge Eating Disorder: Recognition, Diagnosis, and Treatment." *Medscape Mental Health* 2, no. 5 (1997). http://www.medscape.com.

"Treatment of Bulimia and Binge Eating." *Harvard Mental Health Letter* (July 2002).

Tufts University. "Binge Eating Disorder Comes Out of the Closet: Experts Say Leading Obesity Factor Has Long Been Overlooked." *Tufts University Diet & Nutrition Letter* 14, no. 11 (January 1997): 4-5.

ORGANIZATIONS

American Psychiatric Association (APA). Office of Public Affairs. 1400 K Street NW, Washington, DC 20005. (202) 682-6119. http://www.psych.org/.

American Psychological Association (APA). Office of Public Affairs. 750 First St. NE, Washington, DC 20002-4242. (202) 336-5700. http://www.apa.org/.

Eating Disorders Awareness and Prevention. 603 Stewart St., Suite 803, Seattle, WA 98101. (800) 931-2237. http://www.edap.org

National Eating Disorders Organization (NEDO). 6655 South Yale Ave., Tulsa, OK 74136. (918) 481-4044.

Paula Ford-Martin
Teresa G. Odle

Biocytin *see* **Brewer's yeast**

Biofeedback

Definition

Biofeedback, or applied psychophysiological feedback, is a patient-guided treatment that teaches an individual to control muscle tension, **pain**, body temperature, brain waves, and other bodily functions and processes through **relaxation**, visualization, and other cognitive control techniques. The name biofeedback refers to the biological signals that are fed back, or returned, to the patient in order for the patient to develop techniques of manipulating them.

Origins

In 1961, Neal Miller, an experimental psychologist, suggested that autonomic nervous system responses (for instance, heart rate, blood pressure, gastrointestinal activity, regional blood flow) could be under voluntary control. As a result of his experiments, he showed that such autonomic processes were controllable. This work led to the creation of biofeedback therapy. Willer's work was expanded by other researchers. Thereafter, research performed in the 1970s by UCLA researcher Dr. Barry Sterman established that both cats and monkeys could be trained to control their brain wave patterns. Sterman then used his research techniques on human patients with **epilepsy**, where he was able to reduce seizures by 60% with the use of biofeedback techniques. Throughout the 1970s, other researchers published reports of their use of biofeedback in the treatment of cardiac arrhythmias, headaches, **Raynaud's syndrome**, and excess stomach acid, and as a tool for teaching deep relaxation. Since the early work of Miller and Sterman, biofeedback has developed into a front-line behavioral treatment for an even wider range of disorders and symptoms.

Benefits

Biofeedback has been used to successfully treat a number of disorders and their symptoms, including tempromandibular joint disorder (TMJ), chronic pain, **irritable bowel syndrome** (IBS), Raynaud's syndrome, epilepsy, **attention-deficit hyperactivity disorder** (ADHD), migraine headaches, **anxiety**, **depression**, traumatic brain injury, and **sleep disorders**.

Illnesses that may be triggered at least in part by **stress** are also targeted by biofeedback therapy. Certain types of headaches, high blood pressure, **bruxism** (teeth grinding), **post-traumatic stress disorder**, eating disorders, **substance abuse**, and some anxiety disorders may be treated successfully by teaching patients the ability to relax and release both muscle and mental tension. Biofeedback is often just one part of a comprehensive treatment program for some of these disorders.

NASA has used biofeedback techniques to treat astronauts who suffer from severe space sickness, during which the autonomic nervous system is disrupted. Scientists at the University of Tennessee have adapted these techniques to treat individuals suffering from severe **nausea** and **vomiting** that is also rooted in autonomic nervous system dysfunction.

Recent research also indicates that biofeedback may be a useful tool in helping patients with **urinary incontinence** regain bladder control. Individuals learning pelvic-floor muscle strengthening exercises can gain better control over these muscles by using biofeedback. Sensors are placed on the muscles to train the patient where they are and when proper contractions are taking place.

Description

During biofeedback, special sensors are placed on the body. These sensors measure the bodily function that is causing the patient problem symptoms, such as heart rate, blood pressure, muscle tension (EMG or electromyographic feedback), brain waves (EEC or electroencephalographic feedback), respiration, and body temperature (thermal feedback), and translates the information into a visual and/or audible readout, such as a paper tracing, a light display, or a series of beeps.

While the patient views the instantaneous feedback from the biofeedback monitors, he or she begins to recognize what thoughts, fears, and mental images influence his or her physical reactions. By monitoring this relationship between mind and body, the patient can then use these same thoughts and mental images as subtle cues, as these act as reminders to become deeply relaxed, instead of anxious. These reminders also work to manipulate heart beat, brain wave patterns, body temperature, and other bodily functions. This is achieved

ELMER GREEN (1918–)

A life dedicated to science has propelled Elmer Green, Ph.D. into careers as a physicist and a biological psychologist. Both led to his most noted work, the influence on the birth of the biofeedback movement. While the mechanics of moving parts and machinery lured the investigator from LaGrand, Oregon, to his work as a civilian scientist with the Navy in the late 1940s, it was his wife Alyce who caused him to ponder biophysiology and human development. In 1953 she read a book titled *The Human Senses* by Frank Geldard. It was their interests as a couple that led to their continued education at the University of Chicago. In 1957 Green began work for his Ph.D. studies in biopsychology, while Alyce studied for her Master's degree in psychology.

Numerous opportunities, including assisting with the development of a machine for the automated detection of brain damage, led to his position at the Menninger Institute in Topeka, Kansas, in 1964. While there he established the psychophysiology laboratory and the Voluntary Controls Program. It was his treatment of a colleague's wife's headaches that Green became convinced that skin temperature was an autonomic nervous system variable that was responsive to psychophysiologic self-regulation aided by thermal biofeedback. By learning to control temperature he found that headache control could be enhanced. Green's success attracted support by several of the Menninger staff who also began research and use of biofeedback therapy for headaches and hypertension.

The 1960s proved exciting for Green as he, Alyce, and colleague Dale Walters became involved with EEG Biofeedback, and studied the process of meditation—a therapy the Greens had long practiced. In April 1969, Green and his wife organized the Council Grove Conference for the study of the voluntary control of internal states. The conference served as a step toward forming the Biofeedback Research Society, which later became the Biofeedback Society of America, and currently the Association for Applied Psychophysiology and Biofeedback.

Together, Elmer and Alyce Green authored numerous papers, book chapters, and wrote the book, *Beyond Biofeedback* (1977). They lectured throughout the United States and around the world for more than 20 years on multiple topics including EEG biofeedback training and psychophysiologic control.

Green co-founded the International Society For the Study of Subtle Energies and Energy Medicine (ISSSEEM) in 1990 and served as its director. Alyce died in 1994 of Alzheimer's disease. In 2008, 90-year-old Green works as a professional consultant and director emeritus of the Voluntary Controls Program at the Menninger Clinic. He also serves as the science director of the Dove Health Alliance in Aptos, California, and authored a book titled *The Ozawkie Book of the Dead* that was published in 2001.

through relaxation exercises, mental imagery, and other cognitive therapy techniques.

As the biofeedback response takes place, patients can actually see or hear the results of their efforts instantly through the sensor readout on the biofeedback equipment. Once these techniques are learned and the patient is able to recognize the state of relaxation or visualization necessary to alleviate symptoms, the biofeedback equipment itself is no longer needed. The patient then has a powerful, portable, and self-administered treatment tool to deal with problem symptoms.

Biofeedback that specializes in reading and altering brain waves is sometimes called *neurofeedback*. The brain produces four distinct types of brain waves—delta, theta, alpha, and beta—that all operate at a different frequency. Delta, the slowest frequency wave, is the brain wave pattern associated with sleep. Beta waves, which occur in a normal, waking state, can range from 12-35 Hz. Problems begin to develop when beta wave averages fall in the low end (underarousal) or the high end (overarousal) of that spectrum. Underarousal might be present in conditions such as depression or attention-deficit disorder, and

overarousal may be indicative of an anxiety disorder, obsessive compulsive disorder, or excessive stress. Beta wave neurofeedback focuses on normalizing that beta wave pattern to an optimum value of around 14 Hz. A second type of neurofeedback, alpha-theta, focuses on developing the more relaxing alpha (8-13 Hz) and theta waves (4-9 Hz) that are usually associated with deep, meditative states, and has been used with some success in substance abuse treatment.

Through brain wave manipulation, neurofeedback can be useful in treating a variety of disorders that are suspected or proven to impact brain wave patterns, such as epilepsy, attention-deficit disorder, migraine headaches, anxiety, depression, traumatic brain injury, and sleep disorders. The equipment used for neurofeedback usually uses a monitor as an output device. The monitor displays specific patterns that the patient attempts to change by producing the appropriate type of brain wave. Or, the monitor may reward the patient for producing the appropriate brain wave by producing a positive reinforcer, or reward. For example, children may be rewarded with a series of successful moves in a displayed video game.

KEY TERMS

Autonomic nervous system—The part of the nervous system that controls so-called involuntary functions, such as heart rate, salivary gland secretion, respiratory function, and pupil dilation.

Bruxism—Habitual, often unconscious, grinding of the teeth.

Epilepsy—A neurological disorder characterized by the sudden onset of seizures.

Placebo effect—Placebo effect occurs when a treatment or medication with no known therapeutic value (a placebo) is administered to a patient, and the patient's symptoms improve. The patient believes and expects that the treatment is going to work, so it does. The placebo effect is also a factor to some degree in clinically-effective therapies, and explains why patients respond better than others to treatment despite similar symptoms and illnesses.

Raynaud's syndrome—A vascular, or circulatory system, disorder which is characterized by abnormally cold hands and feet. This chilling effect is caused by constriction of the blood vessels in the extremities, and occurs when the hands and feet are exposed to cold weather. Emotional stress can also trigger the cold symptoms.

Schizophrenia—Schizophrenia is a psychotic disorder that causes distortions in perception (delusions and hallucinations), inappropriate moods and behaviors, and disorganized or incoherent speech and behavior.

Temporomandibular joint disorder—Inflammation, irritation, and pain of the jaw caused by improper opening and closing of the temporomandibular joint. Other symptoms include clicking of the jaw and a limited range of motion.

Depending on the type of biofeedback, individuals may need up to 30 sessions with a trained professional to learn the techniques required to control their symptoms on a long-term basis. Therapists usually recommend that their patients practice both biofeedback and relaxation techniques on their own at home.

Preparations

Before initiating biofeedback treatment, the therapist and patient will have an initial consultation to record the patients medical history and treatment background and discuss goals for therapy.

Before a neurofeedback session, an EEG is taken from the patient to determine his or her baseline brainwave pattern.

Biofeedback typically is performed in a quiet and relaxed atmosphere with comfortable seating for the patient. Depending on the type and goals of biofeedback being performed, one or more sensors will be attached to the patient's body with conductive gel and/or adhesives. These may include:

- Electromyographic (EMG) sensors. EMG sensors measure electrical activity in the muscles, specifically muscle tension. In treating TMJ or bruxism, these sensors would be placed along the muscles of the jaw. Chronic pain might be treated by monitoring electrical energy in other muscle groups.

- Galvanic skin response (GSR) sensors. These are electrodes placed on the fingers that monitor perspiration, or sweat gland, activity. These may also be called skin conductance level (SCL) sensors.

- Temperature sensors. Temperature, or thermal, sensors measure body temperature and changes in blood flow.

- Electroencephalography (EEG) sensors. These electrodes are applied to the scalp to measure the electrical activity of the brain, or brain waves.

- Heart rate sensors. A pulse monitor placed on the finger tip can monitor pulse rate.

- Respiratory sensors. Respiratory sensors monitor oxygen intake and carbon dioxide output.

Precautions

Individuals who use a pacemaker or other implantable electrical devices should inform their biofeedback therapist before starting treatments, as certain types of biofeedback sensors have the potential to interfere with these devices.

Biofeedback may not be suitable for some patients. Patients must be willing to take a very active role in the treatment process. And because biofeedback focuses strictly on behavioral change, those patients who wish to gain insight into their symptoms by examining their past might be better served by psychodynamic therapy.

Biofeedback may also be inappropriate for cognitively impaired individuals, such as those patients with organic brain disease or a traumatic brain injury, depending on their levels of functioning.

Patients with specific pain symptoms of unknown origin should undergo a thorough medical examination before starting biofeedback treatments to rule out any serious underlying disease. Once a diagnosis has been made, biofeedback can be used concurrently with conventional treatment.

Biofeedback may only be one component of a comprehensive treatment plan. For illnesses and symptoms that are manifested from an organic disease process, such as **cancer** or diabetes, biofeedback should be an adjunct to (complementary to), and not a replacement for, conventional medical treatment.

Side effects

There are no known side effects to properly administered biofeedback or neurofeedback sessions.

Research and general acceptance

Preliminary research published in late 1999 indicated that neurofeedback may be a promising new tool in the treatment of **schizophrenia**. Researchers reported that schizophrenic patients had used neurofeedback to simulate brain wave patterns that antipsychotic medications produce in the brain. Further research is needed to determine what impact this may have on treatment for schizophrenia.

The use of biofeedback techniques to treat an array of disorders has been extensively described in the medical literature. Controlled studies for some applications are limited, such as for the treatment of menopausal symptoms and premenstrual disorder (PMS). There is also some debate over the effectiveness of biofeedback in ADHD treatment, and the lack of controlled studies on that application. While many therapists, counselors, and mental health professionals have reported great success with treating their ADHD patients with neurofeedback techniques, some critics attribute this positive therapeutic impact to a **placebo effect**.

There may also be some debate among mental health professionals as to whether biofeedback should be considered a first line treatment for some mental illnesses, and to what degree other treatments, such as medication, should be employed as an adjunct therapy.

Training and certification

Individuals wishing to try biofeedback should contact a healthcare professional trained in biofeedback techniques. Licensed psychologists, psychiatrists, and physicians frequently train their patients in biofeedback techniques, or can recommend a specialist who does. In some cases, a licensed professional may employ a biofeedback technician who works under their direct guidance when treating patients.

There are several national organizations for biofeedback therapists, including the Biofeedback Certification Institute of America, which also certifies therapists in the practice.

Resources

BOOKS

Robbins, Jim. *A Symphony in the Brain: The Evolution of the New Brain Wave Biofeedback*. Boston, MA: Atlantic Monthly Press, 2000.

PERIODICALS

Burgio, K.L. et al. "Behavioral vs. Drug Treatment for Urge Urinary Incontinence in Older Women: A randomized controlled trial." *Journal of the American Medical Association* 280 (Dec. 1998): 1995-2000.
Robbins, Jim. "On the Track with Neurofeedback." *Newsweek* 135, no. 25 (June 2000): 76.

ORGANIZATIONS

The Association for Applied Psychotherapy and Biofeedback. 10200 W. 44th Avenue, Suite 304, Wheat Ridge, CO 80033-2840. (303) 422-8436. http://www.aapb.org
Biofeedback Certification Institute of America.10200 W. 44th Avenue, Suite 310, Wheat Ridge, CO 80033. (303) 420-2902.

Paula Ford-Martin

Bioflavonoids

Description

Bioflavonoids, or flavonoids, are a large class of **antioxidants**. They are compounds abundant in the pulp and rinds of citrus fruits and other foods containing **vitamin C**, such as soybeans and root vegetables. Other major sources of bioflavonoids include tea, vegetables such as broccoli and eggplant, **flaxseed**, and whole grains. Bioflavonoids are active ingredients in many herbal remedies. These include **feverfew**, *Tanacetum parthenium*; *Ginkgo biloba*; **licorice** root, *Glycyrrhiza glabra*; **St. John's wort**, *Hypericum perforatum*; and *Echinacea* spp.

Bioflavonoids help maximize the benefits of vitamin C by inhibiting its breakdown in the body. In 1935, Hungarian-American physiologist Albert Szent-Györgyi (1893–1986) demonstrated that an extract he called citrin, made from lemon peels, was more effective than pure vitamin C in preventing scurvy. In 1936, Szent-Györgyi found that citrin was a mixture of bioflavonoids, including the flavone **hesperidin** and a flavonol glucoside. Szent-Györgyi believed that bioflavonoids should be considered vitamins but was not able to substantiate that they were essential nutrients. Still, many researchers and physicians believe that dietary intake of bioflavonoids is beneficial for blood vessel health and possibly for protection against **heart disease**.

Bioflavonoids are categorized in a variety of ways, sometimes with overlapping categories. Types of bioflavonoids include flavones, isoflavonoids, flavanones (such as catechins and naringin), and flavanols.

General use

In their natural state, bioflavonoids are usually found in close association with vitamin C. In treating medical conditions, vitamin C and bioflavonoids enhance the action of each other's compound. Therefore, when taken as supplements, they often should be used in combination to increase effectiveness. In general, all bioflavonoids are potentially useful as antioxidants, antivirals, and anti-inflammatories. Other health benefits of the various bioflavonoids include:

- Preventing nosebleeds, miscarriages, postpartum bleeding, and other types of hemorrhages
- The treatment and prevention of menstrual disorders
- Protecting against cancer and heart disease
- Anticoagulant activity (preventing blood clotting)
- Reducing the occurrence of easy bruising
- Decreasing cholesterol level
- Improving symptoms related to aging
- Protecting against infections
- Counteracting the effects of pollution, pesticides, rancid fats, and alcohol
- Reducing pain
- Improving circulation
- Improving liver function
- Improving vision and preventing eye diseases
- Strengthening the walls of the blood vessels

Major bioflavonoids and their actions

Rutin can be used to treat chronic venous insufficiency (a condition in which blood drains inadequately from a body part), **glaucoma**, **hay fever**, **hemorrhoids**, **varicose veins**, poor circulation, oral herpes, **cirrhosis**, **stress**, low serum **calcium**, and **cataracts**. It is helpful in reducing weakness in the blood vessels and resultant hemorrhages. Rutin can relieve the **pain** from bumps and **bruises**. Rutin may be taken to help reduce serum **cholesterol**. It is useful in treating rheumatic diseases such as **gout**, arthritis,

systemic lupus erythematosus (a chronic disease marked by a rash on the face with a variety of symptoms), and **ankylosing spondylitis** (a condition affecting ligaments in the spine, involving the hips and shoulders). Rutin is most abundant in apricots, buckwheat, cherries, prunes, rose hips, the whitish rind of citrus fruits, and the core of green peppers.

Anthocyanins and proanthocyanidins can be used to treat a number of eye conditions such as cataracts, **night blindness**, diabetic **retinopathy** (a progressive retina disease that is a complication of diabetes), and **macular degeneration** (a hereditary condition causing loss of vision). They are also useful for strengthening the walls of the blood vessels and, therefore, may help prevent bruising, hemorrhoids, varicose veins, and spider veins. These bioflavonoids can help to prevent **osteoporosis** by stabilizing collagen, the major protein in bone. They can reduce cholesterol deposits in arteries and prevent damage to the artery walls. These actions reduce the possibilities of heart disease and strokes. Anthocyanins and proanthocyanidins can produce dilation of blood vessels and prevent **blood clots**. Proanthocyanidins are able to cross the blood-brain barrier to protect the brain from damage by free radicals and infection. Good sources of anthocyanins and proanthocyanidins include blackberries, cranberries, black and **green tea**, raspberries, grapes, eggplant, red cabbage, elderberries, and red wine.

Hesperidin is useful in treating the complaints of **menopause** and in dealing with the viruses that cause herpes, the flu, and certain respiratory ailments. Hesperidin fights allergic reactions by blocking the release of histamine. It may also help reduce **edema** (accumulation of fluid) in the legs. Hesperidin deficiency has been linked to weaknesses in the walls of the blood vessels, pain and weakness in the hands and feet, and leg cramps at night. Hesperidin is found most commonly in the pulps and rinds of citrus fruits.

Ellagic acid helps to inhibit **cancer** by neutralizing the effect of certain carcinogens. It is particularly helpful in reducing the effects of nitrosamines, which are found in tobacco and processed meat products such as bacon and hot dogs. Ellagic acid reduces the effects of the toxic and carcinogenic factors (aflatoxins) produced by *Aspergillus flavus* molds on food. Aflatoxins may cause liver damage and cancer. Ellagic acid diminishes the effects of polycyclic hydrocarbons produced by tobacco smoke and air pollution, as well. Sources of ellagic acid include strawberries, grapes, apples, cranberries, blackberries, and walnuts.

Quercetin is a good antihistamine. It can help reduce the inflammation that results from hay **fever**, **allergies**, **bursitis**, gout, arthritis, and **asthma**. It may lessen other asthma symptoms. Quercetin stimulates **detoxification** in the liver. It strengthens the blood vessels, and is useful in treating **atherosclerosis** (plaque build-up in the arteries) and high cholesterol levels. It may help inhibit tumor formation. Quercetin can be used to treat many of the complications of diabetes. For example, it blocks the accumulation of sorbitol, which has been linked with nerve, eye, and kidney damage in diabetics; and it regulates blood sugar levels. Quercetin inhibits the growth of *Helicobacter pylori,* which is responsible for the development of peptic ulcers. It can also help diminish the effects of the herpes virus, the Epstein-Barr virus (a common virus and a common cause of **mononucleosis**), and the polio virus. Quercetin is found in green tea, onion skins, kale, red cabbage, green beans, tomatoes, potatoes, lettuce, strawberries, cherries, and grapes. It is also found in smaller amounts in many other foods.

Catechins and tannins can be used to stimulate detoxification by the liver and to strengthen the blood vessels. They also help reduce the inflammatory response. Catechins and tannins may help inhibit the formation of tumors. In addition, catechins can be used to inhibit the breakdown of collagen and to treat **hepatitis** and arthritis. Catechins and tannins are both found in green and black teas.

Kaempferols stimulate liver detoxification and strengthen the blood vessels. They may also inhibit tumor formation. Strawberries, leeks, kale, broccoli, radishes, endives, and red beets all are good sources of kaempferols, but kaempferols are very common and found in many plants and foods. Naringen may slow the progression of heart disease and visual degeneration in diabetes. It is a potent anticoagulant that keeps the arteries clear and strong to prevent strokes, heart attacks, and the blindness of diabetes. Naringen is an active ingredient in grapefruits. Genestein is known to be a regulator of estrogen. It is useful in treating disorders of **menstruation** and menopause. Genestein is found in soybeans and soy products.

Preparations

Since bioflavonoids are so widely available in fruits in high concentrations, daily consumption of whole fresh fruits and fresh fruit juices is the best way to get adequate amounts of bioflavonoids. Highly concentrated liquid extracts of some fruits are also available.

KEY TERMS

Antioxidants—Nutrients that protect against oxidation, a chemical reaction that can damage human cells.

Blood-brain barrier—A feature of the brain thought to consist of walls of capillaries that prevent or delay the passage of some drugs and chemicals into the central nervous system.

Free radicals—By-products of the process of energy production in the human body. Free radicals are atoms or groups of atoms with an odd number of electrons. They can damage important cellular components and can be checked by antioxidants.

Precautions

Bioflavonoids are generally safe, even at very high doses. However, pregnant women are advised not to take megadoses of bioflavonoids. Preliminary studies indicated that there may be a link between infant **leukemia** and high doses of bioflavonoids in the mother.

Side effects

Bioflavonoids are not toxic, even at high levels. They are water soluble; therefore, any amount in excess of what is needed by the body is excreted in the urine.

Interactions

Bioflavonoids are usually found in close association with vitamin C, and they enhance its effect. There are no known drug interactions.

Resources

BOOKS

Andersen, Oyvind M., and Kenneth R. Markham, eds. *Flavonoids: Chemistry, Biochemistry, and Applications.* Boca Raton, FL: CRC Press, 2006.

Challem, Jack, and Marie Moneysmith. *User's Guide to Carotenoids & Flavonoids: Learn How to Harness the Health Benefits of Natural Plan Antioxidants.* Laguna Beach, CA: Basic Health, 2005.

Grotewald, Eric. *The Science of Flavonoids.* New York: Springer, 2006.

Patience Paradox
David Edward Newton, Ed.D.

Bioidentical hormone replacement therapy

Definition

Supplementation of hormones that are identical in structure and function to the hormones naturally occurring in the body.

Description

Increasing numbers of women and their physicians are opting for the use of natural, bioidentical hormones to manage the symptoms of **menopause**. This trend has occurred largely as a response to the outcome of several studies which concluded that the risks of using conventional hormone–replacement therapy (HRT) outweighed the benefits. Bioidentical hormone replacement therapy (BHRT) is perceived as a safer alternative for treating menopausal symptoms such as **hot flashes**, **insomnia**, night sweats, poor memory and concentration, and genitourinary symptoms. BHT is also used to help maintain bone density after menopause and prevent **osteoporosis**.

Bioidentical hormones are laboratory–produced hormones that are identical to those found in the human body. They are derived from plant sources, from molecules found in soy (genistein) and wild yam (diosgenin). Although derived from plants, bioidentical hormones are not the same as over–the–counter formulations made from plants. The human body lacks enzymes necessary to convert plant molecules to hormone molecules that are identical to endogenous hormones. The plant products are not hormonally active in their natural form, although they do affect hormone levels as botanical agents. Likewise, bioidentical hormones are not the same as "plant–based" products produced by pharmaceutical companies, which are natural substances converted to synthetics so the product may be patented. These synthetic derivatives have different action and metabolism in the body and are not identical to endogenous hormones.

Conventional hormones are produced by pharmaceutical manufacturers and are available in a limited variety of doses and delivery methods. Conventional HRT are composed of either synthetic estrogen, a synthetic progesterone–like hormone called progestin, or conjugated equine estrogen (CEE). CEE is obtained from the urine of pregnant mares and contains at least 100 different types of estrogen. HRT is often poorly tolerated by women who take them. Between one–third and two–thirds of women discontinue use within the first year due to side effects. Many of the unwanted side effects of conventional HRT are attributable to synthetic progestins, and include weight gain, bloating, breast tenderness and irregular bleeding.

Physicians have prescribed conventional HRT for decades. Estrogen replacement therapy was popularized in the late 1960s, a time in which the predominant perception of menopause was that of a deficiency state. Estrogen was thought to be an elixir of youth, and was given routinely to perimenopausal and menopausal women. Estrogen supplementation was given by itself until it was found in the mid–1970s that increased estrogen in the absence of progesterone caused the uterine lining to thicken, and increased the risk of **uterine cancer**. Subsequently, estrogen has been supplemented in combination with progesterone except in cases where the woman has had a hysterectomy.

Conventional HRT was in widespread use in the United States until studies published between the late 1990s and 2003 revealed serious health risks associated with combined estrogen and progestin HRT. The Women's Health Initiative, a clinical trial with over 16,000 women using HRT, was discontinued prematurely due to participants experiencing an increased risk of **stroke**, cardiovascular disease, **breast cancer** and **dementia**. Negative health outcomes were most significant in women using HRT greater than five years, but many problems occurred within the first year of use. Other large–scale clinical trials such as the Postemenopausal Estrogen/Progestin Interventions (PEPI), the Heart and Estrogen/Progestin Replacement Study (HERS) and the Million Women Study produced similar results, and use of conventional HRT dramatically declined.

Bioidentical hormones have been endorsed by advocates as being safer alternatives to conventional HRT. However, clinical trials confirming their safety are limited with the exception of a few small American and European studies. Further research is needed to confirm that bioidentical hormones are safer than conventional HRT by virtue of being used in smaller doses, having the same mechanism of action, and being more efficiently metabolized and excreted by the body.

Bioidentical hormones are different from conventional hormones in several significant ways. They differ in molecular structure, metabolism, bioavailability, and receptor affinity. The molecular structure of bioidentical hormones is identical to those produced in the body (endogenous). Because they are identical to endogenous hormones, they are metabolized in the same way as hormones made in the body, thereby reducing circulation of potentially toxic metabolic byproducts. For example, synthetic estrogen is slower to be metabolized and excreted than endogenous or bioidentical estrogen. As a result, it has greater potential to damage cells and tissues. Additionally, bioidentical hormones are an exact fit with endogenous hormone receptor sites.

Preparations

Bioidentical hormones can be prepared in many different forms to directly affect target tissues and to enhance absorption and bioavailability. Bioidentical hormones may be delivered in capsules, sublingual pellets, or a variety of transdermal applications. They may be formulated into creams, ointments, or patches. Transdermal application has the benefit of acting directly on target tissue, and may be used for vulvar or vaginal creams to address atrophy and dryness. Prescriptions for bioidentical hormones can be individualized to meet the needs of each woman and compounded in unique doses, combinations, and delivery methods.

Bioidentical hormone replacement preparations can be individually tailored to contain combinations of natural estrogens, progesterone, testosterone and **DHEA**. Each hormone has a unique action in the body, and can be supplemented based on a woman's individual needs as determined by hormone profile testing ordered by her health care provider.

In premenopausal women, estrogen is produced in the ovaries from hormone precursors **androstenedione** and testosterone. After menopause, the majority of estrogen in the body is converted from precursor hormones in the fat tissue, and by the adrenal glands. There are three forms of estrogen that naturally occur in the body: estrone (E1), estradiol (E2) and estriol (E3). Of these forms, estradiol is the most metabolically active, and elevated endogenous levels have been linked to disease.

Estradiol, when used therapeutically, decreases hot flashes and night sweats and improves cognition, mood, sleep and memory. Estriol is a very mild form of estrogen that is elevated during **pregnancy**, and has shown to be protective for breast tissue. It is used therapeutically to treat genitourinary symptoms of low estrogen such as vaginal dryness and urinary tract **infections**. Estrogen is found in very minute amounts in the body, as it is extremely potent and has potentially harmful effects. Elevated estradiol levels are linked with increased incidence of breast and uterine **cancer**. Estrone is the hormone that is produced by hormone conversion in the fat tissue of postmenopausal women, and usually is found in sufficient quantities unless a woman is very thin. Elevated

estrone levels are associated with increased risk of estrogen–dependent cancers.

Estrogen is metabolized in the liver through several phases designed to render it inactive, but keep the byproducts available should they be needed. Estrogen metabolism can follow various pathways to produce three different end products: 2–, 4– and 16–hydroxylated estrogens. When estrogen is metabolized down the 4–hydroxylation pathway, the result is metabolites that are unstable and potentially damaging to cells and tissues.

Progesterone is an estrogen–balancing hormone that modifies the stimulating effect estrogen has on the uterus and arteries. When given alone or in combination with estrogen, progesterone can improve sleep and mood, as well as help strengthen bones. It is important to make the distinction between the biological hormone progesterone and synthetic hormones called progestins found in many conventional HRT formulations. Progestins are similar enough in molecular structure to natural progesterone to stimulate receptors, but do not have the same activity in the body. The American College of Obstetricians and Gynecologists recommend that progestins be prescribed with estrogen to avoid uterine hyperplasia. But while progestins have a beneficial effect on the uterus, they may be harmful to the brain and cardiovascular system. The WHI demonstrated that when medroxyprogesterone, a synthetic progestin, was combined with estrogen in HRT, there was a substantial increase in risk of **heart attack** and stroke, greater than estrogen alone.

Testosterone is prescribed for women to improve libido, build bone and muscle mass. Supplemental testosterone in women who are found to be deficient can improve mood and vitality, as well as help regulate **cholesterol** and blood glucose levels.

DHEA is a precursor androgen hormone that is used as a building block for other hormones, as well as having activity of its own. DHEA works similarly to testosterone to build bone and muscle. DHEA levels may be suppressed from chronic **stress** and exhaustion, which can be detected on hormone profile testing of blood, saliva or urine.

Formulations of BHRT that include estrogen are typically either a two–estrogen (Bi–est) or three–estrogen (Tri–est) formulation. Bi–est compounds are comprised of between 50–80% estriol and 20–50% estradiol. Tri–est formulas typically contain 80% estriol, 10% estradiol and 10% estrone and may be suitable for slim or underweight postmenopausal women who are not producing endogenous estrone. Progesterone may be delivered orally or topically.

KEY TERMS

Bioavailability—The extent to which a drug enters circulation to be usable at receptor sites.

Bioidentical—Identical in chemical structure to that which is naturally occurring in the body.

Endogenous—Produced or originating from the body.

Estradiol—A steroid hormone produced in the ovary, a highly potent form of estrogen.

Estriol—A steroid hormone thought to be the metabolic byproduct of estrone and estradiol. It is produced in higher concentrations during pregnancy.

Estrone—A steroid hormone that is metabolically weaker than estradiol but more potent thatn estriol.

Precautions

The Women's Health Initiative was a large–scale clinical trial with several arms, aimed at studying the effects of conventional hormone replacement therapy. The study evaluating combined estrogen–progestin therapy was discontinued due to the preponderance of negative effects of HRT. Proponents of bioidentical hormone replacement therapy suggest that it is a safer alternative to conventional HRT because it is identical to endogenous hormone in its activity and metabolism. However, further research is needed to fully assess the risks and benefits associated with BHRT. As of early 2008, conservative recommendations for bioidentical hormone therapy limit use to five years or less, using the lowest dose to achieve desired results.

Side Effects

Bioidentical hormone replacement therapy is generally well–tolerated, with fewer side effects than are found with conventional hormone replacement therapy: **headache**, breast tenderness, digestive symptoms, vaginal discharge or spotting. Symptoms to be concerned about include chest **pain**, **dizziness** or fainting, change in speech or vision, breast lumps and abnormal vaginal bleeding.

Interactions

Bioidentical estrogens should be avoided in women with a history of estrogen–dependent cancer. Women with a family history of breast cancer may consider avoiding supplemental estrogens. BHRT may also not be suitable for women with a history of stroke or heart attack, **blood clots** or liver problems.

Resources

BOOKS

Hudson, Tori, ND. *Women's Encyclopedia of Natural Medicine: Alternative Therapies and Integrative Medicine.* Los Angeles, CA: Keats Publishing, 1999.

Lee, John R and Virginia Hopkins. *What Your Doctor May Not Tell You About Menopause: The Breakthrough Book on Natural Hormone Balance.* New York, NY: Time Warner Book Group. 2004.

Lee, John R., Jesse Hanley, MD and Virginia Hopkins. *What Your Doctor May Not Tell You About Perimenopause: Balance Your Hormones and Your Life from Thirty to Fifty.* New York, NY: Time Warner Book Group. 1999.

Love, Susan. *Susan Love's Menopause and Hormone Book: Making Informed Choices.* New York, NY:Three Rivers Press. 2003.

Northrup, Christiane. *The Wisdom of Menopause: Creating Physical and Emotional Health and Healing During the Change.* New York, NY: Bantam Dell. 2003.

PERIODICALS

Anderson, GL, Limacher M, Assaf AR, et al. "Effects of Conjugated Equine Estrogen in Postmenopausal Women with Hysterectomy: the Women's Health Initiative Randomized Controlled Trial." *JAMA*. 2004;291(14):1701–1712.

Cirigliano M. "Bioidentical Hormone Therapy: A Review of the Evidence." *Journal of Women's Health.* 2007 Jun;16(5):600–631.

Eden, JA, NF Hacker, M Fortune. "Three Cases of Endometrial Cancer Associated with "Bioidentical" Hormone Replacement Therapy." *Medical Journal of Australia.* 2007;187(4):244–245.

Hays, B. "Solving the Puzzle of Hormone Replacement." *Alternative Therapies.* 2007;13(3):50–57.

Lewis J.G., H. McGill, V.M. Patton et al. "Caution on the Use of Saliva Measurements to Monitor Absorption of Progesterone from Transdermal Creams in Postmenopausal Women." *Maturitas.* 2002 Jan 30;41(1):1–6.

Moskowitz, D. "A Comprehensive Review of the Safety and Efficacy of Bioidentical Hormones for the Management of Menopause and Related Health Risks." *Alternative Medicine Review.* 2006;11(3):208–223.

Nelson H.D., Humphrey L.L., Nygren P. et al. "Postmenopausal Hormone Replacement Therapy; Scientific Review." *JAMA.* 2002;288:872–881.

North American Menopause Society. "Position Statement: Estrogen and Progesten Use in Peri– and Postmenopausal Women." *Menopause.* March 2007; 14(1):168–182.

Rossouw J.E., G.L. Anderson, R.L. Prentice et al. "Risks and Benefits of Estrogen Plus Progestin in Healthy Postmenopausal Women: Principal Results From the Women's Health Initiative Randomized Trial." *JAMA.* 2002;288:321–333.

Yager, J.D. "Endogenous Estrogens as Carcinogens Through Metabolic Activation." *Journal of the National Cancer Institute Monographs.* 2000; 27:67–73.

ORGANIZATIONS

Women in Balance, P.O. Box 5517, Washington, DC, 20016, http://www.womeninbalance.

Women to Women, P.O. Box 306, Portland, ME, 04112, (800)798 7902, http://www.womentowomen.com.

Diana Christoff Quinn, ND

Biological dentistry *see* **Holistic dentistry**

Biota

Description

Biota, the common name for *Biota orientalis,* is used in Chinese healing and called *bai zi ren.* In English biota is sometimes called oriental arborvitae.

Biota is a slow-growing tree native to China. It grows to a height of about 45 ft (15 m) in moist, well-drained soils throughout East Asia. It tolerates air pollution well and will grow in cities. When cultivated, biota produces an abundant seed crop. The leaves and seeds are used in healing. A yellow dye can be made from the young branches. Many varieties of biota are used for ornamental landscaping.

Biota, the herb, is sometimes confused with *Thuja occidentalis.* **Thuja** is a North American tree in the cedar family that is called American arbor vitae. The leaves of thuja are sometimes used by Western herbalists but are used in very different ways from *B. orientalis.*

General use

Biota is one of the less important of the 50 fundamental herbs of Chinese herbalism. In Chinese herbalism, biota is said to have a neutral nature and a sweet, acid taste. It is associated primarily with the heart and digestive system and is often a component of *shen* tonics.

Biota seeds are used as a sedative, to help disperse **anxiety** and fear, and to alleviate **insomnia**. Other uses are to treat heart palpitations, nervous disorders, night sweats, and **constipation**. Biota is said to be especially helpful for treating constipation in the elderly due to its oily nature.

Biota leaves, either fresh or dried, are used to treat a variety of conditions, including the following:

> **Shen**—One of the five body energies, influencing mental, spiritual, and creative energy. Shen tonics address deficiencies in this type of energy.

- various kinds of bleeding
- bacterial infection
- fever
- cough
- bronchitis
- asthma
- premature baldness
- skin infections
- mumps
- arthritis pain
- dysentery caused by bacteria
- constipation

As an herb, biota has not received much attention from scientists. There have been very few chemical analyses or test-tube studies done on biota leaves or seeds in either Asia or the United States and no reported studies done on humans. Virtually all health claims for this herb are based on its use in **traditional Chinese medicine** and observations of herbalists rather than controlled scientific studies.

Preparations

Biota seeds are prepared by boiling, and extracts are made of the leaves. Commercially most biota is sold as capsules. Most often biota is used as part of a formula or tonic. It is a component of formulas that tend to stimulate the heart and relieve **stress**, **fatigue**, and forgetfulness.

Biota is one ingredient of the cerebral tonic pills called *bu nao wan.* These pills are used to improve concentration and treat conditions such as **Alzheimer's disease**. They are also given to combat restlessness and agitation.

Another common formula that contains biota is ginseng and zizyphus (*tian wang bu xin dan*). This formula treats insomnia and disturbed sleep, nightmares, anxiety, restlessness, forgetfulness, heart palpitations, and hard, dry bowel movements. It is available in both tea and capsule form. Dosage varies considerably depending on the formula and the condition being treated.

Precautions

Some herbal practitioners recommend that biota not be taken by pregnant women.

Side effects

No undesirable side effects have been reported.

Interactions

Biota and other Chinese herbs are often used together with no reported interactions. Since biota has been used almost exclusively in Chinese medicine, there are no studies of its interactions with Western pharmaceuticals.

ORGANIZATIONS

Alternative Medicine Foundation, PO Box 60016, Potomac, MD, 20859, (301) 340-1960, www.amfoundation.org.

American Association of Oriental Medicine, PO Box 162340, Sacramento, CA, 95816, (866) 455-7999, (914) 443-4770, http://www.aaaomonline.org.

Centre for International Ethnomedicinal Education and Research (CIEER), www.cieer.org.

Tish Davidson, A. M.

Biotherapeutic drainage

Definition

Biotherapeutic drainage is a homeopathic method of helping the body eliminate wastes.

Description

Biotherapeutic drainage incorporates homeopathic formulas to clear the body of toxins. Such formulas, referred to as the UNDA numbers, were developed in Europe during the 1920s and 1930s by George Discri, Louis Reuter and Anthoine Nebel. The foundation for the formulas lies in alchemical metallurgy, and the principles of three types of medicine: anthroposophical, homeopathic, and Chinese. The remedies are referred to as the UNDA compounds.

According to the philosophy behind biotherapeutic drainage, clearing the body of toxins opens the pathway for medicines and other treatments to work at lower dosage levels.

UNDA remedies are made from natural plant and animal substances. The remedies prescribed are dependent upon the goal of treatment.

General uses

UNDA therapies are used as alternative therapies for a variety of health conditions, including the following:

- Digestive disorders
- Spasmodic and congestive disorders
- Nasal congestion
- Loss of appetite
- Emotional strain
- Sleep disorders
- Skin irritation, cuts, burns, warts
- Laryngitis, pharyngitis

Precautions

Some UNDA formulations are contraindicated in patients who have a pacemaker or who take cardiac medications. A healthcare professional should be consulted before individuals decide to take these preparations.

Preparations

Products are available in a number of formulations, including **aromatherapy**, drops, oral preparations, and topical applications.

Side effects

Side effects vary by product. Individuals should discontinue use and contact a healthcare provider if signs of an allergic reaction are noted, including **itching**, redness, swelling, difficulty breathing, **hives** or rash.

Resources

OTHER

Thom, Dick. "Biotherapeutic Drainage using the UNDA Numbers." JELD Publications: Portland, 2003. http://www.healingdragon.net.

Rockwell Nutrition. http://www.rockwellnutrition.net.

Rhonda Cloos, RN

Biotin

Description

Biotin is a member of the B complex family, but is not actually a vitamin. It is a coenzyme that works with vitamins. Also known as vitamin H and coenzyme R, it was first isolated and described in 1936. It is water soluble and very unstable; it can be destroyed by heat, cooking, exposure to light, soaking, and prolonged contact with water, baking soda, or any other alkaline substance. The body obtains biotin from foods such as eggs, liver, and cereals. It is also synthesized in the intestines by bacteria.

General use

Biotin is utilized by every cell in the body and contributes to the health of skin, hair, nerves, bone marrow, sex glands, and sebaceous glands. Apart from being a vital cofactor to several enzymes, biotin is essential in carbohydrate metabolism and the synthesis of fatty acids. It is also involved in the transformation of **amino acids** into protein. Biotin is involved with cell growth and division through its role in the manufacture of DNA and RNA, the genetic components of cells.

Adequate biotin is required for healthy nails and hair, and biotin deficiency is known to be a factor in balding and the premature graying of hair. Some practitioners claim that, as part of an orthomolecular regime, it can reverse the graying of hair. When para-aminobenzoic acid (PABA) and biotin are taken together in adequate amounts they can restore hair color. Biotin supplements will also effectively treat weak, splitting nails.

Biotin can be a valuable tool to combat yeast **infections**, which are notoriously difficult to fight. In their book *The Yeast Syndrome*, John Parks Trowbridge and Morton Walker describe how adequate levels of biotin can prevent *Candida albicans* from developing from its yeast-like state into fungal form, in which it sends out mycelium that further invade body organs.

Seborrheic **dermatitis**, or Leiner's disease, which is a non-itchy, red scaling rash affecting infants during the first three months of life, is also treated with biotin and other B complex vitamins.

Biotin has been used in conjunction with other nutrients as part of weight loss programs, as it aids in the digestion and breakdown of fats.

High doses of biotin are sometimes used by the allopathic medical profession to treat diabetes since it enhances sensitivity to insulin and effectively increases levels of enzymes involved in glucose metabolism. Research reported indicates that a combination of **chromium** picolinate and biotin may improve glucose management in 15% of patients who have type 2 diabetes. Biotin is also used to treat patients with **peripheral neuropathy**, a complication of diabetes, and patients with Duchenne muscular dystrophy, who suffer from metabolic deficiencies.

Biotin can be found in beans, breads, **brewer's yeast**, cauliflower, chocolate, egg yolks, fish, kidney, legumes, liver, meat, molasses, dairy products, nuts, oatmeal, oysters, peanut butter, poultry, **wheat germ**, and whole grains.

Preparations

The recommended daily allowance for adults in the United States is 30 mcg. Daily requirements are estimated at 30 mcg for adults and 35 mcg for women who are nursing. Supplementation ranges from 100–600 mcg per day, and can be obtained in the form of brewer's yeast, which contains biotin as part of the B complex, or as an individual biotin supplement.

Recommended dietary allowance of biotin

Age	mcg/day
Children 0-6 mos.	5
Children 7-12 mos.	6
Children 1-3 yrs.	8
Children 4-8 yrs.	12
Children 9-13 yrs.	20
Children 14-18 yrs.	25
Adults ≥ 19 yrs.	30
Pregnant women	30
Breastfeeding women	35

Foods that contain biotin

	mg
Liver, cooked, 3 oz.	27
Egg, 1 cooked	25
Bread, whole wheat, 1 slice	6
Swiss chard, cooked, 1/2 cup	5.2
Salmon, cooked, 3 oz.	4
Chicken, cooked, 3 oz.	3
Cauliflower, raw, 1/2 cup	2
Pork, cooked, 3 oz.	2

mcg = microgram

(Illustration by GGS Information Services. Cengage Learning, Gale)

Precautions

The body needs biotin on a daily basis since it is not stored to any great extent. Biotin requirements increase during **pregnancy** and lactation. Researchers have investigated the need for supplemental biotin during pregnancy. Nearly 50% of pregnant women appear to be deficient in biotin, which could result in birth defects (according to animal studies). Scientists suggest that biotin be included in prenatal multivitamin formulas.

Those taking antibiotics should supplement their **diets** with biotin. Certain individuals are at risk for biotin deficiency, including infants who are fed biotin-deficient formula or who have inherited deficiency disorders, patients who are fed intravenously, and anyone who habitually eats a lot of raw egg whites because they contain a protein called avidin, which prevents the absorption of biotin.

Mild deficiency

Because biotin is synthesized in the gut, deficiency symptoms are rare. Symptoms of deficiency may include weakness, lethargy, grayish skin color, **eczema** (which may appear as a scaly red rash around the nose, mouth, and other orifices), **hair loss**, **cradle cap** in infants, muscle aches, impaired ability to digest fats, **nausea**, **depression**, loss of appetite, **insomnia**, high **cholesterol** levels, eye inflammation, sensitivity to touch, **anemia**, and tingling in the hands and feet.

Extreme deficiency

Symptoms of extreme biotin deficiency include elevation of cholesterol levels, heart problems, and paralysis. When extreme deficiency is a problem, the liver may not be able to detoxify the body efficiently, and depression may develop into hallucinations. Infants may exhibit developmental delay and lack of muscle tone.

Biotin deficiency could result in a loss of immune function, since animal experiments have shown that biotin deficiency leads to a decrease in white blood-cell function. Because biotin is essential to the body's metabolic functions, any deficiency could result in impaired metabolism as well.

Overdose

There have been no reports of effects of overdose of biotin, even at very high doses, primarily because any excess is excreted in the urine.

KEY TERMS

Coenzyme—A non-protein organic compound that plays an essential role in the action of particular enzymes.

Lactobacillus—A bacteria present in the gut of healthy people.

Mycelium—Fine thread-like tendrils that are capable of invading body organs and are sent out by a fungus to seek nutrition.

Peripheral neuropathy—Weakness and numbness of the nerves in the fingers and toes, which may progress up the limbs; often a complication of diabetes.

Side effects

There are no side effects associated with biotin supplementation.

Interactions

Biotin works in conjunction with all the B vitamins, which are synergistic, meaning they work best when all are available in adequate amounts.

Raw egg white contains the protein avidin, which prevents absorption of biotin.

Sulfa drugs, estrogen, and alcohol all increase the amount of biotin needed in the body. In addition, anticonvulsant drugs may lead to biotin deficiency. Long-term use of antibiotics may prevent the synthesis of biotin in the gut by killing off bacteria that help the body produce biotin. Supplements of lactobacillus may help the body make sufficient amounts of biotin after long term antibiotic use.

Resources

BOOKS

Shils, Maurice E., ed. *Modern Nutrition in Health and Disease.* Philadelphia : Lippincott,Williams & Wilkins, 2006.

Zempleni, Janos, ed. *Handbook of Vitamins.* Boca Raton, FL: CRC Press, 2007.

PERIODICALS

Boccaletti, V., et al. "Familial Uncombable Hair Syndrome: Ultrastructural Hair Study and Response to Biotin." *Pediatric Dermatology* (May/June 2007): E14–E16.

Campbell, R. Keith. "A Critical Review of Chromium Picolinate and Biotin." *U.S. Pharmacist* (November 2006): 1–4.

Whatham, Andrew, et al. "Vitamin and Mineral Deficiencies in the Developed World and Their Effect on the Eye and Vision." *Ophthalmic and Physiological Optics* (January 2008): 1–12.

OTHER

Micronutrient Information Center. "Biotin." Linus Pauling Institute. http://lpi.oregonstate.edu/infocenter/vitamins/biotin/. (March 3, 2008).

Patricia Skinner
Teresa G. Odle
David Edward Newton, Ed.D.

Bipolar disorder

Definition

Bipolar, or manic-depressive disorder, is a mood disorder that causes radical emotional changes and mood swings, from manic highs to depressive lows. The majority of bipolar individuals experience alternating episodes of mania and **depression**.

Description

In the United States alone, bipolar disorder afflicts approximately 2.3 million people, and nearly 20% of this population will attempt suicide without effective treatment intervention. The average age at onset of bipolar disorder is from adolescence through the early twenties. However, because of the complexity of the disorder, a correct diagnosis can be delayed for several years or more. In a survey of bipolar patients conducted by the National Depressive and Manic Depressive Association (NDMDA), one-half of respondents reported visiting three or more professionals before receiving a correct diagnosis, and over one-third reported a wait of 10 years or more before they were correctly diagnosed.

The Diagnostic and Statistical Manual of Mental Disorders, Fourth Edition (*DSM-IV*), the diagnostic standard for mental health professionals in the United States, defines four separate categories of bipolar disorder: bipolar I, bipolar II, cyclothymia, and bipolar not-otherwise-specified (NOS).

Bipolar I disorder is characterized by manic episodes, the "high" of the manic-depressive cycle. A bipolar patient experiencing mania often has feelings of self-importance, elation, talkativeness, increased sociability, and a desire to embark on goal-oriented activities, coupled with the characteristics of irritability, impatience, impulsiveness, hyperactivity, and a decreased need for sleep. Usually this manic period is followed by a period of depression, although a few bipolar I individuals may not experience a major depressive episode. Mixed states, where both manic or hypomanic symptoms and depressive symptoms occur at the same time, also occur frequently with bipolar I patients (for example, depression with racing thoughts of mania). Also, dysphoric mania is common (mania characterized by anger and irritability).

Bipolar II disorder is characterized by major depressive episodes alternating with episodes of hypomania, a milder form of mania. Bipolar depression may be difficult to distinguish from a unipolar major depressive episode. Patients with bipolar depression tend to have extremely low energy, retarded mental and physical processes, and more profound **fatigue** (for example, hypersomnia; a sleep disorder marked by a need for excessive sleep or sleepiness when awake) than unipolar depressives.

Cyclothymia refers to the cycling of hypomanic episodes with depression that does not reach major depressive proportions. One-third of patients with cyclothymia will develop bipolar I or II disorder later in life.

A phenomenon known as rapid cycling occurs in up to 20% of bipolar I and II patients. In rapid cycling, manic and depressive episodes must alternate frequently, at least four times in 12 months, to meet the diagnostic definition. In some cases of "ultra-rapid cycling," the patient may bounce between manic and depressive states several times within a 24-hour period. This condition is very hard to distinguish from mixed states.

Bipolar NOS is a category for bipolar states that do not clearly fit into the bipolar I, II, or cyclothymia diagnoses.

Causes and symptoms

The source of bipolar disorder has not been clearly defined. Because two-thirds of bipolar patients have a family history of affective or emotional disorders, researchers have searched for a genetic link to the disorder. Several studies have uncovered a number of possible genetic connections to the predisposition for bipolar disorder. Recent studies emphasize a hereditary connection and early research links several chromosomes, one particularly related to bipolar II, to development of the disorder. A 2003 study found that **schizophrenia** and bipolar disorder could have similar genetic causes that arise from certain problems with genes associated with myelin development in the central nervous system. (Myelin is a white, fat-like

KEY TERMS

Affective disorder—An emotional disorder involving abnormal highs and/or lows in mood. Now termed mood disorder.

Anticonvulsant medication—A drug used to prevent convulsions or seizures; often prescribed in the treatment of epilepsy. Several anticonvulsant medications have been found effective in the treatment of bipolar disorder.

Antipsychotic medication—A drug used to treat psychotic symptoms, such as delusions or hallucinations, in which patients are unable to distinguish fantasy from reality.

Benzodiazepines—A group of tranquilizers having sedative, hypnotic, antianxiety, amnestic, anticonvulsant, and muscle relaxant effects.

DSM-IV—Diagnostic and Statistical Manual of Mental Disorders, Fourth Edition (DSM-IV). This reference book, published by the American Psychiatric Association, is the diagnostic standard for most mental health professionals in the United States.

ECT—Electroconvulsive therapy sometimes is used to treat depression or mania when pharmaceutical treatment fails.

Hypomania—A milder form of mania that is characteristic of bipolar II disorder.

Mania—An elevated or euphoric mood or irritable state that is characteristic of bipolar I disorder.

Mixed mania/mixed state—A mental state in which symptoms of both depression and mania occur simultaneously.

Neurotransmitter—A chemical in the brain that transmits messages between neurons, or nerve cells. Changes in the levels of certain neurotransmitters, such as serotonin, norepinephrine, and dopamine, are thought to be related to bipolar disorder.

Psychomotor retardation—Slowed mental and physical processes characteristic of a bipolar depressive episode.

substance that forms a sort of layer or sheath around nerve fibers.)

Another possible biological cause under investigation is the presence of an excessive **calcium** build-up in the cells of bipolar patients. Also, dopamine and other neurochemical transmitters appear to be implicated in bipolar disorder and these are under intense investigation.

Over one-half of patients diagnosed with bipolar disorder have a history of **substance abuse**. There is a high rate of association between cocaine abuse and bipolar disorder. Some studies have shown up to 30% of abusers meeting the criteria for bipolar disorder. The emotional and physical highs and lows of cocaine use correspond to the manic depression of the bipolar patient, making the disorder difficult to diagnose.

For some bipolar patients, manic and depressive episodes coincide with seasonal changes. Depressive episodes are typical during winter and fall, and manic episodes are more probable in the spring and summer months.

Symptoms of bipolar depressive episodes include low energy levels, feelings of despair, difficulty concentrating, extreme fatigue, and psychomotor retardation (slowed mental and physical capabilities). Manic episodes are characterized by feelings of euphoria, lack of inhibitions, racing thoughts, diminished need

for sleep, talkativeness, risk taking, and irritability. In extreme cases, mania can induce hallucinations and other psychotic symptoms such as grandiose illusions.

Diagnosis

Bipolar disorder usually is diagnosed and treated by a psychiatrist and/or a psychologist with medical assistance. In addition to an interview, several clinical inventories or scales may be used to assess the patient's mental status and determine the presence of bipolar symptoms. These include the Millon Clinical Multiaxial Inventory III (MCMI-III), Minnesota Multiphasic Personality Inventory II (MMPI-2), the Internal State Scale (ISS), the Self-Report Manic Inventory (SRMI), and the Young Mania Rating Scale (YMRS). The tests are verbal and/or written and are administered in both hospital and outpatient settings.

Psychologists and psychiatrists typically use the criteria listed in the *Diagnostic and Statistical Manual of Mental Disorders, Fourth Edition (DSM-IV)* as a guideline for diagnosis of bipolar disorder and other mental illnesses. *DSM-IV* describes a manic episode as an abnormally elevated or irritable mood lasting a period of at least one week that is distinguished by at least three of the mania symptoms: inflated self-esteem, decreased need for sleep, talkativeness, racing thoughts, distractibility, increase in goal-directed activity, or excessive involvement in pleasurable activities that have a high potential for painful consequences. If the mood of the patient is irritable and not elevated, four of the symptoms are required.

Although many clinicians find the criteria too rigid, a hypomanic diagnosis requires a duration of at least four days with at least three of the symptoms indicated for manic episodes (four if mood is irritable and not elevated). *DSM-IV* notes that unlike manic episodes, hypomanic episodes do not cause a marked impairment in social or occupational functioning, do not require hospitalization, and do not have psychotic features. In addition, because hypomanic episodes are characterized by high energy and goal directed activities and often result in a positive outcome, or are perceived in a positive manner by the patient, bipolar II disorder can go undiagnosed.

In late 2001, a study reported at an international psychiatric conference that impulsivity remains a key distinguishing characteristic for bipolar disorder, at least when patients are in manic phases.

Bipolar symptoms often present differently in children and adolescents. Manic episodes in these age groups typically are characterized by more psychotic features than in adults, which may lead to a misdiagnosis of schizophrenia. Children and adolescents also tend toward irritability and aggressiveness instead of elation. Further, symptoms tend to be chronic, or ongoing, rather than acute, or episodic. Bipolar children are easily distracted, impulsive, and hyperactive, which can lead to a misdiagnosis of **attention-deficit hyperactivity disorder** (ADHD). Furthermore, their aggression often leads to violence, which may be misdiagnosed as a conduct disorder.

Substance abuse, thyroid disease, and use of prescription or over-the-counter medication can mask or mimic the presence of bipolar disorder. In cases of substance abuse, the patient must ordinarily undergo a period of **detoxification** and abstinence before a mood disorder is diagnosed and treatment begins.

Treatment

Alternative treatments for bipolar disorder generally are considered to be complementary treatments to conventional therapies. General recommendations for controlling bipolar symptoms include maintaining a calm environment, avoiding overstimulation, getting plenty of rest, regular **exercise**, and proper diet. **Psychotherapy** and counseling are generally recommended treatments for the disease, whether treated alternatively or allopathically. Psychotherapy, such as cognitive-behavioral therapy, can be a useful tool in helping

patients and their families adjust to the disorder and in reducing the risk of suicide. Also, educational counseling is recommended for the patient and family. In fact, a 2003 report revealed that people on medication for bipolar disorder have better results if they also participate in family-focused therapy.

Chinese herbs also may help to soften mood swings. **Traditional Chinese medicine** (TCM) remedies are prescribed based on the patient's overall constitution and the presentation of symptoms. These remedies can stabilize moods, not just treat swings in mood. A TCM practitioner might recommend a mixture called the **Iron** Filings Combination (which includes the Chinese herbs asparagus, **ophiopogon**, **fritillaria**, arisaema, orange peel, polygala, acorus, forsythia, hoelen, fu-shen, scrophularia, uncaria stem, salvia, and iron filings) to treat certain types of mania in the bipolar patient. There are other formulas for depression. A trained practitioner should guide all of these remedies. Compliance can be better with natural remedies if they work. These remedies do not flatten moods and people in manic states do not like to be suppressed.

Acupuncture can be used for treatment to help maintain a more even temperament.

Biofeedback is effective in helping some patients control symptoms such as irritability, poor self control, racing thoughts, and sleep problems. A diet low in **vanadium** (a mineral found in meats and other foods) and high in **vitamin C** may be helpful in reducing depression.

In 2003, a report stated that rhythm therapy, or simply taking steps to go to bed and wake up at consistent times each day, helps some people with bipolar disorder maintain mood stability, especially when faced with psychosocial **stress**.

Recommended herbal remedies to ease depressive episodes may include **damiana** (*Turnera diffusa*), ginseng (*Panax ginseng*), kola (*Cola nitida*), lady's slipper (*Cypripedium calceolus*), **lavender** (*Lavandula angustifolia*), lime blossom (*Tilia x vulgaris*), oats (*Avena sativa*), **rosemary** (*Rosmarinus officinalis*), **skullcap** (*Scutellaria laterifolia*), **St. John's wort** (*Hypericum perforatum*), **valerian** (*Valeriana officinalis*), and vervain (*Verbena officinalis*).

Allopathic treatment

Allopathic treatment of bipolar disorder is usually by means of medication. A combination of mood stabilizing agents with antidepressants, antipsychotics, and anticonvulsants is used to regulate manic and depressive episodes.

Mood stabilizing agents such as lithium, carbamazepine, and valproate are prescribed to regulate the manic highs and lows of bipolar disorder:

- Lithium (Cibalith-S, Eskalith, Lithane, Lithobid, Lithonate, Lithotabs) is one of the oldest and most frequently prescribed drugs available for the treatment of bipolar mania and depression. Lithium has also been shown to be effective in regulating bipolar depression, but is not recommended for mixed mania. Possible side effects of the drug include weight gain, thirst, nausea and hand tremors. Prolonged lithium use may also cause hyperthyroidism (a disease of the thryoid that is marked by heart palpitations, nervousness, the presence of goiter, sweating, and a wide array of other symptoms).

- Carbamazepine (Tegretol, Atretol) is an anticonvulsant drug usually prescribed in conjunction with other mood stabilizing agents. The drug is often used to treat bipolar patients who have not responded well to lithium therapy. Blurred vision and abnormal eye movement are two possible side effects of carbamazepine therapy.

- Valproate (divalproex sodium, or Depakote; valproic acid, or Depakene) is one of the few drugs available that has been proven effective in treating rapid cycling bipolar and mixed states patients. Valproate is prescribed alone or in combination with carbamazepine and/or lithium. Stomach cramps, indigestion, diarrhea, hair loss, appetite loss, nausea, and unusual weight loss or gain are some of the common side effects of valproate.

Because antidepressants may stimulate manic episodes in some bipolar patients, their use is typically short-term. Selective serotonin reuptake inhibitors (SSRIs) or, less often, monoamine oxidase inhibitors (MAOIs) are prescribed for episodes of bipolar depression. Tricyclic antidepressants used to treat unipolar depression may trigger rapid cycling in bipolar patients and are, therefore, not a preferred treatment option for bipolar depression.

Electroconvulsive therapy (ECT), has a high success rate for treating both unipolar and bipolar depression, and mania. However, because of the convenience of drug treatment and the stigma sometimes attached to ECT, ECT usually is employed after all pharmaceutical treatment options have been explored. ECT is given under anesthesia and patients are given a muscle relaxant medication to prevent convulsions. The treatment consists of a series of electrical pulses that move into the brain through electrodes on the patient's head. Although the exact mechanisms behind the success of ECT are not known, it is believed that this electrical current alters the electrochemical processes of the brain, consequently relieving depression. In bipolar patients, ECT often is used in conjunction with drug therapy.

Long-acting benzodiazepines such as clonazepam (Klonapin) and alprazolam (Xanax) are used for rapid treatment of manic symptoms to calm and sedate patients until mania or hypomania have waned and mood stabilizing agents can take effect. Neuroleptics such as chlorpromazine (Thorazine) and haloperidol (Haldol) also are used to control mania while a mood stabilizer such as lithium or valproate takes effect. Clozapine (Clozaril) is an atypical antipsychotic medication used to control manic episodes in patients who have not responded to typical mood stabilizing agents. The drug also has been a useful prophylactic, or preventative treatment, in some bipolar patients.

The treatment rTMS, or repeated transcranial magnetic stimulation, is a relatively new and still experimental treatment for the depressive phase of bipolar disorder. In rTMS, a large magnet is placed on the patient's head and magnetic fields of different frequency are generated to stimulate the left front cortex of the brain. Unlike ECT, rTMS requires no anesthesia and does not induce seizures.

Expected results

While most patients will show some positive response to treatment, response varies widely, from full recovery to a complete lack of response to all treatments, alternative or allopathic. Drug therapies frequently need adjustment to achieve the maximum benefit for the patient. Bipolar disorder is a chronic recurrent illness in over 90% of those afflicted, and one that requires lifelong observation and treatment after diagnosis. Patients with untreated or inadequately treated bipolar disorder have a suicide rate of 15-25% and a nine-year decrease in life expectancy. With proper treatment, the life expectancy of the bipolar patient will increase by nearly seven years and work productivity increases by 10 years.

Prevention

The ongoing medical management of bipolar disorder is critical to preventing relapse, or recurrence, of manic episodes. Even in carefully controlled treatment programs, bipolar patients may experience recurring episodes of the disorder. Patient education in the form of psychotherapy or self-help groups is crucial for training bipolar patients to recognize signs of mania and depression and to take an active part in their treatment program.

Resources

BOOKS

American Psychiatric Association. *Diagnostic and Statistical Manual of Mental Disorders.* 4th ed. Washington, DC: American Psychiatric Press, Inc., 1994.

Whybrow, Peter C. *A Mood Apart.* New York: Harper Collins, 1997.

PERIODICALS

Biederman, Joseph A. "Is There a Childhood Form of Bipolar Disorder?" *Harvard Mental Health Letter.* 13, no. 9 (March 1997): 8.

Bowden, Charles L."Choosing the Appropriate Therapy for Bipolar Disorder." *Medscape Mental Health.* 2, no. 8 (1997). http://www.medscape.com.

Bowden, Charles L. "Update on Bipolar Disorder: Epidemiology, Etiology, Diagnosis, and Prognosis." *Medscape Mental Health.* 2, no. 6 (1997). http://www.medscape.com.

"Family-focused Therapy May Reduce Relapse Rate." *Health & Medicine Week* (September 29, 2003): 70.

Francis, A., J.P Docherty, and D.A. Kahn. "The Expert Consensus Guideline Series: Treatment of Bipolar Disorder." *Journal of Clinical Psychiatry.* 57, supplement 12A (November 1996): 1-89.

Sherman, Carl. "Progress in Bipolar Genetics slow, but promising." *Clinical Psychiatry News.* 29, no. 12 (December 2001): 4.

Sherman, Carl. "Impulsivity a Key Characteristic of Bipolar Disorder." *Clinical Psychiatry News.* 29, no. 11 (November 2001): 35.

"Schizophrenia and Bipolar Disorder Could Have Similar Genetic Causes." *Genomics & Genetics Weekly* (September 26, 2003): 85.

Spete, Heidi. "Rhythm Therapy Can Stabilize Bipolar Disorder Patients." *Clinical Psychiatry News.* (July 2003): 55.

ORGANIZATIONS

American Psychiatric Association (APA). Office of Public Affairs. 1400 K Street NW, Washington, DC 20005. (202) 682-6119. http://www.psych.org/.

National Alliance for the Mentally Ill (NAMI). 200 North Glebe Road, Suite 1015, Arlington, VA 22203-3754. (800) 950-6264. http://www.nami.org.

National Depressive and Manic-Depressive Association (NDMDA). 730 N. Franklin St., Suite 501, Chicago, IL 60610. (800) 826-3632. http://www.ndmda.org.

National Institute of Mental Health (NIMH). 5600 Fishers Lane, Rm. 7C-02, Bethesda, MD 20857. (301) 443-4513. http://www.nimh.nih.gov/.

Paula Ford-Martin
Teresa G. Odle

Birth *see* **Childbirth**

Bites and stings

Definition

A bite is an injury caused by an animal, such as a mammal or insect, that breaks the skin. A sting is a puncture wound made by insects or marine animals. There is often a danger of infection from toxins or venom with bites and stings.

Description

In the United States, dogs surpass all other mammals in the number of bites inflicted on humans. Children face a greater risk than adults, and children under 10 years old are more liable than anyone to suffer serious bites to the face, neck, and head. Cat bites are far less common than dog bites, but they carry a higher risk of infection. Bites from wild animals should be of especial concern due to the risk of **rabies**. More than 70,000 human-to-human bites a year are reported in the United States. Human bites are more infectious than those of any other animal.

The most common invertebrates responsible for bites and stings include lice, bedbugs, fleas, mosquitoes, black flies, fire ants, chiggers, ticks, centipedes, scorpions, spiders, bees, and wasps. Black widows and brown recluse spiders are the two most common poisonous spiders in the United States. The bites of most other spiders in North America cause only minor reactions. Ticks attach themselves to the skin and feed on the blood of animals. Most are relatively harmless, but some carry diseases such as Rocky Mountain spotted **fever** and **Lyme disease**. Now, people worry about the danger or West Nile virus from mosquito bites. Bees and wasps will sting to defend their nests or if they are disturbed. Fifty or more people a year die in the United States after being stung by bees, wasps, or fire ants. Almost all of those deaths are the result of allergic reactions.

The poisonous snakes of the United States are divided into two families, pit vipers (which include rattlesnakes, copperheads, and cottonmouths, also called water moccasins) and the coral snake family. Pit vipers are responsible for about 99% of the poisonous snakebites in the United States. Each year about 8,000 people in the United States fall victim to a venomous snakebite. However, only about 15 of those people die. Most deaths are due to rattlesnake bites. In comparison, coral snakes are responsible for about 25 bites a year in the United States.

Jellyfish, stingrays, sea urchins, sea anemones, barracudas, and coral pose a threat to those who live

KEY TERMS

Antivenin—Antibodies taken from the serum of horses that can be used to neutralize the venom of snakes and insects.

Compress—A cloth used to apply heat, cold, or medications to the skin.

Debridement—The surgical removal of dead tissue.

Edema—An accumulation of excess fluid in the tissues of the body, often due to inflammation or injury.

Electrocardiography—A procedure for measuring heart activity.

Hemorrhaging—Heavy or uncontrollable bleeding.

Necrosis—The death of tissue in response to injury or disease.

Tetanus—A potentially fatal infection of the central nervous system, found in wounds.

or vacation in coastal communities. The majority of stings received from marine animals happen in salt water and are rarely life-threatening.

Causes and symptoms

The typical animal bite results in a laceration, tear, puncture, or crush injury. Cat bites are mostly found on the arms and hands, with deep puncture **wounds** that can reach to muscles, tendons, and bones. Human bites result from fights, sexual activity, and seizures. They may also be due to spousal or child abuse. Children often bite other children, but those bites are hardly ever severe. Human bites are capable of transmitting a wide range of dangerous diseases, including **hepatitis B**, **syphilis**, and **tuberculosis**.

People do not always feel a spider bite. In most cases, spider bites produce only minor symptoms. The first, and possibly only, evidence of a bite may be a mild swelling of the injured area and puncture marks or **blisters**. The affected area may be painful, itchy, or discolored. With more serious bites, there may be severe **muscle cramps** and rigidity of the abdominal muscles shortly after being bitten. Other possible symptoms include excessive sweating, **nausea**, **vomiting**, headaches, fever, **chills**, **edema**, and **dizziness**, as well as problems with breathing, vision, and speech. In addition, a brown spider's bite can lead to necrotic arachnidism, in which the tissue around the bite dies. This can produce an open sore that that can take years to heal completely. The symptoms of bee and wasp stings include **pain**, redness, swelling, and itchiness at the area of the sting. Multiple stings can have much more severe consequences. The danger signs of a severe allergic reaction, called anaphylactic shock, need immediate medical attention. They include nausea, chest pain, abdominal cramps, **diarrhea**, and difficulty swallowing or breathing.

Venomous pit viper bites usually begin to swell within 10 minutes and sometimes are painful. Other symptoms include edema at the wound site, skin blisters and discoloration, weakness, sweating, nausea, faintness, dizziness, bruising, and tender lymph nodes. Severe poisoning can lead to tingling sensations, muscle contractions, an elevated heart rate, rapid breathing, large drops in body temperature and blood pressure, vomiting of blood, and coma. Coral snake bites are painful, and the effects of the venom may include tingling at the wound site, weakness, nausea, vomiting, excessive salivation, and irrational behavior. Nerves can become paralyzed, causing double vision, difficulty swallowing and speaking, and respiratory problems. Poisonous snakes often introduce little or no venom into the victim's body when they bite. The symptoms of these bites are not so severe. However, there is still a danger that the wounds can become infected by harmful microorganisms from the snake's mouth.

Jellyfish venom is delivered by barbs located on their tentacles. These barbs can penetrate the skin of people who brush up against them, even if the jellyfish is dead or the tentacle is severed from the body. Painful and itchy red lesions arise instantly on contact. The pain can continue up to 48 hours. Severe cases may lead to skin necrosis, **muscle spasms and cramps**, vomiting, nausea, diarrhea, headaches, excessive sweating, and other symptoms. In rare cases, jellyfish venom may cause cardiorespiratory failure.

Tail spines are the delivery mechanism for stingray venom. Stingray venom produces immediate, excruciating pain that lasts several hours. They cause deep puncture wounds, which may become infected if pieces of the spines become embedded in them. Sometimes the victim suffers a severe reaction, including vomiting, diarrhea, hemorrhaging, a drop in blood pressure, and cardiac arrhythmia.

Signs of infection in a bite or sting site include redness, pain, swelling, warmth, and a discharge filled with pus. An inflammation of the connective tissue, called cellulitis, may also result. Sometimes systemic, and possibly life-threatening, **infections** develop, especially among those who are immunosuppressed.

Diagnosis

Most bites and stings are minor and do not need to be formally diagnosed. When required, though, diagnosis relies on a physical examination of the victim, information about the circumstances of the injury, and a look at the animal that caused the injury, if possible. It is especially important to retrieve the live animal or carcass of dogs, wild animals, snakes, and spiders for assessment. Information about **tetanus** immunization history and possible **allergies** to venom is important. A physical exam may be required to assess damage caused by deep puncture wounds or severe crush injuries. Chest x rays and electrocardiography may be required to assess severe symptoms. Laboratory tests for identifying the microorganisms may be ordered if there is an infection. Blood and urine tests also may be taken. Testing the blood for hepatitis B and other diseases is always necessary after a human bite, for example. Medical professionals should also look for indications of spousal or child abuse in cases of human bites.

Treatment

Some bites and stings, such as those from venomous snakes, require immediate medical attention, as do a host of others. So often, it is best to check with a medical/emergency practitioner first. Also, once a patient begins treating a bite or sting with an alternative method, if signs of infection or severe allergic reaction appear, he or she should seek immediate medical help.

Homeopathic remedies can be useful for relieving the pain and swelling of bites and stings. If there is a possible allergic reaction, these remedies can be used while awaiting emergency care. *Aconitum* can be helpful, especially if the person feels fearful or panicked after being stung. *Aconitum* should be used while symptoms are intense, and then can be followed a by another remedy, as indicated. *Apis mellifica* is especially useful for bee stings, and it can help to reduce the allergic reaction. *Carbolicum acidum* can also be used to treat an allergic reaction, especially when the person feels sick and weak and has trouble breathing. *Cantharis,Ledum palustre,Hypericum,* and *Urtica urens* are other useful remedies that may be indicated. A 6c or 12c dose of the chosen remedy can be taken every 15 minutes for up to four doses.

Neem, an Ayurvedan remedy, can be used to soothe minor bites and stings as well as to keep insects away. A thick paste can be made from neem powder blended with warm water. It can then be applied to the affected area twice daily. To prevent insect bites altogether, neem oil can be rubbed on exposed skin as a repellant. Another Ayurvedic remedy for soothing insect bites uses the herb cilantro. One cup of the fresh leaves should be mixed with 1/3 cup of water in a blender and strained. The juice should be stored in the refrigerator, and 2 tbsp can be taken three times per day. The pulp should be saved and applied directly to affected areas once or twice daily.

A compress made from meat tenderizer that contains either papain or **bromelain** breaks down the venom of bites and stings. This is because most venom is protein-based. The meat tenderizer functions by breaking down such proteins, which neutralizes the venom. A thick paste can be made using warm water or rubbing alcohol and powdered meat tenderizer and then applied directly to the affected areas for relief. Powdered bromelain or papain can also be used. The typical home's kitchen or medicine cabinet holds quick soothers for bee and wasp stings. Bicarbonate of soda or ammonia can soothe a bee sting and vinegar or lemon juice have been shown to help soothe wasp stings.

Allopathic treatment

Minor animal bites can be treated at home. The wound should be washed with soap and water. Applying pressure to the injured area with a clean towel or sterile bandage can stop bleeding. Antibiotic ointment and a sterile dressing can be applied to the wound if necessary. Alternately, to minimize swelling and infection, ice can be applied to the wound. Bites that do not stop bleeding after 15 minutes with pressure should be seen by a medical professional. Medical attention may also be required if there are signs of infection. People who have been bitten by a cat or by a human should always see a doctor. The same is true for snake bites; bites that are deep or gaping; bites to the head, hands, or feet; and bites that may be in conjunction with broken bones, damaged nerves, or any other major injury. If an unfamiliar animal bites, especially for no apparent reason, rabies may be suspected. A physician should be consulted. Dogs, raccoons, skunks, bats, coyotes, foxes, and ground hogs often carry rabies. In cases of suspected rabies, the victim will be given several injections with rabies vaccine. Diabetics, **AIDS** patients, **cancer** patients, people who have not had a tetanus shot in five years, and anyone else who has increased susceptibility to infection should also seek medical treatment for all bites and serious sting wounds.

Medical treatment may require the removal of dead and damaged tissue. Any patient whose tetanus shots are not up-to-date should receive a booster shot. Some wounds are left open and allowed to heal on their own, while others may require stitches. Antibiotics are usually limited to patients whose injuries or other health problems make them likely candidates for infection. Cat bites and human bites, however, are usually treated with antibiotics. The patient may also require immunization against hepatitis B and other diseases. A follow-up visit could be required.

An ice pack should be applied to the area of a spider bite as soon as it is discovered. Treatment for a serious spider bite may involve the administering of muscle relaxants, antihistamines, antibiotics, pain medication, and possibly a tetanus shot. Areas of necrosis may need debridement and skin grafts. An antivenin is available, but it is not necessary in most cases, and could possibly cause unpleasant side effects.

Most stings can be treated at home. A stinger can be scraped off the skin with a blade, fingernail, credit card, or stiff piece of paper. Tweezers are not recommended, since they may actually push more venom into the wound. The area should then be cleaned and covered with ice. Aspirin and other painkillers, antihistamines, and calamine lotion are good for reducing symptoms. People who experience an allergic reaction, or who are at risk for one, should seek immediate medical attention. People who are allergic should carry emergency kits containing epinephrine to counter anaphylactic shock at all times. Ticks can be carefully removed at home using tweezers. It is important to be sure that the head of the tick is not left embedded in the skin. If symptoms such as fever, rash or pain develop after a tick bite, a physician should be consulted immediately.

Although most snakes are not poisonous, any snakebite should immediately be examined at a hospital. If there is time, the victim should wash the wound site with soap and water, and then keep the injured area still and at a level lower than the heart. The injured person should not have anything to eat or drink, especially alcohol, until an evaluation and treatment is obtained. There is controversy about the use of tourniquets as well as sucking out venom. These should only be done when help is far away and by someone familiar with first aid techniques. Minor rattlesnake bites can be successfully treated without antivenin, as can the bites of copperhead and water moccasins. However, coral snake and the more dangerous rattlesnake bites require antivenin. Other treatment measures include antibiotics to prevent infection and a tetanus booster shot.

When dealing with bites or stings of marine animals, the victim should be kept still. Gloves should be worn when removing stingers. The area should be washed with saltwater and then soaked in very hot water for 30-90 minutes to neutralize the venom. Vinegar and other substances are used to neutralize jellyfish barbs, which are then scraped off. A doctor will usually examine stingray wounds to ensure that no pieces of the spines remain. Anesthetic ointments, antihistamine creams, and steroid lotions are sometimes beneficial. If the bites or stings are severe, they may require emergency care.

Expected results

Most bites and stings require little intervention, and clear up in a few hours or days. Those most at risk of severe problems with bites and stings are very young children, the elderly, those who are immunosuppressed, and people who are allergic to venom. Serious bites and stings require prompt treatment to ensure a favorable outcome. Infected bites may require hospitalization and can be fatal if neglected. In some cases, medication and surgery may be necessary. Some snakebites may result in amputation, permanent deformity, or loss of function in the injured area. People who are allergic to stings may experience a severe, and occasionally fatal, reaction.

Prevention

Insect repellant can help prevent insect bites and stings. Those with concentrated amounts of DEET stay effective longer. Sweet-scented fragrances should be avoided. Wearing white or khaki-colored clothing, including socks and long pants, helps protect the skin from bites or stings. Care and attention should always be used when going into wilderness areas. Posted warnings in swimming areas should be heeded. Unfamiliar animals should not be touched. Dead or dying animals should be avoided, as they may still be able to cause injury. When threatened by a dog, a person should remain still. If an attack seems unavoidable, lying face down with the hands and forearms covering sensitive areas may be the best protection. A rabies vaccine may be taken preventively if there is a high risk of exposure due to work or travel.

Resources

BOOKS

The Burton Goldberg Group. *Alternative Medicine: The Definitive Guide.* Washington: Future Medicine Publishing, 1993.

Bennett, J. Claude and Fred Plum, eds. *Cecil Textbook of Medicine.* Philadelphia: W.B. Saunders, 1996.

PERIODICALS

Kuritzky, Louis. "Comparative Efficacy of Insect Repellents Against Mosquito Bites." *Primary Care Reports* (September 2, 2002):S20.

PERIODICALS

"Pain Relief for Stings can be Found in the Kitchen Cabinet." *Contemporary Pediatrics* (August 2002):129–131.

PERIODICALS

Peterson, Lyle, and Anthony A. Martin. "West Nile Virus: A Primer for the Clinician." *Annals of Internal Medicine* (August 6, 2002):173–177.

OTHER

"Common First Aid Procedures: Bites and Stings." *Columbia University College of Physicians & Surgeons Complete Home Medical Guide.* http://cpmcnet.columbia. edu/texts/guide/hmg14_0004.html#14.6 (January 17, 2001).

Patience Paradox
Teresa G. Odle

Bitter melon

Description

Bitter melon (*Momordica charantia*) is a tropical plant that grows in Asia, Africa, the Caribbean, and South America. It is also known as balsam pear. This annual of the Cucurbitaceae family is a thin, climbing vine with long, stalked leaves that flowers in July or August. The plant bears a long, cucumber-shaped fruit that hangs like a pendulum, with small bumps all over it. The plant, which is green when it is young and yellowish-orange when it is ripe, fruits around September or October. All parts of the plant—the seeds, leaves and vines—are used for medicinal purposes, but the actual fruit of the bitter melon is most

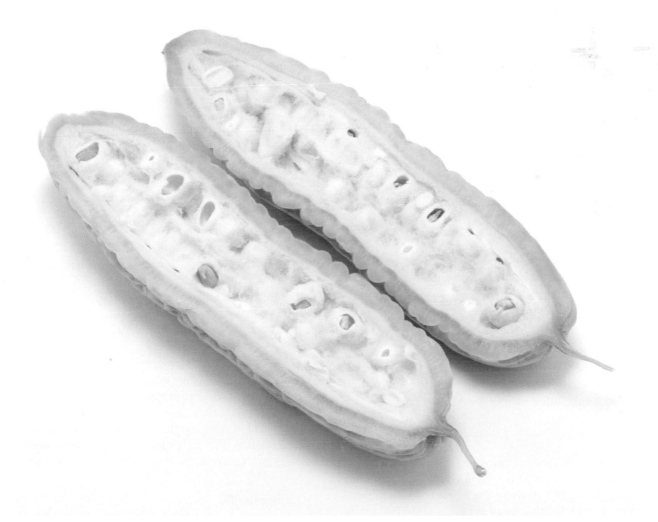

Bitter melon. *(Yiap Pictures / Alamy)*

commonly used. The name of the plant's genus, *Momordica*, is derived from the Latin word for bite, as the seeds of the fruit are serrated and appear as if they have been chewed or bitten.

General use

Bitter melon is used both as a medicine and as a food. It is often added to dishes, for all parts of the plant, as its name suggests, taste very bitter and add an astringent or sour quality to foods. Bitter melon contains a protein, MAP30, that was patented by American scientists in 1996. These scientists stated that MAP30 is effective against tumors, **AIDS**, and other viruses. The plant has been used around the world, from native healers in the Amazon to Ayurvedic doctors in India, to treat diabetes as it is a natural hypoglycemic. In India, the plant is also used in treating **hemorrhoids**, abdominal discomfort, **fever**, warm **infections**, and skin diseases.

Diabetes

Bitter melon has been used to treat **diabetes mellitus**. The plant contains at least three known compounds that significantly lower the body's blood sugar level. The plant's phytochemical composition is a combination of steroidal saponins, charantin, peptides, and alkaloids that contribute to bitter melon's hypoglycemic effects. In the Amazon, the juice of the fruit is used, either alone or in conjunction with a leaf decoction, to treat diabetes. In India, where the plant is called kalara, the leaves are ground up, the juice is extracted, and the extract taken early in the morning for 15 days.

Human immunodeficiency virus (HIV)

The alpha- and beta-momorchardin proteins contained in bitter melon have an inhibiting effect on human immunodefiency virus (HIV) infection, according to a test-tube study published in the *Journal of Naturopathic Medicine*. Bitter melon can be used alone for the treatment of HIV, but it has also been used in combination with other AIDS treatments.

Herpes

True to its antiviral properties, the MAP30 found in bitter melon can also be used by patients with herpes. In a 1982 study of the effects of bitter melon on the herpes simplex virus-1 (HSV-1), MAP30 inhibited the reproduction of the virus, as well as reducing its ability to form plaques (patches of irritated skin).

KEY TERMS

Abortifacient—A substance that induces abortions.

Charantin—A compound with hypoglycemic effects that can be extracted from bitter melon with alcohol.

Emmenagogue—A type of medication that brings on or increases a woman's menstrual flow.

Hypoglycemia—An abnormally low level of glucose in the blood.

Scabies—A skin disease caused by an itch mite that burrows into the skin.

Psoriasis

Bitter melon inhibits the activity of guanylate cyclase, an enzyme that is involved in **psoriasis**.

Skin conditions

Practitioners of **Ayurvedic medicine** have used bitter melon as a treatment for skin diseases, especially **scabies**. The juice is extracted from the leaf and applied externally to the affected area. In **traditional Chinese medicine**, bitter melon is used to treat dry coughs, **bronchitis**, and throat problems. The seeds are used topically for skin swellings caused by **sprains** and **fractures**, and for sores that are slow to heal.

Preparations

Patients who do not mind the extremely bitter taste can eat a small melon. Otherwise, up to 50 ml of fresh bitter melon juice can be taken once a day. Patients who do not want the bitterness of the fresh fruit or fresh fruit juice can take a fresh fruit tincture in 5 ml doses two or three times per day.

Precautions

Bitter melon is an abortifacient, so it should not be taken by women who are pregnant or nursing. It is also a medicinal herb that should not be given to small children and infants due to its hypoglycemic effects. Bitter melon is also an emmenagogue, which means that it brings on or increases menstrual flow in women.

Side effects

If too much bitter melon juice is taken, it can cause mild abdominal **pain** or **diarrhea**.

Interactions

Although bitter melon is commonly used for patients with diabetes, it should be taken with caution. Bitter melon should not be used by diabetic patients who are currently taking such prescription medications as chlorpropamine, glyburide, or phenformin, as well as insulin, for their condition. Bitter melon can increase the effects of these drugs and lead to severe **hypoglycemia**. Patients with diabetes should always take bitter melon under the supervision of a medical or herbal professional.

Resources

ORGANIZATIONS

American Association of Naturopathic Physicians. P. O. Box 20386. Seattle, WA 98112.

American Foundation of Traditional Chinese Medicine (AFTCM). 505 Beach Street. San Francisco, CA 94133. (415) 776-0502. Fax: (415) 392-7003. aftcm@earthlink.net.

Katherine Y. Kim

Bitters

Description

Bitters are herbs and herbal preparations that have a characteristically sharp effect on the palate. The name derives from the Middle English verb *bitan,*, which means "to bite." In the Ayurvedic medical tradition of India, other such groupings of herbs include astringent (e.g. cucumber), salty, pungent (e.g. horseradish or **ginger**), sweet, and sour. Both traditional Chinese and Indian **Ayurvedic medicine** regard the action of bitters as drying. Bitters are also antibacterial, cleansing, detoxifying, germicidal, parasiticidal, stimulating, and tonifying.

While the Chinese and Ayurvedic systems of medicine were familiar with bitters as long ago as 5,000 years, two more recent paths of historical rediscovery and development have contributed substantially to promoting the benefits of bitters. Chronologically, the first of these involves one of the fathers of Western medicine, also regarded as "the father of chemistry," the Swiss physician Paracelsus (1493–1541). Paracelsus is credited with the beginnings of a formula still in use. His development of the formula may have benefited from Marco Polo's travels to China, the opening of the trading route from China known as The Silk Road, and the distribution of commerce through the Venetian trading empire.

A quarter of a century later, the Swedish naturalist and healer, Jonathan Samst, resurrected his family's traditional formula called *elixir ad longam vitam* (elixir for a long life), traceable to the formula of Paracelsus. This mainly European development also branched out to include monasteries, such as the Benedictines, and several European families involved in trade, organized as "Houses." As a result, several Italian, French, and German original bitter herb beverages are commercially available.

The second discovery tradition begins with a German medical doctor, Johann Gottlieb Benjamin Siegert, who in 1820 left Germany to join the South American revolutionary, Simon Bolivar, in winning independence from Spain. Siegert was appointed surgeon general at the military hospital in a trading port town at the mouth of the Orinoco River. The name of this port town, Angostura, is likely familiar to bartenders and gin drinkers. Dr. Siegert, scientifically seeking a more effective means of treating the many wounded who also suffered from **fever** and internal stomach disorders, spent more than four years researching the properties and qualities of local plants and herbs that might be useful to his cause. In 1824, Dr. Siegert, with his privately developed formula called *Amargo Aromatico* (aromatic bitter) used by his patients, family and friends, unwittingly initiated what is today The House of Angostur. This is an industry located on 20 acres in Trinidad, with worldwide distribution.

Bitters include, but are not limited to:

- gentian root (*Gentiana spp.*)
- aloe (Aloe vera syn. *A. barbadensis*)
- wormwood (*Artemisia absinthium*) from which absinthe was made
- dandelion root (*Taraxacum officinale*)
- angelica root (*Angelica archangelica*)
- senna leaves (*Cassia senna*)
- zedoary root (*Curcuma zedoaria*)
- myrrh (*Commiphora molmol*)
- cinchona bark (*Cinchona spp.*)
- turmeric (*Curcuma longa syn. C. domestica*)
- shitetta (*Swertia chirata syn. Ophelia chirata*)
- saffron (*Crocus sativa*)

Other plants may possess the principals and actions of bitters, but are primarily listed in another category. For example, **goldenseal** (*Hydrastis canadensis*) contains the bitter berberine compounds, but is primarily categorized as an astringent.

Alkaloids—A group of plant substances that are basic rather than acidic. They are considered to have strong chemical and pharmacological actions, such as combining with fatty acids to form soap, or combining with acids to form chemical salts used in medicine; may be used in anticancer therapies.

Anthraquinones—A group of plant substances known to produce an irritant laxative effect.

Astringent—Having the characteristic of drawing together or tightening.

Biliary duct disease—Disease of the anatomic duct from the liver, which joins the duct from the gall bladder to form the common bile duct before entering the small intestine.

Crohn's disease—An inflammatory small intestine disease named after the gastroenterologist, Burrill B. Crohn, characterized by symptoms of cramping, especially after meals, and chronic diarrhea of loose, liquid, frequent stools.

Complex sugars—A category of carbohydrate compounds within plants, found to have antiviral and anti-inflammatory effects; they have a more complex structure than the sweet, simple dietary sugars.

Choline and inositol—Two of the vitamins in the B vitamin complex.

Elixir—Similar to a liquid extract, sweetened, and with added aromatic principals, said to be one of the most common forms of liquid herbal medicines for oral consumption.

Extract, or herbal extract—An herbal remedy in which water or alcohol is used to dissolve the medicinally desired components from plant materials. Prepared extracts may be solid or liquid.

Furocoumarins—A kind of compound found in certain foods and plants including celery, limes, and angelica root, known to effect the skin and the immune system; may increase the risk of skin cancer. One source reports that studies with celery lead researchers to conclude that the risk for developing skin cancer is small. Caution, however, is advised, especially with continuous use and significant exposure to sunlight. Fungi were occasionally noted to increase the furocoumarin content of foods.

Furanosesquiterpenes—A sub-class of compounds known as terpenes in the oils of plants and foods that do not contain an alcohol portion. These compounds tend to be found in volatile oils, and are related to the aroma of volatile and essential oils.

Germicidal—Known to kill germs.

Glutathione—Formed from three amino acids (protein building blocks), glutathione is an antioxidant involved in cellular respiration, protection of red blood cells, and the detoxification by the liver of foreign substances.

Irritable bowel syndrome (IBS)—Conditions of the large intestine, which may involve diarrhea and constipation, or alternating bouts of one or the other.

Methionine—A sulfur containing essential amino acids.

N-acetylcysteine (NAC)—A compound amino acid and antioxidant that protects the liver, supports the immune system, and helps break up mucous.

Parasiticidal—Known to kill or eliminate parasites.

Peristalsis—A wave-like action of rhythmic contractions throughout the smooth muscles of the digestive tract, from esophagus to rectum.

Volatile oils—One of the primary chemical characteristics of bitter herbs, these are oils are known for their anti-inflammatory qualities, quick evaporation, and distinctive aromas.

Chemically, the bitter herbs frequently contain volatile oils with anti-inflammatory qualities. Volatile oils evaporate quickly, and have distinctive aromas, forming the chemical basis of **aromatherapy**. Three well-known foods with bitter principles that demonstrate the aromatic characteristic in bitters are coffee, chocolate, and stout beer. Although purveyors and consumers may mask the bitter taste with milk, sugar, or other additives, the bitter action of stimulation of the digestive system remains, and is appreciated by many. In addition to volatile oils, the bitters contain a wide variety of active chemical components, including:

- furocoumarins, also in celery, which stimulate gastric juice secretion and relax the muscles
- complex sugars (complex carbohydrates), which have antiviral and anti-inflammatory effects
- furanosesquiterpenes (a fat in edible oils), with possible antiseptic activity
- anthraquinones, which have an irritant laxative effect

- alkaloids (in chocolate, mildly) with antispasmodic, antibacterial, and pain relieving effects
- other vitamins, minerals, and compounds, some that have demonstrated anticancer effects

General use

For several hundred to several thousand years, the chief medicinal and culinary use of bitter herbs has been to stimulate digestion and improve elimination. This is clearly demonstrated with coffee, chocolate, and stout beer. Nerve endings in the tongue, reacting to the bitter flavor, increase the flow of saliva and trigger a wave-like action of rhythmic contractions throughout the smooth muscles of the digestive tract, from esophagus to rectum. This wave-like action, known as peristalsis, is the means by which food and its non-digestable remainder is moved through the body. The taste of bitters also initiates the flow of stomach, liver, and pancreatic secretions. Bitters, therefore, are known to improve nutrient digestion and absorption. They are regarded as appropriate accompaniments to fatty or heavy meals, which otherwise tend to be digested sluggishly. Bitters are said to tonify and strengthen the digestive system, which may make them useful in the treatment of digestive organs including the stomach, liver, pancreas, and bowels, under the guidance of a healthcare professional.

Bitters also promote circulation. Many anecdotes attest to their usefulness in treating the **pain** of arthritis and rheumatism, animal **bites**, **colic**, **constipation**, and **hemorrhoids**. Their aromatic principals make bitters useful in arousal from fainting. Antiseptic characteristics help in reducing fever, cleansing **wounds**, and the promotion of proper healing. This antiseptic action is a reason why **hops** (*Humulus lupulus*) was used in beer making as a preservative, prior to pasteurization. It is reported that the amount of hops, and therefore the amount of bitterness, is what distinguishes beer from ale and stout (the most bitter). The stimulant action of bitter herbs on the liver, according to one source, makes bitters a first aid remedy for **hangover**. Its purported remarkable effects on gin drinking seem to have contributed to the popularity of Dr. Siegert's Aromatic Bitter in England, and amongst royalty when he first took his product to London in 1862.

Preparations

A number of preparations of bitters are commercially available. Many brand name bitter aperitif (before dinner) and digestif (after dinner) alcoholic beverages and liqueurs have been in use since the mid-1800s. Bitter tonics and extracts, usually in an alcohol base, are available for internal and external use. For internal use, it is recommended that extracts be added to water. Externally, they may be applied on cotton wool as a compress. References to external application also suggest first applying **calendula** (*Calendula officinalis*) ointment or oil, moistening the cotton wool with the bitter herb tonic, and covering with plastic wrap. The ointment or oil prevents drying of the affected area, and the plastic keeps the area warm.

Encapsulations of bitter herbs are now available, which allow consumers to avoid the bitter taste. However, the capsules may be less effective since arousal of the tongue is an initiating physiologic factor in stimulating the digestive system.

Sources recommend that users read label warnings carefully, follow the manufacturer's dosing suggestions, and pay attention to adverse effects, if any, that occur within several hours of taking the bitters.

Precautions

The chief, and almost universal precaution noted with the use of bitter herbal products, is that they are not to be taken internally by children and pregnant or nursing women. Another widely found precaution is avoidance of bitters by persons who have diseases of the gall bladder or the biliary ducts, **irritable bowel syndrome** (IBS), **Crohn's disease**, or other digestive disorders. Some precautions also exist for avoidance if one has kidney disease. Since bitters are known to be drying, caution is also advised regarding dehydration, and avoidance of the simultaneous use or overuse of alcohol products, which are also known to be drying.

Side effects

In general, bitters may cause dehydration in children, and uterine bleeding and miscarriage in women. Individual ingredients may also produce undesirable side effects. For example, **angelica** root may cause hormonal imbalances in children. It may also cause skin sensitivities, especially for persons with **psoriasis**, when used with prolonged exposure to sunlight. **Senna** may cause severe abdominal cramping. Both angelica root and senna are the herbs found in a noted bitter herb tonic. One source advises the universal precaution of paying particular attention to **dizziness**, **nausea**, or skin **rashes**, especially if they occur within several hours of taking a product.

To limit or avoid side effects, sources recommend following the directions of the manufacturer, one's healthcare professional provider, and general health guidelines.

Interactions

The following interactions pertain to the use of bitter herb formulas.

Herb-alternative drug favorable interactions

Formulas using **dandelion** root and leaf as part of the treatment for liver or gall bladder disease, are reported to be facilitated by supplements that contain **methionine**, **choline** and **inositol**, and N-acetylcysteine (NAC). Assistance from a healthcare professional is recommended.

Formulas using dandelion root and leaf as part of the treatment for kidney disease, are reported to be facilitated by supplements. Assistance from a healthcare professional is recommended.

Herb-drug unfavorable interactions

Formulas using any of the berberine compound herbs such as goldenseal, oregon grape root (*Berberis aquifolium*), or **barberry** (*Berberis vulgaris*), for example, are reported to be contraindicated with the use of tetracycline antibiotics.

Formulas using dandelion root or leaf are reported to be contraindicated with **potassium** sparing diuretics, such as amiloride.

Formulas using sedatives such as hops are generally contraindicated with antidepressants, **smoking** cessation prescriptions, or sedatives, and are specifically contraindicated with bupropion and buspirone.

Herb-food unfavorable interactions

No specific unfavorable interactions have been found. However, precautions exist against potential interactions between bitter herb formulas and nonprescription, over the counter (OTC) drugs containing **caffeine** or an alcohol base. Sources recommend following all label advisories.

Resources

BOOKS

Meletis, Chris D., N.D. *Natural Health Magazine, Complete Guide to Safe Herbs.* New York: D.K. Publishing, Inc., 2002.

White, Linda B., and Steven Foster. *The Herbal Drugstore.* Rodale Press, 2000.

OTHER

Angostura, Ltd. "The Story of Angostura Bitters." [cited April 26, 2004]. http://www.angostura.com/test/flash/history.shtml.

Blumenthal, Mark. "A Matter of Taste; Herbal Bitters Can Help Sweeten Up Your Life." *EastWest* 19 (1989) [cited April 26, 2004]. http://galenet.galegroup.com/servlet/HWRC.

Claff, Chester E. A., Jr., Ph.D., "Translator's Guide to Organic Chemical Nomenclature." *Translation Journal, Science and Technology* May 3, 2003 [cited April 26, 2004]. http://accurapid.com/journal/15org.htm.

"Furocoumarins." Committee on Toxicity of Chemicals in Food, Consumer Products and the Environment. *Furocoumarins, Toxicity.* [cited April 29, 2004]. http://www.archive.official-documents.co.uk/document/doh/toxicity/chap-1c.htm.

"Herbal Bitters." *RemedyFind* 2000–2003 [cited April 26, 2004]. http://remedyfind.com/rem.asp?ID = 242.

"The Long Elixir of Life." *Swedish Bitters* [cited April 26, 2004]. http://www.SwedishBitters.com.

"Swedish bitters, ancient herbal remedy, revived." *Better Nutrition for Today's Living* 57 (1995) [cited April 26, 2004]. http://galenet.galegroup.com/servlet/HWRC.

Katy Nelson, N.D.

Black cohosh

Description

Black cohosh (*Cimicufuga racemosa*) is a member of the Ranunculaceae family. Its nicknames of squawroot and snakeroot denote its Algonquian heritage and differentiate it from the common snake root plant (*Aristolochia serpentaria*). It should also not be confused with **blue cohosh** (*Caulophyllum thalictroides*); their only similarity is that both are roots.

Black cohosh grows from a gnarled black root, hence its name; it has a smooth stem and big multiple leaves with jagged edges. In summer, white flowers develop from what are called racemes. These flowers emit a stinky odor. Able to grow to 9 ft (3 m) tall, black cohosh is native to North America and is found on hills and in forests located at high levels. It is found from Ontario, Canada to Maine to the southern states of Georgia and Missouri.

Black cohosh contains several components, as outlined by Phyllis A. Balch in her book *Prescription for Nutritional Healing*:

- actaeine
- cimicifugin
- estrogenic substances
- isoferulic acid
- oleic acid
- palmitic acid
- pantothenic acid

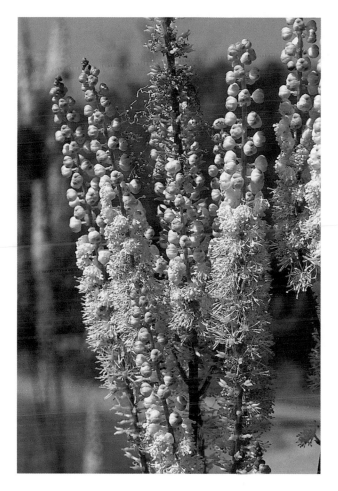

Black cohosh plants. *(©PlantaPhile, Germany. Reproduced by permission.)*

- phosphorus
- racemosin
- tannins
- triterpenes
- vitamin A

General use

Black cohosh has a history of usage for women's health problems, dating back to the Algonquian natives living in the Ohio Valley. However, according to Michael Castleman in his 1991 book *The Healing Herbs*, the Algonquians also boiled the roots in water and drank the concoction for **fatigue**, arthritis, **sore throat**, and a typical occurrence of that time, rattlesnake **bites**. The Eclectic doctors of the 1800s also recommended black cohosh for what they called hysterical diseases, i.e. female reproductive diseases, as well as for fevers, **rashes**, sleeplessness, and **malaria**. A popular patent medicine company of the same era,

the Lydia E. Pinkham's Vegetable Compound, sold a potion containing black cohosh for menstrual complaints.

In the early 2000s, black cohosh is still used for gynecological problems from **menstruation** to **menopause**, with several studies between 1965 and the early 2000s backing up this pattern of usage. A 2002 study of menopausal women in the San Francisco Bay Area found that women taking black cohosh and other herbal remedies for their symptoms reported higher satisfaction with their treatment than women receiving conventional allopathic therapy.

The most famous research was a 1982 open study in which 629 women took 80 mg of black cohosh over a period of six to eight weeks. Over 80% of the women experienced relief from several menopausal symptoms— hot flashes, perspiration, headaches, vertigo, heart palpitations, irritability, sleep disturbances, and **depression**. A later random study focused on 60 women under 40 years of age who had hysterectomies, with one ovary remaining. The women were either given black cohosh or hormone replacement therapy (HRT) of estrogen or estrogen-progestin combinations. Although the HRT met with better results, the study concluded that black cohosh was a favorable natural alternative for post hysterectomy.

A 1998 German clinical study showed that black cohosh has good therapeutic results in treating symptoms of menopause but that black cohosh did not show any hormone-like activity as previously thought. A second German study, published in 2002, reported that black cohosh has antiestrogenic effects.

Because the collective results of a number of studies show synthetic hormone replacement therapy, which contains estrogen, increases **breast cancer** risk by 1–30%, black cohosh is being considered as an alternative. A 1998 study at the University of Bridgeport in Connecticut reviewed eight previous studies of black cohosh as treatment for menopausal symptoms. This study stated that black cohosh is a safe alternative to estrogen replacement therapy (ERT) for women for whom ERT is contraindicated and for women who declined ERT. Some contraindicated conditions from ERT include a history of estrogen-dependent **cancer**, unidentified uterine bleeding, liver disease, gallbladder disease, **endometriosis**, **uterine fibroids**, and **fibrocystic breast disease**.

In a 1999 *in vitro* study at the New York College of Osteopathic Medicine, several herbs, including black cohosh, **hops**, and vitex, were shown to inhibit the growth of T-47D cells. The study concluded that these herbs may be useful in preventing breast cancer.

A 1999–2000 study at Cedars-Sinai Hospital in Los Angeles, California, focused on the efficacy and safety of several traditional phytomedicines, including black cohosh root extract, to treat women's gynecological conditions, such as PMS and menopause. This study concluded that both **dong quai** and black cohosh are safe to use for relieving menopausal symptoms, but only black cohosh showed efficacy. The study stated that information regarding safety for use during **pregnancy** and lactation is limited and suggested pharmacists study scientific literature to help decide the value of recommending these herbs for use.

A 1999 national survey of 500 midwives belonging to the American College of Nurse-Midwives and 48 nurse-midwife education programs was undertaken by the West Virginia University School of Medicine. The purpose was to determine if colleges were educating their students in the use of herbs to stimulate labor. Of the 172 surveys returned, 90 used herbal preparations and 82 did not. Herbal usage was broken down as follows: black cohosh (45%), **evening primrose oil** (60%), blue cohosh (64%), and **castor oil** (93%). Those who used these herbs did so because they are natural, and those who refrained from using them cited the lack of sufficient research about the safety.

In 2007, researchers at the University of Pennsylvania School of Medicine in Philadelphia published a retrospective study of nearly 2,500 women that found a 61% reduction in the risk of getting breast cancer in women who took black cohosh.

In 2006, healthcare regulators in the United Kingdom ordered that all black cohosh products sold in the U.K. contain a warning on the label stating that black cohosh can increase the risk of liver disorders. German health officials followed suit in 2007, asking manufacturers to include a warning in packages of black cohosh stating the risk of liver toxicity. In 2007, the government agency United States Pharmacopia proposed that a similar requirement be placed on the labels of dietary supplements containing black cohosh sold in the United States, warning of potential liver damage. The proposed warning, still under consideration as of early 2008, would state, "Caution: In rare cases black cohosh has been reported to affect the liver. Discontinue use and consult a healthcare practitioner if you have a liver disorder or develop symptoms of liver trouble, such as abdominal **pain**, dark urine, or jaundice." The warning came following several reports in the United States and Europe of liver damage associated with black cohosh use.

Black cohosh can also decrease blood pressure by "opening the blood vessels in the limbs (peripheral vasodilation)" according to a study referred to by Michael Castleman in his book *The Healing Herbs*. A person with **hypertension** should first consult a physician before taking black cohosh.

Other possible benefits of black cohosh are to alleviate **muscle spasms**, reduce **neuralgia** pain, and relieve bronchial **infections** by stopping the compulsion to **cough**. Black cohosh has also been recommended as a glandular tonic.

Preparations

Black cohosh may be taken in capsule, extract, tea, or tincture.

To make a tea, one boils 1/2 tsp powdered black cohosh root for each cup (250 ml) of water for 30 minutes. After it cools, it can be sipped with lemon and honey to mask its bitter taste.

One teaspoon of black cohosh tincture can be taken on a daily basis. Ten to 30 drops of extract mixed in water can be taken daily. Two to five capsules (40 mg/capsule) may be taken daily. The German Commission E recommends taking two 20 mg capsules daily, one in the morning and one at night. These tablets are available under the name Remifemin, a black cohosh extract. A 2002 German study found that these standard dosages are effective for most women and that there is no therapeutic benefit from higher dosages.

Precautions

Black cohosh should not be used during pregnancy except at the time of birth. It should also not be taken by those with a chronic disease or by women taking birth control pills or HRT. Children under 12 years and adults over 62 should start with lower dosages.

The German Commission E recommends taking black cohosh for six months at a time only. However, other studies with animals showed no toxicity problems. It is always best to first consult a health care practitioner.

Side effects

An overdose (over 900 mg/day) could cause **dizziness**, **nausea** and **vomiting**, **diarrhea**, pain in the abdomen, headaches, joint pains, and a lowered heart rate. These conditions could also appear sometimes while a person is taking low dosages of black cohosh. Large dosages can also cause poisoning symptoms.

KEY TERMS

Eclectics—Nineteenth-century herbal scientists in the United States who founded the Reformed Medical School. Their outlook was based on herbal medicines of practitioners in Europe and Asia and uses by Native Americans.

Efficacy—The power to bring about intended results.

Extract—A concentrated form of the herb made by pressing the herb with a hydraulic press, soaking it in water or alcohol, then letting the excess water or alcohol evaporate.

German Commission E—The world standard for regulatation of herbal products.

Hypertension—Another name for high blood pressure, which occurs when blood pressure is above 140/90. Called the silent disease, it often has no symptoms, but if left untreated, it can lead to stroke or a heart attack.

Hysterectomy—Removal of the uterus by surgery either to remove tumors, treat cancer, or precancerous conditions. Surgery is performed through the abdominal wall or through the vagina.

Menopause—Literally means cessation of the menses. Average age of occurrence in women is 51, although it can occur earlier or later.

Menstruation—A monthly occurrence of blood and uterine material discharge from a woman's vagina while she is in her reproductive years.

Oleic acid—Oily acid found in most vegetable and animal oils and fats. Used to make ointments.

Progesterone—Female hormone that prepares the uterus for the fertilized egg. Progesterone is normally produced in the ovaries, except when a woman is pregnant, then it is produced in the placenta. The adrenal glands also produce small amounts of progesterone.

Tannins—Phenolic compounds that occur naturally in plants. Tannins help form proteins, alkaloids and glucosides from a solution. Tannins are found in tea and coffee.

Tincture—Herbs preserved usually in alcohol. The concentration of the herb is usually low, on a strength ratio of 1:10 or 1:5.

Interactions

Women taking black cohosh should not take it together with birth control pills; HRT; such sedatives as diazapam; or blood pressure medications.

Resources

BOOKS

Balch, Phyllis A. *Prescription for Nutritional Healing,* 4th ed. New York: Avery Publishing Group, 2007.

PERIODICALS

Bone, Kerry. "Black Cohosh and Breast Cancer Risk: Benefit Shown." *Townsend Letter: The Examiner of Alternative Medicine* (October 2007): 62(2).

Bone, Kerry. "Black Cohosh Proven Effective in Recent Clinical Trials." *Townsend Letter: The Examiner of Alternative Medicine* (August/September 2006): 42(3).

Hudson, Tori. "Black Cohosh Associated with Breast Cancer Risk Reduction." *Townsend Letter: The Examiner of Alternative Medicine* (August/September 2007): 160.

Hudson, Tori. "Black Cohosh, St. John's Wort, and Menopause Symptons." *Townsend Letter: The Examiner of Alternative Medicine* (January 2008): 117(2).

Rebbeck, Timothy R., et al. "A Retrospective Case-Control Study of the Use of Hormone-Related Supplements and Association with Breast Cancer." *International Journal of Cancer* (April 1, 2007): 1523–1528.

Sego, Sherril. "Black Cohosh." *Clinical Advisor* (June 2006): 104(2).

ORGANIZATIONS

American Institute of Homeopathy, 801 N. Fairfax St., Suite 306, Alexandria, VA, 22314, (888) 445-9988, http://www.homeopathyusa.org.

Australian Homeopathic Association, 6 Cavan Ave, Renown ParkSA, 5008, Australia, (61) 8-8346-3961, http://www.homeopathyoz.org.

Council for Homeopathic Certification, PMB 187, 16915 SE 272nd St., Suite 100, Covington, WA, 98042, (866) 242-3399, http://www.homeopathicdirectory.com.

Homeopathic Medical Council of Canada, 3910 Bathurst St., Suite 202, Toronto, ON, M3H 3N8, Canada, (416) 638-4622, http://www.hmcc.ca.

Office of Dietary Supplements, National Institutes of Health, 6100 Executive Blvd., Room 3B01, MSC 7517, Bethesda, MD, 20892, (301) 435-2920, http://www.ods.od.nih.gov.

Sharon Crawford
Ken R. Wells

Black cumin seed extract

Description

Black cumin seed (*Nigella sativa*)is an annual herbaceous plant and a member of the Ranunculaceae (buttercup) family. The fruit of the plant, the black seeds, accounts for its name. Black cumin seed (also called black seed) should not be confused with the herb, cumin (*Cumunum cyminum*, which is found in many grocery stores.

Considered native to the Mediterranean region, black cumin seed is cultivated in North Africa, Asia, and southeastern Europe. The largest producers of black cumin seed are Egypt, India, Pakistan, Iran, Iraq, and Turkey. Other species, such as Turkish black cumin (*Nigella damascena*), are not used medicinally; and one type, *Nigella garidella*, is even poisonous.

Playfully referred to as "Love in the Mist," the black cumin seed plant has leaves that grow in pairs. The lower leaves are short and supported by slender stems, while the upper leaves generally grow to approximately 4 inches (10 cm) in length. The stalk of the plant, with its bluish white flower petals, can grow up to 18 inches (46 cm) in height while its fruit matures. At first, the seeds (the fruit of the plant) are held in a capsule in the center of the flower. The capsule opens upon maturity, revealing lightly colored seeds. It is only upon their exposure to air that the seeds become black.

Most often, the extract is produced by a process referred to as cold pressing. Temperatures no higher than 140–176°F (60–80°C) are applied to the seeds to help release the oil and preserve its benefits.

Rich with compounds such as nigellone and thymoquinone, black cumin seed is thought to contain over 100 ingredients; many remain unknown. However, experts agree that the most important compounds contained in the extract are the fatty acids and nutrients. Some components of black cumin seed extract are as follows:

- myristic acid
- palmitic acid
- palmitoleic acid
- stearic acid
- oleic acid
- linoleic acid (omega-6)
- linolenic acid (omega-3)
- arachidonic acid
- protein
- thiamin
- riboflavin
- pyridoxine
- niacin
- folacin
- calcium
- iron

KEY TERMS

Prostaglandins—Fatty acid derivatives that are present in many tissues of the body, and affect all organs.

Hypertension—High blood pressure, which occurs when the reading is above 140/90. Called the silent disease, it often has no symptoms, but if left untreated, can lead to stroke or a heart attack.

Hysterectomy—Removal of the uterus by surgery either to remove tumors, treat cancer or precancerous conditions. Surgery is performed through the abdominal wall or through the vagina.

- copper
- zinc
- phosphorous

General use

Black cumin seed has been used for centuries to treat respiratory and digestive problems, parasites, and inflammation. In ancient times, it was a remedy for a variety of health conditions including, colds, **infections**, headaches, and toothaches. The pharoahs' personal doctors are reported to have offered black cumin seed as a digestive aid after large meals. In fact, the extract was found in the tomb of King Tutankhamun, presumably to protect him in the afterlife.

Black cumin was also used as a remedy for skin diseases, dry skin, **dandruff**, and **wounds**.

At one time, black cumin seed was highly valued in Europe, but by the eighteenth century it had lost popularity and was primarily used as a garden decoration. However, black cumin seed extract has regained popularity and is now more widely used as a remedy in Europe and North America.

Many herbalists in current times embrace the healing properties of black cumin seed extract. For example, the extract is sometimes used externally to treat such skin care problems as **psoriasis**, **eczema**, and dry skin, and internally to treat stomach problems, respiratory ailments, and **allergies**, as well as to improve circulation and the immune system. In recent years, the extract has been the subject of immune system research.

One reason that is often given for the medicinal value of black cumin seed extract is its richness in polyunsaturated fatty acids, which help to produce prostaglandin E1. Prostaglandin E1 has many functions in the body, particularly in relation to the immune system, sugar metabolism, skin infections, and **blood clots**. It is also believed to protect the stomach lining.

Experts point out that the medicinal value may be provided by a unique and mysterious synergy (combined action) between the multitude of compounds present in the seeds. In addition, the extract, which is more concentrated than the seeds alone, is said to have greater healing power. A study at Cairo University in Egypt showed a boost in antibacterial activity when the extract was used in combination with antibiotics such as streptomycin and gentamicin. In the same study, it showed additional antibacterial function in combination with erythromycin, tobramycin, doxycycline, and ampicillin, to kill *E. Coli* and the pathogenic yeast, *Candida albicans*. In addition, the study showed that the extract destroyed non-fatal subcutaneous staphylococcal infection in mice.

In 2003, one study noted the antifungal activity of black cumin seed extract against *Candida albicans*. In the study, mice were injected with *Candida albicans*, producing colonies of the organism in their liver, spleen, and kidneys. The researchers found that treatment with black cumin seed extract 24 hours after inoculation inhibited growth of the *Candida albicans*. With continued treatment, the extract significantly decreased the amount of *Candida albicans* found in the kidneys, liver, and spleen.

Aside from verifying its antibacterial and antifungal properties, researchers in recent years have tested the anti-inflammatory and analgesic effects of black cumin seed extract. In 1995, a group of scientists from the Department of Pharmacy at King's College in London found that the extract contains these properties, and is an antioxidant as well. They believe the anti-inflammatory and antioxidant abilities may be linked to ingredients such as thymoquinone and unsaturated fatty acids. Ultimately, the researchers concluded that black cumin seed extract is a justified treatment for rheumatism and related inflammatory diseases.

In 2001, a study performed at the Department of Pharmacology at King Faisal University in Saudi Arabia, reported anti-inflammatory and analgesic activity from the use of black cumin seed extract in animals. Paw **edema** (swelling) was reduced, as was reaction time in response to extreme heat. A 2003 study confirmed the analgesic effects of the extract. Studies in this area are likely to continue well into the future.

Researchers have also investigated and verified the extract's antihistamine activity, focusing on nigellone, an ingredient in black cumin seed extract. One 1993 study found that nigellone acted as an inhibitory agent on histamine (a substance involved in an allergic response, causing widening of blood vessels and tightening of bronchial passages) by inhibiting protein kinase C, known to initiate histamine release. In 2003, another study concluded that black seed oil is an effective treatment for allergies.

Preparations

There are many applications made with black cumin seed extract. It can be found in teas, **cough** syrups, wound salves, compresses, massage oils, and other products. Black seed honey, soap, shampoo, and creams are all available commercially.

The extract has a strong flavor, which is improved by mixing it with honey. Herbal teas also help dilute its strength. As with any product used for medicinal purposes, it is important to read and follow the label instructions and warnings.

Although black cumin seed extract is not normally associated with severe skin irritation, a skin patch test should be conducted before using it for the first time. A small amount of diluted extract is placed on the inside of one elbow and covered with a bandage. After 24 hours, any redness or irritation is indicative of a negative reaction. This test should be done before a person proceeds with more extensive use.

Black cumin seed extract, in these dosages, is used as a remedy for the following conditions:

- Headache. A few drops of the diluted extract are rubbed on the patient's forehead. Some patients may also find it helpful to take 1/2 teaspoon of the extract after breakfast, lunch, and dinner.
- Cough. The dose is 1/2 teaspoon of diluted black cumin seed extract in the morning. A dry cough may require one teaspoon of the extract twice a day, mixed with one cup of coffee or hot tea. The extract can be rubbed on the chest and back for additional relief.
- Common cold. One teaspoon of the extract is mixed with hot lemon tea and honey two or three times a day.
- Diarrhea. One teaspoon of extract is mixed with one cup of yogurt twice a day.

Precautions

Black cumin seed extract is not to be used during **pregnancy**.

Its safety in young children has not been established. Patients with liver or kidney disease are advised not to use this product unless a physician directs them to do so.

Black cumin seed extract is said to lower blood sugar levels; therefore, a diabetic patient is advised to consult with a physician before using.

Side effects

In general, if used as directed, black cumin seed extract is not associated with serious side effects. However, it has been reported that black cumin seed extract has a very low degree of toxicity, and may cause significant negative effects on liver and kidney function. A recommended daily allowance (RDA) has not been established for the extract, so it is wise to consult with a physician before beginning any internal treatment.

Interactions

There does not appear to be a list of serious interactions associated with the use of black cumin seed extract; however, it is recommended that anyone taking prescription drugs seek the opinion of a physician and/or pharmacist before using black cumin seed extract in combination with the prescribed treatment.

Resources

BOOKS

Luetjohann, S. *The Healng Power of Black Cumin.* Twin Trees, WI: Lotus Light Publications, 1998.

Schleicher, P., and M. Saleh. *The Magical Egyptian Herb for Allergies, Asthma, and Immune Disorders.* Rochester, VT: Healing Arts Press, 2000.

PERIODICALS

Albert-Matesz, R. "One of life's tiny treasures." *The Herb Companion* October 2003; 16: 16–25. 1998.

Ali, B. H., and G. Blunden. "Pharmacological and toxicological properties of Nigella sativa." *Phytotherapy Research.* (April 2003): 299–305.

Al-Ghamdi, M.S. "The anti-inflammatory, analgesic, and antipyretic activity of Nigella sativa." *Journal of Ethnopharmacology.* (June 2001): 45–48.

Al-Naggar, T. B., M. P. Gomez-Serranillos, M. E. Carretero, and A. M. Villar. "Neuropharmacological activity of Nigella sativa L Extracts." *Journal of Ethnopharmacology.* (September 2003): 63–68.

Chakravarty, N. "Inhibition of histamine release from mast cells by nigellone." *Annals Allergy.* (March 1993): 237–42.

Hanafy, M. S., and M. E. Hatem. "Studies on the antimicrobial activity of Nigella sativa seed (black cumin)." *Journal of Ethnopharmacology.* (September 1991): 275–8.

Kalus, U., A. Pruss, J. Bystron, A. Smekalova, J. J. Lichius, and H. Kiesewetter. "Effect of Nigella sativa (black seed) on subjective feeling in patients with allergic diseases." *Phytotherapy Research.* (December 2003): 1209–14.

Khan, M. A., M. K. Ashfaq, H. S. Zuberi, M. S. Mahmood, and A. H. Gilani. "The in vivo antifungal activity of the aqueous extract from Nigella sativa seeds." *Phytotherapy Research* (February 2003): 183–6.

OTHER

Blackseedusa.com. "Frequently asked questions." [cited May 14, 2004]. http://blackseedusa.com.

Peles, U. "Prostaglandin." [cited May 14, 2004]. http://www.peles.com/injection.html.

Wagner, H. "Black seed oil." [cited May 14, 2004]. http://www.amazingherbs.com.

Lee Ann Paradise

Black currant seed oil

Description

The black currant, or *Ribes nigrum*, is a deciduous shrub of the Saxifragaceae family. Though all parts of the shrub are used—berries, bark, leaves, and seeds—it is the oil of the seed that is used most commonly today. Black currant seed oil is rich in **essential fatty acids**, which promote and maintain the body's vital functions. Essential fatty acids provide energy, regulate body temperature and metabolism, protect tissues, and insulate nerves. Approximately 17% of black currant seed oil consists of an omega-6 fatty acid, gamma-linolenic acid (GLA). Another 13% consists of an omega-3 fatty acid, alpha-linolenic acid. **Evening primrose oil** is primarily used for its essential fatty acid content, but it contains only about 8% gamma-linolenic acid, half of what is found in black currant seed oil. Because both omega-6 and omega-3 acids are needed in our **diets**, a supplement of black currant seed oil is beneficial. These essential fatty acids are broken down by the body into prostaglandins, the body's regulating substances that block **pain** and govern many other physical functions, especially in proper functioning of the circulatory system.

General use

Because black currant seed oil is so high in gamma-linolenic acid, which makes prostaglandins, it is a highly effective anti-inflammatory herb. The oil is best used for chronic inflammatory conditions, cramps, and aches. It also boosts the immune system, and helps women with their menstrual cycles and **menopause**, while also easing discomforts associated

KEY TERMS

Prostaglandins—A class of fatty acids found in the body that regulate the contraction of smooth muscle, inflammation, body temperature, and many other functions.

with **premenstrual syndrome**. Black currant seed oil is also used to treat skin disorders.

Rheumatoid arthritis

As an anti-inflammatory agent, black currant seed oil works well in **rheumatoid arthritis** patients by decreasing morning stiffness in their joints. The *British Journal of Rheumatology* has noted that black currant seed oil may be so effective in rheumatoid arthritis patients because of a "reduction in the secretion of the inflammatory cytokines 11-1 and TNF-alpha." Cytokines are a source of inflammation. By preventing their production, black currant seed oil offers some relief.

Cardiovascular disorders

Black currant seed oil is beneficial to patients with cardiovascular problems, as prostaglandins counteract the constriction of blood vessels. Two Canadian studies have also showed that **omega-6 fatty acids** lower blood pressure.

Women's health problems

Because prostaglandins regulate the menstrual cycle, black currant seed oil is helpful for women before and during **menstruation**. Gamma-linolenic acid produces anti-inflammatory prostaglandins, as opposed to inflammatory prostaglandins, thus lessening the severity of premenstrual cramps. Gamma-linolenic acid has also been shown to alleviate the symptoms of **depression** and breast tenderness associated with PMS. Menopausal women have also found black currant seed oil to be helpful.

Skin disorders

The anti-inflammatory properties of black currant seed oil are also effective against skin irritations when taken orally. A study at the Skin Study Center in Philadelphia showed that black currant seed oil also helps with dry skin disorders, as the gamma-linolenic acid protects against the water loss that contributes to **itching** and other symptoms associated with dry skin.

Preparations

Black currant seed oil is available in capsule form. When it is taken as a supplement, one to three 500-mg capsules should be taken daily, unless a physician recommends otherwise. The capsules usually contain black currant seed oil, vegetable glycerine and gelatin.

Precautions

There are no known precautions to observe when taking black currant seed oil.

Side effects

Apart from possible allergic reactions, there are no major side effects with black currant seed oil.

Interactions

There are no known interactions between black currant seed oil and standard pharmaceutical preparations.

Resources

OTHER

Grieve, M. *A Modern Herbal*. 1931. Botanical.com. http://www.botanical.com (January 17, 2001).

HealthQuest. 1998-1999. http://www.hquest.com (January 17, 2001).

Katherine Y. Kim

Black haw

Description

Viburnum prunifolium, also known as black haw, is a shrub or small tree with serrated oval leaves. Its white flowers and dark berries occur in clusters. The stem bark of black haw is approved for use in foods in the United States. It is native to the woodlands of temperate and subtropical parts of North America, Europe, and Asia. Its other names are stagbush and American sloe. Black haw belongs to the same genus as *Viburnum opulus*, the guelder rose, which is also known as **cramp bark**. The two are sometimes used interchangeably and have similar properties, but black haw is more specific in its effects on the uterus. The actions of black haw are described as antispasmodic, sedative, astringent, muscle relaxant, cardiotonic, uterine relaxant, and anti-inflammatory.

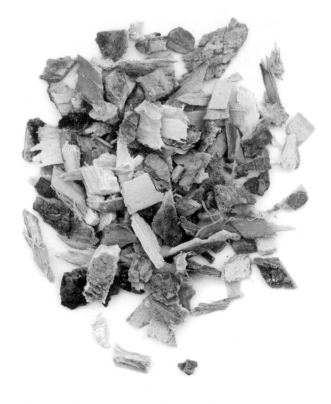

Black haw (Viburnum prunifolium). *(© Geoffrey Kidd / Alamy)*

General use

Black haw has been used traditionally for problems related to the female reproductive tract. It acts as a general antispasmodic that may relax skeletal muscle as well, but is particularly effective on the uterus. As such, it is a potential agent to be included in the treatment of threatened miscarriage, menstrual cramps, false labor, and the afterpains of **childbirth**. The antispasmodic properties of black haw are also reportedly useful for **colic**, bladder spasms, cramping **pain** in the bile ducts, **diarrhea**, and heavy bleeding during **menopause**. Black haw may also have some ability to lower high blood pressure.

The most common use of black haw is as an antispasmodic for menstrual pain. To relax the uterus and relieve menstrual cramping, the most commonly recommended dose is 5 mL (1tsp.) of the tincture in water, taken three to five times daily as needed. Tinctures of black haw are generally prepared by placing an ounce of fresh herb in an ounce of 50% alcohol, and steeping the mixture for six weeks. Alcohol may extract certain chemical components of the herb more or less strongly than water does, so tinctures may exert different levels of activity than teas (generally the least strong preparations) or infusions. Tinctures and other preparations of black haw are commercially available from some herbalists or health food stores.

Black haw is sometimes used to prevent chronic miscarriage. It has been similarly utilized for the condition of irritable uterus occurring in late **pregnancy**. The reported nervine (nerve-calming) effect of black haw may be useful in addition to its spasmolytic properties. One recommended dose for these indications is 1–2 cups of tea per day as soon as pregnancy is diagnosed. Alternatively, the patient may take 0.5 cup per day of an infusion of black haw. A tea can be prepared with 1 tsp of dried herb in 1 cup of boiling water, steeped for up to 20 minutes. An infusion is prepared by putting 1 oz of black haw in a pint jar, filling the jar with boiling water, and steeping for eight hours. This preparation is thought to act as a uterine relaxant but will not prevent a miscarriage due to abnormalities in the fetus or placenta. Women should consult a health care practitioner knowledgeable about herbal use in pregnancy before using black haw or any other herbal remedy when pregnant.

For afterpains following childbirth, 1 oz of black haw or cramp bark can be combined with 0.5 oz of **blue cohosh** root and 0.25 oz of dried **hops** flowers. The mixture of herbs is steeped in a quart of boiling water for eight hours to make an infusion for the relief of uterine pain. This combination is also said to aid milk production and encourage sleep. Small amounts of the infusion are taken as needed.

One of the historical uses of black haw was for the relief of **asthma**. Evidence from contemporary clinical studies does not support this use, although black haw's activity as a smooth muscle relaxant could theoretically relieve bronchoconstriction. On the other hand, some components of black haw, particularly the salicylates, have the potential to trigger an asthmatic reaction in sensitive individuals. Asthma is a serious condition that should be monitored and managed by a health care provider. Conventional medications are available that are generally safe and proven effective to control asthma.

Preparations

The bark of the branches and roots of the plant contain the pharmacologically active ingredients of black haw. These components include salicyclic acid, salicin, oxalic acid, tannins, and scopoletin. The latter ingredient is probably the uterine relaxant. The salicylate constituents would contribute to black haw's anti inflammatory effects. The root bark should be harvested only in the fall. Bark from the branches may be used either in spring or fall.

Fresh plant material from the shrub may be grown or purchased to make teas, tinctures, or infusions. Some of these remedies are described above. These preparations may also be commercially available from professional herbalists or specialty stores.

Precautions

People who are allergic to aspirin could theoretically have a reaction to black haw, as one of its components is a salicylate (compound related to aspirin). Bleeding time may also be prolonged as a result in patients who take high chronic doses of black haw. Patients with a history of **kidney stones** should not use this herb, as the oxalic acid it contains could increase the risk of a recurrence of the disorder.

Some sources say that black haw should not be used in pregnancy. Women should consult a health care practitioner experienced in the use of natural remedies for advice on the use of black haw for the prevention of miscarriage or other possible indications for pregnancy.

Side effects

This species of *Viburnum* has not been well-studied in regard to its efficacy, side effects, or safety, although it has centuries of traditional use in humans.

Interactions

There are no identified interactions of black haw with foods, other herbs, or standard medications.

Resources

BOOKS

Chevallier, Andrew. *The Encyclopedia of Medicinal Plants*. New York: DK Publishing, Inc., 1996.

Jellin, JM, F Batz, and K Hitchens. *Pharmacist's Letter/ Prescriber's Letter Natural Medicines Comprehensive Database*. Stockton, CA: Therapeutic Research Faculty, 1999.

Ody, Penelope. *The Complete Medicinal Herbal*. New York: DK Publishing, Inc., 1993.

Weed, Susun. *Wise Woman Herbal for the Childbearing Year*. Woodstock, NY: Ash Tree Publishing, 1986.

Judith Turner

Black walnut

Description

Black walnut, *Juglans nigra*, is a short-trunked forest tree with a spreading crown that can grow to 100 ft (30 m). It is native to Eastern North America, where it is found from New Brunswick south to

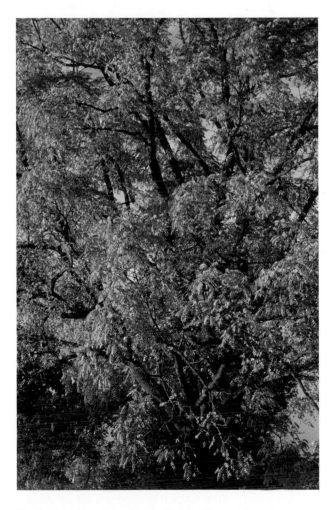

Black walnut tree in autumn. *(© John Glover / Alamy)*

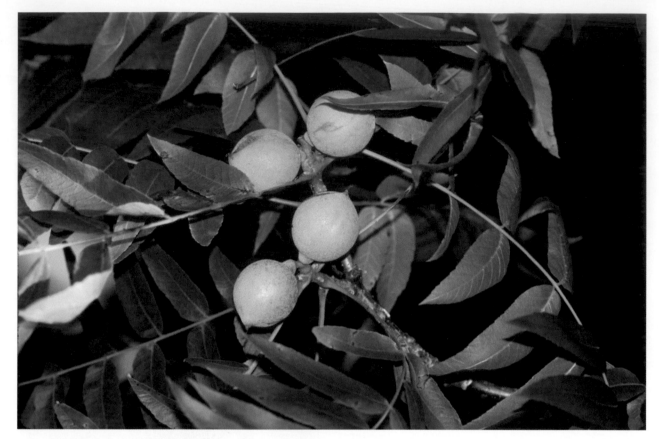

A black walnut tree. *(© Photo Researchers, Inc. Reproduced by permission.)*

Georgia and as far west as Kansas and Minnesota. Although chiefly valued for its decorative fine-grained wood, the tree's bark, root, leaves, and nuts all have medicinal properties. These qualities are similar to those of the closely related *Juglans regia* (better known as English walnut), the tree most commonly used by commercial walnut growers.

General use

The main active ingredients of black walnut are tannins such as galloyglucose and ellagitannins, and juglone (5-hydroxy-alphanapthaquinone). Walnut shells are very rich in **vitamin C**, and betacarotene, B_1, B_2, and B_6 are found in the leaves.

Herbalists use external applications of the plant for a variety of skin complaints including ringworm, **jock itch**, **athlete's foot**, **psoriasis**, **blisters**, **eczema**, scabbing pruritus, varicose ulcers, and even **syphilis** sores. The oil is a traditional hair tonic. Black walnut preparations have also been used for eye **infections** and irritations of the eyelid.

Internally, black walnut extracts are taken for ailments such as **gout**, rheumatism, glandular disturbances,

worms, and parasites. It is also used to stimulate the appetite and as a laxative. Some authors consider it a blood purifier. There is evidence dating back to the 1960s showing that chemical components in the nut may help reduce blood pressure.

An April 2000 report in the *Annals of Internal Medicine* raised hope that walnuts might help reduce harmful LDL **cholesterol**. In a study conducted by a researcher at the Hospital Clinic Provincial in Barcelona, it was reported that substituting 8-11 walnuts a day for olive oil and other fatty foods in the cholesterol-lowering **Mediterranean diet** significantly improved the diet's effectiveness. In fact, the average reduction of LDL cholesterol in walnut dieters was twice that of participants using the traditional Mediterranean diet. However, the walnuts were added to a diet already known to be healthy, so the findings do not necessarily imply that addition of the nuts to a less nutritious diet would have a similar effect.

The ancient Doctrine of Signatures stated that hints to the healing properties of plants could be found in their physical appearance. In accordance with this belief, walnuts, with their convoluted surface,

KEY TERMS

Laminitis—A veterinary term for inflammation in the foot of a horse.

LDL cholesterol—Low-density lipoprotein cholesterol. A blood lipid that increases risk of coronary artery disease.

Mediterranean diet—A low-cholesterol diet that emphasizes vegetables and fish, and limits consumption of red meat and eggs.

Serotonin—A chemical compound that acts as a neurotransmitter, conveying information within the nervous system. Insufficient serotonin is believed to be a cause of depression. Too much serotonin may be responsible for migraines or nausea.

Tannin—An acidic substance often found in plants. Tannins are used for numerous medical purposes and are used to tan leather, color fabrics and ink. They are also used to contribute to the color and flavors of tea.

have long been thought useful in treating brain disorders. Discorides, the ancient Greek author of *De materia medica* which has been the foremost textbook of pharmacology for 16 centuries, considered walnuts to have an excitatory effect on the head. This effect has been attributed to the plant's high levels of serotonin.

In East Asia, dried black walnut is used to treat **cough**, **asthma**, and **bronchitis**. In chronic bronchitis and asthma in older patients, it is given two or three times a day for as long as two months. This is said to improve appetite and sleep patterns. East Asian practitioners also employ the plant in kidney stone remedies to ease **pain**.

The plant has dental applications. Homeopaths use a tincture of black walnut leaves to treat cutting wisdom teeth. In Pakistan, walnut bark is used in toothpaste.

Preparations

Black walnut extract can be bought at health food stores as a liquid or in capsules. Amateur herbalists can also prepare their own black walnut teas or salves. One traditional herbalist quoted in the 1989 book *Herbal Medicine Past and Present* said, "I take a double handful of hulls in boiling water to make a tea. Then I add hog lard and boil again to reduce it to a salve."

The following formula for English walnut leaves is from the 1994 book *Herbal Drugs and Phytopharmaceuticals:* "Making the tea: 1.5 g [1.67 tsp] of the finely chopped [leaves are] put into cold water, heated to boiling, and after three to five minutes passed through a tea strainer, Internally as an adjuvant ... for skin conditions, a cupful of the tea is drunk one to three times a day. For dressings and lotions, a decoction of 5 g [5.6 tsp] drug in 200 ml [3.8 oz (US)] water is used."

Another source recommends an extract produced by boiling black walnut bark in water for 10 or 15 minutes.

According to folklore, drinking a mixture of walnut kernel ash and red wine prevents loss of hair, but also tints it blonde. Another traditional preparation was to gargle with juice from unripened green walnut husks mixed with honey.

Black walnut leaves should be collected, free of leafstalk, early in the summer. The nuts are considered mature four-and-a-half to five months after flowering, and are harvested in the fall. Commercial growers use trunk and limb shakers to remove walnuts when the green, fleshy shucks begin to split and the inner nut is a light tan color. They then use forced-air dryers to reduce the moisture content to 8%.

Precautions

Directions and dosages should be carefully followed, as black walnut contains juglone, a powerful and toxic substance that prevents many plants from growing within the tree's root zone, extending as much as 80 ft (24 m) from a mature black walnut trunk. Juglone is especially strong in the roots, but is also found in the leaves, bark, and wood. Use of black walnut sawdust or wood chips as bedding material for horses has caused laminitis. In high doses, juglone is a kidney and liver toxin. Pollen from black walnut trees (usually shed in May) is a common cause of **allergies** in hypersensitive persons.

In their 1996 book *Botanical Medicine: A European Professional Perspective,* Dan Kenner and Yves Requena warn that black walnut should not be used against a cough involving **fever**.

Juglone can stain the skin yellow, brown, or black. This effect is so pronounced that black walnut oil is used to stain furniture and in artist's pigments.

Side effects

Acknowledging the previous precautions, black walnut generally has no adverse side effects when properly administered in appropriate doses. However, users are advised to consult a health professional before using it.

Interactions

Although interactions are unlikely, it is advisable to see a health professional before using black walnut extracts or capsules.

Resources

BOOKS

D'Amelio, Frank Sr. *Botanicals: A Phytocosmetic Desk Reference.* CRC Press, 1999.

Gruenewald, Joerg, Thomas Brendler, and Christof Jae-nicke, eds. *Physicians' Desk Reference for Herbal Medicines.* Medical Economics Company, Inc., 1998.

Kenner, Dan and Yves Requena. *Botanical Medicine: A European Professional Perspective.* Paradigm Publications, 1996.

PERIODICALS

Zambon, Daniel, et al."Substituting Walnuts for Monoun-saturated Fat Improves the Serum Lipid Profile of Hypercholesterolemic Men and Women." *Annals of Internal Medicine* (April 2000) 132: 533-537.

David Helwig

Bladder cancer

Definition

Bladder **cancer** is a disease in which the cells lining the urinary bladder lose the ability to regulate their growth and start dividing uncontrollably. This abnormal growth results in a mass of cells that form a tumor.

Description

Bladder cancer attacks the urinary bladder, a hollow, muscular organ that stores the urine received from the kidneys until it is excreted out of the body. Bladder cancer is the sixth most common cancer in the United States, and the development of new cases is on the rise. Because of improved diagnosis and treatment, however, the number of deaths from bladder cancer has been decreasing. The disease is almost three times as common among men as women, and the risk of the disease increases with age. Most cases of bladder cancer are found in people in their sixties.

Causes and symptoms

Smoking is considered one of the greatest risk factors for bladder cancer. The risk is probably due to the cancer-promoting substances found in tobacco collecting in the urine, and then becoming concentrated in the bladder while awaiting excretion. Other chemicals, including aniline dyes, beta-naphthylamine, benzadine salts, and mixtures of aromatic hydrocarbons also are believed to be cancer-causing agents. These chemicals are widely used in the rubber, leather, textile, chemical, plastics, petroleum, wood, and paint industries. It may take up to 50 years after the original chemical exposure for bladder cancer to develop. Studies have shown that hormone replacement therapy (HRT), a treatment used by many postmenopausal women, significantly increases the risk of bladder and other cancers.

Frequent urinary tract **infections**, kidney and bladder stones, and other conditions that cause long-term irritation to the bladder may increase the risk of bladder cancer. If there is a past history of tumors in the bladder, there is a strong possibility of their recurrence.

One of the first warning signals of bladder cancer is blood in the urine. Sometimes, there is enough blood to change the color of the urine to yellow-red or dark red. However, during the early stages of bladder cancer there are often no observable symptoms of the disease. Change in bladder habits, such as painful urination, increased frequency of urination, and increased urgency in the need to urinate, are all symptoms of bladder cancer. They are also common symptoms of less serious diseases of the urinary tract and prostate gland.

Diagnosis

Several tests are available to determine whether bladder cancer is present. As a first step, a physician takes a complete medical history to check for any risk factors. He or she then conducts a thorough physical examination to assess all signs and symptoms. Laboratory testing of a urine sample helps rule out the presence of a bacterial infection.

More in-depth tests are used to make a positive diagnosis. The intravenous pyelogram (IVP) is an x-ray examination performed after a dye is injected into the blood stream. It clearly outlines the kidneys, ureters, bladder, and urethra to detect abnormalities in the lining of these organs.

In a procedure known as a cystoscopy, a thin hollow lighted tube is placed into the bladder. If any suspicious masses are seen, a small piece of the tissue can be removed using a pair of biopsy forceps. The tissue is then examined microscopically to verify if cancer is present. Imaging tests such as chest x rays, computed tomography (CT) scans, and magnetic resonance imaging (MRI) may be done to determine if the cancer has spread to other organs.

Treatment

Most alternative treatments for cancer should be used in addition to allopathic treatment. A well-developed treatment plan for cancer should be discussed with an oncologist (cancer specialist) or other physician.

Studies indicate that **garlic** may stop the spread of bladder cancer. It also can help reduce the body wasting and **fatigue** that may accompany cancer, as well as reduce the side effects of radiation and chemotherapy. Practitioners recommend the equivalent of one to two cloves per day.

European **mistletoe**, *Viscum album L.,* is recommended to stimulate the immune system and to kill cancer cells. It also has been reported to reduce tumor size. The most widely available mistletoe extract is sold under the name of Iscador. Iscador is available in Europe only, especially Switzerland. A three-month supply can be purchased and brought back to the United States. Mistletoe often is taken in injectable form and should be administered under a physician's supervision.

High doses of multivitamins have been reported to be useful in decreasing the possibility of the recurrence of bladder cancer. Treatment should be monitored by a qualified healthcare practitioner.

Other complementary and alternative treatments include **guided imagery**, local and general **hyperthermia**, and Chinese herbs. These herbs have been shown effective in controlled trials, particularly as a complement to chemotherapy.

Allopathic treatment

Treatment for bladder cancer depends on the stage of the tumor. The standard modes of treatment are surgery, immunotherapy, radiation therapy, and chemotherapy. Surgery is considered an option only when the disease is in its early stages. If the tumor is small and has not spread to the inner layers of the bladder, surgery can be done without cutting open the abdomen. A cystoscope is placed through the urethra and up into the bladder, and the tumor is removed through it. A high-energy laser beam or other cautery instrument may be introduced through the cystoscope to burn away any remaining cancer.

If cancer has invaded deep into the walls of the bladder, surgery will be done through an incision in the abdomen. Part or all of the bladder and surrounding organs such as the prostate or the uterus, ovaries, and fallopian tubes may have to be removed. If the entire urinary bladder is removed, an alternate place must be created for the urine to be stored before it is excreted. To do this, the ureters are connected to a surgically created opening in the skin, called a stoma. This procedure is called a urostomy. A procedure can create a new bladder (called a neo-bladder) using a portion of the patient's intestine.

Radiation therapy uses high-energy rays to kill cancer cells. It is generally used after surgery to destroy any cancer cells that have not been removed during surgery. In addition, if the tumor is large or is in a location that makes surgery difficult, radiation may shrink the tumor prior to surgery. Radiation is sometimes used together with chemotherapy in place of surgery. Radiation therapy eases **pain**, bleeding, and blockages in cases of advanced bladder cancer.

Chemotherapy uses drugs to destroy cancer cells. Generally a combination of drugs is more effective than any single drug in treating bladder cancer. Medications are either introduced into the bloodstream by injecting them into a vein in the arm, or they may be taken orally in pill form. Anticancer drugs may also be introduced directly into the bladder to treat superficial tumors. Chemotherapy may be given following surgery to kill any remaining cancer cells. Research has shown improved outcomes when bladder cancer patients were given chemotherapy followed by surgery. In a study of 307 patients, those with this combination of therapy lived two years longer than those treated only with surgery.

Immunotherapy, or biological therapy, uses the body's own immune system to fight the disease. In the case of early-stage bladder cancer, *bacille Calmette-Guerin* (BCG), a weakened strain of **tuberculosis**, may be placed directly into the bladder. As the immune system rallies to fight off the tuberculosis, it also attacks and kills cancer cells. This therapy has been shown to be effective in controlling superficial bladder cancer.

New treatments are continuously being investigated. Scientists have made great strides in gene mapping and research in the twenty-first century. A type of gene therapy on experimental animals has produced significant success and human trials have begun on the new technique.

Expected results

If cancer is detected early and is limited to the inner lining of the bladder, it responds well to treatment. Most bladder cancers are first seen at this stage. At least 90% of patients survive five years or more after an initial diagnosis. However, if the disease has spread to nearby tissues, the survival rates drop to 49%, and if the cancer metastasizes to distant organs only about 6% of patients will survive five years or more.

Bladder cancer has a very high rate of recurrence. Even after tumors are totally removed, there is a high chance that new tumors will develop. Therefore, those who have had bladder cancer should have frequent and thorough follow-up care.

Prevention

Those who have a history of bladder cancer, who have been regularly exposed to cancer-causing chemicals, or who have had conditions that cause long-term irritation to the bladder, should undergo regular screening tests for bladder cancer. This regimen will help ensure that the disease is detected in the early stages and treated appropriately.

Avoiding risk factors, such as tobacco, is the best alternative. Appropriate safety precautions should be maintained when working with cancer-causing chemicals. Working with such chemicals should be avoided. Women may want to discuss with their physicians the risks versus benefits of hormone replacement therapy.

Since **stress** and irritation of the bladder may contribute to bladder cancer, the health of the bladder and urinary tract should be carefully maintained.

Caffeine, which is found in coffee, tea, colas, and chocolate, is thought to be a factor in cancer of the lower urinary tract, including the bladder, and should be avoided. It also is important to have adequate fluid intake to flush potential toxins out of the urinary tract. At least six to eight glasses of water as well as fluids such as plain herbal teas and diluted fruit or vegetable juices should be consumed daily. A dropperful (25–30 drops) of a tincture of burdock seed, *Artium lappa,* will help flush the entire urinary tract, relieve bladder irritation and inflammation, and strengthen the bladder.

Resources

BOOKS

Dunetz, Gary N. *Bladder Cancer: A Resource Guide for Patients and Their Families.* Bloomington, IN.: Authorhouse, 2006.

Ellsworth, Pamela, and Brett Carswell. *100 Questions & Answers About Bladder Cancer.* Sudbury, MA: Jones & Bartlett, 2005.

Parker, James N., and Philip M. Parker. *The Official Patient's Sourcebook on Bladder Cancer: A Revised and Updated Directory for the Internet Age.* San Diego: ICON Health Publications, 2002.

Raghaven, Derek, and Kathleen Tuthill. *Bladder Cancer: A Cleveland Clinic Guide.* Cleveland, OH: Cleveland Clinic Press, 2008.

PERIODICALS

Birkhahn, Marc, Anirban P Mitran, and Richard J. Cote. "Molecular Markers for Bladder Cancer: The Road to a Multimarker Approach." *Expert Review of Anticancer Therapy* (December 2007): 1717–1727.

Karak, Fadi El, and Aude Flechon. "Gemcitabine in Bladder Cancer." *Expert Opinion in Pharmacotherapy* (December 2007): 3251–3256.

Madeb, Ralph, et al. "Current State of Screening for Bladder Cancer." *Expert Review of Anticancer Therapy* (July 2007): 981–987.

OTHER

eMedicineHealth. "Bladder Cancer." http://www.emedicinehealth.com/bladder_cancer/article_em.htm (March 3, 2008).

Medline Plus. "Bladder Cancer. National Library of Medicine." http://www.nlm.nih.gov/medlineplus/bladdercancer.html (March 3, 2008).

National Cancer Institute. "Bladder Cancer." http://www.cancer.gov/cancertopics/types/bladder (March 3, 2008).

Patience Paradox
Teresa G. Odle
David Edward Newton, Ed.D.

Bladder infection

Definition

Bladder infection, also called cystitis, refers to infection and inflammation of the urinary bladder. Urethritis is an inflammation of the urethra, which is the passageway that connects the bladder with the exterior of the body. Sometimes cystitis and urethritis are referred to collectively as a lower urinary tract infection, or UTI. Infection of the upper urinary tract involves the spread of bacteria to the kidney and is called pyelonephritis.

Description

The frequency of bladder **infections** in humans varies significantly according to age and sex. The male/female ratio of UTIs in children younger than 12 months is 4:1 because of the high rate of birth defects in the urinary tract of male infants. In adults, the male/female ratio of UTIs is 1:50. After age 50, however, the incidence among males increases due to prostate disorders.

UTIs are common in females. It is estimated that 50% of adult women experience at least one episode of dysuria (painful urination); half of these patients have a bacterial UTI. Between 2 to 5% of women's visits to primary care doctors are for UTI symptoms. About 90% of UTIs in women are uncomplicated but recurrent.

UTIs are uncommon in younger and middle-aged men, but may occur as complications of bacterial infections of the kidney or prostate gland.

In children, bladder infection is often caused by congenital (present at birth) abnormalities of the urinary tract. Vesicoureteral reflux is a condition in which a child cannot completely empty the bladder. It allows urine to remain in or flow backward (reflux) into the partially empty bladder.

Causes and symptoms

The causes of bladder infection vary according to gender because of the differences in anatomical structure of the urinary tract.

Females

Most bladder infections in women are so-called ascending infections, which means that they are caused by bacteria traveling upward through the urethra to the bladder. The relative shortness of the female urethra (1 to 2 in. [3-5 cm] in length) makes it easy for bacteria to gain entry to the bladder, where they multiply. The most common bacteria associated with UTIs in women include *Escherichia coli* (about 80 % of cases), *Staphylococcus saprophyticus*, *Klebsiella*, *Enterobacter*, and *Proteus* species. Risk factors for UTIs in women include:

- Sexual intercourse. The risk of infection increases if the woman has multiple partners.
- Use of a diaphragm for contraception.
- An abnormally short urethra.
- Diabetes or chronic dehydration.
- The absence of a specific enzyme (fucosyltransferase) in vaginal secretions. The lack of this enzyme makes it easier for the vagina to harbor bacteria that cause UTIs.
- Inadequate personal hygiene. Bacteria from fecal matter or vaginal discharge can enter the female urethra because its opening is very close to the vagina and anus.
- History of previous UTIs. About 80% of women with bladder infection develop recurrences within two years.

The early symptoms of bladder infection in women are dysuria (**pain** on urination), urgency (sudden strong desire to urinate), and increased frequency of urination. About 50% of female patients experience **fever**, pain in the lower back or flanks, **nausea** and **vomiting**, or shaking **chills**. These symptoms indicate pyelonephritis, or spread of the infection to the upper urinary tract.

Males

Most UTIs in adult males are complications of kidney or prostate infections. They usually are associated with a tumor or **kidney stones** that block the flow of urine and are often persistent infections caused by drug-resistant organisms. UTIs in men are most likely to be caused by *E. coli* or another gram-positive bacterium. *S. saprophyticus*, which is the second most common cause of UTIs in women, rarely causes infections in men. The symptoms of bladder infection and pyelonephritis in men are the same as in women. Risk factors for UTIs in men include lack of circumcision (the foreskin can harbor bacteria that cause UTIs) and urinary catheterization (the longer the period of catheterization, the higher the risk of UTI).

Hemorrhagic cystitis

Hemorrhagic cystitis, which is marked by large quantities of blood in the urine, is caused by an acute bacterial or viral infection of the bladder. In some cases, hemorrhagic cystitis is a side effect of therapy or treatment with cyclophosphamide. Hemorrhagic cystitis in children is associated with adenovirus type 11. In some cases, hematuria results from athletic training, particularly in runners.

Diagnosis

When bladder infection is suspected, a doctor will first examine the patient's abdomen and lower back to evaluate pain and unusual enlargements of the kidneys or swelling of the bladder. In small children, a doctor will check for fever, abdominal masses, and a swollen bladder.

The next step in diagnosis is collection of a urine sample. The procedure differs somewhat for women and men. Laboratory testing of urine samples can now be performed with dipsticks that indicate immune system responses to infection, as well as with microscopic analysis of samples. Normal human urine is sterile. The presence of bacteria or pus in the urine usually indicates infection. The presence of blood in the urine (hematuria) may indicate acute UTI, kidney disease, kidney stones, inflammation of the prostate (in men), **endometriosis** (in women), or **cancer** of the urinary tract.

Females

Female patients sometimes require a pelvic examination as part of the procedure to diagnose bladder infections. The patient lies on an obstetrical table with feet in stirrups. The doctor may take a vaginal culture smear. The patient often is asked to provide a urine sample. A midstream urine sample of 200 mL is collected to test for bladder infection. Often, just a "clean catch," or midstream sample, is needed without a pelvic exam.

A high bacterial count in the urine sample indicates urethritis. A count of more than 100,000 (10^5 bacteria CFU/mL, or colony-forming units per milliliter) in the midstream sample indicates a bladder or kidney infection. A colony is a large number of microorganisms that grow from a single cell. Bacterial count can be given in CFU or colony forming units.

Males

In male patients, the doctor will cleanse the opening to the urethra with an antiseptic before collecting the urine sample. The first 10 mL of urine are collected separately. The patient then urinates a midstream sample of 200 mL. Following the second sample, the doctor will massage the patient's prostate and collect several drops of prostatic fluid. The patient then urinates a third urine specimen for prostatic culture.

A high bacterial count in the first urine specimen or the prostatic specimen indicates urethritis or prostate infections, respectively. A bacterial count greater than 100,000 bacteria CFU/mL in the midstream sample suggests a bladder or kidney infection. Children may need to be catheterized (a sterile procedure), in which case a culture of 1,000 bacteria CFU/mL is indicative of infection.

Other tests

Women with recurrent UTIs can be given ultrasound exams of the kidneys and bladder together with a voiding cystourethrogram to test for structural abnormalities. (A cystourethrogram is an x-ray test in which an **iodine** dye is used to better view the urinary bladder and urethra.) Voiding cystourethrograms are also used to evaluate children with UTIs. In some cases, computed tomography scans (CT scans) can evaluate patients for possible cancers or other masses in the urinary tract.

Treatment

Diet

Dietary changes that may help to control and prevent bladder infection include:

- Drinking 8–12 glasses of water daily, which helps to wash out bacteria (although this may also dilute antibacterial factors in the urine).
- Acidifying the urine by limiting alkaline foods (dairy, soda, and citrus).
- Following a diet rich in grains, vegetables, and acidifying juices.
- Eliminating foods that irritate the bladder (coffee, black tea, alcohol, and chocolate).
- Eliminating high sugar foods (sweet vegetables, fruits, sugar, and honey).
- Drinking unsweetened cranberry juice to acidify the urine and provide hippuric acid. Cranberry capsules can substitute for the juice.
- Ingesting at least one clove of garlic (or up to 1,200 mg garlic as a tablet) daily for its anti-infective properties.

Herbals and Chinese medicine

Herbals that possess antibacterial, antioxidant, demulcent, astringent, antiviral, antispasmodic, and/ or diuretic properties are useful in treating bladder infection. Herb tinctures have a more rapid effect than teas. Useful herbals include bearberry (*Arctostaphylos uva-ursi*), **buchu** (*Barosma betulina*), **cornsilk** (*Zea mays*), cinnamon, cedar, pipsissewa (*Chimaphilia*), Oregon grape root (*Berberis aquifolia*), **goldenseal** (*Hydrastis canadensis*), marshmallow root (*Althea officinalis*), kava, and birch. A tincture recipe for bladder infection is as follows:

- cornsilk, 2 parts
- bearberry, 2 parts
- *Viburnum prunifolium*, 1 part
- *Valeriana officinalis*, 1 part

The patient should take 5 mL of the tincture three times daily. An infusion of *Archillea millefolium* should be drunk frequently. The patient can take 1.5 g to 3 g of the Chinese patent medicine Qing Lin Wan (Green Unicorn Pill) twice daily.

Supplements

The antioxidant vitamins A, C, and E may be beneficial in treating bladder infection. The patient should take 400–600 IU of **vitamin E** and 300 mg vitamin B$_6$ daily. Ascorbic acid is irritating to the bladder so **vitamin C** should be taken in the form of **calcium** ascorbate, about 6,000 to 20,000 mg per day. **Magnesium** may be helpful in treating renal disease. **Zinc** may boost the immune system.

Homeopathic medicine also can be effective in treating bladder infection. Choosing the correct remedy (based on the patient's symptoms) is always key to the success of homeopathic treatment. Homeopathic remedies for bladder infection include Spanish fly (*Cantharis*), sarsaparilla, stavesacre (*Staphysagria*), and Oregon grape (*Berberis aquifolium*). The correct homeopathic treatment is effective within 12 hours. **Acupuncture** also can be helpful in treating acute and chronic cases of bladder infection.

Allopathic treatment

Medications

Uncomplicated cystitis is treated with antibiotics. These include penicillin, ampicillin, and amoxicillin; sulfisoxazole or sulfamethoxazole; trimethoprim; nitrofurantoin; cephalosporins; or fluoroquinolones. Treatment for women is short-term; most patients respond within three days. Reports have shown that presumed uncomplicated UTIs in women could often be treated over the telephone when the patient reported her symptoms to a nurse who had a series of prepared questions. Men typically do not respond

as well and require seven to 10 days of oral antibiotics for uncomplicated UTIs. Patients of either gender may be given phenazopyridine (Pyridium, Urogesic) or flavoxate (Urispas) to relieve painful urination. Trimethoprim (Trimpex, Proloprim, Primsol) and nitrofurantoin (Furadantin, Macrobid, Macrodantin) are preferred for treating recurrent UTIs in women.

Over 50% of older men with UTIs also suffer from infection of the prostate gland. Some antibiotics, including amoxicillin and the cephalosporins, do not affect the prostate gland. Fluoroquinolone antibiotics or trimethoprim are the recommended drugs for these patients.

Surgery

A minority of women with complicated UTIs may require surgical treatment to prevent recurrent infections. Surgery is also used to treat reflux problems (movement of the urine backwards) or other structural abnormalities in children and anatomical abnormalities in adult males.

Expected outcome

In many cases, alternative medicines can resolve bladder infections quickly. It is important that patients see a doctor if symptoms do not subside after a few days, or if they worsen. The prognosis for recovery from uncomplicated bladder infection is excellent. However, complicated UTIs in males are difficult to treat because they often involve bacteria that are resistant to commonly used antibiotics.

Prevention

Researchers are trying to develop a vaccine for UTIs. A study of women with frequent infections showed that a vaccine administered by a vaginal suppository headed off bladder infections in many of the study participants. A later study used antigens found on the surface of *E. coli* as components of a possible vaccine against UTIs. Although encouraging results were reported, no vaccine has been developed. The following measures may be taken to prevent bladder infection:

- Drinking large amounts of fluid.
- Reducing intake of sugar.
- Urinating frequently and as soon as the need arises.

Women with two or more UTIs within a six-month period are sometimes given prophylactic antibiotic treatment, usually nitrofurantoin or trimethoprim for three to six months. In some cases the patient is advised to take an antibiotic tablet following sexual intercourse.

Other preventive measures for women include:

- Urinating frequently, particularly after intercourse.
- Proper cleansing of the area around the urethra (wiping front to back).
- Acupuncture.

The primary preventive measure specifically for males is prompt treatment of prostate infections. Chronic prostatitis may go unnoticed but can trigger recurrent UTIs. In addition, males who require temporary catheterization following surgery can be given antibiotics to lower the risk of UTIs.

Resources

BOOKS

Iannini, Paul B. *Contemporary Diagnosis and Management of Urinary Tract Infections.* Newton, PA: Handbooks in Health Care, 2003.

Kavaler, Elizabeth. *Seat on the Aisle, Please!: The Essential Guide to Urinary Tract Problems in Women.* New York: Springer, 2006.

Kilmartin, Angela. *The Patient's Encyclopaedia of Urinary Tract Infection, Sexual Cystitis and Interstitial Cystitis.* Chula Vista, CA New Century Press, 2004.

Rane, Abhay. *Urinary Tract Infections.* Jupiter, FL.: Merit Publishing, 2008.

Sadler, Carrie, et al. *Women's Health.* New York: Oxford University Press, 2008.

PERIODICALS

Butrick, Charles W. "Patients With Chronic Pelvic Pain: Endometriosis or Interstitial Cystitis/Painful Bladder Syndrome?" *Journal of the Society of Laparoendoscopic Surgeons* (April/June 2007): 182–189.

Christofi, Nicholas, and Andrew Hextall. "An Evidence-based Approach to Lifestyle Interventions in Urogynaecology." *Menopause International* (December 2007): 154–159.

Theoharides, Theoharis. "Treatment Approaches for Painful Bladder Syndrome/Interstitial Cystitis." *Drugs* (November 2007): 215–235.

OTHER

eMedicineHealth. *Urinary Tract Infections.* http://www.emedicinehealth.com/urinary_tract_infections/article_em.htm

Belinda Rowland
Teresa G. Odle
David Edward Newton, Ed.D.

Bladderwrack

Definition

Bladderwrack is a type of brown seaweed found along the northern coasts of the Atlantic and Pacific oceans, the North Sea, and the Baltic Sea. It has long been used to treat a number of medical conditions, including gastrointestinal problems and **hypothyroidism**, and for the treatment of **wounds**.

Description

The scientific name for bladderwrack is *Fucus vesiculosus*. It is also known by a number of common names, including black tang, rockweed, bladder Fucus, sea **oak**, black tany, cut weed, and rock wrack.

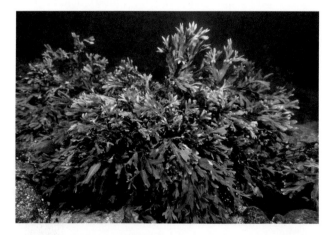

Bladder wrack is a type of seaweed, long used to treat a number of medical conditions, including gastrointestinal problems and hypothyroidism, and for the treatment of wounds. *(Andrew J. Martinez / Photo Researchers, Inc.)*

The most characteristic feature of the bladderwrack is a long thallus (stem) containing air-filled sacs that keep the plant afloat. The thallus is harvested, dried, and used for a variety of medicinal purposes. Bladderwrack's medicinal value probably depends on three primary constituents: **iodine**, alginic acid, and fucoidan. The amount of each constituent present in a sample of bladderwrack differs significantly depending on the area from which the plant is harvested.

Iodine is an essential mineral in the human diet. It is needed to ensure proper functioning of the thyroid. An excess of iodine results in a condition known as **hyperthyroidism**, in which the thyroid is over-active, while a deficiency of iodine results in hypothyroidism, a condition in which the thyroid is less active than normal. Alginic acid acts as a dietary fiber in the human digestive system, contributing to the normal function of the digestive and excretory systems. A form of alginic acid is used in the manufacture of certain antacids that reduce stomach upset and other digestive problems. Other claims have been made for the value of alginic acid, including its use in the healing of wounds and the treatment of some diseases and **infections**. Fucoidan is also a type of dietary fiber with similar value in the human digestive system. Some authorities believe it may have other medical value, as in the reduction of **cholesterol** and blood sugar levels. Little or no scientific evidence exists to support these claims.

Use

Humans have used the ashes produced by burning seaweed as a medicine since at least the 1700s. The procedure involves harvesting seaweed from the oceans and burning it with charcoal. The ashes thus produced are then taken internally or placed on a wound. The primary use of bladderwrack ashes produced in this way was the treatment of goiter. Goiter is a condition that results in the enlargement of the thyroid gland because the body lacks sufficient iodine in the bloodstream. In an effort to produce more iodine, the thyroid grows larger and larger, producing a goiter that may be as large as a grapefruit. Addition of iodine to a person's diet reduces the risk of goiter. A secondary use of bladderwrack ashes was in the treatment of skin disorders.

In 1862, French dermatologist Louis-Victor D. Duchesne-Duparc found that bladderwrack was an effective treatment for overweight and **obesity**. He eventually began making pills containing bladderwrack that he sold as diet aids. That application continued in to the early 2000s to be an important use of bladderwrack. It is an ingredient in a variety of weight-control products, such as the Bio-Mark Weight Control

> ## KEY TERMS
>
> **Goiter**—An enlargement of the thyroid gland caused by insufficient production of iodine.
>
> **Hyperthyroidism**—Excess functioning of the thyroid gland, resulting in overproduction of the thyroid hormones.
>
> **Hypothyroidism**—Reduced functioning of the thyroid gland, resulting in underproduction of the thyroid hormones.
>
> **Thyroid**—An essential gland located at the base of the neck, responsible for a number of important biological functions, including the rate of metabolism.

System, Lee Causey's Slim n' Up, and Starlight International's Natural Trim products. Some alternative therapists have made a number of other claims for the value of bladderwrack, including its ability to relieve the symptoms of rheumatism and arthritis, as an anti-coagulant and anti-estrogen, and as a treatment for **diabetes mellitus**, human immunodeficiency virus (HIV) disease and **AIDS**, and a variety of other diseases.

Effectiveness

As of 2008 no scientific studies on the medical effects of bladderwrack had been reported. At that point, all claims for the beneficial effects of the plant were based on historical and anecdotal evidence. In 2001, the National Toxicology Program (NTP) of the U.S. Department of Health and Human Resources undertook a study of the substance to determine its possible health risks. The study was motivated by concerns over the use of bladderwrack in diet supplements. The supposition had been that bladderwrack's weight-loss effects are caused by iodine present in the plant. That iodine causes the thyroid gland to become more active, thus increasing a person's metabolism, resulting in a lost of weight. However, the level of iodine required to produce this effect is sufficient to produce hyperthyroidism in an individual, a potentially serious health problem. The results of the NTP study were not available as of 2008.

Resources

PERIODICALS

"Seaweed and Soy: Companion Foods in Asian Cuisine and Their Effects on Thyroid Function in American Women." *Journal of Medicinal Food* (March 2007): 90–100.

David E. Newton, Ed.D.

Blessed thistle

Description

Blessed thistle, *Cnicus benedictus* (also known as *Carduus benedictus* and *Carbenia benedicta*), is a member of the Asteracea, or daisy, family. The bitter-tasting, prickly thistles are considered "noxious weeds" when they take root and grow abundantly in open fields and meadows. The presence of this beneficial Mediterranean native, however, indicates fertile ground. The ancient Romans ate the leaf fresh and boiled the root as a vegetable. Thistle was once used as a nutritious fodder for cattle in Scotland, and the leaf, folded between two slices of buttered bread, was eaten with the breakfast meal. In the Middle Ages, thistle was one of the most common European medicinal herbs. Shakespeare wrote about it in his play, *Much Ado About Nothing,* with the advice: "Get you some of this distilled Carduus Benedictus and lay it to your heart; it is the only thing for a qualm." The belief in

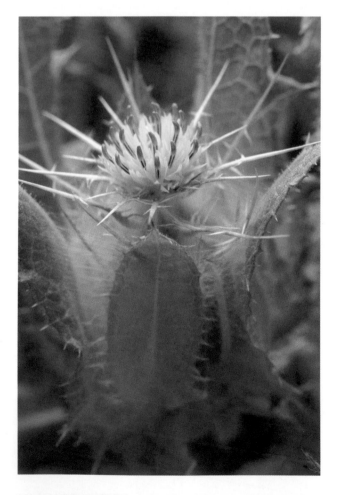

Blessed Thistle (Cnicus benedictus). *(© Arco Images / Alamy)*

thistle as a heart tonic persists. One English herbalist, writing in the mid-twentieth century, declared blessed thistle "Good for all organs of the body, especially the heart and brain." Like many native European herbs, blessed thistle is credited with magical powers. It is said to be effective in exorcism, hex-breaking, and in purification spells. Grown outside the home, this blessed herb is said to attract peace, love, and harmony.

Blessed thistle is also known as holy thistle, St. Benedict thistle, cardin, and spotted thistle. This herbaceous annual has been cultivated for centuries as a medicinal herb. It was a component of many herbal remedies used to combat the plague. The herb was also cultivated in monastery gardens as a cure for smallpox. Its specific name is in honor of St. Benedict, the founder of a holy order of monks.

Other thistles, including *Carduus marianus* or *Silybum marianum,* also sometimes known as holy thistle, Our Lady's **milk thistle**, Marian thistle, and wild **artichoke** have similar medicinal applications, particularly as liver tonics.

Thistles are naturalized throughout North America, found growing wild in sunny locations and stony soils. Blessed thistle grows from a thick taproot first forming a rosette of narrow leaves at ground level. The stems arising from the root are erect and hairy. Dark green, narrow leaves clasp the stem. They are deeply lobed, wavy and toothed on the margins, and veined. Each toothed lobe bears a prickly spine. Even the pale yellow flower heads, blooming at the top of the stem, are covered with prickly spines. The stem is reddish brown and branched reaching to two feet in length. The hardy thistle will self-sow and thrive in good soil. If left to grow wild and uncultivated, thistles may become intrusive.

General use

The entire plant is edible, though the prickly spines can be troublesome. The herb contains B-complex vitamins, **calcium**, **iron**, and **manganese**. Blessed thistle is considered by many contemporary herbalists and in traditional folk use as a tonic, astringent, diaphoretic (increases perspiration), emetic (induces **vomiting**), and stimulant. Both the blessed thistle and milk thistles are recommended as a liver tonic, particularly when the liver disease is brought on by **alcoholism**. It has been used in treatment of **jaundice** and **hepatitis**. A tea from the leaves, taken warm, will increase perspiration, reduce congestion, and help to bring down **fever**. A mild infusion is astringent and may relieve **diarrhea**, but a very strong infusion is emetic and may cause **nausea** and vomiting. Blessed thistle is considered to be one of the best herbs to stimulate the flow of milk in lactating women (lactating women should always consult their physicians before taking this herb), and its emmenagogue action (promotes menstrual discharge) helps to regulate female hormone balance and relieve menstrual **pain**. Blessed thistle has also been used to treat the vaginal discharge known as leucorrhea. The herb is used in the commercial manufacture of herbal **bitters**, and is considered a general tonic and digestive. Its bitter properties increase the flow of bile and other gastric secretions. The herb may stimulate appetite and relieve flatulence. Blessed thistle is said to relieve melancholy and lethargy, and was traditionally fed to mentally ill persons. It acts to increase blood circulation and aids memory. Applied externally in poultice form, blessed thistle is a good treatment for **shingles**, **wounds**, and ulcers. The plant has antimicrobial properties. The essential oil has been shown to have antibiotic action against **infections**, specifically *Staphylococcus aureus* and *S. faecalis*. Blessed thistle has a history in folk use for the treatment of heart ailments, cancers, and as a contraceptive, but these, and other traditional uses, have not been confirmed by research.

Preparations

Collect thistle on a hot and dry mid-summer afternoon, just as the herb begins to bloom. Harvest from the wild in areas where herbicides are not used, or from a cultivated garden patch. The leaves and flowering stems may be hung to dry in a light, airy room away from direct sunlight. Cut the dried herb and store in a clearly-labeled, dark-glass container. Seeds may be gathered in the fall.

Tincture: Combine 4 oz of fresh, or half as much dried, thistle leaf with 1 pt of brandy, gin, or vodka in a glass container. The alcohol should be enough to cover the flowers. The ratio should be close to 50/50 alcohol to water. Stir and cover. Place the mixture in a dark cupboard for three to five weeks. Shake the mixture several times each day. Strain and store in a tightly-capped, clearly labeled, dark glass bottle. A standard dose is 1–2 ml of the tincture three times a day. Tinctures, properly prepared and stored, will retain medicinal potency for two years or more.

Infusion: Use twice as much fresh, chopped herb as dried herb. Steep 1–2 teaspoons of finely chopped fresh or dried thistle per cup of boiled, unchlorinated water for 10–15 minutes. Strain and cover. Drink warm, sweetened with honey if desired. A standard dose is three cups per day. Strong infusions of thistle may cause diarrhea. A prepared herbal infusion will keep for up to two days in the refrigerator and retain its healing qualities.

Precautions

There are no reported incidents of thistle toxicity. However, as with most medicinal herbs, they should not be taken during **pregnancy**. Children under two years should not be given the herb. Lactating women should consult with a qualified herbalist before using the herb. Strong infusions of blessed thistle may cause nausea and vomiting.

Side effects

None reported.

Interactions

None reported.

Resources

BOOKS

PDR for Herbal Medicines. New Jersey: Medical Economics Company, 1998.

Magic And Medicine of Plants. The Reader's Digest Association, Inc. 1986.

Coon, Nelson. *An American Herbal, Using Plants For Healing.* Pennsylvania: Rodale Press, 1979.

Elias, Jason, and Shelagh Ryan Masline. *The A to Z Guide to Healing Herbal Remedies.* Lynn Sonberg Book Associates, 1996, (Wing Books, 1997 edition).

Hoffmann, David. *The New Holistic Herbal, 2nd edition.* Massachusetts: Element, 1986.

Mabey, Richard. *The New Age Herbalist.* New York: Simon & Schuster, Inc., 1988.

McIntyre, Anne. *The Medicinal Garden.* New York: Henry Holt and Company, 1997.

Meyer, Joseph E. *The Herbalist.* Clarence Meyer, 1973.

Murray, Michael T. *The Healing Power of Herbs, 2nd ed.* California: Prima Publications, Inc., 1995.

Phillips, Roger, and Nicky Foy. *The Random House Book of Herbs.* New York: Random House, 1990.

Polunin, Miriam and Christopher Robbins. *The Natural Pharmacy.* New York: Macmillan Publishing Company, 1992.

Thomson, William A. R. *Medicines From The Earth.* San Francisco: Harper & Row, 1983.

Weiss, Gaea, and Shandor Weiss. *Growing & Using The Healing Herbs.* NY: Wing Books, 1992.

OTHER

Grieve, Mrs. M. *A Modern Herbal.* Available at: Botanical.com, http://www.botanical.com/botanical/mgmh/t/thistl11.html.

Clare Hanrahan

Blisters

Definition

Blisters are small, raised lesions where fluid has collected under the skin. They may be caused by an allergic reaction, **burns**, **frostbite**, or by excessive friction or trauma to the skin. Blisters may also be a symptom of a systemic illness, or of a specific skin disorder.

Description

The thin-skinned sac of a blister contains fluid, and in most cases should not be ruptured, as rupturing can introduce infection and slow the healing process. Blisters that contain blood instead of fluid are aptly named blood blisters, and are caused by a rupture of blood vessels beneath the surface of the skin, usually due to trauma.

Causes and symptoms

Blisters can be caused by a number of conditions and environmental agents, including:

- Friction. Rubbing or pinching can cause skin irritation and blistering. Friction blisters frequently occur on the hands and feet.
- Disease. Blisters are symptomatic of skin disorders such as impetigo, incontinentia pigmenti syndrome (IPS), and pemphigus vulgaris. Blisters may also be caused by diseases such as herpes and chickenpox.
- Contact dermatitis. Skin contact with an allergen (e.g., latex, cosmetics, cleaning solutions) can trigger redness, irritation, rash, and blistering of the skin. Blisters also typically appear after skin contact with poison ivy, oak, or sumac.

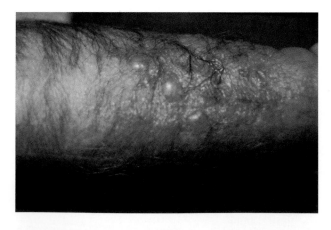

Man with blistered arm from poison ivy. *(Custom Medical Stock Photo. Reproduced by permission.)*

- Burns. Blisters appear in cases of severe sunburn and thermal burns.
- Frostbite. Severely frostbitten skin frequently blisters.
- Trauma. Blood blisters are caused by trauma to the skin.

Other new causes of blisters are discovered by clinicians. In 2002, a report discussed how a newly identified autoimmune blistering disease involving the mucous membranes also increased the risk of some solid cancers.

Diagnosis

Diagnosis and treatment of most minor blisters can typically be made at home by examination of the affected area. Blisters thought to be caused by a systemic illness or disease may require professional diagnosis by a physician, dermatologist, or other healthcare professional. A medical history, physical examination, and further medical testing may be part of the diagnostic procedure.

Treatment

Unless they are hindering movement or are extremely painful due to their size and/or location, blisters should not be ruptured, or "popped," as doing so can introduce bacteria into the wound. If a blister does burst, the extra skin should be left intact. Blisters that are excessively large or painful should only be punctured using antiseptic procedures, preferably by or under the direction of a qualified healthcare professional.

Treatment of blisters depends on their cause. Blisters that are symptomatic of a disease or disorder require treatment of the illness itself. Blisters caused by friction or trauma can be treated by cleansing with mild soap, applying an antiseptic, and covering the area with a sterile bandage. An herbalist, aromatherapist, or holistic healthcare professional may recommend a compress of an antiseptic or anti-microbial herb such as marigold (*Calendula officinalis*), **thyme** (*Thymus vulgaris*), **lavender** (*Lavandula angustifolia*), or **tea tree oil** (*Melaleuca alternifolia*).

The blister should be kept clean and the bandage changed frequently. Blood blisters should be bandaged firmly to apply pressure to the area and prevent further blood vessel ruptures.

Allopathic treatment

Conventional medicine typically follows the same procedures for treating skin blisters. A prescription or over-the-counter antiseptic ointment may be recommended to clean the blistered area.

Impetigo—A bacterial infection of the skin characterized by skin blistering.

Incontinentia pigmenti syndrome (IPS)—An inherited skin disorder characterized by blistered lesions in infancy, which heal but leave uneven pigmentation of the skin.

Pemphigus vulgaris—An autoimmune skin disorder that causes blistering of the skin and mucous membrane.

Expected results

With proper treatment, most minor blisters will heal without complication in a matter of days. More serious blisters caused by severe burns and certain diseases may produce permanent scarring or discoloration of the skin.

Prevention

Friction blisters can be prevented by wearing adequate protection on the area prone to blistering. For example, long distance runners can purchase properly fitting shoes. People who work with their hands or feet can purchase special gloves or shoes and boots. For instance, in 2002, a boot company introduced safety toe footwear for occupational use with enough room for toes to move freely without rubbing against steel–toe caps.

Fair-skinned individuals who are prone to **sunburn** should take extra precautions to avoid skin blistering, such as using a high SPF sunscreen (at least 30 SPF) and wearing a large brimmed hat and long-sleeved, loose clothing in the sun.

Resources

BOOKS

Lawless, Julia. *The Complete Illustrated Guide to Aromatherapy*. Boston, MA: Element Books, 1997.

PERIODICALS

Minter, Stephen G. "Safety Boots to Prevent Blisters." *Occupational Hazards* (May 2002): 106.

Worcester, Sharon. "Risk of Solid Cancers Raised by Blistering Disease (Study of 35 Patients)." *Skin &Allergy News* (June 2002): 45.

Paula Ford-Martin
Teresa G. Odle

Blood clots

Definition

A blood clot is a mass of blood cells and blood components that form to stop the bleeding that occurs when a blood vessel is injured. When a blood vessel is broken, platelets in the blood become sticky and clump together at the site of the injury. They begin to form a mass to stop the flow of blood.

Description

Clotting is the body's normal response to a bleeding injury, a necessary function to prevent a person from losing too much blood. Most blood clots dissolve into the blood when the body has healed the vessel. Blood clots, however, can be potentially dangerous if they occur within healthy blood vessels or if they do not dissolve when their work is done. A *thrombus* is a blood clot that forms along the wall of the heart or a blood vessel. This type of clot can slow blood flow, and if the clot becomes large enough, it may stop the flow of blood in the vessel. An *embolus* is a clot that forms in one area of the body, travels through the bloodstream, and lodges in another vessel in the body. Emboli are less common and more dangerous because they can cause a sudden blockage in blood flow (embolism), which can be fatal. An embolism occurring in an artery will block blood flow to an organ or tissue and can cause tissue damage or death. An embolism in the following locations results in the given condition:

- embolism in a cerebral (brain) artery can cause a stroke
- embolism in a coronary artery can cause a heart attack
- embolism in a pulmonary (lung) artery can cause shortness of breath or death
- embolism in a retinal artery can cause sudden blindness in one eye
- embolism in an artery supplying blood to a limb can cause tissue damage and possibly gangrene
- embolism in any artery leading to an organ can cause loss of that organ's function

Causes and symptoms

Several factors contribute to the formation of blood clots. **Phlebitis** is a condition that may increase abnormal blood clot formation. Blood diseases or other conditions—especially inflammation—that alter the quality of the blood can also affect clot formation.

Both plaque formation in the arteries (**atherosclerosis**) and damaged blood vessels increase the chance of blood clots because they slow blood flow and provide a place for platelets to collect and form a clot. Genetic factors also play a role in predisposition to form blood clots. Diet can have an effect on clot formation as well. **Cholesterol** and saturated fats, which are also implicated in atherosclerosis, can contribute to clot formation. People whose **diets** are low in **essential fatty acids**, vegetables, and fish, and who do not take in proper amounts of nutrients and **antioxidants**, are at a higher risk for clots. Conditions or body positions that slow blood circulation—extended bed rest or sitting in a car or airplane for long periods of time—may cause blood clots to form in the legs. Blood clots can be caused by increased fibrinogen (a blood-clotting factor) due to estrogen in the late stages of **pregnancy** and from long-term use of birth control pills. Other factors include **varicose veins**, **childbirth**, **sickle cell anemia**, **smoking**, **obesity**, liver disease, and cardiovascular disorders.

There may be no obvious symptoms of a blood clot. When symptoms do occur, they often appear suddenly and indicate the location of the clot. Extreme **dizziness** that occurs without warning can indicate a clot in a cerebral artery. Sudden complete or partial blindness in one eye could indicate a clot within the retinal artery. A hard blue bulge in a vein or unexpected **pain** in an arm or leg, along with numbness, weakness, or another sign that blood is not reaching the area, could indicate a blood clot. **Blisters** or ulcers on the skin may occur as well. A clot in an artery near a major organ such as the heart or lung will produce pain or decreased activity in that organ. **Gangrene** (death of tissue) may occur if blood flow to a region is blocked for an extended period of time.

Diagnosis

Patients describe the severity and location of the pain they have been experiencing. A physician may also notice such physical signs of a blood clot as the swelling blue bulge, discoloration of a limb, or an ulcer. Medical personnel check for a missing or lowered pulse or blood pressure in a limb. A Doppler ultrasound examination, angiography, or arteriography may be used to detect the location of the clot. In 2007, the American College of Physicians and the American Academy of Family Physicians endorsed the Wells Prediction Rule for diagnosing venous thromboembolism (a blood clot in a vein rather than an artery). The Wells rule assigns points based on the following conditions in patients:

- Cancer treatment in the previous six months
- Paralysis, paresis, or a plaster cast on the legs or feet
- Recently bedridden for four days or longer or major surgery that required anesthesia within 12 weeks
- Localized tenderness along the deep venous system in the legs, especially the back of the upper legs
- Swelling of the entire leg
- Swelling of the calf of 3 centimeters (1.2 inches) or more compared to a normal calf
- Pitting edema of the leg with symptoms
- Collateral superficial veins in the symptomatic leg

Treatment

Nutritional therapy may include the following: vitamins B_3 (**niacin**), B_6, C, and E; fatty acid and **garlic** supplements; and the minerals **zinc**, **magnesium**, and **manganese**. Herbal remedies may include **cayenne** (*Capsicum frutescens*), other hot peppers, and gingko (*Ginkgo biloba*) to help reduce the protein fibrin, which is a necessary factor in blood clots. **Bilberry** (*Vaccinium myrtillus*), **turmeric** (*Curcuma longa*), and **ginger** (*Zingiber officinale*) help reduce platelets' stickiness, which is essential for clot formation. Onion (*Allium sepa*) and garlic (*Allium sativum*) help reduce fibrin and platelet stickiness. A study by researchers at Brigham and Women's Hospital in Boston reported in 2007 that women who took **vitamin E** supplements reduced their risk of blood clots by 18 percent over women who did not take vitamin E. Several small clinical studies on humans reported that both fresh onions *Allium cepa* and commercial onion extracts actually lower blood cholesterol levels, lower blood pressure, and help prevent the formation of blood clots. Although these studies have been done on only a small number of people, they are consistently supported by additional data from animal and test-tube studies. In addition, many of these properties have been found in garlic, which is a close relative to onion.

Patients who are taking prescribed anticoagulant drugs should consult their doctors before starting vitamin, nutritional, or herbal therapies.

Hydrotherapy treatment for blood clots can include contrast applications. The patient alternates using hot and cold treatments on the body in the area of the clot to increase blood flow. A naturopath will recommend specific remedies based on the symptoms and personality of a particular patient. A remedy for blood clots may include *Hamamelis*. Massage can be helpful if blood clots are a result of poor circulation, although care should be taken if a person suffers from phlebitis, since a clot could mobilize and lodge elsewhere.

Allopathic treatment

Anticoagulant (anticlotting) drugs are usually prescribed for patients with blood clots. The drug streptokinase helps dissolve clots that are already present in the body. Heparin inhibits platelet clumping and can be prescribed after surgery when blood is likely to clot. One promising treatment to prevent clot formation associated with septic shock is a recombinant form of activated human protein C, a natural anticoagulant. Doctors may prescribe aspirin for people who are at risk for having blood clots, although aspirin can injure the stomach lining. Patients may want to ask their doctors about what can be done to minimize damage from aspirin. Surgery is only recommended to remove blood clots that appear to be life-threatening or will cause tissue death if not removed.

Expected results

If a clot goes undetected it is potentially dangerous and can lead to a **stroke**, **heart attack**, or other serious complication. Any sudden unexplained pain or loss of function should be checked by a doctor. If the blood flow to a limb is blocked for an extended period of time, gangrene may set in, and the limb may require amputation. Diet and **exercise** can help prevent future clots.

Prevention

Some risk factors, such as genetically related diseases, cannot be minimized. But minimizing other risk factors helps prevent problems with blood clots. Quitting smoking, maintaining correct weight, and improving **nutrition** can help reduce the risk of problematic blood clotting.

A healthy diet with high-fiber, low-cholesterol foods and plenty of fruits and vegetables can help prevent blood clots and many of the conditions that can lead to blood clots, such as atherosclerosis. In addition, such foods as garlic, ginger, onions, and hot peppers can help reduce platelet stickiness and formation of clots. Fish oils and supplements that add nutrients to the diet are recommended as well.

Moderate exercise helps keep off extra weight and improves circulation, both of which help reduce risk factors for formation of blood clots. Exercise can also reduce the risk of blood clots in women who use birth control pills for long periods of time. Those who must sit for long periods of time—on an airplane, in a car, or

KEY TERMS

Collateral superficial veins—Veins that are readily visible and stick up from the skin surface.

Embolism—Obstruction or blockage in a blood vessel caused by an embolus.

Embolus—A clot that forms in one place in the body and then travels and lodges elsewhere. Emboli is the plural of embolus.

Phlebitis—Inflammation of the blood vessel walls.

Pitting edema—Swelling caused by excess water that can be detected when the skin is pressed with a finger and an indentation remains after the finger is withdrawn.

Thrombus—A clot that forms in the heart or blood vessel and remains there.

Venous thromboembolism—A blood clot in a vein rather than an artery, which, if it breaks free, can travel to a lung.

at work—can help prevent blood clots by wearing loose clothing, walking, and stretching their legs whenever possible. Flexing and releasing the lower body muscles, even while sitting, can help improve circulation as well.

Resources

BOOKS

Schmukler, Alan. *Homeopathy: An A to Z Home Handbook*. Woodbury, MN: Llewellyn, 2006.

PERIODICALS

Allina, Amy. "The FDA Gets It Right—Blood Clots and the Contraceptive Patch." *Women's Health Activist* (January/February 2006): 4.

Compart, Andrew. "WHO Looks at Risks of Blood Clots Among Long-Haul Travelers." *Travel Weekly* (July 9, 2007): 14.

Mohn, Tanya. "Flying and Blood Clots: A Deadly Risk." *New York Times* (November 6, 2007): C5.

Sherman, Carl. "Blood Clots: An Updated Guide from the Experts; Two Primary-Care Organizations Have Issued New Recommendations that Will Enhance Your Ability to Diagnose and Treat Venous Thromboembolism." *Clinical Advisor* (April 2007): 52(4).

Sherman, Carl. "Curtailing Blood Clots: New Recommendations Address the Diagnosis and Treatment of Venous Thromboembolism." *Cortlandt Forum* (May 2007): 72(3).

"Stockings Sharply Reduce Blood Clots." *Harvard Reviews of Health News* (May 11, 2007): N/A.

ORGANIZATIONS

American Association of Acupuncture and Oriental Medicine, PO Box 162340, Sacramento, CA, 95816, (866) 455-7999, http://www.aaaomonline.org.

American Heart Association, 7320 Greenville Ave, Dallas, TX, 75231, (800) 373-242-8721, http://www.americanheart.org.

American Institute of Homeopathy, 801 N. Fairfax St., Suite 306, Alexandria, VA, 22314, (888) 445-9988, http://www.homeopathyusa.org.

Heart and Stroke Foundation of Canada, 222 Queen St., Suite 1402, Ottawa ON, K1P 5V9, Canada, (613) 569-4361, http://www.heartandstroke.ca.

Heather Bienvenue
Ken R. Wells

Blood poisoning

Definition

Blood poisoning, also known as septicemia or sepsis, occurs when the bloodstream becomes infected by bacteria (i.e., staphylococci, streptococci), viruses, or fungi introduced through a wound, **abscess**, or other injury. Septicemia may also originate from a localized infection in the body.

Description

About 100,000 new cases of septicemia occur in the United States each year; approximately two-thirds of the cases are diagnosed in hospitalized patients. Septicemia is an extremely dangerous disorder because it spreads rapidly throughout the body. If bacteria continue to multiply in the bloodstream and the condition progresses to septic shock, blood pressure drops rapidly and organ systems begin to shut down. Septic shock leads to multiple-organ dysfunction syndrome (MODS), and may result in death. Although the mortality rate of patients with sepsis has dropped from 31% in 1979 to 11% in 2004, over 30,000 sepsis patients die in the United States each year. Men are more likely than women to develop sepsis, and the prevalence rate among African Americans is twice the rate seen in Caucasians.

Causes and symptoms

A septic infection can originate in any wound, including **burns**, **cuts**, punctures, scrapes, abscesses, or a soft tissue infection. It can also start as a specific infection such as a **sinus infection** or appendicitis.

Invasive surgical procedures and medical devices, such as catheters, vascular access grafts, and intravenous (IV) lines, also carry a risk of introducing bacteria to the bloodstream if not appropriately cared for and cleaned. A large percentage of septicemia patients acquire the infection in a hospital setting.

Septicemia symptoms include

- elevated white blood cell count
- fever and chills
- rapid breathing
- sudden drop in blood pressure
- tachycardia (a rapid, pounding heartbeat)
- confusion and possible loss of consciousness
- warm, flushed skin
- skin irregularities, such as subcutaneous red lines, swelling, bleeding under the skin, or necrosis (tissue death)

Septic shock can occur when septicemia is not treated adequately or quickly enough. Symptoms of septic shock include:

- severe drop in blood pressure (systolic pressure less than 90 mmHg and/or less than 40 mmHg of the patient's baseline blood pressure)
- organ dysfunction (such as kidney failure) due to reduced blood flow to the organ systems
- loss of consciousness

There are some known risk factors for developing septicemia. These include:

- Having a chronic disorder or disease. The body has a difficult time fighting infection if the immune system is already weakened.
- Use of immunosuppressive drugs. These drugs also weaken the immune system.
- Taking intravenous medications or drugs. Needles can introduce infectious organisms into the bloodstream if not used in a sterile manner.

Diagnosis

There is no specific laboratory test for early diagnosis of septicemia. Blood cultures can sometimes determine the presence of bacteria in the bloodstream once the infection has spread; however, a blood culture requires an incubation time of 24 hours or longer. Given the rapidly progressing nature of septicemia, cultures are more effective for confirming the diagnosis and narrowing the choice of antibiotics, as treatment usually must begin before the cultures are complete. In some cases, septicemia patients may have negative blood cultures. Further analysis of blood samples by a trained hematologist may be required to make a diagnosis. If the infection is thought to have spread from a wound or injury, tissue samples from that site may also be analyzed. Other body fluids, such as urine and sputum, may be cultured for organisms.

Treatment

Septicemia is a potentially fatal, rapidly progressing disease. Any individual who suspects he or she may have septicemia should immediately seek emergency medical care.

Allopathic treatment

Septicemia is treated with a course of intravenous antibiotics. The type of antibiotic used depends on the infectious agent. Blood cultures, wound cultures, and other diagnostic tests will help the healthcare provider select the most effective medication. A catheter is used to drain pus and fluids from abcesses or other sites of infection. Blood pressure medications and fluids are administered to stabilize blood pressure. In cases where the patient is suffering from significant respiratory distress, a ventilator may be required. Further organ support such as dialysis may be administered if the patient progresses to septic shock.

A very promising treatment for sepsis, activated human protein C, has been shown to cut the mortality rate of patients with severe sepsis by 6.1% in the first 28 days after treatment. The drug, also known as drotrecogin alfa, was approved by the FDA in the fall of 2001, and is marketed under the trade name Xigris. It is the only drug approved by the FDA for use specifically in the treatment of severe sepsis. Xigris cannot, however, be given to patients at high risk for active bleeding, including those who have just had surgery, have been diagnosed with an aneurysm or gastrointestinal bleeding, or who are being treated with warfarin (Coumadin) or platelet inhibitors.

Expected results

In 2004, the latest year for which data are available, the mortality rate for patients with septicemia was 11.3%. As the disease progresses to septic shock and organ systems start to be involved, the prognosis worsens. Approximately half of all patients with septic shock die. The patient's overall physical health—especially his or her heart function—has a large bearing on the chance for recovery. Early intervention and aggressive treatment of localized **infections** offer the best chance for survival.

Prevention

Meticulous infection control techniques are the best defense against septicemia. For hospitalized patients

KEY TERMS

Blood culture—A test used to find and identify infectious organisms in the blood. Blood drawn from the patient is placed in a culture medium and the sample is observed for the growth of bacteria. If bacteria grow, they are analyzed for identification.

Hematologist—A physician who specializes in the study of blood and diseases of the blood.

Intravenous—Within a vein.

Subcutaneous—Under the skin.

who are already at a higher risk of contracting the disease, great care should be taken to treat and clean **wounds**, sutures, and burns using sterile techniques in an antiseptic environment. The same rules apply for maintaining such invasive medical devices as intravenous lines, catheters, and gastric and nasal tubes. The use of these devices should be limited whenever possible.

One controversial form of prevention is the use of antibiotic-coated catheters in hospitalized patients. While these catheters appear to be effective in lowering the sepsis mortality rate, some doctors are concerned that their use may also encourage the development of new **strains** of bacteria resistant to antibiotics.

Individuals can take appropriate precautions when treating cuts, scrapes, and other minor wounds at home. Using clean or gloved hands, these injuries should be thoroughly cleansed of dirt and debris with antibacterial soap and water. A sterile compress containing a preparation of naturally antibacterial, antiseptic herbs such as tea tree (*Melaleuca alternifolia*) or **calendula** (*Calendula officinalis*) can also be used to treat the wound site. A medicated cream or analgesic herbal preparation (e.g., **lavender**, or *Lavandula angustifolia*) can soothe associated **pain** and promote healing. A waterproof bandage will protect the wound from dirt and germs. The healing progress should be monitored closely, and a healthcare provider should be contacted immediately should any of the symptoms of septicemia occur.

Resources

BOOKS

Baudouin, Simon V., M.D., ed. *Sepsis.* New York: Springer, 2007.
Septicemia. San Diego: ICON Health Publications, 2005.

PERIODICALS

Juan-Torresa, Antoni, and Stephan Harbarth. "Prevention of Primary Bacteraemia." *International Journal of Microbial Agents* (November 2007): 80–87.

Naber, C. K. "Future Strategies for Treating *Staphylococcus aureus* Bloodstream Infections." *Clinical Microbiology and Infection* (March 2008): 26–34.

Reddy, Srinivas, et al. "Profile of Opportunistic Infections among Patients on Immunosuppressive Medication." *APLAR Journal of Rheumatology* (September 2006): 269–274.

"Septicemia." *Health Statistics from the Americas* (2006): 19–24.

Paula Ford-Martin
Rebecca J. Frey, Ph.D.
David Edward Newton, Ed.D.

Bloodroot

Description

Bloodroot (*Sanguinaria canadensis*) is a perennial plant with a white flower that blooms in early spring. It belongs to the poppy family (*Papaveraceae*) and grows in wooded areas throughout the northeastern regions of the United States and Canada. The leaves are palm-shaped and the flowers have eight to 12 petals. The root is thick and round and 1–4 in (2.5–10 cm) long. The plant generally grows to a height of 6 in (12 cm).

Bloodroot gets its name from its bright red root that, when cut open, oozes a crimson, blood-like juice. Other names for bloodroot are coon root, Indian plant, snakebite, sweet slumber, paucon, red root, and tetterwort.

Native Americans used bloodroot for medicinal, spiritual, and practical purposes. A dye made from the red sap of the root was used as body paint for war dances and ceremonies, as well as to color fabric. It was used medicinally as a remedy for fevers, **cancer**, rheumatism, to induce **vomiting**, and as an oral antiseptic.

General use

The known active components of bloodroot are isoquinoline alkaloids, which have antibacterial,

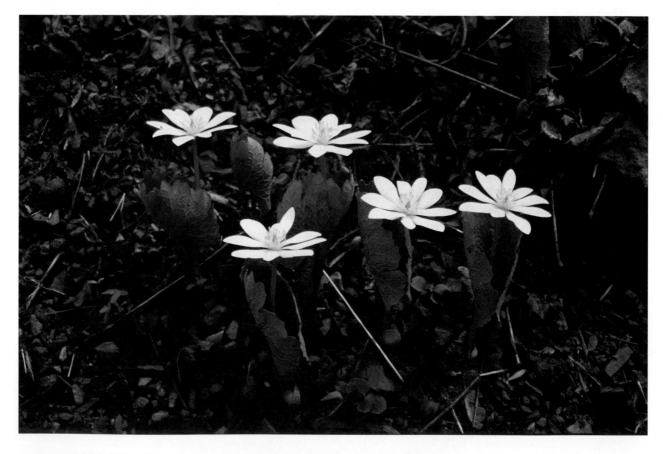

The perennial blood root plant. *(© Photo Researchers, Inc. Reproduced by permission.)*

antimicrobial, expectorant, and antiseptic properties. Sanguinarine, a primary alkaloid of bloodroot, is noted for its ability to destroy bacteria that can cause **gum disease** (gingivitis) and dental plaque. In fact, because of its bacteria-inhibiting properties, sanguinarine is an ingredient in many oral hygiene products such as toothpastes and mouthwashes. Sanguinarine also has pain-relieving qualities. A gargle made from bloodroot can be used to soothe a **sore throat**.

Bloodroot is generally prescribed as an external treatment as it is poisonous if ingested in large amounts. However, bloodroot is a powerful expectorant and has been a primary, albeit rare, internal treatment for chronic **bronchitis**, **croup**, coughs, **asthma**, and other respiratory afflictions. In fact, bloodroot was catalogued as an expectorant in the *Pharmocopoeia of the United States* from 1820 to 1926.

Due to its bacteria-fighting compounds, herbalists often recommend bloodroot as a topical application for skin problems such as chronic **eczema**, fungus, **athlete's foot**, ringworm, venereal **blisters**, and **rashes**.

Bloodroot has a long history of use as a folk remedy for cancer. Native Americans used bloodroot to heal various forms of cancers and tumorous growths. Many modern herbalists prescribe a salve made from the root to remove **warts**, growths, and cancerous tumors. Bloodroot is currently the subject of several studies and experiments, but little scientific research has been performed to substantiate the use of bloodroot as a cure for certain cancers. Some studies have revealed that the alkaloid sanguinarine may inhibit the formation of tumors. However, the safety and effectiveness of its use has not been fully evaluated.

Preparations

The parts used medicinally are the whole plant and root, or rhizome, which is collected in the fall.

Bloodroot is an ingredient in some homeopathic remedies, pharmaceutical preparations, **cough** formulas, toothpaste, and mouthwash. It is also available as a tincture and in dried root form, chopped and in powder.

A salve made from bloodroot can be used to remove warts and other growths.

Precautions

Bloodroot is a potentially toxic herb. Take internally only under the supervision of a health care

professional or qualified herbalist. (Topical use on unbroken skin is generally safe.)

Internal use of this herb should be supervised by a health care professional.

Pregnant or nursing women or women who are trying to conceive should avoid this herb.

Long term internal consumption may contribute to **glaucoma**. Persons with glaucoma should not use bloodroot.

The internal use of bloodroot by children is considered unsafe.

Side effects

Internal doses in excess of 300 mg have been shown to cause vomiting. Higher doses are considered toxic and poisonous.

When taken in excess, bloodroot can also cause **nausea**, impaired vision, intense thirst, **dizziness**, a slowed heart rate, and a burning of the stomach.

Bloodroot contains skin-irritating compounds. When applied topically it may burn the skin or cause the skin to become red.

Interactions

Toothpastes or mouthwashes usually only contain small amounts of sanguinarine and are considered safe for long-term use.

Resources

BOOKS

Chevalier, Andrew. *The Encyclopedia of Medicinal Plants.* DK Publishing Inc., 1996.

Heinerman, John. *Heinerman's Encyclopedia of Healing Herbs and Spices.* Parker Publishing Company, 1996.

Jennifer Wurges

Bloodwort *see* **Yarrow**

Blue-green algae *see* **Spirulina**

Blue gum *see* **Eucalyptus**

Blue cohosh

Description

Blue cohosh *Caulophyllum thalictroides* is a perennial flowering plant that grows in moist forest regions throughout the eastern United States. The plant—also known as squaw root, blue ginseng, papoose root, and yellow ginseng—grows up to 3 ft (1 m) tall, and its greenish yellow flowers turn into small blue berries in autumn. The berries of the plant are toxic and should not be used for medicinal purposes. The root of the plant, harvested in the fall, is the part used medicinally, and it has a bittersweet flavor. Blue cohosh has long been believed to conform to the *doctrine of signatures*, which is an ancient idea that the physical shape of plants gives a clue to their medicinal uses. Blue cohosh has branches that are arranged like limbs in spasm, and the herb has been used to treat **muscle spasms**. It should not be confused with an unrelated herb, **black cohosh**, which has different properties, treatment uses, and side effects.

Blue cohosh has been listed on the threatened list in Rhode Island since 2002 by the USDA Natural Resources Conservation Center. It is also on the watch list in several other states due to over-harvesting and habitat destruction. Efforts were underway in the late 2000s by several environmental organizations, such as the Natural Resources Conservation Center and the non-profit organization, United Plant Savers, to conserve and restore native medicinal plants, such as blue cohosh.

Blue cohosh was widely used by Native Americans to treat a variety of conditions, ranging from parasites to nervous disorders. Native Americans referred to the herb as squaw root or papoose root because of its effectiveness in treating female problems, including easing the **pain** of labor and **childbirth**.

Blue cohosh contains several important minerals, including **potassium**, **magnesium**, **calcium**, **iron**, silicon and **phosphorus**. Active ingredients isolated from the herb, called glycosides, include *caulosaponin* and *caulophyllosaponin*. These compounds have been shown to activate smooth muscle contraction and stimulate uterine contractions to induce labor. Blue cohosh also has been shown to reduce muscle spasms (anti-spasmodic).

General use

Blue cohosh is one of the most commonly recommended herbal preparations used to stimulate labor contractions, particularly by nurse-midwives, according to a 1999 survey conducted by the *Journal of Nurse Midwifery*. Blue cohosh may be used when induction of labor is indicated in specific circumstances, such as when uterine contractions are brief or irregular.

In addition to its use to induce labor, blue cohosh has been indicated for the treatment of menstrual problems, such as **amenorrhea** (absence of menstrual cycles), **dysmenorrhea** (painful periods), and menstrual cramps. Because of its antispasmodic properties, blue cohosh also has been used to treat some cases of **asthma**, **colic**, and nervous coughs, as well as to reduce pain in some cases of **rheumatoid arthritis**.

Blue cohosh is used in **homeopathy**, and the homeopathic remedy made from blue cohosh is called Caulophyllum. It may be used to treat menstrual cramps, PMS, dysmenorrhea, and for support during childbirth. Homeopaths may also use Caulophyllum to treat **gout**, rheumatism, false labor pains, and **gonorrhea**.

Preparations

Blue cohosh is available as dried root, capsules, and in tinctures (liquid extracts). To prepare a tea, one ounce of the root can be added to one pint of water and steeped for half an hour. Two tablespoons of the tea can be taken every two to three hours. The root can be ground into powder, and 3–9 g (0.11–0.32 oz) of it can be taken several times per day. For the herbal tincture, the recommended dosage is 5 drops every 4 hours or 10 drops in hot water every 10 hours.

The homeopathic remedy Caulophyllum is available in tablet, liquid dilution, or tincture form in a wide variety of potencies. Dosing regimens vary among individual practitioners.

Precautions

People diagnosed with **diverticulitis**, gastric ulcers, esophageal reflux, **heart disease**, high blood pressure, or ulcerative **colitis** should not use blue cohosh.

According to the American **Pregnancy** Association (www.americanpregnancy.org), blue cohosh is considered unsafe during pregnancy and should only be taken with extreme caution, under medical supervision. Women who are breastfeeding should not take blue cohosh, as the safety of the herb during lactation is unknown.

Blue cohosh has abortifacient and *emmenagogue* properties, which means it can terminate a pregnancy and stimulate menstrual flow, respectively. Blue cohosh should *never* be used to induce abortion, as it has been shown to cause serious harm to both mother and fetus. One study reported a 21-year-old woman who developed abdominal cramps, heavy sweating, rapid heartbeat, and **nausea** after taking blue cohosh in an attempt to induce abortion.

Caulosaponin is the glycoside compound in blue cohosh that causes the uterus to contract. This compound also causes the blood vessels in the heart to constrict, decreasing the flow of oxygen to the heart, thus having a potentially toxic effect on heart muscle.

The results of several case reports suggest that the use of blue cohosh as an agent for labor induction is unsafe for both the mother and fetus. The earliest case report of harm from a mother's use of blue cohosh was published in 1998. The infant developed congestive heart failure shortly after birth. Additional case reports have shown adverse perinatal events associated with maternal ingestion of blue cohosh, including one infant's inability to breathe spontaneously at birth, resulting in permanent central nervous system hypoxic-ischemic damage, and another infant who had severe congestive heart failure and myocardial infarction at birth, with additional cardiac abnormalities at age two.

Another case report published in the July 15, 2004, issue of the *New Engand Journal of Medicine* described a healthy woman who drank blue cohosh tea to induce labor at 40 weeks gestation, as directed by her obstetrician. The woman had a resulting cesarean section after a failed attempt at vaginal delivery. Within 26 hours of birth, her infant experienced a **stroke**, with focal motor seizures of the right arm. A computed-tomography scan showed an infarct in the cerebral artery. Interestingly, the baby's urine and meconium tested positive for the cocaine metabolite benzoylecgonine, and the mother's bottle of blue cohosh also tested positive for this metabolite. Although the finding should be interpreted with caution, the authors of the case report indicated the causal relationship between the herbal preparation and the infant's condition required further study.

Several systemic literature reviews verify the conclusion from these case reports that there is insufficient data to support the efficacy and safety of blue cohosh for use as an agent to induce labor. Although the body of literature elicits caution regarding the extensive use of blue cohosh during pregnancy, more research is needed to provide definitive conclusions, especially since the data about the dosage, frequency and duration of use in several of these case reports are varied and, in some cases, unclear.

Side effects

In addition to potentially toxic cardiac effects, including perinatal stroke, the side effects of blue cohosh include nausea and **vomiting**, chest pain, headaches, difficulty breathing, tightness in the throat, excessive thirst, skin rash, muscle weakness, and general weakness.

Symptoms of an overdose of blue cohosh resemble those of nicotine poisoning and may include muscle weakness, convulsions, violent stomach cramps, **headache**, loss of coordination, and heart failure.

Interactions

Several herbs are frequently used with blue cohosh in formulas for improving menstrual problems, including false unicorn root, **chasteberry tree**, **angelica**, and rue. To reduce the risk of miscarriage during pregnancy, blue cohosh may be combined with false unicorn root and **cramp bark**. To induce labor, blue cohosh may be taken with black cohosh, under the supervision of a skilled medical professional.

With regard to prescription medications, blue cohosh interferes with the effectiveness of nitrates, calcium channel blockers, and **digitalis** (drugs given to treat high blood pressure and heart disease, including heart failure). It opposes the activity of drugs given to control diabetes. Blue cohosh should not be taken with prescription diuretics as it can intensify their effects and cause a loss of potassium from the body.

Resources

BOOKS

Skendiri, Gazmend. *Herbal Vade Mecum.* Rutherford, NJ: Herbacy Press, 2006.

PERIODICALS

Dugoua J., D. Perri, D. Seely, E. Mills, and G. Koren. "Safety and Efficacy of Blue Cohosh (Caulophyllum Thalictroides) During Pregnancy and Lactation." *Canadian Journal of Clinical Pharmacology* 15, no. 1(January 2008): e66–e73.

Kistin S. J., and A. D. Newman. "Induction of Labor with Homeopathy: A Case Report." *Journal of Midwifery and Women's Health* 52, no. 3 (May 1, 2007): 303–307.

Smith, C. A. "Homoeopathy for Induction of Labour." *Cochrane Database of Systemic Reviews* no. 4 (2007).

OTHER

"HerbalGram." *Journal of the American Botanical Council.* 6200 Manor Rd., Austin, TX 78723. (800) 373-7105. www.herbalgram.org.

Natural Resources Conservation Center, USDA. The PLANTS Database, National Plant Data Center, Baton Rouge, LA 70874-4490. http://plants.usda.gov.

ORGANIZATIONS

American Academy of Clinical Toxicology, 777 East Park Dr., PO Box 8820, Harrisburg, PA, 17105, (717) 558-7847, www.clintox.org.

American Botanical Council, 6200 Manor Rd, Austin, TX, 78723, (800) 373-7105, www.herbalgram.org.

American Herbal Pharmacopoeia, PO Box 66809, Scotts Valley, CA, 95067, (831) 461-6318, www.herbal-ahp.org.

Food and Nutrition Information Center, National Agricultural Library, United States Department of Agriculture. 10301 Baltimore Ave., Room 105, Beltsville, MD, 20705, (301) 504-5414, http://fnic.nal.usda.gov/.

Herb Research Foundation, 4140 Fifteenth St, Boulder, CO, 80304, (303) 449-2265, www.herbs.org.

National Center for Homeopathy, 801 N. Fairfax St., Suite 306, Alexandria, VA, 22314, (703) 548-7790, www.nationalcenterforhomeopathy.org.

Douglas Dupler
Rebecca J. Frey, PhD
Angela M. Costello

Body lice *see* **Lice infestation**

Body odor

Definition

Body odor is the unpleasant smell caused by the mixing of perspiration, or sweat, and bacteria on the skin. Sweat is generally an odorless body secretion. When bacteria multiply on the skin and break down these secretions, however, the resulting by-products may have a strong and disagreeable odor. This odor is often due to poor personal hygiene, but excessive perspiration or some other underlying disease is sometimes involved.

Causes and symptoms

People produce two kinds of sweat, eccrine and apocrine. Eccrine sweat glands secrete a mixture of water, salt (**sodium** chloride), urea, and lactic acid onto the skin. When a person is overheated, sweat seeps over the body, especially where the eccrine glands are numerous. These glands are concentrated in the armpits, the palms of the hands, the soles of the feet, and the forehead. As the sweat dries off, the skin is cooled by the surrounding air. Eccrine glands do not release any tissue cells or cell contents into their watery secretions.

In contrast with eccrine sweat, apocrine sweat is a heavier liquid containing various organic substances, including pheromone hormones. These glands are found mostly under the arms and around the groin. They develop during puberty, and are thought to serve a biological function in sexual attraction. Apocrine glands take their name from the fact that these glands release the apical portion, or tip, of the secreting cell into the liquid along with the other substances.

Sweat is essentially odorless when it is secreted, and the sweat from the eccrine glands remains so. It creates, however, a moist environment in which some of the bacteria that naturally occur on human skin can multiply. These bacteria are attracted to the sweat produced by the apocrine glands, and a strong odor is produced when these substances interact. On the other hand, the eccrine sweat glands may also help to regulate the types of bacteria on the body surface. Researchers in Germany have recently discovered that these glands secrete a peptide that has antimicrobial properties strong enough to kill some disease bacteria.

People who have a condition known as hyperhidrosis tend to sweat excessively, and therefore, they are more likely to develop a strong body odor. Bromhidrosis is the name for a medical condition in which an individual's sweat always has an unpleasant odor.

The human body normally has a slight sweaty or musky odor. Generally, bathing with soap and water, together with the use of deodorants or antiperspirants, is sufficient to prevent a truly unpleasant, unhealthy odor. There are, however, several factors that may contribute to chronic body odor. These include:

- Poor hygiene and inadequate bathing.
- An imbalance in the bacteria that inhabit the gut. Antibiotics may contribute to this condition.
- An inborn error of metabolism or some other problem that may cause about 7% of those suffering from body odor to be unable to digest certain foods. These undigested foods, which are often proteins, cause the body to give off unpleasant odors.
- Certain medications, including bupropion (Wellbutrin), venlafaxine (Effexor), tamoxifen, and pilocarpine (Salagen). These drugs may be responsible for the excretion of odors.
- Such disease conditions as liver disease, kidney disease, diabetes mellitus, a yeast infection, fungal infections, or gastrointestinal disorders may lead to body odor.
- Pathological skin conditions, including cancer, hemorrhoids, and ulcers, may produce unpleasant smelling discharges on the skin or body surface.
- Coffee and other stimulants increase apocrine gland secretion, increasing the possibility of unpleasant odors.
- States of high anxiety and stress that stimulate perspiration may increase the risk of body odors.
- Chain-smoking and heavy drinking. Alcohol and nicotine increase the rate of perspiration.

Diagnosis

Since body odor may be caused by an underlying condition, a thorough medical exam is recommended along with a blood screen and blood chemistry panel.

Treatment

The following remedies are mostly for the topical relief of body odor. For more thorough treatment, the underlying conditions should also be addressed.

- Two or three charcoal capsules per day for several weeks can help absorb waste products and reduce fermentation that may cause body odor.
- Chlorophyll tablets can be taken by mouth to absorb body toxins and odors.
- Sage tea, *Salvia officinalis*, or sage extracts can be taken internally and an undiluted alcohol extract of sage can be applied under the arms.
- Essential oils of rosemary, *Rosmarinus officinalis*, and thyme, *Thymus vulgaris*, can be used under the arms or on the feet.
- Baking soda or body powder will keep affected areas dry and absorb or mask odors.
- The diet should be altered to improve digestion, ensure regular bowel movements, and resolve constipation. There should be an increased intake of fluids to flush the system; six to eight glasses of water should be consumed daily.

Allopathic treatment

Mostly topical treatments are recommended. These include the use of antiperspirants containing chlorhexidine or aluminum chloride applied under the arms, around the groin, on the feet, or under the breasts to relieve odor and wetness. Deodorant preparations that do not contain antiperspirants also work well. Topical antibacterial creams or lotions may also be used. In cases of unrelieved excess sweating, a physician may suggest surgical removal of the sweat glands beneath the armpits.

Prevention

Good hygiene practices are important in preventing body odor. These include regular baths or showers; wearing cotton socks and non-synthetic shoes that breathe; changing the socks once or twice daily; and keeping the feet dry and bare as much as possible. Special foot powders and odor-absorbing shoe inserts may be helpful if foot odor is a particular problem.

Some foods and spices can intensify body odor. Onions, **garlic**, and cumin contain oils that may cause

KEY TERMS

Apocrine—A type of glandular secretion in which the top portion of the secreting cells is released along with the secreted substances.

Blood chemistry panel—A general set of tests measuring substances in the blood that may indicate common diseases.

Bromhidrosis—A medical condition in which a person's sweat always smells unpleasant.

Eccrine—A type of gland that produces a clear watery secretion without releasing cells or cell contents into the secretion.

Hyperhidrosis—A condition in which a person produces excessive amounts of perspiration.

Pheromone hormones—Substances secreted in order to bring out a response from other members of the same species, particularly in regard to sexual arousal.

Topical—Applied on the surface of the body.

odor as they are excreted through the skin. **Caffeine** and nicotine increase sweating and therefore the risk of odor.

Resources

BOOKS

Dollemore, Doug, and the Editors of Prevention Health Books for Seniors. *The Doctor's Book of Home Remedies for Seniors.* New York: St. Martin's Press, 2000.

The Editors of Prevention Magazine Health Books. *The Doctor's Book of Home Remedies II: Simple, Doctor-Approved Self-Care Solutions for 146 Common Health Conditions.* Emmaus, PA: Rodale Press, 2002.

PERIODICALS

Stephenson, Joan. "Sweat Defense." *Journal of the American Medical Association* 286 (December 12, 2001): 2801.

OTHER

HealthWorld Online. http://www.healthy.net.

Patience Paradox
Rebecca J. Frey, PhD

Boils

Definition

Boils are bacterial **infections** of hair follicles and the surrounding skin that form pustules around the follicle. Boils are sometimes called furuncles. When several furuncles merge to form a single deep sore with several "heads," or drainage points, the result is called a carbuncle.

Description

Boils are firm, red swellings about 5–10 mm across that are slightly raised above the skin surface. They are sore to the touch. A boil usually has a visible central core of pus; a carbuncle is larger and has several visible heads. Boils occur most commonly on the face, back of the neck, buttocks, upper legs and groin area, armpits, and upper torso. Carbuncles are less common than single boils; they are most likely to form at the back of the neck. Men are more likely than women to develop carbuncles.

As the infection that causes the boil develops, an area of inflamed tissue gradually forms a pus-filled swelling or pimple that is painful to touch. As the boil matures, it forms a yellowish head or point. It may either continue to swell until the point bursts open and allows the pus to drain, or it may be gradually reabsorbed into the skin. It generally takes between one and two weeks for a boil to heal completely after it comes to a head and discharges pus. The bacteria that cause the boil can spread into other areas of the skin or even into the bloodstream if the skin around the boil is squeezed. If the infection spreads, the patient will usually develop **chills**, **fever**, and swollen lymph nodes. Red lines may appear on the skin running outward from the boil.

Boils and carbuncles are common problems in the general population, particularly among adolescents and adults. People who are most likely to develop these skin infections include those with:

- diabetes, especially when treated by injected insulin
- alcoholism or drug abuse
- recent experience of childbirth, especially women who are breastfeeding their babies
- poor personal hygiene
- crowded living arrangements
- jobs or hobbies that expose them to greasy or oily substances, especially petroleum products
- hair styles requiring frequent use of hair relaxers
- allergies or immune system disorders, including HIV infection

Causes and symptoms

Boils are most often caused by *Staphylococcus aureus* (staph), a bacterium that causes an infection in an oil gland or hair follicle. Although the surface of human skin is usually resistant to bacterial infection, staph can enter through a break in the skin surface, including breaks caused by needle punctures for insulin or drug injections. Hair follicles that are blocked by greasy creams, petroleum jelly, hair relaxers, or similar products are more vulnerable to developing boils. These bacterial skin infections can be spread by shared cosmetics or washcloths, close human contact, or by contact with pus from another boil or carbuncle.

Carbuncles are formed when the bacteria infect several hair follicles that are close together. Carbunculosis is a word that is sometimes used to refer to the development of carbuncles. The abscesses spread until they merge with each other to form a single large area of infected skin with several pus-filled heads. Patients with carbuncles may also have a low-grade fever or feel generally unwell.

Furunculosis is a word used to refer to recurrent boils. Many patients have repeated episodes of furunculosis that are difficult to treat because their nasal passages carry colonies of staph. Skin and anal colonization are fairly common as well. Persistent furunculosis may be an indication of a depressed immune system. A physician should be consulted if boils are a persistent problem in order to determine whether there is an underlying disease such as diabetes, HIV infection, or immune system disorders.

Diagnosis

A diagnosis of boils is usually made on the basis of visual examination of the skin. For the most part, boils are not difficult to distinguish. A doctor can make a culture from pus taken from the boil to confirm the diagnosis and treatment. The patient's nasal discharge may also be tested. In cases of persistent recurrent boils, family members or close contacts may be examined to see if they are carriers of staph.

Treatment

Patient education is an important part of the treatment of boils. Patients need to be warned against squeezing boils because of the danger of spreading the infection into other parts of the skin or bloodstream. It is especially important to avoid squeezing boils around the mouth or nose, because infections in these areas may be carried to the brain, although this happens rarely. Patients should also be advised about keeping the skin clean, washing their hands carefully before and after touching the boil, avoiding the use of greasy cosmetics or creams, and keeping their towels and washcloths separate from those of other family members.

The use of the following supplements is reported to be effective in treating boils: **zinc**, 45 mg per day; **vitamin A**, 50,000 IUs per day for two weeks; **vitamin C**, 1 g three times per day; and beta-carotene, 100,000 IUs per day.

Taking the proper homeopathic medication in the first stages of a boil can bring about early resolution of the infection and prevent pus formation. The most likely choices are **belladonna** or *Hepar sulphuris*. If the boil has already formed, **Mercurius vivus** or **silica** may be recommended to bring the pus to a head.

A variety of herbal remedies can be applied topically to fight infection. These include **essential oils** of bergamot, *Citrus bergamia;* **chamomile**, *Matricaria recutita;* **lavender**, *Lavandula officinalis;* and **sage**, *Salvia officinalis;* as well as **tea tree oil**, *Melaleuca spp.* Application of a paste or poultice containing **goldenseal** root, *Hydrastis canadensis,* is recommended to help kill bacteria and to reduce inflammation. Washing the skin around the affected area with a mixture of goldenseal, *Hydrastis canadensis,* and **witch hazel**, *Hamamelis virginiana,* dissolved in warm water is also recommended.

Allopathic treatment

Boils are usually treated with application of antibiotic creams, following the application of hot compresses. The compresses help the infection to come to a head and drain and are an important part of the treatment regime. Carbuncles and furunculosis are usually treated with oral antibiotics as well as antibiotic creams or ointments. The usual course of oral antibiotics is 5-10 days; however, patients with recurrent furunculosis may be given oral antibiotics for longer periods. Patients with bacterial colonies in their nasal passages are often given mupirocin ointment (Bactroban) to apply directly to the lining of the nose and should wash the area once a month with an antiseptic soap such as Phisohex.

Boils or carbuncles that are very large or that do not resolve may be opened with a sterile needle or surgical knife to allow the pus to drain. Surgical treatment of boils is often painful and usually leaves noticeable scars.

The increase of antibiotic- and biocide-resistant **strains** of *Staphylococcus aureus* has caused growing concern among doctors, as some of these strains are now resistant to disinfectants used to clean endoscopes and other surgical equipment. **Resveratrol**, which is a phytoalexin, or compound formed by plants at the site of a fungal or bacterial invasion, appears to be highly effective in treating boils and other skin infections in humans caused by *S. aureus.*

KEY TERMS

Antiseptic—A substance that works to inhibit the growth and reproduction of bacteria and viruses.

Biocide—Any chemical that works to kill microorganisms and other forms of life by poisoning. Hospital disinfectants are examples of biocides.

Carbuncle—A localized skin inflammation consisting of deep interconnected boils.

Compress—Cloth applied to heat, cold or medication to the skin.

Follicle—The small sac at the base of a hair shaft. The follicle lies below the skin surface.

Furuncle—The medical name for a boil.

Phytoalexin—A type of compound formed in a plant at the site of invasion by microorganisms that helps the plant resist disease. A phytoalexin called resveratrol appears to be useful in treating boils.

Pustule—A small raised pimple or blister-like swelling of the skin that contains pus.

Expected results

Boils usually drain or are reabsorbed in two or three days. Recurrent boils and carbuncles, however, are fairly common. In addition, although the spread of infection from boils is relatively unusual, there have been deaths reported from brain infections caused by squeezing boils on the upper lip or in the tissue folds at the base of the nose.

Prevention

To minimize the risk of developing bacterial skin infections the skin should be kept clean; to avoid spreading the infection, washcloths, towels, and facial cosmetics should not be shared with others. A healthy diet should be maintained and allergic foods should be eliminated. This will ensure that the immune system will be supported, and that boils will be prevented.

Resources

BOOKS

Conn, Rex B., ed., et. al. *Current Diagnosis 9*. Philadelphia: W.B. Saunders, 1997.

Rakel, Robert E., ed. *Conn's Current Therapy*. Philadelphia: W.B. Saunders, 1998.

Tierney, Jr., Lawrence, ed., et. al. *Current Medical Diagnosis & Treatment, 1998*. Connecticut: Appleton & Lange, 1997.

Turkington, Carol A., and Jeffrey S. Dover. *Skin Deep: An A-Z of Skin Disorders, Treatments, and Health*. New York: Facts On File, 1996.

PERIODICALS

Amir, L. "Breastfeeding and *Staphylococcus aureus*: Three Case Reports." *Breastfeeding Review* 10 (March 2002): 15-18.

Chan, M. M. "Antimicrobial Effect of Resveratrol on Dermatophytes and Bacterial Pathogens of the Skin." *Biochemical Pharmacology* 63 (January 15, 2002): 99-104.

Fraise, A. P. "Susceptibility of Antibiotic-Resistant Cocci to Biocides." *Journal of Applied Microbiology* 92 (2002 Supplement): 158S-162S.

Kaur,B. J., H. Singh, and A. Lin-Greenberg. "Irritant Contact Dermatitis Complicated by Deep-Seated Staphylococcal Infection Caused by a Hair Relaxer." *Journal of the National Medical Association* 94 (February 2002): 121-123.

Oliveira, D. C., A. Tomasz, and H. de Lencastre. "Secrets of Success of a Human Pathogen: Molecular Evolution of Pandemic Clones of Methicillin-Resistant *Staphylococcus aureus*." *Lancet Infectious Diseases* 2 (March 2002): 180-189.

Patience Paradox
Rebecca J. Frey, PhD

Bonemeal

Description

Bonemeal is a product created from the waste resulting from the slaughter of animals, especially beef cattle, by meat processors. It is a white powder made by grinding either raw or steamed animal bones. This results in a product that contains the same nutrients necessary for the production of, and maintenance of, bone in both humans and animals.

The composition of bonemeal can vary. **Phosphorus**, in the form of chemical compounds related to phosphates, makes up 20–30% of the powder. In addition to its mineral content, depending upon the amount of tendon and muscle left on the bones, bonemeal can be a fairly good source of protein.

The nutrients typically present in bonemeal include the minerals **calcium**, phosphorus, **iron**, **magnesium** and **zinc**, as well as traces of other elements. Bonemeal, especially when not steamed or cooked, is also rich in vitamins A and D.

General use

Calcium is the most significant nutrient in bone-meal. Calcium is particularly significant to women because of its essential role in the prevention of **osteoporosis**. A 1999 report of the American Dietetic Association and Dietitians of Canada entitled *Women's Health and Nutrition* states that either osteoporosis or osteopenia affects more than 30 million Americans (mostly women).

That same report states that osteoporosis is an irreversible disease process. However, it has been found that increasing bone mass early in life may prevent its occurrence or at least lessen its severity. Bone is living tissue that is, like other cells in the body, in a constant state of buildup and breakdown. This process of bone buildup and breakdown is very dependent upon the amount of calcium taken in. Calcium, especially when ingested along with **vitamin D**, increases bone mass, and can actually sustain the health of bones during the later portions of a woman's life when the body naturally loses bone during **menopause** and old age. It is estimated that menopausal women age 50–60 can lose 10–40% of their bone mass.

It is consistently reported that American women are not meeting even minimum requirements for calcium intake according to the recommendations of the American Dietetic Association (ADA). Although the ADA recommends that people's intake of calcium be consumed via foods rich in this element, such as low-fat dairy foods, it further recognizes that some people cannot eat these foods at all, or cannot take in sufficient quantities to maximize bone health. It therefore concludes that for those persons who cannot consume sufficient calcium rich foods, it will usually be necessary for them to take supplements containing calcium, and sometimes vitamin D as well. Bonemeal provides both of these nutrients. Recent research even reports that calcium supplements can help prevent formation of **kidney stones** when combined with a fairly low animal protein, low salt diet. Doctors once advised a low-calcium diet to prevent kidney stones.

Bonemeal, with its 20–30% phosphate content, is an important organic fertilizer used in gardening of all types. Raw bonemeal works more slowly as a fertilizer than steamed bonemeal. Both work more slowly than other fertilizers, making bonemeal an ideal source of nourishment for bulb plants, such as tulips, crocuses, daffodils, and irises, that are planted several months before growth and blooming occur.

KEY TERMS

Osteopenia—A disease of the bone, characterized by reduced bone mass leading to increased susceptibility to fractures. It is common among teen-aged girls, and is often responsible for fractures of the lower arm.

Ruminant—Any of various hoofed, even-toed, usually horned mammals of the suborder Ruminantia, such as cattle, sheep, goats, deer, and giraffes.

Preparations

Bonemeal tablets are available from health food stores. A typical dose of four tablets per day would commonly contain the following nutrients:

- calcium: 880 mg
- phosphorus: 400 mg
- iron: 1.8 mg
- natural vitamin A: 4,000 units
- natural vitamin D: 400 units
- red bone marrow: 15 mg

Precautions

Phosphates present in bonemeal could potentially be leached into water systems if bonemeal fertilizer is used along shorelines. Phosphates have the capability to drastically alter the chemical makeup of lakes and rivers, and can kill aquatic life if present in sufficient quantities.

Many bonemeal products contain high, even dangerous, levels of lead. Labels should be read carefully to make sure the product has been tested. Unfortunately, preliminary research in the United Kingdom in 2002 found that the bone-boosting effects of calcium supplements did not have the same long-lasting effects of drinking milk.

Resources

PERIODICALS

Affenito, Sandra G., and Jane Kerstetter. "Position of the American Dietetic Association and Dietitians of Canada: Women's Health and Nutrition." *Journal of the American Dietetic Association* 1999.

"Calcium Supplements' Effects Short-lives." *Nutraceuticals International* (January 2002).

"Unrestricted Calcium Intake Protects Against Recurrent Kidney Stones Better than a Restricted Calcium Diet." *Environmental Nutrition* (March 2002): 3.

OTHER

MacDonald, Sarah. *Phosphorus Boosters.* Canada/Nova Scotia Agreement on the Agricultural Component of the Green Plan.

New Zealand Federal Ministry of Agriculture. *Part II: Addressing The Issue.* 1997.

Vitamin Power. "Bone Meal Plus." http://vitaminpower. com/.

Joan Schonbeck
Teresa Odle

Boneset

Description

Boneset (*Eupatorium perfoliatum*) is a common perennial that is native to the eastern United States and Canada, with a range from Nova Scotia to Florida. Other names for boneset are feverwort, sweat plant, and thoroughwort. The Native American name for boneset translates into ague-weed (ague is the name for malarial **fever**). The common name, boneset, comes from break-bone fever, an influenza-like illness causing severe bone **pain** that was treated with *Eupatorium perfoliatum*.

Boneset prefers a damp environment and is found in marshes and meadows, often at the edge of a wooded area. Although boneset can reach a height of 5 ft (1.5 m), it is usually only 2–4 ft (0.6–1.2 m) tall. It has an erect, round, hairy stem that branches at the top. The leaves are large (4–8 in, or 10–20 cm, long), directly across from one another, and are joined at the stem. Lower leaves are large, and they become progressively smaller higher up the plant. They are spear

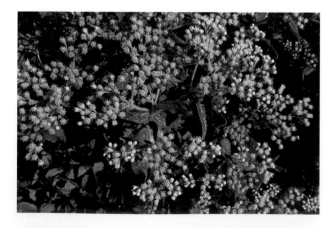

Boneset. *(©PlantaPhile, Germany. Reproduced by permission.)*

shaped with toothed edges and pointy tips, have prominent veins, a rough topside, and a downy, dotted, sticky underside.

Boneset blooms between July and September. Large, numerous, white or purple flower clusters, which appear at the ends of the branches, are comprised of 10–20 florets (small flowers). Boneset has a faint aroma and a very bitter taste.

Constituents and bioactivities

Boneset contains a wide variety of compounds with biological activity that contribute to its medicinal value. Constituents of boneset include:

- sesquiterpene lactones (euccannabinolide, eufoliatin, eufoliatorin, eupafolin, euperfolide, euperfolitin, and helenalin)
- polysaccharides (4-0-methylglucuroxylans)
- flavonoids (astragalin, eupatorin, hyperoside, kaempferol, quercitin, rutin, etc.)
- diterpenes (dendroidinic acid and hebenolide)
- sterols
- volatile oil
- tannic acid
- resin
- gum

Sesquiterpene lactones have antimicrobial, antitumor, and cytotoxic activities. The flavonoid eupatorin has cytotoxic activity. Sesquiterpene lactones and polysaccharides stimulate the immune system. Boneset extracts also activate defense mechanisms against viral **infections**.

Boneset has stimulant, febrifuge (reduces body temperature), laxative (promotes bowel movements), diaphoretic (promotes sweating), bitter, tonic (restores tissue tone), anti-spasmodic (relieves **muscle spasms**), carminative (relieves intestinal **gas**), and astringent (causes skin contraction) activities.

General use

Boneset was used by Native Americans (who later taught the colonists) to treat **influenza**, colds, and other infectious diseases as well as fever, arthritis, and rheumatism. By the eighteenth and nineteenth centuries, European settlers considered boneset to be a cure-all. As a result, boneset was used to treat many different diseases and conditions. It was, perhaps, among the most widely used herbal medicines in the United States. Dried boneset was kept on hand by families, as well as doctors, for immediate use, especially during the flu season.

Boneset is used to treat colds, influenza, fevers, coughs, upper respiratory tract congestion, migraine, **headache**, skin conditions, **worms**, **malaria**, **constipation**, arthritis, muscular rheumatism, **jaundice**, and general debility. Boneset is also used to treat secondary infections that arise during colds or flu. Secondary infections, such as **bronchitis**, **pneumonia**, or **tonsillitis**, are infections that occur while the patient has another illness. Currently, herbalists recommend boneset primarily for relieving the aches and pains associated with fever, clearing congestion, and relieving pain caused by arthritis and rheumatism.

Boneset is considered to be among the best remedies for the flu. Its wide spectrum of activities brings relief to the many symptoms associated with the flu. It helps reduce fever by promoting sweating, reduces aches and pains, and relieves congestion by loosening phlegm and promoting coughing. Boneset also stimulates the immune system, which promotes the destruction of the influenza virus.

Preparations

All above-ground portions of the plant have medicinal value. Boneset is harvested after flowering has begun. The biological activities can be extracted either in water or alcohol, or the plant can be used as the fresh or dried herb. Boneset is used in the dried form and is available commercially as dried flowers and leaves, as a tincture (an alcohol solution), and in tablets and capsules.

Boneset is usually taken as an infusion (tea). To make the infusion, 2-3 teaspoons of dried herb are steeped in one cup of boiling water for 10-15 minutes. To improve boneset's bitter taste, lemon and honey may be added to the infusion, or the infusion may be mixed with a flavorful herbal tea or fruit juice.

Boneset may be taken as soon as flu symptoms appear. To treat influenza, fever, or colds, one cup of hot boneset infusion should be drunk every two hours—up to six cups daily—for two days. Then the dose can be reduced to four cups daily. High doses shouldn't be taken over a long period of time. The tea should be stopped if it has been used for a week and has not helped improve symptoms. To act as a diaphoretic, the patient should remain in bed covered with multiple blankets. Sweating begins after the patient has drunk four to five doses of the hot infusion. Up to four cups may be drunk within six hours; however, the patient should not drink more than six cups within 24 hours. Alternatively, 2-4 ml of the tincture may be taken three times a day.

KEY TERMS

Cytotoxic—An agent that destroys the cells of a specific organ. Anticancer agents are cytotoxic.

Diaphoretic—An agent that induces sweating that is usually used to treat fever.

Perennial—A plant that regrows each year from its roots.

Tonic—An agent that restores normal tone to tissues. Tonics are used to treat indigestion, general debility, and other disorders.

When taken in larger doses, boneset infusion can act as an emetic (causes **vomiting**) and purgative (causes evacuation of the bowels). Boneset infusion is drunk cold, in moderate doses (one-fourth cup), to act as a tonic to treat **indigestion** and general debility.

Boneset may be taken in combination with **cayenne**, **elder** flowers, **ginger**, **lemon balm**, **peppermint**, or **yarrow** to treat influenza. For bronchial conditions, boneset may be taken with **pleurisy** root and elecampane.

Precautions

Fresh boneset contains tremerol, a toxic chemical which can cause rapid breathing and vomiting. Higher doses can cause coma and death. Dried boneset does not contain tremerol. Boneset may cause liver toxicity, so alcoholics and people with liver disease should consult an herbalist before using this herb. Boneset should not be taken for longer than two weeks at a time.

Side effects

Boneset does not generally cause any serious side effects. However, taking large doses of boneset may cause **nausea** or **diarrhea**. Boneset may cause liver toxicity in chronic high doses.

Interactions

As of early 2000, there was no evidence of interactions between boneset and other herbals or conventional medicines.

Resources

PERIODICALS

Sharma, Om P., Rajinder K. Dawra, Nitin P. Kurade, and Pritam D. Sharma. "A Review of the Toxicosis and Biological Properties of the Genus Eupatorium." *Natural Toxins* 6 (1998): 1-14.

OTHER

"Boneset." *A Modern Herbal.* http://www.botanical.com/botanical/mgmh/b/bonese65.html.

"Boneset." *Planet Botanic.* http://www.planetbotanic.com/boneset.htm.

Hoffman, David L. "Boneset." *HealthWorld Online.* http://www.healthy.net/library/books/hoffman/materiamedica/boneset.htm.

Belinda Rowland

Bone spurs

Definition

Bone spurs are abnormal, bony growths at the end of bones. They are most commonly located in the spine or other weight-bearing joints.

Description

Bone spurs may grow on the ends of bones in any part of the body. The spurs have no protective cartilage, as other bones do, and may rub against other bones, blood vessels, or nerves. The spurs may cause slight discomfort or severe **pain**.

Causes and symptoms

Bone spurs have several possible causes. Some are a result of **osteoarthritis**. This condition begins without symptoms from age 20–30, and is marked by the loss of cartilage in the joints. Once the cartilage is gone, there is no cushion to protect the joints from the strain of physical activity or bearing weight. The bones rub together and bone spurs may grow in and around the joints. By the age of 70, almost everyone is afflicted with this condition. Bone spurs can also be found in older adults who have disk problems. As people grow older, the disks in the spinal column can become tough and shrink. The distance between the vertebrae decreases as the disks shrink, and bone spurs, or knobby growths, then appear on the vertebrae. Those who have placed an excessive amount of **stress** on their bodies, such as dancers, athletes, and laborers may develop bone spurs.

Spurs in particular regions of the spine may cause pain in a specific area. Those located in the upper vertebrae of the neck (cervical region) may cause stiffness and pain in the back and neck.

Spurs located in the feet can be particularly painful. Bone spurs occur most often on the heel (**heel spurs**), but can be found on any part of the foot that has been under pressure. This condition can be caused by shoes that fit improperly, excessive use, or heredity.

Most bone spurs cause pain because of their movement against nerves or other bones. Pain or stiffness in the back or neck, or tingling in the hands, arms, or neck, can indicate bone spurs on the spine. Headaches and **dizziness** may also occur, and a person may not be able to keep balanced. A heel spur can cause a sharp pain when weight is placed on one or both feet. If there is a severe, shooting pain in the neck or back with slight movement, this could be a sign of a bone spur pinching a nerve or interfering with muscle movement.

Diagnosis

A medical practitioner may order a computer assisted tomography (CAT) scan or x ray to rule out other causes of back pain and to help locate any existing bone spurs. An electromyography (EMG) can look at the condition of nerves that supply muscles to see if they are affected by bone spurs. Magnetic resonance imaging (MRI) can look at bones, nerves, and disks to check for abnormalities.

Treatment

Exercise and a healthy weight are key ingredients to managing the pain associated with bone spurs. Exercise may be limited by the location of the spur and its effects on movement. Swimming or other forms of water activity, such as water aerobics, may be less stressful for the body, and can also increase flexibility and mobility. Weight loss can also be beneficial in alleviating the pain associated with bone spurs, since

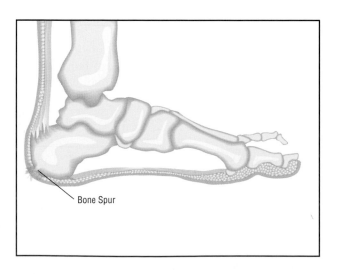

Bone Spur

A bone spur. *(Illustration by GGS Information Services, Inc. Cengage Learning, Gale)*

less weight puts less stress on any joints which are lacking cartilage or plagued with bone spurs.

There are several options for managing the pain caused by bone spurs and increasing movement. A chiropractor may use manipulation and physical therapy to relieve pain associated with bone spurs in the vertebrae. Physical therapy may also increase movement of the affected area. **Acupuncture** can be used to relieve some joint pain. A homeopath will assess more than a patient's physical condition to determine the proper remedy. To prescribe a remedy, a homeopath must have information about the conditions that trigger pain in a patient. **Guided imagery** can help alleviate pain. **Feldenkrais** method can be used to retrain the body's movement when it is inhibited by pain. **Yoga** is another **movement therapy** that can help decrease the stress placed on affected areas, as well as help the body relax and strengthen muscles. **Sodium** in the diet may help break down **calcium** so that it can be resorbed into the blood. Those on a low-sodium diet for health reasons should talk to their doctors before increasing the sodium in their **diets**.

Allopathic treatment

A doctor will usually prescribe anti-inflammatory painkillers, such as aspirin or ibuprofen, to help relieve pain. Resting and keeping pressure off of the affected area can also help diminish the pain. A back or neck brace can provide additional support and relieve pressure. A foam cushion placed in the shoe, with a hole cut out for the spur, can help relieve the pain of a spur on the foot. Severe cases may call for surgery, but this relief may be temporary, since bone spurs can grow back in the same place.

Expected results

Once bone spurs form, patients can use different therapies to manage the pain associated with this ailment and to help improve their range of movement. While surgery may be used to remove a bone spur in severe cases, there is a chance that another could grow to take its place.

Prevention

Maintaining a healthy body weight and reducing stress on one's joints are steps individuals can take to reduce the chance of bone spurs. Exercises which work the muscles of the whole body, such as walking, biking, swimming, and tennis, are recommended for weight loss and muscle strength.

Resources

BOOKS

Somerville, Robert. *The Medical Advisor: The Complete Guide to Alternative & Conventional Treatments.* Alexandria, VA: Time Life Inc., 1996.

PERIODICALS

"Better than aspirin?" *Industry Week* (July 7, 1997): 32.

OTHER

DrKoop.com. *Osteoarthritis.* http://www.drkoop.com. (July 17, 2000).

National Institute of Arthritis and Musculoskeletal and Skin Diseases. *Osteoarthritis.* (May 1, 1999).

Footcare Direct. *Hammertoes/Bone Spurs.* http://www. footcaredirect.com. (July 17, 2000).

Heather Bienvenue

Borage oil

Description

Borage, whose botanical name is *Borago officinalis*, is an annual herb in the Boraginaceae family. There are as many as 2,500 species in this family of plants. The specific designation *officinalis* indicates the herb's inclusion in official listings of medicinal plants. Borage is a wild-growing, hardy native of the Mediterranean region, cultivated and naturalized throughout Great Britain and North America. Traditionally associated with courage, borage was used to flavor the wine for soldiers preparing for battle. The English word "borage" may be derived from the word *borrach*, a Celtic word meaning "a person of courage." In folk tradition throughout its long history of recorded use, borage was believed to dispel melancholy and ease grief and sadness. According to the ancient Greek physician Dioscorides, borage can "cheer the heart and lift the depressed spirits." Common names for the herb include burrage, common bugloss, star flower, tailwort, or beebread. Borage self-seeds freely and flourishes in rich, well-drained soil in full sun. It is a good companion herb in the cottage garden, attracting honey bees and imparting strength and insect resistance to nearby plants, particularly strawberry and tomato.

Borage's silvery-green, oblong to ovate, textured leaves form a basal rosette, then grow alternately up a succulent hollow round stem containing a clear mucilage. The leaves and sprawling branches are covered in bristly white hairs that impart a silvery sheen to the herb and are irritating to the skin on contact. Borage can reach a height of 2 ft (0.6 m), with leaves as long as 5 in (13 cm). The five-petaled star-shaped blue flowers, each with five black anthers, grow in loose, downward-turning clusters at the apex of the stems. Borage may bloom continuously from early spring until frost. The large, brownish-black seeds are three-sided and may be viable for as long as eight years. The roots are shallow and spreading.

General use

Borage seed oil

In contrast to borage's centuries of use as an herb, borage seed oil has only been used for the last 10 years. Borage oil, extracted from the seeds by cold pressing, contains omega-6 **essential fatty acids**, with as much as a 25–30% concentration of gamma linolenic acid (GLA). GLA is a derivative of the **omega-6 fatty acids**. It is an essential fatty acid used by the body to produce prostaglandins, the hormone-like substances in the body that may be out of balance in **premenstrual syndrome** (PMS) or during **menopause**. GLA also appears to reduce the adherence of plaque (abnormal patches of hardened deposits) to artery walls, thus lowering the risk of coronary **heart disease**. GLA helps to relieve PMS, regulate the menstrual cycle, and ease the **hot flashes** and mood swings of menopause.

At present, borage seed oil is best known for its anti-inflammatory properties. The oil has been shown in clinical studies with human subjects to be useful in treating the following conditions:

- rheumatoid arthritis

- atopic eczema

- infantile seborrheic dermatitis

- Raynaud's phenomenon

- Sjögren's syndrome

- juvenile rheumatoid arthritis (JRA)

In addition, the GLA in borage seed oil prevents the formation of **blood clots**, helps to keep cell membranes flexible, and supports the body's immune function.

Other claims for borage seed oil that have not been tested in clinical studies include its use as a remedy for hangovers, as an anti-aging preparation, and as a wrinkle reducer. Various borage oil products that make these claims, however, are readily available over the Internet.

Culinary and medicinal uses

Borage's culinary and medicinal uses have been known for at least 2000 years. Borage is a cooling, cleansing, and refreshing herb with adaptogenic, demulcent, diuretic, expectorant, and anti-inflammatory properties. The entire plant contains mucilage, tannin, essential oil, **potassium**, **calcium**, pyrrolizioline alkaloids, saponins, and **vitamin C**, as well as a high amount of mineral salts. The leaves have been used as an adrenal tonic to balance and restore the health of the adrenal glands following periods of **stress**. A tea made from the leaves and blossoms will also promote lactation, relieve fevers, and promote sweating. The soothing mucilage in borage makes it a beneficial treatment for dry **cough** and throat irritation. Borage tea is also a good remedy to use with such digestive disturbances as **gastritis** and **irritable bowel syndrome**. European herbalists use borage tea to restore strength during convalescence. It may be of particular benefit during recovery from surgery or following steroid treatment. Borage tea is also helpful in clearing up such skin problems as **boils** and **rashes**, and has been used as an eyewash.

About a dozen clinical tests of the medicinal applications of borage in human subjects have been conducted since 1989. In addition, some researchers are now testing the effects of borage on skin cells in animal studies.

Preparations

The leaves, flowers, and seeds of borage have nutritive and medicinal properties. Harvest borage leaves on a dry day, just as the plant begins to blossom. Strip the leaves from the stems and spread out on a tray. The plant has a high water content and the leaves may discolor if dried in direct heat. Place the drying trays in a warm, airy room out of direct sun. When thoroughly dry, store the leaves in dark, tightly-sealed containers. Borage flowers can be collected by gently pulling on the stamen tips to separate the blossom from the green backing attached to the stem. The blossoms may be used fresh, or frozen individually in ice-cube trays for later use.

- Infusion: Place 2 oz (56 g) of fresh borage leaves in a warmed glass container. Bring 2.5 cups (590 ml) of fresh, nonchlorinated water to the boiling point, add it to the herbs. Cover. Allow the tea to steep for 10 minutes, strain, and drink warm. The prepared tea can be stored for two days in the refrigerator. Borage tea may be enjoyed by the cupful up to three times a day. Some herbalists suggest combining borage with

hawthorn berries (*Crataegus oxyacantha*) as a heart tonic.

- Poultice: Chop fresh borage leaves and stems in sufficient quantity to cover the area being treated. Cover the herb with a strip of cotton gauze to hold the poultice in place. The poultice may be soothing and healing to skin inflammations, though the prickly hairs may be irritating.

- Culinary: Borage leaves, eaten fresh, have a crisp, cool taste, reminiscent of cucumber but with a somewhat prickly texture. Borage blossoms are sometimes used as a garnish on salads or crystallized and used to decorate cakes.

- Borage oil is available commercially as bottled oil and in capsule form. One manufacturer offers a package containing 90 capsules for $20. The usual recommended doses of GLA range from 100–300 mg daily (1 tbsp of bottled oil or 1–3 capsules). The dosage and duration of use, however, are best determined by a qualified herbal practitioner.

Precautions

Borage oil has been shown to contain small amounts of such pyrrolizidine alkaloids (PAs) as lycopsamine, amabiline, and thesinine. Some pyrrolizidine alkaloids, particularly unsaturated ones, may be toxic to the liver even in small amounts. Some herbalists stress that use of borage oil should be avoided unless the preparations are certified to be free of these potentially harmful, unsaturated pyrrolizidine alkaloids. In addition, borage oil should be refrigerated after opening to keep it stable, as GLA is damaged in the presence of oxidation. Blending small amounts of **vitamin E** or vitamin C into the oil will also help to slow down the process of oxidation.

The long-term use of herbal borage in medicinal preparations is not recommended.

Side effects

Some minor side effects have been reported when borage preparations are taken internally, even when taken in appropriate forms and in therapeutic dosages. These side effects include bloating, **nausea**, **indigestion**, and **headache**. External contact with fresh borage leaves may cause skin rashes in sensitive persons. Any adverse reactions to borage preparations (or any other herbal products used as dietary supplements) should be reported to the Food and Drug Administration's Center for Food Safety and Applied **Nutrition** (CFSAN), listed under Resources below.

KEY TERMS

Adaptogen—A substance that acts in nonspecific ways to improve the body's level of functioning and its adaptations to stress.

Antioxidant—An agent that helps to protect cells from damage caused by free radicals, the destructive fragments of oxygen produced as a byproduct during normal metabolic processes.

Demulcent—A substance that soothes irritated mucous membranes. Borage contains a mucilage that can be used as a demulcent.

Gamma linolenic acid (GLA)—An essential fatty acid that is found in borage seed oil.

Mucilage—A gummy, gelatinous substance found in the stems of borage that is useful for treating throat irritations.

Raynaud's phenomenon—A vascular disorder in which the patient's fingers ache and tingle after exposure to cold or emotional stress, with characteristic color changes from white to blue to red. Raynaud's phenomenon may be seen in scleroderma and systemic lupus erythematosus.

Sjögren's syndrome—An autoimmune disorder characterized by excessive dryness of the eyes and mouth.

Interactions

Adverse interactions have been reported between borage and three types of prescription medications: anticoagulants (blood thinners), anticonvulsants (drugs to prevent seizures), and anxiolytics (tranquilizers). Borage may prolong bleeding time if taken together with anticoagulant medications. Borage has also been reported to lower the seizure threshold if taken together with anticonvulsant medications. Lastly, borage has been reported to increase the degree of sedation when taken with anxiolytics.

Resources

BOOKS

Bremnes, Lesley. *The Complete Book of Herbs*. New York: Henry Holt, 1995.

Hoffmann, David. *The New Holistic Herbal, 2nd ed*. Boston: Element, 1986.

McIntyre, Anne. *The Complete Woman's Herbal*. London: Dorling Kindersley Limited, 1988.

Ody, Penelope. *The Complete Medicinal Herbal*. New York: Dorling Kindersley, 1993.

PDR for Herbal Medicines. Montvale, NJ: Medical Economics Company, 1998.

Pelletier, Kenneth R., MD. *The Best Alternative Medicine, Part I: Western Herbal Medicine.* New York: Simon & Schuster, 2002.

Tyler, Varro E., Ph.D. *Herbs of Choice: The Therapeutic Use of Phytomedicinals.* New York: The Haworth Press, Inc., 1994.

PERIODICALS

Chung, S., S. Kong, K. Seong, et al. "[Gamma]-Linolenic Acid in Borage Oil Reverses Epidermal Hyperproliferation in Guinea Pigs." *Journal of Nutrition* 132 (October 2002): 3090-3097.

"ShiKai Borage Therapy." (Shopper.) *Contemporary Long Term Care* 25 (September 2002): 43.

Turon, F., P. Bachain, Y. Caro, et al. "A Direct Method for Regiospecific Analysis of TAG Using Alpha-MAG." *Lipids* 37 (August 2002): 817-821.

ORGANIZATIONS

Herb Research Foundation, 1007 Pearl St., Suite 200, Boulder, CO 80302, (303) 449-2265, http://www.herbs.org.

United States Food and Drug Administration (FDA), Center for Food Safety and Applied Nutrition, 5100 Paint Branch Parkway, College Park, MD 20740, (888) SAFEFOOD, http://www.cfsan.fda.gov.

Clare Hanrahan
Rebecca J. Frey, PhD

Boron

Description

Boron is a trace mineral that has gained popularity because of claims that it can strengthen bones, build muscle mass, and boost brain activity. While such macrominerals as **calcium**, **magnesium**, and **potassium** have become household names because they make up over 98% of the body's mineral content, certain trace minerals are also considered essential in very small amounts to maintain health and ensure proper functioning of the body. They usually act as coenzymes, working in conjunction with proteins to facilitate important chemical reactions. While boron is considered essential for plants, it is not known if the mineral is necessary for humans. Evidence has been mounting, however, which suggests boron may be an important micronutrient.

Studies indicate that boron may contribute to the way that calcium (a vital building block of bone) and other minerals are processed by the body. Boron

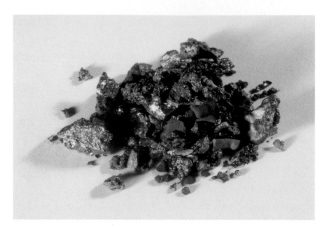

Studies indicate that boron may contribute to the way that calcium (a vital building block of bone) and other minerals are processed by the body. *(Phil Degginger / Alamy)*

appears to increase the amount of calcium absorbed from food and lower the amount excreted by the body. These effects may help to keep bones strong. Boron may also improve mental functioning, strengthen the immune system, boost energy utilization, and affect **cholesterol** production. While the effects of a boron-free diet have not been observed in people, animal studies suggest that a lack of boron can be unhealthy. In one investigation, for example, a boron-deficient diet fed to animals seemed to increase the amount of calcium they lost. It also appeared to have a negative effect on bone development and energy utilization. It is not certain, however, that study results such as this confirm the nutritional importance of boron for human beings. Research is still necessary to determine if boron can produce significant health benefits safely and effectively. The proper dosage of the mineral has not been established.

General use

While not extensively studied, boron has been touted as having a number of beneficial effects. Some people take it to help treat **osteoporosis** or arthritis and to alleviate menopausal symptoms. It has been reported to enhance mental activity, memory, and hand-eye coordination. Some body builders and athletes take boron supplements as a muscle-enhancing agent despite a lack of evidence to support this use. Overall, boron appears to have the most potential as a possible bone-builder and brain booster.

Most of the research suggesting that boron may be helpful for arthritis is indirect and circumstantial. Early studies in sheep and chickens indicated that boron may be useful in helping to treat the disease. There is also an interesting relationship between the incidence of arthritis and boron intake in certain geographical locations. In parts of the world where boron intake is high (intake can range anywhere from 3–10 mg), usually as a result of high boron levels in the soil and water, the number of people who develop arthritis tends to be lower than in areas where people consume less of the mineral. Boron levels in the water and soil are usually highest in arid climates, such as the desert regions of the United States and South America, the Red Sea region of the Middle East, and parts of Australia. There are few human studies of boron in relation to arthritis, although one small investigation in people has suggested that boron may help to relieve symptoms of the disease.

While there is some evidence that boron may be helpful in the treatment of postmenopausal osteoporosis, the mineral does not appear to ease the symptoms associated with **menopause**. In a five-week study involving 46 menopausal women, about 50% of those who received boron supplements experienced more frequent and severe **hot flashes** (as well as night sweats) and generally had an increase in menopausal symptoms. Over one-third of the women who received boron reported that the mineral made no difference in their symptoms. Boron had a beneficial effect in only 15% of the women who took it. These findings suggest that boron may actually aggravate menopausal symptoms more often than it alleviates them.

Researchers from the Grand Forks Human **Nutrition** Research Center, which is affiliated with the United States Department of Agriculture (USDA), investigated the role of boron in brain and psychological function in several studies involving humans and animals. In one study, increasing boron intake in rats receiving a boron-deficient diet seemed to increase mental activity. Studies conducted in people suggested that a lack of boron can decrease mental activity and have a negative effect on hand-eye coordination, the ability to concentrate, and short-term memory. These findings seem to indicate an important role for boron in keeping the brain fit.

The use of boron by body builders stems from its apparent ability to increase testosterone levels. Because testosterone is known to play an important role in the development of muscles, some weight lifters have taken boron supplements because they believe it will increase levels of male hormone and make them stronger. There is no evidence, however, that boron

can increase muscle mass or athletic performance. Boron supplements are generally not considered effective as a muscle-enhancing agent.

Preparations

A recommended daily allowance (RDA) for boron has not been established. The estimated dosage of boron, which is available as an over-the-counter dietary supplement, is generally 3 mg a day. Even without taking supplements, most people get anywhere from 1–3 mg of boron through diet. For this reason, some authorities suggest avoiding boron supplements altogether and eating foods known to contain the mineral. Good sources of boron include fruits especially pears, apples, peaches, grapes, and raisins; leafy vegetables; peanuts and tree nuts; and beans. Beer and wine also contain boron. Drinking water can be a good source of the mineral depending on geographical location. Getting too much of the mineral through food and drink is not considered a significant risk because boron is present only in very small amounts in plants and animals.

Precautions

Boron is not known to be harmful when taken in recommended dosages, although there are some precautions to consider. Boron appears to increase estrogen levels, especially in women receiving estrogen therapy. For this reason, women receiving hormone therapy should talk to their doctors before taking boron supplements. Combining the mineral with estrogen drugs may result in elevated and potentially unhealthy levels of female hormone. However, it is considered safe for women on estrogen therapy to eat boron-containing foods. In fact, many of the fruits and vegetables containing the mineral are believed to contribute to good health.

The long-term health risks associated with taking boron supplements are unknown.

Side effects

When taken in recommended dosages, boron has not been associated with any significant or bothersome side effects. At very high dosages, boron may cause **nausea** and **vomiting**, **diarrhea**, and headaches.

Interactions

Combining boron and estrogen-containing drugs may cause an undesirable increase in estrogen levels.

Resources

BOOKS

Xu, F., et al., eds. *Advances in Plant and Animal Boron Nutrition*. New York: Springer, 2006.

PERIODICALS

Miggiano, G. A., and L. Gagliardi. "Diet, Nutrition, and Bone Health." *Clinical Trial* (January–April 2005): 47–56.

ORGANIZATIONS

Grand Forks Human Nutrition Research Center, 2420 2nd Ave North, Grand Forks, ND, 58202, http://www.gfhnrc.ars.usda.gov.

Greg Annussek
David Edward Newton, Ed.D.

Boswellia

Description

Boswellia is the purified resin made from the gum from the *Boswellia serrata* or *Boswellia carteri* trees. For medicinal purposes, the products of these two trees are used in similar ways.

B. serrata is a moderately large branching tree that grows in the hilly regions of India. It grows to a height of about 12 ft (4 m). The sticky resin, or sap, from the tree is also called Indian frankincense, Indian olibanum, dhup, and salai **guggul**. *B. carteri* is a related tree that grows in parts of North Africa, especially Somalia, and in some parts of Saudi Arabia. The resin from this tree is called frankincense.

General use

Boswellia is a significant herb in the Ayurvedic system of health and healing. **Ayurvedic medicine** is a Hindu-based system of individualized healing that has been practiced in India for more than 2,000 years. It is a complex system that recognizes different human temperaments and body types. Each of these types have different qualities that affect the health and natural balance of the person.

Disease can result from any of seven major causes: heredity, congenital, internal, external trauma, seasonal, habits, or supernatural factors. Disease can also be caused by misuse of the five senses: sight, touch, taste, hearing, and smell. Diagnoses are made through questioning, observation, examination, and interpretation. Health is restored by evaluating the exact cause of the imbalance causing the disease or condition and then prescribing herbs, exercises, diet changes, and/or **meditation** to help restore the natural balance of body, mind, and spirit. Cures are highly individualized, so that the same symptoms may require different remedies in different people.

Boswellia is a guggul. A guggul (sometimes spelled guggal) is a sticky gum resin that comes from the sap of a tree. Ayurvedic healers have used boswellia for centuries to treat arthritis and rheumatism. In traditional Ayurvedic medicine, it has many other uses. These included being used as an antiseptic, expectorant, and diuretic.

In traditional Ayurvedic medicine, many conditions are treated with boswellia. These include:

- arithritis and rheumatism
- asthma
- bronchitis
- diarrhea
- jaundice
- ringworm and other skin diseases
- syphillis
- ulcers
- undescended testicles

Modern usage has focused on the use of *B. serrata*. This is most likely to be used by Western herbalists and found in natural products stores. Modern herbalists use boswellia primarily to treat arthritis and other inflammatory conditions. Boswellia can be taken internally or can be applied as a component of anti-arthritis cream.

Some very promising scientific evidence backs up this traditional use of boswellia. Compounds isolated from boswellia have demonstrated anti-inflammatory in laboratory studies. In experimental animals they reduced swelling as effectively as non-steroidal anti-inflammatory drugs (NSAIDs) such as ibuprofen (Advil, Nuprin, Motrin) and produced none of the side effects such as irritation of the stomach seen with NSAIDs. This could prove important for people who must take anti-inflammatory drugs for a long period of time. Other animal studies have suggested that boswellia lowers **cholesterol** and triglyceride (a type of fat) levels in the blood.

In other controlled human studies, boswellia was shown to decrease the duration of bronchial **asthma**, possibly by blocking formation of the chemicals that cause the blood vessels to contract. It has also been shown to be safe and effective in human studies for the treatment of arthritis.

Preparations

Boswellia is harvested from trees in late October by cutting away a flap of bark 6–8 in (15-20 cm) wide. For about two weeks, the gum is then scraped away from this wound. This material is then purified and used in healing.

Commercially available boswellia is standardized as an extract to a strength of 60–65% boswellic acid. Dosage varies depending on the patient's condition. For example, people with rheumatic conditions might take 150 mg of boswellic acid three times per day. Follow the directions on commercially available tablets. Creams containing boswellic acid can be applied externally.

Precautions

Some herbalists suggest that pregnant women, people with immune system diseases such as **AIDS**, and the frail elderly not take boswellia.

Side effects

Generally boswellia appears to be well tolerated with very few side effects. In rare cases it can cause **diarrhea**, **nausea**, and skin rash.

Interactions

There are few, if any, studies of how boswellia interacts with traditional Western medicines. It has been used for many years in combination with other Ayurvedic herbs without incident. With interest in boswellia high in modern research laboratories, more information on drug interactions is likely to be forthcoming.

Resources

BOOKS

Graedon, Joe, and Teresa Graedon. *The People's Pharmacy Guide to Home and Herbal Remedies.* New York: St. Martin's Press, 1999.

Peirce, Andrea. *The American Pharmaceutical Association Practical Guide to Natural Medicines.* New York: William Morrow and Company, 1999.

PDR for Herbal Medicines. Montvale, New Jersey: Medical Economics Company, 1998.

ORGANIZATIONS

American School of Ayurvedic Sciences, 2115 112th Avenue, NE, Bellevue, WA 98004, (425)453-8002.

The Ayurvedic Institute. P. O. Box 23445, Albuquerque, NM 87112, (505)291-9698.

Tish Davidson

Botanical medicine

Definition

Botanical medicine is a component of the healing arts that draws on the accumulated and developing knowledge of the medicinal properties of plants in the prevention and treatment of disease. Botanical medicine includes:

- medical herbalism, a healing art that relies on the synergistic and curative properties of plants to treat symptoms and disease and maintain health.
- pharmocognosy, the study of the pharmaceutical properties of natural products.
- ethnobotany, the study of the use plants in different cultures.

Botanical medicine is an important component of many traditional medical systems and therapies, including **traditional Chinese medicine** (TCM), **Ayurvedic medicine**, naturopathy, indigenous and shamanic medicine, **homeopathy**, flower essence therapy, and **aromatherapy**. Botanical medicine has survived for many thousands of years in some form and in all cultures throughout the world.

Origins

Plants have been used since prehistoric times as medicinal remedies applied in various ways to provide relief from irritations as minor as a mosquito bite to situations as catastrophic as the plague. In modern medicine, some drugs are derived from plants, and many of these medicines are used in ways that are similar to their traditional uses. Many more drugs in modern medicine, however, are synthetic, and part of the reason for this trend is economic: plants can rarely be patented, so a pharmaceutical company cannot gain the exclusive right to sell a plant-derived medication even after expensive research and marketing. Also, the processing of plants into a medicine cannot be as easily standardized and controlled as the manufacture of synthetic compounds. As a result, the efficacy and safety of only a relative few of the traditionally used botanical remedies have been verified by clinical research. Approximately only 5,000 of the estimated 500,000 known species (including subspecies) of plants have been identified and studied for their medicinal properties.

The knowledge of the healing properties of herbs has been preserved from the time of the clay tablets of the ancient Sumerians more than 5,000 years ago, to the sacred texts and pharmacopoeias of the Hindu and Chinese cultures, to the works of Greek and Roman physicians preserved by Byzantine scholars, to the European folk herbalists and physicians such as Nicholas Culpeper (1616–1654), to the Native American herbalists. One of the earliest records of botanical medicine is the *Pen T'Shao Kang Mu*, a work attributed to China's Yellow Emperor around 2500 B.C. Another is the Ebers papyrus, an Egyptian medical text dating from 1550 B.C. The *Rig-veda*, an ancient Hindu scripture, lists more than 1,000 medicinal plants used in the ancient Ayurvedic system of medicine, already well developed by 1000 B.C.

Theophrastus (327–285 B.C.) is considered the first scientific botanist; he recorded the use of more than 500 medicinal plants. The Greek physician Dioscorides produced what has been called the first true herbal text, or herbal, *De materia medica*, in the first century A.D. In the Middle Ages, the monks in European monasteries worked to preserve this ancient knowledge by copying texts and cultivating extensive gardens of medicinal plants. European folk medicine was passed from generation to generation through oral tradition, and with the introduction in Germany of the printing press in 1439, the information became more widely available in popular printed texts. Colonists brought their herbal knowledge and plant specimens to settlements in North America and learned from the indigenous peoples how to make use of plants native to the New World. The first record of Native American herb use is the manuscript of the Native Mexican physician Juan Badianus in 1552.

The use of herbs for medicinal purposes was developed over the centuries by personal experimentation, local custom, anecdote, and folk tradition. According to the World Health Organization, an estimated 80% of the global population continues to rely on medicinal plant preparations to meet primary healthcare needs. The specific chemical constituents of herbs and their medicinal actions are the subject of ongoing scientific experimentation.

Benefits

Botanical medicines, when administered properly and in designated therapeutic dosages, can be effective, trigger fewer side effects for many patients than pharmaceutical drugs, and are generally less costly than prescription pharmaceutical drugs.

The benefits of botanical medicine may be subtle or dramatic, depending on the remedy used and the illness being addressed. Herbal remedies usually have a much slower effect than pharmaceutical drugs, in part because the active ingredients are less concentrated than in manufactured compounds. Some herbal remedies have a cumulative effect and work slowly over time to restore balance; others are indicated for short-term treatment of acute symptoms. Botanical medicine may be especially beneficial when administered to help with chronic symptoms.

Description

Traditional Chinese medicine

Traditional Chinese medicine (TCM) employs ancient techniques, developed over many thousands of years. Among them are **acupuncture**, **moxibustion**, and herbal formulas. Moxibustion is a process that combines acupuncture with the traditional application of the herb **mugwort**, *Artemisia vulgaris*, known as *Ai ye* or *Hao-shu*. This is a method of heating specific acupuncture points on the body to treat physical conditions, particularly chronic **pain**. When burnt, the mugwort produces a mild heat able to penetrate deeply into the muscle.

TCM also employs specific herbal formulas to restore health and maintain a dynamic balance between two distinct forces known as *yin* and *yang*, particularly with regard to the *qi*. Qi (pronounced "CHEE") is the vital energy flowing along the meridians or energy pathways of the body. The TCM practitioner is a skilled observer who relies on diagnostic techniques, including measuring pulse rate from several positions and noting the general appearance of the patient, including complexion, eyes, nails, hair, tongue, and posture. The assessment not only includes consideration of the patient's symptomatic complaints, but of numerous personal characteristics, including family history, lifestyle, emotional health, environment, diet, and **exercise**. The medicinal herbs prescribed are usually prepared as a formula based on the individual needs of each patient.

Ayurvedic medicine

Ayurvedic literally means the science of life or longevity; Ayurvedic medicine has been practiced in India for more than 5,000 years. This method of healing is concerned equally with the body, mind, and spirit of the person and combines natural therapies to restore balance and harmony. Ayurvedic physicians, like the practitioners of traditional Chinese medicine, use educated observation in diagnosis. In Ayurvedic medicine, there are three basic *doshas*, or metabolic body types. The success of Ayurvedic treatment depends on the proper diagnosis of imbalances in these characteristic aspects.

Ayurvedic medicine emphasizes self-care strategies such as a healthy diet, **yoga**, **meditation**, breathing, and exercises to restore the innate harmony of the body. Taste is an important indicator of the medicinal properties of an herb. Plants are categorized according to six plant essences: sweet, sour, salty, pungent, bitter, and astringent. An understanding of how these plant essences act in the body is a necessary component in Ayurvedic medicine for prescribing herbal remedies.

Indigenous and shamanic medicine

Indigenous and shamanic healing systems rely on extensive folk knowledge of botanical and animal medicine combined with ceremonial ritual in the treatment of disease. The particular form of indigenous medicine is unique to each tribe. The specific herbal remedies are primarily passed on through oral tradition.

Naturopathy

Naturopathic medicine was established in the eighteenth and nineteenth centuries. The naturopathic doctor, or naturopath, uses gentle methods to boost the body's healing, including nutritional supplements, herbal remedies, proper diet, and exercise. The doctor works with the patient to educate the person on ways to restore and maintain a healthy balance in the internal environment that will prevent further illness. Licensed naturopathic doctors pass examinations that include basic clinical botanical medicine competency as well as homeopathy.

Homeopathy

The German physician Samuel Hahnemann (1755–1843) founded Homeopathy in the late eighteenth century. Homeopathy embraces the philosophy of "like cures like." Homeopathy uses extremely diluted solutions of herbs, animal products, and chemicals that are believed to hold a "trace memory" or an energetic imprint of the substance used. Sold as over-the-counter medicine, homeopathic remedies are exempt from government regulations applied to pharmaceuticals. Homeopathic remedies may be sold without proof of safety and efficacy as long as they are labeled with the directions for use and the level of dilution.

Flower essences

The use of flower essences attempts to address a more subtle energy beyond the physical symptoms and to treat the emotional and mental roots of disease. The English physician Edward Bach (1886–1936) developed a method of extracting what he considered the essence of flowers, which he believed had the ability to address a broad range of psychological conditions. This system became known as Bach **Flower Remedies**. This botanical therapy attempts to match the energetic essence of particular flowers with the same energy in the higher self of an individual, thus strengthening the higher energies and promoting self-realization and restoring health. Bach's theory was that the source of all illness could be found in the conflict between the demands of one's higher self, striving to realize its full potential, and the individual personality or ego with its limiting beliefs and actions that obstruct and block this self-realization. The remedies are believed to have a subtle, soul-healing effect based on an instinctual soul rapport with the particular herb.

Aromatherapy

Aromatherapy uses the essential oil of various herbs extracted by steam distillation or cold pressing of flower, leaf, stem, or root to treat various physical and emotional problems. Herbs have long been valued for their healing fragrance. In 1564 the alchemist Giovanni Battista della Porta (1535 or 1538–1615) wrote about methods used to separate **essential oils** from the aromatic distilled waters that had been used in previous centuries. Modern-day aromatherapy was developed by the French chemist Réné-Maurice Gattefossé (1881–1950) in 1937. Aromatherapy identifies the distinct healing properties of various pure essential oils. The small size of the molecules in essential oils enables the chemicals to penetrate tissue easily and to act rapidly on the limbic system, which is believed to be the seat of emotions.

Preparations

The quality of any herbal remedy and the chemical constituents found in the herb depend greatly on the conditions of weather, the soil where the herb was grown, the timing and care in harvesting, and the manner of preparation and storage. Herbs are prepared in a variety of ways depending on the part of the plant that is medicinally active and the results sought. The kinds of herbal preparations are numerous and varied. Some of these preparations are as follows:

- Infusion. Infusion is appropriate for extracting medicinal properties of the leaf, flower, and stem of the plant. Either fresh or dried herb may be used. A standard infusion combines 1 tsp of dried herb, or 2 tsp of chopped fresh herb, per cup of water. Fresh, chlorine-free water is brought to the boiling point in a non-metallic pot, and the herbs are added. A cover prevents the escape of volatile oils. The tea is infused for 10 to 15 minutes, strained, and can be consumed warm or cold. The prepared tea keeps up to two days in the refrigerator.

- Decoction. Decoction is the best method to extract the mineral salts and other healing components from the coarser herb materials, such as the root, bark, seeds, and stem of the plant. One ounce (28 g) of the dried plant materials, or 2 oz (56 g) of fresh plant parts, is added to 1 pint (500 mL) of pure, chlorine-free water in a non-metallic pot. The mixture is brought to a boil, and then the heat is lowered, so the mixture can simmer for about 30 minutes. After straining and covering, a decoction may be refrigerated for up to two days and retain its healing qualities.

- Tincture. Tincture is a method to prepare a concentrated form of the fresh herbal remedy for therapeutic use. These solutions, properly prepared and stored, retain medicinal potency for many years. To prepare a tincture, a clean glass container is packed with chopped fresh or dried herb, and enough good quality brandy or vodka to cover is poured over the herb. The alcohol/water ratio varies, dependent on the plant and the intended extract. The concentration (depending on the herb) is 25 to 90%; often the ratio of alcohol to water is about 50/50. The container then is sealed with an airtight lid. The mixture is left in a darkened place to steep for two weeks and is shaken daily. After straining the mixture through a cheesecloth or muslin bag and pouring it into a dark bottle for storage, it is ready for use. Dosage depends on the herb and its designated use. A standard dosage is .5 to 1 tsp (2–4 ml) of the tincture three times a day. Other fluid extracts may be prepared with glycerin or vinegar.

- Capsule. A capsule is a convenient form for ingesting dried, powdered herbs. Gelatin capsules are available in the standard size 00, which holds 200 to 250 mg of powdered herb. Prepared capsules should be stored in dark glass containers.

- Oil infusion. With this method, the chopped fresh or dried herb is placed in a glass storage container. Enough cold-pressed vegetable oil, such as sunflower or olive oil, is poured into the jar to cover the herb completely. This mixture is sealed and placed on a sunny windowsill for two or three weeks. The infused oil is strained into another jar of the chopped fresh or dried herb. This mixture steeps on a sunny windowsill for another two weeks. After being strained through cheesecloth, this infused oil can be stored in a cool, dark location for future use.

- Ointments. These are prepared with powdered or freshly chopped plant parts combined with melted petroleum jelly, lanoline, beeswax, and vegetable oil. The mixture is simmered in a double boiler for about two hours then strained through cheesecloth and poured into small glass storage containers. Ointments are a spreadable consistency and provide a protective layer for topical application of medicinal herbs to the skin.

- Poultice. A poultice is a hot mixture of the chopped fresh or dry herb that has been boiled briefly and cooled to a tolerable temperature before application to the affected area. A small amount of oil should be applied to the skin before placing the poultice to prevent the herb from sticking. The poultice can be covered with a gauze strip to hold it in place. The poultice can be refreshed every 2 to 3 hours as needed.

- Essential oils. This is the highly concentrated extract of an herb obtained through steam distillation or cold compress methods. Essential oils should be diluted in water or in a nontoxic carrier oil before application to the skin to prevent contact dermatitis (rash) or sensitization. Essential oils are used for topical application, in bath water, and in aromatherapy. The toxicity of the concentrated essential oil varies depending on the chemical constituents of the herb.

The above list is by no means exhaustive. There are many other botanical medicine preparations available.

Precautions

Herbal remedies prepared by infusion, decoction, or alcohol tincture from the appropriate plant part, such as the leaf, root, or flower, are generally safe when ingested in properly designated therapeutic dosages. However, many herbs have specific contraindications for use when certain medical conditions are present. Contraindications also exist for pregnant or breastfeeding women. Some herbs are toxic, even deadly, in large amounts, and there is little research on the chronic toxicity that may result from prolonged use on any others.

Herbal remedies are sold in the United States as dietary supplements. The United States Food and Drug Administration (FDA) regulates dietary supplements, including botanical medicines, under the 1994 Dietary Supplement Health and Education Act (DSHEA). At the time the act was passed, legislators believed that because many dietary supplements come from natural sources such as plants and have been used for hundreds of years by practitioners of complementary and alternative medicine (CAM), these products did not need to be as rigorously regulated as prescription and over-the-counter pharmaceuticals.

DSHEA regulates botanical medicines in the same way that food is regulated. Like food manufacturers, manufacturers of herbal remedies do not have to prove that the remedy is either safe or effective before it can be sold to the public. Manufacturers of conventional pharmaceutical drugs, however, must prove both safety and effectiveness in humans before a new drug is approved for use. With all dietary supplements, the burden of proof falls on the FDA to show that the supplement is either unsafe or ineffective before the remedy can be restricted or banned. Information about an herbal remedy's safety and effectiveness is typically gathered only after people using the product develop health problems or complain that the product does not work. Initially, supplement manufacturers were not required to report consumer complaints of complications or side effects to the FDA. However, beginning in 2007, a federal law requires that all manufacturers of dietary supplements, including botanical products, report consumer complaints of adverse events (negative side effects) to the FDA. This requirement will make accumulating information on the safety of these products faster and easier.

Botanical medicines are required to be clearly labeled with the word "supplement." In addition, the label must show the volume or weight of the contents, the serving size, a list of dietary ingredients and non-dietary ingredients (e.g., artificial color, binders, fillers, flavorings), the name of the manufacturer, packer, or distributor, directions for use, and scientific name of any herbs the product contains.

Unlike conventional drugs, the label for a botanical medicines does not have to show any statements about possible side effects. However, botanical medicines, like all dietary supplements, are not legally allowed to claim that they will cure, treat, mitigate, prevent, or diagnose a specific disease.

Manufacturers of botanical medicines are required to follow federal Good Manufacturing Practices (GMPs) that regulate sanitary and other conditions under which these products are prepared, packaged, and stored. These GMPs, however, are much less stringent than those that regulate the manufacture of pharmaceutical drugs. They do not, for example, assure that the amount of active ingredient in each pill or capsule of an herbal remedy is the same. Some supplement manufacturers try to assure consistency of their product, by confirming that each batch contains the same amounts of active ingredients. This type of standardization is not required by law, and the word "standardized" on the label is not an indication that the product meets any legal requirements as to quality or consistency of contents.

Self-diagnosis and treatment with botanical medicinals may be risky. Consulting a certified clinical herbalist or naturopathic physician is prudent before undertaking a course of treatment. A widely circulated 2002 report stated that patients often fail to inform their physicians about herbal products they are using and that patients do not think of them as medicines. Yet many botanical remedies can interact with allopathic medicines and either cancel their effects or cause adverse effects. For example, **garlic**, ginseng, ginkgo, **feverfew**, **licorice**, and other common remedies have anticoagulant properties that can put patients as risk of bleeding during surgery. Since the 2002 report, traditional physicians have been encouraged to ask patients specifically about herbal remedies, vitamins, minerals, and other supplements they may be taking.

Advances in communication technology have made warnings about herbal remedies more important than ever. The Internet includes many sites with unregulated and often unhealthful advice about use of herbal remedies. Many herbalists and allopathic physicians urge patients to use caution when seeking information on herbal treatments on the Internet. One example of a dangerous herb heavily promoted on the Internet is **ephedra** Ephedra sinica) also known as ma huang. In the late twentieth century, ephedra gained popularity as a weight-loss supplement. The herb can cause life-threatening side effects, and since April 2004, sale of products containing ephedra have been banned in the United States, although this herb is still promoted on some Internet sites.

Essential oils should not be taken internally without expert guidance due to the potential for toxicity even in very small amounts. They are not to be used in any form by pregnant or breastfeeding women without competent medical consultation. Essential oil extracts do not contain the full range of phytochemicals present in the whole plant.

Homeopathic remedies are generally safe because of their extremely diluted nature. These remedies must not be relied upon for treatment of any serious illness or injury. If symptoms persist, other qualified medical help should be sought.

Side effects

Herbs contain many phytochemicals formed in the metabolic process of the plant. These chemicals act on the body in different ways; some of these act on the whole body, whereas others act on a specific organ or system. An herb's effect may be due to a particular chemical in the herb, or it may be due to an interaction among constituents within the plant. Interactions with other herbs, or with pharmacological drugs, is a matter of concern and a growing area of research.

The pure essential oils of aromatic plants, extracted by steam distillation or cold pressing techniques, have been used for more than a century in medicines, food, drink, perfumes, detergents, soaps, cosmetics, in various industrial applications, and in aromatherapy. Some compounds found in plant oils can cause sensitization even in very small amounts. Side effects from external application of some essential oils may include mild skin irritation, such as **itching** and burning; sensitization, which may lead to recurrent mild to severe adverse reactions, such as burning and rash each time the essential oil is used; and phototoxicity, a situation in which certain essential oils react with ultraviolet light and cause reactions from mild skin blotching to severe burning when the skin is exposed to sunlight.

Research and general acceptance

Botanical treatments are generally accepted as part of mainstream medical treatment around the world except in the United States, where herbal remedies are sold as dietary supplements. As of 2008, the branch of the FDA that regulates botanical products under the rubric of dietary supplements is the Center for Food Safety and Applied **Nutrition** (CFSAN). The other U.S. government agency that has some oversight

of botanical preparations is the National Center for Complementary and Alternative Medicine (NCCAM) of the National Institutes of Health, established by an act of Congress in 1998. NCCAM also supports clinical trials and research into botanical products, herbalism, and other alternative therapies that make use of plant-derived products.

In Germany, an expert committee known as the Commission E was established by the government in 1978 to evaluate the safety and efficacy of 300 herbs and herb combinations sold in that country. No equivalent regulatory commission exists in the United States. Several scientific journals, such as the *Journal of Ethnobotany* and the *Journal of Ethnopharmacology* disseminate information or current research on botanical medicines.

Determining the safety or toxicity of essential oils has primarily been accomplished through animal testing. Human trials of essential oils using volunteers have also been conducted. The World Health Organization (WHO), the Council of Europe, and the FDA accomplish some regulation of and guidelines for the use of essential oils, particularly in food. Two sources of information on the safety of essential oils used in aromatherapy are the Research Institute for Fragrance Materials and the International Fragrance Research Association. These organizations evaluate essential oils and publish findings in the journal, *Food and Chemicals Toxicity*.

In homeopathic medicine, the effectiveness of a remedy is "proved" by experimentation and anecdotal reports by famous homeopathic practitioners rather than by any type of organized clinical trials. However, in 1997, homeopathic remedies were tested clinically and an international team of researchers who reviewed more than one hundred controlled studies concluded that the collective results of 26 of these controlled studies indicate that homeopathic remedies produce a somewhat greater benefit than a placebo in the treatment of illness.

Training and certification

Naturopathic physicians are licensed as primary care physicians in many states and complete a four-year graduate level course at a naturopathic medical school. Naturopaths are trained in nutritional medicine, homeopathic medicine, botanical medicine, **hydrotherapy**, psychology, and counseling.

Traditional Chinese medicine practitioners are heir to the benefits of thousands of years of tradition. This ancient system of health care saw a revival in China after efforts by Chinese Nationalists in the 1930s to eliminate traditional Chinese medical practices in favor of Western medical methods. The ancient

KEY TERMS

Alternative medicine—A system of healing that rejects conventional, pharmaceutical-based medicine and accepts the use of dietary supplements and therapies such as herbs, vitamins, minerals, massage, and cleansing diets. Alternative medicine includes well-established treatment systems such as homeopathy, traditional Chinese medicine, and Ayurvedic medicine, as well as current fad-driven treatments.

Complementary medicine—Includes many of the same treatments used in alternative medicine but uses them to supplement conventional drug and therapy treatments, rather than to replace conventional medicine.

Dietary supplement—A product, such as a vitamin, mineral, herb, amino acid, or enzyme, that is intended to be consumed in addition to an individual's diet with the expectation that it will improve health.

Ethnobotany—The study of the plant lore and agricultural practices of a people or culture.

Limbic system—The structures of the brain concerned with emotion and motivation.

Naturopathic medicine—An alternative system of healing that uses primarily homeopathy, herbal medicine, and hydrotherapy and rejects most conventional drugs as toxic.

Pharmacopoeia—A book describing drugs, chemicals, and medicinal preparations, especially one recognized as an authority and serving as a standard.

Sensitization—The process by which the immune system becomes sensitive or hypersensitive to a specific chemical and reaction to it when re-exposed.

Yang—Qualities opposite of yin, such as warmth, activity, light, and activity.

Yin—Qualities opposite of yang, such as cold, stillness, darkness, and passiveness.

way persisted, and traditional Chinese medicine is taught in Chinese medical schools using the traditional medical literature. In the 1990s, China opened its hospitals to U.S. students of acupuncture and Chinese herbology.

Western herbalism is taught in many schools of herbal medicine in the United States, as well as through correspondence and online courses. Certification as a clinical herbalist is not required in the United States, and herbal remedies are widely available without a medical prescription.

Resources

BOOKS

Chevallier, Andrew. *Herbal Remedies.* New York: DK Publishing, 2007.

Foster, Steven, and Rebecca Johnson. *National Geographic Desk Reference to Nature's Medicine.* Washington, DC: National Geographic Society, 2006.

Mayo Clinic Book of Alternative Medicine: The New Approach to Using the Best of Natural Therapies and Conventional Medicine. New York: Time Inc. Home Entertainment, 2007.

PDR for Herbal Medicines, 4th ed. Montvale, NJ: Thompson Healthcare, 2007.

Premla, M. S. *Ayurvedic Herbs: A Clinical Guide to the Healing Plants of Traditional Indian Medicine.* New York: Routledge, 2006.

Yarnell, Eric, and Karen Abascal. *Clinical Botanical Medicine,* 2nd rev. ed. Larchmont, NY: Mary Ann Liebert, 2008.

ORGANIZATIONS

Alternative Medicine Foundation, PO Box 60016, Potomac, MD, 20859, (301) 340-1960, http://www.amfoundation.org.

American Association of Naturopathic Physicians, 435 Wisconsin Ave. NW, Suite 403, Washington, DC, 20016, (202) 237-8150, (866) 538-2267, http://www.naturopathic.org.

American Association of Oriental Medicine, PO Box 162340, Sacramento, CA, 95816, (866) 455-7999, (914) 443-4770, http://www.aaaomonline.org.

American Botanical Council, 6200 Manor Rd, Austin, TX, 7872, (512) 926-4900, http://www.herbalgram.org.

American Holistic Medical Association, PO Box 2016, Edmonds, WA, 98020, (425) 967-0737, http://www.holisticmedicin.org.

American Institute of Homeopathy, 801 N. Fairfax St., Suite 306, Alexandria, VA, 22314, (888) 445-9988, http://homeopathyusa.org.

Flower Essence Society, PO Box 459, Nevada City, CA, 95959, (530) 265-9163, (800) 736-9222, http://www.flowersociety.org., National Center for Complementary and Alternative Medicine Clearinghouse., PO Box 7923, Gathersburg, MD, 20898, (888) 644-6226, http://nccam.nih.gov.

National Center for Homeopathy, 801 N. Fairfax St., Suite 306, Alexandria, VA, 22314, (703) 548-7790, http://www.homeopathic.org/.

National Institute of Ayurvedic Medicine, 375 Fifth Ave., 5th Floor, New York, NY, 10016, (212) 685-8600, http://niam.com/.

Clare Hanrahan
Teresa G. Odle
Rebecca J. Frey, PhD
Tish Davidson, A. M.

Botulism *see* **Food poisoning**

Breast cancer

Definition

Breast cancer is the abnormal growth and uncontrolled division of cells in the breast. These malignant cancer cells form masses (tumors) that invade and destroy surrounding normal tissue. Cancer cells shed from tumors have the ability to spread by way of the circulatory and lymphatic systems from the breast to distant parts of the body, invade other tissues, and form new tumors. This process is called metastasis. If metastasis is not controlled, breast cancer can result in death.

Description

A woman's breast is made up of clumps of cells (glands) that, when stimulated by the proper hormones, secrete milk into a network of small tubes (ducts) that collect the milk and carry it to the nipple. The breast also contains fatty tissue, lymph vessels, and blood vessels. Breast cancer most often begins in the cells that line the ducts (ductal cancer). Groups of glands in breast tissue are called lobules. Cancer can also begin in the lobules (lobular cancer) and much more rarely in other tissues of the breast.

Depending on where in the breast the cancer starts, the disease develops certain characteristics that are used to classify breast cancer into subtypes. Ductal carcinoma begins in the ducts. Lobular carcinoma has a pattern involving the lobules or glands. The more important classification of the disease is related to the tumor's stage or capability to invade and spread, as this characteristic defines the disease as a true cancer. The stage before invasive cancer is called *in situ*, meaning that the early malignancy is located in one spot and has not yet spread. For example, ductal carcinoma in situ is considered a minimal breast cancer.

How breast cancer spreads

The primary tumor begins in the breast itself, but once it becomes invasive, cancer cells may move beyond the breast to the regional lymph nodes. Cells from the tumor also break off and travel through the lymphatic system and blood vessels to other parts of body where they form new tumors. This process is called metastasis.

The lymphatic system carries lymph throughout the body. Lymph is a clear fluid that contains immune system cells that fight infection. It moves through a system of lymph channels and lymph nodes. In the nodes, lymph is filtered, and foreign material and dead cells are removed. Eventually lymph drains into the bloodstream. Nearly all organs in the body have a primary lymph node group filtering fluid that comes from that organ. In the breast, the primary lymph nodes are under the armpit, or axilla. Classically, a primary tumor that begins in the breast first spreads to the regional lymph nodes under the arm. Cancer cells may also invade blood vessels at their site of origin. When cancer cells enter the blood vessels, the circulatory system provides the way for the cancer to spread to distant parts of the body.

Breast cancer tends to follow this progression, although it often becomes widespread early in the course of the disease. By the time one can feel a lump in the breast, it is often 0.4 in (1 cm) in diameter and contains about one million cells. Estimates suggest it may take 1 to 5 years for a tumor of this size to develop. During that time, the cancer cells may be spreading to other parts of body. Favorite sites of distant involvement for breast cancer are the lung, bones, liver, and the skin and soft tissue. The number of regional lymph nodes containing cancer cells remains the single most reliable indicator of whether the cancer has become widely metastasized. Because tests to discover metastasis in other organs may not be sensitive enough to reveal tiny tumors, the evaluation of the axillary nodes for regional metastasis becomes important in making treatment decisions regarding any given case. If breast cancer spreads to other major organs of the body, its presence will compromise the function of those organs. Compromised vital organ function can result in death.

Every woman is at risk for breast cancer. If she lives to be 85, there is a one in eight (12%) chance that she will develop breast cancer at some time during her life. As a woman ages, her risk of developing breast cancer rises dramatically regardless of her family history. The breast cancer risk of a 25-year-old woman is only one out of 19,600; by age 45, it is one in 93. Fewer than 5% of cases are discovered before age 35, and the majority of all breast cancers are found in women over age 50.

The American Cancer Society estimated that about 182,500 new cases of breast cancer would be diagnosed in 2008. About 40,000 women die of breast cancer each year. More cases of breast cancer are being diagnosed because of the increased use of screening mammograms; however, deaths from breast cancer are declining because the disease is being diagnosed in earlier, more treatable stages.

Causes and symptoms

All cancer is thought to occur because of small changes (mutations) in genes. A gene is a small packet of deoxyribonucleic acid (DNA), the genetic master molecule of all cells that is inherited from each parent. Genes control all aspects of development and metabolism. Small changes in the structure of genes can cause changes in proteins that regulate metabolic functions. In healthy cells, cell division is controlled by proteins regulated by genes. Specific genes make proteins that signal healthy cells when to stop dividing. In cancer, the controlling gene(s) is damaged or mutated and does not produce the proteins necessary to signal cells to stop dividing. The mutations that cause breast cancer do not have a single cause. Genetic, environmental, and lifestyle factors all play a role in determining who gets breast cancer. Although men can get breast cancer, women are 100 times more likely to develop the disease.

There are a number of risk factors for the development of breast cancer; however, among experts there is some disagreement about how important each of these factors is. Risk factors include:

- age. 80% of breast cancers are found in women over age 50.
- a family history of breast cancer in mother or sister.
- carrying the BRCA1 and BRCA2 genes. Women with these genes account for 5 to 10% of breast cancer cases and have an 80% chance of developing breast cancer at some time during their life.
- history of abnormal breast biopsies or previous history of breast cancer.
- having first menstruation before age 12 or entering menopause after age 55.
- having no children or having a first child after age 30.
- daily alcohol consumption of two drinks or more.
- obesity and a high fat diet.
- breast exposure to radiation (e.g., in treatment of other cancers).
- postmenopausal hormone replacement therapy (HRT) with a combination estrogen/progesterone drug. Estrogen alone does not appear to increase risk. The longer a woman used HRT, the more her risk increases.

In addition, some other aspects of **nutrition** and lifestyle in Western countries may be responsible for higher rates of breast cancer in these societies. For example, aromatic hydrocarbons in tobacco and certain hydrocarbons in well-done meat may act as carcinogens. Nitrates used in preserving some meat are also suspected of being carcinogens. Breastfeeding for at least one year, an activity performed by only a small percentage of women in industrialized countries, seems to have a protective effect against breast cancer.

Although many factors may increase the risk of developing breast cancer, some women with multiple risk factors never develop the disease, and about 70% of women who get breast cancer have no recognized risk factors. Breast cancer cannot be prevented. Nevertheless, breastfeeding for more than one year, moderate **exercise**, such as walking 10 hours a week, and a diet low in saturated (animal) fats and high in fruits, vegetables, and whole grains have been shown in multiple studies to lower risk of developing breast cancer. These lifestyle choices are endorsed both by alternative and conventional medical practitioners.

Changes in the breast that may indicate breast cancer and should be brought to the immediate attention of a healthcare professional include:

- a lump or thickening in breast or armpit.
- changes in a nipple (thickening, pulling in, bleeding, or discharge).
- dimpled or reddened skin over the breast.
- change in breast size or shape.
- abnormality on a mammogram.

Every lump found in the breast is not cancer. Fibrocystic changes in the breast are extremely common. Fibrocystic condition of the breast is a leading cause of non-cancerous breast lumps. Fibrocystic changes also can cause **pain**, swelling, and discharge from the nipple. Noncancerous (benign) lumps can be either solid or filled with fluid. Signs and symptoms of fibrocystic changes overlap with those of breast cancer. Complete diagnostic evaluation of any significant breast abnormality is essential to differentiate between fibrocystic changes and breast cancer. Certain benign changes in the breast also may be linked to increased risk for breast cancer.

Diagnosis

All women are encouraged to do regular, monthly breast self-examinations, which involves feeling the breasts for any abnormal lumps or pain. A physician will also examine a woman's breasts during routine physical examinations and during regular gynecological examinations.

More than 90% of all breast cancers are detected by mammogram screening. A mammogram is a non-invasive, low-dose x ray that produces a two-dimensional picture of the breast. A typical mammography screening includes two views of each breast, one from above, and one from the side. The test causes no lasting pain, although a woman briefly may feel uncomfortable because her breasts must be compressed to produce an adequate x ray.

Normally, the technologist examines the x-ray films immediately to make sure the x rays are of good quality. A radiologist (doctor who specializes in interpreting x rays) will review the x rays and determine if follow-up tests are needed. The American Cancer Society recommends yearly mammograms for all women over age 40. Women at high risk for breast cancer may begin having mammograms at an earlier age. This test is usually covered by insurance. Mammography is helpful in detecting breast cancer too small to be identified on physical examination. However, 10 to 13% of breast cancer is not detected with mammography. Detection depends in part on the skill of the radiologist reading the x ray. Centers that specialize in mammograms have a better detection rate than general radiologic facilities.

If anything irregular is detected on the mammogram, such as a mass, significant changes from earlier mammograms, abnormalities of the skin, or enlargement of the lymph nodes, additional imaging tests may be done, including a repeat mammogram, magnetic resonance imaging (MRI) of the breast, or a breast ultrasound. None of these is invasive. A breast ultrasound can help distinguish between a fluid-filled cyst and a solid mass. If imaging confirms that a solid lump is present, a biopsy may be done for definitive diagnosis.

Biopsy of the breast is a removal of breast tissue for examination of abnormal cells by a pathologist. Depending on the situation, different types of biopsy may be performed. In an incisional fine needle biopsy, a thin needle is inserted into the abnormal area of the breast, and cells from the area are suctioned into the needle. They are then prepared for microscopic evaluation. Fine needle biopsies are quick procedures done under local anesthetic. A core needle biopsy is an incisional biopsy also done under local anesthesia, only using a larger needle. In excisional biopsy or lumpectomy, the entire lump area and some surrounding tissue is removed for examination.

Once diagnosis is established and before treatment begins, more tests are done to determine if the cancer has spread beyond the breast. These tests are likely to include a chest x ray, blood tests, and liver function tests. Along with the liver function measured by a blood sample, the level of alkaline phosphatase, an enzyme from bone, is also determined. A radionuclear bone scan may be ordered. This test looks at the places in the body to which breast cancer usually metastasizes. A computed tomography (CT) scan also may be ordered. The physician will do a careful examination of the lymph nodes under the armpit (axillary lymph nodes) to assess likelihood of regional metastasis. Sometimes, the physician will remove all the axillary lymph nodes to assess breast cancer stage.

Using the results of these studies, the stage of cancer is defined, which helps establish a treatment protocol and prognosis. In the United States, formal staging is done using the TNM system. This system considers the tumor size and how much it has grown (T), whether the cancer has spread to the lymph nodes (N), and whether it has metastasized (M) to distant sites in the body. Stages are summarized below.

- Stage I. The cancer is no larger than 2 cm and no cancer cells are found in the lymph nodes.
- Stage II. The cancer is no larger than 2 cm but has spread to the lymph nodes or is larger than 2 cm but has not spread to the lymph nodes.
- Stage IIIA. The tumor is larger than 5 cm and has spread to the lymph nodes or is smaller than 5 cm but has spread to the lymph nodes, which have grown into each other.
- Stage IIIB. Cancer has spread to tissues near the breast or to lymph nodes inside the chest wall, along the breastbone.
- Stage IV. Cancer has spread to skin and lymph nodes near the collarbone or to other organs of the body.

Treatment

The best chance for successful treatment is to find breast cancer early. Breast cancer is a life-threatening disease, and a correct diagnosis and appropriate treatment with surgery, chemotherapy, and/or radiation is critical to controlling the illness. Complementary treatments used along with conventional medicine are often successful in moderating side effects and improving the patient's quality of life.

Acupuncture and **guided imagery** may be useful tools in treating pain symptoms and side effects of chemotherapy associated with breast cancer. Acupuncture involves the placement of a series of thin needles into the skin at targeted locations on the body, known as acupoints, in order to harmonize the energy flow within the human body. Guided imagery involves creating a visual mental image of pain. Once the pain can be visualized, the patient can adjust the image to make it more pleasing, and thus more manageable.

Many herbal remedies are available to lessen pain symptoms and chemotherapy side effects such as **nausea**, and to promote **relaxation** and healing. However, breast cancer patients should consult with their healthcare professional before taking any herbal treatments. Depending on the preparation and the type of herb, these remedies may interact with and enhance or diminish the effects of prescribed medications. One herb that is generally regarded as helpful in relieving the nausea that accompanies chemotherapy is **ginger** (*Zingiber officinale*).

Results of a clinical trial performed at the National Cancer Institute of Milan, Italy, indicated that homeopathic remedies of **belladonna** (*Atropa belladonna*) can be useful in relieving the discomfort, warmth, and swelling of the skin associated with radiation therapy for breast cancer. As with all homeopathic remedies, the prescription of belladonna depends on an individual's overall symptom picture, mood, and temperament, and should be prepared by a trained homeopathic professional. When used as a homeopathic remedy, belladonna is administered in a highly diluted form to trigger the body's natural healing response without risk of belladonna poisoning or overdose.

Allopathic treatment

Allopathic treatments offer the best chance of surviving breast cancer. Treatment options include surgery, chemotherapy, radiation, and the use of biotherapeutics. Breast cancer is treated in two ways: locally to eliminate tumor cells from the breast by surgery and radiation and systemically to destroy cancer cells that have traveled to other parts of the body. Systemic therapy includes the use of drugs in chemotherapy, hormonal treatments to reduce the amount of estrogen circulating in the blood, and biotherapeutics to target stray cancer cells.

Surgery

Historically, surgical removal of the entire breast and axillary lymph nodes, along with the muscles down to the chest wall (radical mastectomy), was performed as the preferred therapy for breast cancer. Between 1975 and 2005, surgery remained a primary option, but other therapies rose in importance. Some studies have suggested that breast conserving treatment (as opposed to radical mastectomy) improves the quality of life for women without compromising survival. Ultimately, the extent of surgery depends on the type of breast cancer, whether the disease has spread, and the patient's age and health.

Removing the tumor and a border of normal tissue around it will remove the cancer while saving most of the breast tissue. However, the longer a tumor has been growing in the breast, the more likely it will be that the cancer cells have spread to the lymph nodes. Breast cancer cells are likely to spread to these nodes under the arm or in the chest. During surgery, some of the nodes are removed to check for cancer cells.

The presence of cancer cells in the lymph nodes may require more extensive surgery. If the cancer has spread to the nodes, the patient will need either radiation, chemotherapy, hormone therapy, or a combination of all three after surgery. This supplemental treatment is called adjuvant therapy. Even if no cancer is found in the nodes, radiation almost always follows surgery, and a combination of chemotherapy and radiation offers the best chance of long-term survival.

Surgery can be combined with breast reconstruction (creating a new breast-shaped mound). Patients who want breast reconstruction should tell the surgeon before surgery, since this could change the way the surgeon operates.

Radiation

Once the tumor has been removed, the oncologist (cancer doctor) usually recommends radiation therapy to destroy or shrink any remaining breast cancer cells. Radiation stops cells from dividing. It works especially well on fast-growing cancer cells. Radiation also affects normal cells in the target area. Healthy cells that divide quickly, like those of the skin and hair, are affected the most. Radiation can cause **fatigue**, skin problems, and **hair loss**. Radiation therapy is usually begun post-operatively after surgical **wounds** have healed.

Chemotherapy

Survival after breast cancer surgery is improved by the addition of post-operative chemotherapy. Post-surgical chemotherapy therapy in patients who have no evidence of residual disease is performed on the assumption that some patients have metastases that are too small to be detected. This condition occurs because the surgeon has probably not removed every single cancerous cell. Loose cancer cells, if not killed by chemotherapy, may travel through the circulatory system and form new tumors elsewhere. Chemotherapy may also be given in some circumstances before surgery. Chemotherapy is administered either orally or by injection into a blood vessel and usually involves multiple drugs. It is given in cycles, followed by a period of time for recovery, followed by another course of drugs.

Chemotherapy can produce significant side effects, including nausea and **vomiting**, temporary hair loss, mouth or vaginal sores, fatigue, weakened immune system, and **infertility**. Complementary therapies are often helpful in reducing some of these side effects.

Hormone therapy

Many breast cancers, particularly those originating in post-menopausal women, are responsive to hormones. These cancers have receptors on their cells for the hormone estrogen. Part of the post-surgery primary tumor assessment is evaluation for the presence of estrogen and progesterone receptors. If they are present on the cancer cells, altering the hormone status of the patient will slow tumor growth and have a positive impact on survival. Hormonal status may be changed with drug therapy. The drug tamoxifen binds to estrogen receptors on the cancer cells, so that hormones cannot interact with the cells and stimulate their growth. If the patient has these receptors, tamoxifen is commonly prescribed for five years as an adjunct to primary treatment. In women whose cancer cells have estrogen receptors, tamoxifen reduces the chance of breast cancer reoccurring by about 50%.

Toremifene (Fareston) and fulvestrant (Faslodex) are drugs similar to tamoxifen that target hormone receptors on cancer cells. They are often used when cancer cells are unresponsive to tamoxifen. In addition, a group of drugs called aromatase inhibitors that block the enzymes that produce estrogen in post-menopausal (but not pre-menopausal) women have been used to treat both early and late advanced breast cancer. These drugs include letrozole (Femara), anastrozole (Arimidex), and exemestane (Aromasin). Using these agents has reduced the need for surgical removal of hormone-producing glands, such as the ovary or adrenal, that was sometimes necessary in the past.

BIOTHERAPEUTICS. Biotherapeutics are a type of targeted therapy. Large amounts of antibodies of a single type (called monoclonal antibodies) that react with specific receptors on cancer cells are made in the laboratory. In the patient, they inactivate or destroy those cells containing that specific receptor, but do not react with other cells. Trastuzumab (Herceptin) and lapatinib (Tykerb) target cells that contain a growth protein known as HER/2. Between 15 and 25% of women have breast cancer that responds to these drugs. Bevacizumab (Avastin) is a biotherapeutic used to treat breast cancer that has metastasized. It helps prevent tumors from becoming established by interfering with the growth of blood vessels in the tumor. Without access to nutrients in the blood, the tumors cannot increase in size. Biotherapeutics are typically used in addition to chemotherapy drugs.

Expected results

Lymph node involvement is one of the best indicators of breast cancer survival rates. The ten-year

---

KEY TERMS

Adjuvant therapy—Treatment involving radiation, chemotherapy (drug treatment), hormone therapy, biotherapeutics, or a combination of any of these given after the primary treatment in order to rid the body of residual microscopic cancer.

Antibody—A protein produced by the immune system to fight infection or rid the body of foreign material. The foreign material that stimulates the production of antibodies is called an antigen. Specific antibodies are produced in response to each different antigen and can only inactivate that particular antigen.

Benign—Not malignant, noncancerous.

Biopsy—A procedure in which suspicious tissue is removed and examined by a pathologist for cancer or other disease. For breast biopsies, the tissue may be obtained by open surgery or through a needle.

Complementary therapy—Includes many of the same treatments used in alternative medicine, such as herbal medicine, massage, and focused imaging, but uses them to supplement conventional drug and therapy treatments, rather than to replace conventional medicine.

Homeopathic—Practice that uses very diluted remedies and treatments that cause similar effects to the symptoms they are intended to treat in an effort to stimulate the body's natural immune response system.

Hormones—Chemicals produced by glands in the body that circulate in the blood and control the actions of cells and organs. Estrogens are hormones that affect breast cancer growth.

Hormone therapy—Treating cancers by changing the hormone balance of the body, instead of by using cell-killing drugs.

Lumpectomy—A surgical procedure in which only the cancerous tumor in the breast is removed, together with a rim of normal tissue.

Lymph nodes—Small, bean-shaped masses of tissue scattered along the lymphatic system that act as filters and immune monitors, removing fluids, bacteria, or cancer cells that travel through the lymph system. Breast cancer cells in the lymph nodes under the arm or in the chest are a sign that the cancer has spread and that it might recur.

Malignant—Cancerous.

Mammography—X-ray imaging of the breast that can often detect lesions in the tissue too small or too deep to be felt.

---

survival rate for women with no lymph node involvement is 65 to 80%. If 1 to 3 nodes are involved, the ten-year survival rate is 35 to 65%. If more than four nodes contain cancer, the ten-year survival rate is 13 to 24%. Other factors such as tumor size and whether the cancer is sensitive to biotherapeutics also affect survival rates.

It is typical after breast cancer treatment to be depressed or moody, to cry, lose appetite, or feel unworthy or less interested in sex. If these problems last for an extended time, individual counseling is appropriate. Exercise and **yoga** can help the patient regain strength and flexibility and improve mood. Many women find that attending a support group of breast cancer survivors is helpful during this stage.

Prevention

While breast cancer cannot be prevented, making lifestyle choices that eliminate the risk factors listed above is both prudent and promotes general health and wellbeing. Despite questions about the effectiveness of mammography in detecting breast cancer, regular mammogram screening remains the most effective tool available for detecting breast cancer at an early stage when it is most treatable. A baseline mammogram should be done by age 35, so that this normal x ray can be used to compare to future mammograms. In addition, women should perform breast self-examinations on their breasts at the same time each month. The American Cancer Society (ACS) publishes guidelines recommending how often and at what ages women should have screening mammograms. In 2008 the recommendation was for annual screening mammograms for women beginning at age 40. Very high-risk women with a family history of breast cancer who carry the BRCA1 and BRCA2 genes may want to discuss preventative mastectomy with their physician. As of 2008, preventive surgery remained controversial.

Resources

BOOKS

Geffen, Jeremy R. *The Journey Through Cancer: Healing and Transforming the Whole Person.* New York: Three Rivers Press, 2006.

Kaelin, Carolyn M., Francesca Coltrera, Josie Gardiner, and Joy Prouty. *The Breast Cancer Survivor's Fitness Plan.* New York: McGraw-Hill, 2007.

Link, John S. *Breast Cancer Survival Manual: A Step-by-Step Guide for the Woman with Newly Diagnosed Breast Cancer.*, 4th ed. New York: Henry Holt, 2007.

Visel, Dave *Living With Cancer: A Practical Guide.* New Brunswick, NJ: Rutgers University Press, 2006.

PERIODICALS

Alternative Therapies Magazine. PO Box 627, Holmes, PA 19043-9650. http://www.alternative-therapies.com.

OTHER

"The ABCs of Breast Cancer Guide." *Susan G. Komen Breast Cancer Foundation* 2008. http://cms.komen.org/komen/AboutBreastCancer/TheABCsofBreastCancerGuide/index.htm. (April 6, 2008).

ORGANIZATIONS

Alternative Medicine Foundation, PO Box 60016, Potomac, MD, 20859, (301) 340-1960, http://www.amfoundation.org.

American Association of Oriental Medicine, PO Box 162340, Sacramento, CA, 95816, (866) 455-7999, (914) 443-4770, http://www.aaaomonline.org.

American Cancer Society, 1599 Clifton Road NE, Atlanta, GA, 30329-4251, (800) ACS-2345, http://www.cancer.org.

American Holistic Medical Association, PO Box 2016, Edmonds, WA, 98020, (425) 967-0737, http://www.holisticmedicine.org.

National Cancer Institute Public Inquiries Office, 6116 Executive Blvd., Room 3036A, Bethesda, MD, 20892-8322, (800) 4-CANCER, http://www.cancer.gov.

National Center for Complementary and Alternative Medicine Clearinghouse, PO Box 7923, Gaithersburg, MD, 20898, (888) 644-6226, http://nccam.nih.gov.

Office of Dietary Supplements, National Institutes of Health, 6100 Executive Blvd., Room 3B01, MSC 7517, Bethesda, MD, 20892-7517, (301) 435-2920, http://dietary-supplements.info.nih.gov.

Paula Ford-Martin
Teresa G. Odle
Tish Davidson, A. M.

Breast disease *see* **Fibrocystic breast disease**

Breast-feeding problems

Definition

The term "breast-feeding problems" is used to describe a variety of physical, behavioral, and emotional difficulties with nursing an infant.

Description

Breast-feeding, or nursing, is the practice of nourishing an infant with the milk in the human breast. Full-term babies have a natural suckling instinct, and breast-feeding comes naturally to most as soon as they leave the womb. After delivery, levels of prolactin, the hormone that triggers milk product, begin to rise in the body. At first, babies feed on a nutrient-rich substance known as **colostrum**, which is produced by the breast before milk production begins. New mothers will experience engorgement in the days following the birth of their babies, where breast milk "comes in" and engorges the breasts. After this time, regular feedings and proper breast-feeding techniques usually ensure a healthy milk supply for most babies until it is time to wean. However, breast-feeding can be a complex process and in many cases, there is a problem with the infant's suckling technique, the mother's milk supply, or other factors, and breast-feeding problems result.

Causes and symptoms

Inadequate weight gain and a failure to thrive in nursing infants is the most obvious sign that there is a breast-feeding problem.

A number of factors may interfere with successful breast-feeding. These include:

- Milk supply problems. A variety of factors can cause an inadequate supply in new mothers. Milk production is largely a supply and demand process. If the baby does not feed frequently enough, milk production will adjust itself, going down accordingly. A study published in 2002 showed that women who gave birth to a second child within two years of the birth of their first child produced about 30 percent more breast milk in the first week after birth with their second baby.

- Latching problems. Some babies, particularly pre-term infants, have difficulty suckling. This can be due to an abnormality of the mouth, or simply to a lack of coordination of the jaw muscles. In addition, the mother may not be placing her breast into the infant's mouth properly.

- Scheduling problems. Breastfed infants should be nursed at least once every three hours during the day, and should go no more than five hours at night between feedings. Scheduling also becomes a problem for women who work outside the home, as they often find that their milk flow diminishes after they return to work.

- Nipple and breast problems. Infants may have difficulty latching on to inverted or flat nipples. Other structural problems such as insufficient mammary glandular tissue, may result in reduced milk production. In addition, cracked and sore nipples and breast infections (mastitis) can make nursing painful.

- Retained placenta. If a woman's milk has not "come in" and she continues to experience abnormal bleeding after delivery, she may still be retaining pieces of the placenta within her uterus.

KEY TERMS

Latching—A term used to describe a baby's mouth hold on his or her mother's nipple.

Prolactin—A hormone secreted after delivery which stimulates the production of milk.

- Stomach sleeping. A nursing mother who sleeps on her stomach may experience decreased milk production due to the extended pressure on her breasts.

- Stress and fatigue. New mothers need proper rest in order to produce an adequate milk supply. The ability to relax is also fundamental to proper breast-feeding. Women who are stressed can have difficulty achieving milk "let-down," the sensation of the mammary glands releasing milk.

- Psychological issues. Some women are unable to breastfeed because of preconceived notions about the practice, or ideas instilled by their parents and peers, that have put up a psychological barrier for them. A 2002 study showed that most women are uncomfortable breast feeding in public and may even abandon the practice because they don't want to be shut off from others or feel squeamish about feeding their babies even in front of friends and family members.

Diagnosis

Breast-feeding problems are first determined by an infant's inability to gain weight. Most babies lose some weight in the first week of life. However, they should regain the weight quickly and be back at their birthweight at two weeks of age. An average weight gain of 6–8 oz per week should be maintained through the second or third month. After that, growth charts can demonstrate whether the child is gaining adequate weight.

Once a problem has been established, a healthcare practitioner will ask questions about the baby's feeding schedule and may observe the mother's breast-feeding technique so he or she can determine if an improper latching technique or inadequate suckling is causing the difficulty. Lactation counselors can be helpful in diagnosing these problems. Further physical examination and tests may be necessary to determine if structural breast problems or placental fragments are causing the difficulties.

Treatment

Proper treatment for breast-feeding difficulties depends on the cause of the problem.

Inadequate milk production

Milk production can be boosted in several ways. The easiest way is for the mother to encourage more frequent feedings at the breast. If this is impractical or the baby does not cooperate, milk production can often be increased through intermittent use of a breast pump, a device that expresses milk from the breast. Breast pumps are available in manual and electric models, and can be purchased or rented. Pumped breast milk can be bottled or frozen, and fed by bottle to the baby at a later time, although if milk production is a problem the mother will probably want to put the baby to the breast at every opportunity.

Milk thistle, or *Silybum marianum*, is sometimes prescribed to promote increased breast milk secretion. Although the herb is considered safe for nursing mothers, it should be acquired from a reputable source and prescribed by an herbalist, naturopathic physician, or other healthcare professional familiar with its use.

Each breast contains both foremilk and the richer, fat laden hindmilk. Infants need the nutrients and fat of the hind milk, but must get through the foremilk to reach it. This is why it is important that the mother completely empty one breast before starting the baby on the other one. This can be accomplished by nursing at least 10 minutes per breast. If the baby does not completely empty a breast, the job can be finished with the aid of a breast pump. The next time the mother nurses, she should start the child on the opposite breast.

Latching problems

To ensure proper breast-feeding, the mother should encourage the baby to latch on to the entire nipple, with his or her lips past the outside perimeter of the areola, before starting to suck. The mother will likely have to guide the breast into the baby's mouth, and repositioning may be required.

Practice makes perfect, and sometimes all an infant needs to improve his latching and suckling technique is time. If the baby has a structural problem in his mouth, such as a cleft palate, a breast pump may be required to keep milk production going. In some cases where suckling does not improve, feeding with a supplementary **nutrition** system may be required. The system consists of a feeding bottle containing the mother's own breast-pumped milk, and two tubes that run down from the bottle and attach to the nipples. Milk flows easily from the tubes with a weak sucking action from the baby. Both baby and mother can still maintain closeness while providing the baby with adequate milk flow.

Scheduling problems

Nursing infants who are sleeping through the night without a feeding are probably not getting enough milk. They should go no longer than five hours at night without feeding, and may require waking to ensure they get enough to eat.

Women who have returned to work can use a portable breast pump at least once during the work day to encourage sustained milk flow and to store milk for their babies to eat during their time away from home.

Nipple and breast problems

Liquid **vitamin E** applied regularly to sore or cracked nipples can soothe the **pain** and help the healing process. Women who think they have a breast infection should see their healthcare provider immediately, as they will probably require a course of antibiotics.

Retained placenta

Minor surgery known as a dilatation and curettage (D and C) is usually required to remove pieces of placenta that were retained by the uterus. Once the placenta has been removed, prolactin levels should rise, stimulating milk production.

Stress and fatigue

Relaxation exercises, **yoga**, **meditation**, massage, and **aromatherapy** can all be useful tools for relieving **stress**. Women should establish a quiet, restful environment for nursing. Warm compresses to the breast may also assist in milk let down. If it is feasible, taking naps when the baby is sleeping can help to ease the **fatigue** caused by nighttime feedings.

Psychological issues

Support from family and friends is necessary for any new mother, especially one that chooses to nurse her child. If no familiar support network exists, women may seek help from groups for nursing mothers such as the LaLeche league.

Many hospitals offer mothers and their spouses classes on breast-feeding techniques and nursing issues. Women who have negative feelings about breast-feeding may find classes helpful in overcoming these issues.

Expected results

In most cases, treatment for breast-feeding problems is successful and mother and baby do well. Other women may be able to breastfeed in limited amounts, but require supplementing their child's diet with formula to ensure proper weight gain and adequate nutrition. For a small percentage of women, physical problems or psychological issues may prevent successful nursing altogether.

Prevention

The best way for a new mother to prevent nursing problems is to take care of herself by eating right, drinking plenty of fluids, and staying rested and relaxed. It's important, because breast feeding incidence and duration are both associated with reduced **breast cancer** risk in women, according to a large international study released in 2002.

Resources

BOOKS

Eiger, Marvin S., and Sally Olds. *The Complete Book of Breast-feeding*. New York: Bantam Books, 1999.

Eisenberg, Arlene et al. *What to Expect the First Year*. 2nd edition. New York: Workman Publishing, 1996.

PERIODICALS

"Milk Production and Number of Births (Breastfeeding)." *Special Delivery* (Fall 2002):18.

"Mothers Uncomfortable Breastfeeding in Public." *Australian Nursing Journal* (July 2002):31.

Worcester, Sharon. "Breast-feeding Linked to Reduced Breast Ca Risk (Duration and Incidence)." *OB GYN News* (September 1, 2002):18–21.

ORGANIZATIONS

The LaLeche League. 1400 N. Meacham Rd., Schaumburg, IL 60173-4048. (847) 519-7730. http://www.lalecheleague.org.

Paula Ford-Martin
Teresa G. Odle

Breath therapy

Definition

Breath therapy is an umbrella term that includes a broad range of therapeutic approaches that emphasize the importance of breathing and its potential to affect human health. Most breath therapies employ specific types of breathing exercises, often done in conjunction with other practices. In addition to the ones mentioned here, yoga-like breath therapies include **qigong** and

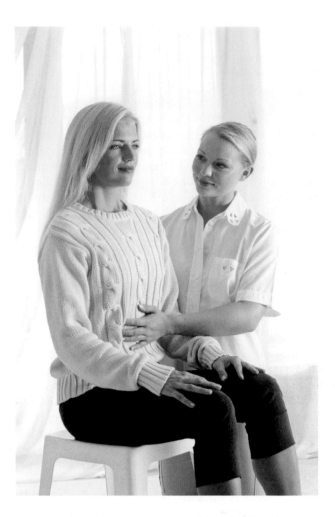

Woman in breathing therapy. *(© mediacolor's / Alamy)*

t'ai chi ch'uan. These Chinese exercises involve breathing and physical movements.

Origins

The therapeutic use of many breath techniques has been explored in various forms since ancient times.

Yoga

Developed thousands of years ago in India, **yoga** in modern times takes many forms. Patanjali, sometimes known as the "Father of Yoga," codified yoga philosophy and technique in his *Yoga Sutras*, written sometime during the last several centuries of the pre-Christian era.

Breathwork

Breathwork refers to a number of different breath-based therapies, most of which were developed after the 1970s. Rebirthing, also known as intuitive breathing, uses breathing techniques (in conjunction with affirmations and other cognitive practices) as a form of **psychotherapy**. The intent is for the person to reexperience and release birth trauma and other emotional and psychological blockages.

Holotropic breathwork

Holotropic breathwork was developed during the mid-1970s by Stanislav Grof and his wife, Christina Grof. Breathwork is done in a group setting, and the goals of the process are wholeness, healing, and wisdom. Experiences such as rebirthing may be the means to those goals, but those experiences are not the purpose of the process, according to the Holotropic Breathwork Web site.

Relaxation response

Herbert Benson of Harvard Medical School began studying the physiological effects of breathing and **meditation** techniques on the human body in the 1960s. This work led him to pinpoint a specific psychophysiological condition said to offer various therapeutic effects. In the 1970s, Benson founded the Mind Body Medical Institute at Harvard. He was later associated with the Benson-Henry Institute for Mind Body Medicine.

Benefits

Most breath therapies are commonly used both to promote general well-being and to address specific psychological, physical, and/or spiritual conditions. General benefits include reduced **stress**, enhanced energy and vitality, and (in the case of yoga and other similar practices) increased flexibility. Breath therapies have also been used to treat a wide range of specific complaints, such as **asthma**, high blood pressure, headaches, and **rheumatoid arthritis**. Breathing exercises have helped some children avoid asthma attacks and improve lung function. Breathing therapy has been used to help reduce anger, exhaustion, hostility, and risk of new heart problems in some people who have had heart surgery. Yoga, in particular, is increasingly being used in the early 2000s as a companion therapy to conventional treatment for such critical illnesses as **cancer**, **heart disease**, and HIV/AIDS.

Breath therapy will not cure those conditions but breath-therapy **relaxation** techniques help to reduce stress and promote a sense of well-being.

Used as a form of psychotherapy, both breathwork and meditation are said to help practitioners address old conflicts, enhance their self-esteem, and achieve greater peace of mind.

In addition to these benefits, spiritual seekers may explore these therapies to achieve higher consciousness.

Description

Yoga

Yoga is based on the belief that mind, body, and spirit are united. Most schools of yoga incorporate breathing exercises (known as pranayama) as one key component, along with physical poses (asanas) and, sometimes, chanting and/or sitting meditation.

One basic form of pranayama is three-level breathing, in which the practitioner first fills the abdomen, then the rib cage, and then the upper chest, before exhaling in reverse order. This action is performed slowly, with inhaled breath taken deep into the body, causing the person to relax. Another breathing technique sometimes used in yogic practice is alternate-nostril breathing, in which air is taken in through one nostril and expelled through the other, often using the hand or a finger to close the unused nostril. A more intensive breathing technique, often associated with the kundalini school of yoga, is the breath of fire. This movement involves pumping the diaphragm to draw in and expel air rapidly. More advanced yogic practice may also involve any number of other breathing techniques.

Breathwork

Various types of breathwork employ a breathing technique originally associated with rebirthing, known as conscious (or circular) connected breath. This technique, performed lying down, involves a continuous cycle of inhaling and exhaling air through the mouth. The person inhales as fully as possible and allows a natural, relaxed exhale, with no pause between intake and release. Holotropic breathwork uses deep and rapid breathing coordinated with dramatic sounds and rhythms to induce psychedelic states.

Relaxation response

Based on his study of the effects of transcendental meditation (a popular approach brought to the West by Maharishi Mahesh Yogi of India), Herbert Benson developed a nonreligious approach to meditation that combines breathing techniques, sitting quietly, and focusing the mind in order to achieve the "relaxation response."

Deep breathing

This technique, also known as belly breathing and relaxed breathing, is somewhat similar to pranayama. The person takes slow, deep breaths to relax. When a person becomes anxious or stressed, the body responds automatically with the fight-or-flight reaction. The body tenses and the heart beats faster. The person breathes from the diaphragm, taking shallow breaths.

The person counteracts this fight-or-flight response by taking deep breaths. The mouth is closed and the person slowly inhales air through the nose. The person holds the air in the lungs for about five seconds. During this time, the inhaled air causes the belly to expand like a balloon. The person releases the air by slowly exhaling it through the mouth. The inhale-exhale cycle is repeated as many times as needed until the person feels calmer.

Precautions

Many breath therapies are intended to be practiced in a safe, controlled environment, under the guidance of a trained facilitator or teacher. As a general rule, it is wise to ask about the training, qualifications, and experience of such facilitators, especially before beginning a rigorous or costly program based on a little-known therapy.

Although breathing is a natural process that is essential to life and breathing exercises are generally taken to be beneficial, some precautions may be advisable. People suffering from asthma or other breathing-related disorders should notify their doctor about any alternative therapy they consider. They should also notify their guide in the therapy of choice about their condition and any medication they take. People suffering from mental disturbances or disorders should be cautious about experimenting with practices designed to induce altered states of consciousness.

Furthermore, it may be necessary to consult a doctor before beginning a physical program such as yoga bodywork. This precaution is especially important for people diagnosed with conditions such as high blood pressure and **osteoarthritis**. While there are yoga classes designed for pregnant women, expectant mothers should first check with their obstetricians.

Side effects

Prolonged, intensive breathing may sometimes create **dizziness** or fainting. Related techniques used in some of the various breath therapies may have other side effects that should be considered before starting a therapeutic program. For example, people doing yoga bodywork may injure themselves or aggravate pre-existing medical conditions.

Research and general acceptance

Deep breathing is accepted by the medical community as an effective method of reducing stress. Furthermore, numerous clinical studies since the 1970s have demonstrated specific benefits associated with various breathing techniques and/or breath-based therapies, particularly certain types of yoga and meditation. Breathing exercises help to reduce stress and may help lower blood pressure and respiratory rate. Yoga bodywork helps to improve a person's flexibility and may help people diagnosed with mild or moderate asthma.

Breath therapy has been researched at the University of California San Francisco's Osher Center for Integrative Medicine. In a randomized controlled trial, the center studied the effect of breath therapy on 36 people diagnosed with chronic lower back **pain**, according to a May 2007 notice on the center's website. The study compared breath therapy and traditional physical therapy. The center charted results at the beginning of the study, six to eight weeks later, and after six months. The center concluded that patients using breath therapy "improved significantly."

Holotropic Breathwork was the subject of several small studies that were described in unpublished dissertations, according to the September 2007 issue of the *Journal of Alternative & Complementary Medicine*. The article authors provided an overview of the studies and concluded with recommendations for the format of future studies. These included selecting an "adequate sample size".

Training and certification

There was no national certification standard for yoga instructors as of February 2008. However, the American Yoga Association website offered recommendations about how to select an instructor. Practitioners of Holotropic Breathwork earn certification in Grof Transpersonal Training. The process requires about 600 hours of residential training that takes at least two years to complete.

Deep breathing can be self-taught and may be supplemented by relaxation CDs and audiotapes.

Resources

BOOKS

Mayo Clinic. *Mayo Clinic Book of Alternative Medicine.* New York: Time Inc. Home Entertainment, 2007.

PERIODICALS

Comarow, Avery. "Embracing Alternative Care: Top Hospitals Put Unorthodox Therapies into Practice." *U.S. News & World Report* January 9, 2008. http://health.usnews.com/articles/health/2008/01/09/embracing-alternative-care.html (February 24, 2008).

Rhinewine, Joseph P., and Oliver J. Williams. "Holotropic Breathwork: The Potential Role of a Prolonged, Voluntary Hyperventilation Procedure as an Adjunct to Psychotherapy." *Journal of Alternative & Complementary Medicine* (September 2007): 771–776.

OTHER

University of California, San Francisco Osher Center for Integrative Medicine. "Randomized Controlled Trial of Breath Therapy for Patients with Chronic Low Back Pain." May 3, 2007. http://www.osher.ucsf.edu/Research/abstract_breath.aspx (February 24, 2008).

ORGANIZATIONS

American Yoga Association, PO Box 19986, Sarasota, FL, 34276, http://www.americanyogaassociation.org.

Association for Holotropic Breathwork International, PO Box 400267, Cambridge, MA, 02140, (617) 674-2474, http://www.breathwork.com.

Benson-Henry Institute for Mind Body Medicine, 824 Boylston Street, Chestnut Hill, MA, 02467, (617) 732-9130, http://www.mbmi.org/home.

Peter Gregutt
Liz Swain

Breema

Definition

Breema is a bodywork technique that has been described as a cross between partner **yoga** and **Thai massage**. The practitioner works with a fully clothed participant on movements that focus on being present in the moment. Nine Universal Principles guide the actions, and the goal of a session is to activate the body's self-corrective reflexes to create a balanced state of energy. Self-Breema is designed for individuals to perform.

Origins

Breema originated in a mountain village in the Near East and was established in the United States with the founding in 1980 of the Breema Center in Oakland, California. Jon Schreiber and a group of colleagues founded the center. Schreiber, a graduate of the Palmer College of **Chiropractic**, served as director after the center opened. He is said to have incorporated Breema into his clinical practice because of its ability to vitalize and heal the body. Schreiber has taught and written about the Breema system since the 1980s.

As of the spring of 2008, Breema classes and workshops were offered at the center and in states ranging from Alabama to West Virginia. Classes and workshops are also held in various countries, including Canada, Argentina, Brazil, Australia and New Zealand, India, Japan, Great Britain, Austria, Denmark, Finland, France, Germany, Italy, the Netherlands, Spain, Switzerland, and Sweden.

Furthermore, the University of Oregon offered Breema classes for college credit, according to the spring 2005 *Well Now* newsletter. Author Hanna Budan wrote that the Breema course was a "unique bodywork and **meditation** class" that helped people remain in the present instead of concentrating on the past or future. That emphasis on connecting mind and body in the present could help students overwhelmed by the stresses of college life, Budan wrote.

Benefits

According to the Breema Center, the primary benefit of Breema is bringing individuals to a level at which they feel nurtured rather than drained by their relationship to their body, surroundings, people, feelings, and other aspects of life. The center maintained that Breema's nurturing atmosphere allows the mind, body, and feelings to become present, receptive, and vital. Secondary benefits that stem from this nurturing include the following:

- renewed vitality
- increased mental clarity and focus
- relief of tension
- increased flexibility
- mental and emotional balance and harmony
- gentle musculoskeletal realignment
- reduced stress
- improved nervous system function
- improved circulation and digestion.

Description

Author Maggie Simon wrote in a 2006 *Share Guide* article that Breema has been described as a cross between partner yoga and Thai massage. However, the aim of Breema was to "nurture an experience of presence," with both practitioner and recipient benefiting form the experience, Simon wrote.

Breema has three important components. They are bodywork, Self-Breema exercises, and the nine Universal Principles of Breema.

Bodywork

Since Breema regards the body as an energy system, the bodywork is intended "to enhance the flow of life energy and bring one to the present," according to information from the center. A person receiving a Breema treatment is fully clothed and either lies or sits on a padded floor.

The recipient works with the practitioner in bodywork described by the center as a harmonious choreography of supported movements, gradual leaning, gentle stretching and bending, holding postures, "nurturing brushes," and rhythmic tapping. Breema treatments are tailored to each recipient at each visit; there is no standard program or sequence. Treatment sessions may last from about 30 minutes to an hour.

Self-Breema exercises

Self-Breema exercises are done individually, so that the person may "experience being both the practitioner and recipient at the same time." The program emphasizes the naturalness of all Self-Breema moves and postures. No muscular force or unusual contortions of the body are involved. Like the bodywork sessions, Self-Breema exercises are customized for each individual to support and balance the flow of life energy through the body, release tension, and increase vitality and dexterity.

Universal Principles

Breema maintains that Universal Principles govern all of life as well as bodywork and health maintenance. Breema's nine Universal Principles are:

- Body comfortable. The body is viewed as an "aspect of a unified whole."
- No extra. Nothing more is needed to express a person's true nature.
- Firmness and gentleness. People who are present manifest both firmness and gentleness simultaneously.
- Full participation. Body, mind, and feelings are united "in a common aim."
- Mutual support. "Giving and receiving support take place simultaneously."
- No judgment. People who come to the present are free from judgment.
- Single moment/Single activity. Each moment is an expression of a person's true nature.

- No hurry/No pause. Neither is found in the "natural rhythm of life energy."
- No force. Letting go of assumptions of separation is letting go of force.

The Breema principles are intended to free people from the conceptual body, defined as "the ideas and images of our body that we carry in our mind." The aim of Breema is "to increase vitality, not to fight sickness, and to create an atmosphere which allows the body to move toward a natural state of balance."

Working with the nine principles of Breema is thought to create a receptive mind, supportive feelings, and a relaxed body. The energy that is usually consumed by conflict between mind and feelings and physical tension becomes available.

Preparations

Breema treatments do not require special preparation other than the wearing of loose and comfortable clothing that allows for free movement.

Precautions

Common sense precautions for any kind of bodywork include seeking advice from a qualified medical practitioner before starting a new program. This precaution is particularly important for people with chronic heart or lung disease, persons recovering from surgery or acute illness, and those with arthritis or other disorders that affect the muscles and joints.

Side effects

As of February 2008, there were no known side effects of Breema therapy in healthy people.

Research and general acceptance

As of February 2008, no published information was available regarding independent scientific studies of Breema.

Training and certification

The Breema Center in Oakland is the world headquarters for training and certifying instructors and practitioners. The center offers a 165-hour practitioner certificate program in Breema bodywork. The coursework encompasses 130 hours of Breema bodywork, 15 hours of anatomy and physiology, and 20 hours of Breema Practitioner Colloquium. The certificate program takes a minimum of six months to complete. The Breema Center is a vocational school licensed by the State of California Bureau for Private

KEY TERMS

Self-Breema—A personalized form of Breema bodywork that the individual performs on his or her own body, without an instructor as partner. It is intended to supplement Breema bodywork treatment sessions with an instructor.

Postsecondary and Vocational Education. To become an instructor, certified Breema practitioners must have years of experience, receive extensive training with Schreiber, and fulfill annual continuing education requirements.

Resources

BOOKS

Schreiber, Jon. *Breema and the Nine Principles of Harmony.* Oakland, CA: Breema Center, 2007.

Schreiber, Jon. *Every Moment Is Eternal: The Timeless Wisdom of Breema.* Oakland, CA: Breema Center, 2007.

PERIODICALS

Budan, Hanna. "Breema: The Art of Being Present." *Well Now* (Spring 2005): 3.

Simon, Maggie. "Understanding Breema." *Share Guide* (September/October 2006): 38–39.

ORGANIZATIONS

Breema Center, 6076 Claremont Ave, Oakland, CA, 94618, (510) 428-0937, http://www.breema.com.

Rebecca Frey
Liz Swain

Brewer's yeast

Description

Brewer's yeast is an ingredient used to ferment sugars to alcohol in the brewing of beer. It consists of the ground, dried cells of *Saccharomyces cerevisiae,* a one-celled plant that is a variety of fungus.

Brewer's yeast is an inactive yeast that has no fermenting or leavening power. Brewer's yeast should not be confused with torula yeast, nutritional yeast, or baker's yeast. These yeasts do not have the same metabolic, physiologic, taxonomic, and genetic properties as brewer's yeast. Brewer's yeast also should not be confused with the yeast that causes vaginal infections, *Candida albicans.*

Brewer's yeast contains all the essential amino acids, 14 minerals, and 17 vitamins. It is one of the best natural sources of the B-complex vitamins thiamin, **riboflavin**, niacin, B_6, **pantothenic acid**, **biotin**, and **folic acid**. It is also high in minerals, including **chromium**, **zinc**, **iron**, **phosphorus**, **magnesium**, and **selenium**. Brewer's yeast is also a good source of protein. It contains approximately 16 g of protein per 30 g of powdered yeast. Brewer's yeast is a good source of RNA, an immune-enhancing nucleic acid that may help in the prevention of degenerative diseases and slowing of the **aging** process.

General use

Vegetarians typically use brewer's yeast as a source of protein, vitamins, and minerals. In addition to being an excellent nutritional supplement, brewer's yeast is often recommended to regulate blood sugar levels, raise HDL **cholesterol** levels, improve the health of the skin, prevent **constipation**, control **diarrhea**, and repel insects in pets.

Brewer's yeast is one of the best sources of the mineral chromium. Two tablespoons of brewer's yeast yields about 120 micrograms (mcg) of chromium, an amount equal to the recommended daily allowance. Chromium plays a role in raising HDL cholesterol levels (the good cholesterol) and is an important factor in regulating blood sugar levels. High levels of chromium increase glucose tolerance.

Diabetes and **hypoglycemia** are two conditions in which blood sugar levels are unstable. Brewer's yeast has been reported to help improve symptoms of diabetes and hypoglycemia, and may act to prevent diabetes from developing in persons with a family history of diabetes and in those who have problems with blood sugar metabolism. Several studies have reported that people with diabetes improve hemoglobin levels, **fasting** glucose levels, and glycemia with brewer's yeast supplementation. However, the authors of a 2007 systemic review of randomized controlled trials published in *Diabetes Care* journal concluded that future studies were needed to address the limitations in the current research before specific health claims can be made about the effects of brewer's yeast on diabetes and hypoglycemia. As more clinical data continue to be published, additional scientific evidence will be available to support health risk reduction claims.

B-complex vitamins are important for healthy skin and nails. Persons deficient in these vitamins may benefit from taking brewer's yeast, as it is rich in B-complex vitamins. A compound derived from brewer's yeast, skin respiratory factor (SRF), reportedly has wound healing properties. SRF has been a component in over-the-counter hemorrhoid remedies for more than four decades. SRF also has been used to treat skin problems. Brewer's yeast has been used in the treatment of **contact dermatitis**, a condition of the skin characterized by red, itchy, and inflamed skin.

Brewer's yeast may help to prevent constipation. Thirty grams of brewer's yeast contains approximately 6 grams of dietary fiber (24% of the recommended daily amount). Fiber is an important part of the diet as it helps increase the bulk of fecal matter, thereby promoting healthy bowels and intestines. Brewer's yeast has also been found to be helpful in cases of diarrhea. The yeast acts to encourage the growth of good bacteria in the intestines.

Generous doses of brewer's yeast may help to prevent cancers such as prostate cancer. When combined with **wheat germ**, brewer's yeast is helpful in preventing heart problems. Brewer's yeast may also be helpful in the treatment of **fatigue**, low energy, or appetite loss.

Pet owners have known about the ability of brewer's yeast to repel ticks and fleas for many years. Wafers that contain brewer's yeast can be given to animals for this purpose. Powdered brewer's yeast may also be sprinkled on the animal's food. The large amounts of **thiamine** in brewer's yeast may repel mosquitoes from humans as well.

Preparations

Brewer's yeast is available at most health food stores in tablets, flakes, and powder form. Brewer's yeast can be added to foods (soups, casseroles, baked goods) to increase their nutritional value. It is also a popular addition to drinks, juices, and shakes, and is marketed as a protein supplement, energy booster, and immune enhancer. The product label will provide instructions on how to take it. Brewer's yeast does not require refrigeration and has a long shelf life.

The quality of brewer's yeast varies depending upon the manufacturer. Some packaged brewer's yeasts are processed to remove the alcohol and/or chemical byproducts that may be left behind in the brewing process. This processing phase lowers the nutritional quality of the yeast. High quality brewer's yeast is grown on molasses or sugar beets and is grown specifically for supplemental purposes. As a result, there is no need for further processing. Brewer's yeast powder is often bitter tasting. Some powders are "debittered."

Brewer's yeast contains higher levels of phosphorus than **calcium**. Too much phosphorus may deplete the body of calcium. To create a balance, some manufacturers add calcium to their brewer's yeast products.

When prescribing brewer's yeast as a food supplement, doctors often recommend a daily dosage of 1–2 tbsp. For a person with diabetes, the recommended dose is 1 tbsp. twice daily.

Ticks and fleas can be prevented by sprinkling powdered brewer's yeast on the animal's food in a dosage of 1 tsp. for cats and 1 tsp. per pound of body weight for dogs.

Precautions

Daily dosage on the product label should not be exceeded.

Those allergic to yeast or susceptible to yeast **infections** should contact their healthcare practitioner before taking brewer's yeast.

Persons with **gout**, vaginal infections, or *Candida albicans* should avoid using brewer's yeast.

Persons with diabetes should consult their healthcare practitioner before using brewer's yeast. Brewer's yeast may interfere with insulin requirements.

The use of brewer's yeast is not appropriate for people who have severely weakened immune systems due to disease or **cancer** treatments, as they can develop serious infections.

Persons with an intestinal disease should not take brewer's yeast.

Brewer's yeast is safe in pregnant or nursing women at doses of 1–2 tbsp. per day.

Side effects

Initial use may cause bloating and **gas**. To lessen these effects, it is best to begin with small amounts of brewer's yeast (less than 1 tsp. daily) and gradually increase to the recommended dosage.

If **nausea** or diarrhea occur, brewer's yeast should be discontinued and the person should follow up with a healthcare practitioner.

Interactions

As of 2008 there were no documented interactions between brewer's yeast and any pharmaceutical drugs or herbal remedies.

Resources

BOOKS

Berdanier C., and J. T. Dywer, eds. *Handbook of Nutrition and Food,* 2nd ed. Boca Raton, FL: CRC Press, 2006.

Huffnagle G. B., and S. Wernick. *The Probiotics Revolution: The Definitive Guide to Safe, Natural Health Solutions Using Probiotic and Prebiotic Foods and Supplements.* New York: Bantam Books, 2007.

PERIODICALS

Balk E. M., A. Tatsioni, A. H. Lichtenstein, J. Lau, and A. G. Pittas. "Effect of Chromium Supplementation on Glucose Metabolism and Lipids: A Systematic Review of Randomized Controlled Trials." *Diabetes Care* 30, no. 8 (August 2007): 2154–2164.

Moyad, M. A. "Brewer's/Baker's Yeast (Saccharomyces Cerevisiae) and Preventive Medicine: Part I." *Urologic Nursing* 27, no. 6 (December 2007): 560–561.

OTHER

Saccharomyces Genome Database. (650) 725-8956. http://www.yeastgenome.org.

ORGANIZATIONS

Alternative Medicine Foundation, PO Box 60016, Potomac, MD, 20859, (301) 340-1960, http://www.amfoundation.org.

American Dietetic Association, 120 South Riverside Plaza, Suite 2000, Chicago, IL, 60606-6995, (800) 877-1600, http://www.catright.org.

Food and Agricultural Organization of the United Nations, http://www.fao.org.

Food and Nutrition Information Center, National Agricultural Library, United States Department of Agriculture, 10301 Baltimore Ave., Room 105, Beltsville, MD, 20705, (301) 504-5414, http://fnic.nal.usda.gov.

International Food Information Council, 1100 Connecticut Ave. NW, Suite 430, Washington, DC, DC, 20036, (202) 296-6540, http://www.ific.org.

Jennifer Wurges
Angela M. Costello

Bromelain

Description

Bromelain, also known as bromelin, is a protein-digesting enzyme extracted from the flesh and stem of the pineapple plant, *Ananas comosus*. Although the people of Guadeloupe introduced Christopher Columbus to the fruit in 1493, Europeans did not recognize the pineapple's beneficial attributes until later. Pineapple had a long history of traditional use among the native peoples of Central and South America. They applied pineapple dressings to **wounds** and skin injuries to reduce inflammation, and eased **stomachaches** and **indigestion** by drinking the juice of the fruit.

Bromelain was first isolated from pineapple juice in 1891 and introduced as a therapeutic supplement in 1957. The active ingredients of bromelain are found in the juice and stem of the pineapple plant, but the stem contains more bromelain than the fruit.

General use

Bromelain is most notable for its effectiveness in the reduction of inflammation and decreasing swelling, but the scope of its benefits continues to increase. As a natural anti-inflammatory enzyme, bromelain has many uses. Arthritis patients may reduce the swelling that causes joint **pain** by taking bromelain. Bromelain may also be helpful for the pain, numbness, tingling, aching, and loss of motor and sensory function in the fingers resulting from **carpal tunnel syndrome** (CTS).

The protease enzyme is beneficial in reducing the clumping of platelets (small platelike bodies in the blood), the formation of plaques in the arteries, and the formation of **blood clots**. All these effects help to prevent and treat cardiovascular disease. Bromelain has also been discovered to have anti-tumor action, as well as helping the body absorb medications.

Although bromelain is often labeled an alternative treatment, mainstream medical research continues to study its effectiveness in the prevention and treatment of hematomas, or localized blood clots. Bromelain has been found useful in the reduction of swelling and congestion in the affected tissue after an athletic injury or surgery. It is commonly used in Germany for this purpose.

Bromelain's anti-clotting activity may be useful in preventing strokes, one of the most feared results of obstructions in the circulatory system. Due to the lack of oxygenated blood flowing to the brain, a **stroke** can cause permanent damage to the affected area of the central nervous system. Bromelain is thought to help maintain healthy cardiac tissue and reduce the risk of stroke by its anti-inflammatory activity. By preventing mild infection or inflammation caused by the fatty substances inside the blood vessels where plaque may form, bromelain helps to reduce inflammation by digesting the byproducts of tissue repair.

Bromelain is helpful to people with colds due to its ability to reduce mucus and keep it moving out of the body. Bromelain has also been shown to reduce the painful inflammation associated with costochondritis, an inflammation of the cartilage that attaches the ribs to the breastbone. In addition, bromelain appears to be beneficial to **asthma** patients. Asthma is caused by spasms of the bronchial passages that restrict the flow of air in and out of the lungs. Taking bromelain may reduce the excess mucus that tends to collect in the respiratory systems of asthma patients. In addition, people who suffer from **hay fever** and similar seasonal **allergies** may also be helped by bromelain's antiinflammatory activity.

Additional benefits of bromelain include reducing the painful symptoms of **varicose veins**, including dull aches, tired legs and feet, and itchy skin.

Research has also shown that bromelain benefits cows as well as humans. Bromelain has been shown to reduce the white blood cell count in cows with mastitis. This reduction increases the quality of their milk. Researchers have found that bromelain works to reduce inflammation by interfering with the synthesis of prostaglandins and other inflammatory substances.

Preparations

Bromelain is available as a dietary supplement that is offered in several different tablet strengths. For **rheumatoid arthritis**, the recommended dosage of bromelain is 250–750 mg, taken two or three times a day between or before meals. In Germany, the standard dosage to reduce swelling after surgery is 80–320 mg daily. The supplement has been found to offer the most benefit when taken on an empty stomach, and its therapeutic effects are also enhanced when taken in higher doses.

Increasing the dosage of bromelain to 400–1,000 mg per day has shown to reduce the symptoms of **angina** pectoris (the severe pain and feeling of constriction about the heart that often radiates to the left shoulder and down the left arm).

Precautions

Bromelain has shown to be generally safe when taken in moderate doses, although a preliminary report links an increased heart rate with the use of the supplement. People with an inflammation of the stomach lining should not use digestive enzyme supplements such as bromelain. In addition, the safe use of bromelain in pregnant or nursing women, small children, and people with kidney or liver disease has not been established.

Side effects

While bromelain can be taken safely without side effects in moderate doses, there are anecdotal reports of allergic reactions to it. Other side effects that have been observed include **nausea**, **vomiting**, **diarrhea**, and menorrhagia (excessively heavy menstrual flow).

Interactions

Because of bromelain's anti-clotting activity, it should not be combined with other blood-thinning medications such as warfarin (Coumadin), heparin, or aspirin. It is also possible that bromelain could cause bleeding problems if it is combined with other complementary therapies that thin the blood, such as **garlic** or gingko biloba.

Resources

PERIODICALS

Petry, Judy J. "Nutritional supplements and surgical patients." *AORN Journal* (June 1997).

Kelly, G.S. "Bromelain: A Literature Review and Discussion of Its Therapeutic Applications." *Alternative Medicine Review* (November 1, 1996).

ORGANIZATIONS

American Botanical Council. PO Box 201660, Austin, TX 78720-1660.

OTHER

HealthWorld Online. http://www.healthy.net (January 17, 2001).

Beth Kapes

Bronchitis

Definition

Bronchitis is an inflammation of the air passages between the nose and the lungs, including the windpipe, or trachea, and the larger air tubes, called bronchi, that bring air into the lungs from the trachea. When bronchitis is mild and brief in duration, it is called acute.

338   GALE ENCYCLOPEDIA OF ALTERNATIVE MEDICINE, 3ʳᵈ EDITION

Chronic bronchitis is recurrent, has a prolonged course, and is often a sign of a serious underlying lung disease.

Description

Acute bronchitis

Bronchitis is an inflammation of the breathing airways accompanied by coughing and spitting up of phlegm. It can be caused by exposure to a cold or the flu, infection, or irritants. Although the symptoms of acute and chronic bronchitis are similar, their causes and treatments are different. Acute bronchitis is most common in winter. It usually follows an upper respiratory infection, and may be accompanied by a secondary bacterial infection. The recovery time for acute bronchitis is usually within two weeks, although the **cough** may persist longer. Like any upper airway inflammatory process, acute bronchitis can increase a person's likelihood of developing **pneumonia**.

Anyone can get acute bronchitis, but infants, young children, and the elderly are more likely to suffer from the disease. Smokers and people with heart or lung diseases have a higher risk of developing acute bronchitis. Individuals exposed to chemical fumes or high levels of air pollution also have a greater chance of developing acute bronchitis.

Chronic bronchitis

Chronic bronchitis is one of a group of diseases that fall under the name *chronic obstructive pulmonary disease,* or COPD. Other diseases in this category include **emphysema** and chronic asthmatic bronchitis. Chronic bronchitis is a major cause of disability and death in the United States. In 2007, the American Lung Association estimated that about 9.5 million Americans suffered from the disease. Chronic bronchitis shows symptoms similar to acute bronchitis, but recurs and is present for at least three months a year. More women than men develop chronic bronchitis. As the number of women who smoke has increased, so has their rate of chronic bronchitis. The number of women with chronic bronchitis is about twice the number of men. Because this disease progresses slowly, middle-aged and older people are more likely to be diagnosed with chronic bronchitis.

Causes and symptoms

Acute bronchitis

Acute bronchitis usually begins with the symptoms of a cold, such as a runny nose, **sneezing**, and dry cough. However, the cough soon becomes deep and painful. Coughing brings up a greenish yellow phlegm or sputum. These symptoms may be accompanied by a **fever** of up to 102°F (39°C). **Wheezing** after coughing is common. About 90% of acute bronchitis is caused by a bacterial infection.

In uncomplicated acute bronchitis, the fever and most other symptoms except the cough disappear after three to five days. Coughing may continue for several weeks. Acute bronchitis is often complicated by a bacterial infection, in which case the fever and a general feeling of illness persist.

Chronic bronchitis

Chronic bronchitis is caused by inhaling respiratory tract irritants; it may also be due to recurrent bouts of acute bronchitis. The most common cause, however, is the irritation of cigarette smoke. The cells that line the respiratory system contain fine, hair-like outgrowths called cilia. Normally, the cilia of many cells beat rhythmically to move mucus along the airways. When smoke or other irritants are inhaled or when there is irritation from repeated dry coughing, the cilia become paralyzed or break off and the airways become inflamed, narrowed, and clogged. This leads to difficulty breathing and can progress to emphysema, which is a life-threatening disease. A mild cough is usually the first visible sign of chronic bronchitis. Coughing brings up phlegm, and may be accompanied by wheezing and shortness of breath.

Diagnosis

General

Initial diagnosis of bronchitis is based on observing the patient's symptoms and health history. The physician will perform a chest examination with a stethoscope, listening for specific sounds that indicate lung inflammation and airway narrowing. A sputum culture may be performed, particularly if the sputum is green or has blood in it, to determine whether a bacterial infection is present and to identify the disease-causing organism so that an appropriate antibiotic can be selected. Occasionally, in diagnosing a chronic lung disorder, the sample of sputum is collected using a procedure called a bronchoscopy.

Chronic bronchitis

A pulmonary function test is important in diagnosing chronic bronchitis and other variations of COPD. The test uses an instrument called a spirometer, which measures the volume of air entering and leaving the lungs. A doctor may do a chest x ray, an electrocardiogram (ECG), and blood tests as well.

Other tests may be used to measure how effectively oxygen and carbon dioxide are exchanged in the lungs.

Treatment

The treatment of chronic bronchitis is complex and depends on the stage of the disease and the presence of other health problems. Lifestyle changes, such as quitting **smoking** and avoiding secondhand smoke or polluted air, are essential first steps. Controlled **exercise** performed on a regular basis is also important.

There are a multitude of botanical and herbal medicines that can be used to treat bronchitis. Examples from **aromatherapy** include **essential oils** of any of the following: benzoin, *Styrax benzoin;* camphor, *Cinnamomum camphora;* **eucalyptus**, *Eucalyptus globulus;* **lavender**, *Lavandula officinalis;* pine, *Pinus sylvestris;* sandalwood, *Santalum album;* and **thyme**, or *Thymus vulgaris.* Any one or combination of these oils should be added to water and inhaled in a warm steam. They can also be dabbed onto a cloth, and the aroma can be inhaled deeply through the nose. A mixture of the essential oils of clove, *Eugenia aromaticum;* cinnamon, *Cinnamomum zeylanicum;* **lemon balm**, *Melissa officianalis;* and lavender, *Lavandula officinalis,* is reported to be particularly effective when taken as a steam inhalation.

Herbalists recommend taking a tea, syrup or tincture of any of the following herbs:

- mullein, *Verbascum thapsus*
- coltsfoot, *Tussilago farfara*
- aniseed, *Pimpinella anisum*
- hyssop, *Hyssopus officinalis*
- elecampane, *Inula helenium*
- garlic, *Allium sativum*

Recommended homeopathic remedies include:

- *Aconite* 6c
- *Kali bichromicum* 6c
- *Phosphorus* 6c

Acupuncture can be useful in preventing chronic bronchitis attacks and in resolving colds that lead to acute attacks.

For a mild case of acute bronchitis, over-the-counter remedies of homeopathic medicine, **traditional Chinese medicine**, and Ayurveda are widely available and quite helpful. Practitioners of these disciplines can be very effective and should be consulted when dealing with more severe or chronic cases. **Hydrotherapy** and massage with tapping and **cupping** is also recommended to loosen mucus, improve breathing, and heighten the immune response to the condition.

Consuming the juice of a lemon squeezed into a cup of water may be consumed to clear out mucus. Hot, spicy foods can help open the air passages. These foods include **garlic**, onions, chili peppers, and horseradish, and should be consumed liberally.

Allopathic treatment

Acute bronchitis

When no secondary infection is present, acute bronchitis is treated in the same way as the **common cold**. Home care includes drinking plenty of fluids, resting, abstaining from smoking, increasing moisture in the air with a cool mist humidifier, and taking acetaminophen (Datril, Tylenol, Panadol) for fever and **pain**. Aspirin should not be given to children because it is associated with seizures in young people. Cough syrups are recommended to reduce coughing, soothe irritation, and increase expectoration of mucus.

It is important for mucus to be cleared from the lungs. Cough suppressants should be limited because they may lead to mucus accumulation in the plugged airways, resulting in a breeding ground for pneumonia bacteria. If the patient is coughing up phlegm, the cough should be allowed to continue to bring up mucus and irritants from the lungs. Cough medicines with expectorants may, therefore, be helpful. Expectorant cough medicines thin the mucus in the lungs, making it easier to cough up and expel. People who are unsure about what types of medications are contained in over-the-counter cough syrups should ask their pharmacist for an explanation.

If a secondary bacterial infection is present, the infection may be treated with an antibiotic. Patients need to take the entire amount of antibiotic prescribed. A number of studies have shown, however, that antibiotics have only limited value in the treatment of acute bronchitis. These studies suggest that, in many cases, a drug is prescribed to make physicians and patients feel as if they are "doing something."

Chronic bronchitis

Drug therapy uses bronchodilators to relax the muscles of the bronchial tubes and allow increased airflow. They can be taken by mouth or inhaled using a nebulizer. Common bronchodilators include albuterol (Ventolin, Proventil, Apo-Salvent) and metaproterenol (Alupent, Orciprenaline, Metaprel, Dey-Dose). Antiinflammatory medications are added to reduce swelling of the airway tissue. Corticosteroids, such as prednisone, can be taken orally or intravenously. Other steroids may be inhaled. Medications are also given to reduce the quantity of mucus. As the disease progresses, the patient may need supplemental

KEY TERMS

Bronchoscopy—An examination of the lungs and airway passages using a flexible fiberoptic instrument.

Emphysema—A disease involving destruction of air sacs in the lungs, so that they do not take in oxygen easily and have the tendency to retain air within the lungs.

Mucus—The slippery secretion of the mucous membranes of the respiratory tract.

Nebulizer—A device that delivers medicine into the airways in the form of a mist.

Phlegm—A thick secretion of mucus that may clog the airway passages; it is produced in response to irritation.

Sputum—Mucus and other substances coughed up from the lungs.

Trachea—A cartilage tube in the area of the throat that carries air to the lungs.

oxygen. A one-time pneumonia vaccination may also be recommended.

In 2002, the United States Food and Drug Administration (FDA) approved a drug therapy for the treatment of chronic bronchitis, as well as other pulmonary diseases. Called Severent Diskus, or salmeterol, the product is a long-acting bronchodilator that can be inhaled twice a day and will last for 12 hours. It works well for patients with the chronic form of bronchitis, but is not intended for use in acute episodes. In 2005, the FDA asked the manufacturers of Severent Diskus to add a warning label to the product indicating that the drug can have lethal effects in some cases and that it should be used only if other treatments have been ineffective.

Expected results

When treated, acute bronchitis normally lasts one to two weeks if no complications occur, although a cough may continue for several more weeks. Unfortunately, there is no cure for chronic bronchitis, and the disease can often lead to or coexists with emphysema. On the whole, all forms of COPD are a leading cause of death.

Prevention

The best way to prevent bronchitis is to avoid becoming a smoker or to stop smoking. Smokers are 10 times more likely to die of COPD than non-smokers. Smokers who stop show improvement in lung function. Other preventive measures include avoiding chemical and environmental irritants, such as air pollution, and maintaining good overall health.

Supplementation with vitamins A, C, and E, **zinc**, and **bioflavonoids**, may also be helpful in preventing recurrence and secondary **infections**. Dairy products, sugary foods, and eggs should be avoided, as they may increase the tendency to form mucus in the lungs.

Resources

BOOKS

Acute Bronchitis—A Medical Dictionary, Bibliography, and Annotated Research Guide to Internet References. San Diego: ICON Health Publications, 2004.

Anzueto, Antonio. *Contemporary Diagnosis and Management of Bronchitis.* Newton, PA.: Handbooks in Health Care, 2006.

Chronic Bronchitis - A Medical Dictionary, Bibliography, and Annotated Research Guide to Internet References. San Diego: ICON Health Publications, 2004.

PERIODICALS

Bush, Andrew, and Anne H. Thomson. "Acute Bronchiolitis." *BMJ* (November 2007):1037–1041.

Fabbri, L. M., et al. "Update in Chronic Obstructive Pulmonary Disease 2005." *American Journal of Respiratory and Critical Care Medicine* (October 2006):1056–1065.

Wenzel, Richard P., and Alpha A. Fowler. "Acute Bronchitis." *New England Journal of Medicine* (November 2006):2125–2130.

ORGANIZATIONS

National Heart, Lung, and Blood Institute Information Center, P.O. Box 30105, Bethesda, MD, 20824-0105.

National Jewish Center for Immunology and Respiratory Medicine, 1400 Jackson Street, Denver, CO, 80206.

Patience Paradox
Teresa G. Odle
David Edward Newton, Ed.D.

Bruises

Definition

Bruises, or ecchymoses, are a discoloration and tenderness of the skin or mucous membranes due to the leakage of blood from an injured blood vessel into the tissues. Pupura refers to bruising as the result of a disease condition. A very small bruise is called a petechia. These often appear as many tiny red dots clustered together, and could indicate a serious problem.

Description

Bruises change colors over time in a predictable pattern, so that it is possible to estimate when an injury occurred by the color of the bruise. Initially, a bruise will be reddish, the color of the blood under the skin. After one to two days, the red blood cells begin to break down, and the bruise will darken to a blue or purplish color. This fades to green at about day six. Around the eighth or ninth day, the skin over the bruised area will have a brown or yellowish appearance, and it will gradually diminish back to its normal color.

Long periods of standing will cause the blood that collects in a bruise to seep through the tissues. Bruises are actually made of little pools of blood, so the blood in one place may flow downhill after awhile and appear in another. For instance, bruising in the back of the abdomen may eventually appear in the groin; bruising in the thigh or the knee will work its way down to the ankle.

Causes and symptoms

Healthy people may develop bruises from any injury that doesn't break through the skin. Vigorous **exercise** may also cause bruises due to bringing about small tears in blood vessels walls. In a condition known as purpura simplex, there is a tendency to bruise easily due to an increased fragility of the blood vessels. Bruises also develop easily in the elderly, because the skin and blood vessels have a tendency to become thinner and more fragile with **aging**, and there is an increased use of medications that interfere with the blood clotting system. In the condition known as purpura senilis, the elderly develop bruises from minimal contact that may take up to several months to completely heal.

The use of nonsteroidal anti-inflammatories such as ibuprofen (Advil) and naproxen (Aleve) may lead to increased bruising. Aspirin, antidepressants, **asthma** medications, and cortisone medications also have this effect. The anti-clotting medications also known as blood thinners, especially the drug Warfarin (Coumadin), may be the cause of particularly severe bruising.

Sometimes bruises are connected with more serious illnesses. There are a number of diseases that cause excessive bleeding or bleeding from injuries too slight to have consequences in healthy people. An abnormal tendency to bleed may be due to hereditary bleeding disorders, certain prescription medications, diseases of the blood such as **leukemia**, and diseases that increase the fragility of blood vessels. If there are large areas of bruising or bruises develop very easily, this may herald a problem. Other causes that should be ruled out include liver disease, **alcoholism**, drug addiction, and acquired immune deficiency syndrome (**AIDS**). Bruising that occurs around the navel may indicate dangerous internal bleeding; bruising behind the ear, called Battle's sign, may be due to a skull fracture; and raised bruises may point to autoimmune disease.

Diagnosis

Bruising is usually a minor problem, which does not require a medical diagnosis. However, faced with extensive bruising, bruising with no apparent cause, or bruising in certain locations, a physician will pursue an evaluation that will include a number of blood tests. If the area of the bruise becomes hard, an x ray may be required.

Treatment

Several types of topical applications are usually recommend to speed healing and to reduce the **pain** associated with bruises. **Vitamin K** cream can be applied directly to the site of injury. Astringent herbs such as **witch hazel**, *Hamamelis virginiana*, can be used. This will tighten the tissues and therefore diminish the bruising. The homeopathic remedy, *Arnica montana*, can be applied as a cream or gel to unbroken skin.

Oral homeopathic remedies may reduce bruising, pain, and swelling as well. *Arnica montana*, at 30 ml (1 oz), taken one to two times per day is highly recommended. For **ledum**, 30 ml (1 oz) one to two times per day is also useful.

Allopathic treatment

A bruise by itself needs no medical treatment. It is often recommended that ice packs be applied on and off during the first 24 hours of injury to reduce the bruising. After that, heat, especially moist heat, is recommended to increase the circulation and the healing of the injured tissues. Rest, elevation of the effected part, and compression with a bandage will also retard the accumulation of blood. Rarely, if a bruise is so large that the body cannot completely absorb it or if the site becomes infected, it may have to be surgically removed.

Expected results

The blood under the skin which causes the discoloration of bruising should be totally reabsorbed by the body in three weeks or less. At that time, the skin color should completely return to normal.

Sometimes, a bruise may become solid and increase in size instead of dissolving. This may indicate blood trapped in the tissues, which may be need to be drained. This is referred to as a hematoma. Less commonly, the body may develop **calcium** deposits at the injury site in a process called heterotopic ossification.

Prevention

Vitamin K promotes normal clotting in the blood, and therefore may help reduce the tendency to bruise easily. Green leafy vegetables, **alfalfa**, broccoli, seaweed, and fish liver oils are dietary sources of vitamin K. Other good foods to eat would be those containing **bioflavonoids**, such as reddish-blue berries. These can assist in strengthening the connective tissue, which will decrease the spread of blood and bruising. **Zinc** and **vitamin C** supplements are also recommended for this.

Resources

BOOKS

Editors of Prevention Magazine Health Books, eds. *The Doctors Book of Home Remedies.* Prevention Health Books, 2000.

Feinstein, Alice, ed. *Prevention's Healing With Vitamins: The Most Effective Vitamin and Mineral Treatments for Everyday Health Problems and Serious Disease.* Prevention Health Books, 1998.

Williams, William J. *Williams' Hematology.* New York: McGraw-Hill, 1995.

Patience Paradox

Bruxism

Definition

Bruxism is the habit of clenching and grinding the teeth. It most often occurs at night during sleep, but may also occur during the day. It is an unconscious behavior or habit perhaps performed to release **anxiety**, aggression, or anger.

Description

Bruxism is one of the oldest disorders known, and approximately one in four adults experience it. It can occur in children and adolescents as well; cases of bruxism in children as young as 24 months have been reported. Most people are not aware of the disorder until their teeth have been damaged.

Causes and symptoms

While bruxism is typically associated with **stress**, it may also be triggered by abnormal occlusion (the way the upper and lower teeth fit together) or crooked or missing teeth. Symptoms of bruxism include: dull headaches, earaches, sensitive teeth, sore and tired facial muscles, and locking, popping, and clicking of the jaw. During a dental examination, a dentist may recognize damage resulting from bruxism, including: enamel loss from the chewing surfaces of teeth, flattened tooth surfaces, loosened teeth, and fractured teeth and fillings. Left untreated, bruxism may lead to tooth loss and jaw dysfunction.

Bruxism also appears to be associated with Rett syndrome, an X-linked neurodegenerative disorder that occurs almost exclusively in girls. It is not known as of 2008 why children with this disorder frequently develop bruxism.

Diagnosis

Medical and dental histories, examinations, and x rays are usually necessary to differentiate bruxism from other conditions that may cause similar **pain**, such as ear **infections**, dental infections, and **temporomandibular joint syndrome** (TMJ). In many cases, untreated bruxism can lead to chronic TMJ due to the stress that prolonged grinding places on the jaw and the temporomandibular joint.

Wearing away of the tooth surface is generally regarded as the most important clinical sign of bruxism. Although there is no universally accepted scale for measuring the degree of tooth wear, a 2002 Dutch study reported on a five-point scale that appears to be a reliable instrument for diagnosing bruxism. The five points are as follows:

- 0 = no wear.
- 1 = visible wear within the tooth enamel.
- 2 = visible wear with dentine exposure and loss of crown height.
- 3 = loss of crown height between 1/3 and 2/3.
- 4 = loss of crown height greater than 2/3.

Treatment

Stress management and **relaxation** techniques, such as hypnosis and **guided imagery**, may be useful in breaking the habit of jaw clenching and teeth grinding. Tight jaw muscles are often relaxed by applying warm compresses to the sides of the face. **Acupuncture** may relieve the jaw tension associated with both bruxism and TMJ. **Massage therapy** and deep tissue

KEY TERMS

Crown—The part of a tooth that is covered by enamel.

Dentine—The hard major portion of a tooth below the enamel.

Enamel—The hard outermost surface of a tooth.

High spot—An area of a tooth or restoration that feels abnormal or uncomfortable because it hits its opposing tooth before other teeth meet.

Night guard—A removable custom-fitted plastic appliance that fits between the upper and lower teeth to prevent them from grinding against each other.

Occlusion—The way upper and lower teeth fit together during biting and chewing.

Rett syndrome—An X-linked disorder of the nervous system found almost exclusively in girls. Children with Rett's syndrome often develop bruxism, for reasons as yet unknown.

Rolfing—Based on the belief that proper alignment of various parts of the body is necessary for physical and mental health, rolfing uses deep tissue massage and movement exercises in an attempt to bring the body into correct alignment.

Temporomandibular joint (TMJ)—The jaw joint formed by the mandible (lower jaw bone) moving against the temporal bone of the skull.

realignment, including **rolfing**, can also assist in releasing the clenching pattern.

Anti-spasmodic herbal preparations which also contain central nervous system relaxant properties, such as **chamomile** (*Matricaria chamomilla*), may be prescribed before bed to prevent grinding while asleep.

Biofeedback, which teaches an individual to control muscle tension and any associated pain through thought and visualization techniques, is also a treatment option for bruxism. In biofeedback treatments, sensors placed on the surface of the jaw are connected to a special machine that allows the patient and healthcare professional to monitor a visual and/or audible readout of the level of tension in the jaw muscles. Through relaxation and visualization exercises, the patient learns to relieve the tension and can actually see or hear the results of their efforts instantly through the sensor readout on the biofeedback equipment. Once the technique is learned and the patient is able to recognize and differentiate between the feelings of muscle tension and muscle relaxation, the biofeedback equipment itself is no longer needed and the patient has a powerful, portable, and self-administered treatment tool to deal with pain and tension.

Allopathic treatment

To prevent further damage to the teeth and jaw, bruxism is treated by placing a removable custom-fitted plastic appliance called a night guard between the upper and lower teeth. Although the clenching and grinding behavior may continue, the teeth wear away the plastic instead of each other.

In some cases, abnormal occlusion may be adjusted and high spots removed so that the teeth fit together in a more comfortable position. Missing teeth may be replaced and crooked teeth may be straightened with orthodontic treatment to eliminate possible underlying causes of bruxism. In cases where jaw muscles are very tight, a dentist may prescribe muscle relaxants.

Expected results

Bruxism may cause permanent damage to teeth and chronic jaw pain unless properly diagnosed and promptly treated. It is considered a major risk factor for the failure of dental implants. The behavior may be eliminated if its underlying causes are found and addressed.

Prevention

Increased awareness in patients prone to anxiety, aggression, or anger may prevent the habit of bruxism from developing.

Resources

PERIODICALS

Baba, K., T. Haketa, and S. Akishige, et al. "Validation of Diagnostic Criteria for Sleep Bruxism." *Journal of Oral Rehabilitation* 29 (September 2002): 872.

Coyne, B. M., and T. Montague. "Teeth Grinding, Tongue and Lip Biting in a 24-Month-Old Boy with Meningococcal Septicaemia. Report of a Case." *International Journal of Paediatric Dentistry* 12 (July 2002): 277-280.

Lobbezoo, F., W. J. Groenink, and A. A. Kranendonk, et al. "A Reliability Study of Clinical Occlusal Tooth Wear Measurements." *Journal of Oral Rehabilitation* 29 (September 2002): 881-882.

Lynch, C. D., and R. J. McConnell. "The Cracked Tooth Syndrome." *Journal of the Canadian Dental Association* 68 (September 2002): 470-475.

Magalhaes, M. H., J. Y. Kawamura, and L. C. Araujo. "General and Oral Characteristics in Rett Syndrome."

Special Care in Dentistry 22 (July-August 2002): 147-150.

Misch, C. E. "The Effect of Bruxism on Treatment Planning for Dental Implants." *Dentistry Today* 21 (September 2002): 76-81.

ORGANIZATIONS

Academy of General Dentistry. Suite 1200, 211 East Chicago Avenue, Chicago, IL 60611.(312)440–4300. http://www.agd.org. agdjournal@agd.org.

American Dental Association. 211 East Chicago Avenue, Chicago, IL 60611. (312)440–2500. http://www.ada.org.

Association for Applied Psychophysiology and Biofeedback. Suite 304, 10200 W. 44th Ave., Wheat Ridge, CO 80033–2840. (303)422–8436. http://www.aapb.org.

Paula Ford-Martin
Rebecca J. Frey, PhD

Bryonia

Description

Bryonia is a toxic plant in the gourd family. There are two species used in healing, *Byronia alba* and *Bryonia diocia*. *B. alba* is most commonly used in homeopathic healing.

Bryonia is a native European perennial climbing vine with red berries, white flowers, and a thick, white, fleshy taproot, or primary root. The root is the part of

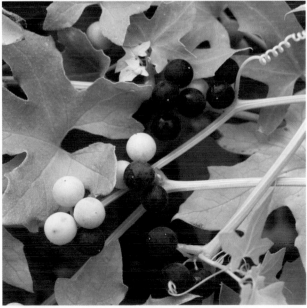

White Bryony. *(© Arco Images / Alamy)*

the plant used in healing. It has a strong, bitter odor and taste and can cause death within hours by inflammation of the digestive system. Bryonia is also called devil's turnip, common bryony, white bryony, or wild **hops**. In **homeopathy** it is abbreviated bry.

General use

Homeopathic medicine operates on the principle that like heals like. This means that a disease can be cured by treating it with products that produce the same symptoms as the disease. These products follow another homeopathic law, the Law of Infinitesimal. In opposition to traditional medicine, the Law of Infinitesimal states that the lower a dose of curative, the more effective it is. To achieve a low dose, the curative is diluted many, many times until only a tiny amount, if any, remains in a large amount of the diluting liquid.

In homeopathic terminology, the effectiveness of remedies is proved by experimentation and reporting done by famous homeopathic practitioners. Bryonia was proved as a remedy by the German founder of homeopathy, Dr. Samuel Hahnemann (1775–1843) in 1834.

In homeopathic medicine, bryonia is used to treat symptoms that develop slowly. These symptoms include feeling lethargic, tired, irritable, extremely thirsty, and feeling excruciating **pain** upon the slightest movement. Psychological symptoms include feeling mentally sluggish. People who need bryonia may fall into a stupor and be confused when called back to reality, especially at night. Some people feel indecisive and restless despite the fact that any movement makes their symptoms worse.

Bryonia is used to treat dry, spasmodic **cough** that causes pain, **influenza** symptoms, and severe headaches that develop slowly. It is also used to treat chronic diseases such as arthritis, painful or swollen joints, and rheumatism.

Other conditions for which homeopathic healers recommend bryonia include inflammation of the chest, **pleurisy**, **pneumonia**, and other lung conditions. Byronia is also said to have an effect on the digestive system. It is used to treat abdominal pain, acute **gastroenteritis**, **diarrhea** (especially diarrhea that is worse in the morning), **nausea**, and **vomiting**.

In homeopathic medicine the fact that certain symptoms get better or worse under different conditions is used as a diagnostic tool to indicate what remedy will be most effective. Symptoms that benefit from treatment with bryonia get much worse with movement. The smallest movement aggravates the person needing bryonia. Symptoms may get worse after eating and drinking, despite the fact that people needing bryonia crave cool drinks and food. Symptoms also get worse in heat and in the summer. People may feel dizzy in the heat and have trouble sleeping. Pain is worse at night and on the right side of the body. Symptoms improve with rest, application of pressure to the painful part of the body, remaining still, and a cool environment.

Homeopathy also ascribes certain personality types to certain remedies. The bryonia personality is said to be insecure about their financial situation, even when they are wealthy, and thus become materialistic. People with the bryonia personality tend to be calculating, clean-living, prudent, and meticulous about details, fitting the stereotype of an accountant or banker.

Outside of homeopathy, bryonia has a long history of folk use. The Greeks used bryony to treat **gangrene**, and in the Middle Ages it was used to treat leprosy. Modern herbalists use bryony to treat painful joints. It may be taken internally, or the leaves may be applied externally to increase blood flow to the painful area. It is also used to treat **asthma**, **bronchitis**, pleurisy, and intestinal ulcers. Some herbalists use it to reduce blood pressure.

Preparations

The root is dug in the autumn, chopped, then pounded into a pulp. For homeopathic remedies, the dried plant material is ground finely then prepared by extensive dilutions. There are two homeopathic dilution scales of dilution, the decimal (x) scale with a dilution of 1:10 and the centesimal (c) scale where the dilution factor is 1:100. Once the mixture is diluted, shaken, strained, then re-diluted many times to reach the desired degree of potency, the final mixture is added to lactose (a type of sugar) tablets or pellets. These are then stored away from light.

Bryonia is available commercially in tablets in many different strengths. Dosage depends on the symptoms being treated.

Homeopathic and orthodox medical practitioners agree that by the time the initial remedy solution is diluted to strengths used in homeopathic healing, it is likely that very few, if any, molecules of the original remedy remain. Homeopaths, however, believe that these remedies continue to work through an effect called potentization that has not yet been explained by mainstream scientists.

Precautions

Bryonia is a poisonous plant and should be used as a folk remedy very, very cautiously. It can cause death. When taken in the extremely dilute doses recommended by homeopaths, it has no toxicity, although some individuals may have a personal adverse reaction to the remedy.

Side effects

When taken in the recommended homeopathic dilute form, no side effects have been reported. When taken in larger doses, bryonia irritates and inflames the digestive system, which may result in death.

Interactions

Studies on interactions between bryonia and conventional pharmaceuticals or other herbs have not been found.

Resources

BOOKS

Chevallier, Andrew. *Encyclopedia of Medicinal Plants*. Boston: DK Publishers, 1996.

Cummings, Stephen, and Dana Ullman. *Everybody's Guide to Homeopathic Medicines*. 3rd edition. New York: Putnam, 1997.

Hammond, Christopher. *The Complete Family Guide to Homeopathy*. London: Penguin Studio, 1995.

Lockie, Andrew, and Nicola Geddes. *The Complete Guide to Homeopathy*. London: Dorling Kindersley, 1995.

Ullman, Robert, and Judyth Reichenberg-Ullman. *Homeopathic Self-Care*. Rocklin, CA: Prima Publishing, 1997.

ORGANIZATIONS

Foundation for Homeopathic Education and Research. 21 Kittredge Street, Berkeley, CA 94704. (510) 649–8930.

International Foundation for Homeopathy. P. O. Box 7, Edmonds, WA 98020. (206) 776–4147.

National Center for Homeopathy. 801 N. Fairfax Street, Suite 306, Alexandria, VA 22314. (703)548–7790.

Tish Davidson

Buchu

Description

Buchu is the bushy shrub known as *Barosma betulina* or *Auguthosma betulina*. It is native to the Cape region of South Africa where it grows wild on sunny hillsides. It is also cultivated in other areas of Africa and in parts of South America. Commercially, buchu is used to enhance black currant flavor in alcoholic beverages such as cassis, a black currant brandy, and as a fragrance in perfumes. The entire plant is strongly aromatic with a spicy odor and mint-like taste.

Buchu grows to a height of about 6 ft (2 m). The small, wrinkled, leathery leaves are used in healing. The leaves have many raised oil glands on their surface that contain the volatile oil that is the chief medicinal component of the plant. Leaves are harvested in the summer when the plant is in bloom and dried for future use. Two related species, *B. crenulata* and *B. serratifolia* are often used interchangeably with *B. betulina*. The Barosma species of buchu should not be confused with Indian buchu (*Myrtus communis*). Barosma buchu leaves are exported commercially from South Africa to Great Britain, Netherlands, and the United States.

General use

Buchu was a traditional folk remedy of the Khoikhoi, a native people of the Cape region of South Africa. The Khoikhoi used buchu as a stimulant, a diuretic, and to relieve bloating.

Buchu was introduced in Great Britain around 1800 and was officially listed as a medicine in the *British Pharmacopoeia* by 1821. British physicians used it to treat inflammations of the urinary system including cystitis, urethritis, and nephritis. South African herbalists still use it to treat these ailments.

Buchu was introduced in the United States shortly after it appeared in Great Britain. By the mid-1800s, it was a popular patent medicine used for treating urinary complaints. In the United States and Germany today, buchu is still used by herbalists as a diuretic. It is recommended to treat symptoms of high blood pressure and is an ingredient in herbal formulas to relieve premenstrual bloating. It is also used as a stomach tonic.

Buchu is believed to have antiseptic properties. German herbalists recommend it as a treatment for irritable bladder, for mild inflammations of the

urinary tract, bladder **infections**, and for prostatitis. American herbalists recommend that compresses soaked in buchu tea be applied to **bruises** to accelerate healing. The tea is also used as a vaginal douche to treat yeast (*Candida*) infections.

The German Federal Health Agency's Commission E was established in 1978 to independently review and evaluate scientific literature and case studies pertaining to herb and plant medications. The E Commission found that buchu's diuretic properties were of the same magnitude as ordinary coffee or tea, which are also diuretics of weaker forms. It declined to recommend buchu as a diuretic.

Some laboratory studies found that buchu extracts did not inhibit the growth of any bacteria that commonly cause urinary tract infections. On the basis of these studies, the E Commission also declined to recommend buchu as a treatment for urinary infections. The United States Food and Drug Administration also declined to approve buchu as an ingredient in non-prescription formulas to relieve premenstrual symptoms.

Preparations

Buchu can be prepared as an infusion, a tincture, or in capsules. An essential oil is produced by steam distillation. The infusion is usually made by steeping 0.5 oz (15 g) of the herb in 2 cups (500 ml) of boiling water. This is drunk two or three times a day. Buchu is also available in commercial herbal teas. Ten to 40 drops of the tincture or extract is taken with water three times a day. Commercial capsules containing 200 mg of the herb are available and are generally taken one to three times daily for a limited time period, usually a week or less.

Buchu is also used in combination with other herbs in commercially available remedies. It is often used in combination with corn silk (*Zea maize*) and **juniper** (*Juniperus communis*) in treatments for cystitis and urinary tract infections, and is combined with **uva ursi** (*Arctostaphylos uva ursi*) in formulas to treat premenstrual bloating.

Precautions

Buchu should not be self-prescribed by people who have **kidney infections**, **pain** during urination, blood in the urine, or any problems with kidney function. Bladder and kidney infections need prompt attention by a medical doctor. Herbalists often recommend that buchu should be avoided by pregnant or breastfeeding women. The volatile oil of buchu contains the compound pulegone that stimulates the uterus to contract and is potentially toxic to the kidneys and liver in excess or over prolonged doses.

Side effects

Due to its diosmin and **essential oils** (diosphenol and pulegone) buchu is a potential kidney and liver irritant in high or prolonged doses. It could also increase the risk of a miscarriage in pregnant women.

Interactions

There has been little scientific study of the interaction of buchu and Western pharmaceuticals. No interactions have been reported nor have there been any reports of herbal interactions.

Resources

BOOKS

Chevallier, Andrew. *Encyclopedia of Medicinal Plants*. Boston: DK Publishers, 1996.

Lawless, Julia. *The Illustrated Encyclopedia of Essential Oils*. Rockport, MA: Element, 1995.

PDR for Herbal Medicines. Montvale, New Jersey: Medical Economics Company, 1998.

Peirce, Andrea. *The American Pharmaceutical Association Practical Guide to Natural Medicines*. New York: William Morrow and Company, 1999.

Tish Davidson

Buckeye *see* **Horse chestnut**

Buckthorn

Description

Buckthorn is the common name for one of several species of shrubs or small trees of the genus *Rhamnus* that are used for medicinal purposes. The two most common species are *R. frangula* and *R. cathartica*.

R. cathartica is also called common or European buckthorn. It was known as a healing herb hundreds of years ago in Anglo-Saxon England, where it was called waythorn, highwaythorn, hartshorn, or ramsthorn. It is also sometimes called purging buckthorn because of its laxative properties. The berries of European buckthorn can be used in healing. The ripe berries of this species are black and the size of a pea.

R. cathartica is a shrubby tree that grows to a height of about 18 ft (6 m). Its twigs are often tipped with small spines, accounting for the "thorn" in its name. Common buckthorn is found throughout Great Britain, continental Europe, and North Africa, where it grows wild in partial sun along the edges of roads and woodlands. It was introduced into North America as an ornamental landscaping plant but has naturalized and become a nuisance plant in much of Canada and the northern United States, where its thick growth crowds out native plants.

R. frangula is shorter, wider, and more shrublike than *R. cathartica*. It grows in damp soil in Great Britain, continental Europe, and parts of Turkey. It was also imported into North America. Bark from the trunk and branches of *R. frangula* is gathered and used in preparing a laxative and a hepatic, or liver medication. *R. frangula* is also called alder buckthorn, black dogwood, frangula bark, alder dogwood, arrow wood, or Persian berries. It is not related to North American dogwood species.

A third species of healing Rhamnus, *R. purshianus*, grows in western North America and is called California buckthorn. Its bark also produces a laxative that is milder than those derived from either of the other two species. Sea buckthorn, *Hippophae rhamnoides*, although it is used in healing and shares a common name with these other species, is not related to the *Rhamnus* buckthorns, nor is it used in the same ways.

General use

All three types of buckthorn are strong laxatives. The berries of *R. cathartica* produce the harshest laxative effect (*cathartica* is a Latin word related to "catharsis," which means purging). The fruit can be used either dried or fresh to treat **constipation** and to

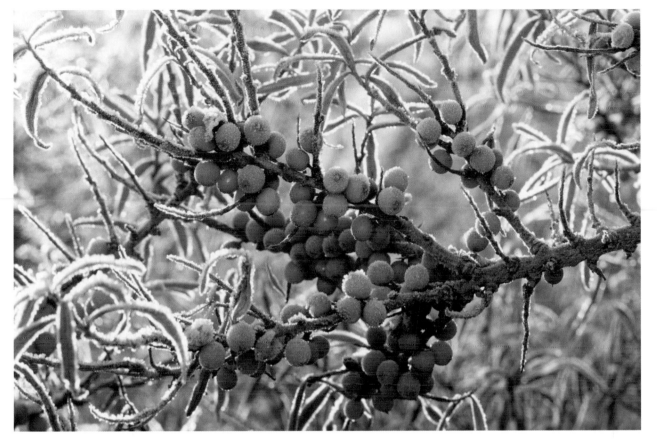

Buckthorn. *(© Arco Images / Alamy)*

soften stools to give relief from **hemorrhoids**, anal fissures, or rectal surgery. The berries are also sometimes mixed with other herbs in "blood purifying" formulas.

The dried bark of *R. frangula* and *R. purshianus* is also used as a laxative. In earlier times it was used to cleanse the gastrointestinal tract before exploratory surgery. Occasionally buckthorn is used in veterinary medicine as a laxative for dogs.

The laxative effect of all these species is well documented. Buckthorn works by causing the large intestine to contract. The contractions shorten the time that waste material remains in the large intestine and allow the formation of softer, moist stools.

In addition to medical uses, buckthorn contains several different pigments used as dyes: yellow from the leaves and bark, green from unripe berries, and blue-gray from ripe berries. *R. frangula* is also a source of high-quality charcoal used for artistic sketching.

Preparations

The berries of *R. cathartica* are harvested when ripe. If used fresh, they can be pressed to yield a bitter,

extremely foul-tasting juice that can be mixed with sugar and flavorings to produce a laxative syrup. The dried berries are powdered, then added to liquid.

The bark of *R. frangula* and *R. purshianus* is harvested in the summer and dried. Young bark is preferred, because the longer the bark is stored, the less potent its laxative properties. Bark used medicinally should be stored *at least* one year before use. Fresh bark acts as an irritant to the gastrointestinal system. A fluid extract or a decoction is then prepared from the bark and mixed with water and flavorings. The ideal dose is the smallest amount necessary to produce soft stools.

Precautions

Buckthorn should not be used by people suspected of having appendicitis or intestinal obstructions, by pregnant or breastfeeding women, the frail elderly, or children under age 12.

Side effects

Buckthorn can cause **nausea**, **vomiting**, and gastrointestinal spasms in large doses or in sensitive

KEY TERMS

Decoction—Decoctions are made by simmering an herb in water, then straining it.

Diuretic—Any substance that increases the production of urine.

Edema—Fluid retention, often leading to swelling in the hands and feet.

Electrolytes—Ions whose movement and balance are essential for proper biochemical functioning of the body.

Hepatic—A drug or medication that acts on the liver.

individuals. Buckthorn causes stool to move more rapidly through the large intestine and allows the body less time to reabsorb fluids and electrolytes. Because of this rapid movement, electrolytes can be lost if stools are too frequent and watery. The long-term use of buckthorn can cause **potassium** imbalances. In rare cases this imbalance can cause heart irregularities, **edema**, and other serious health reactions.

Interactions

Potassium imbalance is worsened by taking thiazide diuretics, corticosteroids, and **licorice** root.

Resources

BOOKS

PDR for Herbal Medicines. Montvale, NJ: Medical Economics Company, 1998.

OTHER

"Plants for the Future: *Rhamnus cathartica* and *Rhamnus frangula*." http://www.metalab.unc.edu (January 17, 2001) .

Tish Davidson

Bugle weed

Description

Bugle weed is the common name given to at least two low-growing flowering ground cover plants which are members of the Ajuga family, *Lycopus europaens* and *Lycopus virginicus*. Ajugas are part of the Lamiaceae, the same grouping to which plants of the mint family belong. Other names by which bugle

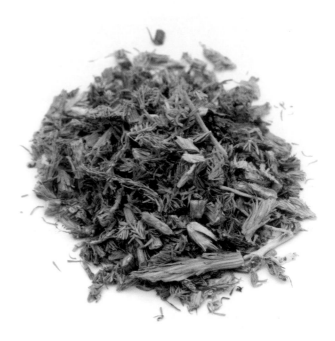

Bugleweed. *(© Geoffrey Kidd / Alamy)*

weed is known include water bugle, sweet bugle, Virginian water **horehound**, and gypsy weed. Bugle weeds usually have shining, oval-shaped leaves that are reminiscent of spinach leaves in appearance and have glandular dots on their underside. This foliage grows thickly along the surface of a spreading transverse root. Bugle weed blooms in spring, typically producing flowers of a startling cobalt blue. Some species, however, have pink or white flowers. Bugle weed flowers are tubular and lipped in appearance, growing in whorls along the erect spikes that rise from the dense foliage.

There are different varieties of bugle weed with varying characteristics:

- *Ajuga genevensis*, or Geneva bugle weed, is one of the taller varieties. It has very dense, dark green leaves, which can grow to 4–5 in (10–12 cm) in length, and produce spikes 6–12 in (15–30 cm) high with either pink or blue flowers in clusters along the spike.

- *Ajuga pyramidalis*, or upright bugle weed, is a bushy, slower-growing plant with very shiny leaves that are slightly puckered. This variety also has bright blue flowers.

- *Ajuga Reptans* is the most common type of bugle weed. It is smaller, with 4–10 in (10–20 cm) spikes, and leaves 2–3 in (5–7.5 cm) in length. Its flowers are the same cobalt blue, and leaves may be either dark green or bronze-colored. There are several highly attractive sub-types in the *A. reptans* grouping. *A. reptans alba* has white flowers; *Atropurpurea* has bronze leaves; burgundy glow bugle weed has three-toned white, green and pink foliage; and several others are combinations of these.

Bugle weed grows in either sun or shade, in well-drained, fairly rich soil. It establishes itself rather quickly and spreads via underground roots. It can become very invasive, and generally provides a mat of dense ground cover that does not permit the growth of weeds or other plants. It can be propagated by dividing the plants.

It is believed that bugle weed is native to the Northern Hemisphere, worldwide. Species of bugle weed are found in Europe, Asia, and North America. Like other members of the Laminaceae or mint family, bugle weed has a mild, pleasant, mint-like aroma when it is freshly picked. It contains flavone glycosides, volatile oils, and tannins.

General use

Beside its horticultural use as an attractive spreading ground cover in rock gardens and other types of gardens, bugle weed is useful medicinally for several different purposes. It is an astringent, and is considered to have sedative qualities as well. It can calm **anxiety** symptoms, including heart palpitations. It is a valued **cough** suppressant. In old herbal remedy books such as Thayer's *Fluid and Solid Extracts*, and even in the more recent *A Modern Herbal*, the authors state that in addition to cough suppression, bugle weed is also useful for healing **tuberculosis** and stopping bleeding from the lungs. It has long been recognized in Western herbal medicine as a cardiac tonic and can actually slow a rapid heart rate and improve the functioning of a weak heart by increasing the strength of the heartbeat. Because of its diuretic properties, bugle weed is useful in removing excess fluid from the body and thus improving circulation. It has been shown to inhibit the body's metabolism of **iodine**, and is helpful for this reason in treating **hyperthyroidism**. Poultices containing bugle weed leaves in combination with other herbs have been found to speed the healing of bruised areas. Lastly, bugle weed is useful in weaning babies as it helps to suppress the production of breast milk.

Preparations

All parts of the bugle weed that grow above ground are used in herbal medicine. It is collected in early spring before the flower buds open. The entire plant is dried and pulverized, and used as a decoction or tea. The tea is made by pouring a cup of boiling water over one teaspoonful of dried bugle weed, and

KEY TERMS

Diuretic—A type of drug that helps remove excess water from the body by increasing the amount lost in urine.

Hyperthyroidism—Overactivity of the thyroid gland and therefore, simultaneous overproduction of thyroid hormones.

Poultice—A soft wet mass of cloth, applied warm or hot to an injured part of the body as a therapeutic measure.

Sedative—A drug or agent that calms or soothes a patient. Bugle weed has sedative qualities.

allowing this mixture to steep for 10–15 minutes. This tea may be taken three times a day. A bugle weed tincture is also available. Poultices are made from the leaves, stems and flower buds, steeped in boiling hot water. Clean white cloth is soaked in this mixture, cooled until warm but not hot enough to burn the patient, and applied to the bruised area.

Precautions

Bugle weed should not be used internally if a person has a thyroid condition unless they have consulted a physician or health care practitioner. Because of bugle weed's influence on thyroid function and its ability to reduce secretions (including breast milk), it should be used only for short periods and prescribed by a trained practitioner.

In addition, plants in the mint family, which includes bugle weed, are high in methyl salicylate. This compound causes **allergies** in some people.

Side effects

The *Complete German Commission E Monographs* includes reports of uncommon cases of long-term high-dosage therapy with bugle weed preparations resulting in enlargement of the thyroid gland. When this herb is used in the treatment of hyperthyroidism, its sudden stoppage can result in an increase in the symptoms.

Interactions

Bugle weed preparations may interfere with the use of radioactive isotopes used in some diagnostic procedures.

Resources

BOOKS

Blumenthal, Mark. *The Complete German E Monographs, Therapeutic Guide to Herbal Medicine,* 1998.

Grieve, M., and C. F. Leyel. *A Modern Herbal: The Medical, Culinary, Cosmetic and Economic Properties, Cultivation and Folklore of Herbs, Grasses, Fungi, Shrubs and Trees With All of Their Modern Scientific Uses.* New York: Barnes and Noble Publishing, 1992.

Hoffman, David, and Linda Quayle. *The Complete Illustrated Herbal: A Safe and Practical Guide to Making and Using Herbal Remedies.* New York: Barnes and Noble Publishing, 1999.

Joan Schonbeck

Bulimia nervosa

Definition

Bulimia nervosa is a serious and sometimes life-threatening eating disorder that mainly affects young women. People with bulimia, known as bulimics, consume large amounts of food, or binge, and then try to

---

Symptoms of bulimia nervosa

Recurrent episodes of binge eating, characterized by eating an excessive amount of food within a discrete period of time and by a sense of lack of control over eating during the episode

Recurrent inappropriate compensatory behavior in order to prevent weight gain, such as self-induced vomiting or misuse of laxatives, diuretics, enemas, or other medications (purging); fasting; or excessive exercise

The binge eating and inappropriate compensatory behaviors both occur, on average, at least twice a week for 3 months

Self-evaluation is unduly influenced by body shape and weight

---

(Illustration by Corey Light. Cengage Learning, Gale)

rid themselves of the food and calories, or purge, through **fasting**, excessive **exercise**, **vomiting**, or use of laxatives. Bulimics often feel that the behavior serves to reduce **stress** and relieve **anxiety**. Because bulimia results from an excessive concern with weight control and self-image, and is often accompanied by **depression**, it is also considered a psychiatric illness.

Description

Bulimia nervosa is a serious health problem affecting many people in the United States. The bingeing and purging activity associated with this disorder can cause severe damage, even death, although the risk of death is not as high as for **anorexia nervosa**, an eating disorder that leads to excessive weight loss.

Binge eating may in rare instances cause the stomach to rupture. In the case of purging, heart failure can result due to loss of vital minerals such as **potassium**. Vomiting causes other serious problems, including acid-related scarring of the fingers if used to induce vomiting, and damage to tooth enamel. In addition, the esophagus, or the tube that brings food from the mouth to the stomach, often becomes inflamed and salivary glands can become swollen. Irregular menstrual periods can also result, and interest in sex may diminish.

Most bulimics find it difficult to stop their behavior without professional help. Many typically recognize that the behavior is not normal, but feel out of control. Some bulimics struggle with other compulsive, risky behaviors such as drug and alcohol abuse. Many also suffer from other psychiatric illnesses, including clinical depression, anxiety, and **obsessive-compulsive disorder** (OCD).

Bulimia nervosa is primarily a disorder of industrialized countries where food is abundant and the culture values a thin appearance. Internationally, the rate of bulimia has been increasing since the 1950s. Bulimia is the most common eating disorder in the United States. Overall, about 3% of Americans are bulimic. Of these 85–90% are female. The rate is highest among adolescents and college women, averaging 5–6%. In men, the disorder is more often diagnosed in homosexuals than in heterosexuals. Some experts believe that number of diagnosed bulimics represents only the most severe cases and that many more people have bulimic tendencies, but are successful in hiding their symptoms. In one study, 40% of college women reported isolated incidents of bingeing and purging.

Bulimia affects people from all racial, ethnic, and socioeconomic groups. The disorder usually begins later in life than anorexia nervosa. Most people begin bingeing and purging in their late teens through their twenties. Men tend to start at an older age than women. About 5% of people with bulimia begin the behavior after age 25. Bulimia is uncommon in children under age 14.

Competitive athletes have an increased risk of developing bulimia nervosa, especially in sports where weight it tied to performance and where a low percentage of body fat is highly desirable. Jockeys, wrestlers, bodybuilders, figure skaters, cross-country runners, and gymnasts have higher than average rates of bulimia. People such as actors, models, cheerleaders, and dancers who are judged mainly on their appearance are also at high risk of developing the disorder. This same group of people is also at higher risk for developing anorexia nervosa. Some people are primarily anorexic and severely restrict their calorie intake while also purging the small amounts they do eat. Others move back and forth between anorectic and bulimic behaviors.

Causes and symptoms

Causes

Bulimia nervosa is a complex disorder that does not have a single cause. Research suggests that some people have a predisposition toward bulimia and that something then triggers the behavior, which then becomes self-reinforcing. Hereditary, biological, psychological and social factors all appear to play a role.

- Heredity: Twin studies suggest that there is an inherited component to bulimia nervosa, but that it is small. Having a close relative, usually a mother or a sister, with bulimia slightly increases the likelihood of other (usually female) family members developing the disorder. However, when compared other inherited diseases or even to anorexia nervosa, the genetic contribution to developing this disorder appears less important than many other factors. Family history of depression, alcoholism, and obesity also increase the risk of developing bulimia.

- Biological factors: There is some evidence that bulimia is linked low levels of serotonin in the brain. Serotonin is a neurotransmitter. One of its functions is to help regulate the feeling of fullness or satiety that tells a person to stop eating. Neurotransmitters are also involved in other mental disorders such as depression that often occur with bulimia. Other research suggests that people with bulimia may have abnormal levels of leptin, a protein that helps regulate weight by telling the body to take in less food. Research in this area is relatively new, and the findings are still unclear.

- Psychological factors: Certain personality types appear to be more vulnerable to developing bulimia. People with bulimia tend to have poor impulse control. They are of often involved in risky behavior such as shoplifting, drug and alcohol abuse and risky sexual activities. People with bulimia have low-self worth and depend on the approval of others to feel good about themselves. They are aware that their behavior is abnormal. After a binge/purge session, they are ashamed and vow never to repeat the cycle, but the next time they are unable to control the impulse to eat and purge. They also tend to have a black-or-white, all-or-nothing way of seeing situations. Major depression, obsessive-compulsive disorder, and anxiety disorders are more common among individuals who are bulimic.

- Social factors: The families of people who develop bulimia are more likely to have members who have problems with alcoholism, depression, and obesity. These families also tend to have a high level of open conflict and disordered, unpredictable lives. Often something stressful or upsetting triggers the urge to diet stringently and then begin binge/purge behaviors. This may be as simple as a family member as teasing about the person's weight, nagging about eating junk food, commenting on how clothes fit, or comparing the person unfavorably to someone who is thin. Life events such as moving, starting a new school, and breaking up with a boyfriend can also trigger binge/purge behavior. Overlaying the family situation is the false, but unrelenting, media message that thin is good and fat is bad; thin people are successful, glamorous, and happy, fat people are stupid, lazy, and failures.

Symptoms

Many people with bulimia will consume 3,000–10,000 calories in an hour. One distinguishing aspect of bulimia is how out of control people with bulimia feel when they are eating. They will eat and eat, continuing even when they feel full and become uncomfortable.

According to the American Anorexia/Bulimia Association, Inc., warning signs of bulimia include:

- eating large amounts of food uncontrollably (bingeing)
- vomiting, abusing laxatives or diuretics, or engaging in fasting, dieting, or vigorous exercise (purging)
- preoccupation with body weight
- using the bathroom frequently after meals
- depression or mood swings

353

- irregular menstrual periods
- onset of dental problems, swollen cheeks or glands, heartburn or bloating

Diagnosis

Bulimia nervosa is officially recognized as a psychiatric disorder in the *Diagnostic and Statistical Manual for Mental Disorders Fourth Edition-Text Revision (DSM-IV-TR)* published by the American Psychiatric Association. The DSM-IV-TR sets guidelines for diagnosing psychiatric illnesses.

According to the standards of the DSM-IV-TR, Bulimia nervosa is diagnosed when most of the following conditions are present:

- Repeated episodes of binge eating followed by behavior to compensate for the binge (i.e. purging, fasting, over-exercising). Binge eating is defined as eating a significantly larger amount of food in a limited time than most people typically would eat.
- Binge/purge episodes occur at least twice a week for a period of three or more months.
- The individual feels unable to control or stop an eating binge once it starts and will continue to eat even if uncomfortably full.
- The individual is overly concerned about body weight and shape and puts unreasonable emphasis on physical appearance when evaluating his or her self-worth.
- Bingeing and purging does not occur exclusively during periods of anorexia nervosa.

Bulimia is treated most successfully when diagnosed early. But because the bulimic may deny there is a problem, getting medical help is often delayed. A complete physical examination in order to rule out other illnesses is the first step toward diagnosis.

Treatment

Alternative therapies may be used as complementary to conventional treatment program for bulimic patients. They include diet, nutritional therapy, herbal therapy, **homeopathy**, **hydrotherapy**, **biofeedback** training, **hypnotherapy**, **massage therapy** and **light therapy**.

Diet

The following dietary changes may be helpful for bulimic patients:

- Eating small but nutritious meals at regularly scheduled hours.
- Avoiding sweet, baked goods or any other foods that may cause craving.

- Avoiding allergenic foods.
- Limiting intake of alcohol, caffeine, monosodium glutamate (MSG), and salty foods.

Nutritional therapy

The following supplements may help improve bulimic symptoms and prevent deficiency of essential vitamins and minerals:

- Multivitamin and mineral supplement to prevent deficiency of essential nutrients.
- Vitamin B complex with C.
- Zinc supplement. Bulimic patients may have zinc deficiency, and zinc is an important mineral needed by the body for normal hormonal activity and enzymatic function.

Homeopathy

A homeopathic physician may prescribe patient-specific remedies for the treatment of bulimia.

Light therapy

Light therapy. Exposure to artificial light, available through full spectrum light bulbs or specially designed "light boxes," may be useful in reducing bulimic episodes, especially during the dark winter months.

Hypnotherapy

Hypnotherapy may help resolve unconscious issues that contribute to bulimic behavior.

Exercise

Yoga, **qigong**, **t'ai chi** or dance not only make patients physically healthier but can also make them feel better about themselves.

Other treatments.

Other potentially beneficial treatments for bulimia include Chinese herbal therapy, hydrotherapy and biofeedback training.

Allopathic treatment

Early treatment of bulimia with a combination of drug and behavioral therapies is necessary to prevent serious health consequences. A comprehensive treatment plan is called for in order to address the complex interaction of physical and psychological problems of bulimia.

Behavioral approaches include individual **psychotherapy**, group therapy, and family therapy. Cognitive behavioral therapy, which teaches patients how to change abnormal thoughts and behavior, is also used. **Nutrition** counseling and self-help groups are often helpful.

Antidepressants commonly used to treat bulimia include desipramine (Norpramin), imipramine (Tofranil), and fluoxetine (Prozac). These medications also may treat any co-existing depression.

In addition to professional treatment, family support plays an important role in helping the bulimic person. Encouragement and caring can provide the support needed to convince the sick person to get help, stay with treatment, or try again after a failure. Family members can help locate resources, such as eating disorder clinics in local hospitals or treatment programs in colleges designed for students.

Expected results

The long-term outlook for recovery from bulimia is mixed. About half of all bulimics show improvement in controlling their behavior after short-term interpersonal or cognitive behavioral therapy with nutritional counseling and drug therapy. However, after three years, only about one-third are still doing well. Relapses are common, and binge/purge episodes and bulimic behavior often comes and goes for many years. Stress seems to be a major trigger for relapse.

The sooner treatment is sought, the better the chances of recovery. Without professional intervention, recovery is unlikely. Untreated bulimia can lead to death directly from causes such as rupture of the stomach or esophagus. Associated problems such as **substance abuse**, depression, anxiety disorders, and poor impulse control also contribute to the death rate.

Prevention

Some ways to prevent bulimia nervosa from developing are as follows:

- If you are a parent, do not obsess about your own weight, appearance, and diet in front of your children.
- Do not tease your children about their body shapes or compare them to others.
- Make it clear that you love and accept your children as they are.
- Try to eat meals together as a family whenever possible.
- Remind children that the models they see on television and in fashion magazines have extreme, not normal or healthy bodies.

KEY TERMS

Binge—To consume large amounts of food uncontrollably within a short time period.

Diuretic—A drug that promotes the formation and excretion of urine.

Neurotransmitters—Certain brain chemicals that may function abnormally in acutely ill bulimic patients.

Obsessive-compulsive disorder (OCD)—A disorder that may accompany bulimia, characterized by the tendency to perform repetitive acts or rituals in order to relieve anxiety.

Purge—To rid the body of food and calories, commonly by vomiting or using laxatives.

- Do not put your child on a diet unless advised to by your pediatrician.
- Block your child from visiting pro-bulimia Web sites. These are sites where people with bulimia give advice on how to purge and support each other's binge/purge behavior.
- If your child is a competitive athlete, get to know the coach and the coach's attitude toward weight.
- Be alert to signs of low self-worth, anxiety, depression, and drug or alcohol abuse and seek help as soon as these signs appear.
- If you think your child has an eating disorder, do not wait to intervene and seek professional help. The sooner the disorder is treated, the easier it is to cure.

Relapses happen to many people with bulimia. People who are recovering from bulimia can help prevent themselves from relapsing by:

- never dieting; instead plan healthy meals
- eating with other people, not alone
- staying in treatment; keep therapy appointments
- monitoring negative self-talk; practicing positive self-talk
- spending time doing something enjoyable every day
- staying busy, but not overly busy; getting at least seven hours of sleep each night
- spending time each day with people you care about and who care about you

Resources

BOOKS

Carlton, Pamela and Deborah Ashin. *Take Charge of Your Child's Eating Disorder: A Physician's Step-By-Step*

Guide to Defeating Anorexia and Bulimia. New York: Marlowe & Co., 2007.

Heaton, Jeanne A. and Claudia J. Strauss. *Talking to Eating Disorders: Simple Ways to Support Someone Who Has Anorexia, Bulimia, Binge Eating or Body Image Issues.* New York, NY: New American Library, 2005.

Kolodny, Nancy J. *The Beginner's Guide to Eating Disorders Recovery.* Carlsbad, CA: Gurze Books, 2004.

The Medical Advisor: The Complete Guide to Alternative & Conventional Treatments. Richmond, VA: TimeLife Education, 1997.

Messinger, Lisa and Merle Goldberg. *My Thin Excuse: Understanding, Recognizing, and Overcoming Eating Disorders.* Garden City Park, NY: Square One Publishers, 2006.

PERIODICALS

Berg, Frances M. "Eating Disorders Affect Both the Mind and Body." *Healthy Weight Journal.* 9/2 (1995): 27-31.

Cismoski, Janet, et al. "Teen Nutrition." *Whose Kids?...Our Kids!* 6 (1995).

Levine, Michael P. "10 Things Men Can Do and Be to Help Prevent Eating Disorders." *Healthy Weight Journal.* 9/1 (1995): 15.

ORGANIZATIONS

American Anorexia/Bulimia Association, Inc, 293 Central Park West, Suite IR, New York, NY, 10024, (212) 501-8351

American Psychological Association, 750 First Street, NE, Washington, DC, 20002-4242, (202) 336-5500, (800) 374-2721, http://www.apa.org.

National Association of Anorexia Nervosa and Associated Disorders (ANAD), P.O. Box 7, Highland Park, IL, 60035, (847) 831-3438, http://www.anad.org.

National Eating Disorders Association, 603 Stewart Street, Suite 803, Seattle, WA, 98101, (206) 382-3587, (800) 931-2237, http://www.edap.org.

Mai Tran

Bunion

Definition

A bunion is an abnormal enlargement of the joint (the first metatarsophalangeal joint, or MTPJ) at the base of the great or big toe (hallux). It is caused by inflammation and usually results from chronic irritation and pressure from poorly fitting footwear.

Description

A displacement of two major bones of the foot (hallux valgus) causes bunions, although not everyone with this displacement will develop the joint swelling

and bone overgrowth that characterize a bunion. One of the bones involved is called the first metatarsal bone. This bone is long and slender, with the big toe attached on one end and the other end connected to foot bones closer to the ankle. This foot bone is displaced in the direction of the four other metatarsals connected with the toes. The other bone involved is the big toe itself, which is displaced toward the smaller toes. As the big toe continues to move toward the smaller toes, it may become displaced under or over the second toe. The displacement of these two foot bones causes a projection of bone on the inside portion of the forefoot. The skin over this projection often becomes inflamed from rubbing against the shoe, and a callus may form.

The joint contains a small sac (bursa) filled with fluid that cushions the bones and helps the joint to move smoothly. When a bunion forms, this sac becomes inflamed and thickened. Inflammation of the bursa is called **bursitis**. The swelling in the joint causes additional **pain** and pressure in the toe.

Bunions can also form on the bones that attach the little toe to the foot (the fifth metatarsal bone). These bunions are called tailor's bunion or bunionette.

Causes and symptoms

Bunions may form as a result of abnormal motion of the foot during walking or running. One common example of an abnormal movement is an excessive amount of **stress** placed upon the inside of the foot. This leads to friction and irritation of the involved structures. Age has also been noted as a factor in developing bunions, in part because the underlying bone displacement worsens over time unless corrective measures are taken.

Wearing improperly fitting shoes, especially those with a narrow toe box and excessive heel height, often causes the formation of a bunion. This forefoot deformity is seen more often in women than men. The higher frequency in females may be related to the strong link between footwear fashion and bunions. In fact, in a recent survey of more than 350 women, nearly 90% wore shoes that were at least one size too small or too narrow. Shoes without proper arch supports contribute to bunions, since they allow the foot to roll inward, or pronate, putting more pressure on the joint of the big toe.

Because genetic factors can predispose people to hallux valgus bone displacement, a strong family history of bunions can increase the likelihood of developing this foot disorder. Various arthritic conditions and several genetic and neuromuscular diseases, such as Down syndrome and Marfan syndrome, cause muscle imbalances that can create bunions from displacement of the first metatarsal and big toe. Other possible causes of bunions are leg-length discrepancies (with the bunion present on the longer leg) and trauma occurring to the joint of the big toe. Persons with flat feet or **gout** are at increased risk for developing bunions.

Symptoms of bunions include the common signs of inflammation such as redness, swelling, and pain. The discomfort is primarily located along the inside of the foot just behind the big toe. Because of friction, a callus may develop over the bunion. If toes overlap, additional rubbing and pain occur. Inflammation of this area causes a decrease in motion with associated discomfort in the joint between the big toe and the first metatarsal. If allowed to worsen, the skin over the bunion may break down causing an ulcer, which also presents a problem of potential infection. (Foot ulcers can be particularly dangerous for people with diabetes, who may have trouble feeling the ulcer forming and healing if it becomes infected.)

Diagnosis

A thorough medical history and physical exam by a physician is always necessary for the proper diagnosis of bunions and other foot conditions. X rays can help confirm the diagnosis by showing the bone displacement, joint swelling, and, in some cases, the overgrowth of bone that characterizes bunions. Doctors will also consider the possibility that the joint pain is caused by or complicated by arthritis (which causes destruction of the cartilage of the joint), gout (which causes the accumulation of uric acid crystals in the joint), tiny **fractures** of a bone in the foot (stress fractures), or infection, and may order additional tests to rule out these possibilities.

Treatment

The first step in treating a bunion is to remove as much pressure from the area as possible. A foam-rubber pad may be worn at night while sleeping to separate the big toe from the other toes. Various taping techniques can be useful to realign the toe and decrease friction and rubbing that may be present. Most patients are instructed to rest or choose exercises that put less stress on their feet, at least until the misalignment is corrected.

Persons with bunions should wear shoes that have enough room in the toe box to accommodate the bunion. High-heeled shoes and tight-fitting socks or stockings should be avoided. Sandals are a good choice. Shoes may be stretched to provide more comfort or customized to relieve pressure on the affected area. Shoes should be removed periodically during the day to give feet a break. Dressings and pads help protect the bunion from additional shoe pressure. Arch supports can reduce the pressure on the bunion. The application of splints or customized shoe inserts (orthotics) to correct the alignment of the big toe joint is effective for many bunions. These can correct the excessive pronation (turning inward) so that the pressure is not continually on the big toe.

Deep friction massage techniques by a physical or massage therapist can be helpful to increase circulation, reduce inflammation, and prevent soft tissue build-up. Physical therapy also provides useful approaches, such as ultrasound, to help retard or reverse the formation of the bunion.

One study found that using an extract from marigold (*Tagetes patula*) with a protective pad led to a reduction in the size and pain of bunions. A used **chamomile** tea bag applied to a bunion may be helpful. Massaging with essential oil of chamomile or with a cream containing chamomile may provide relief. The homeopathic remedy *Calcarea phosphorica* can be useful in balancing the bone formation and remodeling.

Soaking the affected foot in warm water may reduce pain. Elevating the affected foot and applying ice and compression to the bunion can be helpful, especially after **exercise**.

Dietary supplements and dietary changes may help to treat bunions. Vitamins which may be helpful in treating the bursitis associated with bunions include A, B complex, C, and E. Increasing the intake of protein may also be beneficial.

Acupuncture can be useful in treating the symptoms as the spleen meridian is roughly where the pain occurs. Other treatments may help stabilize the foot.

Allopathic treatment

Nonsteroidal anti-inflammatory drugs (NSAIDs) such as ibuprofen (Advil, Motrin), acetaminophen (Tylenol), or naproxen **sodium** (Aleve) may be taken to help reduce bunion pain. Physicians may also use steroid injections with local anesthetic around the bunion to reduce inflammation. Other drugs may be necessary should an infection occur.

If conservative treatments are not successful, surgical removal of the bunion may be necessary to correct the deformity. This procedure is called a bunionectomy, and there are many variations on the operation, which is usually performed by a surgeon who specializes in treating bone conditions (orthopedics) or by one who specializes in treating the foot (podiatry). The procedure chosen depends upon the angle of the bone misalignment, condition of the bursa, and strength of the bones. Most bunionectomies involve the removal of a section of bone and the insertion of pins to rejoin the bone. Sometimes the surgeons may move ligaments (which connect bone to bone in the joint) or tendons (which connect bone to muscle) in order to realign the bones.

Expected results

Often, modifications in footwear allow a good recovery without a need for surgery. If surgery is necessary, complete healing without complications requires approximately four to six weeks. Even after surgery corrects the bone misalignment, patients are usually instructed to continue wearing low-heeled, roomy shoes to prevent the bunion from reforming. Complications of bunions include infection of the bunion and inflammation and arthritic changes in other joints as a result of difficulty in walking.

Prevention

Prevention begins with proper foot wear. Shoes with a wide and deep toe box are best. High-heeled shoes should not be worn for longer than three hours at a time. If a bunion is present and becomes inflamed, the foot should be elevated with the application of an ice pack over the painful area for not more than 20 minutes every other hour. Daily exercise strengthens the muscles of the legs and feet and may prevent bunion formation. Women who wear high-heeled shoes should do calf stretches on a regular basis. Use of arch supports or custom made orthotics can help people whose feet rotate inward as they walk or those with different leg lengths. Stretching the Achilles tendon can counteract stresses on the forefoot.

Resources

BOOKS

Richard B. Birrer, et al. *Common Foot Problems in Primary Care,* 2nd ed. Philadelphia, PA: Hanley & Belfus, Inc., 1998.

PERIODICALS

Cimons, Marlene. "Bothersome Bunions." *Runner's World* 34 (May 1999): 46+.

ORGANIZATIONS

American Orthopedic Foot and Ankle Society. 222 South Prospect, Park Ridge, IL 60068.

American Podiatry Medical Association. 9312 Old Georgetown Road, Bethesda, MD 20814.

OTHER

"Foot Pain." *WebMD.* http://my.webmd.com/content/dmk/dmk_article_40037.

Griffith, H. "Complete Guide to Symptoms, Illness & Surgery." The Putnam Berkley Group, Inc., 1995. Available at: http://www.thriveonline.com.

Belinda Rowland

Bupleurum *see* **Chinese thoroughwax**

Burdock root

Description

Great burdock, *Arctium lappa,* is a coarse biennial herb native to Europe and Asia, and naturalized throughout North America since its introduction by European settlers. This massive herb is thought of as a tenacious weed by many gardeners but it is valued by herbalists worldwide as a medicinal and culinary storehouse. Great burdock may grow as tall as 9 ft (3 m) in its second year. Common burdock, *Articum minus,* a smaller species, is abundant in North America, growing to 5 ft (1.5 m) tall. There are about 10 species of burdock.

Over the centuries, the hardy burdock has acquired many names, including beggar's buttons, bardana, burr seed, clot-bur, clothburr, cocklebur, cockle buttons, fox's clote, great burr, Gypsy rhubarb, happy major, hardock, hareburr, love leaves, personata, philanthropium, thorny burr, and turkey burrseed. In Japan the herb is known as gobo and is cultivated for its somewhat sweet-tasting root, an ingredient in numerous culinary dishes. Gobo has been grown in the United States as a vegetable for soups and salds since the 1980s. In Russia, a common name for the herb is *lapuh*. Most common folk names for this member of the Compositae family refer to the large and prickly seed covers that adhere securely to passersby.

Burdock has a deep primary root producing a large rosette of basal leaves in the first year that may grow as large as 1.5 ft (0.45 m) long and nearly as wide. In the second year of growth, burdock shoots upward with a stout, grooved, branching stem. Leaf stalks are longer than the leaves, and each has a purple hue at the base that extends up the stalk along the inner groove and into the leaf veins. Stalks are hollow in common burdock. Leaves resemble those of rhubarb in size and shape. They are dark green on top and a downy, pale green on the underside. Flower heads are round and thistle-like, with numerous, small purple-hued, funnel-shaped blooms in mid-summer to early fall. Blossoms are surrounded by stiff, prickly, hook-tipped burrs that grasp and hold firmly to clothing and fur.

General use

Burdock's fibrous primary root and rhizome expand to about 1 ft (0.3 m) underground. Most of the herb's medicinal constituents are stored in these underground parts. The entire plant has both nutritive and medicinal uses. The roots contain as much as 45% inulin, as well as alkaloids, essential oil, flavonoids, glycosides, mucilage, polyacetylenes, resin, tannins, and volatile oil. The seeds are rich in vitamins A and B and **essential fatty acids**. Both the seeds and the root have a demulcent quality that is soothing to the mucous membranes of the body. The leaves are generally less potent than the root and seed when used in medicinal preparations.

Burdock is primarily a tonic and alterative herb. The cumulative effect of its use is said to bring a subtle strengthening and cleansing to the entire system. Though most of the therapeutic benefits attributed to this stately herb have not been clinically proven, burdock has been long tested in folk use, and is a safe, if mild, herbal remedy. Burdock has been traditionally used as a blood purifier. It promotes perspiration and the release of toxins from the body. It is helpful in clearing up such skin conditions as **psoriasis** and dry, scaly **eczema**. It works best when used over a period of time. The bitter properties of burdock, particularly noticeable in the dried leaf and seed, stimulate bile secretions. It is a good digestive herb and liver remedy. Burdock's anti-microbial and fungistatic properties have been traced to as many as 14 different

polyacetylene compounds in the root. Burdock has been used to treat **boils**, **canker sores**, carbuncles, **measles**, and **sties**. It will help restore friendly bacteria in the system after antibiotic use, and may bring relief in cases of chronic arthritis and **gout**. Burdock may also help reduce blood sugar levels.

In medieval times burdock was used for more serious problems, such as the treatment of **syphilis** and leprosy. Hildegard of Bingen, a twelfth-century German abbess, considered burdock a valuable remedy for cancerous tumors. Herbalists in other cultures and times, including the Americas, China, India, and Russia have turned to the root of this familiar herb for a folk treatment of **cancer**. The oil of burdock, known as *repeinoe maslo*, used over a period of six to eight months, was said to help stimulate the growth of new hair. A drink prepared with aged wine and fine-shredded, fresh burdock leaves was taken after the bite of a mad dog. A poultice of the fresh leaf, applied to the forehead was used to relieve **headache**. Shredded leaves were also combined with an egg white, beaten until stiff, and the mixture was applied to **burns** to speed healing.

Burdock seeds have also been used in medicinal preparations, particularly to treat psoriasis and to stimulate the digestive process. In Chinese medicine seeds were used as a treatment for feverish colds and **sore throat**.

Burdock has been recently shown to have significant antibacterial and anticandidal activity, which helps to explain its place in folk medicine as a treatment for various infectious diseases. In addition, a team of Asian researchers reported in 2002 that burdock appears to counteract the damaging effects of alcohol on the liver.

Preparations

Burdock root is harvested from the first-year plant in the early fall. Roots are deep and may be difficult to extract. The leaves are best used when fresh, as the dried leaf is bitter. Harvesting is done before the plant flowers.

- Decoction: Burdock's medicinal properties, concentrated in the root, are best extracted by decoction. Add about 1 tsp of thinly-sliced, fresh or dried burdock root per 8 oz of cold water in a glass or ceramic pot. Bring to a boil. Reduce heat and simmer for about 20 minutes. Drink up to three cups daily.

- Poultice: Simmer fresh, chopped burdock leaves for up to five minutes. Drain, squeezing out the liquid. Cool until warm. Apply to the affected area and secure with a clean strip of cotton gauze. A little oil applied to the skin first may keep the poultice from sticking when dry. Prepare a fresh poultice every few hours until the desired relief is obtained.

- Tincture: Combine one part fresh herb to three parts alcohol (50% alcohol/water solution) in glass container. Set aside in dark place. Shake daily for two weeks. Strain through muslin or cheesecloth, and store in dark bottle. The tincture should maintain potency for two years. Standard dosage, unless otherwise prescribed, is 1/2 tsp, three times daily.

- Culinary: Fresh burdock roots are mild tasting and somewhat sweet. They may be peeled and thinly sliced to add to soups, salads, and in a mixture of stir-fried vegetables. The young leaves of the first year plant may be eaten fresh or steamed as a nutritious potherb, and the fresh stalks, peeled and steamed until tender, are also a culinary treat. Burdock root, roasted and ground to a powder, has been used as coffee additive or substitute.

Precautions

Some commercially available burdock leaves and roots have been suspected of being adulterated, on occasion, with the root of the deadly **belladonna** (*Atropa belladonna*) with toxic consequences to unwary users. Consumers of herbal remedies should find a reliable source for medicinal herbs to avoid hazardous mistakes. Pregnant women should not use burdock, as it has a reported action as a uterine stimulant.

Precautions

Medicinal preparations containing burdock should not be used by pregnant or lactating women. Burdock prepared as a vegetable, however, appears to be safe.

Side effects

Large doses of medicinal preparations containing burdock may cause the level of **potassium** in the blood to drop too low. There have also been case reports of people developing an allergic skin rash from touching the leaves and stems of the plant.

Interactions

Burdock has been reported to interact with medications given to control diabetes. Persons with diabetes should consult a physician before taking any herbal preparation containing burdock. In addition, burdock has been reported to intensify the activity of diuretics (drugs given to increase urine output) and lithium.

Burdock may also interfere with the absorption of **iron** and other minerals in the diet. Persons who must take supplemental iron or other dietary minerals should consult their health practitioner before taking burdock.

Resources

BOOKS

PDR for Herbal Medicines. Montvale, NJ: Medical Economics Company, 1998.

Prevention's 200 Herbal Remedies, 3rd ed. Emmaus, PA: Rodale Press, Inc., 1997.

Hoffmann, David. *The New Holistic Herbal,* 2nd ed. Boston, MA: Element, 1986.

Hutchens, Alma R. *A Handbook of Native American Herbs.* Boston, MA: Shambhala, 1992.

McIntyre, Anne. *The Medicinal Garden.* New York: Henry Holt and Company, 1997.

Polunin, Miriam, and Christopher Robbins. *The Natural Pharmacy.* New York: Macmillan Publishing Company, 1992.

Tyler, Varro E., Ph.D. *The Honest Herbal.* New York: Pharmaceutical Products Press, 1993.

Weiss, Gaea and Shandor. *Growing & Using The Healing Herbs.* New York: Wings Books, 1992.

PERIODICALS

Holetz, F. B., G. L. Pessini, N. R. Sanches, et al. "Screening of Some Plants Used in the Brazilian Folk Medicine for the Treatment of Infectious Diseases." *Memorias do Instituto Oswaldo Cruz* 97 (October 2002): 1027-1031.

Lin, S. C., C. H. Lin, C. C. Lin, et al. "Hepatoprotective Effects of *Arctium lappa Linne* on Liver Injuries Induced by Chronic Ethanol Consumption and Potentiated by Carbon Tetrachloride." *Journal of Biomedical Science* 9 (September-October 2002): 401-409.

Rodriguez, P., J. Blanco, S. Juste, et al. "Allergic Contact Dermatitis Due to Burdock (*Arctium lappa*)." *Contact Dermatitis* 33 (August 1995): 134-135.

Strauch, Betsy. "An Herb To Know— Burdock." *The Herb Companion* (Oct./Nov. 1999).

ORGANIZATIONS

American Herbalists Guild. 1931 Gaddis Road, Canton, GA 30115. (770) 751-6021. http://www.americanherbalists guild.com.

Herb Research Foundation. 1007 Pearl Street, Boulder, CO 80302.(303) 449-2265.

Clare Hanrahan
Rebecca J. Frey, PhD

Burns

Definition

Burns are injuries to the tissues caused by heat, friction, electricity, radiation, or chemicals. Such injuries cause the breakdown of body proteins, death of cells, loss of body fluids, and **edema**.

Description

Burns vary depending on the cause, the intensity, and the body parts involved. They are classified by degree, based on the severity of the tissue damage: A first-degree burn causes redness and swelling in the outermost layers of skin called the epidermis. A second-degree burn involves redness, swelling, and blistering. The damage extends beneath the epidermis to the deeper layers of skin, the dermis. A third-degree burn, also called a full-thickness burn, destroys the entire depth of skin, causing significant scarring. Damage also may extend to the underlying fat, muscle, or bone. Third-degree burns require immediate medical attention. Burns are the third leading cause of accidental death in North America.

The severity of a burn is judged by the amount of body surface area (BSA) involved as well as the depth of the burn. A burn is considered to be critical, or major, if a person has third-degree burns on more than 10% of the BSA or second-degree burns covering more than 25% of an adult's BSA, and more than 20% of a child's BSA. Such burns are serious and should be treated in a specialized hospital burn unit. Burns involving the hands, feet, face, eyes, ears, or genitals are considered critical, as well. Moderate burns are defined as first- or second-degree burns covering 15%-25% of an adult's body or 10%-20% of a child's body, or a third-degree burn on 2%-10% BSA. These burns also require medical attention.

Causes and symptoms

Burns may be caused by any encounter, however brief, with heat greater than 120°F (49°C). The source of this heat may be the sun, hot liquids, steam, fire, electricity, friction (rug burns and rope burns,) and chemicals. Signs that the skin has been burned are localized redness, swelling, and **pain**. A blister may develop. The skin may peel, appear white or charred, and feel numb. A burn may trigger a **headache** or **fever**, and extensive burns may induce shock.

Thermal burns are caused by heat sources such as fire, hot liquids, gases or other objects. Radiation burns are usually due to excess exposure to the sun's rays, tanning beds, or x rays. Chemical burns are most likely to come from strong acids, alkalis, phenols, or **phosphorus**. Electrical burns may be quite severe due to the high heat generated by electric currents.

Diagnosis

A physician will diagnose a burn based upon visual examination, and will ask questions to determine the history of contact with possible sources of damage. Depending on the circumstances, there should be an evaluation of the condition of the lungs and breathing, related injuries, evidence of any suspected child abuse, and the extent and location of the burn. Shock and infection are often the results of moderate and major burns, and should be included in any evaluation.

Treatment

A number of herbal remedies, applied topically, can help mild burns heal. These include **aloe**, *Aloe barbadensis* or *Aloe vera*; **St. John's wort**, *Hypericum perforatum; Calendula officinalis;* **comfrey** root, *Symphytum officinale;* and **tea tree oil**, *Melaleuca* spp.

Nutritional support is particularly important for burn victims. Supplementing the diet with vitamins A, C, and E, **zinc** and B-complex, **essential fatty acids** (omega-3 and omego-6), and eating foods high in these nutrients can be very beneficial to the healing process. Proteins and fluid intake should be increased to replace losses. The **traditional Chinese medicine (TCM)** approach recommends foods that remove heat and toxins, nourish yin, and promote the production of body fluids. These foods include mung beans, kidney beans, lima beans, soybeans, cucumbers, potatoes, summer squash, sweet potatoes, and barley. In addition, freshly juiced **ginger**, potatoes, and cucumbers can be applied to burns to reduce pain and swelling. The pulp of fresh pumpkin can be used as a poultice (soft compress applied to the affected area). **Chamomile** tea decreases **anxiety**.

Homeopathic treatment should be given as soon as possible after the onset of the burn injury. **Cantharis** 30c is the most noteworthy remedy for burns. It is recommended to keep **blisters** from forming. A dose can be taken every 15 minutes for up to six doses.

Homeopathic **calendula** mother tincture can be useful to promote the healing of burns. Ten drops should be added to one ounce of water and applied to the burn three times daily. *Arnica montana* 30c can help prevent shock. *Urtica urens* 6c and Causticum 6c may also be useful for burns. Urtica may be applied to the skin as an ointment as well.

Guided imagery can assist with pain control.

Allopathic treatment

Burn treatment usually consists of relieving pain, preventing infection, and maintaining body fluids, electrolytes, and calorie intake while the body heals. Children and the elderly are more vulnerable to complications from burn injuries and require more intensive care. Other factors that influence treatment include associated injuries such as bone **fractures** and smoke inhalation, presence of a chronic disease, a history of abuse, and the occurrence of shock or infection. Moderate and major burns should always be treated by a medical practitioner.

The first act of treating a burn is to stop the burning process. Small thermal burns should be immediately placed in cold water if possible. To avoid infection, the wound should be cleaned with soap and water, and all dirt should be carefully removed. Butter, shortening, or similar salve should never be applied to the burn since it prevents heat from escaping and drives the burning process deeper into the skin. Minor burns should be cleaned gently with soap and water. If the skin is broken or apt to be disturbed, the burned area should be coated lightly with an antibacterial ointment and covered with a sterile bandage. Pain relievers such as aspirin or non-steroidal anti-inflammatory drugs (NSAIDs) may be used as needed. A doctor should be consulted if signs of infection appear: increased warmth, redness, pain, or swelling; pus or similar drainage from the wound; swollen lymph nodes; or red streaks spreading from the burn.

At an accident site, the victim should be immediately removed from the burning process. Clothing should be removed from all affected areas. Any clothing embedded in the burn should not be disturbed. Dry chemicals should be brushed from the skin; burns caused by acids, alkalis, phosphorus, or organic compounds, such as phenols and cresols, should be flushed with water continuously over an extended time.

In cases of moderate and major burn damage, further medical treatment may include assessment of breathing and treatment if the patient's airways or lungs have been damaged; a flush of any chemicals; and the administering of intravenous fluids, since burns may dramatically deplete body fluids. Antibiotic ointments are usually applied to burns, and the patient is also given antibiotics intravenously to prevent infection. A **tetanus** shot may also be given. Dead tissue is surgically removed, or debrided. Once the burned area is cleaned and treated, it is usually covered with sterile bandages. Oral narcotics such as codeine may be required for pain relief. The burn patient may have to undergo physical and occupational therapy. If there is extensive scarring, a skin graft is usually performed.

Expected results

Prognosis is dependent upon the degree of the burn, the amount of body surface covered, whether critical body parts are affected, any additional injuries or complications, and the promptness of medical treatment. The epidermis in first-degree burns regenerates rapidly; not much scarring results unless infection develops. With deeper burns, the process of healing is slow, and scars often develop. This may limit mobility and function, making physical therapy necessary. In some cases, surgery may be advisable to remove scar tissue and restore appearance. Some people, especially young women and people with dark skin, may develop keloids.

Secondary **infections** are common, and may be a major cause of loss of function, disfigurement, and death. Patients with burns over more than 40% BSA, those older than 60 years old, and those with inhalation injuries are at risk for burn injuries that result in death.

Prevention

Burns are commonly received from fires in the home. Properly placed and working smoke detectors in combination with rapid evacuation plans will minimize a person's exposure to smoke and flames in the event of a fire. Children must be taught never to play with matches, lighters, fireworks, gasoline or cleaning fluids.

Burns from scalding with hot water or other liquids may be prevented by setting the water heater thermostat no higher than 120°F (49°C), checking the temperature of bath water before getting into the tub, and turning pot handles on the stove out of the reach of children. Care should be used when removing covers from pans of steaming foods and when uncovering or opening foods heated in a microwave oven.

Sunburns may be avoided by the liberal use of sunscreen. Hats, loose clothing, and umbrellas also provide protection, especially between 10 a.m. and 3 p.m., when the most damaging ultraviolet rays are present.

Burns are often received from electrical appliances. Care should be exercised around stoves, space heaters, irons, and curling irons. Electrical burns may be prevented by covering unused outlets with safety plugs and keeping electrical cords away from infants and toddlers who might chew on them.

Chemical burns may be prevented by wearing protective clothing, including gloves and eye shields. Chemicals should always be used according to the manufacturer's instructions and properly stored when not in use.

Resources

BOOKS

The Burton Goldberg Group. *Alternative Medicine: The Definitive Guide*. Washington: Future Medicine Publishing, 1995.

Lininger, D.C., Skye, editor-in-chief, et al. *The Natural Pharmacy*. California: Prima Health, 1998.

Lockie, Dr. Andrew and Dr. Nicola Geddes. *The Complete Guide to homeopathy: The principles and Practice of Treatment with a Comprehensive Range of Self-Help Remedies for Common Ailments*. London: Dorling Kindersley, Ltd., 1995.

ORGANIZATIONS

Shriners Hospitals for Children. 2900 Rocky Point Drive, Tampa, FL 33607-1435.

OTHER

Health Answers. http://www.healthanswers.com (January 17, 2001).

The Merck Manual. http://www.merck.com/pubs/mmanual/section20/ chapter276/276a.htm (January 17, 2001).

Patience Paradox

Bursitis

Definition

Bursitis is the painful inflammation of one or more bursae, which are padlike sacs found in parts of the body that are subject to friction. Bursae cushion the movements between the bones, tendons and muscles near the joints. Bursitis is most often caused by repetitive movement and is known by several common names, including weaver's bottom, clergyman's knee, housemaid's knee, and miner's elbow, depending on the area of injury.

Description

There are over 150 bursae in the human body. Usually bursae are present from birth, but they may form in response to repeated pressure. Each sac contains a small amount of synovial fluid, a clear liquid that acts as a lubricant. The bursae may become inflamed through traumatic injury, infection, or the development of arthritis. The inflammation then causes **pain** whenever the joint is moved. The most common site for bursitis to occur is the shoulder joint (subdeltoid), but it also is seen in the elbows (olecranon), hips (trochanteric), knees, heels (Achilles), and toes. The affected area may be referred to as "frozen," because movement is so limited. In the knee there are four bursae, and all can become inflamed with overuse.

Causes and symptoms

The most common cause of bursitis is repeated physical activity, but it can flare up for no known

KEY TERMS

Arthritis—Inflammation of a joint that may lead to changes in the joint's structure. It causes pain and swelling. Rheumatoid arthritis is a chronic disease that leads to crippling deformities.

Bursa—A sac that contains synovial fluid and cushions the joints.

Gout—A hereditary metabolic disease that is a form of arthritis and causes inflammation of the joints. It is more common in men.

Kinesiology—The science or study of movement.

Synovia—A clear, somewhat sticky lubricating fluid secreted by membranes that surround the joints.

reason. It can also be caused by trauma, **rheumatoid arthritis**, **gout**, and acute or chronic infection.

Pain and tenderness are common symptoms of bursitis. If the affected joint is close to the skin, as with the shoulder, knee, elbow, or Achilles tendon, swelling and redness are seen and the area may feel warm to the touch. The bursae around the hip joint are deeper, and swelling is not as obvious. Movement may be limited and is painful. In the shoulder, it may be difficult to raise the arm outward from the side of the body. Putting on a jacket or combing the hair, for example, become troublesome activities.

In acute bursitis symptoms appear suddenly; with chronic bursitis, pain, tenderness, and limited movement reappear after **exercise** or strain.

Diagnosis

When a patient has pain in a specific joint, a careful physical examination is needed to determine what type of movement is affected and if there is any swelling present. Bursitis will not show up on x rays, although sometimes there are also **calcium** deposits in the joint that can be seen. Inserting a thin needle into the affected bursa and removing (aspirating) some of the synovial fluid for examination can confirm the diagnosis. In most cases, the fluid will not be clear. It can be tested for the presence of microorganisms, which would indicate an infection, and for crystals, which could indicate gout. In instances where the diagnosis is difficult, a local anesthetic (a drug that numbs the area) is injected into the painful spot. If the discomfort stops temporarily, bursitis is probably the correct diagnosis.

Treatment

Nutritional therapy

Naturopaths and nutritionists emphasize the role of diet as an underlying cause of bursitis. They believe that the faulty use of calcium by the body, **magnesium** deficiencies, and food **allergies** may play a role. Their recommended diet may include the following:

- fresh fruits, vegetables and whole grains
- avoidance of foods that may cause allergies or digestive problems
- multivitamin and mineral supplements
- vitamins A, C and E, selenium, and zinc supplements

Herbal therapy

Herbalists have recommended the following herbs or plant products for treatment of bursitis:

- curcumin (turmeric)
- bromelain (an enzyme found in pineapple)
- ginger
- grape-seed extract
- pine-bark extract
- citrus bioflavonoids

Homeopathy

Homeopathic remedies for bursitis include *Belladonna*, *Bryonia* and *Rhus toxicodendron*.

Hydrotherapy

The application of ice soon after an injury helps decrease the inflammation of acute bursitis. After two days of treatment with ice, however, heat instead of ice is more helpful. A warm heating pad or hot showers or baths can also relieve the symptoms of bursitis.

Acupuncture

Acupuncture has been proven effective in treating hip and shoulder pain caused by bursitis and other conditions.

Chiropractic

Spinal manipulation by a chiropractor may help improve movement in the affected joints by relieving some of the pressure on them.

Body work

Body work starts with adequate rest and massage of the bursitic area. Massage can increase blood circulation in the area, reducing the inflammation and pain. Following the initial phase of body work, patients may participate in **yoga** exercises that help to improve joint mobility and strengthen the muscles surrounding the joints.

Allopathic treatment

Conservative treatment of bursitis is usually effective. The application of heat, rest, and immobilization of the affected joint area is the first step. A sling can be used for a shoulder injury; a cane is helpful for hip problems. The patient can take nonsteroidal anti-inflammatory drugs (NSAIDs) like aspirin, ibuprofen, and naproxen to relieve the pain and inflammation. Once the pain decreases, exercises of the affected area can begin. If the nearby muscles have become weak because of the disease or prolonged immobility, then exercises to build strength and improve movement are best. A doctor or physical therapist can prescribe an effective regimen.

If the bursitis is related to an inflammatory condition like arthritis or gout, then management of that disease is needed to control the bursitis.

When bursitis does not respond to conservative treatment, an injection into the joint of a long-acting corticosteroid preparation like prednisone can bring immediate and lasting relief. The drug is mixed with a local anesthetic and works on the joint within five minutes. Usually one injection is all that is needed.

Surgery to remove the damaged bursa may be performed in extreme cases.

If the bursitis is caused by an infection, then additional treatment is needed. Septic bursitis is caused by the presence of a pus-forming organism, usually *Staphylococcus aureus*. Septic bursitis requires treatment with antibiotics, which can be taken by mouth, injected into a muscle, or injected directly into a vein (intravenously). The bursa will also need to be drained by needle two or three times over the first week of treatment.

Expected results

Bursitis usually responds well to treatment, but it may develop into a chronic condition if the underlying cause is not corrected.

Prevention

Aggravating factors should be eliminated to prevent bursitis. Overexercising or the repetition of a movement that triggers the condition should be avoided. Doing exercises to strengthen the muscles around the joint will also help. When doing repetitive tasks, the patient should take frequent breaks and alternate the repetitive activity with others that use different parts of the body. To cushion the joints, it is a good idea to use cushioned chairs when sitting and foam kneeling pads for the knees. Leaning on the elbows, kneeling, or sitting on a hard surface for a long period of time should be avoided. Not wearing high heels can help prevent bursitis in the heel, as can changing to new running shoes as soon as the old ones are worn out.

Resources

BOOKS

Bennett, J. Claude, and Fred Plum. *Cecil's Textbook of Medicine.* Philadelphia: W. B. Saunders Co., 1994.

Bennett, Robert M. "Bursitis, Tendinitis, Myofascial Pain, and Fibromyalgia." In *Conn's Current Therapy.* Edited by Robert E. Rakel. Philadelphia: W. B. Saunders Co., 1998.

"Bursitis." *The Medical Advisor: The Complete Guide to Alternative and Medical Treatments.* Richmond, VA: TimeLife Inc., 1997.

The Burton Goldberg Group. *Alternative Medicine: The Definitive Guide.* Fife, WA: Future Medicine Publishing, 1995.

Murray, Michael, and Joseph Pizzorno. *Encyclopedia of Natural Medicine,* revised 2nd ed., Rocklin, CA: Prima Health, 1998.

OTHER

Applied Medical Infomatics Inc., 1997. "Bursitis." http:// www.healthanswers.com.

Mai Tran

Butcher's broom

Description

Butcher's broom is the root of the plant *Ruscus aculeatus*. *R. aculeatus* is a common evergreen shrub native to Mediterranean countries. It is related to asparagus. The shrub grows to less than 3 ft (1 m) in height and about the same size in girth in shady, moist, uncultivated ground. Its leaves are small and laced with brown membranes. The root, which is the medicinal part, is fleshy. Butcher's broom has a few small greenish white flowers that mature into red, cherry-sized berries. This herb has spread to many other parts of the world including Great Britain, the United States, and western Asia. Other names for Butcher's broom include kneeholm, knee holly, sweet broom, Jew's myrtle, pettigree, and box holly.

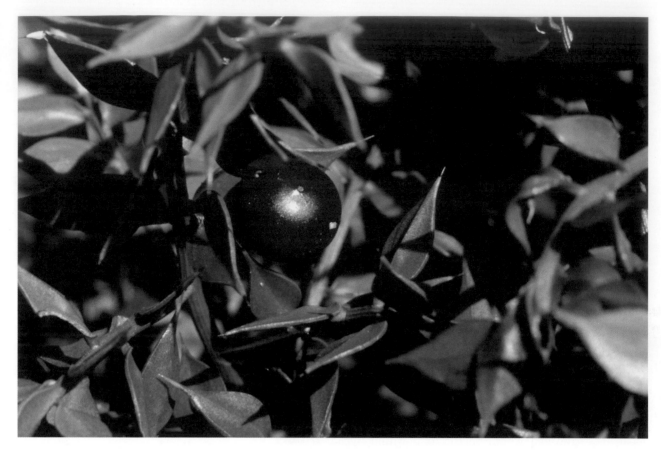

Butcher's broom. *(©PlantaPhile, Germany. Reproduced by permission.)*

General use

Butcher's broom has been used in folk medicine as far back as the first century A.D. In the past, it was used as a laxative and as a treatment for **gout**, **jaundice**, **kidney stones**, and broken bones. It was also used as a diuretic to reduce swelling in the hands and feet, and to reduce inflammation due to arthritis. At one time, the plant was eaten as a vegetable in the United States. The seeds have been roasted and used as a coffee substitute.

Few of these uses survive today. Modern herbalists primarily use butcher's broom as supportive therapy for poor circulation, **hemorrhoids**, varicose vein syndrome, and other manifestations of leaky vein walls and poor venous blood return to the heart. For these conditions, it is taken internally. Although butcher's broom will not cure these conditions, it is used to relieve symptoms such as leg cramps, **pain**, heaviness in the legs, swelling of the legs and feet, and it can strengthen vein walls. Butcher's broom is also used externally as an ointment or suppository to treat **itching** and burning associated with hemorrhoids.

Butcher's broom had been in decline as a medicinal herb until the 1950s. Then researchers discovered that an extract of the root contained two compounds, ruscogenin and neuorscogenin, that could constrict the veins in dogs and other laboratory animals. This improves blood flow and increases the strength and tone of those veins.

Interest in butcher's broom increased. The herb was included in many popular formulations for treating poor leg circulation in Europe (and less so in the United States). A few controlled human studies were conducted. People showed some of the same reactions to the drug as laboratory animals, but the improvements in blood flow were slight, and little was known about the safety of the drug. As a result, the United States Food and Drug Administration (FDA) felt the study data was not conclusive enough to approve butcher's broom as a drug. However, the German Federal Health Agency's Commission E (established in 1978 to independently review and evaluate scientific literature and case studies on herb and plant medications) has approved butcher's broom for use in alleviating the discomforts associated with chronic venous insufficiency.

There is less scientific data about treating hemorrhoids with butcher's broom. Although there are compounds in butcher's broom that constrict blood vessels and reduce inflammation, it isn't clear whether these compounds are effective in ointments and suppositories applied externally to hemorrhoids. Recent research done in Palestine also suggests that extracts of *R. aculeatus* have a mild and selective antifungal property. Although initial studies look promising, more controlled research needs to be done on people to conclusively define the role of butcher's broom in healing.

Preparations

The root of butcher's broom is harvested in the fall and dried before use. It is available in commercial capsules, tablets, and tinctures for internal use, and in ointments and suppositories for external use. Tablets often contain about 300 mg of the dried extract. However, patients should follow package directions or directions from their healthcare provider in using this herb.

Precautions

Not much is known about the safety of butcher's broom, which is one reason why the FDA did not approve its use as a drug. However, no health problems are known to result when this herb is used as directed, and it has been used for centuries. People with high blood pressure should not take butcher's broom. Conditions for which butcher's broom is used can be serious. This herb is intended as supportive therapy for these conditions. People with chronic venous insufficiency should be under the care of a trained doctor.

Side effects

In rare cases, butcher's broom may cause **nausea** and stomach upset. No other side effects have been reported.

Interactions

It is not known how butcher's broom interacts with any other herbs or medicines. Few, if any, scientific studies have been done on its interactions with traditional medications.

Resources

BOOKS

Pierce, Andrea. *The American Pharmaceutical Association Practical Guide to Natural Medicines.* New York: William Morrow and Company, 1999.

PDR for Herbal Medicines. Montvale, New Jersey: Medical Economics Company, 1998.

OTHER

"Plants for the Future: Ruscus aculeatus." http://www.metalab.unc.edu.

Tish Davidson

Buteyko

Definition

Buteyko, also called the Buteyko Method or Buteyko Breathing Technique, is an **asthma** management method based on breathing exercises that reduce airway constriction. The therapy is a learned breathing technique that is designed to slow and lessen the intake of air into the lungs. If practiced over time, it is thought to reduce the symptoms and severity of conditions such as asthma. The technique of shallow, controlled breathing is believed to counteract hyperventilation, a condition referred to as over-breathing.

Origins

The Buteyko method is named after its developer, Russian scientist Konstantin Buteyko. In the 1950s in Moscow, Buteyko was involved in studies of the breathing patterns in sick and healthy people. That involvement started when he was a student at the First Medical Institute in Moscow. During an assignment to monitor the breathing of ill patients, Buteyko noticed that breathing tended to be deeper in patients who were very ill or approaching death. Buteyko discovered that by recording the increases in breathing that he could "form a prognoses on how many days or hours were left before a patient died," according to the Buteyko Education and Training Centre website. Buteyko's findings led to a lifelong interest in how the way people breathe affects health.

After graduating in 1952, Buteyko's research included a study of what happened when healthy people breathed too deeply. According to the website, Buteyko noticed that some experienced **dizziness** and **nausea**. Buteyko, who suffered from **hypertension**, also used himself as a subject. Buteyko theorized that over-breathing could be the cause of some medical conditions. He slowed his breathing and noticed a reduction in hypertension symptoms like headaches and rapid heartbeat.

Buteyko concluded that long-term over-breathing was a cause of imbalance in the body. He called this habit "hidden hyperventilation." Professor Buteyko claimed to cure patients of respiratory disorders by correcting their breathing to more shallow and slower patterns. He also conducted scientific studies on the mechanisms of over-breathing's negative effects on the body.

Buteyko maintained that over-breathing causes an imbalance in the carbon dioxide levels in the body, especially in the lungs and bloodstream. This in turn changes blood oxygen levels and decreases the amount of oxygen that cells receive. Body acidity/alkalinity balance can also be influenced by breathing pattern, and CO_2/O_2 concentrations. Buteyko believed that over time, hyperventilation could **stress** systems of the body including the respiratory, circulatory, and nervous systems.

According to Buteyko, breathing difficulties such as asthma are believed to be symptoms of over-breathing. In addition, he viewed many diseases as the body's reaction to over-breathing. Buteyko also believed that over-breathing was a bad habit that people learned. He cited the prevailing beliefs in Russian society that deep breathing was good for the body and the nerves. He also identified improper breathing habits as being caused by the excess consumption of protein, which requires increased metabolism for digestion and thus deeper breathing. Other causes of improper breathing habits include stress and a sedentary lifestyle.

Buteyko claimed that hyperventilation caused symptoms such as bronchial spasms, excess mucus, nervous problems, dizziness, headaches, and **allergies**. He also theorized that over-breathing was directly linked to many diseases including asthma, hypertension, **heart disease**, strokes, **hemorrhoids**, and **eczema**. Buteyko's philosophy of medicine was that a physician has no right to treat a patient if he or she has not determined the cause of the disease. Only after discovering the root of the disease is it possible to begin recovery.

For Buteyko, deep breathing was the cause of many diseases. He viewed hyperventilation as a bad habit that could be easily replaced with a healthier pattern. He developed a technique to recondition breathing patterns, and supposedly demonstrated success in healing some diseases and conditions with the technique. By January 1, 1967, more than 1,000 people had been treated and reportedly recovered from asthma, hypertension or **angina**.

Buteyko's method met resistance from the mainstream Russian medical system until a 1980 study confirmed the success of a 1968 trial. The earlier trial involved 46 people who were reportedly cured by the Buteyko treatment. However, details about their conditions were not available.

During the 1990s, one of Buteyko's pupils, Alexander Stalmatski, went to Australia to train practitioners in the Buteyko method. He stayed in Australia for six years and then took his teachings to England. In the early 2000s, Australia and England had the largest number of trained Buteyko practitioners. The method also has practitioners in counties including the United States, Canada, and Ireland, and New Zealand.

By 2008, the Buteyko method was promoted as a technique to manage conditions like asthma rather than as a cure for conditions. On the Buteyko Education and Training Centre site, the method is described as "a series of lectures related to breathing" along with techniques and exercises for people to follow. The method no longer includes a diet.

Benefits

The Buteyko breathing technique is a drug-free method for adults and children seeking to manage asthma and other breathing-related conditions. People diagnosed with conditions like asthma use this method to control their breathing and possibly lessen the need for medication. The method is also used for respiratory conditions including **bronchitis**, allergies, **rhinitis**, and **sleep apnea**.

Description

When a person hyperventilates, the individual breathes deeply and quickly. This may cause the level of carbon dioxide in the blood to become too low. When a person begins to hyperventilate, the medically accepted methods of restoring the carbon dioxide level include taking slow, deep breaths; practicing a relaxation technique, or breathing into a paper bag for from five to 15 minutes.

Asthma is a condition that produces inflammation in the airways. The inflammation causes the person to react to triggers such as allergens, dust, and stress. The triggers cause a reaction that produces symptoms such as **wheezing**, coughing, and difficulty breathing.

During an attack, Buteyko maintained that asthma sufferers breathe about twice as fast as people without the condition. The Buteyko method aims to correct the breathing pattern, thereby maintaining balanced body CO_2 and cellular oxygenation levels. With careful and consistent practice of the technique, Buteyko believed that people could retrain their breathing patterns and often improve their symptoms.

In the February 2008 issue of *Better Nutrition*, Emily Kane wrote that the method was "somewhat similar" to breathing into a paper bag when an asthma attack was imminent.

The Buteyko method strives to remove the bad habits of over-breathing and to replace them with new habits of slower, shallower breathing, called "reduced breathing." Emphasis is placed on posture and relaxation in the upper body. Proper breathing technique is one in which the navel and lower rib cage move out slowly during inspiration and move inward during a relaxed expiration. People are taught to avoid breathing through the mouth as much as possible, taking breaths through the nostrils even during **exercise** and sleep.

During training for reduced breathing, the pulse is monitored as a feedback signal: shallow and efficient breathing reduces the pulse and heart rate. During training, there is also attention to what is called a controlled pause, in which breathing stops and the duration of pausing the breath is recorded and extended through practice. In correct Buteyko breathing, the body can maintain a controlled pause of 40 to 60 seconds. For asthma sufferers, the controlled pause is typically five to 15 seconds. However, those training in the technique could result in the controlled pause being held for a longer time.

When the technique is effectively practiced and reduced breathing becomes habitual, Buteyko supporters maintain that fewer allergens are inhaled. They claim that the airways become less dehydrated and irritated. Advocates of this technique believe that mucus and histamine production decreases, inflammation decreases, and breathing becomes easier.

Preparation

People seeking to learn the Buteyko method are encouraged to find a certified practitioner or class. Practitioners give individual and group instruction, with class time ranging from eight to 12 hours. Furthermore, books, videos, and DVDs provide step-by-step instructions in the technique for people who want to learn Buteyko at home.

Precautions

People should consult with their doctor or health practitioner before beginning a Buteyko program. Asthma sufferers learning the Buteyko technique should continue use of their asthma medication, but may taper down with dosages under their doctors' supervision.

Side Effects

No unfavorable side effects to the Buteyko method had been reported as of February 2008.

Research and General Acceptance

The Buteyko method was more prevalent in Australia and England than it was in the United States, as of 2008. Conclusive scientific studies of the method had not been conducted at that time.

As of 2008, there were some indications that Buteyko might help lessen the need for medication, but the technique did not seem to help with lung function. Furthermore, research during the 2000s about the effects of Buteyko produced varied results.

Research included a study described in the December 2003 issue of the *Journal of the New Zealand Medical Association*. The randomized trial involving 34 asthmatics between the ages of 18 and 70 compared people who were taught the Buteyko Breathing Technique to a control group. After six months, researchers concluded that Buteyko was a safe and efficient asthma management technique that merited additional study.

The August 2006 issue of *Thorax* featured information about an Australian study at the University of Sydney, New South Wales. The research involving 57 asthma sufferers compared two breathing exercises: shallow breathing through the nose and non-specific body exercises. After a two-week run-in period, participants did their exercises twice a day and as needed for 30 weeks. Researchers concluded that breathing exercises "may" be helpful for people with mild asthma. However, they found no evidence to favor shallow breathing over the upper-body exercises.

KEY TERMS

Allergen—A foreign substance that causes the airways to narrow and produces symptoms of asthma when inhaled.

Asthma—Respiratory disease characterized by constriction of the airways in the lungs, causing difficulty in breathing.

Training and Certification

Trained instructors may lead individual and group training sessions. Certification classes are available in the United States and other countries.

As of 2008, practitioner certification training was offered jointly through Buteyko International and the Buteyko Clinic of Moscow. The North American affiliate of the international organization, the Buteyko Clinic of Canada, is located in Richmond, a city outside of Vancouver. The clinics schedule training sessions in locations including New York. As of 2008, training cost 2,500 Euros ($3,701.27 in U.S. dollars). The training process included long-distance learning followed by 10 days of practical training with patients at the Buteyko Clinic. Practitioners then taught basic Buteyko for six months to gain practical experience and case studies for the certification process.

Resources

BOOKS

McKeown, Patrick G. *Asthma-Free Naturally: Everything You Need to Know About Taking Control of Your Asthma: Featuring the Buteyko Breathing Method Suitable for Adults and Children.* Harper Thorson, 2005.

PERIODICALS

Kane, Emily. "Balance Your Hormones." *Better Nutrition.* (February 2008): 36–39.
McHugh, Patrick; Aitcheson, Fergus; Duncan, Bruce; Houghton Frank. "A Randomised Controlled Trial of the Buteyko Technique as an Adjunct to Conventional Management of Asthma." *Journal of the New Zealand Medical Association.* (12-Decembers 2003): 1187.
Slader, C.A.; Reddel, H.K.; Spencer, L.M.; Belousova, E.G.; Armour, C.L.; Bosnic-Anticevich, S.Z.; Thien, F.C.; and Jenkins, C.R. "Double Blind Randomised Controlled Trial of Two Different Breathing Techniques in the Management of Asthma." *Thorax.* (August 2006) 651–6.
Thomas, Sandy. "Buteyko: A useful tool in the management of asthma?" *International Journal of Therapy & Rehabilitation.* (October 2004) 476–479.

ORGANIZATIONS

American Lung Association. 61 Broadway, 6th Floor, New York, NY 10006. (212) 315-8700. http://www.lungusa.org.
Asthma and Allergy Foundation of America. 1233 20th Street, NW, Suite 402, Washington, DC, 20036. (800) 727-8462. http://www.aafa.org.
Buteyko Asthma Education USA. 2507 Brewster Road, Indianapolis, IN, 46268. (877) 278-4623. http://www.buteyko-usa.com
Buteyko Clinic of Canada. 9620 Williams Road, Richmond, BC, V7A 1H2, Canada. (604) 723-0479. http://www.buteykointernational.com.
Buteyko Education and Training Centre. http://www.buteyko.com.

Douglas Dupler
Liz Swain

Butternut *see* **Black walnut**

C

Cadmium poisoning

Definition

Cadmium is a metal with an atomic number of 48 and atomic weight of 112.41. In the periodic table of the elements, cadmium is located between **zinc** and mercury. It is used in a large number of industrial applications. In the United States, about 1.2 million pounds of cadmium were used industrially in 2006. Consumption of cadmium has been decreasing significantly because of concerns over health and environmental issues.

The uses for cadmium include:

- component of several metal alloys
- component of solder (metallic cement), particularly solder for aluminum
- electroplating
- nickel plating
- engraving
- cadmium vapor lamps
- nickel-cadmium batteries
- treatment of parasites in pigs and poultry

Cadmium can be very toxic, and is dangerous if swallowed or inhaled. While spontaneous recovery from mild cadmium exposure is common, doses as low as 10 mg can cause symptoms of poisoning. There is no accepted fatal dosage.

Description

The symptoms of ingested cadmium poisoning are:

- increased salivation
- choking
- vomiting
- abdominal pain
- anemia
- painful spasms of the anal sphincter

When cadmium dust or powder is inhaled, the first symptoms are a sweet or metallic taste, followed by throat irritation. Other symptoms that may appear in three to five hours include:

- dry throat
- cough
- headache
- vomiting
- chest pain
- pulmonary edema, a congestive lung condition
- bronchospasm, the abnormal tightening of airways that may be accompanied by wheezing and coughing
- pneumonitis, inflammation of the lung
- muscle weakness
- leg pain

When a person has exposure to cadmium in low doses over a long period of time, symptoms may include loss of sense of smell, **cough**, shortness of breath, weight loss, and tooth staining. Chronic cadmium exposure may cause damage to the liver and kidneys.

Causes and symptoms

The most common cause of cadmium poisoning is lack of proper precautions in places where cadmium is used. In such industries, air quality should be regularly monitored. Cadmium-plated containers should never be used to store acidic foods such as fruit juices or vinegar.

Fossil fuels, such as coal and oil, release cadmium fumes into the air. Chronic cadmium poisoning is also possible through soil or water contamination. This problem may occur with improper disposal of nickel-cadmium batteries used in items such as cameras. Cadmium poisoning has been associated with itai-itai disease in Japan.

Diagnosis

Cadmium poisoning is usually diagnosed by its symptoms, particularly if there is reason to believe that the patient has been exposed to cadmium. Because patients may not request treatment for up to a day following cadmium exposure, diagnosticians should carefully question any patient who shows symptoms consistent with this condition.

Treatment

Other than symptomatic treatment, there are no good options for dealing with cadmium poisoning. Hemodialysis may be used to remove circulating cadmium from the bloodstream, although literature on the subject is scarce. The addition of a chelating agent, particularly ethylenediamine tetraacetic acid (EDTA), will increase the amount of cadmium removed by the dialysate (the fluid used in dialysis to carry substances to or remove from the kidney during hemodialysis).

These treatments are effective only for oral poisoning, and have no demonstrated benefit in cadmium fume inhalation.

Allopathic treatment

There are no generally accepted treatments for the acute effects of cadmium poisoning. Other than dialysis, dimercaptosuccinic acid (DMSA), an oral chelating agent, has been recommended for removal of cadmium from the blood.

Expected results

The prognosis depends on the nature and severity of the cadmium load. Most cases of mild exposure resolve spontaneously after a few days. In other cases, cadmium can lead to permanent damage with shortened lifespan, or even death.

Cadmium may be carcinogenic.

Long-term exposure may also result in bone defects including **osteoporosis**.

Prevention

All work done in areas where cadmium fumes may be present should be well ventilated. Ground water and soil should be checked for cadmium. Cadmium-coated containers should, in general, be avoided. They should never be used with acidic liquids such as fruit juices. Coal and oil-burning utilities should be monitored for cadmium discharge. Nickel-cadmium batteries should be recycled or disposed of as toxic waste.

KEY TERMS

Chelating—A chemical term denoting a compound that has a central metallic ion attached via covalent bonds to two or more non-metallic atoms in the same molecule.

Hemodialysis—A procedure for removing metabolic waste products or toxic substances from the bloodstream.

Itai-itai disease—The first reported cases of cadmium poisoning in the world, seen in Japan in about 1950. The name means "ouch-ouch" and represents the sufferers' screams of pain. The disease caused bone and kidney defects. It was caused by cadmium pollution from mines.

Pneumonitis—Inflammation of lung tissue.

Osteoporosis—A disease in which the bones become extremely porous, are subject to fracture, and heal slowly.

Resources

BOOKS

Beers, Mark H., and Robert Berkow. "Poisoning" in *Merck Manual of Diagnosis and Therapy*. Whitehouse Station, N.J.: Merck Research Laboratories, 2004.

Occupational Safety and Health Administration.*Cadmium*. Washington, D.C.: U.S. Department of Labor, Occupational Safety and Health Administration, 2004.

Scoullos, M. J., et al. *Mercury-Cadmium-Lead Handbook for Sustainable Heavy Metals Policy and Regulation*. New York: Springer, 2002.

Tolcin, Amy C. *Cadmium*. Washington, D.C.: U.S. Geological Survey, 2007.

PERIODICALS

Hung, Yao-Min, and Hsiao-Min Chung. "Acute Self-Poisoning by Ingestion of Cadmium and Barium." *Nephrology Dialysis Transplantation* (May 2004): 1308–1309.

Blanusa, Maja, et al. "Chelators as Antidotes of Metal Toxicity: Therapeutic and Experimental Aspects." *Current Medicinal Chemistry* (November 2005): 2771–2794.

ORGANIZATIONS

Occupational Safety & Health Administration, 200 Constitution Avenue, N.W., Washington, D.C., 20210, http://www.osha.gov/.

Samuel Uretsky, Pharm.D.
David Edward Newton, Ed.D.

Caffeine

Description

Caffeine is a drug that stimulates the central nervous system (CNS). Caffeine is found naturally in coffee, kola seed kernels or nuts (*Cola nidtida*), and a variety of teas. Other foods and beverages, such as chocolate and soft drinks, also contain caffeine, and the drug can be purchased in over-the-counter tablet and capsule form (No Doz, Overtime, Pep-Back, Quick-Pep, Caffedrine, and Vivarin). Some prescription **pain** relievers, medicines for migraine headaches, and antihistamines, also contain caffeine.

General use

Caffeine makes people more alert and less drowsy and improves one's coordination. It is sometimes included in athletes' **diets** to improve physical performance. In addition, one study found that older people who were given a cup of caffeinated coffee in the morning had fewer late-day memory problems than those who were given decaffeinated coffee. Combined with certain pain relievers or medicines for treating **migraine headache**, caffeine enables those drugs to work more quickly and effectively. Caffeine alone can also help relieve headaches. Antihistamines are sometimes combined with caffeine to counteract the drowsiness caused by these drugs. Caffeine is also sometimes used to treat other conditions, including breathing problems in newborns and in young babies after surgery.

Preparations

Kola can be prepared in decoction or tincture form. A decoction is prepared by mixing 1–2 tsp of powdered **kola nut** in a cup of water. After bringing the water to a boil, the decoction should be simmered on low heat for 10 to 15 minutes. Tinctures of kola nut can be purchased at many health food stores or from mail order suppliers. A tincture is an herbal preparation made by diluting the herb in alcohol, glycerin, or vinegar. Dosage of kola tincture varies by formula and the symptoms or illness it is supposed to treat, but an average recommended dosage might be 1–4 mL three times daily. Powdered kola nut and kola tinctures should be stored in airtight containers away from direct light to maintain potency.

For over-the-counter caffeine preparations, adults and children age 12 years and older should take 100–200 mg no more than every three to four hours. In timed-release form, the dose is 200–250 mg

Caffeine content of common dietary and medicinal sources	
Source	**Standard amount in milligrams (mg)**
Bottled beverages (12 oz)	
Red Bull	115.5
Jolt	72
Mountain Dew	55
Diet Coke	45
Dr. Poppor	41
Coca Cola Classic	34
Coffee (8 oz)	
Brewed	80-135
Expresso (2 oz)	100
Instant	65-100
Decaf brew	3-4
Tea (8 oz)	
Iced	47
Brewed	40-60
Instant	30
Green	15
Chocolate	
Dark chocolate bar (1 oz)	20
Hot cocoa (8 oz)	14
Milk chocolate bar (1 oz)	6
Chocolate milk (6 oz)	4
Medications (per tablet)	
Vivarin	200
No-Doz	100
Midol, Maximum Strength	60
Anacin	32
Dristan	16

(Illustration by Corey Light. Cengage Learning, Gale)

Caffeine

once a day. Timed-release forms should not be taken less than six hours before bedtime. Caffeine pills or tablets are typically not recommended for children under 12 years of age.

Precautions

If caffeine is administered in a kola preparation, kola should always be obtained from a reputable source that observes stringent quality control procedures and industry-accepted good manufacturing practices. Consumers should look for the designations "U.S.P." (U.S. Pharmacopeia) or "NF" (National Formulary) on kola nut labeling. Herbal preparations manufactured under USP or NF guidelines meet nationally recognized strength, quality, purity, packaging, and labeling standards as recommended by the United States Food and Drug Administration (FDA).

Persons should avoid taking too much caffeine as an over-the-counter drug. It is important for individuals to consider how much caffeine is being taken in from coffee, tea, chocolate, soft drinks, and other foods. It is advisable to check with a pharmacist or healthcare professional to find out how much caffeine is safe to use.

Caffeine cannot replace sleep and should not be used regularly to stay awake as the drug can lead to more serious **sleep disorders**, such as **insomnia**.

People who use large amounts of caffeine over long periods build up a tolerance to it. When that happens, they have to use more and more caffeine to get the same effects. Heavy caffeine use can also lead to dependence. If an individual stops using caffeine abruptly, withdrawal symptoms may occur, including **headache**, **fatigue**, drowsiness, yawning, irritability, restlessness, **vomiting**, or runny nose. These symptoms can go on for as long as a week. In addition, caffeine dependence is not confined to the adult population. Studies have shown that American teenagers have a high rate of caffeine dependence, partly because they consume large amounts of carbonated beverages that contain caffeine.

If taken too close to bedtime, caffeine can interfere with sleep. Even if it does not prevent a person from falling asleep, it may disturb sleep during the night.

The notion that caffeine helps people become sober after drinking too much alcohol is a myth. In fact, using caffeine and alcohol together is not a good idea. The combination can lead to an upset stomach, **nausea**, and vomiting.

Older people may be more sensitive to caffeine and thus more likely to have certain side effects, such as irritability, nervousness, **anxiety**, and sleep problems. Research also suggest that people with insulin-dependent diabetes should monitor their caffeine intake. One study found that caffeine appears to decrease insulin sensitivity by about 15%.

Allergies

Anyone with **allergies** to foods, dyes, preservatives, or to the compounds aminophylline, dyphylline, oxtriphylline, theobromine, or theophylline should check with a physician before using caffeine. Anyone who has ever had an unusual reaction to caffeine should also check with a physician before using it again.

Pregnancy

Caffeine can pass from a pregnant woman's body into the developing fetus. Although there is no evidence that caffeine causes birth defects in people, it does cause such effects in laboratory animals given very large doses (equal to human doses of 12–24 cups of coffee a day). In humans, evidence exists that doses of more than 300 mg of caffeine a day (about the amount of caffeine in two to three cups of coffee) may cause miscarriage or problems with the baby's heart rhythm. Women who take more than 300 mg of caffeine a day during **pregnancy** are also more likely to have babies with low birth weights. Any woman who is pregnant or planning to become pregnant should check with her physician before using caffeine.

Breast-feeding

Caffeine passes into breast milk and can affect the nursing baby. Nursing babies whose mothers use 600 mg or more of caffeine a day may be irritable and have trouble sleeping. Women who are breast-feeding should check with their physicians before using caffeine.

Other medical conditions

Caffeine may cause problems for people with these medical conditions:

- peptic ulcer
- heart arrhythmias or palpitations
- heart disease or recent heart attack (within a few weeks)
- high blood pressure
- liver disease
- insomnia (trouble sleeping)
- anxiety or panic attacks
- agoraphobia (fear of being in open places)
- premenstrual syndrome (PMS)

KEY TERMS

Arrhythmia—Irregular heart rhythm.

Central nervous system (CNS)—The brain, spinal cord, and nerves throughout the body.

Decoction—An herbal extract produced by mixing an herb in cold water, bringing the mixture to a boil, and letting it simmer to evaporate the excess water. The decoction is then strained and consumed hot or cold. Decoctions are usually chosen over infusion when the botanical or herb in question is a root, seed, or berry.

Palpitation—Rapid, forceful, throbbing, or fluttering heartbeat.

Tinctures—A liquid extract of an herb prepared by steeping the herb in an alcohol and water mixture. Tinctures can also be prepared using vinegar or glycerin, instead of alcohol.

Withdrawal symptoms—A group of physical or mental symptoms that may occur when a person suddenly stops using a drug to which he or she has become dependent.

Side effects

At recommended doses, caffeine can cause restlessness, irritability, nervousness, shakiness, headache, lightheadedness, sleeplessness, nausea, vomiting, and upset stomach. At higher than recommended doses, caffeine can cause excitement, agitation, anxiety, confusion, a sensation of light flashing before the eyes, unusual sensitivity to touch, unusual sensitivity of other senses, ringing in the ears, frequent urination, muscle twitches or tremors, heart arrhythmias, rapid heartbeat, flushing, and convulsions.

Interactions

Using caffeine with certain other drugs may interfere with the effects of the drugs or cause unwanted—and possibly serious—side effects. Certain drugs interfere with the breakdown of caffeine in the body. These include oral contraceptives that contain estrogen, the antiarrhythmia drug mexiletine (Mexitil), the ulcer drug cimetidine (Tagamet), and the drug disulfiram (Antabuse), used to treat **alcoholism**.

Caffeine interferes with drugs that regulate heart rhythm, such as quinidine and propranolol (Inderal). Caffeine may also interfere with the body's absorption of **iron**. Anyone who uses iron supplements should take them at least an hour before or two hours after using caffeine.

Serious side effects are possible when caffeine is combined with certain drugs. For example, taking caffeine with the decongestant phenylpropanolamine can raise blood pressure. Very serious heart problems may occur if caffeine and monoamine oxidase inhibitors (MAO) are taken together. These drugs are used to treat Parkinson's disease and **depression** and other psychiatric conditions. Persons who use caffeine should consult with a pharmacist or physician to find out which drugs can interact with caffeine.

Because caffeine stimulates the nervous system, anyone taking other central nervous system stimulants should be careful about using caffeine.

Resources

BOOKS

Klosterman, Lorrie. *The Facts about Caffeine*. Salt Lake City: Benchmark Books, 2006.

Weinberg, Bennett Alan. *The World of Caffeine: The Science and Culture of the World's Most Popular Drug*. London: Taylor & Francis, 2007.

PERIODICALS

Barrow, Karen. "Wired Nation: Many Teens Are Guzzling Canned Caffeine. What Effect Does This Hyped–up Habit Have on the Body?" *Science World* (November 12, 2007): 22–26.

Boschert, Sherry. "Caffeine, Medications Treat Excessive Sleepiness." *Family Practice News* (November 1, 2005): 74.

Ritchie, K., et al. "The Neuroprotective Effects of Caffeine." *Neurology* (August 2007): 536–545.

Satel, Sally. "Is Caffeine Addictive?—A Review of the Literature." *American Journal of Drug and Alcohol Abuse* (December 2006): 493–502.

ORGANIZATIONS

Office of Dietary Supplements, National Institutes of Health, Building 31, Room 1B25, 31 Center Drive, MSC 2086, Bethesda, MD, 20892-2086, (301) 435-2920, (301) 480-1845, http://odp.od.nih.gov/ods/.

Paula Ford-Martin
Rebecca J. Frey, Ph.D.
David Edward Newton, Ed.D.

Calcarea carbonica

Description

Calcarea carbonica, abbreviated as *Calcarea carb.*, is a homeopathic remedy made from the middle layer of shells. In chemical terms, *Calcarea carbonica* is impure **calcium** carbonate, CaCO₃. Unlike most homeopathic remedies, which are made from substances soluble in water or alcohol, *Calcarea carbonica* must be prepared by a process called trituration. Triturated material is ground or pounded until it is reduced to a fine powder. The discovery of trituration is a tribute to the genius of Samuel Hahnemann (1755–1843), the founder of **homeopathy**. Hahnemann's method of preparing insoluble substances brought about a new therapeutic method.

General use

Homeopathic medicine operates on the principle that "like heals like" which means that a disease can be cured by treating it with substances that produce the same symptoms as the disease, while also working in conjunction with the homeopathic law of infinitesimals. In opposition to traditional medicine, the law of infinitesimals states that the lower a dose of curative, the more effective it is. To achieve a low dose, the curative is diluted many, many times until only a tiny amount remains in a huge amount of the diluting liquid.

Calcarea carbonica is a remedy used more frequently in so-called constitutional prescribing than in treatment of acute conditions. In constitutional prescribing, the homeopathic practitioner selects a remedy to treat the patient's complete symptomatology, based on a careful evaluation of the person's overall health. In homeopathy, constitution includes a person's heredity and life history as well as present lifestyle, environment, and medical history in the narrow sense. Constitutional treatment is based on the assumption that chronic or recurrent illnesses reflect a specific weakness or vulnerability in the patient's total constitution. It is intended to stimulate healing at the deepest levels of the person's emotions and psyche as well as physical characteristics.

Calcarea carbonica is one of the three most important remedies, along with *Lycopodium* and *Sulphur* in the traditional homeopath's medicine chest because all three are antipsoric remedies. The term antipsoric is derived from Hahnemann's theory of miasms. In homeopathy, a miasm is an inherited fundamental weakness or predisposition to chronic diseases. Hahnemann thought that the most ancient and universal miasm, the one that underlay the majority of the chronic illnesses that afflict humans, is the psoric miasm, or Psora. To define a remedy as antipsoric is to say that it is capable of healing a basic source of constitutional vulnerability to disease. Because *Calcarea carbonica* is an antipsoric remedy, it is also a polychrest remedy. Polychrest is the term used in homeopathy for a remedy that has many uses. *Calcarea carbonica* is used to treat a variety of diseases and disorders such as **acne**, arthritis, vaginal discharges in women, night terrors in children, and ringworm on the scalp.

Calcarea carbonica is, in general, considered a "chilly" remedy, appropriate for people who suffer keenly from the cold and have difficulty keeping warm. A homeopathic practitioner who is asking a patient about symptoms will inquire about the circumstances (e.g., light or dark, heat or cold, rest or activity) that make the patient feel better or worse. These factors are called modalities in homeopathy. In terms of modalities, patients who need *Calcarea carbonica* feel worse when they are cold. They may complain of a cold sensation in the abdomen and cold, clammy feet at night. Dampness, activity, and fright also make them feel worse. They feel better when they are warm and lying down.

Other aspects of *Calcarea carbonica* patients that are noted in the homeopathic literature are their tendency to tire easily, to move slowly and sluggishly, to sweat readily, and to have poor muscle tone and swollen lymph nodes. As a rule, they are passive, overweight people with fair or chalky complexions, large heads, and large puffy abdomens. They appear to be bloated rather than solidly muscular. Their perspiration and other body discharges often have a sour smell. Women may have excessively heavy menstrual periods (menorrhagia) and sore breasts before the flow begins. *Calcarea carbonica* patients often crave cold or iced drinks even when they do not have much appetite. By contrast, they may have cravings for indigestible nonfood items (pica), such as coal or chalk. They may dislike milk or meat and complain of headaches and **nausea** after meals.

The intellectual constitution of *Calcarea carbonica* patients is marked by the same slowness and lack of energy that characterizes their physical movements. They may complain of heaviness or sensations of pressure in the head when they are asked to do anything requiring intellectual effort. Children with a *Calcarea carbonica* constitution are slow to teethe and to walk, but they are also likely to be stubborn and strong-willed. Emotionally, *Calcarea carbonica* patients tend to be afraid of the dark, of isolation, of getting sick, and of going insane.

Preparations

Calcarea carbonica is available in tablet form as a single remedy and in a number of combination remedies. Since it is a polychrest remedy, it is manufactured

KEY TERMS

Aggravation—In homeopathy, a temporary worsening or intensification of the patient's symptoms prior to improvement and healing.

Antipsoric—A homeopathic remedy that is an effective constitutional treatment for the psoric miasm. *Calcarea carbonica* is one of three major antipsoric remedies.

Constitutional prescribing—Homeopathic treatment based on a total assessment of the person's life history, heredity, lifestyle, and present environment, as distinct from prescribing based on immediate acute symptoms.

Materia medica—A Latin phrase that means "the materials of medicine." In homeopathy, a *materia medica* is a book that lists the various homeopathic remedies together with the symptoms that they treat.

Miasm—In homeopathy, a hereditary weakness of the constitution and a corresponding predisposition to chronic disease.

Modality—A factor or circumstance that makes a patient's symptoms better or worse. Modalities include such factors as time of day, room temperature, the patient's level of activity, and sleep patterns.

Polychrest—A homeopathic remedy that can be given for a wide variety of diseases and conditions.

Psora—According to Hahnemann, the oldest and most universal miasm, responsible for human vulnerability to the majority of non-venereal chronic diseases.

Trituration—A method of preparing a homeopathic remedy from an insoluble substance by grinding or pounding it into a fine powder. *Calcarea carbonica* is prepared from shells by trituration.

by all major suppliers of homeopathic medicines and can be easily purchased from homeopathic pharmacies or over the Internet.

Precautions

In homeopathy, most precautions about the remedies concern proper storage and administration. Homeopathic practitioners believe that remedies lose their power from exposure to heat, light, or other substances. Guidelines for proper storage of homeopathic remedies include keeping them away from strong sunlight and high temperatures, keeping them in their original containers, and not storing them near perfumes, bleach, or other strong-smelling substances. In addition, patients under the care of a homeopath are instructed to avoid coffee or products containing camphor (e.g., lip balms, chest rubs) during a period of homeopathic treatment and for two days after the last dose. Homeopaths believe that these substances counteract the effects of homeopathic remedies.

Precautions regarding homeopathic remedies also include avoiding contamination of the medicine. The patient should not touch the medicine; it should be dispensed into a cup and tipped directly into the mouth. Homeopathic remedies are not taken with water but allowed to dissolve in the mouth. Patients are asked not to eat or drink for about 20 minutes before and after each dose.

Side effects

Calcarea carbonica, like other homeopathic remedies, has so little of the original substance in the tablets that it is highly unlikely to produce side effects in the usual sense. In addition, because *Calcarea carbonica* is given more often for constitutional treatment than for acute illnesses, it is not as likely to produce the temporary worsening of the patient's symptoms known as aggravation.

Interactions

Homeopathic remedies are so dilute that they are highly unlikely to interact with allopathic medications. However, homeopathic *materia medica* indicates that the remedies can be complementary or incompatible with one another. According to Hahnemann, *Calcarea carbonica* should not be given before *Sulphur*. *Calcarea carbonica* is complementary with **belladonna** but incompatible with **bryonia**.

Resources

BOOKS

Chernin, Dennis. *The Complete Homeopathic Resource for Common Illnesses*. Berkeley, CA: North Atlantic Books, 2006.

Cummings, Stephen, and Dana Ullman. *Everybody's Guide to Homeopathic Medicines*, 3rd ed. New York: Tarcher, 2004.

OTHER

British Homeopathic Library.Hom-Inform. [cited April 20, 2008]. http://www.hom-inform.org.

ORGANIZATIONS

American Institute of Homeopathy, 801 N. Fairfax Street, Suite 306, Alexandria, VA, 22314, (888) 445-9988, http://homeopathyusa.org.

National Center for Homeopathy, 801 N. Fairfax St., Suite 306, Alexandria, VA, 22314, (703) 548-7790, http://www.homeopathic.org/contact.htm.

Rebecca Frey
Tish Davidson, A. M.

Calcium

Description

As the most plentiful mineral in the body, calcium plays a key role in the development and maintenance of bones and teeth. Calcium enables the contraction of muscles, including the function of the body's most important muscle, the heart. It is also essential for normal blood clotting, proper nerve impulse transmission, and the appropriate support of connective tissue.

Almost every segment of the population—women, children, teenagers, men, unborn babies, and the elderly—benefit from calcium in their daily **diets**. The mineral is an important dietary supplement for those who are undergoing significant periods of bone growth, such as in childhood, during **pregnancy**, and while breast-feeding.

Calcium is an effective weapon for the **aging** population as they combat **osteoporosis**. A condition that simply means "porous bones," osteoporosis attacks bones when they are their most vulnerable. As the body ages, bones lose more calcium, and it becomes vital to supplement the diet with calcium in order to encourage bone growth and prevent or slow the process of bone loss.

General use

While the body relies on the presence of calcium for many of its everyday functions, reasons why the mineral should be supplemented in the diet are numerous. Calcium is beneficial to everyone, but research has found that women may benefit more than men. Studies have shown that pregnant women who do not get enough calcium in their diets can increase the bone mineral content of their fetus by as much as 15% by taking 1,300 mg of a calcium supplement per day during their second and third trimesters. For those women who already consume enough calcium, the additional supplements do not have this effect.

Recommended dietary allowance of calcium

Age	mg/day
Children 0-6 mos.	210 (AI)
Children 7-12 mos.	270 (AI)
Children 1-3 yrs.	500
Children 4-8 yrs.	800
Children 9-13 yrs.	900
Children 14-18 yrs.	1,300
Adults 19-50 yrs.	1,000
Adults > 50 yrs	1,200
Pregnant women ≤ 18 yrs.	1,300
Breastfeeding women ≤ 18 yrs.	1,300
Pregnant women ≥ 19 yrs.	1,000
Breatfeeding women 19 ≥ yrs.	1,000

Foods that contain calcium

	mg
Yogurt, plain, 1 cup	415
Cheese, mozzarella, 1.5 oz.	372
Sardines with bones, canned in oil, 3 oz.	324
Cheese, cheddar, 1.5 oz.	305
Milk, any type, 1 cup	300
Yogurt with fruit, 1 cup	245-384
Tofu, firm, with calcium sulfate, 1/2 cup	204
Orange juice, fortified, 6 oz.	200-260
Salmon with bones, canned, 3 oz.	181
Spinach, cooked, 1/2 cup	120
Beans, white, cooked, 1/2 cup	113
Instant breakfast drink, powder, prepared with water	105-250
Cereal, fortified, 1 cup	100-1,000
Bok choy, cooked, 1/2 cup	61
Beans, pinto or red, cooked, 1/2 cup	43
Bread, whole wheat, 1 slice	20

AI = Adequate intake
mg = milligram

(Illustration by GGS Information Services. Cengage Learning, Gale)

Additional research shows that calcium deficiencies lead to preeclampsia during pregnancy, causing high blood pressure, swelling, and weight gain greater than 1 lb (0.5 kg) per day. The risk of preeclampsia is reduced by 45–75% for women who receive calcium supplementation.

Premenstrual syndrome (PMS) is another condition that may be alleviated by the use of calcium supplements. Researchers at the National Institute of Mental Health (NIMH) have concluded that women who take 1,200 mg of calcium per day reduce their overall PMS symptoms by more than 50%. In one study, calcium supplementation led to the reduction of psychological PMS symptoms (such as mood swings) by 45%, food cravings by 54%, and bloating and water retention by 36%.

Some studies have shown that increasing the amount of daily calcium consumed by women may reduce their risk of **stroke**. Women in the 1999 Nurses' Health Study who took more than 400 mg of calcium daily were at the lowest risk for a stroke, while those who consumed more than 600 mg each day did not have an increased benefit. Researchers explain these results by suggesting that the risk of stroke is reduced by calcium from decreased **cholesterol** levels, or by stopping the formation of **blood clots** that cause strokes. More recent studies raise doubts about the 1999 findings, however. In 2008, researchers at New Zealand's University of Auckland reported that calcium supplements actually increased the risk of stroke among postmenopausal women.

For elderly postmenopausal women, the prevention of osteoporosis becomes critical. A number of studies have demonstrated that a low-dose hormone replacement therapy (HRT) combined with calcium and **vitamin D** supplementation is an effective therapeutic option for prevention of osteoporosis. Estriol, which is used in HRT, appears to be helpful in controlling menopausal symptoms.

Calcium alone is frequently prescribed with estrogen at the beginning of **menopause** to treat or prevent osteoporosis. This therapy is recommended to guard against the increased loss of calcium in the bones due to advancing age. As bones lose more calcium they become dense and brittle, and more vulnerable to the attack of osteoporosis. This condition is most common in people over age 70, and in women after menopause, where it may increase the risk of broken hips, ribs, and pelvis, and the weakening of other bones. Increased physical **exercise** is also important for bone strengthening.

On the other hand, although calcium supplementation is useful in lowering the risk of osteoporosis in Western women, more research is needed to determine why the rates of osteoporosis are low in some Eastern societies with low-calcium diets. There is evidence that osteoporosis, like coronary artery disease, is primarily a problem in Western societies. In addition, accumulating evidence that a diet high in fruits and vegetables helps to prevent **fractures** suggests that the level of calcium in the diet is not the only nutritional factor involved in osteoporosis.

Calcium has been shown to be beneficial to the colon. Among persons taking calcium supplements, research points to a modest reduction in the recurrence of colon polyps. Colon polyps are benign tumors that may become cancerous. Researchers believe that calcium binds to carcinogens, preventing abnormal cell growth.

Stemming from its active role in building bone density throughout the body, calcium may prove particularly beneficial for strengthening the jawbone. Researchers have reported that calcium supplementation may prevent periodontal disease, for this reason Periodontal, or gum, disease is an infection caused by bacteria that deposits in pockets between the teeth and gums, and is the leading cause of tooth loss in the United States. As the infection progresses, the jawbone that holds a tooth in place is eventually destroyed, causing the tooth to loosen and fall out. Researchers believe that calcium's overall bone-building role results in the formation of a stronger jawbone that is better able to fight off **gum disease**.

While calcium supplements can be found in many forms, research has shown a promising benefit if it is obtained from dairy foods rather than supplements or leafy greens. Calcium in the form of dairy may actually prevent weight gain. In one study, those who consumed at least 1,000 mg of calcium a day (equaling about three cups, or 750 ml) of skim milk, gained 6–7 lb (about 3 kg) less over two years than those with low-calcium diets. Researchers who conducted the study speculate that calcium probably prevents weight gain by increasing the breakdown of body fat and decreasing its formation. It is important to note, however, that dairy products should be consumed in moderation, as other research has indicated that dairy products are not necessarily a good source of absorbable calcium. In addition, other studies indicate that women are often reluctant to increase their intake of dairy products because they dislike milk, suffer from lactose intolerance, or fear that they will gain too much weight.

Calcium is proving essential to those children around the world stricken by rickets. Rickets is a deficiency condition in children that affects developing cartilage and newly formed bone throughout the body, causing severe deformities. Often thought to be a result of inadequate intake of vitamin D from dietary sources or lack of exposure to sunlight, research has found that children with rickets respond well to calcium supplementation. While rickets is still rare in most developed countries, it remains a problem in many other parts of the world. Researchers conclude that effective treatment for the condition is calcium supplementation alone or in combination with vitamin D. Osteomalacia, or the adult form of rickets, also responds to calcium supplementation.

Evidence is accumulating in the United States that women are not the only group at risk for insufficient dietary levels of calcium. Children and adolescents are also at risk, according to a report from the National Institutes of Health. Researchers found that "only 13.5% of girls and 36.3% of boys ages 12 to 19 in the United States get the recommended daily amount (RDA) of calcium, placing them at serious risk for osteoporosis and other bone diseases" in their adult years. The report listed increased consumption of soft drinks and decreased consumption of milk as contributing to the problem.

Preparations

Calcium may be supplemented in the diet in a variety of ways. Numerous foods are rich in calcium, including dairy products (such as milk, yogurt, and cheese) and leafy green vegetables like turnip greens, broccoli, kale, and collards. Canned salmon, sardines, shrimp, and tofu are also high in calcium. More foods are being fortified with calcium, making it easier to ensure the proper amount of the mineral is consumed. Calcium-fortified foods range from **cranberry** juice cocktail, cereal, and waffles, to orange juice and flour. With almost every segment of the population consuming too little calcium, researchers recommend calcium-fortified foods to increase daily calcium intake.

While the types of foods containing calcium continues to increase, most people still lack enough of the essential mineral. For those who are not getting adequate calcium from foods, supplements are an acceptable alternative. The chemical form of calcium supplements comes in these varieties: carbonate, citrate, lactate, phosphate, chelate, and citrate malate. Supplements are available as tablets, syrup, or suspension. Calcium supplements should be stored at room temperature and away from moisture and sunlight. They should not be stored in the bathroom, and the liquid forms should not be frozen.

Experts state that calcium is best absorbed from the citrate malate form, or the type of calcium found in some juices, but they recommend calcium carbonate for the overall amount of calcium it offers as well as its affordability. Calcium carbonate can be found in antacids, and is absorbed better when taken with meals. Food slows down the time it takes substances to travel through the gut, giving the calcium more time to be absorbed. Absorption is key for the proper functioning of calcium. Sufficient levels of vitamin D and hydrochloric acid in the stomach, and the presence of other minerals such as **magnesium** and phosphorous, are essential for quick absorption.

The body may also be better able to absorb calcium when it is taken along with ingredients extracted from **chicory** root. Research indicates that Raftilin inulin and Raftilose oligofructose, both extracts from chicory root, are dietary fibers that are not digested in the stomach or the small intestine. Instead, they are fermented by bifidobacteria in the colon, beneficially leading to increased calcium absorption throughout the body, with emphasis on bone tissue. Additionally, oligofructose improves the texture and mouth feel while improving taste and fruit flavors in low-fat yogurts. Inulin is used for fat replacement and fiber enrichment of reduced-fat and fat-free sour cream and whipped topping.

There are many ways to ensure calcium is part of a daily diet, but it is important that the recommended daily allowance (RDA), or appropriate dosage of the mineral be followed. The RDA of calcium for adults is 800 mg; pregnant women and young adults should be certain their intake equals 1,200 mg per day. Adults over age 50 should increase their intake to 1,000 mg per day with supplements that include vitamin D.

Calcium supplements may be taken with a large glass of water during or after a meal. Tablets in chewable form must be chewed thoroughly before swallowing, and effervescent tablets should be diluted in cold water or juice before taking. Experts recommend that other medications be taken two hours after any calcium supplement. The simultaneous intake of calcium may interfere with the absorption of other drugs. For best absorption of the mineral, no more than 500 mg of calcium should be taken at one time.

Precautions

When adding calcium supplements to the diet, practitioners recommend that it not be taken within one to two hours of eating bran or whole grain cereals or breads. Large amounts of alcohol or caffeine-containing beverages or tobacco should be avoided. Large amounts of calcium, phosphates, magnesium, or vitamin D in medication or dietary supplements should not be taken unless directed by a physician. Those with **diarrhea**, stomach problems, parathyroid disease, sarcoidosis, or **kidney stones** should consult with their physician before taking calcium.

Side effects

Calcium is typically well tolerated by those who add it to their diets, but if the mineral is taken in high levels it can cause several side effects, including: **nausea, vomiting**, loss of appetite, **constipation**, stomach **pain**, thirst,

KEY TERMS

Carcinogen—Any substance or agent that produces or instigates cancer.

Preeclampsia—A toxemia of pregnancy that causes increasing hypertension, headaches, and swelling of the lower extremities.

Sarcoidosis—A disease of unknown etiology, which causes widespread lesions that may affect any organ or tissue of the body.

Stroke—A hemorrhage into the brain, formation of a clot in an artery, or rupture of an artery that causes sudden loss of consciousness, followed by paralysis.

dry mouth, increased urination, and weakness. While these side effects are rare, a person is even more unlikely to experience the life-threatening symptoms of an irregular or very slow heart beat. If these dangerous symptoms appear while taking calcium, use of the mineral should be discontinued and emergency treatment should be sought. An overdose of a calcium supplement may lead to confusion, irregular heartbeat, **depression**, bone pain, or coma.

Interactions

All over-the-counter (OTC) or prescription medications should be reviewed with a physician before beginning calcium supplementation.

According to the *Complete Guide to Prescription & Nonprescription Drugs,* the following are some of the drugs that may cause possible interactions if taken with calcium:

- alendronate
- anticoagulants
- calcitonin
- calcium-containing medicines
- chlorpromazine
- oral contraceptives
- corticosteroids
- digitalis preparations
- diuretics, thiazide
- estrogens
- etidronate
- iron supplements
- meperidine
- mexiletine
- nalidixic acid
- nicardipine
- nimodipine
- oxyphenbutazone
- para-aminosalicyclic acid (PAS)
- penicillins
- pentobarbital
- phenylbutazone
- phenytoin
- pseudoephedrine
- quinidine
- salicylates

Resources

BOOKS

Krebs, Joachim, and Marek Michalak, eds. *Calcium : A Matter of Life or Death.* Amsterdam: Elsevier Science, 2007.

Weaver, Connie M., and Robert P. Heaney, eds. *Calcium in Human Health.* Totowa, N.J.: Humana Press, 2005.

PERIODICALS

Austin, Steve. "Vitamin D and Calcium Supplementation Reduce Cancer Incidence in Women in a Randomized Trial." *Original Internist* (September 2007): 141–142.

D'Amico, Cara. "Calcium & You: Not Getting Enough Calcium in Your Body Is Bad News for Your Growing Bones. Here's What You Can Do about It." *Scholastic Choices* (April 2007): 22–26.

Kranz, S., P. J. Lin, and D. A. Wagstaff. "Children's Dairy Intake in the United States: Too Little, Too Fat." *Journal of Pediatrics* (July 2007): 642–646.

Lee, Y. H., et al. "Inadequate Dietary Calcium Intake in Elderly Patients with Hip Fractures." *Singapore Medical Journal* (December 2007): 1117–1121.

Park, Yikyung, et al. "Calcium, Dairy Foods, and Risk of Incident and Fatal Prostate Cancer." *American Journal of Epidemiology* (October 2007): 1270–1279.

Walsh, Nancy. "Supplemental Calcium Fails to Prevent Weight Gain." *Family Practice News* (December 2006): 38–39.

ORGANIZATIONS

Food and Drug Administration, Office of Consumer Affairs, HFE–88, Rockville, MD, 20857, http://www.fda.gov/.

Beth Kapes
Rebecca J. Frey, Ph.D.
David Edward Newton, Ed.D.

Calendula

Description

Calendula (*Calendula officinalis*) is also known as garden marigold, holligold, goldbloom, golds, ruddes, Mary bud, bull's eyes, and pot marigold. It is a member of the Asteraceae family. Other members of this plant family include daisies, **arnica**, **chamomile**, and **yarrow**. This bright, flowering herb opens its gold blossoms in the morning and closes them at dusk, or when rain threatens. Calendula is native to Asia and southern and central Europe. Early settlers brought the herb to North America where it has become a garden favorite. It is cultivated throughout the world and valued for its culinary and medicinal uses. The first name, *Calendula*, is from the Latin *kalendae*, the word Romans used to indicate that it bloomed throughout the year in their area. The second name *officinalis* indicates that calendula was included in official lists of medicinal herbs. The common name marigold refers to the blossoms' association with the Virgin Mary.

Calendula is a familiar garden plant with yellow or orange-gold blooms that have a strong and distinctive scent. The plant likes sun and will re-seed from year to year, even in poor soil. The erect, square and branching stems emerge from a taproot to grow up to 2 ft (0.6 m) high. The lower leaves are broad and spatula shaped. Upper leaves may be oblong, are smooth at the edges, and are arranged alternately along the stem. Blossoms may be single or double, are 1–4 in (2.54–10.2 cm) across, and are made of many small florets. The bushy herb blooms continuously throughout the summer. Seeds are crescent to horseshoe shaped with a rough exterior.

General use

Calendula has been used for centuries as a culinary, medicinal, and magical herb. It was believed that calendula could bring protection against dangerous influences. The seventeenth century astrologer and doctor, Nicholas Culpeper, taught that the marigolds were under the influence of the constellation Leo. The flowers, he said were "a comforter of the heart and spirits." The bright yellow blossom of this herb was used to make a dye to color cheese and butter. In the kitchen, leaves and florets were added to sauces, soups, porridge, and puddings for color and medicinal benefit. The dried, powdered blossoms have also been used as a substitute for **saffron** in cooking. During the Civil War, calendula was used to stop the blood flow from battle **wounds**. Calendula blossom preparations continue to be valued as an antiseptic for external application to scrapes, **burns**, **cuts**, or wounds. Local application, in the form of a plant poultice or an infusion soaked in a cloth and applied to a wound, is an effective healing remedy. The Romans valued the herb for its ability to break fevers. During the Middle Ages, calendula used for protection against the plague. In early American Shaker medicine, calendula was a treatment for **gangrene**.

In addition to its first aid uses, calendula also acts as a digestive remedy. An infusion or tincture of the flowers, taken internally, is beneficial in the treatment of ulcers, stomach cramps, **colitis**, herpes viruses, yeast **infections**, and **diarrhea**. An infusion may also be used as an external wash helpful in treating bee **stings**, eye inflammations, **boils** and abscesses, **varicose veins**, **eczema**, **acne**, and as a gargle for mouth sores or a rinse to relieve **toothache**. The flowers have antispasmodic, antimicrobial, and antiviral properties. They improve the circulation of the blood and the lymphatic fluids and aid in elimination of toxins from the body. The juice from the fresh flowers or stem is said to help remove **warts** and help heal mucous membranes and skin. An infusion or tincture of the herb is also helpful in cases of painful or delayed **menstruation**, and the herb is a beneficial ally in the transition to **menopause**. The tincture also has many other uses, such as a topical wash for **diaper rash** in infants, a mouth gargle for sores, a vaginal douche for yeast, an internal soother for inflamed lungs, a topical for **hemorrhoids**, etc.

Despite a large number of studies on the chemical constituents of calendula flowers, the agents responsible for the herb's healing properties haven't been clearly determined. Constituents include saponins, **carotenoids**, resin, bitter principle, essential oil, sterols, flavonoids, and mucilage.

Preparations

Calendula blossoms are harvested when fully open throughout the flowering season. The flower heads are picked on a sunny day after the morning dew has evaporated. The blossoms are then spread on a paper-lined tray to dry in a bright and airy room away from direct sun. The temperature in the drying room should be at least 70°F (21°C). When the blossoms are completely dry, the florets are removed, and the center part of the blossom is thrown away. The dried florets are then be stored in a dark glass container with an airtight lid. The dried herb will maintain medicinal potency for 12 to18 months. The container should be clearly labeled with the name of the herb, the date, and place harvested. The fresh juice of calendula flowers is preserved with 20% alcohol; the traditional tincture contains 50% alcohol.

Infusions are made by placing 2 oz (56.7 g) of fresh or half as much dried calendula blossom florets in a warm glass container. Then 2.5 cups (0.56 kg) of fresh, nonchlorinated water that has been boiled is added to the herbs. The mixture is then covered and steeped for ten to fifteen minutes. Next, the mixture is strained and the tea is drunk warm. The prepared tea will store for about two days in the refrigerator. Calendula blossom tea may be drunk by the cupful up to three times a day, as needed, or applied as an external skin wash.

An ointment is made by mixing dried and powdered calendula florets with olive oil. The combination is then mixed with melted beeswax. Then it is poured into dark glass jars while still warm. The mixture is sealed tightly with a lid when cool.

Precautions

Calendula shouldn't be used during **pregnancy**. It also shouldn't be confused with the French marigold *Tagetes patula*, sometimes grown in gardens as an insect repellant.

Side effects

Calendula is a relatively mild, nontoxic herbal medicine with no known side effects reported.

Interactions

None reported.

Resources

BOOKS

Ody, Penelope. *The Complete Medicinal Herbal*. New York: Dorling Kindersley, 1993.
PDR for Herbal Medicines. New Jersey: Medical Economics Company, 1998.
Phillips, Roger, and Nicky Foy. *The Random House Book of Herbs*. New York: Random House, 1990.
Tyler, Varro E., Ph.D. *Herbs Of Choice, The Therapeutic Use of Phytomedicinals*. New York: The Haworth Press, Inc., 1994.
Tyler, Varro E., Ph.D. *The Honest Herbal*. New York: Pharmaceutical Products Press, 1993.
Weiss, Gaea, and Shandor Weiss. *Growing & Using the Healing Herbs*. New York: Wings Books, 1992.

Clare Hanrahan

Calluses *see* **Corns and calluses**
Camellia sinensis see **Green tea**
Canadensis see **Elder**

Cancer

Definition

Cancer is not a single disease but a group of about 100 diseases characterized by the uncontrolled growth of abnormal cells, many of which form masses (tumors), and the ability of those cells to spread by way of the circulatory and lymphatic systems from the original site to distant parts of the body, invade other tissues, and form new tumors. This process is called metastasis. If metastasis is not controlled, cancer can result in death.

Description

Cancer is the second leading cause of death (after **heart disease**) in the United States. According to the American Cancer Society, in 2008 cancer accounted for one out of every four deaths or over half a million people. In 2008, more than 1.4 million Americans were anticipated to be newly diagnosed with cancer. This number excludes the 1 million Americans who were expected to be diagnosed with basal and squamous cell **skin cancer** (non-melanoma skin cancer) or all those who were to be diagnosed with carcinoma in situ (early cancer that has not spread). In people diagnosed with cancer between 1996 and 2003, the five-year survival rate (people alive five years after they were diagnosed) for all cancers combined was about 66%, although survival rates of different types of cancer vary substantially. The National Health Institute estimated that in 2007 the cost of cancer in the United States was $219.2 billion.

Although cancer can develop in people of any age or race, more than three-quarters of cancers are diagnosed in people over age 55. Although all racial groups are affected by cancer, African American men get cancer at a higher rate than any other racial groups, followed in number by white men, then African American women. In 2008, the most common cancers diagnosed in the United States were non-melanoma skin cancer, **lung cancer**, **colorectal cancer** (cancer of the colon and/or rectum), **breast cancer** (in women), and **prostate cancer** (in men). Cancer of the bladder, non-Hodgkin's lymphoma, melanoma (aggressive skin cancer), kidney, **leukemia** (blood cancer), endometrium (lining of the uterus), pancreas, and thyroid complete the list of major cancers that affect most Americans.

Cancer is thought to occur because of small changes (mutations) in genes. A gene is a small packet of deoxyribonucleic acid (DNA), the master molecule

Cancer-fighting foods

Foods	Effects on cancer
Avocados	May attack free radicals in the body by blocking intestinal absorption of certain fats; may be useful in treating viral hepatitis (a cause of liver cancer)
Beans	May prevent or slow genetic damage to cells, prevent prostate cancer, and lower the risk of digestive cancers
Berries	May help prevent skin, bladder, lung, and breast cancers and slow the reproduction of cancer cells
Cabbage and cauliflower	May slow cancer growth and development and help to reduce the risk of lung, prostate, and bladder cancers
Broccoli	May prevent some types of cancer, including stomach, colon and rectal
Carrots	May reduce a wide range of cancers including lung, mouth, throat, stomach, intestine, bladder, prostate and breast
Chili peppers and jalapeños	May prevent cancers such as stomach cancer
Cruciferous vegetables (broccoli, cauliflower, kale, Brussels sprouts, and cabbage)	May help decrease prostate and other cancers
Dark green leafy vegetables	May reduce the risk of lung and breast cancer
Figs	May shrink tumors
Flax	May reduce the risk of breast, skin, and lung cancer
Garlic	May increase the activity of immune cells that fight cancer and indirectly help break down cancer causing substances. May help block carcinogens from entering cells and slow tumor development. May render carcinogens in the liver inactive May lower risk of a variety of cancers including stomach, colon, lung and skin
Grapefruits	May prevent cancer by sweeping carcinogens out of the body and inhibit the proliferation of breast-cancer cells in vitro
Grapes	May inhibit the enzymes that can stimulate cancer-cell growth and suppress immune response
Kale	May help stop the conversion of certain lesions to cancerous cells in estrogen-sensitive tissues, suppress tumor growth, and block cancer-causing substances from reaching their targets
Licorice root	May prevent the growth of prostate cancer
Mushrooms	May help the body fight cancer and build the immune system
Nuts	May suppress the growth of cancers
Oranges and lemons	May stimulate cancer-killing immune cells like lymphocytes that may function in breaking down cancer-causing substances
Papayas	May reduce absorption of cancer-causing nitrosamines from the soil or processed foods. May minimize cervical dysplasia and certain cancers
Red wine	May inhibit cell proliferation and help prevent cancer
Rosemary	May inhibit the development of breast and skin tumors
Seaweed and other sea vegetables	May help in the fight against breast cancer
Soy products like tofu	May help to prevent breast and prostate cancer by blocking and suppressing cancerous changes
Sweet potatoes	May prevent cancer cells from dividing, reduce the risk of cancer of the stomach, lung, colon, rectum, liver and pancreas, and protect against various types of cancer
Tomatoes	May combat prostate cancer and protect against breast, lung, mouth, stomach, and pancreatic cancer. May reduce risk of breast, prostate, pancreas and colorectal cancer. May prevent cellular damage that leads to cancer.
Tumeric	May inhibit the production of the inflammation-related enzyme cyclo-oxygenase 2 (COX-2), which reaches abnormally high levels in certain inflammatory diseases and cancers, especially bowel and colon cancer
Whole grains	May help decrease the risk of developing most types of cancer

(Illustration by GGS Information Services. Cengage Learning, Gale)

of the cell that is inherited from each parent. Genes control all aspects of development and metabolism. Small changes in the structure of genes can cause changes in proteins that regulate body functions.

One characteristic different types of cancer have in common is unregulated cell growth. In healthy cells, cell division is controlled by proteins regulated by genes. Specific genes make proteins that signal healthy cells when to stop dividing. In cancer, the controlling gene(s) is damaged or mutated and does not produce the proteins necessary to signal cells to stop dividing. Abnormal cells are formed all the time from mutations, but in a healthy individual, the immune system recognizes these cells as abnormal and destroys them. However, some mutant cells may escape destruction and survive to grow into tumors. Cancer cells continue to divide aggressively, often forming a clump called tumor or neoplasm. (Neoplasm means "new growth.") Cells can break off from the tumor, travel through the circulatory system to other parts of the body and lodge

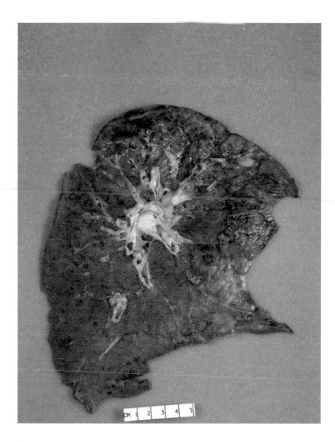

Cancer in the bronchus. (© Medical-on-Line / Alamy)

in new tissues where they begin to grow again and form new tumors.

Tumors are of two types, benign and malignant. A benign tumor is not considered cancer. It is a slow growing tumor that does not spread or invade surrounding tissue, and once removed, it is not likely to recur. A malignant tumor, by contrast, invades surrounding tissue and has the capacity to spread to other parts of the body. Even when the original, or primary, tumor is removed, if the cancer cells have spread (metastasized) or if all the primary tumor cells are not removed or killed, cancer recurs.

Cancers are defined by the type of cell in which they originate and the organ of the body where the primary tumor is located. Carcinomas are cancers that arise in the epithelium (the layer of cells covering the body's surface and lining the internal organs and various glands). About 90% of human cancers are carcinomas. Carcinomas can be subdivided into two types: adenocarcinomas and squamous cell carcinomas. Adenocarcinomas are cancers that develop in an organ or a gland, while squamous cell carcinomas are cancers that originate in the skin. Melanomas are cancers that originate in the skin in the pigment cells

(melanocytes) Sarcomas are cancers of the supporting tissues of the body, such as bone, muscle, and blood vessels. Gliomas are cancers of the nerve tissue and are usually found in the brain and spinal cord. Cancers of the blood arise in the bone marrow and are called leukemias, and cancers of the lymph glands are called lymphomas. These two cancers do not form primary tumors.

Causes and symptoms

Cancer does not have a single identifiable cause. Researchers believe that about three-quarters of all cancers are caused by changes in the cell's DNA that occur because of interaction with the environment. Some cancers are caused by faulty DNA in genes inherited from the individual's parents, however, fewer than 10% of all cancers are clearly hereditary. The most common causes of cancer appear to involve an interaction between the individual's genetics, the environment, and lifestyle choices. These include such factors as tobacco use, exposure to ultraviolet light, radiation, industrial chemicals such as asbestos, and environmental toxins. The cell's DNA is also affected by internal conditions such as inherited mutations (changes in the gene passed from parent to offspring), hormone levels in the body, immune system functioning, and damage caused by cellular metabolism. These internal factors can predispose the individual to developing certain types of cancer. Cancers that are known to have a hereditary link include breast cancer, colon cancer, **ovarian cancer**, and **uterine cancer**. In some cases, scientists have been able to identify defects in specific genes that predispose an individual to developing a certain type of cancer.

Advances in molecular biology and cancer genetics have contributed to the development of several tests designed to assess one's risk of getting cancers. These new techniques include genetic testing to identify mutations in certain genes that have been linked to particular cancers. As of 2008, however, there were limitations to genetic testing and its utility and ethical use appeared ambiguous.

Risk factors

The major risk factors for developing cancer are:

- tobacco use
- alcohol use/abuse
- sexual and reproductive behavior
- specific dietary factors
- exposure to certain infectious agents
- family history of cancer (genetic inheritance)

- occupational exposure to carcinogens
- environmental exposure to carcinogens (pollution)

TOBACCO. Tobacco use is thought to be the cause of about one-third of all cancers and 80 to 90% of lung cancer cases. **Smoking** has also been shown to be a contributory factor in cancers of the upper respiratory tract, esophagus, larynx, bladder, pancreas, and probably liver, stomach, breast, and kidney, as well. Chewing tobacco, snuff, and pipe smoking have been linked to cancers of the mouth and throat. Scientists also have demonstrated that exposure to secondhand smoke can increase the risk of an individual developing cancer. The American Cancer Society estimated in 2008 that about 170,000 cancer deaths annually are directly caused by tobacco use.

ALCOHOL. Heavy consumption of alcohol is a risk factor in certain cancers, such as liver cancer. Alcohol, in combination with tobacco, significantly increases the chances that an individual will develop mouth, pharynx, larynx, and esophageal cancers.

DIET. The American Cancer Society anticipated that about one-third of the cancer deaths in 2008 would be caused by **obesity**, lack of physical **exercise**, and poor **nutrition**. High intake of fat leading to obesity has been associated with cancers of the breast, colon, rectum, pancreas, prostate, gall bladder, ovaries, and uterus.

SEXUAL AND REPRODUCTIVE BEHAVIOR. The human papillomavirus (HPV), which is spread through sexual activity with an infected individual, has been shown to cause cancer of the cervix. In 2007, a vaccine against the virus that causes cervical cancer was introduced. The vaccination process requires three doses of vaccine spread over one year and is paid for by some insurance companies. Having multiple sex partners and becoming sexually active early increases a woman's chance of contracting cervical cancer. In addition, it has also been shown that women who have not had children or who have children late in life have an increased risk for both ovarian and breast cancer.

INFECTIOUS AGENTS. Research scientists believe as of 2008 that about 15% of the world's cancer deaths may be caused by viruses, bacteria, or parasites.

FAMILY HISTORY. Certain cancers such as breast, colon, ovarian, and uterine cancer, tend to run in families. A few cancers, such as the eye cancer retinoblastoma, a specific subtype of colon cancer, and a subtype of breast cancer known as early-onset breast cancer, have definitively been linked to certain genes that can be tracked within a family. It appears that inheriting specific genes makes a person susceptible to certain types of cancers.

OCCUPATIONAL HAZARDS. Certain occupations expose workers to hazards that increase the risk of cancer. For example, asbestos workers have an increased incidence of a specific type of lung cancer. Similarly, a higher likelihood of getting **bladder cancer** is associated with dye, rubber, and gas workers; skin and lung cancer with smelters, gold miners, and arsenic workers; leukemia with glue and varnish workers; liver cancer with PVC manufacturers; and lung, bone, and bone marrow cancer with radiologists and uranium miners.

ENVIRONMENT. Exposure is believed to cause 1 to 2% of all cancer deaths. Ultra-violet radiation from the sun accounts for a majority of melanoma deaths. Other sources of radiation are x rays, radon gas, and ionizing radiation from nuclear material. Environmental pollution can be difficult to pinpoint as a source of cancer because cancer often develops years after exposure. However, researchers have estimated that about 1% of cancer deaths are due to air, land, and water pollution.

Alternative views of cancer causes

Practitioners of systems of alternative medicine tend to disagree with conventional medical findings about the causes of cancer, claiming that environmental pollution and emotional and psychological factors are major causes of the disease. Samuel S. Epstein, professor emeritus of Occupational and Environmental Medicine at the University of Illinois and the chairman of the Cancer Prevention Coalition, is one of the strongest critics of those approaches to preventing and treating cancer accepted by the National Cancer Institute (NCI), the American Cancer Society (ACS), and conventional Western medicine.

Epstein's views echo many of the beliefs of alternative practitioners. He claims that mainstream medicine, driven by politics, profits, and pharmaceutical sales, is not discussing or sufficiently researching some major factors behind cancer or researching ways of preventing those causes. Epstein asserts that a primary cause of cancer is the massive pollution of the air, water, food, and workplace. Epstein believes that the human immune system simply cannot handle all the new carcinogens that have been introduced into the environment since the 1950s. In his view, cancer represents a breakdown of the immune system. Epstein is also a critic of some conventional cancer therapies such as radiation and chemotherapy, claiming that the therapies themselves are highly carcinogenic and are often responsible for recurrent cancer. These views are in line with those held by many alternative medicine practitioners.

Symptoms

Cancer is a progressive disease and goes through several stages with varying symptoms. Some symptoms are produced early and may occur due to a tumor that is growing within an organ or a gland. As the tumor grows, it may press on the nearby nerves, organs, and blood vessels, causing **pain** and some pressure that may be the earliest warning signs of cancer. Other cancers cause general symptoms such as **fatigue** or loss of appetite. Despite the fact that there are different types of cancers with different symptoms, the ACS has established the following seven symptoms as possible warning signals of cancer:

- changes in the size, color, or shape of a wart or a mole
- a sore that does not heal
- persistent cough, hoarseness, or sore throat
- a lump or thickening in the breast or elsewhere
- unusual bleeding or discharge
- chronic indigestion or difficulty in swallowing
- persistent changes in bowel or bladder habits

Many diseases other than cancer can cause these symptoms. However, individuals with these symptoms should be checked promptly, especially if the symptoms have persisted for some time. For all types of cancer, the earlier a cancer is diagnosed and treated, the better the chance of surviving it. Many cancers, such as breast cancer, may not have any symptoms. Screening examinations conducted regularly by healthcare professionals can result in the detection of cancers of the breast, colon, rectum, cervix, prostate, testis, tongue, mouth, and skin at early stages. Some routine screening tests recommended by the ACS are sigmoidoscopy for colorectal cancer, mammography for breast cancer, Pap smear for cervical cancer, and the PSA blood test for prostate cancer. Self-examinations for cancers of the breast, testes, mouth, and skin can also help in detecting the tumors early.

Diagnosis

Diagnosis begins with a thorough physical examination and a complete medical history. The doctor observes, feels, and palpates (applies pressure by touch) different parts of the body in order to identify any variation from the normal size, shape, and texture of the organ or tissue. As part of the physical examination, the doctor inspects the mouth. Focusing a light into the mouth can reveal abnormalities in color, moisture, surface texture, or presence of any thickening or soreness in the lips, tongue, gums, the hard palate on the roof of the mouth, and the throat.

To detect thyroid cancer, the doctor palpates the front and side surfaces of the thyroid gland (located at the base of the neck) to detect any nodules or tenderness. As part of the physical examination, the doctor also palpates the lymph nodes in the neck, under the arms, and in the groin. Many illnesses and cancers cause swelling of the lymph nodes. The doctor may conduct a thorough examination of the skin to look for sores that have been present for more than three weeks and that bleed, ooze, or crust; irritated patches that may itch or hurt; and any change in the size of a wart or a mole.

Examination of the female pelvis is used to detect cancers of the ovaries, uterus, cervix, and vagina. In the visual examination, the doctor looks for abnormal discharges or the presence of sores. Then, using gloved hands the physician palpates the internal pelvic organs such as the uterus and ovaries to detect any abnormal masses. A swab is used to remove mucus and cells from the cervix (a Pap test). This sample is sent to a laboratory for microscopic examination of abnormal cells. Breast examination includes visual observation where the doctor looks for any discharge, unevenness, discoloration, or scaling. The doctor palpates both breasts for masses or lumps.

For males, inspection of the rectum and the prostate is also included in the physical examination. The doctor inserts a gloved finger into the rectum and rotates it slowly to feel for any growths, tumors, or other abnormalities. The doctor also conducts an examination of the testes, in which the doctor observes the genital area and looks for swelling or other abnormalities. The testicles are palpated to identify any lumps, thickening, or differences in the size, weight, and firmness.

If the doctor detects an abnormality on physical examination, or the patient has some symptom that could indicate cancer, the doctor may order diagnostic tests. Laboratory studies of sputum (sputum cytology), blood, urine, and stool can detect abnormalities that may indicate cancer. Sputum cytology is a test in which the phlegm that is coughed up from the lungs is microscopically examined. It is often used to detect lung cancer. A blood test that indicates certain cancers (e.g., prostate cancer) is easy to perform, relatively inexpensive, and practically risk-free. Blood tests can be either specific or non-specific. In certain cancers, the cancer cells release specific proteins (called tumor markers), and blood tests can be used to detect the presence of these markers, which indicate the presence of cancer. However, with a few exceptions, tumor markers are not used for routine screening of cancers because several non-cancerous conditions also produce positive results. Blood tests tend to be more useful in monitoring the effectiveness of the treatment or in following the course of the disease and detecting recurrent disease.

Imaging tests such as computed tomography scans (CT scans), magnetic resonance imaging (MRI), ultrasound, and fiber optic scope examinations help doctors determine the location of the tumor even if it is deep within the body. Conventional x rays are often used for initial evaluation because they are relatively cheap, painless, and easily accessible. In order to increase the information obtained from a conventional x ray, air or a dye (such as barium or **iodine**) may be used as a contrast medium to outline or highlight parts of the body.

The most definitive diagnostic test for cancer is the biopsy, wherein a piece of tissue is surgically removed for microscope examination. Besides confirming a cancer, the biopsy provides information about the type of cancer, the stage it has reached, the aggressiveness of the cancer, and the extent of its spread. Since a biopsy provides the most accurate information, it is considered the definitive diagnostic test.

Diagnosis in alternative treatment often relies on conventional diagnostic tools for determining the type and stage of cancer but will supplement those tools with diagnostic techniques that strive to evaluate the overall mental and physical health of a person in order to treat a person holistically. For example, **Ayurvedic medicine** and **traditional Chinese medicine** place high priorities during diagnosis on the patient's emotional and psychological history, as well as considerations such as lifestyle, relationships, and the degree of social and spiritual support, in order to have insight into the cause and proper treatment of a particular cancer. These alternative practices also have highly developed diagnostic techniques for the body, including **pulse diagnosis**; methods of analyzing the tongue, eyes, skin, hair, and fingernails; palpating and finding abnormalities in various organs; and listening to the breath for clues to the internal environment.

Treatment

Choosing an alternative cancer treatment

A multitude of complementary and alternative treatments are available to help a person with cancer. Complementary treatments are usually integrated with allopathic treatments such as surgery, chemotherapy, and radiation therapy. It is estimated that only about 4% of people with cancer reject all conventional medicine and rely exclusively on alternative medicine. Chemotherapy and radiation treatments are some of the most painful and toxic of conventional

treatments and often have unpredictable, although often successful, results. As a rule, alternative treatments are less invasive, nontoxic, and have minimal side effects, but their efficacy has not been rigorously studied. When used as adjuncts to conventional treatment, many alternative therapies are successful in treating symptoms caused by cancer or conventional cancer treatment (e.g., chemotherapy) but are less successful in curing cancer. Many alternative treatments have been shown to decrease pain and **nausea**, aid in the recovery process, and improve the quality of life of cancer patients.

Alternative treatment of cancer is a complicated arena, and choosing one from the many options can be daunting. When choosing alternative treatment, individuals should evaluate practitioners, therapies, and services delivered by clinics or practitioners, as well as the extent of available documentation and published literature regarding these concerns. In seeking practitioners, patients should evaluate training, credentials, and reputations in the healing community. Referrals from other patients should be requested.

Cancer patients may also consider integrating alternative and conventional therapies, and they may search for traditional and alternative healthcare professionals who are willing to work together during treatment. Such practitioners are knowledgeable and familiar with a broad spectrum of options of treating cancer, including those used by both alternative and conventional medicine. If patients choose a physician who employs and recommends conventional, allopathic methods, that physician should be willing to communicate with patients and the alternative medical provider. An effective practitioner is trustworthy, ethical, and compassionate.

Patients must also evaluate the particular therapy offered by a practitioner or clinic. They should understand how the therapy works and the principles behind it. They need to realistically know the potential risks and benefits of both conventional and alternative therapies, what literature and scientific studies exist for each therapy, and what other patients say about the treatment.

Finally, patients should evaluate the quality of service that the practitioner or clinic offers. Cost, reputation, quality of support personnel, and attention to individual needs are important considerations when evaluating the service dimension of a treatment. Patients choosing an alternative medical practitioner should discuss with their insurance provider what, if any, services are covered under their insurance plan. Many alternative therapies are not covered and must be paid for out-of-pocket.

Types of alternative treatment

Alternative medicine generally views cancer as a holistic problem. That is, cancer represents a problem with the body's overall health and immune system functioning. As such, treatment is holistic as well, striving to strengthen and heal the physical, mental, and spiritual aspects of patients. Alternative cancer treatments may emphasize different basic approaches, which include traditional medicines, psychological approaches, nutritional and dietary approaches, physical approaches, integrated approaches, and experimental programs.

TRADITIONAL MEDICINES. Traditional Chinese medicine uses **acupuncture, acupressure** massage, herbal remedies, and movement therapies such as t'ai chi and chi gong to treat cancer. Some traditional Chinese herbal remedies have been scientifically shown to have anticancer and immune-stimulating properties in the laboratory and in animal studies, although little controlled research has been done on human cancer patients as of 2008. In the late 2000s research continued on many of these remedies.

Ayurvedic medicine uses **detoxification**, herbal remedies, massage, exercise, **yoga**, breathing techniques, and **meditation** as part of its cancer treatment. **Panchakarma** is an extensive detoxification and strengthening program that is recommended for people with cancer and those undergoing chemotherapy or radiation. Panchakarma uses **fasting**, special vegetarian **diets**, enemas, massage, herbal medicines, and other techniques to rid the body of excess toxins and strengthen the immune system. Certain Ayurvedic herbs have been shown to have significant anticancer properties.

Naturopathy and **homeopathy** are traditional Western healing systems that use herbal medicines and various alternative techniques to strengthen the immune system and reduce the pain of cancer treatment. Bodywork therapies such as massage and **reflexology** ease muscle tension and may alleviate side effects such as nausea and **vomiting**. Homeopathy and herbal remedies may alleviate some of the side effects of radiation and chemotherapy. In the United States, the National Center for Complementary and Alternative Medicine (NCCAM) within the National Institutes of Health supervises clinical trials of many complementary and alternative cancer therapies.

PSYCHOLOGICAL APPROACHES. Psychological approaches work with the idea that the mind and emotions can influence the health of the body and diseases such as cancer. In fact, a new field of academic medicine called **psychoneuroimmunology** has developed to study the interactions between mental state and immune system functioning since many studies have indicated that mind and emotions play a role in the health of the body. Psychological approaches are used in conjunction with many conventional cancer programs. Alternative treatments that seek to help patients with the mental and spiritual challenges that cancer poses include **psychotherapy**, support groups, **guided imagery**, meditation, **biofeedback**, and hypnosis. Studies suggest that patients who approach their cancer with positive attitudes and peaceful acceptance have higher survival rates than those who react with negative emotions, such as **depression**, cynicism, or helplessness. Alternative treatments use psychological approaches to help patients overcome the mental and emotional barriers to healing.

PHYSICAL APPROACHES. Physical approaches to cancer include exercise, massage therapies, movement therapies such as t'ai chi and chi gong, breathing techniques, and **relaxation** techniques. These therapies strive to increase immune system response, promote relaxation and **stress** reduction, and reduce side effects of conventional treatments such as pain, nausea, weakness, and physical immobility.

NUTRITIONAL AND DIETARY APPROACHES. Diet is recognized as playing a major role in the risk of developing some cancers. Many nutritionists also believe that cancer patients have heightened needs for diets free of toxic chemicals and full of nutrients such as **antioxidants** that are believed to enhance immune system response. Proper diet and nutrition can improve both a cancer patient's chances for recovery and quality of life during treatment. In some laboratory studies, vitamins such as A, C, and E, as well as compounds such as isothiocyanates and dithiolthiones found in broccoli, cauliflower, and cabbage, and the antioxidant beta-carotene found in carrots, have been shown to have a protective effect against DNA damage. Additionally, **bioflavonoids** and **lycopene** found in **green tea** are thought to play a role in the prevention of cancer.

Dietary approaches to cancer include **vegetarianism**, raw food diets, macrobiotics, the Gerson diet, and the Livingston-Wheeler nutritional program. Cancer diets generally emphasize fresh fruits, vegetables, whole grains, and legumes, and restrict intake of fat, meat, dairy products, sugar, processed foods, and other foods believed to stress cancer patients. Nutritional approaches to cancer include antioxidant and vitamin supplementation and the use of many herbal extracts that have been shown to have anticancer, immune-enhancing, or symptom-reducing properties.

INTEGRATED APPROACHES. Keith Block, a conventional physician and oncologist, integrates many alternative practices into his cancer treatment center affiliated with the Chicago Medical School in Illinois. His program seeks to provide individualized cancer treatment using conventional therapies while integrating alternative healing techniques. Block advocates a special diet (based on vegetarianism and macrobiotics), exercise, psychological support, and herbal and nutritional supplements. Block's program has received acclaim for both treatment success and satisfaction of patients. In 1998, the United States Congress established the National Center for Complementary and Alternative Medicine (NCCAM) under the auspices of the National Institutes of Health. NCCAM supports clinical trials and research into botanical products, herbalism, and other alternative therapies. As more is known and documented about the effectiveness of alternative therapies in treating cancer, an increasing number of traditional physicians are willing to follow Block's example and develop integrated programs for cancer treatment.

EXPERIMENTAL PROGRAMS. Experimental programs offer treatment options that have not been proven to the satisfaction of conventional medical practitioners. Some of these therapies may be harmful, and patients should do research on the safety and effectiveness of the program before agreeing to participate. These programs are not likely to be covered by insurance. Experimental programs are constantly being tried. A few examples are listed below.

Antineoplaston therapy was developed by Stanislaw Burzynski, a Polish physician who began practicing in Houston, Texas. Burzynski has isolated a chemical, deficient in those with cancer, which he believes stops cancer growth, and his treatment has shown some promise.

Joseph Gold, the director of the Syracuse Cancer Research Institute, discovered that the chemical hydrazine sulfate has many positive effects in cancer patients, including stopping weight loss, shrinking tumors, and increasing survival rates.

The Livingston therapy was developed by the late Virginia Livingston, an American physician. She asserted that cancer is caused by certain bacteria that she claimed are present in all tumors. She advocated a detoxification program and special diet that emphasized raw or lightly cooked and primarily vegetarian foods, with special vitamin and nutritional supplements.

The **Gerson therapy** was for years the best-known nutritional therapy for cancer. It is available in two clinics in California and Mexico. It consists of a basic vegetarian diet low in salt and fat, with high doses of particular nutrients using raw fruit and vegetable juices. The Gerson therapy also requires patients to drink raw calf's liver juice, believed to aid the liver, and it advocates frequent coffee enemas, which are claimed to help the body evacuate toxins.

Allopathic treatment

The aim of allopathic (conventional) cancer treatment is to remove all or as much of the tumor as possible and to prevent the recurrence or spread of the primary tumor. Many different conventional medical specialists work together as a team to treat cancer patients. An oncologist is a physician who specializes in cancer care. The oncologist provides chemotherapy, hormone therapy, and any other non-surgical treatment that does not involve radiation. The oncologist often serves as the primary physician and coordinates the patient's treatment plan. The radiation oncologist specializes in using radiation to treat cancer, whereas the surgical oncologist performs the operations needed to diagnose or treat cancer. Gynecologist-oncologists and pediatric-oncologists, as their titles suggest, are physicians involved with treating women's and children's cancers respectively.

Many other specialists also may be involved in the care of a cancer patient. For example, hematologists specialize in disorders of the blood and are consulted regarding blood cancers and bone marrow cancers or when the patient's blood count becomes seriously abnormal during treatment. Tissue samples that are removed for biopsy are sent to a laboratory, where a pathologist examines them to determine the type of cancer and extent of the disease. Hospice nurses tend the terminally ill in their homes or hospice settings. Only some of the specialists who are involved with cancer care have been mentioned above. There are many other specialties, and virtually any type of medical or surgical specialist may become involved with care of the cancer patient should it become necessary.

While patients and healthcare practitioners devise a conventional treatment plan for cancer, the likelihood of curing the cancer has to be weighed against the side effects of the treatment. If the cancer is very aggressive and a cure is not possible, then the treatment is aimed at relieving symptoms and controlling the cancer for as long as possible (palliative treatment). Cancer treatment can take many different forms, and it is always tailored to the individual patient. The decision about which type of treatment is the most appropriate depends on the type and location of cancer, the extent to which it has already spread, the patient's age, sex, general health status, and personal treatment preferences. The major conventional types of medical treatment are: surgery, radiation, chemotherapy, immunotherapy, hormone therapy, and bone marrow transplantation.

Types and uses of surgery

Surgery is the removal of a tumor and some surrounding tissue under general, regional, or local anesthesia. It is the most frequently used cancer treatment. During the course of a cancer, furthermore, surgery can be used for many purposes.

TREATMENT. Treatment of cancer by surgery involves removal of the tumor to cure the disease. Surgery is most effective when a tumor is small and confined to one area of the body (a condition called "cancer in situ"). Along with the tumor, some normal surrounding tissue is also removed to help ensure that no cancer cells remain in the area. The lymphatic system carries lymph throughout the body through. Lymph is a clear fluid that contains immune system cells that fight infection. Since cancer usually spreads via the lymphatic system, adjoining lymph nodes may be examined for cancer cells and sometimes are removed as well.

PREVENTIVE SURGERY. Preventive or prophylactic surgery involves removal of an abnormal looking area that is likely to become malignant. For example, polyps are removed from the colon in people at high risk of developing colon cancer before the polyps can become malignant. The same is done for certain skin growths. Very high-risk women with a family history of breast cancer who carry the BRCA1 and BRCA2 genes may want to discuss preventative mastectomy (breast removal) with their physician. As of 2008, preventive breast surgery remained controversial.

DIAGNOSTIC PURPOSES. The most definitive tool for diagnosing cancer is a biopsy. Sometimes a biopsy can be performed by inserting a needle through the skin and drawing out a sample of cells. At other times, the only way to obtain a tissue sample for biopsy is by performing surgery.

CYTOREDUCTIVE SURGERY. Cytoreductive surgery is a procedure in which the doctor removes as much of the cancer as possible and then treats the remaining area with radiation therapy or chemotherapy or both. It is often done to relieve painful symptoms.

PALLIATIVE SURGERY. The goal of this surgery is to prolong life and to improve the quality of life rather than to cure the cancer. This surgery is performed when the tumor is so large or has spread so much that removing all the cancer is not an option. For example, a tumor in the abdomen may be large enough to press on and block a portion of the intestine, interfering with digestion and causing pain and vomiting.

Debulking surgery may remove a part of the blockage and relieve the symptoms. In tumors that are dependent on hormones, removal of the organs that secrete the hormones is an option. For example, in prostate cancer, the release of testosterone by the testes stimulates the growth of cancerous prostate cells. A man may choose to undergo an orchiectomy (removal of testicles) to slow progress of the disease. Similarly, in a subtype of aggressive breast cancer, removal of the ovaries (oophorectomy) stops the synthesis of hormones by the ovaries and may slow the progression of the cancer.

Radiation

Radiation kills both malignant and normal cells. Radiation, sometimes with other non-surgical treatments, is used when surgery is not possible or desirable. More often, radiation is used in conjunction with surgery and chemotherapy, immunotherapy, and/or hormone therapy. Radiation can be used either before or after surgery and be either external or internal. In the external form, the radiation is aimed at the tumor from outside the body. In internal radiation (brachytherapy), a radioactive substance in the form of pellets or liquid is placed at the cancerous site by means of a pill, injection, or insertion in a sealed container. This procedure helps target the radiation directly to the tumor and spare healthy cells.

Chemotherapy

Chemotherapy is the use of drugs to kill cancer cells; unfortunately, chemotherapy drugs often kill or damage healthy cells, too. Chemotherapy destroys the small clusters of hard-to-detect cancer cells that have spread beyond the primary tumor or loose cancer cells circulating in the body. Chemotherapeutic drugs can be taken either by mouth or intravenously and may be given alone or in conjunction with surgery, radiation, and hormone therapy. They often have side effects that range from uncomfortable to serious.

When chemotherapy is used before surgery or radiation, it is known as primary or neoadjuvant chemotherapy. Neoadjuvant chemotherapy can be used effectively to reduce the size of a tumor before surgery. However, the toxic effects of neoadjuvant chemotherapy are severe. In addition, it may make the body less tolerant to the side effects of other treatments, such as radiation therapy, that follow the surgery.

The more common use of chemotherapy is as an adjuvant therapy that is used to supplement and enhance the effectiveness of other treatments. For example, after surgery, adjuvant chemotherapy can be given to destroy cancerous cells that still remain in the body. Chemotherapy drugs kill both healthy and cancer cells. As of the late 2000s, researchers were working on finding new drugs that are more toxic to cancer cells and less toxic to healthy cells in order to increase the effectiveness of chemotherapy and reduce the side effects.

Immunotherapy

Immunotherapy, also called biologic therapy or biotherapy, uses substances that either stimulate the body's own immune system to destroy cancer cells or provides large quantities of man-made antibodies (disease fighting proteins). This is a type of targeted therapy. Large amounts of antibodies of a single type (called monoclonal antibodies) that react with specific receptors on cancer cells are made in the laboratory. When given to the patient, they inactivate or destroy those cells containing that specific receptor but do not react with or damage other cells. Successful immunotherapy drugs have been developed that target two types of breast cancer cells and one that inhibits the growth of blood vessels into tumors. Without a blood supply, tumors cannot increase in size. Immunotherapy is an area of active research.

Hormone therapy

Hormone therapy is standard treatment for cancers that are hormone-dependent and grow faster in the presence of particular hormones. These include cancer of the prostate, breast, and uterus. Hormone therapy involves blocking the production or action of these hormones. As a result, the growth of the tumor slows down and survival may be extended for several months or years. Tamoxifen, an anti-estrogen breast cancer drug, is the best known of several successful hormone therapy drugs.

Bone marrow transplantation

Bone marrow is the tissue within the bone cavities that contains blood-forming cells. Healthy bone marrow tissue constantly replenishes the supply of blood cells. Sometimes, cancer develops in the bone marrow, resulting in the production of malformed, nonfunctional blood cells. Other times, the drugs or radiation needed to destroy cancer cells also destroys bone marrow cells, reducing the supply of new blood cells to dangerously low levels. Replacing the bone marrow with healthy cells counteracts these effects.

A bone marrow transplant involves the removal of marrow from one person and the insertion of the blood-forming cells in someone else. When bone-

marrow transplantation is used to cure certain blood marrow cancers (leukemias), chemotherapy and radiation must be used to kill all the cancer patient's bone marrow cells. After these cells die, healthy donor bone marrow cells are injected into the cancer patient. In a successful transplant, these cells take up residence in the bones and begin producing healthy blood cells. Bone-marrow transplantation is a complex, often risky, process that involves finding a donor whose cell surface proteins match as closely as possible that of the recipient. Matching is necessary so that the recipient's immune system does not attack and destroy the donor cells as foreign entities.

Cancer treatment and prevention continue to be the focus of a great deal of research. Research into new cancer therapies includes cancer-targeting gene therapy, virus therapy, and the development of drugs that stimulate destruction of cancer cells but not healthy cells. However, all new therapies take years of clinical testing and research before becoming widely available. Individuals interested in volunteering for a clinical trial of a new drug or cancer therapy can find a list of current clinical trials accepting patients at http://www.clinicaltrials.gov. There is no cost to the patient for participating in a clinical trial.

Expected results

The outcome of cancer treatment is affected by many factors, particularly the type of cancer the patient has, the stage of the cancer, the extent to which it has metastasized, and the aggressiveness of the cancer. In addition, the patient's age, general health status, and the effectiveness of the treatment being pursued are important factors. Many cancers are completely curable if detected and treated at their early stages.

To help put into perspective the future course and outcome of a cancer and the likelihood of recovery from it, doctors often use statistics. Five- or ten-year survival rates are the most common measures used. The number refers to the proportion of people with the cancer who are expected to be alive five or ten years after initial diagnosis compared with a similar population that is free of cancer. It is important to note that while statistics can give information about the average survival experience of cancer patients in a given population, they cannot be used to indicate individual prognosis because no two patients are exactly alike.

Alternative medicine rarely is able to cure cancer, but complementary treatment—using alternative therapies in conjunction with traditional medicine—can help to control symptoms and side effects, thus

KEY TERMS

Adjuvant therapy—Treatment involving radiation, chemotherapy (drug treatment), hormone therapy, biotherapeutics, or a combination of any of these given after the primary treatment in order to rid the body of residual microscopic cancer.

Antibody—A protein produced by the immune system to fight infection or rid the body of foreign material. In cancer, malignant cells are treated as foreign entities. Specific antibodies can also be made in the laboratory and used to fight cancer.

Antioxidant—A molecule that prevents oxidation. Antioxidants attach to other molecules called free radicals and prevent the free radicals from causing damage to cell walls, DNA, and other parts of the cell.

Ayurvedic medicine—A 5,000-year old system of holistic medicine developed in India. Ayurvedic medicine is based on the idea that illness results from a personal imbalance or lack of physical, spiritual, social, or mental harmony.

Benign—Mild, nonmalignant, noncancerous.

Biopsy—Surgical removal and microscopic examination of living tissue for diagnostic purposes.

Bone marrow—Spongy material that fills the inner cavities of the bones. All blood cells are produced in the bone marrow.

Carcinogen—Any substance capable of causing cancer.

Chemotherapy—Use of chemicals (drugs) to treat an illness; a therapy used to treat some cancers.

Complementary medicine—Various treatments used in alternative medicine that are used specifically to supplement conventional drug and therapy treatments, rather than to replace conventional medicine.

Epithelium—The layer of cells covering the body's surface (skin) and lining internal organs such as the intestine and various glands.

Holistic—Pertaining to approaches that consider the whole system as opposed to those approaches that analyze or dissect into parts.

Hormone therapy—Treatment that inhibits the production of hormones such as testosterone and estrogen.

Immunotherapy—Treatment that stimulates the body's immune defense system.

Integrative medicine—A medical approach that brings together and uses aspects of conventional and alternative medicines.

Macrobiotics—Special vegetarian diet based on whole grains, legumes, fruits, and vegetables.

Malignant—A general term for cells that can dislodge from the original tumor, invade, and destroy other tissues and organs.

Metastasis—The spread of cancer from its initial site to elsewhere in the body.

Oncologist—Conventional medical doctor who has specialized training in cancer.

Radiation therapy—Treatment using high-energy radiation from x-ray machines, cobalt, radium, or other sources.

Toxin—A general term for something that harms or poisons the body.

Traditional Chinese medicine (TCM)—An ancient system of medicine based on maintaining a balance in vital energy or qi that controls emotions and both spiritual and physical wellbeing. Diseases and disorders result from imbalances in qi (the life force), and treatments such as massage, exercise, acupuncture, and nutritional and herbal therapy are designed to restore balance and harmony to the body.

Tumor—An abnormal growth resulting from a cell that loses its normal growth control restraints and multiplies uncontrollably.

improving the quality of life for people with cancer. Although alternative therapies have sometimes shown unexpected positive results and cures, they may be strongest as preventative or complementary measures.

Prevention

According to alternative practitioners, nutritionists, and conventional physicians, individuals can reduce the risk of developing cancer by following these guidelines:

- Eat a diet high in fruits and vegetables and low in animal fats.
- Have regular screenings for common cancers such as those of the breast, colon, and prostate.
- Exercise vigorously for at least 20 minutes every day or walk moderately for 10 hours a week.

- Keep weight within normal limits; avoid excessive weight gain.
- Avoid tobacco use (including exposure to second-hand smoke).
- Decrease or avoid consumption of animal fats and red meats.
- Avoid excessive alcohol use (more than 1 or 2 drinks per day).
- Avoid exposure to the sun during the midday hours when the sun's rays are the strongest.
- Avoid risky sexual practices such as sex with multiple partners and sex without using a condom.
- Avoid known carcinogens in the environment or work place.
- Strive to maintain sound mental and emotional health, which is believed to help prevent cancer; learn a technique such as yoga, t'ai chi, meditation, or others to reduce stress and promote relaxation; maintain healthy relationships and social support systems.

In addition, refraining from certain activities or drugs that are proven as risk factors for certain cancers can help lower one's cancer risk. For instance, while physicians have long known a small increased risk for breast cancer was linked to use of hormone replacement therapy (HRT), the extensive Women's Health Initiative study released finding in 2003 stated that even relatively short-term use of estrogen plus progestin HRT was associated with increased risk of breast cancer, diagnosis at a more advanced stage of the disease, and a higher number of abnormal mammograms. The longer a woman used HRT, the more her risk increased.

Resources

BOOKS

Bradbury, Robert H., ed. *Cancer*. New York: Springer, 2007.

Geffen, Jeremy R. *The Journey Through Cancer: Healing and Transforming the Whole Person*. New York: Three Rivers Press, 2006.

Visel, Dave. *Living with Cancer: A Practical Guide*. New Brunswick, NJ: Rutgers University Press, 2006.

Weinberg, Robert A. *The Biology of Cancer*. New York: Garland Science, 2007.

OTHER

Alternative Therapies in Health and Medicine. http://www.alternative-therapies.com.

ORGANIZATIONS

Alternative Medicine Foundation, PO Box 60016, Potomac, MD, 20859, (301) 340-1960, http://www.amfoundation. org.

American Association of Oriental Medicine, PO Box 162340, Sacramento, CA, 95816, (866) 455-7999, http://www.aaaomonline.org.

American Cancer Society, 1599 Clifton Rd. NE, Atlanta, GA, 30329-4251, (800) ACS-2345, http://www.cancer.org.

American Holistic Medical Association, PO Box 2016, Edmonds, WA, 98020, (425) 967-0737, http://www.holisticmedicine.org.

National Cancer Institute, (800-4-CANCER), http://www.cancer.gov.

National Center for Complementary and Alternative Medicine Clearinghouse, PO Box 7923, Gaithersburg, MD, 20898, (888) 644-6226, http://nccam.nih.gov.

Office of Dietary Supplements, National Institutes of Health, 6100 Executive Blvd., Room 3B01, MSC 7517, Bethesda, MD, 20892-7517, (301) 435-2920, http://dietary-supplements.info.nih.gov.

Douglas Dupler
Teresa G. Odle
Tish Davidson, A. M.

Cancer, bladder *see* **Bladder cancer**

Cancer, breast *see* **Breast cancer**

Cancer, colorectal *see* **Colorectal cancer**

Cancer, ovarian *see* **Ovarian cancer**

Cancer, uterine *see* **Uterine cancer**

Cancer treatments, biological

Definition

Biological **cancer** treatments, also known as metabolic treatments, work by detoxifying and strengthening the body so that it can overcome cancer cells and metabolize them. This approach is almost always conducted nutritionally, possibly with the aid of nutritional supplements and/or herbs, or by employing **detoxification** procedures such as enemas and **colonic irrigation**.

Origins

It is thought that Paracelsus and Hippocrates cured cancer with biological cures (through food), but it is difficult to verify that they were actually treating cancer, which is commonly regarded as an affliction of modern man. Modern biological cancer therapies began to appear at the beginning of the twentieth century.

The therapy developed by Max Gerson (1881–1959) is probably foremost among the early ones, although Gerson had some equally eminent contemporaries. Gerson's therapy emphasized eating organic foods, using coffee enemas, and detoxifying the body with certain natural supplements. In addition, many alternative health practitioners specialize in the treatment of cancer, although their success rates vary.

Benefits

Biological cancer treatments are non-invasive and do not have the drawbacks associated with chemotherapy and radiation therapy. Unlike biological treatments, conventional medical treatments deplete or completely destroy the body's immune system and can leave patients in a much weakened state.

Biological treatments work by strengthening the immune system so that it can overcome any abnormal condition. A successful biological cancer treatment leaves patients feeling better than they did before they became ill, with all bodily functions effectively harmonized and energy levels raised.

Description

All biological cancer therapies focus on strengthening the human organism so that it can kill the cancer, rather than focusing on the cancer alone, as is the case with allopathic medicine. Therefore, all these therapies promote healthy lifestyle as essential to healing. In particular, this position requires abstaining from processed, denatured foods, and ensuring the absence of pollution and toxins from diet and living environment.

Natural hygiene and other alternative therapies prescribe fresh fruit and vegetables in abundance. The **Gerson therapy** uses fresh juices from organic sources. Especially in the beginning, a vital aspect of the treatment is detoxification, which is the process of encouraging, and sometimes forcing, the body to eliminate toxins stored in the body cells and gastrointestinal tract. In the case of cancer patients, this process can involve a considerable quantity of toxic waste that must be flushed out of the system.

Concurrently with the detoxification process, the treatment aims to provide the organism with plentiful supplies of fresh enzymes and nutrients that allow the body to rebuild itself and renew systems such as the endocrine system and immune system.

When treating most disorders and diseases with natural therapies, the patient is encouraged to undertake a program of **exercise** to enhance the effectiveness of the treatment. However, cancer patients may not be strong enough for such activities, and their bodies need all available strength to fight the cancer. Instead, they are advised to undertake an exercise program only once they are well enough to do so.

Practitioners

Practitioners who have been successful with the treatment of serious disease, particularly cancer, have a reputation for being very tough on their patients. When questioned, many say that unless a cancer patient is prepared to tackle the problem of detoxification seriously and follow the diet without diverting from it, there is little hope that they will be able to overcome the disease. Often patients who are in a weakened state of health need the support of a therapist who is prepared to be firm with them.

MAX GERSON. Gerson's therapy can probably be considered the original biological cancer treatment. In his book *A Cancer Therapy, Results of Fifty Cases*, Gerson documented 50 successfully treated cancer patients. He explains that the cases in his book were the most extensively documented and, therefore, most suitable for the purposes of demonstrating his cure. Gerson believed that chronic illnesses occur as a result of nutritional deficiency as well as toxicity.

To combat deficiencies, this therapy relies mainly on fresh organic juices but includes supplements and strict instructions for lifestyle. A vital aspect of this treatment is the coffee enema he devised to achieve thorough detoxification. In the United Kingdom, a University of Manchester study followed six cancer patients, all with poor prognoses, who adhered to the Gerson regime. Researchers noted that the Gerson program provided both physical and psychological support. The American Cancer Society cautions that adverse reactions may occur when using this form of therapy.

LINUS PAULING. Nobel Prize laureate, Linus Pauling (1901–1994), researched the properties of nutritional supplements in treating disease for many years, and he is generally accepted as the foremost authority on the subject. In 1979, he co-authored with Ewan Cameron the book *Cancer and Vitamin C*. Pauling advocated supplements, in particular megadoses of **vitamin C**, for the treatment of cancer and other degenerative diseases.

The Linus Pauling Institute of Science and Medicine was formed in California in 1979. In 1996, the Linus Pauling Institute at Oregon State University replaced the former organization. Research at the institute has found that diet influences genetic relationships to cancer because certain components of diet have the ability to turn genes on or off. Researchers have also found that elements within cruciferous vegetables such as broccoli, bok choy, and brussels sprouts, contain powerful anti-cancer properties. A number of studies ongoing as of 2008 at the institute sought to expand knowledge in this area.

ANN WIGMORE. Wheatgrass juice and sprouts are the basis for regimen devised by Ann Wigmore (1909–1994). She originally devised this treatment to cure her own chronic diseases, including cancer, and was successful in helping people for decades. The **Wigmore diet** focuses primarily on live foods. Wigmore felt that raw vegetables held more **nutrition** than when cooked and were without the chemical additives that processed foods hold. Her therapy continued into the 2000s to be practiced at the Hippocrates Institute and was adopted by a number of alternative health care practitioners as the basis for their treatment. In the book, *Wheatgrass Nature's Finest Medicine: The Complete Guide to Using Grasses to Revitalize Your Health,* author Steve Meyerowitz writes that wheatgrass, "enhances and maximizes your full healing potential." According to the American Cancer Society, wheatgrass is "generally safe," with only few incidences of reactions such as **nausea**, headaches, **hives**, or swelling of the throat. If individuals experience hives or throat swelling, they should seek emergency medical care, as this may be indicative of a severe allergic reaction.

RANDOLPH STONE. Randolph Stone (1890–1981) developed a system known as **polarity therapy** during his career, which spanned 60 years. Stone believed that health should be measured by an assessment of the human energy field, which is affected, for example, by daily life, nutrition, exercise, touch, sound. Stone recommended a comprehensive regimen consisting of touch therapy (where the practitioner's hands are conduits of energy), diet (a vegetarian diet is emphasized because foods collected in a non-violent way hold more energy), and **yoga** (to tune individuals to their own body). These practices balance health, and so produce satisfactory energy fields.

MICHIO KUSHI. Microbiotics refers to a belief system which states that people are influenced by everything around them, including the environment, foods they eat, and even where they live. Promoting a positive lifestyle is also encouraged in order to keep a good outlook and mental attitude. Possibly the most famous teacher of macrobiotics in the United States, Michio Kushi, wrote *The Cancer Prevention Diet* in collaboration with Alex Jack in 1993. It is a comprehensive guide to the prevention and treatment of cancer with a **macrobiotic diet**.

Therapies

BOTANICAL MEDICINE. There are several different therapies that fit into this category, which encompasses general herbal medicine, Chinese herbalism, and several other ethnic herbal disciplines. A University of Toronto study reported that evidence supports that cancer-preventing abilities exist in botanicals such as **green tea**, Asian ginseng, tomatoes, **garlic**, and soy, and suggested that additional studies be conducted to determine the cancer treatment efficacy of **turmeric**, essiac, **evening primrose oil**, reishi, **mistletoe**, and shiitake. The scientists also suggested that **ginger** may be an effective choice when treating nausea and **vomiting** that sometimes accompanies chemotherapy.

NATURAL HYGIENE. Natural hygiene practitioners have a long history of successfully treating such serious diseases as cancer. This vegetarian diet is designed to maintain a healthy and happy outlook. Rest, fresh air, grains, fruits, and vegetables are encouraged. The American Natural Hygiene Society is a good source of information regarding treatment and practitioners.

AYURVEDIC MEDICINE. This centuries old system of natural medicine originated in India. Arvada has a concept of life force, which is similar to the Chinese chi. It aims to purge the body of undesirable matter and then rebuild it with good nutrition, while at the same time attending to all aspects of the patient's life both physical and spiritual. This system is recognized by the World Health Organization.

MACROBIOTICS. This diet consists mostly of whole grains and vegetables. It is designed in light of a unique philosophy about food that traces its origins to Japanese and Chinese theories.

In general, the charge for various clinics and practitioners varies widely, so it is essential for the patient to discuss fees with the practitioner before treatment.

Preparations

All of these practitioners advocated the use of fresh natural produce, preferably organic, for cancer patients and other people else who want to improve their health. Where herbal remedies or other supplements are prescribed, it is important to ensure that the original formula is purchased, and not a copy. Unscrupulous individuals have been known to pass off unauthentic remedies using the names of well-known practitioners.

Precautions

None of the therapies will be effective if the regimen is not followed in its entirety. No matter how good the quality of organic produce, no benefits will be felt if the patient is still being exposed to environmental pollution, or if detoxification procedures are inadequate. It is for this reason that most practitioners recommend that a cure be taken in the setting of a clinic because all of these details can then become the responsibility of the staff, freeing the patient to concentrate on the business of becoming well.

In fact, many practitioners who treat cancer take their cure so seriously, that they will refuse to treat patients who are not prepared to take all the necessary steps and truly commit themselves to becoming well. They warn that natural cures for cancer are not easy, cancer is a sign that the integrity of the body system has been seriously compromised, and nothing but the strictest regimen is likely to facilitate a return to health. Even so, these therapies remain experimental, and there are no guarantees of a cure.

Side effects

Side effects associated with natural therapies are mild compared to those commonly experienced with allopathic treatments. Cost is one of the main inhibitors of these treatments.

However, in the case of cancer treatment, a healing crisis can be an unpleasant experience. Alternative medicine practitioners believe that all illness is a result of a toxic condition in the body, and cancer, being one of the most serious conditions, is an indication of more serious levels of toxicity. The level of toxicity in the patient means that as the person takes one of these alternative treatments, the body starts to throw off these toxins, the blood system becomes overloaded and the patient experience headaches, fevers, nausea, and in some cases extreme sensitivity to stimuli such as sound and light. It is highly advisable to seek a practitioner to help with detoxification because of these side effects.

Research and general acceptance

Allopathic medicine disapproves most strongly of alternative medicine in its treatments for cancer, and these natural treatments are the subject of much adverse publicity. Alternative practitioners assert that cancer patients should at least have the option of choosing a biological cure for their illness.

Many alternative medicine practitioners recommend that patients compare statistics when deciding

KEY TERMS

Denatured—Food which has been processed and is no longer of benefit to the body.

Detoxification—The process of cleansing the system of accumulated toxins.

Oncologist—Cancer specialist.

on the mode of treatment that is best for them and ask to see documentation.

Training and certification

All of the practitioners named above held advanced degrees, some of them with medical degrees, others with Ph.D.s. The organization *People Against Cancer* specializes in helping people find suitable practitioners and therapies. It also provides practical help regarding the implementation of therapies, can advise on books, and so on.

Resources

BOOKS

Gerson, Charlotte, with Beata Bishop. *Healing the Gerson Way: Defeating Cancer and Other Chronic Diseases.* Carmel, CA: Totality Books, 2007.

Gerson, Max, M.D. *A Cancer Therapy, Results of Fifty Cases.* Del Mar, CA: Totality Books, 1977.

Meyerowitz, Steve. *Wheatgrass Nature's Finest Medicine: The Complete Guide to Using Grasses to Revitalize Your Health,* 7th ed. Great Barrington, MA: Sproutman, 2006.

PERIODICALS

Molassiotis, A., and P. Peat. "Surviving Against All Odds: Analysis of 6 Case Studies of Patients with Cancer who Followed the Gerson Therapy." *Journal of Integrative Cancer Therapies* 6, no. 1 (March 2007): 80–88.

OTHER

"Epigenetics: Providing a New View of Diet and Cancer." Oregon State University News and Communication Services. July 25, 2007. http://oregonstate.edu/dept/ncs/newsarch/2007/Jul07/cancerinhibition.html. (April 6, 2008).

ORGANIZATIONS

American Cancer Society, 1599 Clifton Road NE, Atlanta, GA, 30329-4251, (800) 227-2345, http://www.cancer.org.

American Holistic Medicine Association, http://www.holisticmedicine.org/index.html.

American Natural Hygiene Society, PO Box 30630, Tampa, FL, 33630, (813) 855-6607, http://www.anhs.org/.

American Polarity Therapy Association, PO Box 19858, Boulder, CO, 80308, (303) 545-2080, http://www.polaritytherapy.org.

Kushi Institute, PO Box 7, Becket, MA, 01223, (413) 623-5741, http://www.macrobiotics.org.

Linus Pauling Institute, Oregon State University 571 Weniger Hall, Corvalis, OR, 97331-6512, (541) 737-5075, http://lpi.oregonstate.edu/.

Patricia Skinner
Rhonda Cloos, R.N.

Canker sores

Definition

Canker sores are small sores or ulcers that appear inside the mouth. They are painful and often recur from once every few years to almost continually. Canker sores are known medically as apthous ulcers or apthous stomatitis.

Description

Canker sores occur on the inside of the mouth, usually on the inside of the lips, cheeks, and/or soft palate. They can also occur on the tongue and in the throat. Often, several canker sores will appear at the same time and may be grouped in clusters. They are painful and sensitive to touch. The average canker sore is about one-quarter inch in size, although they can occasionally be larger. The sores may last for weeks at a time and leave a scar. The initial symptom is a tingling or mildly painful **itching** sensation in the area where the sore will appear. After one to several days, a small red swelling appears, which eventually becomes a grayish ulcer with a red ring of inflammation surrounding the sore. Canker sores can be very painful, especially if they are touched repeatedly (e.g., by the tongue). They last for one to three weeks.

Approximately 20% of the United States population is affected with recurring canker sores, and more women than men get them. Women are more likely to have canker sores during their premenstrual time.

Canker sores may be confused with cold sores caused by the herpes simplex virus because the appearance of both is similar. However, herpes **infections** occur most commonly on the outside of the lips, on the hard palate, and on the gums, whereas canker sores usually occur on the soft tissues inside the mouth. Unlike canker sores, herpes cold sores are infectious.

KEY TERMS

Inflammation—A localized reaction to tissue injury or damage, usually characterized by pain, swelling, and redness.

Skin lesion biopsy—A procedure in which a sliver of tissue from the skin is removed in order to examine it and establish a diagnosis.

Ulcer—A site of damage to the skin or mucous membranes characterized by the formation of pus and the death of tissue. It is frequently accompanied by inflammation.

Causes and symptoms

The exact cause of canker sores is unknown. There seems to be at least some link to immune reactions. There may also be a genetic tendency to develop canker sores. Accidental injuries to the mouth from vigorous toothbrush scrapes, poorly fitted dentures, braces, or self-inflicted **bites** may give rise to canker sores. They can also be triggered by **stress**, dietary deficiencies, hormonal changes, and food **allergies**. **Sodium** lauryl sulfate, which is an ingredient in many toothpastes, may contribute to the development of canker sores by stripping the mucous coating inside the mouth.

Diagnosis

Canker sores are diagnosed by observation of the sore. A distinction between canker sores and cold sores should be made because the latter is infectious. Other disorders of the mouth may need to be ruled out as well; a skin lesion biopsy may be required for further diagnosis.

Treatment

Many alternative therapies for canker sores try to heal the existing sores and prevent their recurrence. Several herbal remedies may be helpful in the treatment of existing sores. These include:

- calendula (*Calendula officinalis*)
- chamomile (*Matricaria recutita*)
- goldenseal (*Hydrastis canadensis*)
- licorice (*Glycyrrhiza glabra*)
- myrrh (*Commiphora molmol*)
- peppermint (*Mentha peperita*)
- slippery elm (*Ulmus fulva*)

The herbs can be made into a strong tea. Compresses soaked in the tea can be applied directly to the mouth, or the tea can be swished in the mouth for several minutes.

The deglycyrrhizinated (DGL) form of **licorice** root, *Glycyrrhiza glabra,* is soothing to the mucous membranes of the mouth and can shorten the healing time for canker sores. The powdered DGL should be mixed with warm water to make a thin paste that can be used twice daily. It should be swirled in the mouth for several minutes and then spit out.

B-complex vitamins, **folic acid**, and **iron** (taken separately or combined in a multivitamin) can help prevent recurrent outbreaks, since canker sores are often associated with deficiencies in these nutrients.

Canker sores often occur during stressful times. **Relaxation** techniques such as **meditation, guided imagery**, and **acupressure** may help prevent or lessen the severity of outbreaks.

Allopathic treatment

Since canker sores heal themselves in most cases, treatment usually isn't necessary. Topical anesthetics, such as lidocaine and similar remedies, may be used for **pain** relief. Corticosteroid ointments may be used to reduce inflammation and speed healing. A protective paste, like Orabase, can be used to prevent irritation of the sores by teeth, dental appliances, or fluid intake.

Severe cases may be treated with the antibiotic tetracycline. This is not recommended for children, however, because it may permanently discolor any teeth that are still forming. Chemical or physical cautery or low-powered laser treatments may also be used to decrease severe pain. Ulcers tend not to recur where a laser has been used.

Expected results

Canker sores tend to heal spontaneously. The pain usually decreases within a few days, and other symptoms resolve in one or two weeks. If symptoms last longer, if there are increasing numbers of outbreaks, or if the pain is severe, a doctor should be consulted.

Prevention

Good oral hygiene is necessary to prevent recurrent outbreaks as well as secondary bacterial infections during an outbreak. This includes regular brushing, flossing, and regular trips to the dentist. Dentures, braces, and fillings should be rechecked and possibly refitted. Toothpastes containing sodium lauryl sulfate should not be used.

Identifying food allergens and making dietary changes may help prevent outbreaks. Spicy foods should also be avoided because they may serve as irritants.

Resources

BOOKS

Larsen, D.E., ed. *Mayo Clinic Family Health Book.* New York: William Morrow, 1996.

Schlossberg, D. *Current Therapy of Infectious Disease.* St. Louis: Mosby, 1996.

OTHER

DrKoop.com. http://www.drkoop.com/conditions/ency/article/000998.htm (January 17, 2001).

The Merck Manual. http://www.merck.com/pubs/mmanual/section9/chapter105/105b.htm (January 17, 2001).

MotherNature.com. http://www.mothernature.com/ency/concern/canker_sores.asp (January 17, 2001).

Patience Paradox

Cannabis sativa see **Marijuana**

Cantharis

Description

Cantharis is a homeopathic remedy obtained from the insect *Lytta vesicatoria*; common names are Spanish fly or blister beetle. This beetle lives on **honeysuckle** and olive trees in western Asia and southern Europe. It is bright green and about 0.5 in (1.3 cm) in length. Other names for cantharis include: *Cantharis vesicator,* N.O. Insecta, and coleoptera.

The Spanish fly produces a toxic substance called cantharidin. Cantharidin is a strong poison that primarily affects the urinary tract and causes burning **pain** and **vomiting**. Cantharidian is caustic and causes skin blistering. Since **homeopathy** is based on the Law of Similars, a doctrine that says to treat a symptom with a diluted remedy that produces the same symptom in stronger amounts, this homeopathic remedy is used for illnesses that have burning pain as a symptom. Because cantharis is a member of the animal kingdom, its activity excites the passions of animals. As such, cantharis is indicated for anger that is very severe with fits of rage. Likewise, cantharis is indicated for conditions of the body that are extreme, ie. pain that is stabbing, burning, and sharp.

KEY TERMS

Cantharidin—The irritating poison produced by Spanish fly that serves as the active ingredient in cantharis. Because of cantharidin, high doses of cantharis are highly toxic.

Cystitis—Painful inflammation of the urinary bladder caused by infection, irritation, allergy, or other causes.

Homeopathy—A therapeutic system in which diseases are treated with agents that cause a similar set of symptoms in healthy persons. A "like treats like" philosophy.

General use

Homeopathic remedies are chosen based upon the specific set of symptoms and traits displayed by each patient. In general, cantharis is used to treat conditions characterized by burning pain and strong thirst but no urge to drink. Conditions for which cantharis is indicated will typically worsen rapidly.

Cantharis is primarily used to treat cystitis, which is inflammation of the urinary bladder because of infection or irritation. It is also used to treat **burns** and **blisters**. Spanish fly was traditionally used as an aphrodisiac (increases sexual desire). It was also used to remove **warts**, treat baldness, increase loss of fluids (acting as a diuretic), and for rheumatic problems (inflammation and degeneration of the joints).

Mental symptoms treated with cantharis

Homeopathy treats a person's whole being, mental and physical. The patient who needs cantharis can be confused and have odd ideas, may be maniacal and demonstrate raging fury or sexual frenzy, or may loose consciousness. The cantharis patient may be restless and excitable. He or she may be extremely thirsty but have difficulty swallowing. Also, the patient may have no appetite and a strong avoidance of food. Other mental problems that can be treated with cantharis include: excessive desire for sex (nymphomania), severe **anxiety**, screaming, querulousness (constant complaining), and insolence (being overbearing).

Physical symptoms treated with cantharis

The intense urge to urinate and burning pain are key symptoms for cantharis. Cantharis is indicated for the patient who experiences rapid and intense inflammation of the urinary system. There is lower abdominal and lower back pain. The severe burning pain associated with the urinary tract makes the patient afraid to urinate. There is a frequent and urgent need to urinate, however, only small amounts (drops) of urine are passed. The urine may contain blood. The patient may experience hydrophobia (fear of water) and, although extremely thirsty, cannot drink water or even tolerate seeing or hearing water. A severe, stabbing **headache** may be present and the patient may avoid bright light.

Cantharis is also used to treat burns or skin conditions that resemble burns. It is used for **sunburn**, blisters, skin eruptions, and insect **bites**. Symptoms associated with burns for which cantharis is indicated include blister formation, searing pain, and relief upon application of a cold compress. This remedy can relieve the pain associated with second or third degree burns. Cantharis is indicated for blisters that are burning and **itching** and feel better upon application of a cold compress.

The patient feels better at night and in the morning. Also, warmth, gentle massage, and lying flat on the back make the patient feel better. Passing **gas** and burping make the patient feel better. The patient feels worse in the afternoon, during movement, and by drinking cold water or coffee.

Other physical symptoms or conditions treated with cantharis include:

- irritation of the digestive system causing a bloated stomach
- burning diarrhea
- colitis (inflammation of the colon)
- loss of appetite
- burning feeling in the throat
- considerable thirst without the desire to drink
- pleurisy (inflammation of the membrane surrounding the lungs)
- nighttime burning feeling on the bottom of the feet
- ice-cold hands with hot, red fingernails
- swelling and rash with pus on the hands
- stings with black centers
- erysipelas (infection of lymph ducts)
- fast spreading skin infection
- eczema
- dandruff
- shingles (herpes zoster)
- eye inflammation
- tongue inflammation
- neuralgia (nerve pain)

Preparations

Homeopathic canthous is prepared from the entire beetle, dried and powdered. It is commercially available as a homeopathic liquid or tablet. Because of the toxic nature of cantharis, the tincture (an alcoholic extract) requires a doctor's prescription.

Cystitis is treated with 30C of homeopathic cantharis every half hour, with up to six doses. Minor burns are treated with 30C of cantharis every 15 minutes for four doses. Blisters are treated with 6C of cantharis four times a day until the pain disappears. Burns may be treated locally with water containing a few drops of cantharis tincture. **Shingles** may be treated with an ointment made with 3X of cantharis.

Precautions

Large doses of cantharidin (the poison produced by the Spanish fly found in cantharis) can cause a burning pain in the stomach and throat, difficulty swallowing, violent vomiting, **diarrhea**, frequent urges to urinate, and possibly convulsions and coma.

Side effects

Excessive doses of cantharis may cause symptoms of cantharidin toxicity including burning pain, vomiting, and frequent urge to urinate.

Interactions

The **belladonna**, **phosphorus**, mercurius, **sepia**, and sulphur homeopathic remedies may be used to complement the activity of cantharis. Homeopathic remedies that serve as antidotes are **aconite**, **apis**, camphora, kali nit., and **pulsatilla**. Cantharis serves as an antidote for the homeopathic remedies alcohol, camphora, and vinegar. Homeopathic coffea and cantharis are incompatible.

Resources

BOOKS

Lockie, Andrew, and Nicola Geddes. *The Complete Guide to Homeopathy: The Principles and Practice of Treatment with a Comprehensive Range of Self-Help Remedies for Common Ailments.* New York: Dorling Kindersley, 1995.

Lodkie, Andrew, and Nicola Geddes. *The Women's Guide to Homeopathy: The Natural Way to a Healthier Life for Women.* New York: St. Martin's Press, 1994.

ORGANIZATIONS

American Foundation for Homeopathy. 1508 S. Garfield, Alhambra, CA 91801.

Homeopathy Educational Services. 2124B Kittredge Street, Berkeley, CA 94704. (510)649-0294. mail@homeopathic.com.

National Center for Homeopathy. 801 N. Fairfax Street, Suites 306, Alexandria, VA 22314.

OTHER

Clarke, John Henry. "Cantharis." *A Dictionary of Practical Materia Medica.* http://www.homeoint.org/clarke/c/canth.htm.

Belinda Rowland

Car sickness *see* **Motion sickness**

Carbuncles *see* **Boils**

Cardamom *see* **Grains-of-paradise fruit**

Carnitine

Description

Carnitine is an amino acid that is essential for babies and nonessential for others. In this context, essential means it must be obtained in the diet. Non-essential types of **amino acids** can be synthesized to some extent within the body. The kidney is able to form carnitine from the amino acids **lysine** and **methionine**, in addition to **iron** and vitamins B_6, **niacin**, and C. The function of carnitine is to mobilize long-chain fatty acids into the powerhouse of the cell, where they are used for energy. Carnitine is necessary for infants to grow and develop normally.

General use

The strongest indication for supplemental carnitine is a genetic defect that causes a deficiency. It may also be inadequately manufactured by babies, particularly those who are premature or have a low birth weight.

Abnormally low levels of carnitine are most commonly associated with a few rare genetic diseases. Symptoms of inadequate carnitine can include confusion, heart **pain**, muscle weakness, and **obesity**. Poor consumption of the nutrients required in order to synthesize carnitine also sometimes results in deficiency. These nutrients include lysine, methionine, **vitamin C**, iron, niacin, and vitamin B_6 (**pyridoxine**). Anyone with a protein deficient diet may have inadequate levels of the building blocks for carnitine. Lysine and methionine are likely to be lacking in a strict vegan diet, although some fortified grains are available. Those who are under severe or chronic health **stress** are also at higher risk. People who have had surgery, severe **burns**, or wasting illnesses require higher protein levels, and might benefit from a supplement. The use of supplements containing D-carnitine has the potential to cause L-carnitine deficiency.

The heart is the most carnitine-rich organ in the body, and there are several heart or circulatory conditions that may benefit from more carnitine than is normally in the diet. Carnitine appears to help the heart, a muscle that requires a lot of energy, function better. One of the primary heart problems that can be helped by carnitine supplementation is **angina** (heart pain due to decreased oxygen because of coronary artery disease). Two studies using L-carnitine, and one using L-propionyl-carnitine, have demonstrated a reduction in symptoms of this condition. When carnitine is added to the treatment plan, it can potentially reduce some of the other medications used to control angina. However, reducing medication for angina patients should be supervised and guided by a healthcare provider.

Intermittent claudication is a condition that develops in some people with severe **atherosclerosis**. Walking becomes painful as a result of decreased blood flow to the legs. Most studies have shown significant improvement in the distance walked without pain when a supplement of L-propionyl-carnitine was used. The dose used in one study was 0.07 oz (2 g) per day.

When used along with traditionally prescribed medications, carnitine may improve survival rates after a **heart attack**. Other benefits, including lowering the heart rate, blood pressure, and lipid levels occurred in treated groups. The dose and type used in one study was 0.14 oz (4 g) per day of L-carnitine.

Most studies of carnitine used to improve athletic performance have not shown any benefit.

Supplementation may have some minimal effects on Alzheimer's patients; some study groups had slightly slower rates of deterioration. These results remain questionable and further study is needed.

There is some evidence that the use of supplemental L-carnitine, at a dose of approximately 500-1000 mg three times per day, may help to lower levels of serum **cholesterol**. However, this regimen would be expensive, and there are other effective and less expensive supplements available. These include **garlic**, red yeast rice, niacin, high fiber **diets**, and soy proteins.

A condition known as **chronic fatigue syndrome** (CFS) causes a number of potentially debilitating symptoms, including severe **fatigue**, muscle pain, and **depression**. Carnitine may prove helpful in alleviating the symptoms of CFS, perhaps by increasing the efficiency of energy production. One small study used a dose of 0.1 oz (3 g) of L-carnitine per day.

Undocumented claims for the health benefits of carnitine include treatment of Down's syndrome, muscular dystrophy, some forms of male **infertility**, chronic obstructive pulmonary disease (COPD), and alcoholic fatty liver disease. Carnitine has also been said to reduce the toxicity of AZT, a medication for **AIDS**.

Preparations

Carnitine is found primarily in meats, but may also be found in avocados, breast milk, dairy products, and tempeh. In the body, it can be synthesized in the kidney from lysine and methionine. Supplements are available in capsules, but are generally quite expensive.

Several forms of oral carnitine are available, including L-carnitine, D-carnitine, and DL-carnitine. The latter two forms are often found in over-the-counter nutritional products and supplements. They are associated with more adverse effects. Products containing D-carnitine and DL-carnitine should be avoided. L-acetyl-carnitine and L-propionyl-carnitine are acceptable alternative formulations that may be recommended for specific conditions.

Precautions

Women who are pregnant or may become pregnant should not take carnitine supplements. Breast-feeding mothers should also avoid them, since they may not be safe for infants in this situation. Babies requiring a supplement due to low birth weight or pre-term conditions should have it prescribed and monitored by a healthcare provider. Those with food allergies to proteins are at risk of adverse reactions to carnitine. People who have chronic liver disease are at risk of having high carnitine levels due to their illness and should not take carnitine supplements.

Side effects

L-carnitine taken by mouth has been known to cause gastrointestinal symptoms, including **nausea**, **vomiting**, cramps, and **diarrhea**. DL-carnitine is sometimes associated with a syndrome of severe weakness and wasting of muscle, particularly in patients with kidney disease who have been on long-term hemodialysis.

Interactions

Valproic acid, a drug sometimes used to treat seizures, is more likely to cause toxicity if the patient under treatment has a carnitine deficiency. The drug may cause decreased carnitine levels. A healthcare provider should be consulted regarding the advisability of taking supplemental carnitine under those circumstances. Supplements of carnitine may increase the effects of the anticoagulant medication warfarin.

Resources

BOOKS

Balch, James, and Phyllis Balch. *Prescription for Nutritional Healing.* New York: Avery Publishing Group, 1997.

Bratman, Steven, and David Kroll. *Natural Health Bible.* Prima Publishing, 1999.

Griffith, H. Winter. *Vitamins, Herbs, Minerals & Supplements: The complete guide.* Arizona: Fisher Books, 1998.

Jellin, Jeff, Forrest Batz, and Kathy Hitchens. *Pharmacist's Letter/Prescriber's Letter Natural Medicines Comprehensive Database.* California: Therapeutic Research Faculty, 1999.

Pressman, Alan H., and Sheila Buff. *The Complete Idiot's Guide to Vitamins and Minerals.* New York: Alpha books, 1997.

Judith Turner

Carotenoids

Description

The term carotenoid refers to a family of about 600 different plant pigments that function as **antioxidants**. The yellow, orange, and many of the red pigments in fruits, vegetables, and plant materials are usually carotenoids. In the autumn, when deciduous

Carotenoids	
Carotenoid	Food sources
Alpha-carotene	Carrots Collard greens Peas Plantains Pumpkin Tangerines Tomatoes, raw Winter squash
Beta-carotene	Broccoli Cantaloupe Carrot juice Carrots Dandelion greens Kale Pumpkin Spinach Turnip greens Sweet potatoes Winter squash
Beta-cryptoxanthin	Carrots Corn, yellow Nectarines Orange juice Oranges Papaya Pumpkin Red bell peppers Tangerines Watermelon
Lutein and zeaxanthin	Broccoli Brussels sprouts Collard greens Corn, yellow Dandelion greens Kale Mustard greens Peas Pumpkin Spinach Summer squash Turnip greens Winter squash
Lycopene	Baked beans, canned Catsup Grapefruit, pink Marinara sauce Sweet red peppers Tomato juice Tomato paste and puree Tomato soup Tomatoes, raw Vegetable juice cocktail Watermelon

(Illustration by GGS Information Services. Cengage Learning, Gale)

trees prepare for winter and stop their chlorophyll production, the green color of the leaves fade and the orange, yellow, and red colors of the carotenoids in the leaves are revealed before the leaves die and fall to the ground. Plants appear to produce carotenoids to protect their stems and leaves from the energy of the sun.

Ultraviolet (UV) wavelengths can generate molecules called free radicals that can damage living cells. Free radicals are molecules, or fragments of molecules, that are unstable and highly reactive. Free radicals are produced as the result of a normal molecule's losing or gaining an electron. In normal, stable molecules, electrons associate in pairs. However, radiation from the sun can result in the removal of an electron from a molecule and the formation of a free radical. Carotenoids as antioxidants limit free radical damage by donating electrons to quench, or neutralize, the oxidant radicals.

In human **nutrition**, carotenoids, as antioxidants, serve to protect cells from the danger of free radicals that may be produced by the body during metabolism or by cigarette smoke, sunlight, radiation, pollutants, or even **stress**. Tens of thousands of free radicals are created in the body every second. When a free radical captures an electron from another molecule, a new free radical is created as the second molecule has a lone, unpaired electron. This new free radical seeks to capture another electron and become normal again. This continual process of forming free radicals becomes a chain reaction. Unless quenched, these free radicals can damage DNA, fats, and proteins. However, the body has a defense against free radicals. With proper nourishment, the body can make sufficient quantities of antioxidant enzymes and substrates for those enzymes that can facilitate the quenching of free radical reactions by antioxidants. These enzymes include superoxide dismutase, catalase, and **glutathione** peroxidase. In addition to these enzymes produced by the body, antioxidant nutrients taken into the body through foods or through dietary supplements also can surrender electrons to the free radicals without adding to the chain reaction, thus terminating the free radical reactions. Antioxidant nutrients include vitamins A, C, and E, **bioflavonoids**, lipoic acid, and carotenoids.

There are many other minor dietary carotenoids that most likely provide significant health benefits. A diet that includes many types of fruits and vegetables is important for supplying those nutrients and their associated health benefits.

Despite the large number of carotenoids in nature, only about 50 are present in foods that people in the United States eat, and only about 14 of those have been identified in blood, an indication of what is absorbed in the human body. All carotenoids are fat-soluble compounds, meaning that they can dissolve in fats and oils but not in water. The carotenoid family consists of smaller families of pigments called carotenes and xanthophylls. Carotenes are hydrocarbons, containing only carbon and hydrogen atoms, while xanthophylls also contain oxygen. The carotenes have been studied more than the other carotenoids. The ones of most interest in human nutrition are beta-carotene, alpha-carotene, and **lycopene**. Important xanthophylls include **lutein**, astaxanthin, zeaxanthin, and cryptoxanthin.

Five individual carotenoids (beta-carotene, alpha-carotene, lycopene, lutein, and beta-cryptoxanthin) were added to the National **Cancer** Institute's Diet History Questionnaire as a result of the increasing acceptance of the many health benefits of carotenoids. The carotenoids appear to reduce the risk of some forms of cancer, cardiovascular disease, and eye degeneration. As of 2008, continued research was anticipated to provide scientific evidence to confirm many of the health effects and to identify additional benefits of carotenoids.

Beta carotene

As one of the most common carotenoids, beta-carotene is the most well-known and well-studied carotenoid. It is found in carrots, pumpkins, peaches, and sweet potatoes. Beta-carotene is the primary precursor to **vitamin A** and is often called pro-vitamin A. With the aid of dioxygenase enzymes, the human body can split one molecule of beta-carotene into two vitamin A molecules. Vitamin A has many vital functions in the human body, including being involved in (1) the growth and repair of body tissues, (2) the formation of bones and teeth, (3) the resistance of the body to infection, and (4) the development of healthy eye tissues. Vitamin A deficiency symptoms include **night blindness**; dry eyes; dry, rough skin; impaired bone growth; and susceptibility to respiratory **infections**. Vitamin A is a fat soluble vitamin, can be stored in the body long-term, and can reach toxic levels over time if amounts above recommended levels (10,000 IU for adults and only 6,000 IU for pregnant women) are ingested. Too much vitamin A can cause headaches, vision problems, **nausea**, **vomiting**, an enlarged liver or spleen, birth defects, and even death at very high levels. Beta-carotene is a better source of vitamin A than vitamin A supplements because it is only converted to vitamin A on an as-needed basis; excess beta-carotene is stored in the body and, unlike vitamin A, is not toxic when taken in amounts in excess of body needs. Beta-carotene also improves immune function, increases lung capacity, reduces DNA damage, may provide protection from the sun, and may lessen the risks of some types of cancer. However, for people who drink and smoke excessively, beta-carotene may increase the risk of **lung cancer**.

Alpha carotene

Alpha-carotene, another common carotenoid, is typically found in the same foods as beta-carotene. It is similar to beta-carotene in structure, with one of the ring structures being beta-ionone. However, the other ring is different, so one molecule of alpha-carotene yields only one molecule of vitamin A. Alpha-carotene has been found to have powerful anticancer properties in cell-culture studies.

Lycopene

Lycopene is often the most common carotenoid in the American diet because it is found in tomato products, including pizza and spaghetti sauce. It is also present in lesser amounts in watermelon, pink grapefruit, guava, and apricots. Lycopene does not produce vitamin A. However, lycopene in tomato juice and spaghetti and pizza sauces has been associated with a lower risk of **prostate cancer** in men. Several clinical trials have shown that lycopene supplementation reduces the risk of prostate cancer as well as slows its progression. It has also been shown to reduce the risk of **osteoporosis**.

Cooked tomato sauces are associated with greater health benefits, compared to uncooked tomatoes because the lycopene in cooked tomatoes is more easily absorbed. Also, since lycopene is fat-soluble, absorption increases when it is mixed with oil in the sauces. Uncooked tomatoes also have health benefits, though to a lesser degree, especially when they are used in a salad with an oil-based dressing or in a sandwich with fat-containing meat. Lycopene may help in the prevention of other cancers as well as protect against heart attacks. In the late 2000s research continued on the potential health benefits of lycopene.

Lutein

Lutein, which is almost as common as beta-carotene in the American diet, and zeaxanthin are xanthophylls found in kale, spinach, broccoli, corn, **alfalfa**, and egg yolks. Both are components of the macula of the eye, a small area in the center of the retina responsible for detailed vision. These carotenoids may prevent and slow **macular degeneration**, a leading cause of blindness in the elderly. As antioxidants, they reduce the amount of free radical damage to the macula. Lutein may also help prevent the formation of **cataracts**, reduce the risk of **heart disease**, and protect against **breast cancer**.

Astaxanthin is a minor carotenoid that serves as a pigment in aquatic animals such as salmon, trout, and Antarctic krill (small shrimp-like crustaceans that feed on algae and that serve as a food source for other sea animals such as whales). Astaxanthin is a strong antioxidant that appears to enhance the immune system and protect against cancer. It also may protect against UVA light, a wavelength of ultraviolet light that can cause **sunburn** and **skin cancer**.

Beta-cryptoxanthin

Cryptoxanthin is a minor carotenoid found in peaches, papayas, tangerines, and oranges. Cryptoxanthin is second to beta-carotene in the amount of dietary carotene converted to vitamin A. Along with other carotenoids it forms an antioxidant barrier in the human skin. It also appears to protect women from cervical cancer.

General use

Although not classified as essential nutrients, carotenoids are important substances in human food sources, especially in fruits, vegetables, and plant greens, that provide many health benefits. In addition, some are precursors to vitamin A. A diet that includes many types of fruits and vegetables is important for supplying the essential carotenoids and their associated health benefits. The more common carotenoids also are available as dietary supplements.

Preparations

Beta-carotene, lutein, and lycopene are sold as individual carotenoid supplements. Beta-carotene is available in two forms, natural and synthetic. The natural form is preferred to the synthetic, as the natural form appears to be a stronger antioxidant. Algae are an abundant source of beta-carotene and are used to produce supplements. Their presence in a supplement is usually identified on the label as *Dunaliella salina* or as some related type of algae. *D. salina* produces 10 to 100 times more beta-carotene than carrots. It grows in areas with strong sunlight, high temperatures, and salty water, environments in which antioxidants are greatly needed for protection from free radicals. A dose for adults for beta-carotene may range up to 10 to 15 mg, or 25,000 IU, daily.

Lutein is prepared from marigold petals as either free lutein or lutein ester. Both forms are absorbed well by the body, though preliminary research showed that lutein ester may be assimilated slightly better and be retained slightly longer than free lutein. For general health, 4 to 6 mg of lutein should be satisfactory. For those at risk for macular degeneration, 30 to 40 mg daily may be useful.

Carotenoids

Lycopene supplements are prepared from tomatoes. A typical daily dose is 4 mg, which is the amount in one large ripe tomato. Zeaxanthin is not available as a supplement. However, the body can convert some lutein to zeaxanthin. Also lutein supplements usually contain some zeaxanthin.

Mixed carotenoid supplements are available, with different formulations. For example, one typical formula contains mostly beta-carotene, with smaller amounts of lutein, zeaxanthin, and cryptoxanthin. Another type contains less beta-carotene but a higher percentage of alpha-carotene. Mixed carotenes may also be included in some multi-vitamin and multi-oxidant supplements. Labels of supplements should be read carefully to determine the types of carotenoids present and their dosages.

A person consuming the typical American diet obtains only about 1.5 mg of carotenoids per day. The Recommended Dietary Allowance (RDA), as established by the United States National Research Council for the purpose of evaluating **diets**, for vitamin A is 1,000 RE (retinol equivalents), or 6 mg of beta-carotene. The USRDA, established by the United States Food and Drug Administration as a consumer convenience for labeling purposes, is 5,000 IU of vitamin A, or 3 mg of beta-carotene. The United States Department of Agriculture and the National Cancer Institute have suggested that perhaps 5 to 6 mg of carotenoids should be a dietary target.

To enhance dietary health benefits, it may be useful to supplement a diet high in fruits and vegetables with an additional 10 to 15 mg of carotenoid supplements per day. Those with poor diets may consider supplementation with 25 mg of supplementation per day. Since it is not possible to put every beneficial carotenoid in a supplement, the best way to obtain a wide variety of carotenoids is to eat a diet containing an assortment of carotenoid-containing foods.

As of 2008 research had not answered the question of whether individuals require additional vitamin A if they are taking beta-carotene supplements. Vitamin A is only available in foods of animal origin, so vegetarians should consider using vitamin A supplements. Persons with diseases such as diabetes may not be as efficient in converting beta-carotene into vitamin A, so they may need to get some from their diet or from supplements.

Precautions

A study conducted to investigate the effects of **vitamin E** and beta-carotene on the incidence of lung

cancer and other cancers in male smokers indicated that, in the subjects who were heavy smokers and also were heavy drinkers, beta-carotene supplements appeared to increase adverse health effects, including a slight increase in cancer. Another study of smokers indicated that high supplemental doses of beta-carotene and vitamin A increased the risk of lung cancer (though in former smokers, beta-carotene and vitamin A decreased the chances of developing lung cancer). Therefore, the use of beta-carotene supplements and vitamin A is not recommended for those who smoke or drink heavily. In the late 2000s, additional studies were conducted on the effects of beta-carotene supplementation.

Side effects

Ingesting high doses of beta-carotene can result in a benign orange coloration of the skin, especially on the palms of the hands and soles of the feet. This discoloration can be reversed with reduced dosage or discontinued use of beta-carotene for one month, with continued use at a lower dose thereafter.

Interactions

Carotenoids seem to work best together in a complementary and synergistic manner to provide antioxidant and other health benefits; they also seem to work well with other antioxidants. Therefore, the use of a mixed carotenoid supplement in combination with a multi-antioxidant formula, along with a diet rich in a variety of fruits and vegetables, is most desirable.

Carotenoid supplements are readily assimilated by the body, but to optimize absorption, they should be taken with the highest fat-content meal of the day.

As of 2008, research had not determined how the consumption of one type of carotenoid as a supplement may affect the absorption of other carotenoids. One study showed that beta-carotene reduced the absorption of canthaxanthin, another showed that beta-carotene reduced the levels of lutein in the body, while other studies showed that beta-carotene actually increased levels of other carotenoids in the body. In the late 2000s, research was ongoing in the search to identify potential interactions.

Resources

BOOKS

Challem, Jack, and Marie Moneysmith. *User's Guide to Carotenoids & Flavonoids: Learn How to Harness the Health Benefits of Natural Plant Antioxidants.* North Bergen, NJ: Basic Health, 2005.

Duyff, Roberta Larson. *American Dietetic Association Complete Food and Nutrition Guide.* Hoboken, NJ: Wiley, 2006.

PERIODICALS

Rao, Leticia. "More than Minerals." *Alive: Canadian Journal of Health & Nutrition* 298 (August 2007): 52–53.

ORGANIZATIONS

Alternative Medicine Foundation, PO Box 60016, Potomac, MD, 20859, (301) 340-1960, http://www. amfoundation.org.

Food and Nutrition Information Center, National Agricultural Library, United States Department of Agriculture, 10301 Baltimore Ave., Room 105, Beltsville, MD, 20705, (301) 504-5414, http://fnic.nal.usda.gov.

International Carotenoid Society, http://www.carotenoid society.org.

International Food Information Council, 1100 Connecticut Ave. NW, Suite 430, Washington, DC, 20036, (202) 296-6540, http://www.ific.org.

National Center for Complementary and Alternative Medicine. National Institutes of Health, 9000 Rockville Pike, Bethesda, Maryland, 20892, (888) 644-6226, http://www.nccam.nih.gov.

Office of Dietary Supplements, National Institutes of Health, 6100 Executive Blvd., Room 3B01, MSC 7517, Bethesda, MD, 20892-7517, (301) 435-2920, http://ods.od.nih.gov.

Judith Sims
Teresa Norris
Angela M. Costello

Carpal tunnel syndrome

Definition

Carpal tunnel syndrome is a disorder caused by compression at the wrist of the median nerve supplying the hand, causing numbness and tingling.

Description

The carpal tunnel is an area in the wrist where the bones and ligaments create a small passageway for the median nerve. The median nerve is responsible for both sensation and movement in the hand, in particular the thumb and first three fingers. When the median nerve is compressed, an individual's hand will feel numb.

Women between the ages of 30 and 60 have the highest rates of carpal tunnel syndrome. Research has demonstrated that carpal tunnel syndrome is a significant cause of missed work days due to **pain**. A 2007 report issued by the United States Bureau of Labor Statistics indicated that that during 2006, private industry saw more than 13,000 cases of carpal tunnel syndrome involving missed work days.

Causes and symptoms

Compression of the median nerve in the wrist can occur during a number of different conditions, particularly those conditions which lead to changes in fluid accumulation throughout the body. Because the area of the wrist through which the median nerve passes is very narrow, any swelling in the area leads to pressure on the median nerve. This pressure ultimately interferes with the nerve's ability to function normally. **Pregnancy**, **obesity**, certain thyroid conditions, diabetes, and certain pituitary abnormalities all predispose

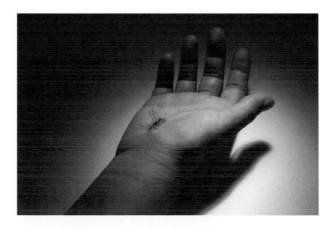

A hand with stitches after surgery for carpal tunnel syndrome. *(Chuck Goodenough / Alamy)*

a person for developing carpal tunnel syndrome. Other conditions that increase the risk for carpal tunnel syndrome include some forms of arthritis, kidney failure, and various injuries to the arm and wrist (including **fractures**, **sprains**, and dislocations). Furthermore, activities that require repeatedly bending the wrist inward toward the forearm can predispose to carpal tunnel syndrome. Certain jobs that require repeated strong wrist motions carry a relatively high risk of carpal tunnel syndrome. Injuries of this type, referred to as repetitive-motion injuries, are more frequent among secretaries who do a lot of typing, people working at computer keyboards or cash registers, factory workers, and some musicians.

Symptoms of carpal tunnel syndrome include numbness, burning, tingling, and a prickly pin-like sensation over the palm surface of the hand and into the thumb, forefinger, middle finger, and half of the ring finger. Some individuals notice a shooting pain that goes from the wrist up the arm or down into the hand and fingers. With continued median nerve compression, an individual may begin to experience muscle weakness, making it difficult to open jars and hold objects with the affected hand. Eventually, the muscles of the hand served by the median nerve may begin to grow noticeably smaller (atrophy), especially the fleshy part of the thumb. Untreated, carpal tunnel syndrome may result in permanent weakness, loss of sensation, or even paralysis of the thumb and fingers of the affected hand.

A 2008 study conducted by the National Institute of Neurological Disorders and **Stroke** examined the link between educational intervention and reduction in the number of cases of carpal tunnel syndrome.

Diagnosis

The diagnosis of carpal tunnel syndrome is made in part by checking to see whether the patient's symptoms can be brought on by holding his or her hand with the wrist bent for about a minute. Wrist x rays are often taken to rule out the possibility of a tumor causing pressure on the median nerve. A physician examining a patient suspected of having carpal tunnel syndrome performs a variety of simple tests to measure muscle strength and sensation in the affected hand and arm. Further testing might include electromyographic or nerve conduction velocity testing to determine the exact severity of nerve damage. These tests involve stimulating the median nerve with electricity and measuring the resulting speed and strength of the muscle response, as well as recording the speed of nerve transmission across the carpal tunnel. A 2002 report stated that three medical organizations had concluded that electrodiagnostic studies were the preferred methods of diagnosing carpal tunnel syndrome, offering the highest degrees of sensitivity and specificity.

Treatment

Carpal tunnel syndrome is initially treated with splints, which support the wrist and prevent it from flexing inward into the position that exacerbates median nerve compression. Some people get significant relief by wearing such splints to sleep at night, whereas others need to wear the splints all day, especially if they are performing jobs that **stress** the wrist.

The activity which caused the condition should be avoided whenever possible. Also, the actions of making a fist, holding objects, and typing should be reduced. The patient's work area should be modified to reduce stress on the body. This modification may be achieved by correct positioning and with ergonomically designed furniture. Performing hand and wrist exercises periodically throughout the day may be beneficial.

Researchers found that the carpal ligament can be lengthened or released without surgery through osteopathic manipulation and weight loading. Combining the two gives additional benefit because manipulation lengthens the ligament at one end and weight loading increases the length at the other end. Patients can be taught a stretching **exercise** for self-manipulation of the ligament.

A National Institute of Health (NIH) panel concluded that traditional **acupuncture** may be a useful alternative or complementary treatment for carpal tunnel syndrome. Studies have shown that both laser acupuncture and microamp transcutaneous electrical nerve stimulation (TENS) can significantly reduce the pain associated with carpal tunnel syndrome. Both of these therapies are painless. Greater than 90% of the patients treated reported no pain or pain that had been reduced by more than half. Patients in this study were also using Chinese herbal medicines, deep acupuncture (including needle acupuncture), **moxibustion**, and omega-3 **fish oil** capsules. All patients were able to return to work and the pain of most patients remained stable for up to two years. Persons over the age of 60 years had poorer responses.

A 1995 study conducted at the University of Pennsylvania School of Medicine concluded that **yoga** alleviated symptoms in persons suffering from carpal tunnel syndrome. A later study by Australian researchers also found that yoga was among effective non-surgical treatments. The list also included oral steroids, splints, ultrasound, and carpal bone immobilization.

Some studies have shown that persons with carpal tunnel syndrome are deficient in vitamin B$_6$ (**pyridoxine**) and that supplementation with this vitamin is beneficial. Carpal tunnel syndrome should improve within two to three months by taking 100 mg three times daily. Patients should consult with their physician when taking high doses of this vitamin.

Chinese and homeopathic remedies include:

- arnica; 30c dose
- astra essence
- Rhus toxicodendron; 6c dose
- Ruta graveolens; 6c dose

Allopathic treatment

Ibuprofen or other nonsteroidal anti-inflammatory drugs may be prescribed to decrease pain and swelling. Diuretics may be used if the syndrome is related to the menstrual cycle. When carpal tunnel syndrome is more advanced, steroids may be injected into the wrist to decrease inflammation.

The most severe cases of carpal tunnel syndrome may require surgery to decrease the compression of the median nerve and restore its normal function. Such a repair involves cutting the ligament that crosses the wrist, thus allowing the median nerve more room and decreasing compression. This surgery is done almost exclusively on an outpatient basis and is often performed without the patient having to be rendered unconscious. Careful injection of numbing medicines (local anesthesia) or nerve blocks (the injection of anesthetics directly into the nerve) create sufficient numbness to allow the surgery to be performed painlessly, without the risks associated with general anesthesia. Recovery from this type of surgery is usually quick and without complications.

In 2002, researchers in the Netherlands reported that after studying about 80 patients over two years, surgery proved more successful than nighttime splints in freeing up compressed nerves of patients with carpal tunnel syndrome. Many patients in the splint group ended up choosing the surgery option after several months of wearing splints.

Expected results

Without treatment, continued pressure on the median nerve puts the patient at risk for permanent disability in the affected hand. Alternative medicines have been shown to reduce pain. Most people are able to control the symptoms of carpal tunnel syndrome with splinting and anti-inflammatory agents. For those who go on to require surgery, about 95% have complete cessation of symptoms.

KEY TERMS

Carpal tunnel—A passageway in the wrist, created by the bones and ligaments of the wrist, through which the median nerve passes.

Electromyography—A test in which a nerve's function is examined by stimulating the nerve with electricity and then measuring the speed and strength of the corresponding muscle's response.

Ergonomic—The science of correlating a person's body and the person's workplace in order to facilitate the efficient use of human energy.

Median nerve—A nerve that runs through the wrist and into the hand. It provides sensation and some movement to the hand, the thumb, the index finger, the middle finger, and half of the ring finger.

Prevention

Avoiding or reducing the repetitive motions that put the wrist into a bent position may help to prevent carpal tunnel syndrome. People who must work long hours at a computer keyboard, for example, may need to take advantage of advances in ergonomics and position the keyboard and computer components in a way that increases efficiency and decreases stress. Taking frequent breaks is important. Wearing fingerless gloves may help to maintain flexibility and warmth in the hands. Early use of a splint may also be helpful for persons whose jobs put them at risk of carpal tunnel syndrome.

Resources

BOOKS

Montgomery, Kate. *End Your Carpal Tunnel Syndrome without Surgery*. Elkhart, IN: Sports Touch, 2007.

ORGANIZATIONS

Association for Repetitive Motion Syndromes, PO Box 514, Santa Rosa, CA, 95402, (707) 571-0397, http://www.certifiedpst.com/arms/.

National Institute of Neurological Disorders and Stroke, PO Box 5801, Bethesda, MD, 20824, (800) 352-9424, (301) 496-5751, http://www.ninds.nih.gov/index.htm.

U.S. Bureau of Labor Statistics, Postal Square Building, 2 Massachusetts Ave. NE, Washington, DC, 20212-0001, http://www.bls.gov/.

Teresa G. Odle
Rhonda Cloos, RN

Cartilage supplements

Description

Cartilage is a type of dense connective tissue found in humans and other animals. Bluish-white or gray in color, the semi-opaque tissue has no nerve or blood supply of its own. Cartilage supplements come from such animal sources as cattle, sheep, sharks, and chickens. Bovine cartilage supplements are derived from the windpipes of cows, whereas the cartilage from the heads and fins of sharks is used for shark cartilage supplements.

General use

Both shark and bovine cartilage supplements have been proposed as treatments for **cancer**. In addition, a compound derived from cartilage called **chondroitin** has been publicized as a useful treatment for **osteoarthritis**. Cartilage preparations are available as pills, powders, or liquids for oral dosage. They can also be given as enemas, topical applications, or intravenous or intramuscular injections.

Bovine cartilage supplements

Beginning in the 1950s, the physician John F. Prudden noticed that bovine cartilage could enhance wound healing in animals. Prudden then injected an extract of bovine cartilage into a **breast cancer** patient whose tumor had ulcerated her skin. The patient's tumor ultimately disappeared, and she lived for 12 years before dying of other causes. In 1985, Prudden published the first of several scientific papers on the subject.

Prudden asserted that the anticancer ingredients in bovine cartilage are mucopolysaccharides, which are complex sugar molecules that help fight cancer by stimulating the patient's immune system. Prudden also stated that these large sugar molecules act on tumor cell membranes by blocking mitosis (cell division). Other proposed explanations of the effectiveness of bovine cartilage include the inhibition of protease, which is an enzyme that helps to break down proteins, and the blocking of the formation of enzymes that break down collagen proteins. Bovine cartilage is also reported to reduce the rate of new blood vessel growth in tumors, called angiogenesis. Although numerous bovine cartilage supplements have been made available for immunostimulation or to fight cancer, there is little scientific evidence of their effectiveness. Most positive reports on tumor response and the survival of cancer patients after cartilage treatment are anecdotal. As of 2008 there had been very few scientific studies on the use of bovine collagen in humans, and those that had been done had not shown it to be an effective treatment.

Shark cartilage supplements

The use of shark cartilage to treat cancer is based on the claim that it blocks angiogenesis or the development of new blood vessels that tumors need to survive. Judah Folkman, a researcher at Harvard Medical School in the 1970s, developed the theory of angiogenesis. Dr. Folkman's proposal that tumors, much like a normal organ or mass of cells, require a supply of blood to deliver nutrients for growth, later became closely linked to the treatment of cancer with shark cartilage.

In 1983, William Lane, motivated by Folkman's research, began investigating the possible link between shark cartilage and its ability to starve tumors with an antiangiogenetic mechanism. In 1993, Lane published his book *Sharks Don't Get Cancer*, making shark cartilage one of the leading alternative cancer therapies, with the vast majority of the cartilage market since that time comprised of shark cartilage.

The use of shark cartilage as an alternative treatment has been opposed by wildlife experts who say that use of the substance threatens the shark population. Estimates vary widely on the number of sharks killed each year to make cartilage products, but most put the number at greater than 100,000. Further research has also shattered the myth that sharks do not get cancer. A variety of studies on sharks since the popularization of shark cartilage as a cancer fighter have documented that sharks do, in fact, get cancer, and cases of cancer of the cartilage have even been documented.

Both shark and bovine cartilage have been used to treat a wide variety of cancers, including tumors of the breast, ovary, cervix, prostate, rectum, colon, stomach, kidney, and brain. The U.S. Food and Drug Administration (FDA) maintains that both types of cartilage can be tested as potential cancer therapy in clinical trials but must be sold strictly as dietary supplements. Dietary supplement manufacturers are also prohibited from making specific claims that the supplements can cure disease. Dietary supplements are not regulated in the same way as drugs, which means that products can vary widely in the amount of cartilage contained in the supplement and the purity of the cartilage.

While some laboratory studies have shown positive results from both bovine and shark supplements as a treatment for cancer, continued research as of 2008 was being conducted to determine their effectiveness. Some studies indicate that the proposed antiangiogenetic effects of shark cartilage are ultimately destroyed by digestion, and the substance therefore is unlikely to be effective when taken orally as a pill. There is some evidence that a liquid shark cartilage extract called AE-941 (Neovastat) may be effective at slowing blood vessel growth. As of 2008 Neovastat was approved by the FDA as an investigational drug approved for use in clinical trials, and clinical trials were underway to test its effectiveness.

Chondroitin sulfate

Chondroitin is best known to the general public as a remedy for osteoarthritis, which is a form of arthritis caused by wearing away or degeneration of the cartilage that cushions the ends of bones. It is thought that the drying out of cartilage tissue in osteoarthritis is a major cause of tissue destruction. Chondroitin sulfate is given together with **glucosamine**, a compound that is a building block of cartilage. The chondroitin helps to attract and hold fluid within cartilage tissue. Tissue fluid keeps cartilage healthy in two ways: it acts as a shock absorber within the joints of the body, thus protecting cartilage from being worn away by the bones, and it carries nutrients to the cartilage.

The evidence for the use of chondroitin is mixed. Although many early studies showed significant positive effects on osteoarthritis, later studies, which tended to be larger and have patients with more advanced osteoarthritis, showed little to no effect. A meta-analysis published in 2007 in the *Annals of Internal Medicine* analyzed 20 previous studies and concluded that there was little or no evidence that chondroitin had a positive effect on osteoarthritis. However, the authors did not take into account studies that combine glucosamine and chondroitin, which some evidence shows may work better than chondroitin alone.

Preparations

Shark and bovine cartilage supplements are available in capsule form, while shark is also sold as a powder and liquid. Shark supplements are made from ground-up shark skeletons (mainly the fins and head), while bovine supplements are prepared from the cartilage taken from cow bones and the windpipe. Chondroitin sulfate can be taken orally as a pill, powder, or liquid. It can also be administered by injection. Oral preparations of chondroitin, by itself or in combination with glucosamine, are available in the United States as over-the-counter (OTC) dietary supplements. They can be purchased over the Internet, at pharmacies, health food stores, and many grocery stores.

The recommended dosage of shark and bovine cartilage varies depending on the person and individual need. General guidelines indicate that the recommended dose of shark cartilage is 1 g daily per kilogram of body weight—the equivalent to almost 70 g per day for a 150-pound individual. With observed shrinkage of the tumor, the dosage may be lowered. The recommended bovine cartilage dosage per day is 9 g. With both supplements, patients must keep taking the same dose and include the supplements in their **diets** for life. Because the supplements must be taken over the long term, they can be prohibitively expensive. Individuals considering taking cartilage supplements should carefully consider the long-term cost of doing so.

Precautions

While cartilage supplements do not appear to be harmful, individuals who are considering them as a cancer treatment should never use them as the only form of therapy and should consult a doctor before taking them. Individuals who are considering chondroitin as a treatment for joint **pain** should be careful not to diagnose themselves. They should check with their physician to be sure that the pain is caused by osteoarthritis. Some conditions, including **Lyme disease**, **gout**, **bursitis**, and **rheumatoid arthritis**, can also cause pain in the joints. Although chondroitin may be helpful in treating osteoarthritis, it is not useful for these other conditions. Chondroitin has not been studied in children or in pregnant or nursing women.

Side effects

Both shark and bovine cartilage supplements show little or no side effects when taken at the appropriate dosage levels. Individuals who are allergic to seafood or shellfish should not take shark cartilage supplements. Some patients have reported an allergic reaction to traces of bovine protein or other side effects that include a bad taste in the mouth, **fatigue**, and **nausea**. Shark cartilage can cause hypercalcemia (excessive amounts of **calcium** in the body) when taken at the recommended daily dose of 70 g per day. This dosage results in 14 times the amount of calcium recommended by the United States Recommended Daily Allowance (USRDA). Some patients taking

KEY TERMS

Angiogenesis—The development of new blood vessels, specifically those that supply tumors with blood and nutrients for growth.

Chondroitin—A complex carbohydrate found in human and animal cartilage that is used to treat several physical disorders, most importantly arthritis.

Glucosamine—A complex carbohydrate composed of glucose and an amino acid called glutamine. It is an important building block of cartilage and is often taken together with chondroitin as a treatment for osteoarthritis.

Mucopolysaccharide—An older term for a class of large sugar molecules that are found in cartilage and other forms of connective tissue. Mucopolysaccharides are called glycosaminoglycans.

chondroitin have been known to experience nausea and **gas** or bloating.

Interactions

Chondroitin sulfate is not known to cause any significant interactions with other medications. One researcher, however, has suggested that chondroitin might increase the effect of anticoagulant drugs and should probably not be used in combination with them. No scientific studies have been done as of 2008 to investigate possible interactions of cartilage supplements with medications and other supplements. Individuals should always consult a doctor or pharmacist before beginning to take a new supplement.

Resources

BOOKS

Bales, Peter. *Osteoarthritis: Preventing and Healing without Drugs.* Amherst, NY: Prometheus Books, 2008.

Barrow, Colin, and Fereidoon Shahidi, eds. *Marine Nutraceuticals and Functional Foods.* Boca Raton, FL, CRC Press, 2008.

Columbus, Frank, ed. *Arthritis Research.* New York: Nova Biomedical Books, 2005.

PERIODICALS

Loprinzi, Charles L., et al. "Evaluation of Shark Cartilage in Patients with Advanced Cancer." *Cancer* 104, no. 1 (July 1, 2005): 176–183.

Reichenbach, Stephan, et al. "Meta-analysis: Chondroitin for Osteoarthritis of the Knee or Hip." *Annals of Internal Medicine* 146, no. 8 (April 17, 2007): 580–590.

ORGANIZATIONS

National Cancer Institute, 6116 Executive Blvd., Room 3036A, Bethesda, MD, 20892-8322, (800) 4-CANCER, (800) 332-8615, http://www.cancer.gov.

National Center for Complementary and Alternative Medicine (NCCAM), National Institutes of Health, 9000 Rockville Pike, Bethesda, MD, 20892, http://www.nccam. nih.gov.

Beth Kapes
Teresa G. Odle
Helen Davidson

Castor oil

Description

Castor oil is a natural plant oil obtained from the seed of the castor plant. The castor seed, or bean, is the source of numerous economically important products as one of the world's most important industrial oils, and was one of the earliest commercial products. Castor beans have been found in ancient Egyptian tombs dating back to 4000 B.C. According to the Ebers Papyrus, an Egyptian medical text from 1500 B.C., Egyptian doctors used castor oil to protect the eyes from irritation. The oil from the bean was used thousands of years ago in facial oils and in wick lamps for lighting. Castor oil has been used medicinally in the United States since the days of the pioneers. Traveling medicine men in the late 1800s peddled castor oil, often mixed with as much as 40% alcohol, as a heroic cure for everything from **constipation** to **heartburn**. It was also used to induce labor. At the present time, castor oil is used internally as a laxative and externally as a castor oil pack or poultice.

The castor plant, whose botanical name is *Ricinus communis*, is native to the Ethiopian region of east Africa. It now grows in tropical and warm temperate regions throughout the world and is becoming an abundant weed in the southwestern United States. Castor plants grow along stream banks, river beds, bottom lands, and in almost any warm area where the soil is well drained and with sufficient nutrients and moisture to sustain growth. They are annuals that can grow 6–15 ft (1.8–5 m) tall in one season with full sunlight, heat, and moisture. The tropical leaves, with five to nine pointed, finger-like lobes, may be 4–30 in (10–76 cm) across. Flowers occur on the plant (which is monoecious, meaning that there are separate male and female flowers on the same individual), during most of the year in dense terminal clusters, with female flowers

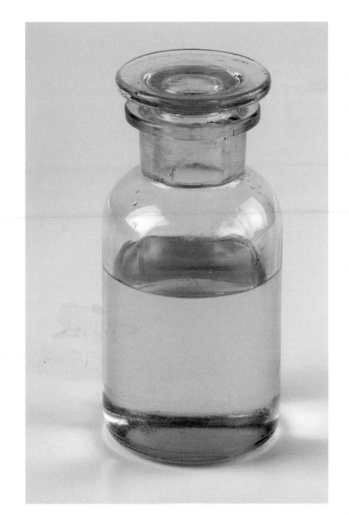

Castor oil. The castor plant (Ricinus communis) is native to the Ethiopian region of east Africa. It now grows in tropical and warm temperate regions throughout the world and is becoming an abundant weed in the southwestern United States. *(Bon Appetit / Alamy)*

The name "castor" was given to the plant by English traders who confused its oil with the oil of another shrub, *Vitex agnus*—Castus, which the Spanish and Portuguese in Jamaica called agno-casto. The scientific name of the plant was given by the eighteenth-century Swedish naturalist Carolus Linnaeus. *Ricinus* is the Latin word for tick; apparently Linnaeus thought the castor bean looked like a tick, especially a tick in engorged with blood, with the caruncle of the bean resembling the tick's head. *Communis* means "common" in Latin. Castor plants were already commonly naturalized in many parts of the world by the eighteenth century.

There are several cultivated varieties of the castor plant, all of which have striking foliage colorations. The castor plant grows rapidly with little care and produces lush tropical foliage. Its use as a cultivated plant should be discouraged because its seeds or beans are extremely poisonous. Children should be taught to recognize and avoid the plant and its seeds, especially in the southwestern United States where it grows wild near residential areas. Flower heads can be snipped off of castor plants as a protective measure.

The active poison in the castor bean is ricin, a deadly water-soluble protein called a lectin. The ricin is left in the meal or cake after the oil is extracted from the bean, so castor oil does not contain any of the poison. The seed is only toxic if the outer shell is broken or chewed. Humans and horses are most susceptible to ricin, although all pets and livestock should be kept away from the castor seed. It has been estimated that gram for gram, ricin is 6,000 times more deadly than cyanide and 12,000 times more deadly than rattlesnake venom. A dose of only 70 micrograms, or one two-millionth of an ounce (roughly equivalent to the weight of a single grain of table salt) is enough to kill a 160-pound person. Even small particles in open sores or in the eyes may be fatal. As few as four ingested seeds can kill an adult human. Lesser amounts may result in **vomiting**, severe abdominal **pain, diarrhea**, increased heart rate, profuse sweating, and convulsions. Signs of toxicity occur about 18–24 hours after ingestion. Ricin seems to cause clumping (agglutination) and breakdown (hemolysis) of red blood cells, hemorrhaging in the digestive tract, and damage to the liver and kidneys.

Ricin has attracted considerable attention as of early 2003 because of its association with terrorist groups. Although ricin cannot easily be used against large groups of people, it has been used to assassinate individuals by injection. The Centers for Disease Control and Prevention (CDC) considers ricin a "B"-list

just above the male flowers. Each female flower consists of a spiny ovary, which develops into the fruit or seed capsule, and a bright red structure with feathery branches (stigma lobes) to receive pollen from the male flowers. Each male flower consists of a cluster of many stamens that shed pollen that is distributed by wind. The spiny seed pod or capsule is composed of three sections, or carpels, that split apart at maturity. Each carpel contains a single seed. As the carpel dries and splits open, the seed is ejected, often with considerable force. The seeds are slightly larger than pinto beans and are covered with intricate mottled designs, none of which have exactly the same pattern due to genetic variations. At one end of the seed is a small spongy structure called the caruncle, which aids in the absorption of water when the seeds are planted.

bioterrorism agent, meaning that it is relatively easy to make and is considered a moderate threat to life.

On the positive side, ricin is being investigated as a tool for **cancer** treatment. A promising use is the production of an immunotoxin in which the protein ricin is joined to monoclonal antibodies. The ricin-antibody conjugate, which is produced in a test tube, should theoretically travel directly to the site of a tumor, where the ricin can destroy the tumor cells without damaging other cells in the patient.

General use

Internal uses

Castor oil is a strong and effective cathartic or purgative (laxative), with components in the oil that affect both the small and large intestines. It has been used to clear the bowels after **food poisoning** and to relieve constipation. It is sometimes used in hospitals to prepare the patient's abdomen for x rays of the colon or kidneys. Castor oil is classified as a stimulant laxative, also known as a contact laxative. This type of laxative encourages bowel movements by acting on the intestinal wall, increasing the muscle contractions that move along the stool mass. Stimulants are a popular type of laxative for self-treatment, but unfortunately are more likely to cause side effects. There are milder types of laxatives that may be more useful for inducing regularity and treating constipation. Generally laxatives should be used to provide short-term relief only, unless otherwise directed by a doctor.

Castor oil is frequently used in animal experiments to test the effects of new medications on the gastrointestinal tract.

If castor oil has been prescribed by a doctor, his or her instructions for the timing and quantity of doses should be followed. For self-treatment, users should follow the manufacturer's instructions. At least 6–8 glasses (8 oz each) of liquids should be taken each day to soften the stools. Castor oil is usually taken on an empty stomach for rapid effect. Because results usually occur within two to six hours, castor oil is not usually taken late in the day. The unpleasant taste of castor oil may be improved by chilling it in the refrigerator for at least an hour. It may then be stirred into a glass of cold orange juice. Flavored preparations of castor oil are also available.

External uses

Castor oil is also used topically to treat **corns**. The oil is applied once or twice daily directly to the corns, which are surrounded with adhesive-backed corn aperture pads made of felt to hold the oil. The corns are then covered with hypoallergenic silk tape. After soaking with the castor oil, the corns will be softened for removal with a pumice stone. Castor oil can be used in a similar manner to remove **warts**. Castor oil is also used to treat ringworm, abscesses, **bruises**, dry skin, **dermatitis**, **sunburn**, open sores, and other skin conditions. Additional less well-known uses of castor oil include hair tonics, cosmetics, and contraceptive creams and jellies.

For menstrual cramping, especially when fibroids may be present or when flows are heavy, castor oil packs may be placed on the abdomen for up to an hour. The packs are made by soaking square or rectangular pieces of cotton, cotton flannel, or undyed wool 2–4 in (5–10 cm) thick with 4–6 oz (118–177 ml) of castor oil. The pack is folded over once or twice, placed directly on the abdomen, and covered with plastic wrap. Over the pack, a water bottle or a heating pad on a low setting may be used to keep the pack warm. After use, the skin may be cleansed with a warm solution of baking soda and water (2 tsp of baking soda to 1 qt water). Some herbal therapists maintain that castor oil packs may aid in shrinking small fibroids. Castor oil packs have also been used in the treatment of many other diseases and disorders, including breast pain, digestive tract problems, abscesses, **hemorrhoids**, **wounds**, and **gallstones**.

Nonmedical uses

Castor oil and its derivatives also are used in many industrial products, including paint and varnish, fabric coatings and protective coverings, insulation, food containers, soap, ink, plastics, brake fluids, insecticidal oils, and guns. It is a primary raw material for the production of nylon and other synthetic resins and fibers, and a basic ingredient in racing motor oil for high-performance automobile and motorcycle engines. Castor oil is also used as a fuel additive for two-cycle engines, imparting a distinctive aroma to their exhaust. Even though it is malodorous and distasteful, it is the source of several synthetic flower scents and fruit flavors.

Preparations

Castor oil for medicinal purposes is pressed from the seeds of the castor plant and is slightly yellow or colorless. It has a lingering nauseating aftertaste, even though **peppermint** or fruit juices are sometimes added as flavor enhancers in an attempt to disguise its disagreeable taste. Castor oil is available in both oil and emulsified liquid preparations.

Precautions

Castor oil should not be used by a pregnant woman, as it can cause contractions. Castor oil should not be used if a patient is hypersensitive to the castor bean; or has an intestinal obstruction, abdominal pain, cramping, bloating, soreness, **nausea**, vomiting, fecal impaction, or any signs of appendicitis or an inflamed bowel. It should not be used by anyone for more than a week unless a doctor has ordered otherwise. Overuse of a laxative may lead to dependence on it. Any sudden changes in bowel habits or function that last longer than two weeks should be checked by a doctor before using a laxative.

Children up to the age of six should not take a laxative unless prescribed by a doctor. In older adults, the use of castor oil may worsen weakness, lack of coordination, or **dizziness** and light-headedness.

External overexposure to castor oil may result in a slight local skin irritation. The irritated area should be washed with soap and water.

Side effects

Side effects of castor oil that require medical attention include:

- confusion
- irregular heartbeat
- muscle cramps
- skin rash
- unusual tiredness or weakness

There are other less serious side effects that are less common and may go away as the patient's body adjusts to the castor oil. These side effects include belching, cramping, diarrhea, and nausea. If they do continue or are bothersome, the person should check with a doctor. In addition, because castor oil causes a complete emptying of the contents of the intestine, patients should be advised that they may not have another bowel movement for two to three days after a dose of castor oil.

Interactions

Patients should not take castor oil within two hours of taking other types of medicine, because the desired effect of the other medicine may be reduced. Patients who are taking **digitalis**, digoxin, or a diuretic should consult their physician before taking castor oil, as the castor oil may intensify the effects of these drugs by causing the body to lose **potassium**.

Resources

BOOKS

McGarey, William G. *The Oil That Heals: A Physician's Successes with Castor Oil Treatments.* A.R.E. Press, 1993.
Wilson, Billie Ann, et al. *Nurses Drug Guide 1995.* Norwalk, CT: Appleton & Lange, 1995.

PERIODICALS

Layne, Marty. "Castor Oil: A Great Home Remedy for Bumps, Bruises and Cuts." *Natural Life* (July-August 2002). 14-15.
Lyall, Sarah. "Arrest of Terror Suspects in London Turns Up a Deadly Toxin." *New York Times*, January 8, 2003.
Rahman, M. T., M. Alimuzzaman, S. Ahmad, et al. "Antinociceptive and Antidiarrhoeal Activity of *Zanthoxylum rhetsa.*" *Fitoterapia* 73 (July 2002): 340-342.
Sandvig, K., and B. van Deurs. "Transport of Protein Toxins Into Cells: Pathways Used by Ricin, Cholera Toxin and Shiga Toxin." *FEBS Letter* 529 (October 2, 2002): 49-53.

ORGANIZATIONS

Centers for Disease Control and Prevention (CDC). 1600 Clifton Road, Atlanta, GA 30333. (404) 639-3311. http://www.cdc.gov.
National Digestive Diseases Information Clearinghouse. National Institute of Diabetes and Digestive and Kidney Disease. National Institutes of Health. 2 Information Way. Bethesda, MD 20892-3570. (310) 654-3810.

Judith Sims
Rebecca J. Frey, PhD

Cataracts

Definition

A cataract is a cloudiness or opacity in the normally transparent crystalline lens of the eye. This cloudiness can cause loss of vision and may lead to eventual blindness.

Description

The human eye has several parts. The outer layer of the eyeball consists of a transparent dome-shaped cornea and an opaque white sclera, which is a fibrous membrane. The cornea and sclera help protect the eye. The next layer contains the iris, pupil, and ciliary body. The iris is the colored part of the eye; the pupil is the small dark round hole in the middle of the iris. The pupil and iris allow light into the eye. The ciliary body contains muscles that help the eye to focus. The lens lies behind the pupil and iris. It is covered by a cellophane-like capsule. The lens is normally transparent, elliptical in shape, and somewhat elastic. This elasticity allows the lens to focus on both near and far objects. The lens is attached to the ciliary body by fibers (zonules of Zinn). Muscles in the ciliary body act on the zonules, which then change the shape of the lens. This changing of shape is called accommodation. As people age, the lens hardens and accommodates less easily, which makes it harder for the person to see close objects. This hardening of the lens generally occurs around the age of 40 and continues until about age 65. The condition is called presbyopia. It is a normal condition of **aging**, generally resulting in the need for reading glasses.

The lens is made up of approximately 35% protein and 65% water. As people age, the proteins in the lens begin to degenerate. Changes in the proteins, water content, enzymes, and other chemicals may contribute to cataract formation.

The major parts of the lens are the nucleus, the cortex, and the capsule. The nucleus is in the center of the lens, the cortex surrounds the nucleus, and the capsule is the outer layer. Opaque areas can develop in any part of the lens. Cataracts, then, can be classified according to location (nuclear, cortical, or posterior subcapular cataracts). The density and location of the cataract determines the extent of vision affected. If the cataract forms in the area of the lens directly behind the pupil, the person's vision may be significantly impaired. A cataract that occurs on the outer edges or side of the lens will cause less impairment.

Cataracts in the elderly are so common that they are considered a normal part of the aging process. People between the ages of 52–64 have a 50% chance of developing a cataract, while at least 70% of those 70 and older are affected. Cataracts associated with aging (senile or age-related cataracts) most often occur in both eyes, with each cataract progressing at a different rate. At first, these cataracts may not affect vision. If the cataract remains small or at the periphery of the lens, the visual changes may be minor.

Cataracts that occur in people other than the elderly are much less common. Congenital cataracts occur very rarely in newborns. Genetic defects or an infection or disease in the mother during **pregnancy** are among the causes of congenital cataracts. One condition called blue cataracts is inheritance-linked and affects primarily Tibetans and some other Asians. Traumatic cataracts may develop after an injury or foreign body damages the lens or eye. Systemic illnesses such as diabetes may result in cataracts. Cataracts can also occur secondary to other eye diseases—for example, an inflammation of the inner layer of the eye (uveitis) or **glaucoma**. Such cataracts are called complicated cataracts. Toxic cataracts result from chemical toxicity, such as steroid use. Cataracts can also result from exposure to the sun's ultraviolet (UV) rays.

Causes and symptoms

Studies have been conducted to determine whether diet or the use of vitamins might have an effect on the formation of cataracts in older people. Although debate continues in the 2000s, several studies reported in late 2001 that a diet rich in certain **carotenoids** may protect against development of cataracts. Likewise, there has been considerable interest in the use of antioxidant supplements as a protection against cataracts. Such antioxidant vitamins as vitamins A, C, E, and beta-carotene protect body tissues against free radicals, which are byproducts of oxidation. **Vitamin C**, in particular, has shown the strongest impact on lower rates of cataracts. Some vitamins are marketed specifically for the eyes. Patients should speak to their doctors about the use of such vitamins.

Studies also have linked changes in lens proteins to cataract formation. Soluble proteins in the lens begin to condense and form clumps, leading to cataracts. Researchers have identified mutations in genes that likely lead to protein changes resulting in juvenile cataracts. The next step is to study a possible genetic relationship to formation of age-related cataracts as well.

The National Eye Institute reports a definitive link between **smoking** and cataracts, and a 2004 report from the surgeon general also indicates such a link. Alcohol intake has been implicated in cataract formation. Some studies have determined that a diet high in fat increases the likelihood of cataract formation, while eating more foods rich in **antioxidants** lowers the risk. A study conducted in the United Kingdom and reported in the literature in 2004 showed no connection between dietary intake of vitamin C and cataract reduction. More research is needed to determine if diet, alcohol consumption, or vitamins have any connection to the formation of cataracts. Research was underway in 2008 to determine a link between sunlight exposure and cataract development.

Cataracts may have the following symptoms:

- gradual, painless onset of blurry, filmy, or fuzzy vision
- poor central vision
- frequent changes in eyeglass prescription
- changes in color vision
- increased glare from light, especially oncoming night-time headlights
- second-sight improvement in near vision (no longer needing reading glasses), but a decrease in distance vision
- poor vision in sunlight
- the presence of a milky whiteness in the pupil as the cataract progresses

Diagnosis

Both ophthalmologists and optometrists may detect and monitor cataract growth and prescribe prescription lenses for visual deficits. Only an ophthalmologist, however, can perform cataract extraction.

Cataracts are easily diagnosed from the reporting of symptoms, a visual acuity examination using an eye chart, and by a physician or optometrist's examination of the eye. Shining a penlight into the pupil may reveal opacities or a color change of the lens even before the patient develops visual symptoms. A slit lamp, which is basically a large microscope, allows the doctor to examine the front of the eye and the lens and to determine the location of the cataract.

Some other diagnostic tests may be used to determine if cataracts are present or how much improvement the patient may have after surgery. These tests include a glare test, potential vision test, and contrast sensitivity test.

Treatment

Because free radicals have been implicated as a cause of cataracts, alternative therapies emphasize the importance of a healthful diet, nutritional supplements, and/or herbal remedies to prevent and slow down the progression of cataracts.

Nutritional therapy

A naturopathic doctor or a nutritionist may recommend the following dietary changes:

- Reduce consumption of salty or fatty foods. Diabetics should also limit their intake of milk and other dairy products.
- Increase intake of foods that are high in beta-carotene: peaches, apricots, berries, carrots, and leafy green vegetables. Beta-carotene and other antioxidants can protect against or slow down the development of cataracts.
- Stop cigarette smoking and avoid exposure to secondhand smoke.
- Eat a diet rich in fruits and vegetables with high concentrations of vitamin C. Take supplemental vitamin C (1 g three times daily) and vitamin A (25,000 IU per day).
- Take supplemental beta-carotene (25,000–100,000 IU per day) and selenium (400 mcg per day). Low selenium levels may increase the risk of cataracts.
- Increase intake of L-cysteine (400 mg per day), L-glutamine (200 mg per day), and L-glycine (200 mg per day). These three amino acids may be beneficial to some cataract patients.
- Add other supplements: zinc, lutein, riboflavin, and cod liver oil.

Herbal therapy

Two herbal remedies may help protect the eyes against cataracts:

- Bilberries (40–80 mg daily). Early research indicates that eating bilberries may halt cataract progression.
- *Hachimijiogan.* Animal studies suggest that this ancient Chinese herbal formula may protect the eyes against cataracts by increasing the glutathione content of the lens.

Allopathic treatment

Cataracts that cause no symptoms or only minor visual changes may not require any treatment. An ophthalmologist or optometrist should continue to monitor and assess the cataract at scheduled office visits. Stronger prescription eyeglasses or contact lenses may be helpful.

Cataract surgery is the only option for patients whose cataracts interfere with vision to the extent of affecting their daily lives. The most frequently performed surgery in the United States, this procedure improves vision in over 90% of patients. Some people assert that a cataract should be ripe before being removed; a ripe or mature cataract means that the lens is completely opaque. Most cataracts are removed before they reach that stage. Sometimes cataracts need to be removed so that the doctor can examine the back of the eye more carefully. Patients with diseases that may affect the eye may require cataract surgery for this reason. Advances in cataract surgery make possible a surgical incision of as little as three millimeters in length and may require no stitches. The procedure takes only a few minutes, and patients often return to work in a few days. If cataracts are present in both eyes, only one eye at a time should be operated on. Healing occurs in the first eye before the second cataract is removed, sometimes as early as the following week. A final eyeglass prescription is usually given about four to six weeks after surgery. Patients may still need reading glasses. The overall health of the patient needs to be considered in making the decision to operate. Age alone, however, need not preclude effective surgical treatment of cataracts; people in their 90s can benefit from cataract surgery.

The natural human lens filters out blue wavelength light, which may damage the retina. The intraocular lenses utilized in the early 2000s to replace the natural lens in cataract surgery possess the ability to filter such light.

Patients are given antibiotic drops to prevent infection and steroids to reduce inflammation after surgery. An eye shield or glasses during the day protect the eye from injury while it heals. At night, the patient should wear an eye shield. The patient returns to the doctor the day after surgery for assessment, with several follow-up visits over the following two months to monitor the healing process.

Expected results

The success rate of cataract extraction is very high, with a good prognosis. Visual acuity of 20/40 or better may be achieved. If an extracapsular cataract extraction is performed, a secondary cataract may develop in the remaining back portion of the capsule one to two years after surgery. Yttrium aluminum garnet (YAG) capsulotomy is most often used to treat this type of cataract. Yttrium aluminum garnet refers to the name of the laser used for this procedure. The laser beam makes a small opening in the remaining back part of the capsule, allowing light through.

Complications occur in a small percentage (3–5%) of surgical cataract extractions. **Infections**, swelling of the cornea (**edema**), bleeding, **retinal detachment**, and the onset of glaucoma have been reported. Any haziness, redness, decrease in vision, **nausea**, or **pain** should be reported to the surgeon immediately.

Prevention

Preventive measures emphasize wearing glasses with a special coating to protect against UV rays. Dark lenses alone are not sufficient. The lenses must protect against UV light (specifically, UV-A and UV-B). Antioxidants and herbal remedies may also provide some protection by reducing free radicals that can damage lens proteins. A study published in 2008 found that females who ingested a higher intake of lutein/zeaxanthin and **vitamin E** showed less risk of developing cataracts. A healthful diet rich in sources of antioxidants, including citrus fruits, sweet potatoes, carrots, green leafy vegetables, and/or vitamin supplements may be helpful. When individuals take certain medications, such as steroids, they may need more frequent eye exams. Patients should speak to their doctors to see if medications may affect their eyes.

Resources

BOOKS

Cataract and Refractive Surgery: Essentials in Ophthalmology. Edited by Thomas Kohnen and Douglas D. Koch. New York: Springer, 2006.

PERIODICALS

Christen, William G., et al. "Dietary Carotenoids, Vitamins C and E, and Risk of Cataract in Women." *Archives of Ophthalmology* 126, no. 1 (2008): 102–109.

ORGANIZATIONS

American Academy of Ophthalmology (National Eyecare Project), PO Box 429098, San Francisco, CA, 94142-9098, (800) 222-EYES, http://www.eyenet.org.

American Optometric Association, 243 North Lindbergh Blvd., St. Louis, MO, 63141, (314) 991-4100, http://www.aoanet.org.

Lighthouse, 111 East Fifty-ninth St., New York, NY, 10022, (800) 334-5497, http://www.lighthouse.org.

National Eye Institute, 2020 Vision Place, Bethesda, MD, 20892-3655, (301) 496-5248, http://www.nei.nih.gov.

Prevent Blindness America, 500 East Remington Rd., Schaumburg, IL, 60173, (800) 331-2020, http://www.prevent-blindness.org.

Mai Tran
Teresa Norris
Rhonda Cloos, RN

Catmint *see* **Catnip**

Catnip

Description

Catnip, or *Nepeta cataria*, is a flowering herb valued for its healing properties in a wide range of maladies. Catnip is indigenous to Europe and is now naturalized throughout the United States. It can be identified by the dozens of small white flowers with small purple spots covering its flowering, spiky top. The aromatic herb is a member of the Lamaciae or mint family; in England it is sometimes called catmint. Catnip is harvested in the summer and fall, and dried for medicinal use.

General use

Both the flowering tops and the leaves of the catnip plant are used for medicinal purposes. Catnip is used to treat a variety of symptoms and illnesses, including:

- Gastrointestinal distress. Catnip has carminative properties, which means that it is helpful in preventing gas and related nausea, colic, and diarrhea.
- Muscle cramps. The herb's antispasmodic properties promote relaxation of the gastrointestinal muscles, the uterus (for menstrual cramps), and other tight or sore muscles.
- Nervous disorders. Catnip can be used as a sedative to relieve stress, ease anxiety, relieve the symptoms of migraines and tension headaches, and promote general relaxation.

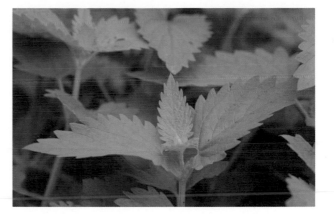

Both the flowering tops and the leaves of the catnip plant are used for medicinal purposes. Catnip is used to treat a variety of symptoms and illnesses. *(©InsideOutPix / Alamy)*

- Cold or flu with fever. Catnip is a diaphoretic, which means that it promotes sweating. This property makes it a valuable remedy in treating patients with feverish conditions, including influenza, colds, and bronchitis.
- Cuts and scrapes. Catnip is an astringent, and can be applied externally to cuts and scrapes to stop bleeding and promote healing.

Preparations

Catnip is most commonly taken as an infusion, or tea. The herb can be purchased in tea bags or in loose, dried form. Tea bag infusions can be prepared according to package directions. When using the dried form of the herb, place 10 tsp of catnip in a piece of muslin or cheesecloth, in an infuser, or loose, and submerge it in one liter of boiling water. After steeping the mixture in a covered container for ten minutes, strain the infusion before drinking. The infusion should be steeped in a covered pot to prevent the volatile oils in the catnip from escaping through evaporation.

A second method of infusion is to mix the loose catnip with cold water, bring the mixture to a boil in a covered pan or teapot, and then strain the infusion before drinking. Two to three cups of the catnip infusion can be taken daily. The remaining infusion should be stored in a well-sealed bottle and refrigerated to prevent bacteria and other micro-organisms from contaminating it.

Catnip can be mixed with such other herbs as **boneset** (*Eupatorium perfoliatum*), **elder** (*Sambucus nigra*), **yarrow** (*Achillea millefolium*), and **cayenne** (*Capsicum annuum*) in an infusion for treating colds.

Astringent—A substance that constricts or binds skin cells.

Carminative—A preparation that helps to expel gas from the stomach and bowel.

Diaphoretic—A substance or medication given to induce or promote sweating.

Diuretic—A medication or substance that increases urine output.

Infusion—A herbal preparation made by adding herbs to boiling water and then steeping the mixture to allow the medicinal herb to infuse into the water.

Tincture—A liquid extract of an herb prepared by steeping the herb in an alcohol and water mixture.

Volatile oil—A component of aromatic botanicals that gives herbs their characteristic odor and may possess therapeutic properties. Volatile oils vaporize or evaporate quickly when heated and exposed to air.

Catnip is also available in tincture form to take by mouth or apply topically. A tincture is an herbal preparation made by diluting the herb in alcohol. A catnip tincture or crushed catnip can be applied to a compress to treat **cuts** and scrapes.

Loose catnip and catnip in tea bags should be stored in an airtight container in a cool location out of direct sunlight to retain potency. Careful storage also prevents the catnip from absorbing odors and moisture.

Precautions

Catnip should always be obtained from a reputable source that observes stringent quality control procedures and industry-accepted good manufacturing practices. Botanical supplements are regulated by the FDA; however, they currently do not have to undergo any approval process before reaching the consumer market. Herbs are presently classified as nutritional supplements rather than drugs. Legislation known as the Dietary Supplement Health and Education Act (DSHEA) was passed in 1994 in an effort to standardize the manufacture, labeling, composition, and safety of botanicals and supplements. In January 2000, the FDA's Center for Food Safety and Applied **Nutrition** (CFSAN) announced a ten-year plan for establishing and implementing these regulations by the year 2010.

Although there are no known side effects or health hazards associated with recommended dosages of catnip preparations, pregnant women, women who breastfeed, and individuals with chronic medical conditions should consult with their healthcare professional before taking catnip or any other herb.

Side effects

Catnip has diuretic properties, and may increase the frequency and amount of urination. It can also cause an upset stomach in some individuals.

Because of the sedative qualities of catnip, individuals taking the herb should use caution when driving or operating machinery.

Interactions

There are no reported negative interactions between catnip and other medications and herbs, although certain drugs with the same therapeutic properties as catnip may enhance its effects.

Resources

BOOKS

Hoffman, David. *The Complete Illustrated Herbal*. New York: Barnes & Noble Books, 1999.
Medical Economics Corporation. *The PDR for Herbal Medicines*. Montvale, NJ: Medical Economics Corporation, 1998.

ORGANIZATIONS

Office of Dietary Supplements. National Institutes of Health. Building 31, Room 1B25. 31 Center Drive, MSC 2086. Bethesda, MD 20892-2086. (301) 435-2920. Fax: (301) 480-1845. http://odp.od.nih.gov/ods/ (Includes on-line access to International Bibliographic Information on Dietary Supplements (IBIDS), a database of published international scientific literature on dietary supplements and botanicals).

Paula Ford-Martin

Cat's claw

Description

Cat's claw is a large woody vine indigenous to the Amazon rain forest of South America. The herb earns its name from the curved thorns on the vine that resemble the claws of a cat. Also known by its Spanish equivalent *uña de gato,* cat's claw has a long history of use as a folk medicine by native peoples to treat intestinal complaints, **asthma**, **wounds**, **cancer**, tumors, arthritis,

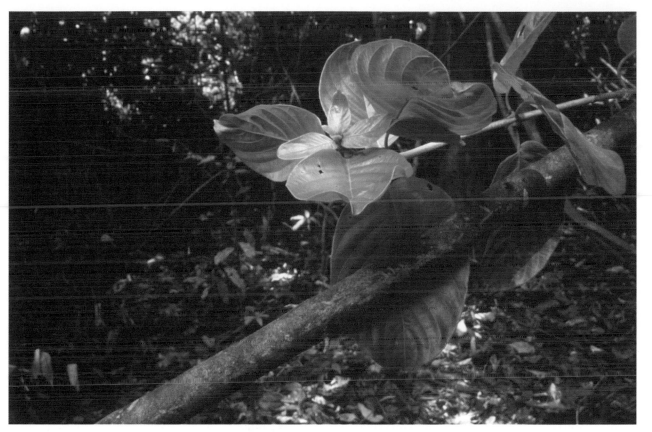

The botanical herb Cat's claw. *(©) Photo Researchers, Inc. Reproduced by permission.)*

inflammations, diabetes, irregularities of the menstrual cycle, fevers, ulcers, dysentery, and rheumatism. They have also utilized the herb as a kidney cleanser, blood cleanser, and contraceptive.

Two species of cat's claw are found in the rain forest: *Uncaria tomentosa* and *Uncaria guianensis*. Although these species are similar in appearance and have been used in many of the same ways, research on *Uncaria tomentosa* has revealed it to be more valuable as a therapeutic agent.

General use

Cat's claw has been called one of the most important botanical herbs found in the rain forest and is used as a cleansing and supportive herb of the immune system, cardiovascular system, and intestinal system. Although research on cat's claw began in the 1970s, it didn't gain worldwide attention until the 1990s, when studies showed it to be a possible treatment for Acquired Immune Deficiency Syndrome (**AIDS**) and Human Immunodeficiency Virus (HIV) infection; cancer; and other ailments. Cat's claw is reported to enhance immunity and heal digestive and intestinal

disorders. It has been used to treat many other ailments including **acne**, **allergies**, arthritis, asthma, candidiasis, chronic **fatigue**, chronic inflammation, **depression**, **diabetes mellitus**, environmental toxicity and poisoning, Epstein-Barr virus (EBV), **fibromyalgia**, **hemorrhoids**, herpes, **hypoglycemia**, **systemic lupus erythematosus** (SLE), menstrual disorders and hormone imbalances, parasites, **premenstrual syndrome** (PMS), tumors, upper respiratory **infections**, viral infections, and wounds.

One unfortunate effect of recent interest in and use of cat's claw has been its virtual extinction in parts of the rain forest. According to the Herb Research Foundation, the government of Peru has had to outlaw the export of all wild cat's claw plants. Almost all cat's claw root and bark used for commercial preparations as of 2003 comes from cultivated plants.

Although the stem bark of cat's claw has some medicinal activity, the root is three to four times more active than the stem bark. The strength of the active components in cat's claw is quite variable; it depends on the time of year that the plant is harvested.

The active compounds in cat's claw include alkaloids, triterpenes, phytosterols, and proanthocyanidins. Researchers have isolated unique alkaloids in the bark and roots that activate the immune system by increasing white blood cell activity. Rynchophylline, one of the alkaloids isolated from cat's claw, has antihypertensive properties that may be beneficial in lowering the risk of strokes and heart attacks by reducing heart rate, lowering blood pressure, increasing circulation, and lowering blood **cholesterol** levels.

Researchers have also discovered substances in cat's claw that have antitumor, antileukemic, antioxidant, antimicrobial, antibacterial, anti-inflammatory, antiviral, and diuretic properties. Dr. Brent W. Davis has studied cat's claw for a number of years and has described it as "the opener of the way" in reference to its ability to treat many bowel, stomach, and intestinal complaints including **diverticulitis**, leaky and irritable bowel syndromes, **gastritis**, ulcers, hemorrhoids, **Crohn's disease**, and **colitis**.

Cat's claw's anti-inflammatory actions have been effective in relieving the stiffness and swelling prevalent in arthritis, rheumatism, and joint **pain**. An Austrian study published in 2002 found that cat's claw significantly reduced joint tenderness and swelling in a sample of 40 patients with **rheumatoid arthritis**, with only minor side effects and no interactions with the patients' other arthritis medications. A recent study done in Peru indicates that the anti-inflammatory effects of cat's claw are stronger in extracts made with alcohol than in water-based solutions.

Studies of the therapeutic benefits of cat's claw on cancer have produced several interesting findings. Cat's claw's immunostimulating properties have been shown to enhance the function of white blood cells to attack and digest carcinogenic substances and harmful microorganisms that may inhibit the growth of cancer cells and tumors. Used as an adjunct treatment to chemotherapy and radiation, cat's claw has shown promise in diminishing side effects such as **hair loss**, **nausea**, skin problems, infections, and weight loss.

Clinical studies have tested Krallendon, an immune-boosting extract of cat's claw, in the treatment of AIDS patients and persons who are HIV-positive, either as a single treatment or in conjunction with the AIDS drug azidothymidine (AZT). Results showed that Krallendon was able to deter the reproduction of the AIDS virus, stop growth of cancerous cells, and activate the immune system. In addition, painful side effects resulting from the AZT treatment were diminished. Cat's claw's antioxidant properties help protect cells from environmental substances such as smoke, pesticides, pollution, alcohol, x rays, gamma radiation, ultraviolet light, rancid food, and certain fats. The herb also helps prevent the spread of free radicals, protecting cells from mutating and developing into tumors.

Preparations

Cat's claw is available in health food stores and herb shops in several forms: dry extract, crushed bark, capsule, tablet, tea, and tincture.

To prepare the tea, boil 1 g (0.4 oz) of the bark in 1 cup of water for 10–15 minutes. Strain the mixture before drinking. A suggested dose is one cup of tea three times daily.

Tincture dosage: 1–2 ml up to two times daily. Children over two years of age and adults over 65 should begin use with mild doses and increase strength gradually if needed.

Precautions

Cat's claw is not recommended for pregnant or nursing women or for women who are trying to conceive. Children under the age of two should not take cat's claw. Persons with a health condition should consult a qualified herbalist before taking cat's claw.

Side effects

European studies have reported low toxicity in the use of cat's claw, even when taken in large doses. The only noted side effect was **diarrhea**. In 2001, however, one case study was reported from South America of a patient with lupus developing kidney failure after taking cat's claw extracts.

Interactions

Cat's claw should not be combined with hormonal drugs, insulin, or vaccines. It may cause the immune system to reject foreign cells, so persons who have received organ or tissue transplants should not use this herb. The dosage may need to be reduced when taken with other herbs.

Cat's claw has also been reported to potentiate, or intensify, the effects of antihypertensives (medications given to control high blood pressure). Persons taking such drugs should use cat's claw only on the advice of a physician.

Resources

BOOKS

Elkins, Rita. *Cat's Claw (Una de Gato): Miracle Herb from the Rain Forest of Peru.* Woodland Publishing, 1996.

Jones, Kenneth. *Cat's Claw: Healing Vine of Peru.* Sylvan Press, 1995.

Steinberg, Phillip N. *Cat's Claw: The Wondrous Herb from the Peruvian Rainforest.* Healing Wisdom Publications, 1996.

PERIODICALS

Aguilar, J. L., P. Rojas, A. Marcelo et al. "Anti-Inflammatory Activity of Two Different Extracts of *Uncaria tomentosa* (Rubiaceae)." *Journal of Ethnopharmacology* 81 (July 2002): 271-276.

Blumenthal, Mark. "Una de Gato (Cat's Claw) Rainforest Herb Gets Scientific and Industry Attention." *Whole Foods* (October 1995): 62, 62, 66, 68, 78.

Craig, Winston J. "A Closer Look at Cat's Claw." (Herb Watch). *Vibrant Life* 18 (September-October 2002): 38-39.

Mur, E., F. Hartig, G. Eibl, and M. Schirmer. "Randomized Double-Blind Trial of an Extract from the Pentacyclic Alkaloid-Chemotype of *Uncaria tomentosa* for the Treatment of Rheumatoid Arthritis." *Journal of Rheumatology* 29 (April 2002): 678-681.

ORGANIZATIONS

Herb Research Foundation. 1007 Pearl St., Suite 200, Boulder, CO 80302. (303) 449-2265. www.herbs.org.

Southwest School of Botanical Medicine. P. O. Box 4565, Bisbee, AZ 85603. (520) 432-5855. www.swsbm.com.

Jennifer Wurges
Rebecca J. Frey, PhD

Caveman diet *see* **Paleolithic diet**

Cayce systems

Definition

The Cayce Health System, or Cayce systems, combine an extensive and varied assortment of treatments for hundreds of physical conditions, diseases, and disabilities into a holistic approach to health and healing. The fundamental concepts are based on information provided in psychic readings by Edgar Cayce (1877–1945) for thousands of individuals with a wide array of symptoms and ailments.

Origins

Often regarded as the father of modern **holistic medicine**, Edgar Cayce was born near Hopkinsville, Kentucky on March 18, 1877. He allegedly began exhibiting paranormal abilities as a child, for example memorizing his school lessons by sleeping with his head on his textbooks. At age 24, after undergoing hypnosis during which he prescribed successful treatment for his own months-long bout of **laryngitis** that had baffled his doctors, Cayce began to dispense his readings. He gave these readings while he was in a trance-like state, leading to his designation as "The Sleeping Prophet." Over the course of his lifetime, Cayce gave readings on diverse subjects, including health, religion, dream interpretation, world affairs, and business. Although some early readings were lost, at his death in 1945 more than 14,000 separate Edgar Cayce readings on over 10,000 topics had been stenographically transcribed. Almost 9,000 readings address medical ailments.

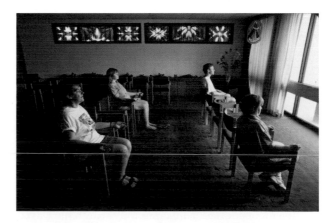

Meditation taking place in a Cayce meditation room, Virginia Beach, Virginia. *(Photo Researchers, Inc. Reproduced by permission.)*

Benefits

Cayce's holistic approach addresses the body, mind, and spirit connection. The information offered in his readings is aimed at treating the whole person and helping people develop a self-awareness and responsibility for improving their own physical health and spiritual well-being.

Cayce's readings focus on addressing the root cause of an ailment rather than simply alleviating the symptoms. Almost all of his physical readings address diet and **nutrition**. He felt that providing the body key building materials it needs to do its work is crucial, as is **detoxification**. Poor eliminations are the most cited cause of disease in Cayce's readings. He also addresses various systemic imbalances in the nervous, circulatory, and glandular systems, and acid/alkaline imbalances. Infection, **stress**, attitudes, and emotions are also central to his disease explanations.

Recommendations comprise an extensive variety of therapies too numerous to list here. They include conventional medicines and surgeries as well as alternative therapies such as electrotherapy, **osteopathy**, and massage. Readings often recommend herbs, chemical concoctions, color and light therapies, colonics, **castor oil**, and taking on responsible, healthful attitudes and behaviors such as dietary changes and **prayer**. Cayce even developed some original appliances to deliver his prescribed treatments.

Proponents of Cayce's therapies claim healings ranging from routine to miraculous. Critics argue that many recommended therapies lack rigorous scientific research and evaluation, and attribute "cures" to factors other than Cayce's alleged psychic perception of medical needs.

Description

Cayce systems combines Cayce's insights with Cayce-oriented health practitioners, lay persons, organizations, training programs, researchers, and health products. Treatment protocols are individualized for each patient. Clinicians may follow several different treatment modalities, emphasizing the uniqueness of each individual patient and inclination of the clinician. This integration of treatment modalities is a principal concept of the Cayce approach. Establishing healthy habits and attitudes are also central. Self-responsibility such as self-care and home care modalities (e.g., dietary changes, massage, etc.) is often incorporated. Clinicians may search the Cayce readings for the case most closely matching their patient's condition or medical diagnosis. However, most readings were given for a specific individual's complaint. Interpreting the readings is not always a straightforward task, since many subjects apparently had more disorders than the one addressed in the reading. Treatment may require experimentation and the Association for Research and Enlightenment (A.R.E.) Health and Rejuvenation Research Center (HRRC) recommends that it should be undertaken and evaluated under the care of a physician trained in the Cayce approach.

As in Cayce's original recommendations, a wide range of therapeutic tools and treatments may be used. These may generally be arranged under the following categories:

- Manual therapy is therapeutic use of hands to diagnose and treat illness. The Cayce system relies heavily on traditional osteopathic applications together with modern chiropractic, physical medicine and massage therapy.
- Electrotherapy includes several appliances and techniques such as the wet cell battery, radial appliance, violet ray appliance, ultraviolet ray lamp, sinusoidal, x-ray, and magnetic therapy.
- Diet/Nutritional therapy focuses on acid/alkaline balance and food combining with special diets for strengthening the blood, body, and nerves.
- Hydrotherapy (therapeutic use of water) includes colon therapy (irrigations), fume and steam baths, sitz baths, Epson salt baths, and various packs.
- Pharmacology relies heavily on natural remedies such as herbal medicine and dietary supplements.
- Mental therapy covers a broad range of psychological and psychosocial techniques such as cognitive-behavioral therapy, visualization, hypnosis, and environmental therapy.
- Spiritual healing includes interventions such as prayer, meditation, and laying on of hands.

Research and general acceptance

The Cayce transcripts are housed in the A.R.E. and are available for general research. The library also has a collection of circulating files on various health conditions. Numerous books organize information from the Cayce readings. As of 2000, the HRRC is conducting research projects including **energy medicine**, manual therapies, acid/alkaline balance, and the nervous system. The HRRC also offers individual research protocols enabling individuals to apply Cayce principles at home. They solicit anecdotal evidence on successful applications of Cayce modalities, invite clinicians using Cayce modalities to document outcomes, and conduct historical research on osteopathic textbooks. They also team with the Meridian

EDGAR CAYCE (1877–1945)

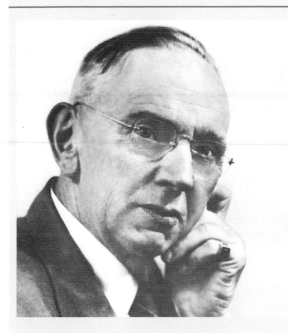

(Betmann/CORBIS. Reproduced by permission.)

Edgar Cayce was born on March 18, 1877, in Hopkinsville, Kentucky, the son of a businessman. He grew up in rural Kentucky and received only a limited formal education. He was a member of the Christian Church (Disciples of Christ). As an adult he began a career as a photographer.

Cayce's life took a radically different direction in 1898, after he developed a case of laryngitis. He was hypnotized by a friend and while in the trance state prescribed a cure that worked. Neighbors heard of the event and asked Cayce to do similar "readings" for them. In 1909 he did a reading in which he diagnosed and cured a homeopathic physician, Dr. Wesley Ketchum. During the next years Cayce gave occasional sittings, but primarily worked in photography.

In 1923, theosophist Arthur Lammers invited Cayce to Dayton, Ohio, to do a set of private readings. These readings were noteworthy because they involved Cayce's initial exploration of individual past lives. These readings encouraged Cayce to leave photography and become a professional. Among his early supporters was businessman Morton Blumenthal, who gave financial backing for Cayce Hospital (1928) and a school, Atlantic University (1930). Unfortunately, Blumenthal was financially destroyed by the Great Depression and both enterprises failed.

In 1932 Cayce organized the Association for Research and Enlightenment (ARE). With the resources generated by the association, complete records of all the readings for the next 12 years were made. These formed a huge body of material, and Cayce's readings were later indexed, cross-referenced, and used as the basis of numerous books.

Cayce died in 1945, and his son Hugh Lynn Cayce continued the work of the association and promoted the abilities of his father. Cayce's work became known by a large audience outside the psychic community in 1967 through a biographical book by Jess Stern, *Edgar Cayce, The Sleeping Prophet.*

Institute (a non-profit organization dedicated to researching Cayce health information) to look at specific illnesses.

Training and certification

Four levels of certification are offered for Cayce systems. As described on the A.R.E. website, Cayce home health therapists help patients apply Cayce information in their home settings. Cayce physiotherapists have passed certifications in general manual therapy, **hydrotherapy**, energy medicine, and the basic Cayce diet. Cayce health case managers are certified in providing information and support services (e.g., assessment, service planning, referrals, and advocacy). Cayce physicians, in additional to being licensed by their state boards, are certified in applying Cayce system principles and techniques.

Resources

BOOKS

Bolton, Brett. *An Edgar Cayce Encyclopedia of Foods for Health and Healing*. Virginia Beach, A.R.E. Press. 1996.

Karp, Reba A. *Edgar Cayce Encyclopedia of Healing*. New York, Warner Books. 1986.

McGarey, William A. *Physician's Reference Notebook*. Virginia Beach, A.R.E. Press. 1998.

Read, Anne, Carol Ilstrup, and Margaret Gammon. *Edgar Cayce on Diet and Health*. New York, Hawthorne. 1969.

Reilly, Harold J. and Ruth Hagy Brod. *The Edgar Cayce Handbook for Health Through Drugless Therapy*. New York, Macmillan. 1975.

Stearn, Jess. *Edgar Cayce: The Sleeping Prophet*. Virginia Beach, A.R.E. Press, 1997.

Sugrue, Thomas. *There is a River*. Virginia Beach, A.R.E. Press. 1988.

ORGANIZATIONS

The Association for Research and Enlightenment, Inc. 215 67th St., Virginia Beach, VA 23451. (757) 428-3588 or (800) 333-4499. are@edgarcayce.org. http://www.are-cayce.com/index.htm.

Health and Rejuvenation Research Center A division of the Association for Research and Enlightenment, Inc. 215 67th Street Virginia Beach, VA 23451-2061. (757) 428-3588 ext. 7340. hrrc@are-cayce.com.

Meridian Institute 1853 Old Donation Parkway, Suite 1 Virginia Beach, VA 23454. (757) 496-6009. http://www.meridianinstitute.com meridian@meridianinstitute.com.

Kathy Stolley

Cayenne

Description

Cayenne (*Capsicum frutescens, C. annum*) is a stimulating herb that is well known for its pungent taste and smell. Cayenne is a popular spice used in many different regional styles of cooking, but it has also been used medicinally for thousands of years.

The name cayenne is derived from a Tupi word, "kyinha," which means "hot pepper." The cayenne plant produces long red peppers and grows to a height of 2–6 ft (0.5–2 m). The plant is native to tropical areas of America and is cultivated throughout the world in tropic and subtropic climate zones. Most of the cayenne supply in the United States is imported from India and Africa.

Cayenne is a member of the genus *Capsicum*. Other species of this genus include Tabasco pepper, African pepper, Mexican chili pepper, bell pepper, pimento, paprika, and bird pepper. Cayenne is often referred to as chili, which is the Aztec name for cayenne pepper.

The main medicinal properties of cayenne are derived from a chemical called capsaicin. Capsaicin is the ingredient that gives peppers their heat. A pepper's capsaicin content ranges from 0–1.5%. Peppers are measured according to heat units. The degree of heat determines the pepper's value and usage. Generally, the

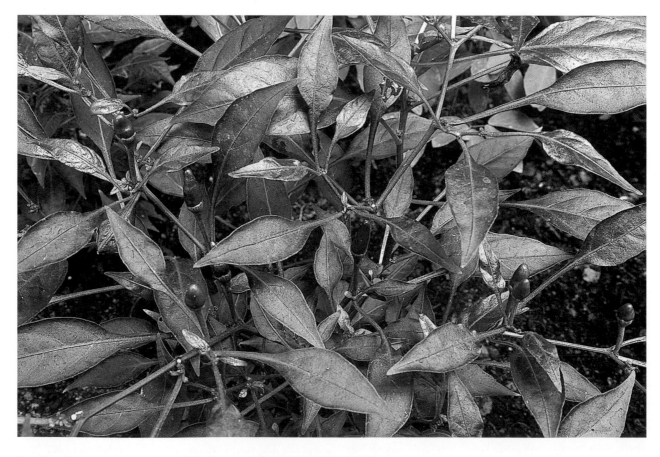

Cayenne pepper plants. (*©PlantaPhile, Germany. Reproduced by permission.*)

hotter the pepper, the more capsaicin it contains. In addition to adding heat to the pepper, capsaicin acts to relieve **pain** and reduce platelet stickiness. Other constituents of cayenne are vitamins C and E and **carotenoids**.

Cayenne has anti-inflammatory, antioxidant, antiseptic, diuretic, analgesic, expectorant, and diaphoretic properties. The dried ripe fruit and seeds of the plant are used for medicinal purposes. Cayenne is available in many forms, including capsules, ointments, liniments, tinctures, creams, oils, and dried powders.

Origin

Cayenne was originally grown in Central and South America in pre-Columbian times. It was cultivated in Mexico 7,000 years ago and in Peru 4,000 years ago. For 9,000 years, Native Americans have used cayenne as a food and as a medicine for stomach aches, cramping pains, **gas**, and disorders of the circulatory system. Cayenne was brought to Europe in the fifteenth century by Christopher Columbus. From Europe, cayenne was transported to tropical regions around the world, where it is now grown.

General use

Today, cayenne is used worldwide to treat a variety of health conditions, including weak digestion, chronic pain, **shingles**, **heart disease**, **sore throat**, **headache**, high **cholesterol**, poor circulation, and **toothache**.

Indian Ayurvedic, Chinese, Japanese, and Korean medicines use cayenne to treat many different conditions. One Ayurvedic remedy for pain combines cayenne and mustard seeds into a paste to be applied to the affected area. **Ayurvedic medicine** also utilizes cayenne to treat gas and poor digestion. Chinese medicine employs cayenne for digestive ailments. An ointment or tincture made from cayenne is used in China and Japan to heal **frostbite** and myalgia (muscle pain). The German Commission E has approved cayenne in the treatment of painful **muscle spasms**, arthritis, rheumatism, **neuralgia**, lumbago, and chilblains.

Digestive aid

Cayenne is used as a digestive aid throughout India, the East Indies, Africa, Mexico, and the Caribbean. When taken internally, cayenne soothes the digestive tract and stimulates the flow of saliva and stomach secretions. These secretions contain substances that help digest food.

Cayenne is also used to relieve **constipation**, as it stimulates gastric secretions, thereby activating a sluggish gastrointestinal tract.

Circulatory helper

Many people take cayenne internally to treat and prevent heart disease. The intake of cayenne has been found to have a positive effect on the circulatory system. Cayenne may reduce the risk of **heart attack**. It has been shown to lower cholesterol levels and the risk of **blood clots**. Studies have shown cayenne to lower blood pressure. A study in India showed that cayenne prevented a rise in liver and serum cholesterol levels when taken with dietary cholesterol.

Pain relief

Cayenne is a proven remedy for the temporary relief of pain, both external and internal. Its analgesic effect acts to distract sensory nerves from the irritation or pain, which results in a temporary abatement of pain. The capsaicin in cayenne depletes substance P, a chemical that sends pain signals to the brain from the local nervous system. When there is a lack of substance P, the sensation of pain diminishes because it cannot reach the brain.

Capsaicin has been approved by the United States Food and Drug Administration (FDA) for the pain of shingles, an adult disease that is caused by the virus that leads to chicken pox in children. Such over-the-counter (OTC) creams as Zostrix or Hcet contain capsaicin and are applied externally to treat rheumatic and arthritic pains, cluster headaches, diabetic foot pain, **fibromyalgia**, and postherpetic nerve pain. These creams usually contain 0.025–0.075% capsaicin.

Research has helped to quantify capsaicin's pain relieving effects. Creams containing the compound lowered pain in arthritis sufferers' hands by 40% when used four times a day. Seventy-seven percent of people with pain from long-term shingles had reduced pain after using the cream for four months. Researchers also found that capsaicin-containing cream is less expensive and safer than other painkillers used for the same conditions.

Other conditions

Cayenne can be an effective remedy for relieving congestion and coughs. It thins mucus, thus improving the flow of body fluids. It is also used to boost energy and relieve stress-related **fatigue** and **depression**. Late in the 1990s, British journals reported that people taking cayenne daily increased their fat metabolism and had decreased appetites. In addition, cayenne can be used as a treatment to prevent thumb sucking and nail biting in children.

Other uses

Research has suggested a number of other possible uses for cayenne. One study showed that the herb causes a reduction in human **prostate cancer** cells transplanted into experimental mice. Canadian researchers report that mice with a form of diabetes were cured of the disease after treatment with capsaicin.

Preparations

- Internal dosage: Cayenne should be taken internally as directed by an experienced practitioner.
- Creams: The creams should be used as directed. Generally creams must be applied three or four times per day for two to three weeks before their effects are felt.
- Oil: Cayenne oil may be rubbed on **sprains**, swelling, and sore muscles and joints to relieve pain. It should not, however, be applied to open **cuts** or broken skin.
- Tea: To ease gas and stomach cramps or to help promote digestion, a tea may be made by adding 0.25 tsp of cayenne to one cup of hot water. When taken as a hot tea, cayenne will induce sweating. Taken as a cold tea, cayenne works as a diuretic, increasing urination. Cayenne teas, however, should not be given to children.
- Toothache: Chewing on a hot pepper may provide temporary relief from toothache.
- Cold feet: Ground cayenne added to talcum powder or cornstarch can be placed inside a pair of socks. The cayenne causes the blood vessels under the skin of the feet to dilate, thus stimulating extra blood flow and providing warmth to the feet.
- Sore throat: To treat a sore throat, cayenne may be combined with **myrrh** and gargle as needed. This mixture can also be used as an antiseptic mouthwash. This treatment should not be given to children.

Precautions

To avoid irritating sensitive tissues, heating pads or hot compresses should not be placed on areas of the skin where cayenne has been applied.

Cayenne should not be applied to an area for longer than two days since the heat may cause nerve damage. It may be applied to the same location after four days have passed.

KEY TERMS

Analgesic—A pain-relieving substance.

Capsaicin—A colorless, bitter compound that is present in cayenne and provides its heat.

Chilblains—Redness and swelling of the skin caused by exposure to the cold.

Commission E—A committee formed in Germany in 1978 to evaluate the efficacy and safety of herbs used in traditional medical practice.

Diaphoretic—A substance that promotes sweating.

Diuretic—A substance that increases urination.

Expectorant—A substance that increases the coughing up of mucus.

Lumbago—Lower back pain caused by rheumatoid arthritis, muscle strain, osteoarthritis, or a ruptured spinal disk.

Cayenne should not come into contact with mucous membranes, eyes, open **wounds**, or sensitive areas.

Hands should be washed after using cayenne, or gloves should be worn when applying it externally.

Persons with an active gastrointestinal ulcer should not use cayenne internally without consulting a physician.

Side effects

Cayenne may irritate the mouth, throat, eyes, and open wounds. Drinking a glass of milk may relieve burning in the mouth and throat caused by consumption of cayenne. The protein in the milk helps to counteract the capsaicin.

Large internal doses of cayenne may produce **vomiting** and/or stomach pain.

Interactions

Asthma patients who are taking theophylline should consult a physician before taking cayenne. Cayenne may increase the amount of theophylline absorbed by the patient's system, possibly leading to toxicity.

Resources

BOOKS

De, Amit Krishna, ed. *Capsicum: The Genus Capsicum.* Boca Raton, FL: CRC Press, 2003.

McKenna, Dennis J., Kenneth Jones, and Kerry Hughes. *Botanical Medicines: The Desk Reference for Major Herbal Supplements,* 2nd edition. Binghamton, NY: Haworth Press, 2002.

PERIODICALS

Binshtok, Alexander M., Bruce P. Bean, and Clifford J. Woolf. "Inhibition of Nociceptors by TRPV1-mediated Entry of Impermeant Sodium Channel Blockers." *Nature* (October 4, 2007): 607–610.

Mori, Akio, et al. "Capsaicin, a Component of Red Peppers, Inhibits the Growth of Androgen-independent, p53 Nutant Prostate Cancer Cells." *Cancer Research* (March 2006): 3222–3229.

Razavi, Rozita, et al. "TRPV1 Sensory Neurons Control ß Cell Stress and Islet Inflammation in Autoimmune Diabetes." *Cell* (December 15, 2006): 1123–1135.

Szolcsányi, J. "Forty Years in Capsaicin Research for Sensory Pharmacology and Physiology," *Neuropeptides* (December 2004): 377–384.

Jennifer Wurges
Teresa G. Odle
David Edward Newton, Ed.D.

Ce bai ye *see* **Thuja**

Cedar, red *see* **Red cedar**

Celiac disease

Definition

Celiac disease occurs when the body reacts abnormally to gluten, a protein found in wheat, rye, barley, and oats. Gluten causes an inflammatory response in the small intestine, which damages the tissues and results in impaired ability to absorb nutrients from foods.

Description

Celiac disease—also called sprue, nontropical sprue, gluten sensitive enteropathy, celiac sprue, and adult celiac disease—may be discovered at any age. Researchers believe that a combination of genetic and environmental factors trigger the disease. Environmental events that may provoke celiac disease in those with a genetic predisposition to the disorder include surgery or a viral infection.

The disorder is more commonly found among white Europeans or those of European descent. The exact incidence of the disease is uncertain. Estimates vary from one in 5,000 to as many as one in every 300 individuals with this background. An estimated 3 million Americans have celiac disease but only about 3% of these have been diagnosed, according to the American Academy of Allergy, **Asthma**, and Immunology. An Italian study followed patients with type 1 (juvenile) diabetes and reported that celiac disease was 20 times more common among these patients than in the general population, yet often goes undetected in these children. The study authors recommended celiac disease screening programs for children recently diagnosed with type 1 diabetes.

Causes and symptoms

Celiac disease is caused by an inflammatory response of the small intestine. The exact mechanism of the disorder is not clearly understood, but it is known that both heredity and the immune system play a part. When food containing gluten reaches the small intestine, the immune system begins to attack a substance called *gliadin*, which is found in the gluten. The resulting inflammation causes damage to the delicate finger-like structures in the intestine, called *villi*, where food absorption actually takes place.

The most commonly recognized symptoms of celiac disease relate to the improper absorption of food in the gastrointestinal system. The patient has **diarrhea** and fatty, greasy, unusually foul-smelling stools. The patient may complain of excessive **gas** (flatulence), distended abdomen, weight loss, and generalized weakness.

Not all patients have these problems. Unrecognized celiac disease may cause or contribute to a variety of other conditions. The decreased ability to digest, absorb, and utilize food properly (malabsorption) may cause **anemia** from **iron** deficiency or easy bruising from a lack of **vitamin K**. Poor mineral absorption may result in **osteoporosis**, which may lead to bone **fractures**. **Vitamin D** levels may be insufficient and bring about a softening of bones (osteomalacia), which produces **pain** and bony deformities. Defects in the tooth enamel, characteristic of celiac disease, may also occur. Celiac disease may be discovered during medical tests performed to investigate failure to thrive in infants or lack of proper growth in children and adolescents. People with celiac disease may also experience lactose intolerance because they do not produce enough of the enzyme lactase, which breaks down the sugar in milk into a form the body can absorb.

A distinctive skin rash called *dermatitis herpetiformis* may be the first sign of celiac disease. Approximately 10% of patients with celiac disease have this

Gluten-free diet

Ingredients/foods to avoid	May contain gluten	Foods allowed
Barley	Baking powder	Amaranth
Bran (wheat or oat)	Beans, baked	Beans, dried, unprocessed
Bulgur	Bouillon cubes	Buckwheat
Cake meal	Candy	Cassava
Couscous	Cheese sauces and spreads	Cheese, aged
Emulsifier	Chips, potato and tortilla	Corn
Farina	Chocolate drinks and mixes	Eggs, unprocessed
Flavoring	Coffee substitutes	Fish, unprocessed
Flour, enriched, durum, graham, semolina	Cold cuts	Flax
Gluten	Communion wafers	Fruits and juices, fresh, frozen or canned
Hydrolyzed plant protein	Corn cakes, popped	Herbs and spices, pure
Kamut	Egg substitutes, dried eggs	Ketchup
Malt and malt flavoring	French fries	Legumes
Matzo meal	Fruits, dried	Meats, unprocessed
Oatmeal and oat bran	Fruit-flavored drinks	Milk
Oats, rolled	Fruit pie fillings	Millet
Rye	Gravy	Mustard
Semolina	Hot dogs and other processed meats	Nuts, unprocessed, and nut flours
Seitan	Matzo	Olives
Soy sauce or soy sauce solids	Mayonnaise	Pickles, plain
Soy	Milk drinks	Potatoes and sweet potatoes
Spelt	Nuts, dry roasted	Quinoa
Stablizer	Peanut butter	Rice, wild rice, Indian rice
Starch, modified, or modified food starch	Pudding mixes	Sago
Triticale	Rice, brown	Seeds, unprocessed
Vegetable gum	Rice crackers and cakes	Soy flour
Vegetable protein	Rice mixes	Soy sauce, gluten-free
Vinegar, malt	Salad dressings	Sorghum
Wheat	Sauces	Tapioca
Wheat berries	Seasoning mixes	Tomato paste
Wheat bran	Sour cream	Vegetables without gluten-containing additives
Wheat, cracked	Soy nuts	Vinegar, apple, cider, and distilled white
Wheat germ	Syrup	Yucca
Wheat protein and hydrolyzed wheat protein	Teas, flavored and herbal	
Wheat starch	Turkey, self-basting	
Whole wheat	Vegetables in sauces	
	Yogurt, flavored or frozen	

(Illustration by GGS Information Services. Cengage Learning, Gale)

rash, but it is estimated that 85% or more of patients with the rash have the disease.

Because of the variety of ways celiac disease can manifest itself, it is often not discovered promptly. The condition may persist without diagnosis for so long that the patient accepts a general feeling of illness as normal. This circumstance may lead to further delay in identifying and treating the disorder.

Diagnosis

About 97% of people who have celiac disease are undiagnosed. Much of this is because of incorrect diagnosis by physicians when symptoms are presented, according to Peter H. R. Green, a professor of medicine and director of Columbia University's Celiac Disease Center. Green reports that many doctors think diarrhea is always present in celiac disease when, in fact, it is only present in about half of the cases. Also, Green asserts that physicians are taught in medical school that celiac disease is a rare condition, so they often do not consider it when diagnosing a patient with its symptoms. Green made his remarks in an address at the 2007 meeting of the American Academy of Allergy, Asthma, and Immunology in San Diego.

If celiac disease is suspected, a blood test that looks for the antibodies that the immune system produces in celiac disease is ordered. Some experts advocate not just evaluating patients with symptoms, but using these blood studies as a screening test for high-risk individuals, such as those with relatives known to have the disorder. An abnormal result points towards celiac disease, but further tests are needed to confirm the diagnosis. Other tests may be ordered to look for nutritional deficiencies. For example, doctors may order a test of iron levels in the blood because low levels of iron (anemia) may accompany celiac disease.

Doctors may also order a test for fat in the stool, since celiac disease prevents the body from absorbing fat from food.

The next step is a biopsy of the small intestine. This procedure is usually performed by a gastroenterologist, a physician who specializes in diagnosing and treating bowel disorders. It is generally performed in the office or in an outpatient department in a hospital. The patient remains awake but is sedated. A narrow tube is passed through the mouth, down through the stomach, and into the small intestine. A small sample of tissue is taken and sent to the laboratory for analysis. If it shows a pattern of tissue damage characteristic of celiac disease, the diagnosis is established.

Treatment

The treatment for celiac disease is a **gluten-free diet** (GFD). This may be easy for the doctor to prescribe, but difficult for the patient to follow. Gluten is present in any product that contains wheat, rye, barley, or oats. It helps make bread rise and gives many foods a smooth, pleasing texture. In addition to the many obvious places gluten can be found in a normal diet, such as breads, cereals, and pasta, there are many hidden sources of gluten. These include ingredients added to foods to improve texture or enhance flavor and products used in food packaging. Gluten may even be present on surfaces used for food preparation or cooking.

Fresh foods that have not been artificially processed, such as fruits, vegetables, and meats, are permitted as part of a GFD. Gluten-free foods can be found in health food stores, mail-order companies, and in some supermarkets. Help in dietary planning is available from support groups for individuals with celiac disease. Many cookbooks on the market are specifically designed for those on a GFD. In the late 1990s and 2000s, an increasing number of gluten-free products came on the market, including breads, baking products, pasta, baby foods, and even gluten-free beer. However, the cost of gluten-free products can run two to three times the cost of comparable products that contain gluten. A gluten-free diet can add $100 a week to the grocery bill for a family of four, according to a 2007 estimate from the Food Institute.

Treating celiac disease with a GFD is almost always completely effective in alleviating symptoms. Secondary complications, such as anemia and osteoporosis, resolve in almost all patients. People who have experienced lactose intolerance related to their celiac disease usually see those symptoms subside as well.

Allopathic treatment

Both complementary and allopathic healthcare practitioners generally agree that a gluten-free diet is the best treatment for celiac disease. Several studies have reported that **lipase**, in combination with other pancreatic enzymes, enhances the benefits of a gluten-free diet for people with celiac disease. The enzyme lipase is used by the body to break down dietary fats (lipids), especially triglycerides, into a form that can be absorbed in the intestines. Lipase supplements usually contain other enzymes that help digest carbohydrates and protein. In the United States, the supplement pancreatin contains lipase, amylase, and proteases. A government standard is used to rate lipase supplements and is denoted as USP units. The standard government measurement for pancreatin is 25 USP units of amylase, 2 USP units of lipase, and 25 USP units of protolytic (protease) enzymes. So a lipase supplement that states on the label that it is "9X pancreatin" means that it is nine time stronger than the government standard. Lipase supplements are usually made from enzymes found in animals, although there are a few supplements that use lipase and other pancreatic enzymes derived from plants. Pancreatin supplements usually contain 6,000 LU (lipase activity units) of lipase. The recommended dosage for adults is one to two capsules or tablets three time a day. Dosages for children should be determined by a pediatrician.

A small number of patients develop a refractory type of celiac disease, for which the GFD no longer seems effective. Once the diet has been thoroughly assessed to ensure no hidden sources of gluten are causing the problem, medications may be prescribed. Steroids or immunosuppressant drugs are often used to try to control the disease.

Expected results

The physician will periodically recheck the level of antibody in the patient's blood after a diagnosis of celiac disease has been made. After several months on a GFD, the small intestine of the patient is biopsied again. If the diagnosis of celiac disease was correct, healing of the intestine will be apparent. Most experts agree that it is necessary to follow these steps in order to be sure of an accurate diagnosis.

Patients with celiac disease must keep a strict GFD as long as they live. Although the disease may have symptom-free periods, silent damage continues to occur if the diet is not followed. Patients who do not follow their **diets** run higher risks of serious complications like gastrointestinal cancers, iron–deficiency

KEY TERMS

Antibodies—Proteins that provoke the immune system to attack particular substances. In celiac disease, the immune system makes antibodies to a component of gluten.

Gluten—A protein found in wheat, rye, barley, and oats.

Lipase—An enzyme that is used by the body to break down dietary fats (lipids), especially triglycerides, into a form that can be absorbed in the intestines.

Pancreas—A large elongated glandular organ near the stomach. It secretes juices into the small intestine, and the hormones insulin, glucagon, and somatostatin into the bloodstream.

Villi—Tiny, finger-like projections that enable the small intestine to absorb nutrients from food.

anemia, and decreased bone mineral density. Celiac disease cannot be outgrown or cured, according to medical authorities.

Once the diet has been followed for several years, individuals with celiac disease have similar mortality rates to the general population. However, about 10% of people with celiac disease develop a **cancer** involving the lymphatic system (lymphoma).

Prevention

There is no way to completely prevent celiac disease. However, the key to decreasing its impact on overall health is early diagnosis and strict adherence to the prescribed diet. Interestingly, a 2002 study of Swedish children found that the gradual introduction of gluten-containing foods into an infant's diet while they are still being breast-fed can reduce the risk of celiac disease, at least in early childhood.

Resources

BOOKS

Bower, Sylvia Llewelyn. *Celiac Disease: A Guide to Living with Gluten Intolerance.* New York: Demos Medical, 2006.

Green, Peter H. R., and Rory Jones. *Celiac Disease: A Hidden Epidemic.* New York: Collins, 2008.

Libonati, Cleo J. *Recognizing Celiac Disease: Signs, Symptoms, Associated Disorders & Complications.* Ambler, PA: GFW, 2007.

PERIODICALS

Brunk, Doug. "Underdiagnosis of Celiac Disease Continues." *Internal Medicine News* (August 15, 2007): 32.

Corbet, Kelly. "The Gluten Question: What You Need to Know." *Delicious Living* (October 2007): 49(3).

Cotliar, Sharon. "No Wheat, No Worries." *People Weekly* (June 11, 2007): 143.

Johnson, Kate. "Diet Role Debated in Asymptomatic Celiac Disease." *Family Practice News* (April 1, 2007): 38.

Presutti, John R., et al. "Celiac Disease." *American Family Physician* (December 15, 2007): 1795.

Turner, Lisa. "6 Simple Tricks for Living Gluten-Free: A Diagnosis of Celiac Disease or Gluten Intolerance Doesn't Mean You Have to Give Up Your Favorite Foods and Treats. Replacing Problem Ingredients and Following a Gluten-Free Diet Are Easier than You Think." *Better Nutrition* (October 2007): 50(4).

ORGANIZATIONS

Canadian Celiac Association, 5170 Dixie Rd., Suite 204, Mississauga, ON, L4W 1E3, Canada, (800) 363-7296, http://www.celiac.ca.

Celiac Disease Foundation, 13251 Ventura Blvd., Suite 1, Studio City, CA, 91604-1838, (818) 990-2354, http://www.celiac.org.

National Institute of Diabetes and Digestive and Kidney Diseases, Bldg. 31, Room 9A06, 31 Center Dr., MSC 2580, Bethesda, MD, 20892, (800) 891-5390, http://www.niddk.nih.gov.

National Pancreas Foundation, 363 Boylston St., 4th Floor, Boston, MA, 02116, (866) 726-2737, http://www.pancreasfoundation.org.

Paula Ford-Martin
Ken R. Wells

Cell salt therapy

Definition

Cell salt therapies use a set of specific minerals, also known as the 12 tissue salts, to correct symptoms arising from metabolic deficiencies. They are very similar to **homeopathy**, and may be prescribed by a homeopathic doctor.

The 12 cell salts are as follows:

- *Calcarea fluor* (calcium fluoride)
- *Calcarea phos* (calcium phosphate)
- *Calcarea sulph* (calcium sulfate)
- *Ferrum phos* (iron phosphate)
- *Kali mur* (potassium chloride)
- *Kali phos* (potassium phosphate)
- *Kali sulph* (potassium sulfate)

- *Magnesia phos* (magnesium phosphate)
- *Natrum mur* (sodium chloride)
- *Natrum phos* (sodium phosphate)
- *Natrum sulph* (sodium sulfate)
- *Silicea* (silica)

Origins

Cell salt therapy was developed by a German physician, W. H. Schussler, in the 1870s. Schussler studied cremated human bodies, and found that these 12 substances made up the bulk of the remains. From this finding he theorized that these 12 so-called tissue salts are responsible for the harmonious functioning of the human organism. Disease follows when a person becomes deficient in any of the 12 salts. Schussler recommended that patients take the salts in pill form to cure a variety of disorders. He believed that the salts provided adequate **nutrition** to the cells. If cell nutrition was adequate, then cell metabolism would be normal, and the body would be healthy. However, Schussler's pills were not direct nutritional supplements as we would understand them today. He followed the principles of homeopathy, which works somewhat to the reverse of modern medicine, in that the smaller the dose, the more effective it is believed to be. Cell salts are prepared like homeopathic medicines, by a process of continued dilution and shaking or pounding (succussion).

Benefits

Practitioners of cell salt therapy believe the minerals to be effective against a variety of ailments. For example, *Calcarea fluor* is thought to be essential to vascular health; it is given to patients with circulatory diseases or such conditions as **varicose veins, hemorrhoids**, and hardening of the arteries. *Ferrum phos* is used to treat colds, flu, and inflammation. *Kali phos* is used to treat **body odor**, as well as mental problems. Other salts treat other disorders, from cramps to **gout** to skin problems. Some are prescribed for general healing; that is, to restore general health to a person without any overriding specific disease.

Preparations

Cell salts may be derived from inorganic sources, though they can also be derived from plants. The salts are made into pills which are extremely dilute, following the principles of homeopathy. The salts are crushed into fine particles, and the particles go through a series of dilutions, then are molded into tablets. The patient does not swallow the tablet, but allows it to dissolve on the tongue.

Precautions

Though the cell salt pills are extremely dilute, practitioners believe them to be quite potent. Practitioners advise people to take cell salts only under the advice of a homeopathic physician. The cell salts are not intended to be a complete treatment, but only one part of a treatment plan devised by a knowledgeable practitioner.

Side effects

Because of the extremely dilute nature of cell salt pills, side effects are unlikely. Traditionally trained medical doctors would consider them placebos.

Research and general acceptance

Cell salt therapy, like homeopathy, is not based on scientific research but on provings. Provings are basically anecdotal evidence gathered from volunteers. This method of testing the efficacy of remedies was devised by Samuel Hahnemann, the German physician who originated homeopathy. Within the field of homeopathy, cell salt therapy is considered a sister therapy or perhaps a subset of homeopathy. Homeopaths prescribe cell salts, sometimes in conjunction with other remedies.

Training and certification

Cell salts are available as over-the-counter remedies, and patients are able to treat themselves if they wish. An understanding of cell salts can be gained from reading Schussler's work, or from comprehensive guides to homeopathy. Cell salt therapy may be administered by a homeopathic doctor. Rules governing the practice of homeopathy vary from state to state. Homeopaths in the United States can become certified through the Council for Homeopathic Certification. This requires at least 500 hours of training in homeopathy through a school or seminars, plus a written examination. Certification is also offered to practitioners who have apprenticed for at least 2,000 hours with a certified homeopath. Other qualifications may also be necessary, such as having taken a course in CPR (cardiopulmonary resuscitation) and human anatomy.

Resources

BOOKS

Cummings, Stephen, and Ullmann, Dana. *Everybody's Guide to Homeopathic Medicines.* New York: Jeremy P. Tarcher/Putnam, 1996.

PERIODICALS

Stehlin, Isadora. "Homeopathy: Real Medicine or Empty Promise?" *FDA Consumer* (December 1996): 15.

ORGANIZATIONS

National Center for Homeopathy. 801 North Fairfax Street, Suite 306. Alexandria, VA 22314. (703) 548-7790.

Angela Woodward

Cell therapy

Definition

Cell therapy is the transplantation of human or animal cells to replace or repair damaged tissue and/or cells.

Origins

The theory behind cell therapy has existed for several hundred years. The first recorded discussion of the concept of cell therapy was written by Phillippus Aureolus Paracelsus (1493–1541), a German-Swiss physician and alchemist in his *Der grossen Wundartzney* (Great Surgery Book, 1536): "the heart heals the heart, lung heals the lung, spleen heals the spleen; like cures like." Paracelsus and many of his contemporaries agreed that the best way to treat an illness was to use living tissue to restore the ailing. In 1667, at a laboratory in the palace of Louis XIV, Jean-Baptiste Denis (1640–1704) attempted to transfuse blood from a calf into a mentally ill patient. Since blood transfusion is, in effect, a form of cell therapy, this could be the first documented case of this procedure. However, the first recorded attempt at non-blood cellular therapy occurred in 1912 when German physicians attempted to treat children with **hypothyroidism**, or an underactive thyroid, with thyroid cells.

In 1931, Paul Niehans (1882–1971), a Swiss physician, became known quite by chance as "the father of cell therapy." After a surgical accident by a colleague, Niehans attempted to transplant a patient's severely damaged parathyroid glands with those of a steer. When the patient began to rapidly deteriorate before the transplant could take place, Niehans decided to dice the steer's parathyroid gland into fine pieces, mix the pieces in a saline solution, and inject them into the dying patient. Immediately, the patient began to improve and, in fact, lived for another 30 years.

Cell therapy as alternative medicine practitioners practice it is quite different from embryonic stem cell research performed in government-regulated laboratories by traditionally trained scientists. Embryonic stem cells are cells taken from an embryo before they have differentiated (specialized) into such specific cell types as muscle cells, nerve cells, skin cells, for example. In laboratory test tube and animal experiments, stem cells often can be manipulated to differentiate into specific types of cells that have the potential to replace differentiated cells in damaged organs. For example, in early 2008, researchers at the Diabetic Research Institute at the University of Miami in Florida were able to convert embryonic stem cells into insulin-producing cells and use them to treat insulin-dependent diabetes in mice. Embryonic stem cells have great potential to treat a wide range of diseases and disorders, but they were as of 2008, for the most part, still in the test tube and animal research stage of development. Because of the ethical questions raised when embryos are destroyed by the harvesting of stem cells, the Bush administration placed restrictions on human stem cell research. As of 2008, much stem cell research was being carried out in other countries, especially Thailand, South Korea, and China, where fewer restrictions are placed on obtaining human stem cells for experimentation.

Cell therapy as it is carried out by alternative medical practitioners most often follows the "like heals like" theory and uses fully differentiated adult cells from the same type of organ that the practitioner is trying to heal. Cells may come from humans but are more likely to come from animals. Practitioners of this type of cell therapy believe that when these differentiated cells are injected into the body of an ill person, the body transports them to the site of the organ to be healed and the injected cells heal the organ. This theory challenges accepted findings about how the body's immune system attacks and destroys foreign cells.

Benefits

Alternative practitioners of cell therapy claim that it has been used successfully to rebuild damaged cartilage in joints, repair spinal cord injuries, strengthen a weakened immune system, treat autoimmune diseases such as **AIDS**, and help patients with neurological disorders such as Alzheimer's disease, Parkinson's disease, and **epilepsy**. They further claim that the therapy has shown positive results in the treatment of a wide range of chronic conditions such as arteriosclerosis, congenital defects, and **sexual dysfunction**. The therapy also has been used to treat **cancer** patients at clinics in Tijuana, Mexico. Few of these applications have been supported by controlled human clinical studies. Some of the diseases and disorders that alternative practitioners claim to be able to cure through cell therapy are now the target of researchers doing scientifically rigorous, regulated embryonic stem cell research.

Description

Cell therapy as practiced by alternative healers is, in effect, a type of organ transplant that has also been referred to as live cell therapy, xenotransplant therapy, cellular suspensions, glandular therapy, or fresh cell therapy. The procedure involves the injection of either whole fetal xenogenic (animal) cells (e.g., from sheep, cows, pigs, and sharks) or cell extracts from human tissue. The latter is known as autologous cell therapy if the cells are extracted from and then transplanted back into the same patient. Several different types of cells can be administered simultaneously.

In accord with Paracelsus's theory that "like cures like," the types of cells that are administered correspond in some way with the organ or tissue in the patient that is failing. No one has shown how cell therapy works as of 2008, but proponents claim that the injected cells travel to the similar organ from which they were taken to revitalize and stimulate that organ's function and regenerate its cellular structure. In other words, the cells are not species specific, but only organ specific. Supporters of cellular treatment believe that embryonic and fetal animal tissue contains active therapeutic agents distinct from vitamins, minerals, hormones, or enzymes that aid in healing.

Preparations

There are several processes to prepare cells for use. One procedure involves extracting cells from the patient and then culturing them in a laboratory setting until they multiply to the level needed for transplantation back into the same patient. Another procedure uses freshly removed fetal animal tissue that has been processed and suspended in a saline (salt water) solution. The preparation of fresh cells then may be either injected immediately into the patient or preserved by being freeze-dried or deep-frozen in liquid nitrogen

before being injected. Injected cells may or may not be tested for pathogens, such as bacteria, viruses, or parasites, before use.

Precautions

Patients undergoing cell therapy treatments that use cells transplanted from animals or other humans run the risk of cell rejection, in which the body recognizes the cells as a foreign substance and uses the immune system's T-cells to attack and destroy them. There are also cases in which injection of animal cells into humans has caused an allergic reaction. In addition, there is the risk of the cell solution transmitting bacterial, viral, or fungal infection or parasites to the patient.

Many forms of legitimate stem cell therapy in the United States were still experimental procedures as of 2008. A list of FDA-approved clinical trials involving stem cells can be found at http://www.clinicaltrials. gov. Patients should approach any alternative cell therapy treatments with extreme caution, inquire about their proven efficacy and legal use in the United States, and should only accept treatment from a licensed physician. The physician should educate the patient completely on the risks and possible side effects involved with cell therapy. These same cautions apply for patients interested in participating in clinical trials of cell therapy treatments.

Side effects

Because cell therapy encompasses a wide range of treatments and applications and many of these treatments were still experimental as of 2008, the full range of possible side effects of the treatments is not yet known. Anaphylactic shock (severe allergic reaction that can result in death), immune system reactions, and encephalitis (inflammation of the brain) are just a few of the reported side effects in some patients.

PAUL NIEHANS (1882–1971)

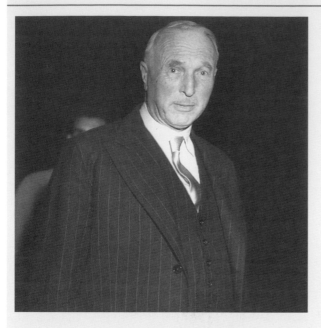

(AP/Wide World Photos. Reproduced by permission.)

Paul Niehans was born and raised in Switzerland. His father, a doctor, was dismayed when he entered the seminary, but Niehans quickly grew dissatisfied with religious life and took up medicine after all. He first studied at Bern, then completed an internship in Zurich.

Niehans enlisted in the Swiss Army in 1912. When war erupted in the Balkans, Niehans set up a hospital in Belgrade, Yugoslavia. The war provided him the opportunity to treat numerous patients, gaining a firsthand knowledge of the body and its workings.

Since 1913, Niehans had been intrigued with Alexis Carrel's experiments concerning the adaptive abilities of cells, though Niehans himself specialized in glandular transplants and by 1925 was one of the leading glandular surgeons in Europe.

Niehans referred to 1931 as the birth year of cellular therapy. That year, he treated a patient suffering from tetany whose parathyroid had been erroneously removed by another physician. Too weak for a glandular transplant, the patient was given injections of the parathyroid glands of an ox, and she soon recovered. Niehans made more injections, even experimenting on himself, and reported he could cure illnesses through injections of live cells extracted from healthy animal organs. He believed adding new tissue stimulated rejuvenation and recovery.

Niehans treated Pope Pious XII with his injections and was nominated to the Vatican Academy of Science following the pope's recovery.

Niehans remained a controversial figure throughout his life. As of 2008, the Clinique Paul Niehans in Switzerland, founded by his daughter, continued his work.

Research and general acceptance

Cell therapy as it is practiced by alternative healers is generally rejected as effective by the traditionally trained scientific community. Most of the claims made for these therapies are based on anecdotal evidence and are not backed by controlled clinical trials. Whereas some mainstream stem cell therapy procedures have shown some success in clinical studies, others were largely unproven as of 2008 including cell therapy for cancer treatment. Until large, controlled human clinical studies are performed on cell therapy procedures, they will remain fringe treatments.

Training and certification

Cell therapy should only be performed by a licensed physician with experience in prescribing and administering the treatment. Surgical cell therapy procedures, such as the arthroscopic surgery involved in chondrocyte cell therapy, should only be performed by a surgical specialist.

Resources

BOOKS

Steenblock, David, and Anthony G. Payne. *Umbilical Cord Stem Cell Therapy: The Gift of Healing from Healthy Newborns.* Laguna Beach, CA: Basic Health Publications, 2006.

PERIODICALS

Pollack, Andrew. "Stem Cell Therapy Controls Diabetes in Mice." *New York Times* February 21, 2007. http://www.nytimes.com/2008/02/21/health/research/21stem.html (April 12, 2008).

ORGANIZATIONS

Alternative Medicine Foundation, PO Box 60016, Potomac, MD, 20859, (301) 340-1960, http://www.amfoundation.org.

American Holistic Medical Association, PO Box 2016, Edmonds, WA, 98020, (425) 967-0737, http://www.holisticmedicine.org.

Center for Cell and Gene Therapy. Baylor College of Medicine, One Baylor Place N1002, Houston, TX, 77030, (713) 798-1246, http://www.bcm.edu/genetherapy.

Paula Ford-Martin
Teresa G. Odle
Tish Davidson, A. M.

Cellulite

Definition

Cellulite is a popular term to describe fat deposits under the skin. It is characterized by a dimpled or orange-peel appearance due to structural changes underneath the skin's top layer. Cellulite is a perfectly normal and harmless condition, however, it is a cosmetic concern of many people, especially women.

Description

Cellulite is a normal occurrence resulting from uneven fatty deposits, mostly below the waistline. In women, fat is arranged in large chambers underneath a fairly thin layer of skin. These chambers are separated by columns of collagen fibers. In obese (overweight) persons, too much fat is being stuffed into these chambers, causing the pitting and bulging of the skin. In addition, as women age, the fibers shrink and thicken, pulling the skin downward. This results in a quilt-like appearance on the skin surface, especially in areas such as the buttocks, thighs, or hips. Most women develop cellulite as they age, regardless of their race. According to some studies, as many as 95% of women over age 30 develop some form of cellulite in their body.

Female hormones (estrogen, and to a lesser extent, progesterone) play important roles in the formation of cellulite. Estrogen stimulates the storage of fat, which is needed for **menstruation**, **pregnancy**, and lactation. In addition, during the later phases of pregnancy, estrogen also causes the breakdown of collagen fibers to relax the cervix, making it possible for a woman to deliver her baby. This collagen breakdown sets the stage for the formation of cellulite. Progesterone may also contribute to the cellulite problem by weakening veins and causing water retention and weight gain.

Cellulite is mostly a women's problem. Due to different body physiques, men tend to have lower percentages of body fat, while women have higher percentages. In addition, men tend to accumulate fat in the abdominal area while women have fat deposits mostly in the buttocks and thighs. Men have thicker skin and the chambers are smaller and more tightly-held together. Therefore, cellulite is not often found in men.

Causes and symptoms

Many scientists believe cellulite, as well as **obesity**, is mostly predetermined by the genes that the persons

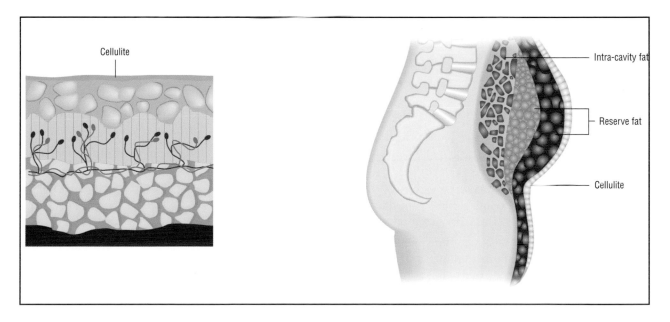

A close-up of cellulite deposits found beneath the top layer of skin. (Illustration by GGS Information Services, Inc. Cengage Learning, Gale)

carry. However, environmental as well as behavioral factors are also believed to have some effects on the development of cellulite.

The following factors are thought to contribute to the development of cellulite:

- Being overweight. Though cellulite also appears on thin people, excess weight makes cellulite worse.

- Pregnancy. Cellulite problems get worse with each successive pregnancy. During pregnancy, estrogen and progesterone levels are high. As a result, pregnant women have increased fatty deposits, weight gain, water retention, and weakened fiber structure. The most effective ways for women to get rid of body fat and cellulite and get back to pre-pregnancy shape are breast-feeding and exercise.

- Aging. As women age, skin sags and wrinkles. In addition, the body's energy requirement lowers, thus, there is more fat accumulation.

- Poor blood circulation. When there is impaired blood flow to the fat-storage area, collagen fibers are damaged due to lack of oxygen and accumulation of toxic wastes. The fibers shrink and thicken, resulting in the quilted appearance of the fat chambers. In addition, because oxygen is needed to burn fat for energy, fat in these poorly oxygenated areas is the last to be used. This is also why cellulite is so difficult to eliminate. Poor blood circulation is often caused by sedentary lifestyles, smoking, and high caffeine consumption.

- Poor lymph drainage. The lymphatic system acts like a sewage system, filtering out and carrying away cellular wastes and toxins. If it is impaired, toxic products accumulate and inflate these fat cells, causing cellulite.

- Lack of exercise. Cellulite may be caused by impaired blood circulation and poor muscle tone underneath the skin, which are caused by sedentary lifestyles.

- High fat and sugar consumption. This often leads to excess caloric and fat intake, which causes increases in body fat and thus, cellulite.

- Food allergy. Food allergy causes a variety of symptoms including food craving, weight gain, bloating and water retention, all of which worsen cellulite.

- Highly processed foods that contain preservatives, artificial sweeteners and other additives. Heavy consumption of prepackaged foods causes build up of these toxins in the body.

- Yo-yo dieting. Yo-yo dieting causes a woman to lose fat in the upper body while increasing fat deposits in the buttocks, thighs, and hips. Therefore, this practice tends to make cellulite problems worse than before dieting.

- Sun exposure. Prolonged exposure to the sun accelerates the skin-aging process.

Diagnosis

There are high-tech methods developed to determine the presence and extent of cellulite such as ultrasound and electrical impedance, which are expensive and unnecessary. However, a woman can determine for herself if she has cellulite using the skin-pinch and roll technique. First, a woman sets up a reference point for later comparisons. Using her fingers, a woman should gently pinch a large fold of skin in an area not known for having cellulite. Then she should do the same with skin in the buttock, thigh or hip areas. Comparing the first pinch with later experiences, she should see if there are signs of cellulite such as skin thickening, dimpling, broken veins, cold skin, and lumpiness.

Treatment

Exercise

The best solutions to cellulite problems involve reducing subcutaneous fat through diet and **exercise**. Working out for at least 30 minutes five times a week firms up the skin by increasing muscle tone and keeping connective tissue fibers healthy. Exercise also increases blood circulation to these problem areas.

Diet

Dieting has to be combined with regular exercise to be effective in controlling or reducing cellulite. The following dietary changes are recommended:

- Drinking lots of water. Water cleanses the digestive system and flushes toxins out of the body.

- Eating a low-fat, low-sugar, high-fiber diet with emphasis on fruits, vegetables, and whole grains.

- Refraining from smoking. Smoking causes poor blood circulation and contributes to premature aging of the skin.

- Avoiding highly processed foods, caffeine, and alcohol.

- Avoiding salty foods. Salty foods increase water retention and make cellulite appear worse.

- Maintaining a normal, healthy body weight. Obesity increases fatty deposits and makes cellulite much worse.

Body massage

Massage with or without anti-cellulite cream may have some limited benefits by improving blood circulation and **lymphatic drainage**. Regular massage also helps maintain smoother skin.

Herbal supplements

There are many herbal products on the market for the treatment of cellulite. Products such as Cellasene do not offer any therapeutic benefits. Cellasene is a popular herbal mixture of fucus vesiculous, **grape seed extract**, **sweet clover**, **ginkgo biloba**, borage, **lecithin**, and **fish oil**. Its manufacturer claims that the herbal combination works by increasing the rate the body **burns** fat cells for energy. Many medical experts remain doubtful of its claim of effectiveness. A recent study shows that it may be just another fad product that has no therapeutic value.

There are several products, though, such as *Centella asiatica* (**gotu kola**) and *Aesculus hippocastanum* (**horse chestnut**) that may help improve the appearance of cellulite. These herbs improve the underlying integrity of the skin by making the connective tissue fibers stronger and more elastic.

Allopathic treatment

Liposuction is the most widely used treatment for cellulite. Fat cells are removed by suctioning through a cut or excision in the buttocks or thigh. Then some of these fat cells are redeposited into areas of dimpling to smooth out the contour. While liposuction significantly reduces total amount of fat in the body immediately, it may not significantly improve skin appearance. In other words, liposuction may or may not remove the dimpling or unevenness under the skin. Nor does it make leathery, wrinkling skin look taut and young. Even when it is effective, liposuction is only a temporary quick-fix solution. As long as there is excessive caloric and fat intake, the excess energy will be stored as fat and cellulite will certainly reappear, albeit probably in other parts of the body.

Liposuction is a surgical procedure. Therefore, it does carry some potentially severe consequences and complications. **Pain** and **edema** (fluid accumulation) occur in most patients. It may take up to six months for the edema to completely go away. Skin dimpling may look even worse immediately after surgery, however, the unevenness will smooth out over time. Surgical complications such as **infections**, uncontrollable bleeding, fatal **blood clots**, and inadequate or excessive fat removal (leaving behind flabby skin folds) may also occur.

Expected results

Liposuction is not a generally recommended treatment for cellulite because it is an invasive, potentially life-threatening procedure. It can sometimes produce satisfying results but it is not a cure for cellulite. Repeat liposuction is often required because as long as there is excess caloric or fat intake, there will be fatty deposits in the body. Unless there are significant changes in lifestyle and diet, cellulite will reappear.

A 2002 study showed that a combination of ultrasound-assisted liposuction followed by mechanical massage (endermologie) proved more effective than either technique used alone in reducing cellulite. Women with the best results also added exercise into their post-operative routine.

Fat-dissolving lotions and creams are not proven effective in treating cellulite. Herbal cellulite-dissolving products do not result in loss of body fat, as they often claim. At most, products such as Cellasene may be able to make the dimpling from cellulite become less noticeable. Further, when several ingredients are combined in these creams, it is difficult for investigators to determine which ingredient might be responsible for any reduction in the appearance of cellulite.

The most effective treatment for cellulite remains diet and exercise. Adhering to a low-fat, **high-fiber diet** and regular exercise will make the body as fit and trim as it can be. These are long-term solutions that also provide many additional health benefits including prevention of **heart disease** and **cancer** and slowing the **aging** process.

Prevention

Cellulite is a normal occurrence in the human body and predetermined by genetics. Some women will naturally have more cellulite than others. However, diet and exercise can keep the body fit and trim.

Resources

BOOKS

Dancey, Elizabeth. *The Cellulite Solution.* USA: St. Martin's Press, 1996.

Murray, Michael T., and Joseph E. Pizzorno. "Cellulite." *Encyclopedia of Natural Medicine, revised 2nd ed.* Rocklin, CA: Prima Publishing, 1998.

The Burton Goldberg Group. "Cellulite." *Alternative Medicine: The Definitive Guide.* Tiburon, CA: Future Medicine Publishing, Inc., 1999.

PERIODICALS

Bernstein, Gerald. "Liposuction: Liposuction of the Thigh." *Dermatologic Clinics* 17 no.4 (October 1999): 849-863.

Bolivar de Souza, Pinto E., P.J.I. Erazo, F.S.A. Prado Filho, et al. "Superficial Liposuction." *Aesthetic Plastic Surgery* 20 (1996): 111-122. In Year Book of Dermatologic Surgery, 1997.

"Dermatologists Shed Light on Treatments for Cellulite." *Obesity, Fitness & Wellness Week* (September 21, 2002): 8.

Lis-Balchin M. "Parallel Placebo-Controlled Clinical Study of a Mixture of Herbs Sold as a Remedy for Cellulite." *Phytother Res* 13 no.7 (Nov 1999): 627-629.

Scheck, Anne. "Dual Lipoplasty, Endermologie Approach Offers Successful Cellulite Reduction." *Cosmetic Surgery Times* (July 2002): 22.

ORGANIZATIONS

The American Society of Plastic and Reconstructive Surgeons (ASPRS). 444 East Algonquin Road, Arlington Heights, IL 60005. (800) 228-9900. http://www.plasticsurgery.org

OTHER

Srinivasan, Kalpana. "FTC Eyes Cellulite Supplement: Can Manufacturer Substantiate Claims?" *Dr. Koop.com* http://abcnews.go.com/sections/living/DailyNews/cellulitepill990527.html.

Mai Tran
Teresa G. Odle

Cerebral palsy

Definition

Cerebral palsy (CP), or static encephalopathy, is the name for a collection of movement disorders caused by brain damage that occurs before, during, or shortly after birth. A person with CP is often also affected by other conditions caused by brain damage.

Description

The affected muscles of a person with CP may become rigid or excessively loose. The person may lose control of muscles or have problems with balance and coordination. A combination of these conditions is also possible. Those with CP may be affected primarily in the legs (paraplegia or diplegia) or in the arm and leg of one side of the body (hemiplegia) or all four limbs may be involved (quadriplegia).

A person with CP may also be affected by a number of other problems, including a seizure disorder, visual deficits, hearing problems, mental retardation, learning disabilities, and **attention-deficit hyperactivity disorder**. None of these conditions is necessarily part of CP, although they may accompany the disorder.

CP affects approximately 500,000 children and adults in the United States and is diagnosed in about 10,000 newborns and young children each year. It is not an inherited disorder, and as of 2008 there was no way to predict with certainty which children would develop CP. It is not a disease and is not communicable. CP is a nonprogressive disorder, which means that symptoms neither worsen nor improve over time. However, manifestation of the symptoms may become more severe over time. For example, rigidity of muscles can lead to contractures and deformities that require a variety of interventions.

Causes and symptoms

Causes

Cerebral palsy is caused by damage to the motor control centers of the brain. When the nerve cells (neurons) in these regions die, the appropriate signals can no longer be sent to the muscles under their control. The resulting poor control of these muscles causes the symptoms of CP.

The brain damage leading to CP may be caused by lack of oxygen (asphyxia), infection, trauma, malnutrition, drugs or other chemicals, or hemorrhage. In most cases it is impossible to determine the actual cause, although premature birth is recognized as a significant risk factor. It was once thought that difficult or prolonged delivery was responsible for many cases of CP, but many researchers have come to believe that the great majority of cases result from brain damage occurring before birth. The same injury that damages the motor areas can harm other areas as well, leading to problems commonly associated with CP.

If brain cells do not get enough oxygen because of poor circulation, they may die. Defects in circulation in the developing brain may cause CP in some cases. Asphyxia during birth is also possible, and about half of newborns known to have suffered asphyxia during birth (perinatal asphyxia) develop CP. However, asphyxia during birth is usually considered a symptom of an underlying neurological problem in a newborn, rather than its cause, and the resulting CP may be another sign of that problem. Asphyxia after birth can be caused by choking, poisoning (such as from carbon monoxide or barbiturates), or near-drowning.

The fetal brain may be damaged by an infection contracted by the mother. **Infections** correlated with CP include **rubella** (German **measles**), toxoplasmosis (often contracted from cat feces), cytomegalovirus (a herpes virus), and HIV (the virus that causes **AIDS**). Encephalitis and **meningitis**, which are infections of the brain and its coverings, can also cause CP when contracted by infants.

Physical trauma to the pregnant mother or infant may cause brain damage. Blows to the infant's head, as from a motor vehicle accident, violent shaking, or other physical abuse can damage the infant's brain. Maternal malnutrition may cause brain damage, as can the use of drugs, including cocaine or alcohol. Although these factors may cause CP, they may be more likely to cause mental retardation or other impairments.

Incompatibility between the Rh blood types of mother and child was once a major cause of athetoid CP, one type of movement impairment seen in cerebral palsy patients. In some cases, this incompatibility can cause the mother's defense (immune) system to attack and destroy the child's blood cells during **pregnancy**, a condition called erythroblastosis fetalis. High levels of a blood cell breakdown product called bilirubin in a child's circulation, leading to yellowish pigmentation of the skin caused by bile (**jaundice**), can result in brain damage. This condition is rare as of 2008 due to testing procedures that identify potential Rh incompatibility and treatment that prevents the mother's immune system from attacking the child's blood cells. Jaundice can be treated with special lights that help the breakdown of bilirubin. Blood transfusions for the child are also possible in extreme cases. Despite the virtual elimination of this cause of CP in the last part of the twentieth century, CP rates have not declined, largely because of the increase of survival of premature babies.

Prematurity is one of the most significant risk factors for CP. About 7% of babies weighing less than three pounds at birth develop CP, and the risk increases dramatically as weight falls. Prematurity may increase the risk of CP because of the increased likelihood of hemorrhaging in the brain associated with low birth weight. Brain hemorrhage is most common in babies weighing less than four pounds at birth, and the risk increases as weight decreases. The hemorrhage may destroy brain tissue, either through asphyxia or release of toxic breakdown products.

Researchers in Sweden reported in 2002 that babies conceived through in vitro fertilization (IVF) were 3.7 times more likely to have CP than babies conceived naturally. In part, this correlation can be attributed to a higher rate of twins, low birth weight, and premature births associated with IVF babies, but some single births also have higher rates of CP.

Symptoms

The symptoms of CP are usually not noticeable at birth. As children develop in the first 18 months of life, however, they progress through a predictable set of developmental milestones. Children with CP will develop these skills more slowly due to their motor impairments, and delay in reaching milestones is usually the first symptom of CP. The more severe the CP, the earlier the diagnosis is usually made.

Selected developmental milestones, and the ages at which a child typically acquires them, are given below. There is some cause for concern if the child does not acquire the skill by the age shown in parentheses:

- sits well unsupported, 6 months (8–10 months)
- babbles, 6 months (8 months)
- crawls, 9 months (12 months)
- finger feeds, holds bottle, 9 months (12 months)
- walks alone, 12 months (15–18 months)
- uses one or two words other than dada/mama, 12 months (15 months)
- walks up and down steps, 24 months (24–36 months)
- turns pages in books, removes shoes and socks, 24 months (30 months)

Children do not consistently favor one hand over the other before 18 months, and doing so may be a sign that the child has difficulty using the other hand. This same preference for one side of the body may show up as an asymmetric crawling effort, or continuing to use only one leg for the work of stair climbing after age three.

It must be remembered that children normally progress at somewhat different rates, and slow initial accomplishment is often followed by normal development. There are also other causes for delay in reaching some milestones, including problems with vision or hearing. Because CP is a non-progressive disease, loss of previously acquired milestones indicates that CP is not the cause of the problem.

The impairments of CP become recognizable in early childhood. The type of motor impairment and its location are used as the basis for classification. There are five generally recognized types of impairment:

- Spastic: Muscles are rigid, posture may be abnormal, and fine motor control is impaired.

- Athetoid: Movements tend to be slow, writhing, involuntary.

- Hypotonic: Muscles are floppy, without tone.

- Ataxic: Balance and coordination are impaired.

- Dystonic: Impairment is mixed.

The location of the impairment usually falls into one of three broad categories:

- Hemiplegia: One arm and one leg on the same side of the body are involved.

- Diplegia: Both legs are involved and arms may be partially involved.

- Quadriplegia: All four extremities are involved.

A person with CP may be said to have spastic diplegia, or ataxic hemiplegia, for instance. CP is also termed mild, moderate, or severe, although these are subjective categories with no firm boundaries.

Loss of muscle control, especially of the spastic type, can cause serious orthopedic problems, including **scoliosis** (spine curvature), hip dislocation, or contractures. Contracture is shortening of a muscle, caused by an imbalance of opposing force from a neighboring muscle. Contractures begin as prolonged contractions but can become fixed or irreversible without regular range of motion exercises. A fixed contracture occurs when the contracted muscle adapts by reducing its overall length. Fixed contractures may cause postural abnormalities in the affected limbs, including clenched fists, tightly pressed or crossed thighs, or equinus. In equinus, the most common postural deformity, the foot is extended by the strong pull of the rear calf muscles, causing the toes to point. The foot is commonly pulled inward as well, a condition called equinovarus. Contractures of all kinds may be painful and may interfere with mobility and normal activities of daily living, including hygiene tasks.

As noted, the brain damage that causes CP may also cause a large number of other disorders. These may include:

- mental retardation
- learning disabilities
- attention-deficit hyperactivity disorder (AD-HD)
- seizure disorder
- visual impairment, especially strabismus (cross-eye)
- hearing loss
- speech impairment

These problems may have an even greater impact on the child's life than the physical impairment of CP, although not all children with CP are affected by other problems. About one-third of children with CP have moderate to severe mental retardation, one-third have mild mental retardation, and one-third have normal to above average intelligence.

Diagnosis

The tracking of developmental progress is the most important test the physician has in determining whether a child has cerebral palsy. Most children with CP can be confidently diagnosed by 18 months. However, diagnosing CP is not always easy because variations in child development may account for delays in achieving milestones and even children who are obviously delayed may continue to progress through the various developmental stages, attaining a normal range of skills later on. Serious or prolonged childhood illness may cause delays that are eventually recovered.

Evidence of other risk factors may aid the diagnosis. The Apgar score, evaluated immediately after birth, measures a newborn's heart rate, cry, color, muscle tone, and motor reactions. Apgar scores of less than three out of a possible 10 are associated with a highly increased indication of CP. Presence of abnormal muscle tone or movements may signal CP, as may the persistence of infantile reflexes. A child with seizures or congenital organ malformation has an increased likelihood of CP. Ultrasound examination, a diagnostic technique that creates a two-dimensional image of internal body structures, may help to identify brain abnormalities, such as enlarged ventricles (chambers containing fluid) or periventricular leukomalacia (an abnormality of the area surrounding the ventricles), which may be associated with CP.

X rays, magnetic resonance imaging (MRI) studies, and computed tomography (CT) scans are often used to look for scarring, cysts, expansion of the cerebral ventricles (hydrocephalus), or other brain abnormalities that may indicate the cause of symptoms. Blood tests and genetic tests may be used to rule out other possible causes, including muscular dystrophy (a disease characterized by the progressive wasting of muscles), mitochondrial (cellular) disease, and other inherited disorders or infections.

Treatment

A number of people with cerebral palsy, both children and adults, have found systematic relief and enhanced quality of life from a combination of alternative and complementary treatments, including nutritional therapy, **craniosacral therapy**, bodywork, herbal therapy, **homeopathy**, and **acupuncture**.

General recommendations

Pregnant women should avoid cleaning cat litter, which may contain toxoplasma parasite. This organism causes severe brain damage or death in the unborn fetus. Unprotected sex increases risk of contracting sexually transmitted diseases such as **genital herpes**, which can infect the unborn child. Women should also be vaccinated before getting pregnant to prevent measles and rubella, which can cause severe brain damage to the fetus. They should avoid taking certain drugs, **smoking**, or drinking alcohol. Cocaine, heroine, nicotine, and alcohol are toxic to the developing fetal brain.

Nutritional therapy

The following dietary adjustments have been recommended to alleviate some symptoms in patients with cerebral palsy:

- Those with CP should avoid potential allergenic foods. Allergic foods are believed to worsen symptoms in many CP patients.
- CP patients should also avoid preservatives and food additives such as MSG (which are potentially toxic to the brain) by eating fresh and unprocessed foods such as whole grains, vegetables, beans, fruits, nuts, and seeds.
- To improve muscle tone, CP patients should supplement their diets with magnesium, thiamine, pyridoxine, vitamin C, and bioflavonoids. Alternatively, they can take daily multivitamin/mineral supplements that can provide all these helpful nutrients and make sure they are getting adequate protein in diet or supplements.

Osteopathy

Craniosacral therapy, a special form of osteopathic treatment, may be successful in preventing cerebral palsy if performed right after a difficult labor or delivery by forceps. This manipulation of bones of the newborn's skull may prevent **stress** and distortion of the child's head occurring during traumatic delivery. Craniosacral therapy is less successful, however, in established cerebral palsy in an older child.

Bodywork

Bodywork such as massage, **reflexology**, **Feldenkrais**, or **Rolfing** can help improve blood circulation and muscle tone and reduce **muscle spasms** in patients with cerebral palsy.

Other therapies

Other potentially helpful treatments include acupuncture, homeopathy and herbal therapy, and dance and **music therapy**. Although still not proven in clinical trials, hyperbaric **oxygen therapy** (HBOT) has been used to alleviate many symptoms of CP. It provides pure oxygen at higher-than-normal pressure in an enclosed chamber and is more commonly known for treating divers with compression sickness. A 2007 review of six studies on the use of HBOT to treat patients with CP found some level of improvement in motor skills but concluded that additional research was needed.

Allopathic treatment

Cerebral palsy cannot be cured, but many of the disabilities it causes can be managed through planning and timely care. Treatment for a child with CP depends on the severity, nature, and location of the impairment, as well a child's associated problems. Optimal care of a child with mild CP may involve regular interaction with only physical and occupational therapists, whereas care for a more severely affected child may include a speech-language therapist, special education teacher, adaptive sports therapist, nutritionist, orthopedic surgeon, and neurosurgeon.

Parents of a child newly diagnosed with CP are not likely to have the necessary expertise to coordinate the full range of care their child will need. Support groups for parents of physically or mentally impaired children can be significant sources of both practical advice and emotional support. Many cities have support groups that can be located through the United Cerebral Palsy Association or a local hospital or social service agency. Children with CP are also eligible for special education services. The diagnosing doctor should refer parents to the local school district for these services. Even children aged birth to three years are eligible through early intervention programs.

Influence of CP on development

Cerebral palsy may restrict a child's ability to reach for and grasp objects, to move about, to explore the properties of toys, and to communicate with others, which are all central activities in the child's growth and development. Therefore, the disease inhibits acquisition of motor skills, knowledge of the world, and social competence. The family can do much to overcome these restrictions by adapting the child's environment to meet his or her needs and providing challenges within the child's abilities to accomplish. The advice and direction of an occupational therapist can be critical to promoting normal development of the child with CP.

Posture and mobility

Spasticity, muscle coordination, ataxia, and scoliosis are all significant impairments that affect the posture and mobility of a person with cerebral palsy. Physical therapists work with the family to maximize the child's ability to move affected limbs, to develop normal motor patterns, and to maintain posture. Adaptive equipment may be needed, including wheelchairs, walkers, shoe inserts, crutches, or braces. The need for adaptive equipment may change as the person develops or as new treatments are introduced.

SPASTICITY. Spasticity causes muscles to shorten, joints to tighten, and postures to change. Spasticity can affect the ability to walk, use a wheelchair, and sit unaided; it can prevent independent feeding, dressing, personal hygiene care, or other activities of daily living. Contracture and dislocations are common consequences of spasticity.

Mild spasticity may be treated by regular stretching of the affected muscles through their full range of motion. Such activities are conducted at least daily. Moderate spasticity may require bracing to keep a limb out of the abnormal position or serial casting to return it to its normal position. Ankle-foot braces (orthoses) made of lightweight plastic are often used to increase a child's stability and to promote proper joint alignment.

Spasticity may also be treated with muscle relaxing drugs, including diazepam (Valium), dantrolene (Dantrium), and baclofen (Lioresal). A variety of experimental surgeries have been tried for people with cerebral palsy to control spasticity. Many of these procedures have not proven effective.

Ataxia and coordination

Ataxia, or lack of balance control, is another factor affecting mobility. Physical therapy is an important tool for helping the child with CP maximize balance. Coordination can be worsened if one member of a muscle pair is overly strong; bracing or surgical transfer of the muscle to a less overpowering position may help.

SCOLIOSIS. Scoliosis, or spine curvature, can develop when the muscles that hold the spine in place become either weak or spastic, which can cause **pain** and interfere with normal posture and internal organ function. Scoliosis may be treated with a trunk brace. If this proves unsuccessful, spinal fusion surgery may be needed to join the vertebrae together, which keeps the spine straight.

Seizures

Seizures occur in 30 to 50% of children with CP. Seizures may be treated with drugs, most commonly carbamazepine (Tegretol) or ethosuximide (Zarontin). A combination of a ketogenic diet and **fasting** may also be used to control seizures. Although the need for antiseizure medication is temporary in some children, it may be required throughout life for others.

Strabismus

Strabismus, or squinting and lack of parallelism in the eyes, occurs in nearly half of all people with spastic CP. Strabismus may be treated with patching and corrective lenses. When these treatments do not work, the condition may be treated with either surgery on the eye muscles causing the problem or by injection of botulinum toxin.

Nutrition

Due to poor muscle coordination, CP children may not take in adequate **nutrition** for full growth and development, worsening the results of the disorder. Careful attention to nutritional needs and nutritional supplements is required. Poor swallowing coordination may lead to aspiration, or inhaling of food or saliva. A speech-language therapist may be able to teach the person more effective movement patterns to avoid aspiration. In severe cases, a gastrostomy tube may be required to provide adequate nutrition directly into the digestive system while preventing aspiration.

Other common medical problems

Drooling, dental caries (cavities), and **gum disease** are more common in people with CP than in the general population, partly because of reduced coordination and increased muscle tightness in the mouth and jaw. Each of these conditions can be prevented to some degree, either through behavioral changes alone or in combination with drug therapy. **Constipation** is more common as well and may be treated through dietary changes or with enemas or suppositories when necessary.

Communication

Poor coordination of the tongue and mouth muscles can also affect speech. Children may benefit from picture boards or other communication devices that allow them to point to make their desires known. For school-age children or older persons with CP, there are a large number of augmentative communication devices, including shorthand typing programs and computer-assisted speech devices. A speech-language therapist can offer valuable advice on the types of equipment available.

Education

The school best suited for the child with CP is determined by the presence and degree of mental impairment and physical impairment, as well as the facilities available in the area. Inclusion, or mainstreaming the child in a regular public school classroom, may work well for the child with mild physical impairment. Separate classrooms or special schools may be needed for more severely impaired children. Schooling for disabled students in the United States is governed by the Individuals with Disabilities Education Act (IDEA) at the federal level and state special education rules at the local level. An educational specialist within the school system or from a community social services agency may be able to help the family navigate the various bureaucratic pathways that will ensure the best schooling available.

The process of developing an educational plan for a child with CP begins with an assessment of the child's needs. The assessment is carried out under state guidelines by a team of medical professionals. After the assessment, the school district works with the parents and others involved in the child's education and treatment to develop an Individualized Educational Plan (IEP). The IEP states the child's specific needs for special instruction and indicates what services will be provided. The special services may be as simple as allowing extra time to travel between classes or as extensive as individualized instruction, adapted classroom equipment, and special testing procedures. More information about assessments and IEPs is available through the National Information Center for Children and Youth with Disabilities. The United

Cerebral Palsy Association is another resource for advocacy, information, and legal rights.

Behavioral and mental health services

The child with CP may have behavioral problems or emotional issues that affect psychological development and social interactions. These problems may require special intervention or treatment, including behavior modification programs or individual and family counseling. Attention-deficit hyperactivity disorder is common in children with CP and may require behavioral, educational, and medical intervention.

Expected results

Cerebral palsy can affect every stage of maturation, from childhood through adolescence to adulthood. At each stage, indiviuals with CP and their caregivers must strive to achieve and maintain the fullest range of experiences and education consistent with each person's abilities. The advice and intervention of professionals is invaluable for many people with CP.

Although CP is not a terminal disorder, it can affect a person's lifespan by increasing the risk of infection, especially lung infections. Poor nutrition can contribute to the likelihood of infection. People with mild cerebral palsy may have near-normal lifespans. The lifespan of those with more severe forms, especially spastic quadriplegia, is often considerably shortened. However, over 90% of infants with CP survive into adulthood.

Cerebral palsy is one of the diseases for which stem cell research holds the greatest promise. Stem cell research makes use of very primitive cells with the ability to develop into any one of the specialized cells found in the body. As of 2008, extensive research had been conducted on the production and use of stem cells, but no successful application of stem cells for any specific disease in humans had been accomplished.

Prevention

The cause of most cases of CP is unknown, but it became clear in the 1990s that birth difficulties are not to blame in most cases. Developmental problems before birth, usually unknown and generally undiagnosable, are responsible for most cases. Although the incidence of CP caused by Rh factor incompatibility has declined markedly, the incidence of CP as a consequence of prematurity has increased because of the increasing success of medical intervention in keeping premature babies alive.

The risk of CP can be decreased through good maternal nutrition, avoidance of drugs or alcohol during pregnancy, and prevention or prompt treatment of

KEY TERMS

Ataxic—A condition in which balance and coordination are impaired.

Athetoid—The type of CP that is marked by slow, writhing, involuntary muscle movements.

Attention-deficit/hyperactivity disorder—A behavioral disorder marked by inattentiveness, hyperactivity, and impulsivity.

Augmentative communication devices—Computers, picture boards, and other devices that increase the ability to communicate, either with or without speech.

Contracture—Shortening of a muscle caused by an imbalance of force between opposing muscles.

Diplegia—Paralysis of corresponding parts on both sides of the body.

Dorsal rhizotomy—A surgical procedure that cuts nerve roots to reduce spasticity in affected muscles.

Dystonic—Describes the condition dystonia, in which fine motor control is confused.

Equinovarus—A condition in which the foot is typically pulled inward.

Equinus—A common postural deformity, in which the foot is extended by the strong pull of the rear calf muscles, causing the toes to point.

Hemiplegia—Paralysis of one side of the body.

Hypotonic—Describes the condition hypotonia, in which fine motor control is floppy, without tone.

Individualized educational plan (IEP)—A plan that guides the delivery of services to a child with special education needs.

Ketogenic diet—A specialized diet designed to increase the blood levels of breakdown products known as ketone bodies. For unknown reasons, this diet aids in seizure control.

Perinatal asphyxia—Lack of oxygen that occurs before, during, or around the time of birth.

Quadriplegia—Paralysis of all four limbs.

Serial casting—A series of casts designed to gradually move a limb into a more functional position, as opposed to doing it all at once with one cast, as would be done in setting a broken bone.

Spastic—Describes a condition in which the muscles are rigid, posture may be abnormal, and fine motor control is impaired.

Tenotomy—Surgical procedure that cuts the tendon of a contractured muscle to allow lengthening.

infections. In the 2000s research suggested that **magnesium** sulfate may reduce the risk of CP in mothers taking it for the medical treatment of preeclampsia and preterm labor.

Resources

BOOKS

Hinchcliffe, Archie. *Children with Cerebral Palsy: A Manual for Therapists, Parents, and Community Workers*, 2nd ed. Thousand Oaks, CA: Sage, 2007.

Martin, Sieglinde. *Teaching Motor Skills to Children with Cerebral Palsy and Similar Movement Disorders: A Guide for Parents And Professionals*. Bethesda, MD: Woodbine House, 2006.

Miller, Freeman. *Physical Therapy of Cerebral Palsy*. New York: Springer, 2007.

Miller, Freeman, and Steven J. Bachrach. *Cerebral Palsy: A Complete Guide for Caregiving*, 2nd ed. Baltimore: Johns Hopkins University Press, 2006.

PERIODICALS

Beckung, E., et al. "The Natural History of Gross Motor Development in Children with Cerebral Palsy Aged 1 to 15 Years." *Developmental Medicine & Child Neurology* (October 2007): 751–756.

McDonagh, Marian S., et al. "Systematic Review of Hyperbaric Oxygen Therapy for Cerebral Palsy: The State of the Evidence." *Developmental Medicine & Child Neurology* (December 2007): 942–947.

"Spastic Hemiplegia." *Developmental Medicine & Child Neurology* (January 2008): 71–75.

Subasi, Feryal, et al. "Factors Affecting Oral Health Habits among Children with Cerebral Palsy: Pilot Study." *Pediatrics International* (December 2007): 853–857.

ORGANIZATIONS

National Information Center for Children and Youth with Disabilities, PO Box 1492, Washington, DC, 20013-1492, (800) 695-0285, http://www.nichcy.org/.

United Cerebral Palsy Association, 1660 L St. NW, Suite 700, Washington, DC, 20036-5602, (800) USA-5-UCP, http://www.ucpa.org.

Mai Tran
Teresa G. Odle
David Edward Newton, Ed.D.

Cerebral vascular insufficiency

Definition

Cerebral vascular insufficiency is defined as insufficient blood flow to the brain. The most common cause of decreased blood flow is **atherosclerosis** of the arteries that supply blood to the brain.

Description

Cerebral vascular insufficiency is a common condition in the older population of developed countries due to the high prevalence of atherosclerosis. The artery affected in most cases of this disease is the carotid artery, which carries most of the brain's blood supply.

Causes and symptoms

A **stroke**, caused by reduced blood and oxygen supply, may be an indication of severe blockage in the carotid artery. Less severe blockage may still cause "mini-strokes" or transient ischemic attacks (TIAs), which can cause symptoms of **dizziness**, ringing in the ears, blurred vision, and confusion. Any of these problems could indicate cerebral vascular insufficiency.

Diagnosis

Diagnosis of cerebral vascular insufficiency is based upon the presence of one or more of the following symptoms:

- blurred vision
- depression
- vertigo (dizziness)
- headache
- lack of vigilance
- senility
- short-term memory loss
- ringing in the ears (tinnitus)

The diagnosis is confirmed by using an ultrasound exam to analyze blood flow to the brain.

Treatment

EDTA chelation therapy

EDTA (ethylene-diamine-tetra-acetic acid) **chelation therapy** involves intravenous or oral administration of EDTA, a compound which pulls out plaque components and helps to break it down. EDTA can improve blood flow and relieve symptoms associated with atherosclerotic vascular disease. It may be necessary to take vitamin and mineral supplements during EDTA therapy to avoid certain deficiencies, so a health practitioner should be consulted before beginning therapy, and a qualified EDTA chelation specialist should be consulted for intravenous therapy.

Aortic glycosaminoglycans (GAGs)

A natural medicine which can be helpful is an extract of aortic glycosaminoglycans (GAGs), a mixture which is naturally present in the human aorta. Significant improvements in both symptoms of cerebral vascular insufficiency and blood flow have been noted when aortic GAGs are added to the diet. An effective dosage of aortic GAGs is 100 mg daily and should be used for at least six months after a stroke or TIA, after consultation with a health practitioner.

Ginkgo biloba

In well-designed studies, **ginkgo biloba** (*Ginkgo biloba*) extract (GBE) has displayed an ability to reduce major symptoms of cerebral vascular insufficiency, including short-term **memory loss**, vertigo, **headache**, ringing in ears, lack of vigilance, and **depression**. A consultation with a practitioner or doctor is recommended before beginning a ginkgo biloba regimen.

Properties of GBE helpful for cerebral vascular insufficiency:

- Neutralizes free radicals.
- Makes blood more available in ischemic areas through dilation.
- Inhibits platelet-activating factor (PAF) as an alternative for those allergic to aspirin.
- Increases the rate at which information is transmitted at the nerve cell level, improving vigilance and mental performance.

Coleus forskohlii

Many of the properties of **coleus** (*Coleus forskohlii*) prove helpful for this condition. Coleus is a vasodilator, an agent that widens or dilates blood vessels to allow more blood flow. The use of coleus as a treatment for high blood pressure indicates its usefulness in cerebral vascular insufficiency and resulting stroke. Its ability to retard platelet activation and accumulation indicate that it may be helpful in preventing atherosclerotic events.

Spinal manipulative therapy

In one study, some patients receiving soft tissue therapy, **trigger point therapy**, postisometric **relaxation** of spasmed muscles (a technique used for relaxation of muscle tension), and spinal manipulation to partially dislocated vertebrae experienced improvement of cerebral vascular insufficiency symptoms such as vertigo, **fatigue**, and sleep disturbances, and improved cerebral circulation. However, patients who were initially diagnosed with an early form of cerebral vascular insufficiency with vascular disturbances in the neck area or vertebral artery syndrome had their symptoms worsen during manipulative treatment.

A person with these diagnoses should not undergo spinal manipulation.

Allopathic treatment

Vasodilators help to treat the symptoms of cerebral vascular insufficiency and arteriosclerosis by increasing the blood flow in veins and arteries. *Isoxsuprine* is a vasodilator that relaxes blood vessels, making them wider and allowing blood to flow through them more easily. Other treatments that are becoming more common are carotid angioplasty (surgical repair of the arteries that pass up the neck and supply the head) and stenting. (A stent is a device that is used to keep open a tubular structure, like a blood vessel.)

If a person has severe cerebral vascular insufficiency, including frequent TIAs or past stroke and severe (about 70%) blockage, carotid endarterectomy may be necessary. This surgery involves the surgical removal of the atherosclerotic plaque from the carotid artery.

Expected results

Physicians who use EDTA chelation treatment claim great success; however EDTA chelation therapy has not been FDA approved for treatment of atherosclerosis. People considering this therapy may want to do some research and talk with their doctors or an EDTA chelation specialist.

Carotid endarterectomy is a surgery which may have serious complications, including strokes, which may cause permanent neurological damage or death. However, for people with severe cerebral vascular insufficiency this may be the best option. A person with this condition should talk with his or her doctor about the risks and benefits of surgery.

Any treatment for vascular disease caused by atherosclerosis should include an evaluation of diet and other factors to prevent re-blocking of the arteries. Improved diet and **exercise** can help a perzson's long term outlook for this condition.

Prevention

Measures taken to prevent **hypertension** and reduce **cholesterol** and atherosclerosis will also help prevent cerebral vascular insufficiency. Proper diet and lifestyle may not only protect against atherosclerosis, but may also reverse blockage in the arteries. A low-fat diet including vegetables, grains, legumes, and soybean products along with cold water fish and some poultry (no red meat) in addition to **stress** reduction

---

KEY TERMS

Arteriosclerosis—Any hardening of the arteries.

Atherosclerosis—Hardening of the arteries characterized by plaque buildup.

Endarterectomy—A procedure in which the diseased inner portions of an artery, including any deposits, are removed.

Free radicals—Atoms in the body that carry an unpaired electron. Thought to promote the formation of arterial plaque in atherosclerosis.

Homocysteine—An amino acid in the blood, too much of which is related to a higher risk of vascular disease.

Ischema—Local anemia due to mechanical obstruction, mainly arterial narrowing, of the blood supply.

Vigilance—Attentiveness or alertness.

---

techniques and exercise can reduce atherosclerosis. Other important factors are controlling high blood pressure and diabetes and avoiding tobacco. Homocysteine, an amino acid the human body produces that is related to atherosclerosis, may be reduced through dietary reform as mentioned above and supplementation of **folic acid**, B_6(pyridoxine), and B_{12}. Gingko biloba may also be taken as a supplement for its properties mentioned above.

Resources

BOOKS

Goldberg, Burton. *Alternative Medicine: The Definitive Guide.* Tiburon, CA: Future Medicine Publishing, Inc., 1999.

ORGANIZATIONS

American College for Advancement in Medicine. 23121 Verdugo Drive, Suite 204, Laguna Hills, CA 92653. http://www.acam.org.

Life Extension Foundation. 995 SW 24th Street, Fort Lauderdale, FL 33315. (954) 766-8433, (877) 900-9073. http://www.lef.org.

National Institute of Neurological Disorders and Stroke. Bethesda, MD 20892. http://www.ninds.nih.gov/index.htm.

OTHER

Oral chelation for improved heart function. http://www.kirlian.org/life_enhancement_products/oralchelation.html. July 25, 2000.

Melissa C. McDade

Cervical dysplasia

Definition

Cervical dysplasia is a term to describe the appearance of abnormal cells on the cervix.

Description

The cervix is an organ in the female reproductive system, located at the lower end of the uterus and separating it from the vagina. When a woman is pregnant, the cervix seals off the uterus to carry the developing fetus. During **childbirth**, the cervix dilates to allow the baby to pass through. The cervix resembles a small mound with a dimple in the middle.

The cervix has two types of cells. The outer part of the cervix near the vagina is covered with squamous epithelial cells, and the cervical canal is lined with epithelial cells that secrete mucous during ovulation. The border between these two types of cells is called the transformation zone, which changes shape and position with age, especially if a woman carries a **pregnancy**. Women's health providers may closely examine the transition zone to watch for problems in both types of cells. Young women are particularly at risk for problems affecting the transition zone, because early in life the transition zone is exposed on the face of the cervix, making it more vulnerable to exposure of viruses and other agents.

The cervix is susceptible to exposure of sexually transmitted **infections** (STIs) including the human papillomavirus (HPV), as well as other problems including cervicitis, infections and **cancer**. Cervical dysplasia is considered a precancerous condition, because cells of the cervix have abnormalities. The abnormal cells are characterized as mild, moderate or severe dysplasia. Cervical dysplasia is treatable when detected early, and only a very small percentage of cases will develop into cervical cancer.

Causes and Symptoms

Cervical dysplasia is believed to be caused by a confluence of factors, the most significant of which is the presence of HPV infection. Human papillomavirus is a group of viruses that include over 120 different **strains** or types. More than 30 of these are sexually transmitted, and are further subdivided into "high–risk" and "low–risk" types. Low–risk HPV infections may cause mild abnormalities of cervical cells or **genital warts**. Infection with high–risk strains of HPV may cause abnormalities of cervical cells, and may lead to cancer of the cervix or other parts of the genitalia of both females and males. There are at least thirteen high–risk types of HPV. HPV types 16 and 18 are correlated with about 70% of invasive cervical cancer. High–risk strains are present in 93–100% of cases of cervical cancer. The low risk strains 6 and 11 are the most common infections causing condylomata, or genital **warts**.

Infection with the human papillomavirus is extremely common. According to the United States Center for Disease Control (CDC), approximately 20 million people are infected with HPV and over 6 million acquire new infections annually. The CDC data estimates that at least 80% of women will contract a genital HPV infection by the time they are fifty years old. Prevalence of HPV infection peaks in the age group 20–24 years, age 15–19 years has the next highest prevalence. Incidence declines after age 30. HPV infections are either transient or persistent. A study of sexually active college–age women showed that 70% of newly infected women clear the infection within 12 months, and 90% cleared the infection within 24 months. Clearance in older women is 50–80%. Transient infections can cause mild abnormalities of cervical cells, whereas persistent infections cause more severe cell abnormalities.

There are several concomitant variables that increase risk of cervical dysplasia. Sexual behaviors associated with increased risk of dysplasia are: greater than three sexual partners, first intercourse under age twenty, history of other STIs, and not using barrier methods to protect against sexually transmitted infections (condoms, dental dams). HPV transmission occurs in both heterosexual and homosexual partnerings and safer sex precautions using barrier methods can reduce risk.

Another risk factor for developing cervical dysplasia is **smoking**. Women who smoke have a two–fold increased risk of developing cervical cancer. Nicotine, a known carcinogen found in cigarettes, has been found in high concentration in the cervical cells of women who smoke. The risk of smoking appears to be dose–dependent, with severity of dysplasia increasing with the number of cigarettes smoked each day. Smoking more than ten cigarettes daily increases the risk of high–grade dysplasia. Exposure to second–hand smoke is also considered an increased risk.

Additional co–factors in the development of cervical dysplasia and cervical cancer are nutrient deficiencies, oral contraceptive use for five years or longer, more than two pregnancies carried to term, and a compromised immune system. Deficiencies of **vitamin A**, **vitamin C** and **folic acid** have all been found to correlate with cervical dysplasia. Oral contraceptives, in addition to depleting several nutrients, have been found to increase severity of abnormal cellular changes in women with high–risk HPV infection. Both the use of oral contraceptives and the number of full–term pregnancies appear to increase risk by promoting the progression of dysplasia to cervical cancer when HPV is present. Risk of cervical cancer increases slightly with each pregnancy carried to term, due to the effects that pregnancy has on the transformation zone of the cervix. A woman who has been pregnant and given birth seven times has nearly four–fold increased risk of cervical cancer. Additionally, impaired immune function will increase cervical cancer risk due to diminished immune activity needed to clear the HPV infection.

Cervical dysplasia is generally asymptomatic, which means that most women are not aware of the condition by experiencing symptoms. To detect cervical dysplasia, women must rely on diagnostic tests.

Diagnosis

The Pap test is the primary screening tool for detecting cervical dysplasia or cervical cancer. Since its development in the 1950s, screening for abnormal cervical cells with the Papanicolaou (Pap) test has reduced deaths from cervical cancer in the U.S. by over 70%. Incidence of cervical cancer has declined by at least 50% since 1960 in populations of American women who get regular Pap tests, because abnormal cell changes are detected and treated earlier.

It is recommended that women get Pap tests annually beginning at age 21, or within three years of first becoming sexually active, whichever comes first. Women should continue being tested annually until age 65, at which point their health provider can determine how frequently they should continue being screened for cervical cancer. The Pap test is performed by doctors, nurses, midwives and other clinical health care providers. To prepare for the test, a woman must avoid sexual intercourse, using contraceptive foam or jelly, douching, and using tampons or medications vaginally for one to two days. During a speculum examination, the health care provider will insert a small brush and spatula into the cervix to collect a sample of cells.

In 1996, the FDA approved the use of a liquid preparation for Pap testing that has replaced the previous slide method. The advantages of this test are increased sensitivity for abnormal cell changes, and the ability to reflexively test for the presence of high–risk HPV if abnormal cells are found. As of early 2008, there is no comparable test for HPV in males.

For definitive diagnosis of cellular changes, a colposcopic examination and biopsy may be necessary. Colposcopy is a tool for examining the cervix under magnification, often using an iodine–based solution to evaluate for abnormal cells. Biopsy of any abnormal tissue changes on the face of the cervix will be taken during the colposcopic examination, along with a sample of the cells in the endocervical canal. Cell changes on the Pap test are classified according to the grade of abnormality and correlate with different guidelines for management. The lowest category is called ASC–US, which stands for Atypical Squamous Cells of Undetermined Significance, meaning that abnormal cells were found but the significance of these findings is unclear. Of women diagnosed with ASC–US on Pap tests, 75% did have higher grades of dysplasia on further workup, but 10–20% had moderate to severe dysplasia. For ASC–US and mild cases of cervical dysplasia called Low–grade Squamous Intraepithelial Lesion (LSIL), reflex testing for high–risk HPV is often done. Practitioners may choose to monitor these patients with Pap tests every three to six months to determine if the condition will improve on its own, as these cases are usually indicative of a transient HPV effect. Women diagnosed with High–grade Squamous Intraepithelial Lesions (HSIL) may have moderate to severe dysplasia, typically caused by persistent HPV infection and more likely to progress.

Treatment

Conventional treatment guidelines are different depending on the grade of abnormal tissue. A procedure known as loop electrosurgical exicision procedure (LEEP) employs a small wire loop with electrical charge to destroy abnormal cells. An alternative surgical procedure called conization may be used, in which a surgeon removes a cone–shaped segment of the cervix. Less common treatments to destroy abnormal cells of the cervix are freezing them with cryosurgery, or burning them with trichloroacetic acid.

There are several natural therapies that can be utilized for cervical dysplasia in conjunction with conventional management. **Nutrition**, dietary supplements and **botanical medicine** can support the immune system in resolving the HPV infection and restoring health to cervical cells. Lifestyle modifications such as avoidance of smoking, alcohol, **caffeine** and sugar reduce co–factors for dysplasia that inhibit immune function. **Stress** management and **exercise** are also important in maintaining immune system health.

Nutritional therapy for dysplasia consist of a diet predominantly vegetarian and low in fat, emphasizing whole grains, fresh fruits and vegetables, nuts and legumes. Decreasing animal proteins from meat and dairy will reduce intake of hormones and steroids that can exacerbate hormone imbalances. Further nutritional support includes the supplementation of B–complex vitamins, particularly folic acid, vitamin B6 and vitamin B12. Vitamins A, C and E are recommended, as are minerals **selenium** and **zinc**.

Because estrogen plays a role in the progression of cervical dysplasia, treatment targeting hormone balance may be helpful. Phytoestrogens like soy and flax seeds can be incorporated into the diet for hormone balance. **Green tea** extract inhibits growth of precancerous cells on the cervix and is beneficial when used both orally and topically to the cervix. Vaginal suppositories are available that combine anti viral and immune support botanicals with potent nutrients, and have been shown to support healing of the cervical tissue in dysplasia. Botanicals such as **thuja**, ligusticum and **usnea** are used to inhibit viral proliferation, and immune modulating herbs include **Echinacea** and **goldenseal**. Cruciferous vegetable compounds indole–3–carbinol (I3C) and diindolylmethane (DIM) are indicated for cervical dysplasia because they both protect against cancer and support healthy estrogen metabolism. Supplemental I3C and DIM can be used therapeutically to help reverse cellular abnormalities of the cervix.

Prognosis

Cervical dysplasia caused by HPV infection and other co–factors often clears up completely without any medical intervention. In 50% of cases HSIL resolves without conventional treatment. Untreated HSIL may progress to non–invasive cancer known as carcinoma in situ, or to invasive cervical cancer. Invasive cervical cancer has a 92% survival rate if caught and treated early, and survival is nearly 100% for non–invasive cases of cervical cancer.

Prevention

Prevention of cervical dysplasia includes reduction of risk by using safer sex practices with barrier methods, avoiding cigarette smoke and maintaining healthy diet and lifestyle habits. Women diagnosed with dysplasia may consider avoiding use of oral contraceptives. The Pap test continues to be an important tool in prevention of severe cervical dysplasia and

---

KEY TERMS

Cervix—The lower end or "neck" of the uterus, separating the womb from the vagina.

Conization—Surgical removal of a cone–shaped piece of tissue from the cervix

Dysplasia—Abnormality in the size, shape or organization of cells that may be precancerous.

Human papillomavirus—Over 120 types of viruses, about 30 of which are sexually transmitted and cause genital warts and cervical cell changes. HPV types 16, 18, 31, 33, 35, 39, 45, 51, 52, 56, 58, 68 and 82 are considered high–risk as they are associated with pre–cancerous dysplasia.

Lesion—An area of abnormal tissue.

Neoplasia—The development of new, abnormal tissue.

Squamous epithelial cells—The flat cells that make up the surface layer of skin and mucous membranes.

---

cervical cancer. The greatest incidence of cervical cancer is in women who had never been screened or who had not had a Pap test in the last five years.

In 2006, the FDA approved a vaccine for HPV, (Gardasil, developed by Merck & Co.) designed to protect users from four strains of HPV: low–risk strains 6 and 11, and high–risk strains 16 and 18. A bivalent vaccine for HPV 16 and 18 is also being developed (manufacturer GlaxoSmithKline). Gardasil, administered in a series of three injections within a six month period, has been approved for use in females aged 9 to 26 years. It appears that the vaccine is most effective in protecting against HPV infection in females who have not yet become sexually active. It is notable that HPV 16 and 18 correlate with approximately 70% of cases of invasive cervical cancer, and the vaccine does not confer complete protection against HPV and cervical cancer. No long–term data is available on the efficacy of the vaccine in providing ongoing protection against HPV.

As of early 2008, the vaccine is not being targeted to males, although males are carriers of HPV and are susceptible to genital warts and, rarely, genital cancers from high–risk HPV. After its placement on the market in 2006, several states moved to mandate the Gardasil vaccine for preadolescent girls, a controversial decision that has since been overturned in at least one state.

Resources

BOOKS

Hudson, Tori, N.D. *Women's Encyclopedia of Natural Medicine: Alternative Therapies and Integrative Medicine for Total Health and Wellness.* New York: McGraw–Hill, 2008.

PERIODICALS

Ahn, W.S. S.W. Huh, C.K. Kim, et al. "Protective Effects of Green Tea Extracts (Polyphenon E and EGCG) on Human Cervical Lesions." *European Journal of Cancer Prevention.* 2003;12(5):383–390.

Berek, JS. "Bethesda III, ACS, ACOG and ASCCP Guidelines for Cervical Cancer." *OBG Management* September 2003; Supplement, 16–21.

The Females United to Unilaterally Reduce Endo/Ectocervical Disease (FUTURE II) Study Group. "Quadrivalent Vaccine against Human Papillomavirus to Prevent High–Grade Cervical Lesions." *The New England Journal of Medicine.* 2007;356(19):1915–1927.

Fey, M.C., M.W. Beal. "Role of Human Papillomavirus testing in Cervical Cancer Prevention." *Journal of Midwifery & Women's Health.*2004;49(1):4–13.

Giulian, A.R., L. Sedjo, D.J. Roe, et al. "Clearance of Oncogenic Human Papillomavirus (HPV) Infection: Effect of Smoking." *Cancer Causes and Control.* 2002;13 (9):839–846.

Mao, C. L.A. Koutsky, K.A. Ault, C.M. Wheeler, et al. "Efficacy of Human Papillomavirus–16 Vaccine to Prevent Cervical Intraepithelial Neoplasia." *Obstetrics & Gynecology* 2006;107(1):18–27.

Muller, C.Y. "The Role of HPV: Cervical Dysplasia and Cancer, DNA Testing, and Vaccine Trials." *OBG Management.* September 2003; Supplement, 9–15.

Saslow, D., C.D. Runowicz, D. Solomon, et al. "American Cancer Society Guideline for the Early Detection of Cervical Neoplasia and Cancer." *CA: Cancer Journal of Clinicians* 2002;52(6):342–362

Thorne Research, Inc. "Indole–3–Carbinol." *Alternative Medicine Review* 2005;10(4):336–342.

Zeligs, M.A. "The Cruciferous Choice: Diindolylmethane or I3C? Phytonutrient Supplements for Cancer Prevention and Health Promotion." *Chemico–Biological Interactions.* 1998;110(1–2):1–5

ORGANIZATIONS

American College of Obstetricians and Gynecologists (ACOG), 409 12th Street, SW, P.O. Box 96920, Washington, DC, 20090-6920, http://www.acog.org.

Quit Smoking, Center for Disease Control and Prevention, 1600 Clifton Road NE, Atlanta, GA, 30333, (800) 311-3435, (404) 498-1515, http://www.cdc.gov/tobacco/quit_smoking/.

Smokefree.gov, in affliliation with the National Cancer Institute, CDC, National Institutes of Health, Department of Health and Human Services, and USA.gov, 1-800-QUITNOW (1-800-784-8669), TTY 1-800-332-8615, http://www.smokefree.gov/.

Diana Christoff Quinn, ND

CFS *see* **Chronic fatigue syndrome**

Chakra balancing

Definition

Chakra balancing is based on the ancient Indian belief in a series of seven *chakras*, or energy centers. Chakra is the Sanskrit word for wheel. These energy centers are believed to be located at specific points between the base of the spine and the top of the skull. Some esoteric systems include additional chakras, said to extend beyond the physical body into the human auric field. Each chakra is believed to relate to particular organs of the body, ailments, colors, elements, and emotions. However, different systems or sources that use the idea of chakras may disagree about the details. The concept of chakras plays a key role in two ancient Indian healing systems (**ayurvedic medicine** and **yoga**) that are popular today. In recent decades, however, many modern therapies (like **polarity therapy**, **therapeutic touch**, process **acupressure**, core energetics, and **color therapy**) have also incorporated the idea of chakras into their own visions of healing. Various approaches may be used to "balance" the chakras. Chakra balancing is believed to promote health by maximizing the flow of energy in the body, much as a tune-up enables a car to operate at peak efficiency.

Origins

Yoga

Chakras are part of the ancient belief system associated with yoga. These traditions were handed down orally for thousands of years before being codified by Patanjali in his *Yoga Sutras*, several centuries before Christ.

Ayurveda

The ancient healing science of ayurveda is based on a collection of scriptures known as *vedas* (a Sanskrit word meaning knowledge or wisdom). Ayurveda literally means "life knowledge." It remained the predominant form of health care in India until the British colonial government tried to suppress it during the nineteenth century. Over the last half-century, however, a modernized form of ayurveda has gained considerable popularity in India. More recently, traditional ayurveda has been popularized in the West by such high-profile advocates as Deepak Chopra.

Benefits

Balancing the chakras is believed to promote general health and well-being by ensuring the free flow of life energy (also known as *prana* or *qi*) throughout the body. It is believed that blockages in the flow of this vital energy will eventually result in mental, emotional, and/or physical illness. By removing such blockages and maximizing energy flow, practitioners are said to enable body, mind, and spirit to function optimally. Some alternative practitioners, such as medical intuitives, say they can "read" a patient's chakras to detect imbalances and diagnose problems. This is also sometimes done using a pendulum.

Description

Yoga

Just as the various forms of yoga attempt to mediate between the physical and spiritual realms, so the chakras are believed to operate as energy transformers. They are often shown as circles, spaced at intervals along the spine, or sometimes as funnels of energy. Specific chants or sounds associated with the different chakras are used in some yogic **meditation** practices as tools for healing and spiritual evolution.

Each of the seven chakras is said to have specific physiological and metaphysical functions that relate to both the nature of the associated blockages and to the physical problems they produce.

- Base/root chakra (muladhara). The first chakra, located at the base of the spine, is linked with basic survival and with the adrenal glands. It is associated with the color red and the earth element.
- Second chakra (svadisthana). Thought to reside in the genital region, this chakra is linked with sexuality and with the reproductive system. It is associated with the color orange and the water element.
- Third chakra (manipura). Situated near the navel, this chakra is linked with the pancreas and the solar plexus. It is associated with the color yellow, the fire element, and power in the world.
- Heart chakra (cnahata). The fourth chakra, associated with the heart and the immune system, is believed to be the seat of love and compassion. It is associated with the color green and the air element.
- Throat chakra (visuddha). The fifth chakra, situated in the throat area, is associated with the thyroid gland, the color blue, and communication.

- Brow/forehead chakra (ajna). The sixth chakra, also known as the "Third Eye," is said to reside in the forehead. It is associated with hormonal production, the color indigo, and intuition.
- Crown chakra (saha srara). The seventh chakra, located at the top of the skull, is associated with elevated spiritual consciousness, the pineal gland, and the color violet.

Precautions

In recent decades, yoga has gained widespread acceptance in the West as a tool for **relaxation**, **stress** reduction, increased flexibility and energy. However, there is no generally recognized scientific evidence for the existence of either chakras or prana.

Side effects

Although the concept of chakra balancing is harmless, any of the many contemporary therapies that include chakras may also use specific treatments or practices with potential side effects. Anyone exploring such therapies should be cautious and keep his or her healthcare provider informed of these therapies.

Research and general acceptance

Although there is a growing body of research documenting the positive effects of yoga and meditation, chakras have not been measured by scientific instruments. Support for the concept is based on anecdotal rather than scientific evidence.

Resources

BOOKS

Cassileth, Barrie R. *The Alternative Medicine Handbook.* New York: W.W. Norton & Company, 1998.

Pond, David. *Chakras for Beginners: A Guide to Balancing Your Chakra Energies.* Saint Paul: Llewellyn Publications, 1999.

Woodham, Anne, and David Peters. *DK Encyclopedia of Healing Therapies.* New York: DK Publishing, 1997.

Peter Gregutt

Chamomile

Description

Chamomile is a traditional medicinal herb native to western Europe, India, and western Asia. It has become abundant in the United States, where it has

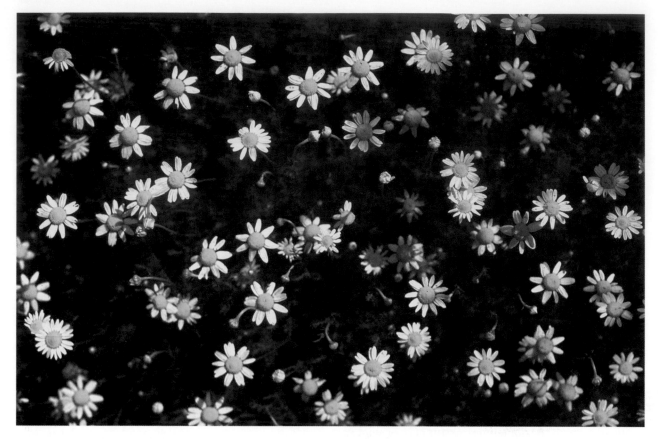

A field of chamomile. *(© Scott Camazine/Photo Researchers, Inc. Reproduced by permission.)*

escaped cultivation to grow freely in pastures, corn-fields, roadsides, and other sunny, well-drained areas. The generic name, chamomile, is derived from the Greek, *khamai*, meaning "on the ground," and *melon*, meaning "apple." The official medicinal cha-momile is the German chamomile *Matricaria recutita*. Chamomile was revered as one of nine sacred herbs by the ancient Saxons. The Egyptians valued the herb as a cure for **malaria** and dedicated chamommile to their sun god, Ra. Two species of this sweet-scented plant, Roman chamomile and German chamomile, have been called the true chamomile because of their similar appearance and medicinal uses.

Roman chamomile *Chamaemelum nobile* is a member of the *Asteraceae*, or daisy family. It is a hardy, low-growing, perennial. Because of the creep-ing roots and compact, mat-like growth of this species it is sometimes called lawn chamomile. Roman cha-momile releases a pleasant, apple scent when walked upon. It was used as a strewing herb during the middle ages to scent the floors and passageways in the home and to deter insects. The Spanish call the herb *manza-nilla*, or "little apple." This fragrant evergreen is a garden favorite. It is also called the physician herb

because of its beneficial effect on other herbs as a companion in the garden. Blossoms grow singly on long stalks attached to the erect, branching, hairy stems. The tiny, daisy-like flowers, blooming May to September, have a small, yellow, solid cone sur-rounded by white rays. The leaves are twice divided and have a feathery appearance. They are light green and somewhat shiny.

German chamomile *Matricaria recutita*, or *Cha-momilla recutita* is a hardy, self-seeding annual herb. It has long been cultivated in Germany to maximize its medicinal properties. The hollow, bright gold cone of the blossom is ringed with numerous white rays. The herb has also been called scented mayweed, and Bald-er's eyelashes, after Balder, the Norse God of Light. German chamomile is also a sprawling member of the *Asteraceae* family, as it closely resembles the Roman chamomile.

Dyer's chamomile *Anthemis tinctora*, also known as yellow chamomile, or golden marquerite, is valued for its use primarily as a dye plant. This native of southern and central Europe is also found in Britain and North America, where it grows wild in many places. It closely resembles the other species, but does not have the medicinal properties of Roman and German chamomile. This species may be biennial or perennial. Both the disk and the rays of the blossom are golden yellow, yielding a distinctive dye that varies from a bright yellow to a more brownish-yellow tint. The type of mordant used influences the color produced. Dyer's chamomile is hardy and can grow to three feet, spreading out as wide as it is high. The branched stems are erect and woolly, with leaves that can grow to three inches long.

General use

The aromatic flower heads and herba (leaves) of both Roman and German chamomile are used medicinally. They are highly scented with volatile, aromatic oil, including the heat-sensitive Azulene, which is the blue chamomile essential oil. The phytochemical constituents in chamomile also include flavonoids, coumarins, plant acids, fatty acids, cyanogenic glycosides, **choline**, tannin, and salicylate derivatives. This bittersweet herb acts medicinally as a tonic, anodyne, antispasmodic, anti-inflammatory, antibacterial, antiallergenic, and sedative. Traditionally, a mild infusion of the herb has been safely used to calm restless children, and to ease **colic** and teething **pain** in babies. It is also effective in relieving acid **indigestion** and abdominal pain. Its carminative properties relieve intestinal **gas**, and it helps in cases of **diarrhea**, **constipation**, and peptic ulcers. The herbal tea can ease symptoms of colds and flu by relieving **headache** and reducing **fever**. The infusion is also helpful to treat **toothache**, arthritis, **gout**, and premenstrual tension. It may also be used in douche preparations, or sitz baths. As an external wash in strong infusion, or decoction, or as part of a hot compress, the herb can soothe **burns** and scalds, skin **rashes**, and sores. Chamomile can be used in a douche, as a gargle for mouth ulcers, as a soothing eye wash for **conjunctivitis**, and as a hair rinse to brighten the hair. Chamomile blossoms may also be used as an herbal aromatic treatment, providing a tonic lift with its pleasing scent. This use of chamomile is especially popular among Hispanics living in the southwestern United States, who use the herb at significantly higher levels than the rest of the population.

Preparations

Chamomile is most often prepared as an infusion of the blossoms of German chamomile, and less commonly of Roman chamomile. Traditionally the tiny blossoms are picked on midsummers' eve. The best time to harvest is on a sunny day when the mass of blossoms is at its fullness in the morning. Harvesting

KEY TERMS

Anodyne—A medicinal herb that relieves distress or soothes pain.

Coumarin—A chemical compound found in plants that breaks down red blood cells.

Decoction—A plant extract obtained by boiling the water in which plant parts have been soaked and then straining out the plant materials.

chamomile blossoms can be painstaking work, requiring a gardner's best patience. Pinch off the flower head, leaving the stem. Fresh or dried blossoms may be used in herbal preparations.

Blossoms to be dried for storage should be spread singly on a screen or mat and placed in a well-ventilated place, out of direct sun, with a temperature close to 95°F (35°C). The rapid drying will preserve much of the volatile oil and other medicinal properties. A few blossoms go a long way with this pleasant and safe herbal ally. Store dried blossoms in tightly sealed, glass containers, away from light. They will maintain potency for about one year. Chamomile is prolific, and the plant blossoms frequently throughout the summer. Sometimes two or three harvests can be made in one season.

Chamomile tea may be made from an infusion of blossoms prepared as a tisane, for a single, soothing cup, or in a larger quantity for use throughout the day. Chamomile combines well with mints, such as **lemon balm** (*Melissa officinalis*) or **spearmint** (*Mentha spicata*), combined in equal quantity. For a tisane, use 1 tsp of dried blossoms, or 1.5 tsp of freshly picked flowers in a warm cup. Heat water to the boiling point and pour over the blossoms in glass container. Cover, and infuse for 3–5 minutes. Let strain. Be careful not to oversteep chamomile, lest it lose its delicate flavor to a bitter edge. Standard dose is up to three cups per day. The prepared tea will keep for a day or two in the refrigerator.

To prepare a chamomile decoction, which is a stronger preparation, let the plant parts steep in a covered nonmetallic pot for at least ten minutes. The decoction may be used as a skin wash, hair rinse, mouth wash, or to bathe **wounds**.

An extract of the essential oil can be prepared by placing 2 oz (57 g) of fresh blossoms into a glass container and covering the plant with 0.5–1 pt (0.24–0.47 l) of olive oil. Place the mixture on a sunny window sill for about one week. Strain and store in a dark container with a tight-fitting lid. The oil remains potent for up to one year. It is best when applied warm.

Precautions

Chamomile has been used over the centuries and is generally considered a safe and gentle herbal remedy that may be used daily as a calming tea. Persons who may be allergic to such pollen-bearing plants as chamomile would be wise to experiment with this herbal remedy with some caution.

Side effects

The moderate internal use of chamomile preparations has no known side effects; however, some herbalists warn that the herb, when taken internally in excessive doses, can induce **vomiting** and produce vertigo (**dizziness**). With regard to the external use of chamomile preparations, a small number of persons experience mild skin irritation.

Interactions

There are no contraindications for using this gentle, healing herb. Chamomile does combine well with other herbs that enhance its pleasant and medicinal qualities.

Resources

BOOKS

Gladstar, Rosemary. *Herbal Healing for Women.* New York: Simon & Schuster, 1993.

Hoffman, David. *The New Holistic Herbal.* Boston, MA: Element Books, Inc., 1992.

McIntyre, Anne. *The Medicinal Garden.* New York: Henry Holt and Company, 1997.

McVicar, Jekka. *Herbs for the Home.* New York: Viking Penguin, 1995.

PERIODICALS

Rivera, J. O., M. Ortiz, M. E. Lawson, and K. M. Verma. "Evaluation of the Use of Complementary and Alternative Medicine in the Largest United States-Mexico Border City." *Pharmacotherapy* 22 (February 2002): 256-264.

Schempp, C. M., E. Schopf, and J. C. Simon. "Plant-Induced Toxic and Allergic Dermatitis (Phytodermatitis)." [Article in German] *Hautarzt* 53 (February 2002): 93-97.

Clare Hanrahan
Rebecca J. Frey, PhD

Charcoal, activated

Description

Activated charcoal is a fine, black, odorless, and tasteless powder. It is made from wood or other materials that have been exposed to very high temperatures in an airless environment. It is then treated, or activated, to increase its ability to adsorb by reheating with oxidizing **gas** or other chemicals to break into a very fine powder. Activated charcoal is pure carbon specially processed to make it highly adsorbent of particles and gases in the body's digestive system.

Activated charcoal has been used since ancient times to cure a variety of ailments including poisoning. Its healing effects have been well documented since as early as 1550 B.C. by the Egyptians. However, charcoal was almost forgotten until 15 years ago when it was rediscovered as a wonderful oral agent to treat most overdoses and toxins.

General use

Activated charcoal's most important use is for treatment of poisoning. It helps prevent the absorption of most poisons or drugs by the stomach and intestines. In addition to being used for most swallowed poisons in humans, charcoal has been effectively used in dogs, rabbits, rats and other animals. It can also absorb gas in the bowels and has been used for the treatment of gas or **diarrhea**. Charcoal's other uses, such as for the treatment of viruses, bacteria, bacterial toxic by-products, snake venoms and other substances by adsorption, have not been supported by clinical studies. By adding water to the powder to

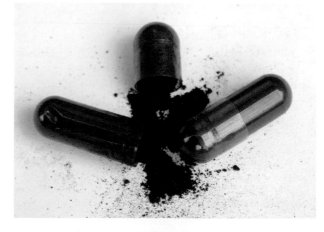

Activated charcoal is pure carbon specially processed to make it highly adsorbent of particles and gases in the body's digestive system. *(julie woodhouse / Alamy)*

make a paste, activated charcoal can be used as an external application to alleviate **pain** and **itching** from **bites and stings**.

Poisons and drug overdoses

It is estimated that one million children accidentally overdose on drugs mistaken as candies or eat, drink, or inhale poisonous household products each year. In the year 2000, the American Association of Poison Control Centers said that more than 1,142,000 calls had been received in centers around the country regarding poison exposures to children under six years of age. Activated charcoal is one of the agents most commonly used for infants and toddlers exposed to poison. It can absorb large amounts of poisons quickly. In addition, it is non-toxic, may be stored for a long time, and can be conveniently administered at home. Charcoal works by binding to irritating or toxic substances in the stomach and intestines. This prevents the toxic drug or chemical from spreading throughout the body. The activated charcoal with the toxic substance bound to it is then excreted in the stool without harm to the body.

When poisoning is suspected the local poison control center should be contacted for instructions. They may recommend using activated charcoal, which should be available at home so that it can be given to the poisoned child or pet immediately. For severe poisoning, several doses of activated charcoal may be needed. A 2002 study showed that in some cases, charcoal could be administered at home sooner than in the emergency room, and was beneficial for children who had ingested poisonous mushrooms. However, the study concluded that more research was needed to be sure that home-administered doses were accurate and the best solution for other types of poisoning.

Intestinal disorders

In the past, activated charcoal was a popular remedy for gas. Even before the discovery of America by Europeans, Native Americans used powdered charcoal mixed with water to treat an upset stomach. Now charcoal is being rediscovered as an alternative treatment for this condition. Activated charcoal works like a sponge. Its huge surface area is ideal for soaking up different substances, including gas. In one study, people taking activated charcoal after eating a meal with high gas-producing foods did not produce more gas than those who did not have these foods. Charcoal has also been used to treat other intestinal disorders such as diarrhea, **constipation**, and cramps. There are few studies to support these uses and there are also concerns that frequent use of charcoal may decrease absorption of essential nutrients, especially in children.

KEY TERMS

Antidote—A remedy to counteract a poison or injury.

Adsorption—The binding of a chemical (e.g., drug or poison) to a solid material such as activated charcoal or clay.

Other uses

Besides being a general antidote for poisons or remedy for gas, activated charcoal has been used to treat other conditions. Based on its ability to adsorb, or bind to other substances, charcoal has been effectively used to clean skin **wounds** and to adsorb waste materials from the gastrointestinal tract. In addition, it has been used to adsorb snake venoms, viruses, bacteria, and harmful materials excreted by bacteria or fungi. However, because of lack of scientific studies, these uses are not recommended. Activated charcoal, when used together with other remedies such as **aloe** vera, **acidophilus**, and **psyllium**, helps to keep symptoms of ulcerative **colitis** under control. While charcoal shows some anti-aging activity in rats, it is doubtful if it can do the same for humans.

Preparations

For poisoning

Activated charcoal is available without prescription. However, in case of accidental poisoning or drug overdose an emergency poison control center, hospital emergency room, or doctor's office should be called for advice. In cases where both syrup of **ipecac** and charcoal are recommended for treatment of the poison, ipecac should be given first. Charcoal should not be given for at least 30 minutes after ipecac or until **vomiting** from ipecac stops. Activated charcoal is often mixed with a liquid before being swallowed or put into the tube leading to the stomach. Activated charcoal is available in liquid form in 30 g bottles. It is also available in 15 g container sizes, as slurry of charcoal pre-mixed in water, or in a container to which water or soda is added. Keeping activated charcoal at home is a good idea so that it can be taken immediately when needed for treatment of poisoning.

For acute poisoning, the dosage is as follows:

- Infants (under 1 year of age): 1 g/kg.
- Children (1-12 years of age): 15-30 g or 1-2 g/kg with at least 8 oz of water.
- Adults: 30-100 g or 1-2 g/kg with at least 8 oz of water.

For diarrhea or gas

A person can take charcoal tablets or capsules with water or sprinkle the content onto food. The dosage for treatment of gas or diarrhea in adults is 520 to 975 mg after each meal and up to 5 g per day.

Precautions

Parents should keep activated charcoal on hand in case of emergencies.

Charcoal should not be taken together with syrup of ipecac, as the charcoal will adsorb the ipecac. Charcoal should be taken 30 minutes after ipecac or after the vomiting from ipecac stops.

Some activated charcoal products contain sorbitol. Sorbitol is a sweetener as well as a laxative, therefore, it may cause severe diarrhea and vomiting. These products should not be used in infants.

Charcoal may interfere with the absorption of medications and nutrients such as vitamins or minerals. For uses other than for treatment of poisoning, charcoal should be taken two hours after other medications.

Charcoal should not be used to treat poisoning caused by corrosive products such as lye or other strong acids or petroleum products such as gasoline, kerosene, or cleaning fluids. Charcoal may make the condition worse and delay diagnosis and treatment. In addition, charcoal is also not effective if the poison is lithium, cyanide, **iron**, ethanol, or methanol.

Parents should not mix charcoal with chocolate syrup, sherbet, or ice cream, even though it may make charcoal taste better. These foods may prevent charcoal from working properly.

Activated charcoal may cause swelling or pain in the stomach. A doctor should be notified immediately should this occur. It has been known to cause problems in people with intestinal bleeding, blockage or those people who have had recent surgery. These patients should talk to their doctor before using this product.

Charcoal may be less effective in people with slow digestion.

Charcoal should not be given for more than three or four days for treatment of diarrhea. Continuing for longer periods may interfere with normal **nutrition**.

Charcoal should not be used in children under three years of age to treat diarrhea or gas.

Activated charcoal should be kept out of reach of children.

Side effects

Charcoal may cause constipation when taken for overdose or accidental poisoning. A laxative should be taken after the crisis is over.

Activated charcoal may cause the stool to turn black. This is to be expected.

Pain or swelling of the stomach may occur. A doctor should be consulted.

Interactions

Activated charcoal should not be mixed together with chocolate syrup, ice cream or sherbet. These foods prevent charcoal from working properly.

Resources

BOOKS

Blumenthal, Mark. *Linden Charcoal*. The Complete German Commission E Monographs, Therapeutic Guide to Herbal Medicines, American Botanical Council, Boston: Integrative Medicine Communications, 1998. Accessed online. http://home.mdconsult.com.

Cooney, David. *Activated Charcoal: Antidote, Remedy, and Health Aid*. Brushton, NY: TEACH Services, Inc., 1999.

Lacy Charles F., Lora L. Amstrong, Naomi B. Ingrim, and Leonard L. Lance. *Charcoal*. The Drug Information Handbook Pocket Version: 1998-1999, Hudson, OH: Lexi-Comp Inc., 1998.

Roberts. *Activated Charcoal*. Clinical Procedures in Emergency Medicine, Philadelphia, PA: W. B. Saunders Company, 1998: 726-8. Accessed online. http://home.mdconsult.com.

Wilson, Billie A., Margaret T. Shannon, and Carolyn L. Stang. *Charcoal, Activated (Liquid Antidote)*. Nurses Drug Guide 2000, Stamford, CT: Appleton & Lange, 2000.

PERIODICALS

Bond, C. Randall. "Activated Charcoal in the Home: Helpful and Important or Simply a Distraction." *Pediatrics* (January 2002) : 145.

Mai Tran
Teresa G. Odle

Chasteberry tree

Description

The chasteberry tree, whose botanical name is *Vitex agnus castus*, belongs to the Verbenaceae family. The fruit is also called chasteberry, vitex, or monk's

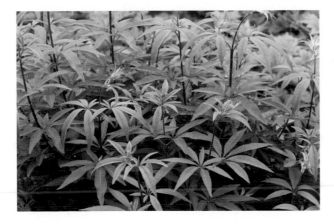

Chasteberry tree (Vitex agnus castus) foliage. This plant is used in herbal medicine to treat female reproductive disorders and menstrual difficulties. *(Adrian Thomas / Photo Researchers, Inc.)*

pepper. The terms "chasteberry" and "vitex" are used interchangeably below.

The chasteberry tree can grow to a height of 22 ft (6.71 m) and can be found on wet banks of rivers in southern Europe and the Mediterranean area. It is also grown as an ornamental plant in the United States. Although the red-black berry is the most used part, the leaves contain the highest amount of flavonoids—up to 2.7%, with the blue-violet flowers a close second at 1.5%. The berries contain nearly 1% flavonoids, including casticin, kaempferol, isovitexin, orientin and quercatagetin.

Surprisingly, in spite of chasteberry's use for hormonal problems, it does not contain plant estrogen. Instead, the chasteberry tree contains:

- androstenedione, epitestosterone, hydroxyprogesterone, progesterone and testosterone in the flowers and leaves
- iridoid glycosides, such as aucubin and agnuside, in the berries
- essential oil, which includes cineol and pinene monoterpenes, as well as castine, citronellol, eucalptol, limonene, linalool and sesquiterpenes (Chasteberry's spicy aroma is derived from its essential oil.)
- vitricine, an alkaloid

General use

Chasteberry was used by the ancient Greeks and Romans as well as by medieval monks to lower sexual desire. The Greeks and Romans also used it to keep away evil. Hippocrates used chasteberry to treat injuries. Dioscorides advised its application for inflamed wombs, diseases of the spleen and lactation. European nuns used chasteberry for women's hormonal problems, and this latter application is chasteberry's main function today. It is considered a uterine tonic.

Chasteberry acts as a balancer, not only in female hormonal problems, but also with regard to libido. Therefore, chasteberry can act as both an aphrodisiac and an anaphrodisiac. It can normalize hormonal imbalances; treat **amenorrhea** or dysmenorrhoea; and act to increase or suppress lactation.

Chasteberry works by helping the pituitary gland to raise progesterone levels. Chasteberry induces the pituitary gland to free a lutcinizing hormone and stop a follicle-stimulating one. Chasteberry is sometimes called a support for female hormones from **menstruation** to **menopause**.

PMS problems are usually caused by low progesterone levels in relation to the estrogen level. Taking the progesterone-laden vitex can relieve many PMS symptoms, as was shown in a 1997 double-blind clinical study. One hundred and seventy-five women randomly received daily doses of a standard vitex capsule (3.5–4.2 mg), a placebo, or two **pyridoxine** capsules (100 mg each) to measure the alleviation of such PMS symptoms as bloating, irritability, **depression**, breast tenderness, weight gain, skin problems, and digestive problems. In the efficacy part of the study, 77.1 % of subjects taking vitex reported improvement in their symptoms, compared to only 60.6% in the pyridoxine group.

Some studies show that chasteberry can both increase and decrease prolactin levels in the body. Too much prolactin is related to amenorrhea (no menstrual periods) and breast tenderness associated with PMS; too little prolactin can mean reduced milk production. In one study featuring 100 nursing mothers, those who took chasteberry had more milk than those who took a placebo. In another clinical study of PMS associated with high prolactin levels, vitex balanced not only prolactin levels but the menstrual cycle itself. According to David L. Hoffman, taking vitex after stopping birth control pills can regulate cycles and therefore increase the likelihood of **pregnancy**. Another writer has described her own situation of stopping birth control pills and having no periods for two and a half years until she started taking chasteberry. German studies also show that vitex may also help prevent a miscarriage.

Chasteberry is also used to treat fibroid cysts, especially cysts in smooth muscle. Vitex has been said to be effective in stopping the heavy bleeding of

KEY TERMS

Agnuside—The active ingredient in chasteberry.

Amenorrhea—The abnormal absence of menstrual periods.

Anaphrodisiac—A substance or medication that suppresses sexual desire.

Dopamine—A neurotransmitter that acts within certain brain cells to regulate movement and emotions.

Essential oil—Oil from a herb, obtained by steam distilling or cold pressing, then mixed with a vegetable oil or water. It has many functions, including use with massage or as an inhalant.

Extract—A concentrated form of the herb made by pressing the herb with a hydraulic press, soaking it in water or alcohol, then letting the excess water or alcohol evaporate.

Flavonoids—Plant pigments that have a variety of effects on human physiology. The casticin, kaempferol, isovitexin, orientin and quercatagetin contained in chasteberry are flavonoids.

Melatonin—A hormone secreted by the pineal gland that helps to regulate biorhythms.

Perimenopause—The time span just before a woman reaches menopause. It usually begins when a woman is in her 40s and may produce many of the symptoms associated with menopause.

Pyridoxine—Another name for vitamin B_6.

Tincture—An alcohol-based extract prepared by soaking plant parts.

perimenopause and reduce the **hot flashes** in menopause itself. It is used extensively in England for this purpose. Also, chasteberry's antiandrogenic influence can help to reduce **acne** in teenagers of either sex.

Preparations

Chasteberry may be taken as a tincture, an extract, a tea or in capsules. The usual dosage is 200 mg of the berry, with a standardized amount (0.5%) of the active ingredient agnuside. The recommended dosage varies with the ailment being treated, and should be decided upon in conjunction with a health care practitioner.

Tincture and extracts of chasteberry are mixed with water or juice, 10–30 drops per drink. They should be taken up to three times daily.

Chasteberry tea is made from 1 tsp of ripe berries to 1 cup (250 ml) of boiling water. The tea must be steeped for 10–15 min and should be drunk three times daily.

According to one naturopathic physician, the usual dosage of extract of chasteberry is 175–225 mg on a daily basis. Capsules are available in doses from 40–400 mg. The capsules are usually taken one to three a day about one hour before breakfast to increase their absorption. If taken before bedtime, chasteberry may aid in sleeping as well as increase the secretion of **melatonin** in the early morning. Because chasteberry acts slowly in the body, it can take from one to six months to see permanent results. These results should continue even after use of chasteberry is discontinued. To increase milk production, women are advised to take chasteberry the first 10 days after giving birth.

Chasteberry may be taken in conjunction with Vitamin B_6 for PMS.

Precautions

Some practitioners of alternative medicine recommend that pregnant women should abstain from taking chasteberry. German research indicates that chasteberry is safe for the first three months of pregnancy, but is unsafe after that time as it might start the flow of milk too early.

Herbal experts may also advise patients with **breast cancer**, **uterine cancer**, or pituitary tumors not to take chasteberry. It is always best to check with your health care provider first.

Because chasteberry does not contain plant estrogens, it should not be used as a substitute for hormonal replacement therapy, or HRT. Women who are concerned about the possible side effects of HRT should consider fo-ti or other herbs shown to have measurable estrogen-like activity, such as **licorice** and **hops**.

Side effects

Chasteberry rarely has side effects but a few have been reported: allergic **rashes**; minor headaches and **nausea** when first taking chasteberry; changes in the length of the menstrual period; and increased bleeding. The alcohol in chasteberry tinctures may cause some gastric irritation if taken on an empty stomach. This situation can be avoided by mixing the tincture in water, by taking half the tincture before breakfast and half after lunch, or by taking capsules.

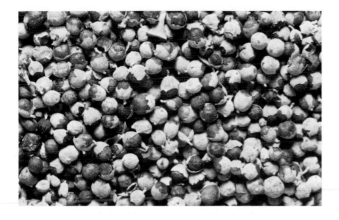

Chasteberry, also known as monk's pepper, is recommended as an herbal treatment for premenstrual syndrome.
(© TH Foto / Alamy)

Interactions

Chasteberry should not be combined with such synthetic hormones as those contained in birth control pills or hormone replacement therapy. The latter includes Premarin and Provera.

Drugs that act on a neurotransmitter in the brain called dopamine may either affect or be affected by vitex. These include medications for **Parkinson's disease** (L-dopa, Parlodel); psychosis (Haldol); **smoking** cessation (Zyban); and depression (Wellbutrin).

Resources

BOOKS

Ali, Elvis et al. *The All-In-One Guide to Natural Remedies and Supplements.* AGES Publications, 2000.

Balch, James F., MD, and Phyllis A. Balch, CNC. *Prescription for Nutritional Healing, 2nd ed.* New York: Avery Publishing Group, 1997.

Landis, Robin, with Karta Pukh Singh Khalsa. *Herbal Defense.* New York: Warner Books, Inc., 1997.

Murray, Michael, ND. *Encyclopedia of Nutritional Supplements.* Rocklin, CA: Prima Publishing, 1996.

Murray, Michael, ND. *The Healing Power of Herbs, 2nd ed.* Rocklin, CA: Prima Publishing, 1995.

PERIODICALS

Oerter Klein, K., M. Janfaza, K. A. Wong, and R. J. Chang. "Estrogen Bioactivity in Fo-Ti and Other Herbs Used for Their Estrogen-Like Effects as Determined by a Recombinant Cell Bioassay." *Journal of Clinical Endocrinology and Metabolism* 88 (September 2003): 4077–4079.

ORGANIZATIONS

National Center for Complementary and Alternative Medicine (NCCAM) Clearinghouse. P.O. Box 7923, Gaithersburg, MD 20898-7923. (888) 644-6226. http://nccam.nih.gov.

U. S. Food and Drug Administration (FDA). 5600 Fishers Lane, Rockville, MD 20857. (888) 463-6332. http://www.fda.gov.

OTHER

Herb World News Online, Herb Research Foundation. http://www.herbs.org.

Whole Health Products. http://wholehealthproducts.com, 2000.

Sharon Crawford
Rebecca J. Frey, PhD

Chelated minerals

Description

Chelated minerals are specially formulated mineral supplements designed to improve absorption of these essential nutrients by the body. What makes a mineral a chelated compound is the bonding of the mineral to nitrogen and the ligand that surrounds the mineral and protects it from interacting with other compounds. Although some people believe that chelated minerals are absorbed more efficiently within the body, studies have shown no significant difference between chelated and nonchelated forms.

General use

The importance of minerals

Minerals are vital to health because they are the building blocks that make up muscles, tissues, and bones. They also are important components of many life-supporting systems and activities and are important to hormones, oxygen transport, and enzyme systems.

Minerals participate in the chemical reactions that occur inside the body. These nutrients may work as cofactors or helpers in enzyme reactions. As cofactors, minerals help enzymes function properly. Minerals may also work as catalysts to initiate and speed up these enzymatic reactions.

Minerals are the electrolytes that the body needs to maintain normal body fluids and the acid-base balance. As electrolytes, minerals act as gatekeepers to control nerve signal movements throughout the body. Because nerves control muscle movements, minerals also regulate muscle contraction and **relaxation**.

Many minerals, such as **zinc**, **copper**, **selenium**, and **manganese**, act as **antioxidants**. They protect the body against the damaging effects of free radicals (reactive molecules). They scavenge or mop up these highly reactive radicals and change them into inactive, less harmful compounds. In so doing, these minerals help prevent **cancer** and many other health problems such as premature **aging**, **heart disease**, autoimmune diseases, arthritis, **cataracts**, **Alzheimer's disease**, and diabetes.

There are two kinds of minerals: major (or macro) minerals and trace minerals. Major minerals are those that the body needs in large amounts. The major minerals include **calcium**, **phosphorus**, **magnesium**, **sodium**, **potassium**, **sulfur**, and chlorine. They are needed to build muscles, blood, nerve cells, teeth, and bones. They are also essential electrolytes that the body requires to regulate blood volume and the acid-base balance.

Unlike the major minerals, trace minerals are needed only in tiny amounts. Even though they can be found in the body in exceedingly small amounts, they are also very important. These minerals participate in most chemical reactions in the body. They are also needed to manufacture important hormones. Trace minerals include **iron**, zinc, **iodine**, copper, manganese, fluorine, **chromium**, selenium, molybdenum, and **boron**.

Why supplements are used

Some studies have shown that mineral supplements are needed because most Americans do not get adequate amounts of minerals in their **diets**. In the 2000s, increasing numbers of people take chelated minerals daily to ensure that the body has enough of these nutrients to function properly. Many healthy people take minerals to boost their body's immune system and to achieve maximal levels of energy and mental alertness.

Treatment and prevention of diseases

People take individual minerals to prevent or treat certain diseases and conditions. The benefits/uses of key minerals and the optimum daily intake (ODI) of each mineral are given below. ODI is the amount most people require to function at their best level.

CALCIUM (ODI=1,000–1,500 MG). Calcium supplements are commonly used for the prevention and treatment of **osteoporosis** (a bone thinning disease). However, calcium supplements also provide other benefits as well. Studies have shown that calcium may also be effective in treating high blood pressure and relieving symptoms of leg cramps and arthritis. It may also prevent colon cancer.

Calcium supplements may be contaminated with lead, which is highly toxic. A study by the Department of Environmental Toxicology, University of California, Santa Cruz, indicates that for calcium supplements, chelation may be a bad idea. They found that non-chelated calcium supplements had lower levels of lead contamination than the chelated products.

PHOSPHORUS (ODI=200–400 MG). Phosphorus is an important mineral for humans. However, because Americans often exceed their phosphorus intake due to high consumption of sodas and meat, phosphorus supplements are neither necessary nor recommended. Excessive consumption of phosphorus accelerates bone loss leading to osteoporosis.

MAGNESIUM (ODI=500–750 MG). Magnesium supplements have been used to promote healthy teeth and bones, treat **muscle spasms**, relieve premenstrual **pain**, and lower high blood pressure in patients with low magnesium levels. Magnesium has also been used to prevent premature labor and low birth weight.

ZINC (ODI=22.5–50 MG). Zinc is one of the most frequently used supplements. A strong antioxidant, zinc protects the body against damaging free radicals and boosts the body's immune system. It helps heal **burns** and **wounds**, offers some protection against common **infections** such as colds or flu, and helps prevent cancer. It may be effective in the prevention and/or treatment of age-related **macular degeneration** (an eye disease), **infertility**, **hair loss**, **anorexia nervosa** (an eating disorder), **prostate enlargement**, and common skin problems such as **acne**.

IRON (ODI=15–25 MG FOR MEN; 18–30 MG FOR WOMEN). Iron supplements are most often prescribed to treat iron deficiency **anemia**. Iron is also used to increase energy and mental sharpness.

COPPER (ODI=0.5–2 MG). Copper deficiency is relatively rare due to the abundance of it in natural food sources and in drinking water. Because of the potential risk of severe toxicity, copper is best taken as part of a multivitamin-mineral formula.

MANGANESE (ODI=15–30 MG). Supplements of this trace mineral have been used to prevent cancer, to improve blood sugar control, and to treat arthritic symptoms.

CHROMIUM (ODI=200–600 MICROGRAMS OR MCG). This trace mineral may help prevent or treat low blood sugar levels and diabetes. It may also offer protection against heart disease by lowering blood **cholesterol** levels.

SELENIUM (ODI=50–400 MCG). A good antioxidant, selenium may help protect the body against cancer, premature aging, and degenerative diseases such as heart disease and arthritis.

IODINE (ODI=UP TO 150 MCG). Iodine is sometimes used to prevent goiter, an iodine deficiency disease.

POTASSIUM (ODI=99–300 MG). Potassium supplements are most often prescribed to treat potassium deficiency caused by chronic diuretic use. Diuretics are products that increase the urine that is excreted.

BORON. There is no ODI for boron; however, 3 to 6 mg of boron may be helpful in preventing osteoporosis and improving symptoms of **osteoarthritis**.

Prevention of drug-induced side effects

Mineral supplements are used to prevent drug-induced mineral deficiencies. A mineral deficiency sometimes occurs after prolonged use of certain drugs. For example, patients who receive diuretics such as hydrochlorothiazide or furosemide for high blood pressure often have low potassium levels. The condition is so common that doctors routinely prescribe potassium supplements together with diuretics. Because high potassium levels are toxic to the body, patients should not take more potassium than their doctor has ordered.

Preparations

One major problem associated with mineral supplements has been poor absorption. Traditional forms of mineral supplements, the mineral salts, are very inexpensive. However, they do not absorb well into the body. Most of the minerals contained in these tablets pass right through the body rather than being absorbed into the blood.

Chelation has been used as a means of improving absorption of minerals from supplements, but the value of this method is limited at best. Generally, chelated minerals are not absorbed more than 5% more effectively than unchelated supplements. This minor benefit rarely justifies the higher prices charged for chelated products. The poor absorption of minerals is taken into account when the daily diet recommendations are developed, so that the recommended intake should be enough of the mineral to provide the levels that are actually desired.

Precautions

People should remember several guidelines when using chelated mineral supplements.

- Mineral supplements are not substitutes for a healthy diet. In addition, they are not absorbed well by a malnourished body. Therefore, it is important to adhere to a low-fat, high-fiber diet. People should eat plenty of fruits and vegetables and limit consumption of caffeine, alcohol, red meat, processed foods, and foods high in fat or sugar.

- A naturopath or a nutritionist may recommend one or several individual supplements for short-term treatment for a specific mineral deficiency. However, if continued for too long, this diet may upset the mineral balance in the body and cause deficiencies of other minerals. For general good health, it is best to use multiple vitamin and mineral supplements with the minerals in the form of chelates.

- Because of potential interactions between minerals (such as calcium, iron, or zinc) and other herbal supplements or medications, people should inform their doctor about all supplements they are taking.

- Unlike vitamins, minerals are easily overused and can have toxic effects. People should not take minerals at dosages exceeding the recommended ODI.

Side effects

The following are some of the adverse effects associated with high-dose individual mineral supplementation.

- Copper: Copper toxicity, a serious condition, causes abdominal pain, nausea, vomiting, diarrhea, dizziness, general fatigue, headache, depression, insomnia, and poor brain function.
- Fluorine: High fluorine levels in the body may cause stomach ulcers and increase the risk of bone cancer.
- Iron: Iron toxicity causes nausea, vomiting, and abdominal pain. Too much iron in the diet has been associated with increased risk of infections and cancer.
- Zinc: Excessive zinc supplementation may cause copper deficiency, nausea, and vomiting.
- Potassium: Potassium toxicity can occur if a person takes more than 18 g of supplement per day. Symptoms of potassium toxicity include irregular heart beat, muscle fatigue, and heart failure.
- Selenium: Symptoms of selenium toxicity include hair loss, brittle fingernails, skin irritation, nausea, fatigue, garlic odor on the breath, and increased risk of infections.

Interactions

Foods increase absorption of minerals. Therefore, mineral supplements should be taken with food for better absorption.

Minerals such as calcium, iron, manganese, magnesium, copper, or zinc can bind to many drugs when taken together and can decrease their effectiveness.

KEY TERMS

Chelate—A chemical compound in which a metal is bonded to one or more organic groups.

Free radical—An atom, molecule, or ion with an odd number of unbonded electrons.

Optimum daily intake (ODI)—The amount of a supplement that provides the greatest value to a person.

Therefore, mineral supplements should be taken two hours before or two hours after any of the following medications:

- ciprofloxacin
- ofloxacin
- tetracycline
- doxycycline
- erythromycin
- warfarin
- mineral oil

Resources

BOOKS

Card, David R. *12 Essential Minerals for Cellular Health: An Introduction to Cell Salts.* Prescott, AZ: Hohm Press, 2007.

Jeep, Robin, and Richard Couey. *The Super Antioxidant Diet and Nutrition Guide: A Health Plan for the Body, Mind, and Spirit.* Charlottesville, VA: Hampton Roads, 2008.

Smith, Pamela Wartian. *What You Must Know about Vitamins, Minerals, Herbs, & More: Choosing the Nutrients that Are Right for You.* Garden City Park, NY: Square One, 2008.

Vohora, S. B., and Mohammad Athar. *Mineral Drugs: Used in Ayurveda and Unani Medicine.* New Delhi: Narosa Publishing House, 2007.

PERIODICALS

Greenwald, Peter, et al. "What Is the Efficacy of Multivitamin: Multimineral Supplements in Chronic Disease Prevention in the General Population of Adults?" *American Journal of Clinical Nutrition* (January 2007): 3148–3175.

ORGANIZATIONS

American Association of Naturopathic Physicians, 4435 Wisconsin Ave. NW, Suite 403, Washington, DC, 20016, (202) 237-8150, (866) 538-2267, http://www.naturopathic.org.

National Center for Complementary and Alternative Medicine, NCCAM Clearinghouse, National Institute of Health, PO Box 7923, Gaithersburg, MD, 20898, (888) 644-6226, http://nccam.nih.gov.

Samuel Uretsky, Pharm.D.
David Edward Newton, Ed.D.

Chelation therapy

Definition

Chelation therapy is an intravenous treatment designed to bind heavy metals in the body in order to treat heavy metal toxicity. Proponents claim it also treats coronary artery disease and other illnesses that may be linked to damage from free radicals (reactive molecules).

Origins

The term chelation is from the Greek root word "chele," meaning "claw." Chelating agents were originally designed for industrial applications in the early 1900s. Probably the best known of chelating agents is ethylenediamine tetraacetic acid (EDTA). During World War II the potential of chelating agents for medical therapy was realized. The initial intent was to develop antidotes to poison **gas** and radioactive contaminants. The need for widespread therapy of this nature did not materialize, but more practical uses were found for chelation. During the 1950s, EDTA chelation therapy became standard treatment for people suffering from **lead poisoning**. Patients who had received this treatment claimed to have other health improvements that could not be attributed to the lead removal only. Especially notable were comments from those who had previously suffered from intermittent claudication (**pain** in the legs accompanied by limping) and **angina**. They reported suffering less pain and **fatigue**, with improved endurance, after chelation therapy. These reports stimulated further interest in the potential benefits of chelation therapy for people suffering from **atherosclerosis** and coronary artery disease.

Benefits

The benefits of EDTA chelation for the treatment of lead poisoning and excessively high **calcium** levels are undisputed. The claims of benefits for those suffering from atherosclerosis, coronary artery disease, and other degenerative diseases are more difficult to prove. Reported uses for chelation therapy include treatment of angina, **gangrene**, arthritis, **multiple sclerosis**, **Parkinson's disease**, **psoriasis**, and **Alzheimer's disease**. Some practitioners also claim improvement for people experiencing diminished sight, hearing, smell, coordination, and sexual potency.

Description

If the preparatory examination suggests that there is a condition that could be improved by chelation therapy, and there is no health reason why it should not be used, then the treatment can begin. The patient is generally taken to a comfortable treatment area, sometimes in a group location, and an intravenous line is started. A solution of EDTA together with vitamins and minerals tailored for the individual patient is given. Most treatments take three to four hours, as the infusion must be given slowly in order to be safe. The number of recommended treatments is usually between 20 and 40. They are given one to three times a week. Maintenance treatments can then be given at the rate of once or twice a month. Maximum benefits are reported to be attained after approximately three months after a treatment series. The cost of therapy is considerable, but it is a fraction of the cost of an expensive medical procedure such as cardiac bypass surgery. Intravenous **vitamin C** and mercury chelation therapies are also offered.

Preparations

A candidate for chelation therapy should initially provide a thorough medical history and under go a physical examination to define the type and extent of clinical problems. Laboratory tests are done to determine whether there are any conditions present that may prevent the use of chelation. Patients who have preexisting hypocalcemia, poor liver or kidney function, congestive heart failure, **hypoglycemia, tuberculosis**, clotting problems, or potentially allergic conditions are at higher risk for complications from chelation therapy. A Doppler ultrasound may be performed to determine the adequacy of blood flow in different regions of the body.

Precautions

It is important for people who receive chelation therapy to seek medical personnel who are experienced in the use of this treatment. Treatment should not be undertaken before a good physical, lifestyle evaluation, history, and necessary laboratory tests are performed. The staff must be forthcoming about test results and should answer all questions the patient may have. Evaluation and treatment should be individualized and involve assessment of kidney function

before each treatment with chelation, since the metals bound by the EDTA are excreted through the kidneys.

Although EDTA binds harmful, toxic metals such as mercury, lead, and cadmium, it also binds some essential nutrients of the body, such as **copper, iron**, calcium, **zinc**, and **magnesium**. Large amounts of zinc are lost during chelation. Zinc deficiency can cause impaired immune function and other harmful effects. Supplements of zinc are generally given to patients undergoing chelation, but it was not known as of 2008 whether this is adequate to prevent deficiency. Also, chelation therapy does not replace proper **nutrition, exercise**, and appropriate medications or surgery for specific diseases or conditions.

Side effects

Side effects of chelation therapy are reportedly unusual but are occasionally serious. Mild reactions may include irritation at the infusion site, skin reactions, **nausea, headache, dizziness**, hypoglycemia, **fever**, leg cramps, or loose bowel movements. Some of the more serious complications reported have included hypocalcemia, kidney damage, decreased clotting ability, **anemia**, bone marrow damage, insulin shock, thrombophlebitis with embolism, and even in rare cases death. However, some doctors believe that the latter groups of complications occurred before the safer method for giving chelation therapy was developed.

Research and general acceptance

EDTA chelation is a highly controversial therapy. The treatment is approved by the United States Food and Drug Administration (FDA) for lead poisoning and seriously high calcium levels. However, for the treatment of atherosclerotic **heart disease**, EDTA chelation therapy is not endorsed by the American Heart Association (AHA), the FDA, the National Institutes of Health (NIH), or the American College of Cardiology. The AHA reports that there are no adequate, controlled, published scientific studies using currently approved scientific methods to support this therapy for the treatment of coronary artery disease. However, a pooled analysis from the results of more than 70 studies showed positive results in all but one. In 2002, the American College of Advancement in Medicine pledged its full support to a $30 million federal study aimed at determining the safety and efficacy of chelation therapy in patients with heart disease. Scheduled to begin in 2008, the five-year clinical trial was anticipated to involve more than 2,000 people at about 100 sites around the country.

Training and certification

The American Board of Chelation Therapy (ABCT) provides minimum standards for members administering chelation. Diplomates have passed written and oral tests and received supervision of treatment in order to become certified.

One professional group that makes recommendations for treatment methods is the American College for Advancement in Medicine (ACAM). If contacted, the organization will mail out a directory of doctors who are members and follow their methods. ACAM also offers chelation therapy workshops.

Resources

BOOKS

Hawken, C. M. *Chelation Therapy for Cardiovascular Health*. Chapmanville, WV: Woodland Press, 2007.

PERIODICALS

Barton, James C. "Optimal Management Strategies for Chronic Iron Overload." *Drugs* (May 2007): 685–700.

"Deaths Associated with Hypocalcemia from Chelation Therapy: Texas, Pennsylvania, and Oregon, 2003–2005." *Morbidity and Mortality Weekly Report* (March 3, 2006): 204–207.

Payne, Krista A., et al. "Clinical and Economic Burden of Infused Iron Chelation Therapy in the United States." *Transfusion* (October 2007): 1820–1829.

OTHER

"Chelation therapy." American Heart Association. [cited March 19, 2008]. http://www.americanheart.org/presenter.jhtml?identifier=4493.

Green, Saul. "Quackwatch: Chelation therapy." July 24, 2007 [cited March 19, 2008]. http://www.quackwatch.com/01QuackeryRelatedTopics/chelation.html.

ORGANIZATIONS

American College for Advancement in Medicine (ACAM), 24411 Ridge Route, Suite 115, Laguna Hills, CA, 92653, (949) 309-3520, http://www.acamnet.org/site/.

American Heart Association, National Center, 7272 Greenville Ave., Dallas, TX, 75231, (800) 242-8721, http://www.americanheart.org/.

Judith Turner
Teresa G. Odle
David Edward Newton, Ed.D.

Chelidonium

Description

Chelidonium majus is an herb of the Papaveraceae (poppy) family. Its long thin stems support yellow blooms that contain four petals measuring about 1 inch. The plant is native to Europe, Western Asia, and North Africa. It is found growing in damp areas and wild gardens along roads and other open spaces, in close proximity to human life. The entire plant is considered poisonous. However, its medicinal properties may be beneficial in the proper dosages. Isoquinoline alkaloids within the plant possess both toxic and therapeutic properties. The plant's orange juice, known as greater celandine, has been used for medicinal purposes for thousands of years.

General Use

In ancient times, the greater celandine portion of the plant was used as a treatment for eye conditions, particularly **cataracts**. Among the isoquinoline alkaloids inherent in greater celandine are allocriptine, berberine, chelidonine, and spartaine. These constituents enable the herb to serve as a mild sedative, antispasmodic, and as a muscle relaxant in the bronchial tubes, intestines, and other internal organs. Chelidonine lowers blood pressure, whereas spartaine causes blood pressure to rise.

Benefits of Chelidonium

In 1985, Germany's Commission E approved Chelidonium for the treatment of **indigestion**.

Greater celandine is used in Western and Chinese medicine for its properties as an antispasmodic, diuretic, and analgesic (**pain** reducer). It is used in the treatment of respiratory conditions such as **asthma**, **bronchitis**, and **whooping cough** (pertussis). It has also been used to treat **jaundice**, **gallstones**, and the pain associated with gallbladder disease, although there is some controversy regarding these uses.

Cheladonium is also used in the treatment of stomach ulcers and may possess anti-cancer and anti-microbial abilities. In a study released in 2002, greater celandine showed anti-tumor properties when given in ultra-low doses to mice that had liver **cancer**.

The plant's yellow latex component is used to treat skin conditions such as **eczema**, **corns**, and **warts**. Due to its use with the latter, it was once called wartweed.

Preparations

Chelidonium must be taken under professional supervision because of the potential for liver toxicity. Under proper medical supervision, extracts standardized to 4 g of chelidonine per capsule may be taken by mouth three times a day. An alternative is the preparation of a mixture of 1–3 ml tincture and water. The liquid concoction may be sipped slowly over a 10 to 30 minute period prior to meals. The external topical preparation is made of concentrated tinctures of the yellow latex. In regards to wart treatment, herbalists suggest applying the latex to the area and allowing it to dry in place.

A semi-synthetic injectable form of chelidonium is available in Europe and Mexico under the trade name, Ukrain. As of 2008, Ukrain was not approved by the U.S. Food and Drug Administration.

Precautions

Chelidonium must be used with caution and taken only under professional direction because of its potential for toxicity to the liver. It is not to be used by women who are pregnant or breastfeeding or by children under age 12. In certain countries, restrictions ban its use. Its use should be discontinued and a healthcare professional consulted immediately if signs of an allergic reaction are present, including **itching**, redness, swelling, tightness of the chest or throat, or difficulty breathing.

At the 1998 meeting of the American Association for the Study of Liver Diseases, a German report highlighted cases of liver toxicity related to greater celandine. The following year, the final report was published, documenting 10 cases. Researchers found that the 10 patients, all taking greater celandine, acquired mild to severe **hepatitis**. Following discontinuation of the greater celandine, the individuals recovered quickly. Their liver enzymes subsequently returned to normal levels. Greater celandine was added to the list of herbs that cause acute hepatitis.

KEY TERMS

Isoquinoline alkaloid—Natural compound found in plants that may be toxic to humans and animals, but also possesses therapeutic qualities.

Side effects

Chelidonium causes the urine to take on a bright yellow color. High doses of the herb may lead to drowsiness. It may irritate the respiratory tract, causing bouts of aggressive and powerful coughing or difficulty breathing. Other potential side effects are an allergic reaction, skin irritation, and stomach upset.

Interactions

At the time of publication, *chelidonium majus* has no known drug interactions.

Resources

OTHER

PeaceHealth. Locations throughout Oregon, Washington, and Alaska. http://www.peacehealth.org.
Plants for a Future. http://www.pfaf.org/.

ORGANIZATIONS

Memorial Sloan-Kettering Cancer Center, 1275 York Ave., New York, NY, 10065, (212) 639-2000, http://www.mskcc.org.
Third Age, Inc, 25 Stillman St., Suite 102. , San Francisco, CA, 94107-1309, http://www.thirdage.com.

Rhonda Cloos, RN

Chemical poisoning

Definition

Chemical poisoning is a major public health concern. Approximately 95% of all accidental or intentional poisonings are due to chemicals. Nearly 90% of these cases occur at home. Infants, toddlers, and small children are at the greatest risk for accidental (acute) poisoning. In 2006, poison control centers received about 2.5 million calls about poison exposures, more than a million of which involved children younger than age 6. Chronic exposure is chemical poisoning that occurs slowly and insidiously over a prolonged period of time. Many chronic, degenerative diseases have been linked to environmental pollution or poisoning. The list may include **cancer**, **memory loss**, **allergies**, **multiple chemical sensitivity**, **chronic fatigue syndrome**, **infertility** in adults, learning and behavioral disorders, developmental abnormalities, and birth defects.

Description

Of the millions of natural and synthetic chemicals in existence, approximately 3,000 are known to cause significant health problems. In many cases, the type and severity of danger posed by a chemical is a matter of dispute among experts. Accidental acute chemical poisoning involving common household or garden products is easy to diagnose and treat, as long as it is recognized early enough. By contrast, chronic poisoning due to daily exposure to chemicals is more difficult to diagnose and the extent of damage is more difficult to assess. Toxic chemicals can be found everywhere— in homes, around homes on private property, at work, on the playground—even in foods and drinking water. Some result from illegal dumping. However, many chemical poisonings occur insidiously by the supposedly harmless chemicals that people bring into their homes or office to make their lives more comfortable.

Household poisons

Because of the huge amounts of toxic chemicals that can be found inside homes, scientists have come to believe the home—not the office or the freeway—is the most contaminated place of all. Any chemicals found inside the house can be accidentally ingested by small children. Daily exposure to chemicals indoors may also cause significant health risks. Major chemical poisons inside homes include volatile organic compounds, lead, radon, carbon monoxide, and the various substances in household cleaners and carpet.

VOLATILE CHEMICALS. Indoor air pollution is caused by volatile chemicals, those which evaporate at room temperature. When people use products that contain these volatile substances, the chemicals are trapped inside their homes, and they can reach levels thousands of times higher than exist outdoors in the air. Chronic exposure to polluted air may cause lung **infections**, headaches, **nausea**, mental confusion, **fatigue**, **depression**, and memory loss. In addition, it may cause damage to an unborn fetus and increase the risk of developing cancer. The following are some of the most common volatile substances found inside the home:

- trichloroethane (spray cans, insulation, spot removers)
- tetrachloroethylene (dry-cleaning solutions)
- formaldehyde (glue, foam, preservatives, plywood, fabrics, insulation)
- para-dichlorobenzene (pDCB) (mothballs, air fresheners)
- toluene (solvents, cleaning fluids, wood finishing products)
- benzene (gasoline)
- xylene (paints, finishing products)
- acetone (nail polish remover)
- styrene (foam, carpets, adhesives)
- carbon tetrachloride (dry cleaning solutions, paint removers)
- perchloroethylene (cleaning solvents)

LEAD AND OTHER HEAVY METALS. Lead is a very toxic chemical, especially to small children. **Lead poisoning** can cause learning disabilities and behavioral problems in children. Lead poisoning in pregnant mothers can cause fetal abnormalities, brain damage, and impaired motor skills in babies. Lead is found in leaded paint (in old houses) and is sometimes present in pesticides, pottery and china, artist's paint, and products used for hobbies and crafts. Also harmful are other heavy metals, such as mercury and cadmium.

RADON. Radon is an odorless **gas** produced from the radioactive decay of uranium. It is believed to be the most common cause of **lung cancer** after **smoking**. In the outdoor environment, radon gas is usually too well-dispersed to reach dangerous levels. It is far more dangerous indoors, where ventilation tends to be inadequate, in places such as basements, where radon can seep from the soil and accumulate to dangerous concentrations. Radon testing is the only way to discover if a home is contaminated.

CARBON MONOXIDE. In closed areas, carbon monoxide (CO) is the most lethal gas produced by a burning heat source. Sources of CO are gas heat, fireplaces, or idling cars. A CO detector is needed in all homes because this gas is odorless, colorless, and deadly.

CHEMICALS TRAPPED INSIDE CARPETS. Carpets contain many chemicals capable of causing nerve damage. These neurotoxic chemicals include acetone, benzene, toluene, phenol, xylene, decane, and hexane.

HOUSEHOLD CLEANERS. The following are neurotoxic chemicals commonly found in household cleaners:

- chlorine (dishwasher detergents)
- ammonia (antibacterial cleaning agents)
- petroleum (dish soaps, laundry detergents, floor waxes)

MEDICINES. Medicines are one of the most common causes of accidental and intentional (suicide) poisonings. Drugs most commonly involved are aspirin, acetaminophen, sedatives, any psychoactive drug if the patient is prone to impulsive, suicidal action (e.g., antidepressants), anti-seizure drugs, **iron** pills, vitamins/mineral supplements containing iron, and cardiac drugs, such as digoxin and quinidine.

Yard chemicals

Yard materials that can be toxic to humans and pets include:

- Insecticides. Toxic chemicals that can be found in insecticide preparations include lindane, arsenic, lead, malathion, diazinon, and nicotine.
- Rodenticides (chemicals that kill mice or rats). Rodenticides often contain very toxic chemicals, such as sodium fluoroacetate, phosphorus, thallium, barium, strychnine, methyl bromide, and cyanides.
- Herbicides (chemicals that kill weeds). Herbicides contain carbaryl and diazinon, which increase the risk of childhood brain cancer.

The regulatory status of some of these chemicals varies from country to country and state to state. Critics often call for a ban on chemicals that are especially toxic or otherwise dangerous. For example, in the late 2000s, lindane was approved for use in the United States and many other countries. However, a worldwide campaign was working to have the chemical banned because of its toxicity.

Occupational hazards

Workers are often exposed to toxic effects of various chemicals in their working environment:

- Polluted air. Workers in poorly ventilated plants that manufacture paints, insecticides, fungicides, pesticides.
- Radiation. Workers in poorly constructed nuclear chemical plants.
- Contaminated environment. Miners who labor underground.
- Obnoxious fumes. Fire fighters who are exposed to toxic fumes.
- Skin contact with toxic chemicals. Crop pickers who have exposure to sprayed insecticides.

Toxic chemicals in foods

Highly processed or prepackaged foods use various chemical additives to make these foods look more attractive, taste better, or store for longer periods of time. Harmful substances that can be found in foods include:

- Monosodium glutamate (MSG), a common flavoring agent. Excessive consumption of MSG may cause hyperactivity, memory loss, or other types of brain damage. It is often associated with the so-called Chinese restaurant syndrome characterized by headaches, nausea, vomiting, palpitations, and flushing of skin, due to the MSG content in the food.
- Artificial sweeteners, such as aspartame or saccharin. These sweeteners can cause a variety of health problems, including headaches (migraines included), dizziness, seizures, depression, nausea, and vomiting, and abdominal cramps. Their use may be associated with hyperactivity in children. Whether they increase risk of cancer was unknown as of 2008. Pregnant women should avoid using these sweeteners.
- Artificial colors. Color additives can be found in a variety of foods, including cereals, juices, candy, frozen foods, ice cream, cookies, pizza, salad dressings, and soft drinks. Children and adults alike may be exposed to cancer-causing artificial colors such as Red numbers 8, 9, 19, and 37, or Orange number 17.
- Preservatives. Many of the preservatives found in foods are very hazardous. Nitrates, common preservatives in cured and luncheon meats and canned products, are known to cause cancer. In addition, a pregnant woman who consumes large amounts of nitrates (for example, through eating hot dogs or salami) unknowingly increases risk of brain damage in her unborn child. Synthetic antioxidants are used in prepackaged foods to prevent food spoilage. Common synthetic antioxidants, such as butylated hydroxyanisole (BHA) and butylated hydroxytoluene (BHT), can be found in cereals, baking mixes, or instant potatoes. These products are known to cause brain, liver, and kidney damage, as well as respiratory problems.
- Food contaminants. Health-promoting foods such as fruits and vegetables may contain dangerous herbicide and pesticide residues on their surfaces. Fish in contaminated lakes or rivers may contain mercury, dioxin, PCBs, or other harmful chemicals. Babies of mothers who consume contaminated fish during pregnancy have lower birth weight, smaller heads, developmental delays, and lower scores on tests of baby intelligence.

Air pollution and environmental contamination

Air pollution can cause or worsen lung or heart diseases and increase risk of cancer. Chemicals that most often cause pollution in the air and water supply include asbestos, carbon monoxide, hydrogen sulfide, lead, nitrogen oxides, halogenated hydrocarbons, and pesticides.

Causes and symptoms

Acute poisoning

The following events are possible causes for acute poisoning:

- Accidental ingestion of household products. This problem primarily affects children under the age of five.
- Medication errors. Such errors occur most often among elderly people. Sometimes hospital staff makes the error; at other times, the patient gets confused about or cannot read directions regarding the identity or dosage of drugs.
- Suicide.
- Excessive alcohol or drug abuse.

The following signs and symptoms indicate the possibility of acute chemical poisoning:

- difficulty breathing
- changes in skin color
- headaches or blurred vision
- irritated eyes, skin, or throat
- sweating
- dizziness
- breath odor: bitter almond (cyanide poisoning), garlic odor (arsenic poisoning)
- nausea, vomiting, diarrhea
- unusual behavior
- difficulty walking or standing straight

Chronic poisoning

COMMON ROUTES OF EXPOSURE TO TOXIC CHEMICALS. Individuals may accumulate toxic amounts of a chemical in their body through daily exposure to the chemical. Common routes of exposure include:

- inhalation of the poisonous gas
- consumption of contaminated food, water, or medications
- contact with toxic or caustic chemicals in the eyes, skin, or through contaminated clothing
- pregnant mother's exposure to toxic chemicals during pregnancy, especially during the first trimester

EFFECTS OF TOXIC CHEMICALS ON DEVELOPING FETUSES AND CHILDREN. Toxic chemicals can have devastating effects on developing fetuses and young children. The following diseases and conditions are linked to chronic exposure to home and environmental pollution:

- miscarriages and spontaneous abortions
- low birth weight
- premature births
- stillbirths
- birth defects
- sudden infant death syndrome (SIDS)
- developmental delays
- poor motor coordination
- attention-deficit hyperactivity disorder (ADHD)
- aggressive behavior
- learning disabilities
- speech and language problems
- autism
- sensory deficits
- allergies and chemical sensitivity in childhood and in later years
- asthma, hay fever, and sinusitis
- cancer in childhood, adulthood, and in subsequent generations
- poorly functioning organs and systems
- weakened immune system and increased risk of infections

The following chronic diseases and conditions may occur in adults as a result of cumulative chemical poisoning:

- fatigue
- headaches
- skin rashes
- aches and pains
- generalized weakness
- asthma
- increased risk of infection
- depression and irritability
- liver diseases, such as jaundice (yellowing of the skin and eyes), inflammation of the liver (hepatitis), and cirrhosis (a chronic degenerative disease of the liver)
- lung diseases
- heart diseases
- cancer
- decreased life expectancy
- sick building syndrome
- Gulf War syndrome (due to nerve agent and pesticide exposure)

Diagnosis

Acute poisoning

In many cases, the identity of the poison is known to the patient or the parents of the affected child. The role of the physician is to determine what treatment (if any) is necessary based on the type and amount of toxic substance exposure, the identity of the chemical, and patient's signs and symptoms.

Chronic poisoning

Chronic environmental poisoning is more difficult to diagnose. To find out if environmental pollution is causing an illness, a physician conducts a thorough physical exam of the patient. The doctor also obtains a thorough medical history with detailed information concerning the food and water sources, as well as the nature of the patient's work or place of residence. Laboratory tests may include blood and urine tests and hair sample analysis. In addition, liver and kidney function tests are conducted to see if these organs are affected. The doctor also inquires about other diseases the patient may have developed in the recent past.

Treatment

Alternative treatments are not appropriate for acute chemical poisoning. When an emergency poisoning occurs, especially in children, parents are encouraged to call a toll-free hotline that is staffed 24 hours a day at 1-800-222-1222. However, alternative treatments may be useful in treating chronic exposure to toxic chemicals. The specific treatment plan depends on the type of poison by which a person is affected. Generally speaking, most treatments involve identifying the offending chemical and avoiding future exposures to it. A healthy diet, nutritional supplements and/or **detoxification** therapy are also helpful. Detoxification therapy is especially effective for the liver, which is the organ that metabolizes most toxins.

Detoxification diet

Naturopaths sometimes recommend patients suspected of chronic chemical poisoning to follow a detoxification (detox) diet for at least several months. Pregnant women, small children, or very frail people should avoid taking this diet. A detox diet has the following characteristics:

- Low fat intake to increase fat mobilization (moving fat from storage to be used for energy). Limited consumption of olive oil and vegetable oils is allowed.
- Limited intake of sugar and highly processed foods and avoidance of alcohol, caffeine, and tobacco.
- High fiber consumption to absorb the toxic chemicals and eliminate them from the body.
- Limited consumption of red meat. The bulk of protein intake should come from vegetable sources, such as legumes and tofu, as well as fish from unpolluted waters.
- Strong emphasis on organic fruits and vegetables (and their juices) with detoxification effects. These include papayas, apples, pears, strawberries, dark green leafy vegetables, carrots, beets, and garlic. Antioxidant foods, such as broccoli, cauliflower, kale, yams, tomatoes, peaches, watermelon, hot peppers, green tea, red grapes, citrus fruits, soybeans, and whole grains are also recommended.
- Increased water intake to at least eight glasses of water per day to help eliminate waste from the body.
- Dietary supplementation with high potency multivitamin/mineral products.

Exercise

Exercise to the point of perspiration helps eliminate toxins from the body. Daily walking for 30 minutes is helpful and appropriate for most people.

Herbal therapy

Milk thistle (*Silybum mariannum*) is a powerful antioxidant that protects the liver and assists in the detoxification process by increasing **glutathione** supply in the liver. Glutathione is the enzyme primarily involved in the detoxification of many toxic chemicals in the environment, such as solvents, pesticides, and heavy metals.

Traditional Chinese medicine

Depending on a patient's specific condition, an expert Chinese herbalist may prescribe herbal remedies that can help remove toxins from the body and improve liver function.

Homeopathy

For homeopathic therapy, patients should consult a homeopathic physician who can prescribe specific remedies based on knowledge of the underlying cause.

Fasting

Fasting is an ancient way of detoxification and is very efficient. During three-day fasting, patients take supplements and drink four glasses of juice a day to assist the cleansing process and to prevent exhaustion. Supplements recommended are those that include **antioxidants**, such as vitamins C and E, **selenium**, zinc, and **magnesium**. For patients suspected of significant poisoning, a naturopath may also prescribe milk thistle to aid the detoxification process and provide support for the body. The patient may also consider consuming a food fast, where only food that is simple to digest is consumed. For example, ultraclear hydrolyzed rice is simple to digest and is also hypoallergenic.

Allopathic treatment

Acute poisoning

For acute poisoning, individuals should call 911, a local poison control center, or 1-800-222-1222 immediately. The toll-free number is a national hotline begun in 2002 by the American Association of Poison Control Centers to provide 24-hour poison treatment and prevention services. If a child is suspected of eating or drinking hazardous chemicals, parents should look for the container and call for instructions. Patients or parents of the poisoned child should wait for instructions before administering syrup of **ipecac**, **activated charcoal**, or anything else by mouth. Treatment of a particular poison depends on the identity of the poison and how the poison is absorbed by the body.

INHALED POISONS. Treatment of inhaled poison includes bringing the patient out and away from the area contaminated with poisonous gas. The patient should be given oxygen and other respiratory support as necessary.

SKIN AND EYE CONTAMINATION. If a person's skin comes into contact with toxic chemicals, the contaminated clothing should be removed, the chemical carefully brushed off the skin, and the body flushed with running water to dilute the poison. The **wounds**, if any, should be covered with sterile gauze or cloth and the patient transferred to the hospital for treatment of chemical burn. If toxic or caustic chemicals get in the eyes, the affected person should remove glasses or any contact lenses immediately, rinse the eyes well with clean water or normal saline solution, and go to the emergency room for further treatment or observation.

INGESTED POISONS. Depending on the specific type of ingested poisons, syrup of ipecac, activated charcoal, and/or gastric lavage can be used.

In many cases of accidental poisoning, syrup of ipecac can be used effectively. When swallowed, it irritates the stomach and induces **vomiting**. As of 2008, syrup of ipecac was considered the safest drug for treating poisoning and was often the most effective. Syrup of ipecac can be used for most ingested poisons. However, syrup of ipecac should not be used if the suspected poison is strychnine, a corrosive substance (strong acids or lye), petroleum products (gasoline, kerosene, paint thinner, or cleaning fluids), or certain prescription drugs, such as antidepressants or sustained-release theophylline. In addition, it should not be used in patients who are unconscious or seizing.

Activated charcoal is also an effective treatment for many chemical poisons. It absorbs poisons quickly and in large amounts. In addition, it is nontoxic, may be stored for a long time, and can be conveniently administered at home. Charcoal works by absorbing irritating or toxic substances in the stomach and intestines. This action prevents the toxic drug or chemical from spreading throughout the body. The toxic drug or chemical and the activated charcoal are excreted in the stools without harming the body.

If both syrup of ipecac and charcoal are recommended for treatment of the poison, ipecac should be given first. Charcoal should not be given for at least 30 minutes after ipecac or when vomiting from ipecac stops. Activated charcoal is often mixed with a liquid before being swallowed or put into the tube leading to the stomach. Activated charcoal is available in liquid form in 30 g bottles. It is also available in 15 g container sizes, as slurry of charcoal premixed in water, or in a container to which water or soda is added.

Charcoal should not be used to treat poisoning caused by corrosive products, such as lye or other strong acids or petroleum products such as gasoline, kerosene, or cleaning fluids. Charcoal may make the condition worse and delay the diagnosis and treatment. In addition, charcoal is not effective if the poison is lithium, cyanide, iron, ethanol, or methanol.

Gastric lavage may also be used to treat chemical poisoning. This procedure is performed by medical professionals in emergency rooms only. Lavage fluids (saline water or water) are given through a large tube down the patient's throat and the stomach contents are pumped out. This procedure is repeated until most of the toxic substance is removed. Then a specific antidote for the chemical or activated charcoal is given to absorb the rest.

Sometimes, antidotes are available to neutralize poison and render it harmless. The following are common antidotes:

- naloxone: for morphine, methadone, or heroin overdose
- atropine: for organophosphate (insecticide) poisoning

- acetylcysteine: for acetaminophen (Tylenol) toxicity
- digoxin immune fab (Digibind): for digoxin toxicity

Chronic chemical poisoning

Treatment of chronic chemical poisoning involves identifying and eliminating the source of poison from the patient's environment, followed by symptomatic treatment of the condition. **Chelation therapy** can be used to remove heavy metals, such as lead, iron, mercury, **copper**, nickel, zinc, cadmium, beryllium, and arsenic. This treatment uses chelating agents, such as ethylenediamine tetraacetic acid (EDTA) and dimethylsuccinate (DMSA) to bind and precipitate metals and remove them from the body.

Expected results

Depending on the severity of the poisoning, the affected person may have total or partial recovery. If the rescue effort comes too late, a patient may die of acute chemical or drug poisoning. For those affected by chronic exposure to environmental poisoning, recovery depends on the severity of the poisoning, the ability to stay away from the offending agent, and appropriate diagnosis and treatment. Total recovery can occur in many patients.

Prevention

Some strategies to avoid poisoning are:

- Avoid eating contaminated fish, especially that which comes from known contaminated areas or a lot of big fish, such as shark, swordfish, or tuna, which tend to contain higher amounts of mercury than smaller fish. Pregnant women should not consume more than 7 oz of tuna per week. Mercury can cause brain damage in the developing fetus.
- Do not paint or remodel a home while pregnant or when children are still small. Paint may contain chemicals that can harm a fetus and cause learning disabilities in small children.
- Limit use of chemicals inside the house as much as possible and instead use natural benign alternatives, such as baking soda (as cleaner, deodorizer), distilled white vinegar (as cleaner), essential oils (as fragrances), lemon juice (as cleaner), and liquid soaps (as detergents).
- Increase ventilation of the house.
- Consider installing tile or wood floors in new homes instead of new carpet.
- Have the house tested for radon.
- Eat organic foods. Otherwise, to better remove toxins, wash fruits and vegetables carefully before eating with a mild acid solution, such as diluted vinegar.

- Avoid toxic chemical exposure as much as possible if pregnant.
- Keep all medications, petroleum products, and cleaning products locked and away from small children. Install child-proof locks or gates to prevent children from finding poisons.
- Avoid mixing household cleaning products. Non-toxic chemicals when mixed together can release toxic gases or cause an explosion.
- Keep all chemicals in original containers, properly identified and stored away from foods.
- Only use chemicals in well-ventilated areas to avoid breathing in fumes. Use adequate skin, eye, and respiratory protection.
- Never put household chemicals in food or beverage containers.
- Avoid smoking or lighting a candle near household chemicals such as cleaning solutions, hair spray, paints or paint thinner, or pesticides.
- Dispose all hazardous chemicals properly according to the manufacturer's instructions.

Resources

BOOKS

Chapman, Anne. *Democratizing Technology: Risk, Responsibility, and the Regulation of Chemicals.* London: Earthscan Publications, 2007.

Howd, Robert A., and Anna M. Fan. *Risk Assessment for Chemicals in Drinking Water.* New York: Wiley Interscience, 2007.

Penney, David G., ed. *Carbon Monoxide Poisoning.* London: Informa Healthcare, 2007.

Stranks, Jeremy. *The A-Z of Food Safety.* Abingdon, England: Thorogood, 2007.

Van Leeuwen, C. J., and T. G. Vermeire, eds. *Risk Assessment of Chemicals: An Introduction*. New York: Springer, 2007.

PERIODICALS

Cooper, Kelli, et al. "Public Health Risks from Heavy Metals and Metalloids Present in Traditional Chinese Medicines." *Journal of Toxicology and Environmental Health: Part A* (January 2007): 1694–1699.

Isman, Murray B. "Botanical Insecticides: for Richer, for Poorer." *Pest Management Science* (January 2008): 8–11.

Peter, John Victor, John L. Moran, and Petra L. Graham. "Advances in the Management of Organophosphate Poisoning." *Expert Opinion on Pharmacotherapy* (July 2007): 1451–1464.

Schier, Joshua G., et al. "Strategies for Recognizing Acute Chemical-associated Foodborne Illness." *Military Medicine* (December 2006): 1174–1180.

OTHER

"Case Definitions for Chemical Poisoning." Centers for Disease Control and Prevention. [cited March 18, 2008]. http://www.bt.cdc.gov/chemical/casedef.asp.

"Chemical Poisoning and Syrup of Ipecac." University of Maryland Medical Center. January 25, 2008 [cited March 18, 2008]. http://www.umm.edu/non_trauma/chempois.htm.

ORGANIZATIONS

Agency for Toxic Substances and Disease, 1825 Century Blvd., Atlanta, GA, 30345, (800) 232-4636, http://www.atsdr.cdc.gov/.

American Academy of Environmental Medicine, 6505 E. Central Ave., #296, Wichita, KS, 67206, (316) 684-5500, http://www.aaemonline.org.

American Association of Poison Control Centers, 3201 New Mexico Ave., Suite 330, Washington, DC, 20016, (800) 222-1222, http://www.aapcc.org/.

Environmental Protection Agency, Ariel Rios Building. 1200 Pennsylvania Ave. NW, Washington, DC, 20460, (202) 260-7751, http://www.epa.gov/.

Mai Tran
Teresa G. Odle
David Edward Newton, Ed.D.

Cherry bark

Description

Cherries are members of the botanical genus *Prunus*, which is a member of the *Rosaceae* (or rose) family. Cherries can be a shrub or a tree, and are believed to have originated in the Caucasus mountain region between Europe and Asia.

Cherries are divided into two broad groups: sweet *(Prunus avium)* and sour *(Prunus cerasus)*. Varieties of the cherry are widely distributed throughout temperate regions of the world and have been cultivated for thousands of years. Roman historian Pliny reported that sour cherries were introduced to ancient Rome as part of a victory celebration after the defeat of the Parthians at a place called Cerasus.

From the simple division of sweet and sour cherries, classification of the various cherry types has grown increasingly complex through the years. Today, there are literally hundreds of varieties due to their long record of cultivation and crossbreeding.

Cherry trees have been used widely for their fruit, eaten fresh and used in cooking. Both the fermented fruit and the crushed pits are used in making the European liqueur, kirsch. The tree is also a source of wood used in making high-quality furniture. The stalks from some of these cherry varieties have been used medicinally as an astringent, however, it is widely accepted that the cherry tree bark used in herbal medicine comes from the wild cherry (listed now as *Prunus serotina*, but in nineteenth century herbal books is listed as *Prunus virginianus*).

The wild cherry is a native of North America. It is found in central and northern parts of the United States, as well as in cooler, nondesert parts of the Southwest. Wild cherry trees characteristically grow to a height of 50-80 ft (15.2-24.4 m), with a trunk width of 2-4 ft (0.6-1.2 m). The leaf of the wild cherry is oval, with a minutely serrated edge, and is more pointed toward the tip. Its leaves are approximately 3 in (7.6 cm) in length, dark green and shiny on top, and paler and fuzzy on the underside. Small, white, petaled flowers appear along the stems before the leaves in early spring. Pea-sized, purplish black fruits that are bitter develop and ripen by late summer.

The outer bark of the wild cherry tree is dark gray to black, very rough to the touch, and breaks away easily from the trunk. Even though the bark from the roots, trunk, and branches has medicinal properties, it is the root bark that is the most beneficial. Beneath a cherry root's dark outer covering, the interior is a dusky reddish color. It has an almond-like aroma that evaporates when dried, but re-emerges when the bark is crushed or dissolved. Its tastes astringent and bitter. Its chemical constituents include cyanogenic glycosides, starch, resin, tannin, gallic acid, fatty matter, lignin, red coloring material, as well as **calcium**, **potassium**, and **iron** salts.

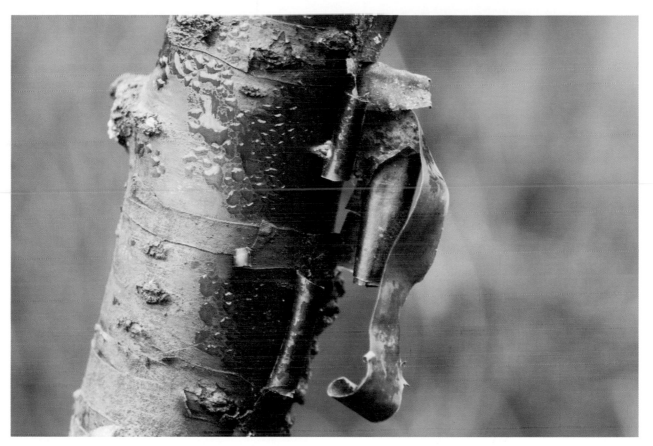

Cherry bark. *(O.D. vande Veer / Alamy)*

General use

Wild cherry bark has a strong sedating effect on the **cough** reflex and is particularly useful to treat dry, nonproductive coughs in respiratory conditions. Because of its antispasmodic qualities, it has been used with other herbs to treat **asthma**. It is given for spasmodic cough to enhance **relaxation** and resting or at night to reduce cough and enhance sleep. Its astringent properties make it useful as a bitter, taken to stimulate sluggish digestion and the appetite. A cold infusion of wild cherry bark has been noted to soothe eye inflammation.

Preparations

Bark is collected in the autumn by carefully stripping away small sections. The outer wild cherry bark is then removed and the lighter colored, reddish interior cortex is dried, but not in direct sunlight. Once thoroughly dried, it must be stored in airtight containers away from light. Because it deteriorates so rapidly, it is more beneficial if used when still fresh and must be newly collected each year. The fragments of inner bark crush easily to make a powder. This powdered cherry bark can then be dissolved in either alcohol or water. A cough remedy is made by dissolving 4 oz (113 g) of the bark in 4 oz (120 ml) of water for several hours. The solution is then strained, and honey is added to sweeten to taste. Boiling cherry bark is not recommended since this decreases the medicinal properties. Cherry bark can also be used to make a tincture and lozenges.

Precautions

Coughing is a normal and helpful reaction to airway or lung irritation. It is designed to expel harmful substances (such as excess phlegm or irritants) from the lungs. Suppressing a cough, then, can actually prevent or postpone recovery. It is persistent coughing that needs treatment. It is also important for potential users to remember that a cough is merely a symptom of some other illness, as are digestive problems. Wild cherry bark preparations should not be taken for an extended period of time. They should only be used for temporary relief of symptoms. A doctor should be consulted for persistent cough or digestive problems.

Side effects

Wild cherry bark preparations can cause sedation, especially if recommended dosage is exceeded.

Interactions

None known.

Resources

BOOKS

Grieve, M., and C.F. Leyel. *A Modern Herbal: The Medical, Culinary, Costmetic and Economic Properties, Cultivation and Folklore of Herbs, Grasses, Fungi, Shrubs and Trees With All of Their Modern Scientific Uses.* Barnes and Noble Publishing, 1992.

Hoffman, David, and Linda Quayle. *The Complete Illustrated Herbal: A Safe and Practical Guide to Making and Using Herbal Remedies.* Barnes and Noble Publishing, 1999.

ORGANIZATIONS

Hobbs, Christopher. *Herbal Advisor.* http// www.AllHerb.com.

Joan Schonbeck

Cherry, wild *see* **Wild cherry**

Chest pain *see* **Angina**

Chickenpox

Definition

Chickenpox (varicella) is a common and extremely infectious childhood disease that also occasionally affects adults. It produces an itchy, blistery rash that typically lasts about a week and is sometimes accompanied by a **fever** or other symptoms.

Description

About four million Americans contract chickenpox each year, resulting in roughly 5,000-9,000 hospitalizations and 100 deaths. Chickenpox is caused by the varicella-zoster virus (a member of the herpes virus family), which is spread through the air or by direct

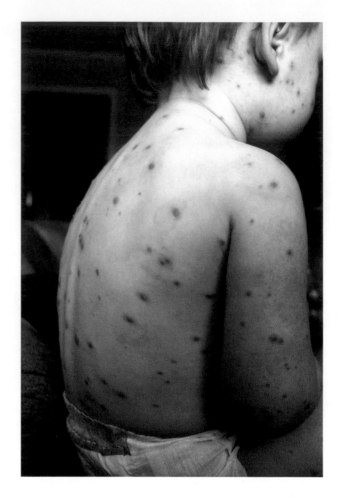

Child with chickenpox. *(© Janine Wiedel Photolibrary / Alamy)*

contact with an infected person. Once someone has been infected with the virus, symptoms appear in about 10-21 days. The period during which infected people can spread the disease is believed to start one or two days before the rash appears until all the **blisters** have formed scabs, usually four to seven days after the rash breaks out. For this reason, doctors recommend keeping children with chickenpox away from school for about a week.

Chickenpox has been a typical part of growing up for most children in the industrialized world (although this may change because of the new varicella vaccine). The disease can strike at any age, but by ages nine or 10 about 80-90% of American children have already been infected. U.S. children living in rural areas and many foreign-born children are less likely to be immune. Because almost every case of chickenpox leads to lifelong protection, adults account for less than 5% of all cases in the United States. Study results reported by the Centers for Disease Control and Prevention (CDC) indicate that more than 90% of

American adults are immune to the chickenpox virus. Adults, however, are much more likely than children to suffer dangerous complications. More than half of all chickenpox deaths occur among adults.

Causes and symptoms

A case of chickenpox usually starts without warning or with only a mild fever and a slight feeling of unwellness. Within a few hours or days small red spots begin to appear on the scalp, neck, or upper half of the trunk. After a further 12-24 hours the spots typically become itchy, fluid-filled bumps called vesicles, which continue to appear for the next two to five days. In any area of skin, lesions of a variety of stages can be seen. These blisters can spread to cover much of the skin, and in some cases may also be found inside the mouth, nose, ears, vagina, or rectum. Some people develop only a few blisters, but in most cases the number reaches 250-500. The blisters soon begin to form scabs and fall off. Scarring usually does not occur unless the blisters have been scratched and become infected. Occasionally a minor and temporary darkening of the skin (called hyperpigmentation) is noticed around some of the blisters. The degree of itchiness can range from barely noticeable to extreme. Some chickenpox sufferers also have headaches, abdominal **pain**, or a fever. Full recovery usually takes five to 10 days after the first symptoms appear. The most severe cases of the disease tend to be found among older children and adults.

Some groups are at risk for developing complications, the most common of which are bacterial **infections** of the blisters, **pneumonia**, dehydration, encephalitis, and **hepatitis**. Immediate medical help should always be sought when anyone in these high-risk groups contracts the disease. These include:

- Infants. Complications occur much more often among children less than one year old than among older children. The threat is greatest to newborns, who are more at risk of death from chickenpox than any other group. Children born to mothers who contract chickenpox just prior to delivery face an increased possibility of dangerous consequences, including brain damage and death. If the infection occurs during early pregnancy, there is a small (less than 5%) risk of birth defects.
- Immunocompromised children. Children whose immune systems have been weakened by a genetic disorder, disease, or medical treatment usually experience the most severe symptoms of any group. They have the second-highest rate of death from chickenpox.

- Adults and children 15 and older. The typical symptoms of chickenpox tend to strike this group with greater force.

Diagnosis

Where children are concerned, especially those with recent exposure to the disease, diagnosis can usually be made at home, by a school nurse, or by a doctor over the telephone if the child's parent or caregiver is unsure that the disease is chickenpox. A doctor should be called immediately if:

- The child's fever goes above 102°F (38.9°C) or takes more than four days to disappear.
- The child's blisters appear infected. Signs of infection include pus drainage or excessive redness, warmth, tenderness, or swelling.
- The child seems nervous, confused, unresponsive, or unusually sleepy; complains of a stiff neck or severe headache; shows signs of poor balance or has trouble walking; finds bright lights hard to look at; is having breathing problems or is coughing a lot; is

complaining of chest pain; is vomiting repeatedly; or is having convulsions. These may be signs of Reye's syndrome or encephalitis, two rare but potentially very dangerous conditions.

Treatment

Treatment focuses on reducing symptoms of chickenpox. The patient should drink plenty of fluids and eat simple, nutritious foods. Soups (especially mung bean), herbal teas, and fruit juices are good choices.

Applying wet compresses or bathing the patient in cool or lukewarm water once a day can help the itch. Adding four to eight ounces of baking soda or one or two cups of oatmeal to the bath is helpful. Only mild soap should be used and patting, not rubbing, is recommended for drying the patient. The patient should not scratch the blisters as this can lead to infection or scarring. For babies, light mittens or socks on the hands can help guard against scratching. If mouth blisters are present, cold drinks and soft, bland foods can make eating less painful.

Supplements

Vitamin A may help to heal skin. **Vitamin C** and bioflavinoids help to reduce fever and stimulate the immune system. **Zinc** also stimulates the immune system and promotes healing, however, it can cause **nausea** and **vomiting**. **Calcium** and **magnesium** help to relieve restlessness and sleeping difficulties. Magnesium has a laxative effect at high doses.

Herbals and Chinese medicine

The following herbals are ingested to treat chickenpox:

- Echinacea and goldenseal (*Hydrastis canadensis*) support the immune system and soothe skin and mucous membranes. Echinacea is also an antiviral.
- Chamomile tea is a sleep aid.
- Chinese cucumber (*Trichosanthes kirilowii*) root tea is used to relieve symptoms of chickenpox.
- Elder flower, peppermint, and yarrow reduce fever.
- Garlic has antiviral activity.
- Mullein (*Verbascum thapsus*) treats chickenpox.
- Yin Qiao Jie Du Wan (Honeysuckle and Forsythia Pill).
- Ban Lan Gen Chong Ji (Isatis Infusion).

The following herbals are used externally to treat chickenpox:

- Aloe leaf, calendula, and plantain relieve the itching of the chickenpox rash.
- Turmeric powder mixed with lime juice treats chickenpox rash.
- Garlic clears skin infection.

Other remedies

Homeopathic remedies are selected on a case by case basis. Some common remedy choices are **apis**, aconitum, **belladonna**, **calendula**, antimonium tartaricum, pulsatilla, *Rhus toxicodendron*, and sulphur.

The **acupressure** points Four Gates, Large Intestine 11, Spleen 10, and Stomach 36 help alleviate symptoms associated with chickenpox.

Allopathic treatment

Treatment usually focuses on reducing discomfort and fever. Because chickenpox is a viral disease, antibiotics are ineffective. Antibiotics may be prescribed if the blisters become infected. Calamine lotion helps to reduce itchiness. Painful genital blisters can be treated with an anesthetic cream recommended by a doctor or pharmacist.

Fever and discomfort can be reduced by acetaminophen (Tylenol) or other medications that do not contain aspirin. *Aspirin (or any aspirin- containing medications) must not be used with chickenpox, because it increases the chances of developing Reye's syndrome.* The best idea is to consult a doctor or pharmacist if one is unsure about which medications are safe.

Immunocompromised chickenpox sufferers are sometimes given the antiviral drug acyclovir (Zovirax). Zovirax also lessens the symptoms of chickenpox in otherwise healthy children and adults.

Expected results

Most cases of chickenpox run their course within a week. The varicella-zoster virus lies dormant in the nerve cells, where it may be reactivated years later by disease or age-related weakening of the immune system. The result is **shingles** (herpes zoster), a very painful rash and nerve inflammation, that strikes about 20% of the population, particularly people 50 and older.

Prevention

A substance known as varicella-zoster immune globulin (VZIG), which reduces the severity of chickenpox symptoms, is available to treat persons at high risk of developing complications. It is administered by injection within 96 hours of known or suspected exposure to the disease.

A vaccine for chickenpox (Varivax) has been found to prevent the disease in 70-90% of the vaccinated population, to reduce the severity of disease in the remaining cases. CDC and the American Academy of Pediatricians recommend vaccination of all children (with some exceptions) at 12-18 months of age. For older children, up to age 12, the CDC recommends vaccination when immunity cannot be confirmed. Vaccination is also recommended for any older child or adult considered susceptible to the disease, particularly those who face a greater likelihood of severe illness or transmitting infection. A single dose of the vaccine is sufficient for children up to age 12; older children and adults receive a second dose four to eight weeks later.

Resources

BOOKS

Pattishall, Evan G., III. "Chickenpox." In *Primary Pediatric Care.* edited by Robert A. Hoekelman, et al. St. Louis: Mosby, 1997.

Ying, Zhou Zhong, and Jin Hui De. "Common Diseases of Pediatrics." In *Clinical Manual of Chinese Herbal Medicine and Acupuncture.* New York: Churchill Livingston, 1997.

PERIODICALS

Kump, Theresa. "Childhood Without Chickenpox? Why Parents Are Still Wary of This New Vaccine." *Parents.* (April 1996): 39-40.

Napoli, Maryann. "The Chickenpox Vaccine." *Mothering.* (Summer 1996): 56-61.

Shapiro, Eugene D., and Phillip S. LaRussa. "Vaccination for Varicella—Just Do It!" *Journal of the American Medical Association* 278 (1997): 1529-1530.

ORGANIZATIONS

Centers for Disease Control and Prevention. National Immunization Hotline. 1600 Clifton Rd. NE, Atlanta, GA 30333. (800) 232- 2522 (English). (800) 232-0233 (Spanish). http://www.cdc.gov.

OTHER

Centers for Disease Control and Prevention."Prevention of Varicella: Recommendations of the Advisory Committee on Immunization Practices (ACIP)." http://aepo-xdv-www.epo.cdc.gov/wonder/prevguid/m0042990/M0042990.asp. (12 December 1997).

Zand, Janet. "Chickenpox." *HealthWorld Online.* http://www.healthy.net/library/books/smart/chcknpox.htm.

Belinda Rowland

Chickweed

Description

Chickweed (*Stellaria media*) is a member of the Caryophyllaceae, or carnation, family. There are about 25 species of *Stellaria*, including some native varieties, growing abundantly in the wild in North America. Chickweed is a European native that has naturalized throughout the world in fertile, mineral-rich soil. It thrives in shady, moist locations in gardens, near human habitations, and on the edge of woods. The herb is often found growing under the shade of **oak** trees. Chickweed is a persistent annual. It self-seeds and may produce as many as five generations within one season.

The genus name *Stellaria* refers to chickweed's tiny, white, star-shaped flowers. The common name refers to the herb's appeal to birds and barnyard fowl, particularly young chickens. Other common names include Indian chickweed, stitchwort, starwort, white bird's eye, chick wittles, satin flower, adder's mouth, mouse ear, starweed, passerina, tongue grass, and winter weed. Chickweed has been used for centuries. The nutritious herb was fed to caged birds and rabbits. It was also traditionally prepared as an early spring tonic, eaten fresh or steamed, to cleanse the kidneys and liver. English physician Nicholas Culpeper described chickweed as "a fine soft pleasing herb under the dominion of the Moon."

Chickweed is a juicy, succulent, low-growing, and delicate herb which grows from a slender taproot. The straggly, weak stems may stretch along the ground for two feet or more forming dense mats only a few inches off the ground. The light-green, oval, and entire leaves grow in opposite pairs about an inch apart along the smooth and branching stem. A single line of fine white hairs grow along one side or the other of the thin stems, alternating at the node of each pair of leaves. Stems are slightly swollen at the joints. Leaves appear stalkless at the growing tip but the older leaves develop stalks at least as long as the attached leaf. At night the half-inch long leaves close in on each other to protect the developing buds. The tiny white flowers grow singly in the leaf axils of the upper leaves. The five petals are deeply incised, and smaller than the pointed green sepals. Blossoms open in the sun and close on cloudy, gray days and throughout the night hours. Minuscule seed capsules, with a barely-perceptible toothed edge, follow the blossoms. In damp weather the "teeth" swell, effectively closing the capsule to protect the ripening seed. The tiny yellow-orange seeds continue to ripen even after the herb is harvested. Chickweed self-seeds freely in cool, moist habitats.

General use

The entire chickweed plant is edible. The stems and leaves are used in medicinal preparations. Herbalists, however, disagree about the medicinal potency of chickweed. One writer, a professor of pharmacognosy, dismissed chickweed as a "worthless weed" and an "ineffective herb." Other writers and herbalists praise the diminutive herb for providing "optimum nutrition" and for its "unsurpassed" ability to cool fevers and **infections**. The English physician Nicholas Culpeper, writing in the seventeenth century, credited chickweed as beneficial for "all pains in the body that arise of heat." Taken as an infusion, chickweed acts internally to cool inflammation of the digestive and respiratory system. It has been used to treat **bronchitis**, **pleurisy**, **colitis**, **gastritis**, **asthma**, and **sore throat**. The herb's diuretic action helps eliminate toxins from the system and reduce retention of fluids. Chickweed contains mucilage, saponins, **silica**, coumarins, flavonoids (including glycoside rutin), triterpenoids, and carboxylic acids. The herb is rich in minerals, including **copper** and **iron**, and vitamins A, B, and C.

Gathered fresh, chickweed is beneficial in poultice form to ease rheumatic **pain** and to treat **boils** and abscesses. The herb can also be used to draw out splinters and the stingers of insects and to dissolve **warts**. Its vulnerary (wound-healing) action speeds the healing of **cuts** and **wounds**. Its emollient qualities soothe **itching** and irritation of **eczema** or **psoriasis**. An infusion of chickweed may be added to bath water for soothing relief of inflamed skin. Chickweed also provides relief to swollen and painful **hemorrhoids**.

Another species of chickweed, *S. dichotoma*, known as *yin chai hu* is used in Chinese medicine to stop nosebleed, to reduce heavy menstrual bleeding, and to bring down fevers. The species *S. alsine* is also used in Chinese medicine as a medicinal remedy for treating colds, snakebites, and even traumatic injury.

Preparations

Gather chickweed from young plants before or during flowering and throughout the year. Snipping the stems will encourage growth of new branches for later harvest. The freshly harvested herb will keep for several days if refrigerated. The fresh herb may be eaten in salads, or very lightly steamed as a potherb. Chickweed has a somewhat bland taste, so other edible greens may be added to the pot to enhance the flavor.

- Infusion: Place 2 oz of fresh chickweed leaves and stems in a warmed glass container. Bring 2.5 cups of fresh, nonchlorinated water to the boiling point and

add it to the herbs. Cover and infuse the tea for about 10 minutes. Strain and drink warm. The prepared tea will store for about two days in a sealed container in the refrigerator. Chickweed tea may be enjoyed by the cupful up to three times a day. A strong infusion may be used as a skin wash or bath additive to soothe itching and inflamed skin.

- Poultice: Chop fresh chickweed leaves and stems in sufficient quantity to cover the area being treated. Sprinkle the herb with water and place over the area. Cover the herbal mass with a strip of wet cotton gauze to hold the poultice in place. When gathering the older, tougher plant, the herb may be simmered either in water alone or in a 50/50 mixture of water and vinegar for about five minutes. Apply to the skin after the mixture has sufficiently cooled.

- Tincture: Combine four ounces of finely-cut fresh or powdered dry herb with one pint of brandy, gin, or vodka, in a glass container. The alcohol should be enough to cover the plant parts. Place the mixture away from light for about two weeks, shaking several times each day. Strain and store in a tightly-capped, dark glass bottle. A standard dose is 1–4 ml of the tincture three times a day.

Precautions

The wind-blown pollen of chickweed may aggravate **hay fever**. Chickweed is considered safe for all external applications. There was a report in 1980 of "temporary paralysis" after ingestion of large amounts of the infused herb, however there are no other documented reports of toxicity. The *PDR For Herbal Medicines* reports no health hazards when this herb is taken "with the proper administration of designated therapeutic dosages."

Side effects

None reported.

Interactions

None reported.

Chicory

Resources

BOOKS

Duke, James A. *The Green Pharmacy*. Emmaus, Penn.: Rodale Press, 1997.

Hutchens, Alma R. *A Handbook Of Native American Herbs*. Boston: Shambhala Publications, Inc., 1992.

McIntyre, Anne. *The Medicinal Garden*. New York: Henry Holt and Company, 1997.

Ody, Penelope. *The Complete Medicinal Herbal*. New York: Dorling Kindersley, 1993.

PDR for Herbal Medicines New Jersey: Medical Economics Co., 1998.

Polunin, Miriam, and Christopher Robbins. *The Natural Pharmacy*. New York: Macmillan Publishing Company, 1992.

Tyler, Varro E. *Herbs of Choice, The Honest Herbal*. New York: Pharmaceutical Products Press, 1993.

Weiss, Gaea, and Shandor Weiss. *Growing & Using The Healing Herbs*. New York: Wings Books, 1992.

Clare Hanrahan

Chicory

Description

Chicory (*Cichorium intybus*) is an herb and root that has been known for its curative benefits since the first century A.D.. It is a member of the Asteraceae family. A scraggly plant with blue flower heads, chicory flourishes in the wild, as well as in gardens all over the world. It may be found in Europe, the Near East, northern and southern Africa, Australia, New Zealand, and North and South America.

The dried leaves and roots of the chicory plant are collected in autumn for medicinal purposes. When flowering, the whole plant is collected and dried. With a height that may reach up to 5 ft (1.5 m), chicory can be recognized by its oblong leaves that resemble a crosscut saw or slit, with numerous stiff hairs on the underside. Chicory, whose common names include succory, chicory root, chicory herb, blue sailors, wild chicory, or hendibeh, is well known for its bitter taste and use as a coffee substitute.

General use

The ancient Egyptians ate large amounts of chicory because it was believed that the plant could purify the blood and liver, while others have relied on the herb for its power to cure "passions of the heart." Chicory continues to be a popular herbal remedy due to its healing effects on several ailments.

KEY TERMS

Biodegradable—Capable of being broken down by the actions of living organisms. Inulin from chicory roots can be used to produce biodegradable substances used in industry.

Diuretic—A medicine or agent that increases the body's output of urine.

Infusion—A liquid extract of an herb or other plant prepared by steeping or soaking the plant material in water. Chicory can be taken at home as an infusion.

Inulin—A starchlike complex sugar obtained from chicory roots that is used to improve the texture of processed foods.

Prebiotic—A type of nondigestible substance found in chicory and some other plants that supports the growth and activity of beneficial bacteria in the colon.

Premenstrual syndrome (PMS)—A group of symptoms that occur several days prior to the beginning of menstruation, including irritability, emotional tension, anxiety, and mood changes such as depression, headache, breast tenderness with or without swelling, and water retention. Symptoms usually subside shortly after the onset of the flow.

Sedative—A drug or agent that calms or soothes. Chicory by itself has a sedative effect on the body.

Chicory is taken internally for the following disorders.

- jaundice
- spleen problems
- gallstones
- rheumatism
- gout
- loss of appetite

In addition, the leaves of chicory may also be used as compresses to be applied externally to ease skin inflammations and swellings.

According to folklore, chicory was recommended as a laxative for children, and it is also believed to increase the flow of bile. As a mild diuretic, it increases the elimination of fluid from the body, leading to its use as a treatment for rheumatism and **gout**.

Women who suffer from **premenstrual syndrome** (PMS) may find that regular use of chicory root as a bitter and a liver tonic may assist in maintaining hormone balance and lessening the symptoms of PMS. In addition, altering the diet by eating a "bitter" salad that includes fresh **dandelion**, chicory, and sorrel is believed to strengthen the liver and discourage the growth of candida.

Chicory also supports the body's ability to absorb **calcium**, a nutrient that helps build and maintain strong teeth and bones. Raftilin inulin and raftilose oligofructose are fibers extracted from chicory root that cannot be digested by the small intestine. Instead, they are fermented by bacteria in the large intestine, leading to the increased absorption of calcium and other minerals. Oligofructose is an example of a prebiotic, or nondigestible food ingredient that benefits health by supporting the growth of one or several types of bacteria in the colon.

A study published in 2002 indicates that inulin appears to lower the risk of colon **cancer**. The precise nature of its protective effects is not yet known, however.

In addition to enhancing digestive processes, chicory helps to keep the liver healthy. The inclusion of chicory root supplements in the diet supports the proper metabolism of **cholesterol**.

Preparations

While the medicinal uses of chicory are numerous, the plant is also often used as a food additive, as a flavoring agent, and in meals. Inulin can be used to improve the texture of processed foods as well as sweeten them. It can also be used to make biodegradable nonfood substances with many industrial applications. This versatility is important to environmentalists because chicory is a renewable natural resource.

Wild and cultivated chicory leaves may be added to salads or sautéed and served alone. Moreover, the roasted and ground root of the plant is a common addition to coffee in Europe and in the United States.

Studies have shown that chicory complements coffee when it is used as a supplement due to its lactucin and lactucopicrin. These two substances are responsible for the bitter taste of chicory, and may serve to counteract the stimulating effects of **caffeine**. Chicory by itself actually has a sedative action on the central nervous system.

Chicory is available over the counter in bulk as green leaves and dried roots. To prepare the herb as a tea, also known as an infusion, for home use: steep 1 tsp (5 ml) rootstock or dried herb with 0.5 cup (4 fl oz) water and strain after 10 minutes. To treat **jaundice**,

spleen problems, **gallstones**, or **gastritis**, drink 8-12 oz (225-350 ml) of chicory tea per day.

As a dietary supplement, 1 tsp (5 ml) of juice from chicory stems may be squeezed by hand and taken in milk or water three times a day.

Precautions

Chicory has shown to be safe for a variety of medicinal uses and as a food source. There are no necessary precautions to observe when including the herb in the diet.

Side effects

There are no known health hazards or side effects when chicory is added to the diet. The only possible minor side effect is skin irritation. If the hands become irritated after handling chicory, it is best to cover them with gloves and treat the affected area as needed.

Resources

BOOKS

The Editors of Time-Life Books. "Chicory." *The Medical Advisor: The Complete Guide to Alternative & Conventional Treatments*. Richmond, VA: Time-Life Inc., 1996.

Fleming, Thomas. "Cichorium Intybus." *PDR for Herbal Medicines, First Edition*. Montvale, NJ: Medical Economics Company Inc., 1998.

PERIODICALS

Chow, J. "Probiotics and Prebiotics: A Brief Overview." *Journal of Renal Nutrition* 12 (April 2002): 76-86.

Crawford, Sharon. "High Herbs: For Plant Medicine Go to the Mountains." *Alive* (May 31, 1997): 44–45.

Franck, A., "Technological Functionality of Inulin and Oligofructose." *British Journal of Nutrition* 87 (March 2002): Supplement 2, 287-291.

Pool-Zobel, B., J. Van Loo, et al. "Experimental Evidences on the Potential of Prebiotic Fructans to Reduce the Risk of Colon Cancer." *British Journal of Nutrition* 87 (March 2002): Supplement 2, 273-281.

Stengler, Mark. "Blast Cholesterol." *Alive* (June 30, 1999): 20–21.

Stevens, C. V., A. Meriggi, and K. Booten. "Chemical Modification of Inulin, a Valuable Renewable Resource, and its Industrial Applications." *Biomacromolecules* 2 (Spring 2001): 1-16.

ORGANIZATIONS

American Botanical Council. P. O. Box 201660. Austin, TX 78720-1660.

Beth Kapes
Rebecca J. Frey, PhD

Chigong *see* **Qigong**

Childbirth

Definition

Childbirth, or parturition, is the process of labor that dilates the cervix and includes the delivery of the baby and placenta through the birth canal.

Description

Most babies are born following approximately nine calendar months of **pregnancy**. Delivery between 37–42 weeks of gestation is considered normal and full-term. A baby born prior to 37 weeks of gestation is considered premature, or preterm. After 42 weeks, a baby is considered postterm. Both preterm and post-term deliveries are considered higher risk deliveries.

Labor occurs in three stages. The first is the dilation of the cervix, the second is the delivery of the baby, and the third is the expulsion of the placenta. Approximately 25 percent of babies born in the United States, however, are surgically delivered by Caesarean section. This procedure can be necessary and even life-saving, but many medical experts believe that Caesarean sections are performed too frequently and could be reduced through better management of labor and a more informed public.

At one time, "once a Caesarean, always a Caesarean" meant a woman could not deliver vaginally after having a Caesarean, but as of 2008 that is no longer true for everyone. Part of the reason is that the Caesarean surgery is performed differently, and women can heal from it sufficiently to have a subsequent birth vaginally. In fact, more and more women choose vaginal birth after Caesarean (VBAC). Having a sympathetic, informed caregiver and preparation helps achieve this goal for some women.

The first stage of labor is the time the cervix must reach full dilation. It includes latent (early), active, and transition phases. The latent phase of labor, when the cervix progresses from being closed to 3 cm open, may last for days or longer. For some women, latent labor is not a distinguishable phase, and for others it leads immediately into active labor. The latent phase is often exciting for the mother, who wonders if her baby is finally going to be born. Contractions during this phase are not very painful. Active labor ensues around the time the cervix reaches 3 cm dilation and continues until approximately 7 cm dilation. At this stage, labor contractions are powerful and require the mother's concentration. The length of this stage is also variable and is usually longer for first-time mothers than for those having subsequent babies. Active labor is followed by transition, the shortest and most intense stage of labor, when many women express feelings of despair or not being able to continue. At the end of transition, the cervix is fully dilated to 10 cm and pushing can begin.

The second stage of labor is pushing the baby out through the vagina (birth canal). Contractions are generally less frequent than in the first stage of labor but are very strong and long lasting. Many women find it a relief to be able to push. In the unmedicated mother, pushing is reflexive and instinctual. The pressure of the baby's head on stretch receptors in the maternal pelvis triggers the urge to push. First-time mothers generally push for about 60 minutes; subsequent births require an average of only 15 minutes.

The third stage of labor is the delivery of the placenta, which often goes unnoticed by the mother who is attending to her newborn. After the baby is delivered, the uterus should continue to contract in order to push out the placenta. The placenta functioned to bring the baby nourishment from the mother throughout the pregnancy and return the child's waste products to the mother to be excreted. If contractions become sluggish or stop before the placenta is delivered, breastfeeding the baby can trigger the release of the hormone oxytocin to stimulate the uterus to contract again. Alternatively, artificial oxytocin (pitocin) can be given by injection.

Causes and symptoms

The onset of spontaneous labor may be marked by irregular contractions, not very different from the Braxton-Hicks contractions that are common throughout late pregnancy. In approximately 10 percent of spontaneous labors, rupture of membranes ("water breaking") may occur before the onset of contractions. Since prolonged rupture of membranes prior to delivery presents a risk of infection, the care provider for the mother should be contacted regardless of whether she is experiencing contractions.

Even experienced mothers sometimes have difficulty recognizing when labor begins, as prelabor may occur on and off for days or longer before settling into a regular pattern. In general, the contractions associated with labor will gradually become more frequent, more regular, longer, and stronger. Walking or changing activity will not alter them. These contractions are effective at changing the cervix, which will become appreciably lower, thinner, and more dilated. By contrast, contractions of prelabor stay about the same intensity and frequency. A change of activity will often make them disappear. These contractions may be uncomfortable and may even cause some mild cervical changes, but they do not change on an hourly basis.

Diagnosis

For women who choose to deliver in a hospital, a diagnosis of active labor is generally made if contractions are regular and strong, and the cervix is effacing and/or dilating noticeably on an hourly basis. A woman who arrives at the hospital reporting regular contractions who has no complicating factors is generally observed for at least an hour to see whether her labor will progress. Monitors that fit around the abdomen measure the fetal heart rate and the nature of the contractions. A nurse checks the position and station of the baby, as well as the effacement, dilation, and position of the mother's cervix. Admission is generally made regardless of progress if the water has broken (rupture of membranes) or if complications exist. These may include high maternal blood pressure, more than one fetus, fetal distress, abnormal fetal presentation, or excessive bleeding. Women delivering before 37 weeks or after 42 weeks of gestation are also well-advised to deliver in a hospital.

Treatment

For a routine, uncomplicated labor and delivery, the primary treatment required is assistance with comfort measures. What each mother finds comforting is individual. At some point during the pregnancy, it is a good idea to make a list of methods to try to relieve **pain** during labor, in the event that one or two favored techniques do not work: A mother who generally enjoys massage may suddenly discover that it is distracting to be touched during active labor, or a woman who plans to rely on medication could have an epidural that does not take or be laboring too quickly for it to be allowed. Having a list of comfort measures on hand is useful and reassuring for most laboring women. Reassurance is important, as relieving **stress** during labor allows it to progress more quickly and with less pain. Many women find it helpful to employ an experienced doula, or birth assistant, to provide comfort, reassurance, and information.

Fear of the unknown can certainly contribute to increased pain. Expectant parents should learn all they can about the process of childbirth. Many good reference books are available. Taking Lamaze classes lends a personal touch, and many couples enjoy the camaraderie of sharing the learning experience with other expectant families. Even though labor can take unexpected turns, being aware of the options at each stage

lends some perception of control. Making a list of birth preferences can be helpful in defining what the parents desire at the birth, but flexibility is important to avoid disappointment if every expectation is not met.

Acupuncture

A skilled acupuncturist may be able to offer some relief of labor pain, particularly for women who have previously found **acupuncture** to be helpful with other types of pain.

Massage therapy

Some women find massage or **therapeutic touch** to be quite relaxing during labor. Contractions are sometimes felt intensely in the back, and a combination of massage and counterpressure can offer relief. Foot massage may also be comforting, both during pregnancy and during labor. Laboring women report a great temptation to tense the abdomen against a contraction. The contraction will be more effective and less painful with effleurage (light stroking) of the area, and a verbal reminder to let the abdomen hang heavy and relax. The jaw area is also frequently clenched and benefits from **relaxation**. Gentle touch and massage of any area that appears tense will help to relieve stress. This is a good technique to practice before labor begins.

Music

The sounds of a favorite piece of music can be an excellent aid to relaxation. Instrumentals are generally preferable to singing. Soothing sounds or tunes that evoke happy memories are helpful. Some women enjoy tapes of nature sounds.

Hydrotherapy

A warm tub or shower may be one of the most underestimated methods of relieving the pain of labor. Warmth encourages muscle relaxation, which in turn decreases **anxiety**. The water in a tub also supports the mother's body. In a jetted tub, position and water pressure can be adjusted to soothe areas that are cramping or painful. This may be particularly comforting for back labor. In a birthing pool or large tub, the mother is free to move around and find a position that optimizes her comfort. The relaxation brought on by water can make for a shorter, more comfortable labor.

Aromatherapy

Some **essential oils** are particularly recommended during birth for those women who enjoy the scents. They can be added to a diffuser or a crock-pot of water in the birthing area, emitted from a scented candle, or concentrated drops of the scent can be placed on the pillow and bed linens. Clary **sage** and **lavender** are popular choices, but any scent that is pleasant to the mother may be used.

Visualization

The use of visualization, or **guided imagery**, can be powerful to promote relaxation and the progress of labor. One exercise that can be practiced in advance of labor is choosing a place or image that the mother associates with comfort, security, and serenity. This place can be imagined and explored at any time to help relieve stress. If the details of this visualization are shared with someone who will be present during labor, that person can help to evoke those feelings during times of pain or stress. Another popular visualization is that of a flower blooming. The cervix can be envisioned as a flower bud that gradually opens to allow the baby to descend. Other scripts for guided imagery can be practiced to relieve stress and reduce pain.

Increasingly, women (not in high-risk pregnancies) desire a more low-tech approach to labor and choose a nurse midwife to assist them rather than a physician. For thousands of years, midwives have given women support and care through the birthing process. In 2004, a nurse-midwife rather than a physician attended about 8 percent of births, which is approximately twice the number in 1989. Nurse-midwives are committed to helping meet mothers' individual needs and to give them freedom of choice during birth. They work to provide a natural childbirth and to help the woman prevent complications before, during, and after the birth. Those wishing to use midwives should check with the obstetrician and also determine if the midwife is certified (CNM). More and more obstetrician practices also employ or work with nurse-midwives.

Allopathic treatment

Modern pain relief for childbirth generally involves the use of medication. Although medication has evolved from the days of mothers being put under so-called twilight sleep for a normal vaginal birth, the use of chemical pain relief is not without risk.

One of the most common pain relief methods during labor is the epidural. This technique involves the injection of anesthetic medication through a catheter into the epidural space in the back. Epidurals often provide excellent relief of pain from contractions, episiotomy, and perineal repair. They do not impair the mother's mental alertness, although she may sleep if labor to that point has been long and arduous. The disadvantages of epidurals include possible prolonging of labor, impaired ability to push, inability to move around, possible need for bladder catheterization and accompanying risk of infection or injury, maternal low blood pressure, maternal **fever**, spinal **headache** from inadvertent injection into the subdural space, and patchy or ineffective blocks. Low blood pressure can result in **nausea** and **dizziness**, as well as fetal distress. Supplemental oxygen may be given to the mother to alleviate this effect. Allergic reactions to the anesthetic agents occur rarely. The woman who wishes to have an epidural needs to have IV access, IV fluids in advance to help prevent low blood pressure, and fetal monitoring. The woman's inability to move around and change positions because of the tubes and wires can impede the progress of labor. If labor slows, it may be augmented by the injection of pitocin. Assisted delivery via forceps or vacuum extractor may be necessary if the mother finds herself unable to push effectively.

Injectable narcotic pain medications are also available. They can be given by either intramuscular (IM) or intravenous (IV) routes. When given intravenously, the effects are felt sooner and are shorter in duration. These medications are more likely to affect the fetus and are generally not given late in labor. Some women say that their pain is not greatly diminished but that they are better able to rest between contractions. Others experience side effects, such as nausea, **vomiting**, and dizziness that they feel negate any benefit that they get from the medication.

Prevention

Techniques that are used to prevent pregnancy are known as contraception. Some methods require a prescription, including those involving hormones, diaphragms, cervical caps, or intrauterine devices (IUDs). Hormonal birth control is available as a daily pill, an injection, a patch, a vaginal ring, or an implant. Consultation with a healthcare professional will determine the appropriateness of these methods. Conditions including clotting diseases, **breast cancer**, and liver disease will preclude hormonal forms of birth control. Significant side effects may occur even in women who are good candidates for these methods. Timing of taking the daily birth control pills is important, and back-up methods should be available if doses are missed. Diaphragms and caps are barriers used next to the cervix along with a spermicide. For diaphragms and caps, the typical pregnancy rate lies between 20 and 40 percent, according to the U.S. Food and Drug Administration (FDA). If these two methods are always used correctly, the pregnancy rates fall to 6 to 26 percent. The IUD is a uniquely long-term device. It is placed by a medical professional and, depending on the type, can retain effectiveness for as long as 10 years. It is not recommended for women who have ever had **pelvic inflammatory disease** or for those who are not in a mutually monogamous relationship. The pregnancy rate for IUD users is from 0.6 to 2 percent, according to the FDA.

Several popular forms of birth control are non-prescriptive. Barrier method materials, such as condoms, foam, and spermicides are available over the counter. Condoms have the distinction of being the only type designed for males. Used correctly, they are highly effective in preventing pregnancy. They have no side effects, and latex varieties have the additional advantage of providing some protection against sexually transmitted diseases. Average pregnancy rates are around 14 percent for typical users, but fall to 3 percent when they are always used correctly, according to the FDA.

Periodic abstinence, sometimes called natural family planning, requires training and attentiveness to physical signs. A variety of methods are available and may include monitoring of cycle days, basal body temperature, cervical mucus characteristics, and other symptoms related to the timing of ovulation. Effectiveness can be as great as 99 percent, according to the FDA, but it requires significant commitment for the couple to faithfully monitor signs and abstain from intercourse for at least one week of every cycle. Women with irregular cycles or unreliable signs have the most unplanned pregnancies with these methods.

Resources

BOOKS

Dick-Read, Grantly, and Michel Odent. *Childbirth Without Fear: The Principle and Practice of Natural Childbirth,* 4th rev. ed. London: Pinter & Martin, 2005.

Schwegel, Janet, ed. *Adventures in Natural Childbirth: Tales from Women on the Joys, Fears, Pleasures, and Pains of Giving Birth Naturally.* New York: Marlowe & Company, 2005.

ORGANIZATIONS

Association of Labor Assistants and Childbirth Educators (ALACE) (formerly Informed Birth & Parenting), PO. 390436, Cambridge, MA, 02139, (888) 222-5223, http://www.alace.org/.

International Childbirth Education Association (ICEA), PO Box 20048, Minneapolis, MN, 55420, (952) 854-8660, http://www.icea.org.

Judith Turner
Teresa Norris
Leslie Mertz, Ph.D.

Childhood nutrition

Definition

Childhood **nutrition** involves making sure that children eat healthy foods to help them grow and develop normally, as well as to prevent **obesity** and future disease.

The traditional or mainstream approach to good childhood nutrition is to follow suggestions based on dietary guidelines that are appropriate for a child's age and development level and that have been developed and recommended by government, research, and medical professionals. The guidelines include selections from different food groups to provide the vitamins and minerals young bodies need for natural growth and activity. The U.S. Department of Agriculture's (USDA's) Food Guide Pyramid recommends how many servings a day a child should eat of each food group, such as milk, vegetables, fruits, fats, and meats. The Food Guide Pyramid asserts that by sticking closely to the guidelines, parents can ensure their children get a well-balanced diet that supplies the vitamins, minerals and calories they need to support growing bodies and active lifestyles. However, in this age of what has been called "advanced medicine," there are those who seek to understand why so many among us, especially children, suffer from so much serious illness.

Minimum nutrient and calorie levels for school lunches

(school week averages)

	Preshcool	Grades K–6	Grades 7–12
Calories	517	664	825
Total fat (percentage of total food energy)	*1	*1, 2	*2
Saturated fat (percentage of actual total food energy)	*1	*1, 3	*3
RDA for protein (g)	7	10	16
RDA for calcium (mg)	267	286	400
RDA for iron (mg)	3.3	3.5	4.5
RDA for vitamin A (RE)	150	224	300
RDA for vitamin C (mg)	14	15	18

*1 The Dietary Guidelines for Americans recommends that after 2 years of age, children should gradually adopt a diet, that by about 5 years of age, contains no more than 30 percent of calories from fat.

2 Not to exceed 30 percent over a school week

3 Less than 10 percent over a school week.

"RE" refers to "retinol equivalent," a measure of the vitamin A activity in foods.

(Illustration by GGS Information Services. Cengage Learning, Gale)

Origins

Humans, unlike plants, cannot manufacture the nutrients they need to function. Each culture over centuries has developed its own traditional diet. In modern-day western civilization, many of these **diets** have developed into convenient, fatty and sugary foods, leading to obesity even in children and teens.

Advice on nutritional choices predates recorded language, but the first science-based approach to a healthy diet probably began just over 100 years ago. W. O. Atwater, the first director of the Office of Experiment Stations in the U.S. Department of Agriculture (USDA) and a pioneer in the field of nutrition investigation, developed some of the components needed for a food guide. He created food tables with data on protein, fat, carbohydrate, mineral matter, and fuel value for common foods.

Food guides with food groups similar to those used today first appeared in USDA publications in 1916 and were developed by nutrition specialist Caroline L. Hunt. Interestingly, the first daily food guide was published under the title *Food for Young Children*. In the early 1930s, the Depression economic restraints on families and the USDA responded with advice on how to select affordable healthy foods. In 1941, the Food and Nutrition Board of the National Academy of Sciences released the first recommended dietary allowances (RDAs) for calories and essential nutrients. The nine nutrients included on the list were protein, **iron**, **calcium**, vitamins A, C, and D, thiamin, **riboflavin**, and **niacin**.

Throughout the years following the release of the first guidelines, recommendations were debated and revised. The new food guide was first presented in 1984 as a *food wheel*. The USDA first used a pyramid to represent the food groups in 1992 after intensive research on the most effective way to visually communicate healthy eating by portion and food choice. Although it has been modified over the years, the pyramid has continued to represent the food groups.

Annemarie Colbin was brought up on a European vegetarian diet before she came to the United States in 1961. In her search for optimum health and the ability to control how one feels by what one eats, she became a professional cook, lecturer, founder of the Natural Gourmet Cookery School in New York City, and author of best-selling books *Food and Healing, The Book of Whole Meals,* and *The Natural Gourmet,* as well as articles appearing in the *New York Times* and *Cosmopolitan.*

In Chapter One of *Food and Healing,* Colbin looks at the health of children and she points out that:

- A child born today can expect to live 26 years longer than a child born in 1900, but a person who has already reached 45 today can expect to live only four or five years longer than a person born in 1900.

- The following childhood problems that were rare in 1900 are now so prevalent that they are called "the new morbidity (an unsound, gruesome condition)": learning difficulties, behavioral disturbances, speech and hearing difficulties, faulty vision, serious dental misalignment.

- The average child loses three permanent teeth to decay by age 11, eight or nine by age 17, and 94% of adolescents have cavities in their permanent teeth.

- Among children, tuberculosis is on the rise

- By the mid-1980s, cancer as a killer of children and adolescents was surpassed by only accidents and violence.

Colbin cites statistics linking children to emotional disorders and violence, indicating that at any given time, as much as a quarter of our population is estimated to suffer from depression, **anxiety**, or other emotional disorders; that suicide is the ninth leading cause of death for all age groups; and that there may be as many as four million cases of child abuse every year, at least 2,000 of which result in death. She then states, "All this violence is no longer viewed as purely

Causes, risks, and prevention of childhood obesity

Causes

Increased consumption of sugary beverages with a decreased consumption of milk

Super-size portions in fast food restaurants

More meals eaten away from home and use of prepared foods in the home

Increased snacking between meals and fewer meals eaten together as a family

Heavy advertising of high-sugar high-fat foods to children

Decrease in children carrying their lunch to school from home

Poor eating habits such as skipping breakfast and later snacking on high fat, sugary foods

More time spent watching television or using the computer

Fewer children walking to school

Fewer physical education requirements at school and decreased recess in grades 1-5

Fear of crime, which limits outdoor activities of children

Increase in teen access to cars

Inherited tendency toward weight gain or having at least one obese parent

Eating in response to stress, boredom, and loneliness and/or poor sleeping habits

Medical conditions, such as Prader-Willi syndrome, hypothyroidism, mental illness, binge eating disorder, or taking certain medications

Risks

Type 2 diabetes

High blood pressure (hypertension)

Cardiovascular disease

Gallbladder disease

High cholesterol

Fat accumulation in the liver (fatty liver/liver disease)

Sleep apnea

Early puberty; early start of menstruation in girls

Eating disorders

Joint pain and degenerative joint disease

Sleep apnea

Depression

Increased anxiety and stress

Low self-esteem

Exposure to social prejudice and discrimination

Prevention

Serve a healthy variety of foods and keep healthy snacks on hand

Choose low-fat cooking methods such as broiling or baking

Eliminate junk snack food and sugary beverages from the house

Eat meals together as a family rather than grabbing something quick on the run

Limit visits to fast-food restaurants

Plan family activities that involve physical activity, such as hiking, biking, or swimming

Encourage children to become more active such as walking to school, biking to friends' houses, walking the dog or mowing the lawn

Limit television and computer time

Avoid using food as a reward

Pack healthy homemade lunches on school days

Encourage school officials to eliminate soda machines on campus, bake sales, and fundraising with candy and cookies

Set realistic goals for weight control and reward children's efforts

Model the eating behaviors and active lifestyle you would like your child to adopt

(Illustration by Corey Light. Cengage Learning, Gale)

Healthy snack foods for children

- Applesauce cups (unsweetened)
- Apples or pears and low-fat cheese
- Baby carrots and celery
- Bagels pizzas with tomato sauce and melted low-fat cheese
- Baked potato chips or tortilla chips with salsa
- Cereal, dry or with low-fat milk
- Cucumber or zucchini slices
- Dried fruits such as raisins, apple rings, or apricots
- Fresh fruit
- Fruit canned in juice or light syrup
- Fruit juice
- Fruit salad
- Frozen fruit bars
- Frozen grapes
- Low-fat chocolate milk
- Low-fat frozen yogurt with fresh berries
- Low-fat yogurt with fruit
- Nonfat cottage cheese with fruit
- Popcorn, air popped or low-fat microwave
- Pretzels (lightly salted or unsalted) and a glass of low-fat milk
- Raw vegetable sticks with low-fat yogurt dip, cottage cheese or hummus
- Rice cakes with peanut butter
- Smoothies with low-fat milk or yogurt and sliced bananas or strawberries
- String cheese and fruit (canned or fresh)
- Vanilla wafers, gingersnaps, graham crackers, animal crackers or fig bars and a glass of milk
- Whole-grain crackers or English muffin with peanut butter
- Whole-wheat crackers with cheese or peanut butter

(Illustration by GGS Information Services. Cengage Learning, Gale)

psychological. A growing body of research links mood, violent behavior, and even criminal behavior with various physiological imbalances: an over-active thyroid, an excess of testosterone (male hormones), **allergies**, low blood sugar. **Lead poisoning**, vitamin deficiencies, and of course alcohol and drugs all alter physiology as well as mood. Behavioral problems have even been associated with a lack of natural light, insofar as light plays a vital role in the metabolism of calcium, a mineral widely regarded as 'nature's tranquilizer.'"

Based on these statistics and many more that she cites, Colbin contends that proper nutrition plays a key role in disease prevention. She indicates that she sees three major errors in our contemporary assumptions about health and illness: the belief that physiological symptoms such as headaches, fevers, etc. are mistaken reactions of the body to normal stimuli; the belief that surgical intervention or chemical substances, natural or artificial in origin, can restore health by stopping the disease process; and the belief that dietary habits are unrelated to symptoms or illnesses. Although the last belief is slowly changing, it has a long way to go. For example, she points out, many people are still buying antacids for digestive distress without changing their diet.

Benefits

The Food Guide Pyramid and other healthy eating recommendations generally apply to children age two and older. When used as a starting point for planning family meals and snacks, applying these sensible recommendations to children's daily diets can encourage good eating habits at an early age. This will help children develop mentally and physically according to growth charts and other measurements set by pediatricians (physicians who specialize in caring for children) and will help prevent future problems with overeating or with eating disorders. Many nutritional experts agree that if children eat a balanced diet that includes all of the recommended food groups, they will not need to take vitamin/mineral supplements. Also, eating a balanced diet with a variety of foods will give children the energy they need to stay physically active, which is important to their growth and mental health, and in keeping obesity in check.

Description

In spite of recommendations, the diet quality of most children is not what it should be. The USDA surveyed American children ages two to nine in 1998 and found that up to 8% of them had a poor diet, while as many as 80% of those ages seven to nine had a diet that needed improvement. The Centers for Disease Control (CDC) defines childhood obesity at a level above the 95th percentile of body mass index for the child's age group. Body mass index (BMI) is a measurement system used to assess if a child (or adult) is underweight, overweight, or at risk for becoming overweight. Pediatricians use height and weight measurements taken at a child's regular checkup to determine his or her BMI. To help guide parents and others in making good nutritional choices, maintain a healthy BMI, and keep children healthy, the American Medical Association (AMA) suggests the following food choices for children based on the USDA guidelines.

Children two to five years of age

The AMA and USDA recommend food guidelines for young children similar to those for older children and adults, but with smaller portions. When looking at a range of portion sizes, parents and those who care for young children should choose smaller portion sizes for children age two or three, and slightly larger portions for children who are age four or five. Daily recommendations include:

- four to five servings of breads, cereals, rice, pasta
- two or more servings of vegetables
- two or more servings of fruit

- three to four servings of dairy products
- two or three servings of meat, fish, poultry, legumes (beans, lentils, peas)

After age two, a child needs less fat than an infant— about 30% of daily calories. After age three, fiber becomes more important in a child's diet and can impact future heart health.

Calcium requirements steadily increase as children get older, from 500 mg a day at age three to 800 mg a day at age four to eight. There is more calcium in the body than any other mineral. Calcium works together with **phosphorus** (two parts calcium to one part phosphorus) for healthy bones and teeth and works together with **magnesium** (two parts calcium to slightly over one part magnesium) to prevent cardiovascular (blood vessels of the heart) and other degenerative diseases. In order for calcium to be absorbed by the body, it must also have sufficient amounts of vitamins C, D and A. In addition to food sources, an hour of sunshine each day can also provide a child with his/her daily **vitamin D** requirement.

Children six to twelve years of age

By the time children reach age five or six, they begin to tell parents what foods they like. Parents and those who care for children can help select foods from each recommended group that a child will enjoy. Calorie requirements and portion sizes increase as children get older: between ages six and ten, boys and girls need between 1,600 and 2,400 calories each day. During puberty and adolescent growth between ages 10 and 12, girls need about 200 more calories a day. Boys will begin needing about 500 more calories a day after age 12. The following servings per day are recommended for children ages six to twelve:

- six to 11 servings of breads, cereals, rice, pasta
- three to five servings of vegetables
- two to four servings of fruit
- three or four servings of dairy products
- two or three servings of meat, fish, poultry, legumes

By age six, children still need only about 30% of calories from fat. Nutritionists say that by adding five to the child's age, parents can estimate the number of fiber grams a child needs each day. Calcium requirements continue to rise, from 800 mg a day at ages four to eight to 1,300 mg each day for children beginning at age nine.

Preparations

Getting children to eat the right foods is easy if they develop good eating habits at a young age and if they are offered a variety of healthy foods. Many

books, magazines, and web sites offer tips on making healthy foods interesting. Some foods children like from each food group are suggested below.

- breads, cereals, and pastas including whole grain breads, unsweetened cereals, unrefined rice, whole grain crackers, cornbread, rice cakes
- vegetable servings from cooked or raw vegetables such as asparagus, beets, broccoli, carrots, corn, green and red peppers, green beans, kale, peas, pumpkin, squash, sweet potato, tomato, zucchini, or vegetable juice
- good fruit choices such as apples, applesauce, bananas, cantaloupe, apricots, peaches, unsweetened fruit cocktail, plums, grapefruit, kiwi, nectarines, strawberries, watermelon, and fresh fruit juices
- milk, low-fat yogurts and cheeses are good dairy sources, as are low-fat cottage cheese, custard, ice milk, and occasional ice cream servings
- meat, fish, poultry, and legume choices include lean meats, dried beans, peanut butter, shellfish, dried peas, lentils, tofu, and reduced-fat cold cuts

To reduce fat in a child's diet, parents can switch to low-fat or non-fat milk; remove skin from poultry or trim fat from red meat; reduce use of margarine and butter; use low-fat cooking methods such as baking, broiling, and steaming; and serve foods rich in fiber.

Fresh salads can improve fiber in diet, as can adding oat or wheat bran to baked foods. Good, easy-to-assimilate sources of calcium for children, besides milk and cheeses, are tofu made with calcium sulfate; soup made with fish, fowl or beef bones and one tablespoon of wine vinegar to draw out the calcium into the broth; canned salmon and sardines with bones; sesame seeds and tahini (ground sesame seed butter); beans and nuts; calcium-fortified fresh orange juice; greens, especially broccoli, collards, kale, mustard, turnip tops, **parsley**, watercress and **dandelion**; and cooked sea vegetables if children like them.

In *Food and Healing,* Annemarie Colbin explains what sugar is and why it causes so much damage to the health of children and adults. White sugar, like white rice and white flour, goes through an industrial refining process: its juice is extracted from sugar cane, then filtered and boiled until it has been separated from all of its water, minerals, vitamins, protein and fiber, all of which the body needs to digest and metabolize the sugar. Because it lacks those nutrients, refined sugar becomes what Colbin calls a "naked carbohydrate," and so the body will draw them from other foods in the same meal or the body's tissues. Thus when refined white sugar is consumed, there is loss of stored B vitamins, calcium, phosphorus, iron, and other nutrients from the body. The loss of calcium stored in teeth weakens them and makes them more susceptible to bacterial attack/cavities. Also, this nutrient loss from refined sugar consumption can produce hunger for the missing nutrients and provoke great sugar-eating binges. On food labels, sugar is often identified as lactose, maltose, fructose, sucrose, and others. Glucose is the name of sugar found in the blood.

Colbin points out that if you eat meat, you need to digestively balance it with white sugar and vice versa, and that serious problems arise when the amount of sugar eaten is more than the amount needed to balance the meat. Sugar is as addictive as a drug because eating a small amount creates a desire for more sugar and because quitting sugar "cold turkey" brings on withdrawal symptoms that can last for an extended period of time. Typical withdrawal symptoms include strong cravings, **fatigue**, depression, mood swings, and sometimes headaches. Excessive sugar consumption is believed to be involved in such very common problems as **hypoglycemia** or hyperinsulinism, diabetes, **heart disease**, dental caries, high **cholesterol**, obesity, **indigestion**, **myopia** (nearsightedness), seborrheic **dermatitis**, **gout**, genetic narrowing of pelvic and jaw structures, crowding and malformation of teeth, hyperactivity, lack of concentration, depression, and anxiety.

Colbin notes that these problems result when the sugar intake provides more "naked carbohydrates" than are needed to balance the animal protein intake. Since white flour also provides additional "naked carbohydrates," only a small amount of sugar can create an excess amount in the body.

It is important that children eat three meals a day and not skip breakfast. Studies have shown that children and teens who skip breakfast have more trouble concentrating, do not perform as well in school, and often later develop heart disease. Obesity is common in children who skip breakfast.

While the obesity problem in today's youth can be blamed on a number of factors, including larger food portions for adults and children, convenient salty and sugary snack foods, and cheap and convenient fast food, much attention has been focused on the role of the nation's schools. There are fewer physical education classes due to more emphasis on academic classes. Those gym classes that remain do not include enough activities that interest the children, say some experts. School lunches generally have not provided healthy or balanced nutrition but instead have consisted of highly refined, processed foods that are full of additives and simple carbohydrates, which do not provide good nutrition or energy. In addition, many schools also offer "snack bars" or vending machines with sodas and sugary, fatty, or salty snacks. Many children choose these snacks over prepared school lunches.

To counter this problem in schools, the Healthy Schools Summit was held in October 2002. It consisted of representatives from more than 30 national education, fitness, nutrition, and health organizations, as well as 450 school administrators, government leaders, food service directors, counselors, dietitians, nurses, and health and fitness teachers. Since that time, many school districts around the country have been working to improve their physical education programs and to remove or change the selections in vending machines and snack bars on school campuses. Parents can look into lunchtime option at their children's schools or pack healthy lunches from home with foods their children like to ensure they eat well while at school.

Children who are very active and participate in organized sports need a particularly healthy diet. For extended energy, they should eat many complex carbohydrates, such as unrefined rice, whole grain pasta and bread, and whole grain cereal. While all children need to drink plenty of water, those who participate in sports need to drink even more. Some experts say an easy formula to remember is one cup of fluid for every one-half hour of physical activity.

At home, some parents choose convenient snack and fast foods because often, both parents work long hours. Today's youth eat bigger portions, spend more time in front of the television instead of engaged in physical activity, and are growing accustomed to less nutritional foods. Many experts say that getting children up off the couch and watching their snack choices helps. Also, many sources can help parents find healthier alternatives to fast food meals for their families. Suggestions include cooking healthy meals on weekends and freezing them for busy weekdays and looking for cookbooks or online sources of quick and healthy recipes. Simply cooking with less fat and using baking, roasting or poaching methods instead of frying makes meals healthier for everyone. Also, offering children healthy snacks to last them until mealtime will keep them from reaching for poor snack choices and make them less likely to overeat at the evening meal.

For a variety of reasons, some children follow vegetarian diets. Some people are concerned that a vegetarian diet is harmful for children, but generally, if a child aged two or older still follows the recommended Food Guide Pyramid and makes good food choices, a vegetarian diet can be healthy. In fact, 2% of children ages six to 17 never eat meat, fish, or poultry. If a vegetarian child needs a vitamin or mineral supplement, a physician or professional nutritionist can help determine the proper level of supplement needed.

Precautions

Parents are sometimes cautioned by nutritional experts not to turn mealtimes and eating into a battle of wills. Offering a variety of healthy choices allows children to select favorite foods from among those that are good for them and to balance foods containing a number of vitamins and minerals. Research in 2004 showed that taste for certain foods probably develops while people are still infants. In fact, infants in the study who had been exposed to the flavor of carrots through their mothers' breast milk later ate more of a carrot-flavored cereal that those who had not been exposed to carrots as infants. The researchers said that encouraging children to eat more fruits and vegetables as early as possible was helpful.

Many physicians and medical researchers have cautioned parents not to turn to fad diets for their children's weight problems. Many of the diets and diet products on the market have not been proven by clinical studies to be effective in the long term for adults and therefore they certainly have not been proven safe or effective as a solution to weight problems in children. The best solution for childhood obesity is a combination of activity, a balanced diet that follows the AMA/USDA guidelines for food groups and portions, and involvement of a physician, dietician, or other trained professional as needed. A further caution concerning dieting is the concern that as young children enter adolescence, too much worry about weight and appearance can cause social anxieties and lead to eating disorders such as anorexia and bulimia.

When changing a young child's diet, it should be done slowly, particularly when introducing fiber, and with the help of a physician, dietician, or nutritionist. Too much fiber can interfere with the body's absorption of vitamins and minerals.

Children who do not eat enough food and do not get enough nutrition suffer from severe undernourishment, or malnutrition. Each year, more than six million children under the age of five years die around the world as a result of hunger. Malnutrition can also make a child more susceptible to a number of diseases. Worldwide, it is estimated that food insecurity affects 815 million households, mostly in developing countries. However, in 2003, a report showed that at least 10% of U.S. households don't have enough food and about 3% report hunger at home. In this case, it is not the sort of hunger a person feels when they eat a late lunch but the kind of painful sensation someone gets from repeated or involuntary lack of food.

There are parents and health professionals, both traditional and alternative, who feel children should have vitamin/mineral supplements to stay healthy. However, there are also parents and health professionals who believe that when children eat a balanced diet of wholesome foods, they seldom need vitamin supplements; that individual vitamins and minerals should be taken, like medicine, when a deficiency has been created by a diet imbalance; and that when such a deficiency has been corrected, they should be discontinued.

If children are not eating a healthy diet and are being given a vitamin/mineral supplement, it is important to keep chewable vitamins out of reach of young children, as their appealing taste may be irresistible and dosage needs to be controlled according to directions. Children with poor appetites or erratic eating habits also may benefit from vitamins and minerals. It is best to check with a pediatrician, dietician or nutritionist for dosing.

Some parents and health professionals feel that vegetarian children may benefit from vitamin/mineral supplementation because they may lack some iron and **zinc** normally obtained through meat products and/or fish. Other substantial sources of iron are eggs, whole-grain breads and cereals, leafy and other vegetables, potatoes, fruit and milk. Foods containing **vitamin C** (broccoli, Brussels sprouts, collards, kale, parsley, sweet peppers, strawberries, grapefruit, melons, tangerines, potatoes, and more) will increase absorption of iron in non-animal foods. Vegetarian sources of zinc are eggs, legumes, and whole grains. Zinc deficiency has been found in populations whose intake is derived solely from cereal sources, but in recent studies, vegetarians had adequate zinc levels. Those children who avoid dairy products, although it is difficult to get enough, may get calcium from broccoli, leafy green vegetables like kale, canned salmon and sardines including the bones, and soy products. If a child's physician or qualified nutritionist feels a supplement is necessary, he/she should recommend the dosage.

Children often don't recognize feelings of thirst and have to be encouraged to drink before becoming thirsty. If a child's urine is clear or the color of pale lemonade, he or she is drinking enough fluids. Dark urine the color of apple juice indicates too little fluid and the child is in danger of dehydration or heatstroke.

Side effects

Only the fat-soluble (capable of being dissolved in fat or oil) vitamins A, D, K and E have side effects that are potentially, though rarely, toxic (poisonous).

In their book *The Real Vitamin & Mineral Book*, Sheri Lieberman and Nancy Bruning state, "The facts are that only a few vitamins and minerals have any known toxicities, all of which are reversible, with the exception of vitamin D. Anything can be harmful if you take enough of it—even pure water. But vitamins and minerals are among the safest substances on earth. The amounts needed to become toxic are enormous." They add that being on medication or having a medical condition can influence vitamin/mineral requirements and indicate that when one's physician is not well-versed in nutrition, it is ideal to have him or her work with a qualified nutritionist.

With regard to vitamin D, they indicate, "According to several studies, up to 1,000 IU per day of vitamin D appears to be safe. Both the beneficial and adverse effects of exceeding this amount are controversial. Overdosing of vitamin D is *irreversible and may be fatal*. Symptoms of too much vitamin D are **nausea**, loss of appetite, **headache**, **diarrhea**, fatigue, restlessness, and calcification of the soft tissues (insoluble lime salts in tissue) of the lungs and the kidneys, as well as the bones." Vitamin D (400 IU) is usually sold with **vitamin A** (5,000 IU) in a tiny tablet or capsule.

Lieberman and Bruning say that active vitamin A from fish liver oil or synthetic palmitate is stored in the liver; that 15,000 IU would cause problems in infants; but that 100,000 IU of active vitamin A would have to be taken daily for months before any signs of toxicity (state of being poisonous) appear. Vitamin A in the form of beta-carotene can be taken without any risk of toxicity.

At doses of 800–1,200 IU per day, Lieberman and Bruning found no well-documented toxicity of **vitamin E**. At doses of over 1,200 IU per day, adverse effects such as flatulence, diarrhea, nausea, headache, heart palpitations, and fainting have been reported, but were completely reversible when dosage was reduced.

Vitamin K is easily obtained by the body from a healthy diet and deficiencies are rare, especially in children. It is given prophylactically to newborn infants to prevent hemorrhage and before surgery to people with blood-clotting problems. Lieberman and Bruning describe the major effect of too much vitamin K as an **anemia** where red blood cells die more quickly than usual and cannot be replaced by the body.

Some children have severe food allergies. It is important to watch for signs of allergies in very young children in particular, since they are eating many foods for the first time. Signs of food allergies can range from mild to severe. A child may, for instance, eat peanuts or shellfish and immediately show signs of a severe reaction, such as swelling and trouble breathing. Other food allergies may be less obvious but may occur from common foods found in many everyday products such as milk, eggs, wheat, or soy. If a child appears to have a severe reaction and has trouble breathing, the parent or caregiver should seek immediate medical attention, since the allergic reaction may be serious. If a child has ongoing problems such as **eczema** or other allergic reactions or signs of intolerance to foods, the parent may choose to seek help from a registered dietician and/or an allopathic physician who specializes in allergies. The allopathic physician may test the child first to determine the source of the allergies. The dietician will work with the family to help plan ways to meet nutritional needs while avoiding foods that cause allergic reaction or intolerance.

The parent of an allergic child can also choose to seek help from a homeopathic or naturopathic physician.

Andrew Weil, M.D., author of *Spontaneous Healing*, a *New York Times* number one bestseller that sold well over one million copies, believes that the body can heal itself and believes allergies are learned responses of the immune system to environmental agents that are not necessarily harmful. Weil says treatment should focus on calming an over-reactive immune system in order to alleviate allergy symptoms. Allergies can and are frequently "healed." However, traditional allergy medications tend to be "more or less" toxic to the body and can increase an allergic response over time.

To increase the likelihood of spontaneous healing, Dr. Weil made the following recommendations. Dietary modification to reduce allergic responses: following a low-protein diet; cutting down on animal protein in general; eliminating cow's milk and products made from it because they are known to irritate the immune system; and eating organically grown foods as much as possible to avoid agricultural chemicals that cause immune system reaction. Regular use of **quercetin**, a natural product from buckwheat and citrus fruits, that stabilizes cell membranes that release histamine, which is involved in many allergic reactions. Quercetin is a preventative and Dr. Weil recommends it be used regularly. The recommended dose is 400 mg twice a day between meals. For **hay fever**, the freeze-dried extract of the herb stinging **nettle**, one to two capsules every two to four hours as needed, he says will control symptoms with none of the toxicity of antihistamines or steroids. He also recommends a safe nasal spray, Nasalcrom, which works like quercetin. In the home, environmental methods like installing air filters can reduce allergic effects on and relieve the immune system. And finally, some allergic reactions indicate that high brain levels are involved in misdirected immune system response, and mind/body intervention is suggested.

Research and general acceptance

The AMA has based many of its food choices on the Dietary Guidelines for Americans, which were developed through research by the U.S. Department of Agriculture and the U.S. Department of Human Services. Input for the guidelines comes from a number of resources, including national surveys from the Centers for Disease Control (CDC).

As for children and the general public, accepting the importance of nutrition is another story. A 2003 study from the American Dietetic Association reported that preteens and their parents weren't concerned about preteens' weight being a health risk. Children and parents related obesity more to food than to physical activity and many overweight children said they didn't have much opportunity for physical activity.

Training and certification

Qualified dieticians and nutritionists may have a bachelor's, master's or a doctoral degree in nutrition and dietetics from an accredited college. They are also required to constantly update their knowledge with continuing education. Through the American Dietetic Association, these professionals can gain certification in their fields, including a certificate of training in childhood and adolescent weight management. Pediatricians obtain M.D. or D.O degrees and some specialize in childhood diseases and treatment. In the field of alternative medicine, parents may choose to seek treatment from naturopaths and homeopaths.

Andrew Weil, M.D. in *Spontaneous Healing* points out the benefits of **naturopathic medicine**. "Naturopathy comes from the old tradition of European health spas with their emphasis on hydro (water) therapy, massage, and nutritional and herbal treatment." Naturopaths are well trained in the sciences and have more experience with nutritional and herbal medicine than many allopathic physicians. Naturopathy is based on a general philosophy that focuses on the body's natural healing potential in an attempt to circumvent the use of drugs and surgery; however, naturopathic physicians may focus on different methods, using such therapies as **acupuncture**, bodywork, herbalism, and **homeopathy**. They are licensed in only a few states in the United States, mostly in the West. According to Dr. Weil, "Good naturopaths are worth consulting for childhood illnesses, recurrent upper respiratory **infections** and sinusitis, gynecological problems, and all ailments for which conventional doctors have only suppressive treatments. Naturopaths can be valuable as advisors to help people design healthy lifestyles." To find a naturopathic physician in their area, parents can contact the American Association of Naturopathic Physicians, 601 Valley Street, Suite 105, Seattle, Washington 98109, (206) 298-0126.

With regard to homeopathy, Dr. Weil also has positive feedback for the discipline. Homeopathy is a system that has a two hundred year old history. Homeopaths use diluted natural remedies to work on the body's energy field and encourage healing. Homeopathic physicians can be M.D.s, osteopaths, naturopaths, chiropractors, or lay persons. If a parent wishes to consult an alternative practitioner for homeopathic advice, the National Center for Homeopathy can be contacted at 801 North Fairfax Street, Suite 306, Alexandria, Virginia 22314, (703) 548-7790.

Resources

BOOKS

Colbin, Annemarie. *Food and Healing*. New York: Ballantine Books, 1986, 1996.

Colbin, Annemarie. *The Book of Whole Meals*. New York: Ballantine Books, 1983.

Colbin, Annemarie. *The Natural Gourmet*. New York: Ballantine Books, 1989.

Dufty, William. *Sugar Blues*. New York: Warner Books, 1978.

Estella, Mary. *Natural Foods Cookbook*. New York: Harper & Row, 1985.

Hewitt, Jean. *The New York Times Natural Foods Cookbook*. New York: Avon Books, 1972.

Kordich, Jay. *The Juiceman's Power of Juicing*. New York: Warner Books, 1993.

Lappe, Frances Moore. *Diet for a Small Planet*. New York: Ballantine Books, 1991.

Lieberman, Sheri , and Nancy Bruning. *The Real Vitamin and Mineral Book*. New York: Avery Publishing Group, Inc., 1990.

Mindell, Earl, Ph.D, R.Ph. *Vitamin Bible for the 21st Century*. New York: Warner Books, 1999.

Walker, Norman W., D.Sc. *Fresh Vegetable and Fruit Juices*. Prescott, Arizona: Norwalk Press, 1970.

Weil, Andrew, M.D. *Spontaneous Healing*. New York: Ballantine Books, 1995.

PERIODICALS

Berler, Ron. "The Problem is Big: More Kids than Ever are Overweight. We'll Tell You About the Crisis, Offer Some Solutions, and Explain Why Controlling Your Weight Can Make You a Better Athlete." *Sports Illustrated for Kids* (October 1, 2003): 60.

"Food Insecurity." *Pediatrics* (February 2003): 357–358.

"Kids Don't Think Obesity is a Health Problem." *Nutrition Today* (July-August 2003): 115–116.

McCook, Alison. "Food Taste Acceptance 'Programmed' in Infancy." *Reuters Health* (April 5, 2004).

ORGANIZATIONS

American Academy of Pediatrics. 141 Northwest Point Boulevard, Elk Grove Village, IL 60007-1098. (888) 227-1770. http://www.aap.org/family.

American Herbalists Guild. P.O. Box 1683. Soquel, CA 95073. 408-464-2441.

American Holistic Medical Association. 5728 Old McLean Village Drive. McLean, VA 22101-3906. (703) 556-9728.

International Food Information Council. 1100 Connecticut Avenue, NW, Suite 430, Washington, DC, 20036. (202) 296-6540. http://www.ific.org.

KidsHealth/Nemours Foundation. 4600 Touchton Road East, Building 200, Suite 500, Jacksonville, FL 32246. http://www.kidshealth.org.

U.S. Department of Agriculture and U.S. Department of Health and Human Services. (888) 878-3256. http://www.usda.gov/FoodAndNutrition.

OTHER

BMI For Children and Teens. National Center for Chronic Disease Prevention and Health Promotion. [cited June 16, 2004]. http://www.cdc.gov/nccdphp/dnpa/bmi/bmi-for-age.htm.

Healthy Food Choices: Six to 12 Years. American Medical Association. [cited June 16, 2004]. http://www.medem.com.

Healthy Food Choices: Two to Five Years. American Medical Association. [cited June 16, 2004]. http://www.medem.com.

Report Card on the Diet Quality of Children Ages Two to Nine. Publication of the USDA Center for Nutrition Policy and Promotion. [cited June 16, 2004]. http://www.cnpp.usda.gov.

Ruth Ann Carter

Chili pepper *see* **Cayenne**

Chills

Definition

Chills is the common name for a feeling of coldness accompanied by shivering and possibly **fever**.

Causes and symptoms

Chills may occur for the following reasons:

- Exposure to extremely low outside temperature.
- Insufficient protection from cold temperature or weather.
- Age, as newborns and elders are intolerant of cold temperature.
- Anemia, particularly in women who frequently complain of cold intolerance. The condition is frequently found in females of reproductive age due to significant monthly blood loss during menses.
- Stress or poor health condition.
- Malnutrition. Poor diet and/or B-complex vitamin deficiency often makes a person more sensitive to cold temperature.
- Hypothyroidism. Hypothyroidism is one of the most common reasons for cold intolerance in women.
- Diabetes.
- Poor immune function as in AIDS or cancer patients. In these patients, chills and shivering may be signs of

infections (most likely), tumors, drug-induced fever, or malnutrition.

- Infections. Chills and fever are often caused by the common cold or viral infections. However, they may also be due to something more serious such as cystitis (bladder infection), septicemia (blood infections), pneumonia, meningitis, malaria or tuberculosis.
- Medications. Certain medications such as beta interferons can cause chills as side effect.
- Unknown infections or diseases.

Diagnosis

Those suffering from chills should investigate possible causes if the symptoms persist or are accompanied by fever and/or night sweat. They may be a sign or symptom of a serious condition and may require medical attention. A doctor can make accurate diagnosis of underlying diseases through detailed questioning about the chills, accompanying symptoms if any, patient's diet, daily **stress**, and lifestyle. In addition, doctors may order blood tests for **anemia**, **hypothyroidism**, or **infections** if these conditions are suspected.

Treatment

Alternative treatment of chills includes protecting oneself from inclement weather conditions, drinking warm teas, and making appropriate dietary changes. Ayurvedic treatment might include fomenation therapy, called *svedana*, to aggravate the fatty tissue and force excess sweat out of the body. Svedana is used to relieve bodily stiffness, heaviness, and coldness.

In **traditional Chinese medicine**, those complaining of chills should follow a diet of "warming" foods and avoid "cold" foods. Reference to cold or warming does not mean the actual temperature of the food, but its internal effect. In general, the Chinese recommend cooked rather than cold, raw foods for this condition. The Ayurvedic formula for producing internal heat is *trikodu*, made of equal parts of **ginger**, black pepper, and long pepper (pippali, native to India and Java), and alleviating coldness and stagnation in the body.

Nutritional therapy

The following dietary changes are recommended to help prevent chills and cold intolerance:

- Limiting alcohol and caffeine intake and refraining from smoking tobacco products. These chemicals increase cold intolerance.
- Drinking warm tea with or without herbs such as ginger (a warming herb used in Chinese and Native American medicine) or chamomile.

- Taking daily multiple vitamin/mineral supplement or B-complex vitamins with C. People who are deficient of B-vitamins often are sensitive to cold temperature.

Allopathic treatment

Persons should consult their doctors if cold intolerance is severe or if chills are often followed by persistent fever or night sweats. They may be signs or symptoms of serious conditions or infections. Hypothyroidism or poor thyroid function should also be ruled out in women complaining of cold sensitivity.

If cold intolerance is accompanied by other signs and symptoms of thyroid deficiency such as lethargy, **obesity**, and **depression**, persons should consult their doctor for treatment of hypothyroidism. Thyroid supplement may be necessary.

Patients should also be concerned if chills frequently occur with fever. Fever may be the body's response to infections. Persistent chills, night sweat, fever, and rapid weight loss should be brought to a doctor's attention. They may be symptoms of **cancer** or infections such as **AIDS** or **tuberculosis**. Chills and fever in immunodeficient patients are often signs of infections that can be serious in patients with weakened immune systems.

Fever and chills can often be treated with over-the-counter medication such as acetaminophen or ibuprofen. Aspirin should not be given to a child for fear of Reye's syndrome. Patients should be given soups, fruit juices, or water to replace fluid loss due to fever. If fever is high (more than 104°F [40°]), occurs in newborns (less than three months old) or lasts longer than 48 hours, a physician should be contacted.

Prevention

Wearing appropriate clothes for the weather, eating nutritious foods, and taking dietary supplements may help prevent chills in some people.

Resources

BOOKS

The Burton Goldberg Group. "Chills." In *Alternative Medicine: The Definitive Guide*. Tiburon, CA: Future Medical Publishing, Inc., 1999.

Yoder, Ernest. "Disorders due to Heat and Cold." In *Cecil Textbook of Medicine*, 2nd ed. Philadelphia: W.B. Saunders Company, 2000.

ORGANIZATIONS

National Cancer Institute. Building 31, Room 10A24, 9000 Rockville Pike, Bethesda, MD 20892. (800) 422-6237.

OTHER

Strange, Carolyn J. "Fighting the (I'm) Cold War." *iVillage.com*. http://onhealth.com/women/columnist/item,46788.asp.

PDQ. "Fever, Chills and Sweats." *CBS Health Watch*. http://cbs.medscape.com.

Mai Tran

Chinese angelica *see* **Dong quai**

Chinese bupleurum *see* **Chinese thoroughwax**

Chinese foxglove root

Description

Chinese **foxglove** root is a perennial herb found in northern China. It grows 6-8 in (15-20 cm) tall and has long oval leaves that are covered with fine hairs, fluted flowers that are reddish orange tinted with purple, and a round fruit. The root is thick and reddish yellow. Chinese foxglove root is collected in the fall. Its Latin name is *Rehmannia glutinosa* and it is also called *Rehmannia chinensis*.

General use

In China, Chinese foxglove root is used as a remedy for many different ailments: blurred vision, chronic **fever**, **constipation**, heart palpitations, hearing problems, **hot flashes**, **insomnia**, light-headedness, **low back pain**, menstrual irregularity and uterine bleeding (especially after **childbirth**), night sweats, restlessness, and stiff joints. It is also used to combat the effects of **aging**. Its effectiveness in treating these ailments has not been verified.

Preparations

Chinese foxglove root is washed and dried in the sun. It is sold in large, fleshy brownish-yellow chunks and tastes sweet and moist. The root is used in two stages of preparation: dried and cooked. To make dried Chinese foxglove root, called *sheng di huang* or dry Rehmannia, the fresh root is removed from the sand, washed well, then dried in the sun during the winter. Cooked Chinese foxglove root, called *shu di huang* or cooked Rehmannia, is prepared by steaming the fresh root until it is cooked, letting it dry, then steaming and drying it again several times. Cooking Chinese foxglove root is said to enhance the herb's properties as a blood tonic. To combat the effects of aging, the root is prepared with cardamon so that it is easier to digest and use as a tonic. The raw form of the root is a cooler herb and used for symptoms of heat. The cooked root is more of a blood tonic.

Chinese medicine practitioners also make special preparations of Chinese foxglove root for specific ailments. It can be mixed with gelatin for coughing and **vomiting** blood, **nosebleeds**, and bleeding from the uterus. It can be mixed with **cornus** and **Chinese yam** or freshwater turtle shell as a remedy for symptoms such as forgetfulness, insomnia, and lightheadedness. Rehmannia is the main ingredient in the Chinese six flavor Rehmannia tonic used for ailments and discomfort such as frequent urination, **infertility**, **impotence**, and weak and painful knees.

Both cooked Chinese foxglove root and the raw version are available in Chinese pharmacies, Asian markets, and some Western health food stores. There are no formal guidelines for recommended doses of Chinese foxglove root.

Precautions

People who have digestive problems, especially those who tend to have **gas** or become bloated, should use Chinese foxglove root with care; the cooked root can swell the belly and cause loose stools. There is no information available on what happens to people who take an overdose of Chinese foxglove root.

Side effects

The use of Chinese foxglove root can cause **diarrhea**, **nausea**, and abdominal **pain**. Many Chinese herbalists include **grains-of-paradise fruit**, a kind of cardamon, in their Chinese foxglove root preparations to prevent these side effects.

Interactions

No interactions due to use of Chinese foxglove root have been reported.

Resources

BOOKS

Reid, D. *A Handbook of Chinese Healing Herbs*. Boston: Shambhala Publications, Inc., 1995.

Sifton, David W., ed. *The PDR Family Guide to Natural Medicines & Healing Therapies*. New York: Three Rivers Pr., 1999.

OTHER

China-Med.net. Traditional Chinese Medicine. "Radix Rehmanniae." Paracel@clarityconnect.com. http://www.china-med.net/herb_search.html. (May 2000).

Lori De Milto

Chinese gentiana *see* **Gentiana**

Chinese massage

Definition

Chinese massage is the name for a family of massage therapies practiced within **traditional Chinese medicine**. In traditional Chinese practice, massage is one of the fundamental treatment modalities, along with dietary regulation, herbal medicine, acupuncture/moxibustion, and therapeutic **exercise**.

Origins

The history of massage as a part of Chinese medical treatment dates back about 4,000 years. Written massage textbooks began to appear as early as the fourth century B.C., along with the earliest Chinese medical texts. Massage appears to have developed alongside both therapeutic exercise (**qigong**) and **acupuncture**, as it depends on the same understanding of the meridians and the flow of qi in the human body. The type of massage known as qi healing, or curing with external qi, was developed by master teachers of qigong.

Benefits

Chinese massage is not intended to be an experience of pampering or **relaxation**. It is a form of deep tissue therapy that conveys the following benefits:

- speeding the healing of injuries and clearing bruises
- stimulating blood circulation and regulating the nervous system
- removing scar tissue
- easing emotional distress
- curing some conditions affecting the internal organs
- increasing flexibility in the joints and improving posture
- relieving chronic pain
- maintaining wellness and functioning as a form of preventive care
- improving athletic performance
- strengthening the body's resistance to disease

The fact that some forms of Chinese massage do not require extensive training and can be used at home is another benefit of this modality.

Description

Theoretical background

The techniques of Chinese massage are inseparable from the philosophical belief system that underlies traditional Chinese medicine. Chinese massage is holistic in its orientation, which means that massage is understood to affect the patient's entire being, not just his or her physical body.

Several concepts are important in understanding all the major forms of Chinese massage, including *qi*, *jing luo*, *xue*, and *jin*.

Qi, sometimes spelled chi or ki, is the basic life energy animating the universe as well as human beings. The word can be translated into English as "breath" or "air." Qi can be transferred or transmuted. In humans, the digestive tract extracts the qi from food, whereas the lungs extract it from the air. When these two forms of qi meet in the bloodstream, they form human qi, which then circulates throughout the body.

The meridians or channels (*jing luo*) are a network of energy pathways that link and balance the various organs. The meridians have four functions: to connect the internal organs with the exterior of the body and connect the person to the environment and the universe; to harmonize the yin and yang principles within the body's organs and Five Substances; to distribute qi within the body; and to protect the body against external imbalances related to weather. When the *jing luo* are blocked so that qi and blood cannot circulate, the person experiences physical **pain**.

The acupoints (*xue*) are locations on the body where qi tends to collect and can be manipulated or redirected. They are connected to different body organs through the meridians.

The soft and connective tissues (*jin*) and the joints all affect the flow of qi along the meridians. Thus, one function of Chinese massage is to relax the patient's *jin*.

In general, Chinese massage emphasizes movement and communication. The basic purpose of massage is to restore free movement to the patient's qi and blood. Chinese massage therapists use a range of techniques to accomplish this goal: they press, knuckle-roll, squeeze, knead, dig, drag, pluck, tweak, hammer, push, stretch, vibrate, knock, and even tread on the body with their feet. Massage accomplishes its purpose in three ways: it activates the activity of qi and blood, it regulates their movement and disperses stagnation, and it removes external causes of blockage (cold and damp). Since Chinese practitioners regard massage as affecting all dimensions of the patient's being, they think of it as involving communication between the therapist's qi and the patient's qi. In *Tui na* massage, the patient is allowed or even encouraged to talk while the therapist is working. This practice often helps the patient to release stored-up feelings.

Tui na massage

Tui na massage takes its name from two Chinese words that mean "push and pull." It requires the controlled use of very deep but constantly moving pressure, repeated hundreds of times. The practitioner pushes hard with the ball of the thumb then rubs lightly around the area being treated. A therapist using this form of massage might spend as much time on one of the patient's joints or limbs as a Western therapist would spend massaging the entire body. *Tui na* is used to treat a wide variety of conditions that would require a team of physiotherapists,

chiropractors, and physicians specializing in sports medicine to treat in the West. One Chinese medical book lists over 140 conditions that can be treated with *Tui na*, including disorders of the internal organs as well as **sprains**, pulled muscles, arthritis, and **sciatica**, a pain in the lower back and back of the thighs.

Chinese pediatric massage

Chinese pediatric massage, or *xiao er tui na*, is a form of *Tui na* massage adapted to the special needs of children from birth to 12 years of age. The Chinese believe that a child's energy system is different from an adult's because children have fewer physical and emotional barriers in place. Their qi is therefore more accessible to treatment. The acupoints and techniques used in pediatric massage are different from those used with adults. Massage oil, typically **sesame oil**, is often used with children. The sessions are much shorter than those for adults, usually only 15 to 20 minutes, but they may be repeated several times a day for children who are seriously ill. Pediatric massage is used to treat such chronic conditions as **asthma**, **bedwetting**, and nightmares as well as teething, **colic**, **nausea**, **fever**, **constipation**, and the **common cold**. Parents often learn the basic techniques of pediatric massage as preventive health care for their children or to treat minor illnesses.

An mo massage

An mo is a type of massage used for health maintenance and to restore vitality. Its name means "press and stroke" in Chinese. It can be used at home but is also part of **martial arts**, qigong, and athletic training. *An mo* differs from *Tui na* massage in that it is a full-body balanced treatment. *An mo* combines yang techniques to break up stagnant qi and activate its flow, followed by yin techniques to soothe and calm the body. *An mo* has a set pattern of movements and techniques that the therapist follows, but these can be adjusted to the patient's needs. A session of *An mo* massage may last as long as two hours, particularly if there is a strong qi communication between the therapist and the patient.

Dian xue massage (acupressure)

Dian xue, or "point press," is familiar to many Westerners as **acupressure**. It uses the same acupoints on the body as acupuncture but relies on pressure from the fingers rather than needles. *Dian xue* can be used by massage therapists to stimulate two different acupoints, one with each hand, while the area of the body between the points is stretched or twisted to maximize the flow of qi. *Dian xue* can be given in the home and is sometimes used by acupuncturists when needles cannot be used.

Qi healing massage

The Chinese name of this form of massage is *wai qi liao fa*, or "curing with external qi." In qi healing, a qigong master who has practiced the art for many years transmits qi directly to the patient. Qi healing massage represents one strand of Chinese traditional practice in which healers passed on their own discoveries of the healing arts only to their closest disciples.

Preparations

Chinese massage is usually given with the patient lying on one side on a couch or seated on a chair or stool. The patient typically wears thin cotton clothing, particularly if the massage is being given in a public hospital or clinic. In smaller communities, the practitioner may work directly on the patient's skin. Touching the skin directly is thought to improve communication with the patient's qi; it also allows the application of herbal preparations to the skin.

Tui na massage is preceded by taking a full case history using the traditional four examinations of Chinese medicine (verbal interview; visual observation, which includes close examination of the tongue; listening to the patient's breathing and coughing; and touching, which includes taking twelve separate pulses). The massage therapist uses the information from the four examinations to identify the root complaint, the underlying pattern causing it, and the principles that will govern the treatment.

Precautions

Apart from giving a case history prior to receiving *Tui na* massage, no special precautions are necessary.

Side effects

Side effects are usually limited to some soreness, particularly after the first session of *Tui na* massage. This discomfort usually goes away after several more sessions. Pediatric massage is said to have few or no side effects. On rare occasions, patients have experienced headaches or mild stomach upset. These side effects are attributed to the imbalance or stagnation in the patient's qi prior to treatment.

Research and general acceptance

Between 1985 and 2005, Chinese massage became widely accepted in the West. A growing number of Western practitioners studied Chinese massage and

obtained their training and certification from centers of traditional Chinese medical education. As of 2008, numerous alternative treatment centers in the United States offered Chinese massage along with Western forms of bodywork. Still another indication of the wider acceptance of Chinese forms of treatment is the emergence of hybrid massage therapies that combine Chinese techniques with those derived from other Oriental traditions of massage or from Western practices.

Training and certification

In China, massage is part of the curriculum of traditional Chinese schools of medicine, since it is an important aspect of primary health care. Graduates of these schools must pass rigorous examinations and government licensing procedures before setting up their practices. In addition, it is common for Chinese physicians to visit other practitioners as patients in order to learn about specialized techniques for treating specific conditions with massage. Last, many Chinese physicians come from families that have produced several generations of healers; younger practitioners often learn the techniques of massage from older family members. The master/apprentice model of teaching is still followed in traditional Chinese medical training in the twenty-first century.

In the United States, the Accreditation Commission for Acupuncture and Oriental Medicine (ACAOM) is the national accrediting agency, recognized by the U.S. Department of Education, that accredits acupuncture and Oriental medicine master degree level programs. The ACOM represents more than 50 schools and colleges with accredited or candidacy status.

The National Certification Commission for Acupuncture and Oriental Medicine (NCCAOM) is the only nationally recognized certification program available to qualified practitioners of acupuncture and Oriental medicine. NCCAOM certification is a requirement for licensure in most states. NCCAOM certifications are offered in acupuncture, Chinese herbology, Oriental medicine and Asian bodywork therapy.

The American Organization for the Bodywork Therapies of Asia (AOBTA) and the American Association of Acupuncture Oriental Medicine (AAAOM) are professional organizations that represent practitioners of Oriental medicine. These groups support appropriate credentialing, define scope of practice and educational standards, and provide training, professional development, and networking resources to their members.

KEY TERMS

Acupoint—A point or site on the body where qi tends to accumulate. Acupoints are pressed or manipulated in Chinese massage in order to activate or redirect the patient's qi.

An mo—A form of Chinese massage that treats the whole body and emphasizes balancing yin and yang techniques in the treatment. Its name means "press and stroke" in Chinese.

Dian xue—The Chinese name for acupressure. This form of massage can be done at home as well as by a trained therapist.

Qi—The Chinese word for life energy. Since traditional Chinese medicine understands pain to be the result of blocked or stagnant qi, all forms of Chinese massage are intended to restore free movement to the patient's qi and blood.

Tui na—A form of Chinese massage that focuses on a part of the patient's body in order to treat injuries and chronic pain. Its name literally means "push and pull" in Chinese.

Resources

BOOKS

Maciocia, Giovanni. *The Foundations of Chinese Medicine: A Comprehensive Text for Acupuncturists and Herbalists,* 2nd ed. Philadelphia: Churchill Livingstone/Elsevier, 2005.

Yang, Jwing-Ming. *Qigong Massage: Fundamental Techniques for Health and Relaxation,* 2nd ed. Boston: YMAA Publication Center, 2005.

ORGANIZATIONS

Alternative Medicine Foundation, PO Box 60016, Potomac, MD, 20859, (301) 340-1960, http://www.amfoundation.org.

American Association of Acupuncture Oriental Medicine, PO Box 162340, Sacramento, CA, 95816, (866) 455-7999, (916) 443-4770, http://www.aaaomonline.org.

American Organization for the Bodywork Therapies of Asia (AOBTA), Laurel Oak Corporate Center, Suite 408, 1010 Haddenfield-Berlin Rd., Voorhees, NJ, 08043, (856) 782-1616, http://www.aobta.org/.

Accreditation Commission for Acupuncture and Oriental Medicine (ACAOM), Maryland Trade Center #3, 7501 Greenway Center Dr., Suite 760, Greenbelt, MD, 20770, (301) 313-0855, http://www.acaom.org.

National Center for Complementary and Alternative Medicine. National Institutes of Health, 9000 Rockville Pike, Bethesda, MD, 20892, (888) 644-6226, http://www.nccam.nih.gov.

National Certification Commission for Acupuncture and Oriental Medicine (NCCAOM), 76 South Laura St., Suite 1290, Jacksonville, FL, 32202, (904) 598-1005, http://www.nccaom.org/.

Rebecca Frey
Angela M. Costello

Chinese medicine *see* **Traditional Chinese medicine**

Chinese system of food cures

Definition

The Chinese system of food cures regards dietary regulation as preventive medicine as well as a corrective measure to be undertaken when one falls ill. Diet is one of four major treatment modalities in **traditional Chinese medicine**, the other three being acupuncture/moxibustion, herbal medicine, and massage, plus remedial physical **exercise**.

Origins

The selection of foods in the diet as part of a lifelong program of health maintenance and treatment of illness has been a part of Chinese medicine from its beginnings. The first extensive written Chinese medical treatises (as the West understands the term) date from the Han dynasty (206 B.C.–A.D. 220), but the use of food as preventive medicine probably goes several thousand years further back. Legends says that tribal shamans and holy men who lived as hermits in the mountains of China as early as 3500 B.C. practiced what was called the "Way of Long Life." This regimen included a diet based on herbs and other plants, **qigong** exercises, and special breathing techniques that were thought to improve vitality and life expectancy.

After the Han dynasty, the next great age of Chinese medicine was under the Tang emperors, who ruled from A.D. 608 to A.D. 906. The first Tang emperor established China's first medical school in A.D. 629. This period produced China's earliest expert on dietary therapy, Sun Simiao. He specialized in the treatment of diseases caused by malnutrition and wrote several works on diet and health. Sun Simiao's principle of using diet and lifestyle changes as the first line of treatment for illness has governed traditional Chinese practice ever since. According to Sun Simiao, only when dietary treatment is not enough to cure the patient should the doctor turn to **acupuncture** and herbal medicines.

Benefits

The benefits of traditional Chinese dietary treatment are many years of vigorous good health. According to the *Nei Jing*, China's oldest medical classic, the metaphor is that human beings are constituted to live for a hundred years, barring accidents or violence. Diet and good digestion are considered the most important ways to maintain physical strength and vitality.

Description

Chinese food cures are based on the philosophical principles of Taoism and its teachers' observations about nature. Some of its concepts are difficult for Westerners to understand because they rely on symbols and images rather than scientific measurements and theories. In general, Chinese medicine regards the human organism as an integrated entity within itself and as linked to the family, society, and the natural order by a pattern of symbolic connections.

The cosmic and natural order

In early Chinese philosophy, the Tao, or universal first principle, generated a duality of opposing principles that underlie all the patterns of nature. These principles, yin and yang, are mutually dependent as well as polar opposites. Yin represents everything that is cold, moist, dim, responsive, slow, heavy, and moving downward or inward; while yang represents heat, dryness, brightness, activity, rapidity, lightness, and upward or outward motion. The dynamic interaction of these two principles is reflected in the cycles of the seasons, the human life cycle, and other natural phenomena.

In addition to yin and yang, Taoist teachers also believed that the Tao produced a third force, primordial energy or chi (also spelled *qi* or *ki*, the Japanese term). The interplay between yin, yang, and chi gave rise to the Five Elements of water, wood, fire, earth, and metal. These entities are all reflected in the structure and functioning of the human body.

The human being

Traditional Chinese physicians did not learn about the structures of the human body from dissection (although they did perform some animal studies) because they thought that cutting open a body insulted the person's ancestors. Instead they built up an understanding of the location and functions of the major

organs over centuries of observation, and then correlated them with the principles of yin, yang, chi, and the Five Elements. Thus wood is related to the liver (yin) and the gall bladder (yang); fire to the heart (yin) and the small intestine (yang); earth to the spleen (yin) and the stomach (yang); metal to the lungs (yin) and the large intestine (yang); and water to the kidneys (yin) and the bladder (yang). The Chinese also believed that the body contains Five Essential Substances, which include blood, spirit, vital essence (a principle of growth and development produced by the body from chi and blood), fluids (all body fluids other than blood, such as saliva, spinal fluid, sweat, etc.), and chi.

A unique feature of traditional Chinese medicine is the meridian system. Chinese doctors viewed the body as regulated by a network of energy pathways called meridians that link and balance the various organs. The meridians have four functions: to connect the internal organs with the exterior of the body, and connect the person to the environment and the universe; to harmonize the yin and yang principles within the body's organs and Five Substances; to distribute chi within the body; and to protect the body against external imbalances related to weather (wind, summer heat, dampness, dryness, cold, and fire).

The composition and use of foods

Chinese food cures operate within this system of cosmic principles, symbolic correlation of internal organs with the five elements, and the meridian system. Food serves several functions in traditional Chinese medicine. It supplies nutritional energy to the body to replenish chi. It is also used by the body to produce vital essence and blood. Lastly, foods can be chosen to regulate the balance of yin and yang and the five elements within the body and to direct the flow of chi to different parts of the body.

Chinese medicine classifies foods according to four sets of categories:

- Temperature. Foods are classified as cold or cool (yin); or warm or hot (yang).
- Taste. There are five tastes correlated with the Five Elements: sour (wood); bitter (fire); sweet (earth); pungent (metal); and salty (water).
- Direction of action. Pungent, salty, and bland foods are thought to have an ascending or floating action that redirects chi upward, while sour, bitter, and sweet foods are thought to have a descending or sinking action that moves the chi downward.
- The organ or meridian affected by the food.

Chinese medicine uses foods to keep the body in internal harmony and in a state of balance with the external environment. In giving dietary advice, the Chinese physician takes into account the weather, the season, the geography of the area, and the patient's specific imbalances (including emotional upsets) in order to select foods that will counteract excesses or supply deficient elements. Basic preventive dietary care, for example, would recommend eating yin foods in the summer, which is a yang season. In the winter, by contrast, yang foods should be eaten to counteract the yin temperatures. In the case of illness, yin symptom patterns (**fatigue**, pale complexion, weak voice) would be treated with yang foods, while yang symptoms (flushed face, loud voice, restlessness) would be treated by yin foods. In addition, cravings for specific foods or flavors point to deficiencies to be remedied. Thus someone who wants a lot of hot drinks probably has a "cold" illness, while someone who refuses beverages has a "damp" disease.

Chinese medicine also uses food as therapy in combination with exercise and herbal preparations. One aspect of a balanced diet is maintaining a proper balance of rest and activity as well as selecting the right foods for the time of year and other circumstances. If a person does not get enough exercise, the body cannot transform food into chi and vital essence. If they are hyperactive, the body consumes too much of its own substance. With respect to herbal preparations, the Chinese used tonics taken as part of a meal before they began to use them as medicines. Herbs are used in Chinese cooking to give the food specific medicinal qualities as well as to flavor it. For example, **ginger** might be added to a fish dish to counteract the cold of the fish. Food and medical treatment are closely interrelated in traditional Chinese medicine. A classical Chinese meal seeks to balance not only flavors, aromas, textures, and colors in the different courses that are served, but also the energies provided for the body by the various ingredients.

Preparations

A traditional Chinese physician will examine a patient carefully before giving advice about diet. The diagnosis is based on four types of examination: visual observation, which includes examining the shape, color, and coating of the tongue as well as observing the complexion and taking the pulse; listening to the voice and breathing; inquiring about the patient's symptoms, food preferences, emotions, bowel habits, and sleeping patterns; and palpating (feeling) the patient's abdomen and key points along the meridians. The doctor will suggest changes in diet that will return the patient to inner balance and harmony with the environment according to the patterns he detects.

Precautions

The most important precaution for Westerners who are interested in Chinese food therapy is to consult an experienced practitioner of Chinese medicine. The system is complex and based on principles that differ from Western systems of thought. These factors make self-evaluation quite difficult.

Side effects

There are no known side effects from using the Chinese system of food cures as part of a wellness program under the guidance of an experienced practitioner.

Research and general acceptance

Research in the West has been largely confined to study of the herbs used in traditional Chinese medicine as distinct from food cures. Alternative practitioners in the West, however, have shown considerable interest in incorporating Chinese food cures into other systems, including **color therapy** and women's folk medicine. One school of color therapy classifies foods as yin or yang according to their color and recommends certain color combinations to correct energy imbalances in the body.

Training and certification

In contemporary China, traditional medicine is practiced alongside Western methods of diagnosis and treatment. Some Chinese medical schools still offer courses in Chinese medicine. Practitioners of traditional medicine must pass rigorous examinations and be licensed by the government. They usually obtain their clinical experience by serving apprenticeships under experienced doctors.

Resources

BOOKS

Chiazzari, Suzy. "Color and Food." In *The Complete Book of Color*. Part 3. Boston: Element Books Inc., 1999.

Reid, Daniel P. *Chinese Herbal Medicine*. Boston: Shambhala, 1993.

Stein, Diane. "Chinese Healing and Acupressure." In *All Women Are Healers: A Comprehensive Guide to Natural Healing*, chapter 4. Freedom, CA: The Crossing Press, 1996.

Svoboda, Robert, and Arnie Lade. *Tao and Dharma: Chinese Medicine and Ayurveda*. Twin Lakes, WI: Lotus Press, 1995.

ORGANIZATIONS

American Foundation of Traditional Chinese Medicine (AFTCM). 505 Beach Street, San Francisco, CA 94133. (415) 776-0502. Fax: (415) 392-7003. aftcm@earthlink.net.

Rebecca Frey

Chinese tea *see* **Green tea**

Chinese thoroughwax

Description

Chinese thoroughwax is an herb that is often called bupleurum, referring to the scientific naming of the species *Bupleurum chinense* and *Bupleurum falcatum*. Another name for the herb is hare's ear, and in **traditional Chinese medicine** the herb is called chai-hu.

Chinese thoroughwax (bupleurum) is a perennial flowering plant that grows from one to three feet tall. The leaves are long and slender, and the plant has yellow flowers in the summer months. It grows naturally in China, Japan, and Korea, and in other countries in northern Asia and northern Europe. The root of the plant is pale red, and is the part that is used medicinally. It tastes slightly bitter and pungent, and is believed to have cooling properties in the body.

One of the major herbs in traditional Chinese medicine, Chinese thoroughwax is used in several traditional formulas for liver problems, fevers, and inflammation. Chinese herbalists prescribe it for conditions that are associated with stagnation of qi, or chi (life energy), in the liver. Chinese thoroughwax is a major ingredient in a widely used Oriental medicinal formula called *shosaikoto* in Japanese, which also contains **Korean ginseng**, **licorice** root, **ginger** root, and other herbs. The Chinese name for the formula is *xiao chai hu tang*. This formula is almost 2,000 years old and is used in situations when someone gets a cold or flu but never completely recovers like some kinds of **chronic fatigue syndrome**.

Bupleurum has received attention most recently by researchers in China and Japan. Several studies that have shown significant findings have been translated into English. Professor Shibata of Tokyo University isolated a substance in Chinese thoroughwax he termed *saikogenin*, which is in a class of biologically active chemicals called saponins. In laboratory tests, saikogenin has shown potent anti-inflammatory properties, which recommend it for treating skin **infections** and other disorders in which inflammation and swelling are problematic. Saikogenin has been shown to increase the effectiveness of cortisone drugs, which are pharmaceutical steroids prescribed for arthritis, **asthma**, inflammation and other conditions. Bupleurum significantly increased the action of the cortisone drug prednisone in some laboratory tests. Another benefit of bupleurum is that it has been shown to protect the adrenal glands from the damaging effects of cortisone drugs.

Bupleurum extract has been shown in human studies to improve the symptoms of **hepatitis**, or viral infection of the liver. Other studies have pointed to its effectiveness as an antipyretic (fever-reducing agent), a mild tranquilizer, an antibiotic and antiviral agent, and as an immune system stimulant. A Japanese study published in 2002 suggests that bupleurum may be effective in the treatment of gastric ulcers. Chinese thoroughwax has also been shown to increase the efficiency of the chemotherapy drug 5-FU. It should be noted that Chinese thoroughwax has been generally most effective in tests when used in conjunction with other herbs in traditional Chinese herbal formulas.

General use

Traditional Chinese medicine recommends Chinese thoroughwax for chest congestion, respiratory problems, and for **chills** and fevers, including those associated with **malaria** and blackwater **fever**. It is used to treat fevers that have associated symptoms of excessively high dosages.

Side effects

Chinese thoroughwax can cause nausea, dizziness, sweating, and intestinal discomfort when taken in excessively high dosages.

Preparations

Chinese thoroughwax is available as dried root and capsules in herb stores, health food stores, and Chinese markets. It is also available in several formulated Chinese medicines. To prepare a daily serving of tea, 3–12 g of the dried root can be simmered for over an hour in a quart of water. For more extreme cases of fever and hepatitis, two servings of the tea can be drunk daily.

Chinese thoroughwax (including xiao chai hu tang) are used for **cancer** treatment and as herbal support during chemotherapy.

Some medicinal formulas containing Chinese thoroughwax can be taken as an herbal supplement with corticosteroid drugs, to reduce the risks of damage to the adrenal glands. Some Chinese thoroughwax is used in tonics to strengthen the lungs and sense organs, and to tone the leg muscles. Chinese thoroughwax is used to strengthen the liver and to treat liver problems, such as hepatitis and alcohol-related liver damage (**cirrhosis**).

For women, Chinese thoroughwax is used in formulas to regulate menstrual cycles in cases of **amenorrhea** (loss of menstrual cycle), to reduce the symptoms of PMS, and as a tonic for the female reproductive system. Chinese thoroughwax can be taken as an herbal supplement with corticosteroid drugs, to reduce the risks of damage to the adrenal glands.

bitter taste in the mouth, irritability, **nausea**, and abdominal pains, and is sometimes prescribed for **dizziness** and vertigo that occur with chest **pain**. Chinese thoroughwax is used in tonics to strengthen the lungs and sense organs, and to tone the leg muscles. Chinese thoroughwax is used to strengthen the liver and to treat liver problems, such as hepatitis and alcohol-related liver damage (**cirrhosis**).

KEY TERMS

Interferon—A protein produced by animal cells that have been invaded by a virus. It has been reported to cause negative interactions with bupleurum.

Qi, or chi—Universal life energy, according to traditional Chinese medicine, that is found in the body, air, food, water, and sunlight.

Saikosaponins—Chemical compound found in bupleurum that have anti-inflammatory effects.

Traditional Chinese medicine—Ancient Chinese healing system involving acupuncture, herbal remedies, dietary therapies, and other healing techniques.

Interactions

Chinese thoroughwax is frequently prescribed with licorice root and Korean ginseng. In the traditional and often used Oriental medicine called *shosaikoto* in Japanese or *xiao chai hu tang* in Chinese, Chinese thoroughwax is blended with licorice, jujube fruit, ginger root, Korean ginseng, Chinese **skullcap** root, and half summer root (*Pinellia ternata*). Herbalists often recommend that Chinese thoroughwax be combined with lycii berries to counteract its drying effects in the body. For cases of vertigo and chest pain, and as a liver tonic, bupleurum can be taken with **white peony root**, bitter orange fruit, and licorice. For **menstruation** problems, bupleurum may be combined with white peony and mint.

Bupleurum has been reported to have negative interactions with interferon, which is a protein produced by animal cells when they are invaded by a virus. Interferon is frequently used to treat hepatitis, and patients who are receiving interferon for this disease should not take herbal formulations containing bupleurum.

Resources

BOOKS

Lu, Henry C. *Chinese Herbal Cures.* New York: Sterling, 1994.

Reid, Daniel. *Chinese Herbal Medicine.* Boston: Shambhala, 1996.

Teeguarden, Ron. *Chinese Tonic Herbs.* New York: Japan Publications, 1995.

PERIODICALS

Matsumoto, T., X. B. Sun, T. Hanawa, et al. "Effect of the Antiulcer Polysaccharide Fraction from *Bupleurum falcatum L.* on the Healing of Gastric Ulcer Induced by Acetic Acid in Rats." *Phytotherapy Research* 16 (February 2002): 91–93.

Park, K. H., J. Park, D. Koh, and Y. Lim. "Effect of Saikosaponin-A, a Triterpenoid Glycoside, Isolated from *Bupleurum falcatum* on Experimental Allergic Asthma." *Phytotherapy Research* 16 (June 2002): 359–363.

ORGANIZATIONS

American Association of Oriental Medicine. 5530 Wisconsin Avenue, Suite 1210, Chevy Chase, MD 20815. (301) 941-1064. http://www.aaom.org.

Rocky Mountain Herbal Institute. P. O. Box 579, Hot Springs, MT 59845. (406) 741-3811. http://www.rmhiherbal.org.

Douglas Dupler
Rebecca J. Frey, PhD

Chinese wolfberry *see* **Lycium fruit**

Chinese thoroughwax

Chinese yam

Description

Chinese yam (*Dioscorea opposita*) is a root that is used in **traditional Chinese medicine**. The Chinese pharmaceutical name for this herbal is *Rhizoma dioscoreae*. Other names for Chinese yam include *dioscorea* and *shan yao*. Chinese yam is native to China, Japan, Korea, and Taiwan, where it can be found growing wild on hill slopes and in valleys. It is also propagated for medicinal and dietary uses.

The genus name *Dioscorea* is dedicated to the Greek physician and naturalist, Dioscorides. There are between 600 and 800 different species of *Dioscorea*, making it one of the largest genera of the plant kingdom. Many species in this genus are grown and collected for their medicinal properties. Sweet potatoes are often called yams, although they are different plants.

The Chinese yam plant is a climbing vine that supports itself by coiling around the branches of other vegetation. The plant can be 9.75 ft (3 m) high and 5 ft (1.5 m) wide. Chinese yam has heart-shaped leaves and it produces small white flowers which have a cinnamon-like aroma. Small tubers (called tubercles) form in the axials (the angles between the leaves and the stem). These pea-sized tubercles are harvested in the late summer or early fall and are used to propagate the plant.

Chinese yam plants take three or four years to reach maturity, although fairly large roots may be harvested from well developed plants after the first year. Chinese yam is a spindle-shaped, thick, hard root or tuber that is white on the inside. However, cultivated forms from China or Japan may have different root shapes. The yam may be up to 3 ft (about 1 m) in length. Chinese yam is dug up in the winter. After the rough bark is removed, the root is washed and allowed to dry in either the shade or the sun. The dried root is rehydrated in water and then cut into slices.

Chinese yam contains large amounts of mucilage. Mucilage is a thick, slimy substance produced by plants. It has a soothing effect on mucous membranes, such as the tissues that line the respiratory passages. This may explain why Chinese yam is effective at **relieving cough**.

General use

Traditional Chinese medicine classifies Chinese yam as neutral and sweet. It serves to tonify and

augment the spleen and stomach; augment the lung yin and tonify the lung qi; and stabilize, tonify, and bind the kidneys. Chinese yam enters through the spleen, lung, and kidney channels (meridians). It is used as a tonic (restores tone to tissues). Chinese yam is used to treat weak digestion with **fatigue** and **diarrhea**, general weakness, frequent urination, decreased appetite, leukorrhagia (excessive vaginal discharge), premature ejaculation, the symptoms associated with diabetes, and chronic **wheezing** (whistling sound caused by breathing difficulty) and coughing.

Chinese yam should not be taken if the patient's symptoms include abdominal swelling and **pain**.

Preparations

Chinese yam may be found in dried or fresh form or as a powder. It is available in Asian food stores, Chinese pharmacies, and may be found in certain health food stores.

Chinese yam is taken by mouth for all indications. A tea (infusion) may be prepared by steeping slices of the root in boiling-hot water. The dosage is 10–30 g of root or 6–10 g of powder.

Combinations

It is common in traditional Chinese medicine to mix herbs to treat specific sets of symptoms. Chinese yam may be combined with the following to treat certain symptoms as shown:

- poria and white attractylodes for loose, watery stools.
- codonopsis root for general weakness, fatigue, and poor appetite.

KEY TERMS

Mucilage—A thick, slimy, adhesive substance produced by certain plants. It consists of gum that is dissolved in the plant's juices.

Tonic—An agent that restores normal tone to tissues. Tonics are used to treat indigestion, general debility, and other disorders.

Traditional Chinese medicine—The medicine practiced in China since ancient times which utilizes herbal remedies, acupuncture, cupping, and other treatment modalities.

Tubercles—Small, pea-sized tubers that grow on *Dioscorea* plants in the angles between the leaves and the stem. They are used in the cultivation of Chinese yam.

- Chinese foxglove root and cornus for lightheaded-ness, forgetfulness, insomnia, and related symptoms.
- ginseng (ren shen), white atractylodes rhizome (bai zhu), and poria (fuling) for weakness of the spleen and stomach characterized by poor appetite, lassitude (exhaustion, weakness), and diarrhea.
- white atractylodes rhizome, poria, and euryale seed (qian shi) for excessive dampness because of defi-ciency of the spleen characterized by white leukor-rhagia and lassitude.
- phellodendron bark (huang bai) and plantain seed (che qian zi) for excessive dampness changing into heat characterized by yellow vaginal discharge.
- dogwood fruit (shan zhu yu) and dodder seed (tu si zi) for deficient kidneys characterized by lower back pain and leukorrhagia.
- astragalus root (huang qi), trichosanthes root (tian hua fen), pueraria root (ge gen), and fresh rehmannia root (sheng di huang) for the thirst, excessive drink-ing and eating, lassitude, and frequent urination associated with diabetes.
- dogwood fruit and prepared rehmannia root (shu di huang) for frequent nighttime urination because of deficient kidneys.
- bitter cardamon (yi zhi ren) and mantis egg case (sang piao xiao) for frequent urination because of deficient kidneys.
- glehnia root (sha shen), schisandra fruit (wu wei zi), and ophiopogon root (mai dong) for deficient lungs characterized by chronic cough

Precautions

Species of *Dioscorea* that are edible have opposite leaves (leaves on the stem are directly across from one another), whereas species that are poisonous have alternate leaves (leaves on the stem are not directly across from one another).

Women who are pregnant or lactating should consult with a physician before using Chinese yam.

Side effects

There are no side effects associated with the use of Chinese yam.

Interactions

Chinese yam should not be taken with kan-sui root. As of mid-2000, there were no indications of any interactions between Chinese yam and any drug or other herbal medicine.

Resources

BOOKS

"Chinese Yam." In *The Alternative Advisor: The Complete Guide to Natural Therapies and Alternative Treatments.* Alexandria, VA: Time-Life Books, 1999.

OTHER

Decne. "Dioscorea batatas." http://www.gardenbed.com/D/1402.cfm.

"Rhizoma Dioscoreae." http://www.healthlink.us-inc.com/publiclibrary/htm-data/htm-herb/bhp623.htm.

Belinda Rowland

Chiropractic

Definition

The term chiropractic is from Greek words *cheir* meaning hand and *praxis* meaning action. Chiroprac-tic is a system of treatment grounded in the principal that the body can heal itself when the skeletal system is correctly aligned and the nervous system is function-ing properly. To achieve this proper function and alignment, practitioners uses their hands or an adjust-ing tool to perform specific manipulations, most com-monly of the spine. When the bones of the spine are not correctly articulated, resulting in a condition known as subluxation, the theory is that nerve trans-mission is disrupted and causes **pain** and illness man-ifested in the back as well as other areas of the body.

Chiropractic is one of the most popular alterna-tive therapies currently available. According to the National Institutes of Health's National Center for Complementary and Alternative Medicine, about 20% of Americans report having used chiropractic care at least once. Chiropractic treatment is covered by many insurance plans, including Medicare. The most common reason for seeking chiropractic care is for pain in the lower back. According to the American Chiropractic Association, lower back pain accounts for about 43% of chiropractic visits. In addition, many people seek chiropractic care for a variety of other problems, including ear **infections**, **dysmenor-rhea**, infant **colic**, migraine headaches. Patients also visit chiropractors with complaints of pain or injury to the neck, middle back, arms, or legs.

Origins

Spinal manipulation has a long history in many cultures. However, Daniel D. Palmer (1845-1913) all communication from the brain to the rest of the body passes through the spinal canal and areas that are poorly aligned or under **stress** can cause physical symptoms both in the spine and in other areas of the body. Thus, the body has the innate intelligence to heal itself when unencumbered by spinal irregularities causing nerve interference. After his success with Lillard, other patients began coming to Palmer for care and responded well to adjustments. This success resulted in Palmer's further study of the relationship between an optimally functional spine and normal health.

Palmer founded the first chiropractic college in 1897. His son, B. J. Palmer, continued to develop chiropractic philosophy and practice after his father's death. B. J. and other faculty members were divided over the role of subluxation in disease. B. J. saw it as the cause of all disease. The others disagreed and sought a more rational way of thinking, thus broadening the base of chiropractic education. From 1910 to 1920, many other chiropractic colleges were established. Other innovators, including John Howard, Carl Cleveland, Earl Homewood, Joseph Janse, Herbert Lee, and Claude Watkins also helped to advance the profession.

The theories first developed by the Palmers received somewhat broader interpretation in the late 2000s. Many chiropractors believe that back pain can be relieved and health restored through chiropractic treatment even in patients who do not have demonstrable subluxations. Scientific development and research of chiropractic is gaining momentum, with controlled, scientific studies of chiropractic techniques becoming increasingly common. The National Center for Complementary and Alternative Medicine has even targeted funding to help increase the number of chiropractors participating in research.

Many people besides the Palmers have contributed to the development of chiropractic theory and technique. Some have gone on to create a variety of procedures and related types of therapy that have their roots in chiropractic, including McTimoney-Corley chiropractic, craniosacral manipulation, naprapathy, and **applied kinesiology**. **Osteopathy** is a related holistic discipline that utilizes spinal and musculoskeletal manipulation as a part of treatment, but osteopathic training is more similar in scope to that of a medical doctor.

Benefits

Many people experience back pain at some time in their lives. Depending on the cause and severity of the condition, options for treatment may include physical

founded modern chiropractic theory in the 1890s. A grocer and self-taught magnetic healer, Palmer applied his knowledge of the nervous system and manual therapies to unusual situations. One renowned story concerns Harvey Lillard, a janitor in the office where Palmer worked. The man had been deaf for 17 years, ever since he had sustained an injury to his upper spine. Palmer performed an adjustment on a painful vertebra in the region of the injury and Lillard's hearing was reportedly restored. Palmer theorized that

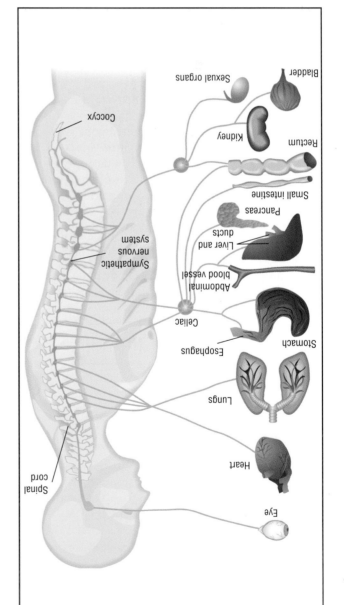

Points on the spine that correspond to various organs and their functions according to chiropractic medicine. *(Illustration by GGS Information Services, Inc. Cengage Learning, Gale)*

therapy, rest, medications, surgery, or chiropractic care. Chiropractic is not believed to carry the risks of surgical or pharmacologic treatment. Practitioners use a holistic approach to health, which is appreciated by many patients. The goal is not merely to relieve the present ailment, but to analyze the cause and recommend appropriate changes of lifestyle to prevent the problem from recurring. Chiropractors generally believe in performing a risk/benefit analysis before use of any intervention. The odds of an adverse outcome are extremely low. Chiropractic is often less expensive than many more traditional treatment methods such as outpatient physical therapy. Relief from some neuromuscular problems is immediate, although a series of treatments is likely to be required to maintain the improvement. Spinal manipulation is often considered an excellent option for acute lower back pain and may also relieve **neck pain** and other musculoskeletal pain. Although many instances of back pain subside eventually with no treatment at all, chiropractic treatment can significantly shorten the time required for improvement. Some types of **headache** can also be successfully treated by chiropractic.

Description

Initial visit

An initial chiropractic exam often includes a history and a physical. The patient is asked about the current complaint, about any chronic health problems, about family history of disease, dietary habits, medical care received, and any medications currently being taken. Further, the chiropractor asks how long the patient has had the problem, how it has progressed, and whether it resulted from an injury or occurred spontaneously. The chiropractor also asks for details of how the injury occurred. The physical exam evaluates by observation and palpation whether the painful area has evidence of inflammation or poor alignment. Range of motion may also be assessed. In the spine, either hypomobility (fixation) or hypermobility may be a problem. Laboratory analysis is helpful in some cases to rule out serious infection or other health issues that may require referral for another type of treatment. Many practitioners also take x rays during the initial evaluation

Manipulation

When spinal manipulation is employed, it is generally done with the hands, although some practitioners may use an adjusting tool. A classic adjustment involves a high velocity, low amplitude thrust that produces a usually painless popping noise and improves the range of motion of the joint that was treated. The patient may lie on a specially designed, padded table that helps the practitioner achieve the proper positions for treatment. Some adjustments involve manipulating the entire spine, or large portions of it, as a unit; others are small movements designed to affect a single joint. Stretching, traction, and slow manipulation are other techniques that can be employed to restore structural integrity and relieve nerve interference.

Length of treatment

The number of chiropractic treatments required varies depending on several factors. Generally longer-term treatment is needed for conditions that are chronic, severe, or occur in conjunction with another health problem. Patients who are not in overall good health may also have longer healing times. Some injuries will inherently require more treatments than others. Care is usually given in three stages. Initially, appointments are more frequent with the goal of relieving immediate pain. Next, the patient moves into a rehabilitative stage to continue the healing process and help to prevent a relapse. Finally, the patient may elect periodic maintenance, or wellness treatments, along with lifestyle changes if needed in order to stay in good health.

Follow-up care

Discharge and follow-up therapy are important. If an injury occurred as a result of poor fitness or health, a program of **exercise** or **nutrition** should be prescribed. Home therapy may also be recommended, involving such treatments as anti-inflammatory medication and applications of heat or ice packs. Conscious attention to posture may help some patients avoid sustaining a similar injury in the future, and the chiropractor is be able to advise the patient of any poor postural habits that require correction.

Types of practitioners

Some practitioners use spinal manipulation to the exclusion of all other modalities and are known as straight chiropractors. Others integrate various types of therapy such as massage, nutritional intervention, or treatment with vitamins, herbs, or homeopathic remedies. They may also embrace ideas from other health care traditions. This group is known as mixers. The vast majority of chiropractors, perhaps 85%, fall in this second category.

Preparations

Patients should enter the chiropractic clinic with an open mind, which will help to achieve maximum results.

Precautions

Chiropractic is not an appropriate therapy for all problems. Many diseases and conditions require medication or surgery. Although there are many conditions of the spine that are amenable to manipulative treatment, it is not appropriate for **fractures**. The chiropractor should be informed in advance if the patient is taking anticoagulants or has **osteoporosis** or any other condition that may weaken the bones. Other circumstances that contraindicate chiropractic care are detected in the history and physical exam. Down syndrome, some congenital defects, some types of **cancer**, and a variety of other diseases and conditions may preclude spinal manipulation. On rare occasions, a fracture or dislocation may occur during manipulation. There is also a risk of a **stroke** occurring as a result of spinal manipulation, although this risk is extremely low. Estimates put the risk at no more than 2.5 occurrences per one million treatments.

Side effects

It is not uncommon to have local discomfort in the form of aches, pains, or spasms for a few days following a chiropractic treatment. Some patients may also experience mild headache or **fatigue** that resolves quickly.

Research and general acceptance

As recently as the 1970s, the American Medical Association (a national group of medical doctors) was quite hostile toward chiropractic. AMA members were advised that it was unethical to be associated with chiropractors. Later that changed and as of 2008, many allopathic or traditionally trained physicians enjoyed cordial referral relationships with chiropractors. There remained, however, strong debate over which diseases and conditions can be successfully treated using chiropractic.

Although some members of the medical community continue to have reservations about chiropractic, it seems to be favored by a significant section of the general population. A study published in the October 2007 volume of the *Journal of Occupational & Environmental Medicine* found that 89% of workers experiencing occupational **low back pain** began visiting a chiropractor within 30 days after the onset of pain.

Although studies such as this one show how popular chiropractic care is with the general population, scientists and medical researchers continue to conduct studies to determine which treatments are really effective.

A July 2006 study took 235 subjects who were seeking care for low back pain and randomly assigned them to either chiropractic care or to physical therapy. The study found that, in general, those who received chiropractic care had a larger reduction in pain. The study did find, however, certain subgroups, such as those with recurrent pain, improved more with physical therapy. This type of complexity may help to explain why some studies find that chiropractic intervention has a very high success rate in treating low back pain, and other studies find that it is not effective.

In addition to treating low back pain, there is some anecdotal evidence that recommends chiropractic treatment for ailments unrelated to musculoskeletal problems, but as of 2008 there was not enough research-based data to support this. By contrast, a chiropractor may be able to treat problems and diseases unrelated to the skeletal structure by employing therapies other than spinal manipulation.

Although many chiropractors limit their practice to spine and joint problems, others claim to treat disorders that are not closely related to the back or musculoskeletal system. These include **asthma**, bedwetting, **bronchitis**, coughs, **dizziness**, **dysmenorrhea**, **earache**, fainting, headache, hyperactivity, **indigestion**, **infertility**, migraine, **pneumonia**, and issues related to **pregnancy**. There is not a significant body of scientific evidence showing that chiropractic care is successful in treating these conditions. There are, however, at least three explanations sometimes given for why chiropractic may be successful in treating these

DANIEL PALMER (1845–1913)

Chiropractic inventor, Daniel David Palmer, was born on March 7, 1845, in Toronto, Ontario. He was one of five siblings, the children of a shoemaker and his wife, Thomas and Katherine Palmer. Daniel Palmer and his older brother left Canada with a tiny cash reserve in April 1865. They immigrated to the United States on foot, walking for 30 days before arriving in Buffalo, New York. They traveled by boat through the St. Lawrence Seaway to Detroit, Michigan. There they survived by working odd jobs and sleeping on the dock. Daniel Palmer settled in What Cheer, Iowa, where he supported himself and his first wife as a grocer and fish peddler in the early 1880s. He later moved to Davenport, Iowa, where he raised three daughters and one son.

Palmer was a man of high curiosity. He investigated a variety of disciplines of medical science during his lifetime, many of which were in their infancy. He was intrigued by phrenology and assorted spiritual cults, and for nine years he investigated the relationship between magnetism and disease. Palmer felt that there was one thing that caused disease. He was intent upon discovering this one thing, or as he called it: the great secret.

In September 1895, Palmer purported to have cured a deaf man by placing pressure on the man's displaced vertebra. Shortly afterward Palmer claimed to cure another patient of heart trouble, again by adjusting a displaced vertebra. The double coincidence led Palmer to theorize that human disease might be the result of dislocated or luxated bones, as Palmer called them. That same year he established the Palmer School of Chiropractic where he taught a three-month course in the simple fundamentals of medicine and spinal adjustment.

Palmer, who was married six times during his life, died in California in 1913; he was destitute. His son, Bartlett Joshua Palmer, successfully commercialized the practice of chiropractic.

---

conditions. One is that the problem could be linked to a nerve impingement, as may be possible with bed-wetting, dizziness, fainting, and headache. In a second group, chiropractic treatment may offer some relief from complicating pain and spasms caused by the disease process, as with asthma, bronchitis, coughs, and pneumonia. The discomforts of pregnancy may also be relieved with gentle chiropractic therapy. A third possibility is that manipulation or use of soft-tissue techniques may directly promote improvement of some conditions. One particular procedure, known as the endonasal technique, is thought to help the eustachian tube to open and thus improve drainage of the middle ear. The tube is sometimes blocked off due to exudates or inflammatory processes, which can cause earaches. Some headaches also fall in this category, as skilled use of soft tissue techniques and adjustment may relieve the muscle tension that may initiate some headaches.

Dysmenorrhea, hyperactivity, indigestion, and infertility are said to be relieved as a result of improved flow of blood and nerve energy following treatment. Evidence for this is anecdotal at best, but manipulation is unlikely to be harmful if causes treatable by other modalities have been ruled out.

For conditions such as cancer, fractures, infectious diseases, neurological disease processes, and any condition that may cause increased orthopedic fragility, chiropractic treatment alone is not an effective therapy and may even be harmful in some cases.

Chiropractic treatment should never be sought to the complete exclusion of traditional medical therapies. Those who have known circulatory problems, especially with a history of thrombosis, should not have spinal manipulation.

Training and certification

Chiropractors are licensed by the state in which they practice. Matriculation at a certified school of chiropractic requires at least two years of science-based undergraduate work, and most applicants have completed a bachelor's degree. Chiropractic college is an additional four-year program and graduates receive a DC (doctor of chiropractic) degree. Chiropractic education emphasizes anatomy, physiology, diagnostic skills, neurology, and radiology. As of the year 2008, there were 18 chiropractic colleges in the United States. Following graduation, the doctors must pass both national board and state board exams in order to be licensed. A minimum number of continuing education hours per year may be required in some states to maintain licensure. Practitioners may also opt for a program to become a diplomate of a more specialized group. Requirements for these groups vary considerably, from a program similar to a traditional residency down to some that require a minimal number of hours of continuing education. Some of the specialties offered are radiology, orthopedics, sports injuries, nutrition, neurology, and internal medicine. Most chiropractors do not specialize.

Resources

BOOKS

Gatterman, Meridel I., and Ron Kirk. *Chiropractic, Health Promotion, and Wellness.* Sudbury, MA: Jones & Bartlett, 2007.

Haldeman, Scott, et al., eds. *Principles and Practice of Chiropractic.* New York: McGraw-Hill Medical, 2005.

Kanan, Joseph. *Living Pain Free through Chiropractic and Trigger Point Therapy.* Apple Valley, MN: Center Path, 2006.

Weintraub, Michael I., Ravinder Mamtani, and Marc S. Micozzi, eds. *Complementary and Integrative Medicine in Pain Management.* New York: Springer, 2008.

PERIODICALS

Bronfort, Gert, et al. "Evidence-Informed Management of Chronic Low Back Pain with Spinal Manipulation and Mobilization." *Spine Journal* 8, no. 1 (January/February 2008): 213–226.

Klotter, Julie. "Chiropractic and Migraines." *Townsend Letter: The Examiner of Alternative Medicine* 292 (November 2007): 37.

Stevens, Gerald L. "Behavioral and Access Barriers to Seeking Chiropractic Care: A Study of 3 New York Clinics." *Journal of Manipulative and Physiological Therapeutics* 30, no. 8 (October 2007): 566–573.

ORGANIZATIONS

American Chiropractic Association, 1701 Clarendon Blvd., Arlington, VA, 22209, (703) 276-8800, http://www.amerchiro.org/.

Judith Turner
Teresa G. Odle
Helen Davidson

Chlamydia

Definition

Chlamydia is the most common sexually transmitted disease in the United States. More than a million new cases of the diseases were reported in 2007, the most ever for a sexually transmitted disease in the United States. The disease is caused by a bacterium called *Chlamydia trachomatis.* The following areas in the body can be affected:

- cervix
- fallopian tubes, which carry ova (eggs) from the ovaries to the uterus
- urethra, which carries urine from the bladder to outside the body
- epididymis, a small organ attached to the testicles that is responsible for sperm production
- prostate gland, a gland at the base of the penis that provides nutrients for sperm
- anus
- throat
- eyes

In addition, *Chlamydia trachomatis* also causes lung and eye **infections** in newborns whose mothers have a chlamydial infection during the last part of their **pregnancy**.

Description

Chlamydia is most often found in sexually active adolescents aged 15 to 19. Data gathered by the Centers for Disease Control (CDC) suggest that sexually active girls in this age group may account for up to 40% of chlamydial infections.

According to the CDC, approximately 40% of women infected with chlamydia develop **pelvic inflammatory disease** (PID). If untreated, 18% of women with PID have chronic inflammatory **pain**. In addition, chlamydia may cause extensive damage to the fallopian tubes. Scarring can block the tube and prevent the egg from being fertilized. As a result, one of every five women with PID is unable to conceive. Tube scarring may also cause the fertilized egg to be trapped inside the tube, unable to reach the uterus. When the fertilized egg develops inside the tube rather than in the uterus, the condition is called tubal pregnancy. The condition is potentially fatal if the tube ruptures. In the United States, tubal pregnancy is the number one cause of death of women in early pregnancy.

Causes and symptoms

Cause

Chlamydia is caused by a bacterial parasite called *Chlamydia trachomatis.* The organism lives inside humans, who act as hosts. It is dependent on humans for energy because it is unable to produce energy for itself. *C. trachomatis* often causes genital and urinary tract infections in sexually active men and women.

Mode of transmission

A person can become infected with *C. trachomatis* in the following ways:

- having sex (oral, genital, or anal) with an infected partner
- sharing infected sex toys

- passing through the infected birth canal of a mother who has chlamydia
- experiencing an episode of sexual abuse (in children)

Risk factors

The following are risk factors for contracting chlamydia infections:

- Age. Young sexually active people aged 15 to 19 are most frequently affected.
- Race. Blacks contract this disease more often than whites or Hispanics.
- Marital status. Chlamydia is most often found in single women. Married women have the lowest risk.
- Behavioral factors. Douching increases risk of chlamydial infections. Smoking also increases one's risk of contracting this disease. Those who have sex with many different partners or with strangers are at high risk. Also at increased risk are those who have unprotected sex with partners of unknown disease status. Previous induced abortions also increase a woman's chance of getting this disease.
- Socio-economic status. Poor, uneducated women living in big cities are more often affected by this disease.
- Postpartum period. Increased risk of contracting chlamydia is observed during the period immediately after giving birth or undergoing an induced abortion. This risk arises because the cervix is not entirely closed, allowing a greater chance for infection.

Symptoms

Approximately 75% of women do not have symptoms. If a woman has symptoms, they typically develop one to three weeks after she is infected. Her symptoms may include:

- burning pain during urination
- more frequent urination
- abnormal vaginal discharge
- dull pelvic pain
- bleeding between periods and after sexual intercourse
- menstrual bleeding that is heavier than usual
- more painful periods

Chlamydia infection in men may develop in the urethra, epididymis, and/or the prostate. Approximately 50% of infected men do not have any symptoms. If a man has symptoms, they tend to develop one to three weeks after he is infected. His symptoms may include:

- burning pain during urination
- more frequent urination

- white or yellow discharge from the penis
- redness at the tip of the penis
- itchy or irritated urethra (urethritis)
- pain and swelling in the testicles (epididymitis)
- pain between the scrotum and anal area and difficult and frequent urination (prostatitis)

On rare occasions, chlamydia infection in men and women can develop outside the genital areas. These patients may have infections at the following sites:

- eyes (due to a contaminated hand touching the eyes): itching, redness and itching of the eyelids
- throat (following oral sex with infected men): throat irritation or no symptoms
- anus (following anal intercourse with infected men): rectal bleeding, mucous rectal discharge, diarrhea, and pain with bowel movement.

Diagnosis

Diagnosis is based on patients' history, laboratory testing for *C. trachomatis*, and physical examination for men and pelvic examination for women to determine if the patient is infected and/or the extent of infection.

There are several tests available for chlamydial infection. They often require swipes from the infected site or urine samples. Tests for chlamydia include:

- Cell culture test. This old test is reliable but requires 48 to 72 hours to complete. In the early 2000s, it was being replaced by faster and more convenient tests. In 2001, the U.S. Food and Drug Administration (FDA) recommended routine screening for chlamydia among sexually active young women. One year later, the administration approved a test called Thin-Prep, a new type of Pap smear that allows doctors to screen for chlamydia, gonorrhea, and the human papillomavirus at the same time women have annual pap exams for cervical cancer.
- Direct fluorescent antibody (DFA) staining. This test is faster than the traditional culture test.
- Enzyme immunoassay (EIA). This test is easy to perform and faster than the traditional culture test but is not as accurate.
- DNA probe. This test is expensive but is more specific and convenient than culture, EIA, or DFA tests. Genital swipe samples are not necessary. Urine tests can provide accurate results.
- Nucleic acid amplification (PCR and LCR) tests. These tests look for genetic material of the organism. These are the tests of choice because they are the

most sensitive (more than 90% accurate) and the most specific. They are also convenient because they can be performed on urine samples and do not require a pelvic exam.

Treatment

Alternative therapy should be complementary to antibiotic therapy. Because of the potentially serious nature of this disease, patients should first consult an allopathic physician to start antibiotic treatment for infections. Traditional medicine is better equipped to quickly eradicate the infection while alternative treatments can help the body fight the disease and relieve symptoms associated with this disease. Some alternative treatments include nutritional therapy, herbal remedies, **traditional Chinese medicine**, and **homeopathy**.

Nutritional therapy

The following dietary changes may be helpful:

- Following a low-fat, high-fiber diet. The diet should include a variety of fresh fruits and vegetables. These foods contain high amounts of phytonutrients and essential vitamins that help keep the body strong and stimulate the immune system to fight infections.
- Limited intake of fat, sugar, highly processed foods, caffeine, and alcohol, which depresses the immune function.
- Taking a multivitamin/mineral supplement daily.
- Drinking cranberry juice. Cranberry juice helps prevent urinary tract infections.
- Taking acidophilus pills to prevent yeast infections while on antibiotics.
- Eating fresh garlic or taking garlic pills to help fight infection.

Herbal treatment

Echinacea and berberine-containing herbs such as **saw palmetto** (*Serenoa repens*) and **goldenseal** are natural antibiotics. These herbs can assist the action of prescription antibiotics.

Traditional Chinese medicine

An experienced Chinese herbalist typically prepares an herbal mixture based on a patient's specific condition and symptoms.

Homeopathy

A homeopathic practitioner may prescribe a patient-specific remedy to help reduce some of the symptoms associated with disease. Remedies for chlamydial symptoms include *Cannabis sativa*, *Cantharis*, and *Salidago virga*.

Allopathic treatment

Once detected, chlamydia can be easily treated with antibiotics. However, if not detected early enough, scarring of fallopian tubes (and resulting **infertility**) may not be preventable. The two most commonly used drugs are azithromycin and doxycycline. Azithromycin is more expensive but much more convenient to administer. Only one dose is needed to treat the disease. Doxycycline is cheaper but needs to be taken twice a day for more than seven days. Because patients tend to stop taking drugs after a few days, doxycycline is not as effective as azithromycin. Therefore, many doctors prefer to give azithromycin. Patients are advised to refrain from sex for a full week after taking azithromycin or until they finish doxycycline treatment.

An infected person should contact all partners within the last two months so that they can be tested for chlamydia.

Infected pregnant women should be given erythromycin for seven days, instead of other drugs, because this drug is safer during pregnancy.

Follow-up testing is done four weeks after drug treatment to see if the infection is eradicated. If tests continue to be positive, the patient is given another course of antibiotics.

Expected results

A woman's prognosis depends on the duration of infection, whether the infection has spread through the uterus and the fallopian tubes, and the number of previous chlamydial infections. If detected early, the disease can be completely cured with antibiotic treatment in seven days. However, if left untreated, chlamydia can spread through the uterus to the fallopian tubes and cause chronic pelvic inflammatory disease. Infertility may occur as a result of serious damage to the female reproductive tract. Potentially fatal tubal pregnancy is also a risk.

Prevention

Prevention is the most important means of stopping the spread of this disease. The following practices are recommended to prevent the spread of this and other sexually transmitted diseases:

- Abstinence. Abstinence is the only sure way to prevent chlamydia and other STD infections.

KEY TERMS

Abstinence—Choosing not to engage in a certain action, such as sex.

Infertility—Inability to have children, which may occur as a result of pelvic infections.

Nongonococcal urethritis (NGU)—A sexually transmitted urethral infection that is not gonorrhea.

Pelvic Inflammatory Disease (PID)—An infection of the uterus, fallopian tubes, and/or ovaries.

Tubal pregnancy—A fertilized egg that implants in the fallopian tube instead of inside the uterus, which often occurs as a result of sexually transmitted infections such as Chlamydia; also known as ectopic pregnancy.

- Monogamy. Having a mutually monogamous relationship with an uninfected partner reduces the chance of getting STD infections.

- Avoiding a sexual relationship with an unknown partner or a partner whose infection status is unknown.

- In having sex with an unknown partner, using a barrier contraceptive such as a condom (for men) or diaphragm (for women) is recommended. However, condoms (or diaphragms) are not 100% effective against chlamydia or other STDs.

- Refraining from douching.

- Avoiding sex soon after giving birth or undergoing an induced abortion.

- Getting tested for chlamydia at yearly pelvic examinations.

Resources

BOOKS

Aral, Sevgi O., and John M. Douglas, eds. *Behavioral Interventions for Prevention and Control of Sexually Transmitted Diseases*. New York: Springer, 2007.

Brequet, Amy. *Chlamydia*. New York: Rosen, 2006.

Holmes, King K., et al. *Sexually Transmitted Diseases*. New York: McGraw Hill Professional, 2007.

Marr, Lisa. *Sexually Transmitted Diseases*, 2nd ed. Baltimore: Johns Hopkins University Press, 2007.

PERIODICALS

Bissell, Mary. "Chlamydia Screening Programs: A Review of the Literature. Part 2: Testing Procedures and Educational Interventions for Primary Care Physicians." *Canadian Journal of Human Sexuality* (March 2006): 13–22.

Hafner, Louise M., and Celia McNeilly. "Vaccines for Chlamydia Infections of the Female Genital Tract." *Future Microbiology* (February 2008): 67–77.

McKay, Alexander. "Chlamydia Screening Programs: A Review of the Literature. Part 1: Issues in the Promotion of Chlamydia Testing of Youth by Primary Care Physicians." *Canadian Journal of Human Sexuality* (March 2006): 1–10.

Skidmore, Sue, Sarah Randall, and Harry Mallinson. "Testing for Chlamydia Trachomatis: Self-test or Laboratory-based Diagnosis?" *Journal of Family Planning and Reproductive Health Care* (October 2007): 231–232.

OTHER

"Chlamydia." Womenshealth.gov. May 2005 [cited March 18, 2008]. http://www.4women.gov/faq/stdchlam.htm.

"Chlamydia: CDC Fact Sheet." Centers for Disease Control and Prevention. [cited February 3, 2008]. http://www.cdc.gov/std/Chlamydia/STDFact-Chlamydia.htm.

ORGANIZATIONS

CDC National STDs Hotline, (800) 227-8922, (800) 342-2437

NIH National Institute of Allergy and Infectious Diseases, NIAID Office of Communications, 31 Center Dr. (MSC-2520), Building 31, Room 7A50, Bethesda, MD, 20892-2520, http://www.cdc.gov/nchhstp/.

Mai Tran
Teresa G. Odle
David Edward Newton, Ed.D.

Chlorella

Description

Chlorella is a type of single-cell green algae. It is a major component of phytoplankton, which are very small free-floating aquatic plants found in plankton. Chlorella is a popular food supplement, especially in Japan, and is sold as a nutritional supplement in the United States, Canada, and other parts of the world. There are several species of chlorella, but those most commonly found in supplements are *Chlorella vulgaris* and *Chlorella pyrenoidosa*.

General use

Chlorella contains high levels of chlorophyll, protein, **iron**, vitamins C and B_{12}, **beta carotene**, and 19 **amino acids**.

Several studies have indicated that chlorella may be effective in treating some types of **cancer**, high **cholesterol**, **hypertension** (high blood pressure), and **fibromyalgia** syndrome, and in boosting the immune

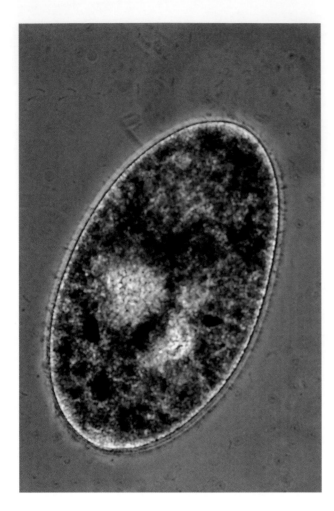

This ciliate protozoan Paramecium bursaria, a green slipper animalcule, gets its color from symbiotic algae Chlorella. (PHOTOTAKE Inc. / Alamy)

system and detoxifying the body. As is often the case with alternative therapies, there are several studies that dispute the effectiveness of chlorella in treating these medical conditions.

The ability of chlorella to fight cancer cells has been shown in several scientific studies, although the exact mechanisms by which it works were not known as of 2008. Several scientists believe chlorella stimulates the activity of T-cells—important components of the immune system—and macrophages, which are large cells that protect against infection by removing waste products, harmful microorganisms, and other toxins from the bloodstream. Increasing the production of T-cells and macrophages increases interferon levels in the body, enhancing the immune system's ability to fight invading substances such as viruses, bacteria, and chemicals. Interferon is an immune-related protein produced by the body that performs antiviral and anti-tumor activities.

Studies in laboratory animals suggest some substances in chlorella may reduce bone marrow suppression in patients taking the anticancer drug fluorouracil. In this interaction, chlorella may increase the white blood cell and platelet counts, which reduces the risk of infection and bleeding, respectively.

Studies have also shown chlorella can significantly reduce cholesterol levels in laboratory animals. As of 2008 studies were underway to determine if chlorella has the same effect on human cholesterol levels.

Chlorella may help reduce blood pressure in some people with hypertension (high blood pressure). A study reported in the March 2003 issue of *Original Internist* indicated that treatment with 10 grams of chlorella daily for three months significantly improved blood pressure in 25% of the patients involved.

In a 2000 study, patients with fibromyalgia syndrome (a disorder that causes muscle aches, **fatigue**, and **sleep disorders**) were treated with high doses of chlorella. After two months, the study found significant benefits from chlorella treatment.

Clinical studies of laboratory animals have also shown that chlorella can protect against gamma radiation and other toxic drugs and chemicals, including dioxin. In the intestines, it can deactivate heavy metals such as cadmium, lead, and mercury.

The benefits of chlorella have been disputed. According to an equivocal article about chlorella on the American Cancer Society Web site, there is no scientific evidence showing chlorella's effectiveness against cancer or any other disease. Limited laboratory and animal research suggests that the algae may have some anticancer properties. One investigation concluded that a protein extract from one type of chlorella prevented the spread of cancer cells in mice. Another study of mice suggested that the extract decreased the side effects of chemotherapy treatment without affecting the potency of anticancer medications.

Preparations

Chlorella is available in various forms, including capsule, tablet, softgel, powder, and liquid. It is found as a supplement alone or in a combination with other green food extracts such as wheat grass, **barley grass**, and **spirulina** (a nutritionally rich microorganism). Capsules and tablets are available in doses of 200 to 500 milligrams (mg). There is no standard dosage, but some herbalists recommend 3 grams (g) per day.

KEY TERMS

Algae—A mainly waterborne organism that produces energy from light and chlorophyll.

Amino acids—A group of organic compounds that are vital to living cells.

Cadmium—A heavy metal.

Chlorophyll—A green plant pigment found in plants, algae, and some bacteria. Chlorophyll is responsible for capturing the light energy needed for photosynthesis.

Cholesterol—A compound found in animal tissue, blood, and fats, high levels of which in the blood are linked to clogged arteries, heart disease, and gallstones.

Diabetes—A metabolic disorder in which the body produces insufficient insulin or is unable to effectively use normal amounts because of insulin resistance. Type 1 diabetes typically manifests in children as a pancreatic deficiency; Type 2 (adult onset diabetes) is usually a consequence of chronic blood sugar dysregulation.

Dioxin—A toxic chemical produced in the manufacture of some pesticides and herbicides.

Fibromyalgia syndrome—Also called fibromyalgia, a disorder that causes muscle aches, fatigue, and sleep disorders.

Fluorouracil—An anticancer drug.

Gamma radiation—High energy electromagnetic waves emitted in some nuclear reactions.

Hypertension—High blood pressure.

Insulin—A hormone that helps muscle and fat cells take up and sugars, starches, and other foods for conversion into energy the body needs.

Interferon—An immune protein produced by cells in the body to fight viral infections.

Macrophages—Large cells that protect against infection by removing waste products, harmful microorganisms, and other toxins from the bloodstream.

Phytoplankton—Very small free-floating aquatic plants found in plankton.

Plankton—A mass of tiny animals and plants floating in the sea or in lakes, usually near the surface.

Platelet—The smallest kind of blood cell, usually found in large quantities, that plays an important part in blood clotting. Also called thrombocytes.

Spirulina—A nutritionally valuable organism that is rich in vitamins, minerals, essential fatty acids, and antioxidants.

T-cells—A type of white blood cell that plays an important role in the immune system and in combating viral infections and cancers.

Ulcerative colitis—An inflammation in the walls of the bowel that causes internal sores, called ulcers, on the lining of the bowel.

Warfarin—A blood-thinning drug, known by the brand name Coumadin.

Precautions

Pregnant and breastfeeding women are advised to use caution and follow the advice of their healthcare professional, since the effects of chlorella have not been studied for these two groups. Caution may also be advised for persons known to be sensitive or allergic to **iodine**.

Side effects

Although chlorella appears to be safe, no research as of 2008 in humans had been conducted to determine if the supplement causes any negative side effects. Also, no studies had been done regarding the consequences of long-term use. Mild side effects that have been reported include bloating and **nausea**, which usually disappear after a few days of use. Some people using chlorella have had allergic reactions and adverse reactions to sunlight. Allergic reaction symptoms include

difficulty breathing, chest **pain**, **hives**, rash, and itchy or swollen skin. If any of these reactions occurs, the person should seek medical care immediately.

Interactions

Persons taking the blood-thinning drug warfarin (Coumadin) are advised to completely avoid chlorella or use caution and follow the advice of their healthcare professional because some chlorella supplements contain high amounts of **vitamin K** that may affect the inhibition of **blood clots**.

Resources

BOOKS

McCauley, Bob. *Achieving Great Health: How Spirulina, Chlorella, Raw Foods, and Ionized Water Can Make You Healthier than You Have Ever Imagined*. Lansing, MI: Watershed Wellness Center, 2005.

Sandoval, David. *The Green Foods Bible: Everything You Need to Know About Barley Grass, Wheatgrass, Kamut, Chlorella, Spirulina, and More.* Topanga, CA: Freedom Press, 2007.

ORGANIZATIONS

Alternative Medicine Foundation, PO Box 60016, Potomac, MD, 20859, (301) 340-1960, http://www.amfoundation.org.

Office of Dietary Supplements, National Institutes of Health, 6100 Executive Blvd., Room 3B01, MSC 7517, Bethesda, MD, 20892-7517, (301) 435-2920, http://ods.od.nih.gov.

Ken R. Wells
David Edward Newton, Ed.D.

Cholecalciferol *see* **Vitamin D**

Cholesterol

Definition

Cholesterol, a fatty substance found in animal tissue, is an important component of the human body. It is manufactured in the liver and carried throughout the body in the bloodstream. Problems can occur when excess cholesterol causes accumulation of plaque on blood vessel walls, which impedes blood flow to the heart and other organs. The highest cholesterol content is found in meat, poultry, shellfish, and dairy products.

Description

Cholesterol has both good effects and bad effects. It is necessary for digesting fats, making hormones, building cell walls, and it participates in other processes for maintaining a healthy body. The body contains two forms of cholesterol: high-density cholesterol (HDL), the so-called good cholesterol, and low-density cholesterol (LDL), the so-called bad cholesterol. The total amount of HDL and LDL is called the total cholesterol. A third type of fatty material found in the body, triglycerides, is a simple form of fat with health effects related to those of cholesterol.

The American Heart Association estimated in 2008 that 106.7 million American adults, roughly one-half of the adult population, have elevated cholesterol levels. High LDL is a major contributing factor for **heart disease**. The cholesterol forms plaque in the heart's blood vessels that restricts or blocks the supply

Types of cholesterol

Types	Levels (mg/dl)
Total cholesterol:	
Desirable	<200
Borderline	200 to 240
Undesirable	>240
HDL cholesterol:	
Desirable	>45
Borderline	35 to 45
Undesirable	<35
LDL cholesterol:	
Desirable	<130
Borderline	130 to 160
Undesirable	>160
Ratio of total cholesterol to HDL cholesterol:	
Desirable	<3
Borderline	3 to 4
Undesirable	>4

(Illustration by Corey Light. Cengage Learning, Gale)

of blood to the heart and causes **atherosclerosis**, which can lead to a **heart attack**, resulting in damage to the heart and possibly death.

The U.S. population as a whole is at some risk of developing high LDL cholesterol. Specific risk factors include a family history of high cholesterol, **obesity**, heart attack or **stroke**, **alcoholism**, and lack of regular **exercise**. The chances of developing high cholesterol increase after the age of 45. One of the primary causes of high LDL cholesterol is too much fat or sugar in the diet, a problem especially prevalent in the United States. Cholesterol is also produced naturally in the liver and overproduction may occur even in people who limit their intake of high cholesterol food. Low HDL and high triglyceride levels also are risk factors for atherosclerosis.

Dietary cholesterol

Food	Cholesterol (mg)
Beef liver, cooked, 3 oz	331
Beef sweetbreads, cooked, 3 oz.	250
Squid, cooked, 3 oz.	227
Egg, whole, large	212
Shrimp, cooked, 3 oz.	166
Ice cream, gourmet, 1 cup	90
Salmon, baked, 3.5 oz.	87
Lamb chop, cooked, 3 oz.	75
Chicken breast, cooked, 3 oz.	72
Beef, round, cooked, 3 oz.	71
Beef, sirloin, cooked, 3 oz.	71
Pork chop, cooked, 3 oz.	71
Chicken, dark meat, cooked, 3 oz.	70
Beef, rib eye, cooked, 3 oz.	65
Ham, regular, cooked, 3 oz.	50
Tuna, water packed, drained, 3.5 oz.	42
Milk, whole, 1 cup	33
Butter, 1 tbsp.	31
Ice cream, light, 1 cup	31
Cheese, cheddar, 1 oz.	30
Scallops, cooked, 3 oz.	27
Hot dog, beef, 1 frank	24
Cheese, reduced fat, 1 oz.	6
Yogurt, part skim, 1 cup	6

(Illustration by GGS Information Services. Cengage Learning, Gale)

Causes and symptoms

There are no readily apparent symptoms that indicate high LDL or triglycerides, or low HDL. A simple blood test can reveal a problem. However, one general indication of high cholesterol is obesity. Another is a high-fat diet. Research has shown that both genetic factors and diet contribute to cholesterol levels.

Diagnosis

High cholesterol is often diagnosed and treated by general practitioners or family practice physicians. In some cases, the condition is treated by an endocrinologist or cardiologist. Total cholesterol, LDL, HDL, and triglyceride levels as well as the cholesterol to HDL ratio are measured by a blood test called a lipid panel. The cost of a lipid panel is typically covered by health insurance and HMO plans, including Medicare, providing there is an appropriate reason for the test. Home cholesterol testing kits are available over the counter, but these test only for total cholesterol. The results should be used only as a guide, and if the total cholesterol level is high or low, a lipid panel should be performed by a physician. In most adults the recommended levels, measured by milligrams per deciliter (mg/dL) of blood, are: total cholesterol, less than 200; LDL, less than 130; HDL, more than 40;

triglycerides, less than 200; and cholesterol to HDL ratio, four to one. However, the recommended cholesterol levels may vary, depending on other risk factors such as **hypertension**, a family history of heart disease, diabetes, age, alcoholism, and **smoking**.

Doctors wonder why some people develop heart disease whereas others with identical HDL and LDL levels do not. Some studies indicate it may be due to the size of the cholesterol particles in the bloodstream. A test called a nuclear magnetic resonance (NMR) LipoProfile exposes a blood sample to a magnetic field to determine the size of the cholesterol particles. Particle size also can be determined by a centrifugation test, in which blood samples are spun to allow particles to separate and move at different distances. The smaller the particles, the greater the chance of developing heart disease. This test allows physicians to treat patients who have normal or close to normal results from a lipid panel but abnormal particle size.

Treatment

U.S. guidelines in the late 2000s for management of cholesterol levels were established in a 2004 report of the National Cholesterol Education Program of the National Heart, Lung, and Blood Institute, American College of Cardiology Foundation, and American Heart Association. According to that report, the primary goal of cholesterol treatment is to lower LDL to under 160 mg/dL in people without heart disease and who are at lower risk of developing it. The goal in people with higher risk factors for heart disease is less than 130 mg/dL. In patients who already have heart disease, the goal is under 100 mg/dL. Also, since low HDL levels increase the risks of heart disease, the goal for all patients is an HDL level of more than 35 mg/dL.

In both alternative and conventional treatment of high cholesterol, the first-line treatment options are exercise, diet, weight loss, and stopping smoking. Other alternative treatments include high doses of **niacin**, **soy protein**, **garlic**, algae, and the Chinese medicine supplement Cholestin (a red yeast fermented with rice).

Diet and exercise

Since a large number of people with high cholesterol are overweight, a healthy diet and regular exercise are probably the most beneficial natural ways to control cholesterol levels. In general, the goal is to substantially reduce or eliminate foods high in animal fat. These foods include meat, shellfish, eggs, and dairy products. Several specific diet options are beneficial. One is the vegetarian diet. Vegetarians typically get up to 100% more fiber and up to 50% less cholesterol from their food than non-vegetarians. The vegetarian low-cholesterol diet consists of at least six servings of whole grain foods, three or more servings of green leafy vegetables, two to four servings of fruit, two to four servings of legumes, and one or two servings of non-fat dairy products daily.

A second diet is the Asian diet, with brown rice being the staple food. Other permitted foods include fish; vegetables, such as bok choy and bean sprouts; and black beans. This diet includes one weekly serving of meat and very few dairy products. The food is flavored with traditional Asian spices and condiments, such as **ginger**, chilies, **turmeric**, and soy sauce.

Another regimen is the low glycemic or diabetic diet, which may raise the HDL (good cholesterol) level by as much as 20% in three weeks. Low glycemic foods promote a slow but steady rise in blood sugar levels following a meal, which increases the level of HDL. They also lower total cholesterol and triglycerides. Low glycemic foods include certain fruits, vegetables, beans, and whole grains. Processed and refined foods and sugars are avoided.

Exercise is an extremely important part of lowering bad cholesterol and raising good cholesterol. It should consist of 20 to 30 minutes of vigorous aerobic exercise at least three times a week. Exercises that cause the heart to beat faster include fast walking, bicycling, jogging, roller skating, swimming, and walking up stairs. Various aerobic programs are available at gyms or on videocassette.

Garlic

A number of clinical studies have indicated that garlic can offer modest reductions in cholesterol. A 2006 summary of those studies concluded that garlic appears to have the potential for reducing the level of substances such as LDL associated with heart disease but that further studies were needed to confirm this relationship.

Cholestin

Cholestin first became available in the over-the-counter market in 1997 as a cholesterol-lowering dietary supplement. It is a processed form of red yeast fermented with rice, a traditional herbal remedy used for centuries by the Chinese. Two studies released in 1998 showed Cholestin lowered LDL cholesterol by 20 to 30%. It also appeared to raise HDL and lower triglyceride levels. Although the supplement contains hundreds of compounds, the major active LDL-

lowering ingredient is lovastatin, a chemical also found in the prescription drug Mevacor. The FDA banned Cholestin in early 1998 but a federal district court judge lifted the ban a year later, ruling the product was a dietary supplement, not a drug. As of 2008, it remained unclear how the substance works. Patients may want to consult with their physician before taking Cholestin. No serious side effects have been reported, but minor side effects, including bloating and **heartburn**, have been reported. As of 2008, the FDA had not approved the use of Cholestin for any disease, and many questions remained about its efficacy in treating coronary problems.

Other treatments

A study released in 1999 indicated that blue-green algae contains polyunsaturated fatty acids that lower cholesterol levels. The algae, known as alga *Aphanizomenon flos-aquae* (AFA) is available as an over-the-counter dietary supplement. As of 2008, only one study had confirmed the results of the initial 1999 research, and questions remained as to the value of AFA in treating cholesterol problems. Niacin, also known as nicotinic acid or vitamin B_3, has been shown to reduce LDL levels by 10 to 20% and to raise HDL levels by 15 to 35%. It can also reduce triglyceride levels. But because an extremely high dose of niacin (2–3 grams) is needed to treat cholesterol problems, it should be taken only under a doctor's supervision so that in monitoring use, he or she can watch for possible toxic side effects. Niacin can also cause flushing when taken in high doses. Soy protein with high levels of isoflavones has been shown to reduce bad cholesterol by up to 10%. A daily diet that contains 62 mg of isoflavones in soy protein is recommended and can be incorporated into other diet regimens, including vegetarian, Asian, and low glycemic.

Allopathic treatment

Various prescription medicines are available to treat cholesterol problems. These include statins such as lovastatin (Mevacor), fluvastatin (Lescol), pravastatin (Pravachol), simvastatin (Zocor), cervastatin (Baycol), and atorvastatin (Lipitor) to lower LDL. A group of drugs called fibric acid derivatives are used to lower triglycerides and raise HDL. These include gemfibrozil (Lopid), clofibrate (Atromid-S), and fenofibrate (Tricor).

A new class of drugs was identified late in 2001 that work differently from the statin drugs. These drugs rely on compounds that bind to a sterol that regulates protein (called SCAP) and speeds up removal of cholesterol from the plasma (the fluid

KEY TERMS

Atherosclerosis—A buildup of fatty substances in the inner layers of the arteries.

Estrogen—A hormone that stimulates development of female secondary sex characteristics.

Glycemic—The presence of glucose in the blood.

Hypertension—Abnormally high blood pressure.

Legumes—A family of plants that bear edible seeds in pods, including beans and peas.

Lipid—Any of a variety of substances that, along with proteins and carbohydrates, make up the main structural components of living cells.

Polyunsaturated fats—Non-animal oils or fatty acids rich in unsaturated chemical bonds not associated with the formation of cholesterol in the blood.

part of the blood). Doctors decide which drug to use based on the severity of the cholesterol problem, side effects, and cost.

Expected results

High cholesterol is one of the key risk factors for heart disease. Left untreated, too much bad cholesterol can clog the blood vessels, leading to chest **pain (angina)**, **blood clots**, and heart attacks. Heart disease is the number one killer of men and women in the United States. By reducing LDL, people with heart disease can prevent further heart attacks and strokes, prolong and improve the quality of their lives, and slow or reverse cholesterol buildup in the arteries. In people without heart disease, lowering LDL can decrease the risk of a first heart attack or stroke.

Prevention

The best way to prevent cholesterol problems is through a combination of healthy lifestyle activities, a primarily low-fat and **high-fiber diet**, regular aerobic exercise, not smoking, and maintaining an optimal weight. But for people with high risk factors for heart disease, such as a family history of heart disease, diabetes, and being over the age of 45, these measures may not be enough to prevent high cholesterol. In the late 2000s research continued on the effectiveness of existing anti-cholesterol drugs for controlling cholesterol levels in people who do not meet the criteria for high cholesterol, but no definitive results were yet available.

Resources

BOOKS

American Heart Association's Low-Fat, Low-Cholesterol Cookbook: Delicious Recipes to Help Lower Your Cholesterol, 4th ed. New York: Clarkson Potter, 2008.

O'Neil, Edward T. *High Blood Cholesterol: Description and Bibliography.* Hauppauge, NY: Nova Science, 2007.

Rinzler, Carol Ann, and Martin W. Graf. *Controlling Cholesterol for Dummies,* 2nd ed. Indianapolis, IN: For Dummies, 2008.

Rubin, Jordan. *The Great Physician's Rx for High Cholesterol.* Nashville, TN: Thomas Nelson, 2007.

Steinberg, Daniel. *The Cholesterol Wars: The Cholesterol Skeptics vs. the Preponderance of Evidence.* Burlington, MA: Academic Press, 2007.

PERIODICALS

Das, Undurti N. "Beneficial Actions of Polyunsaturated Fatty Acids in Cardiovascular Diseases: But How and Why?" *Current Nutrition & Food Science* (February 2008): 2–31.

"New Study Identifies Genes Involved in Regulating Cholesterol Levels." *Pharmacogenomics* (February 2008): 137–139.

Rahman, K., and G. M. Lowe. "Garlic and Cardiovascular Disease: A Critical Review." *Journal of Nutrition* (March 2006): 736S–740S.

Suryadevara, Ramya S., Richard H. Karas, and Jeffrey T. Kuvin. "Use of Extended-release Niacin in Clinical Practice." *Future Lipidology* (February 2008): 9–16.

ORGANIZATIONS

National Cholesterol Education Program, NHLBI Information Center, PO. Box 30105, Bethesda, MD, 20824-0105, (301) 592-8573, http://www.nhlbi.nih.gov.

Ken R. Wells
Teresa G. Odle
David Edward Newton, Ed.D.

Choline

Description

Choline is an organic compound that functions as an important nutrient. It is found in many animal tissues, either by itself or combined with **lecithin**. In 1998, the United States Food and **Nutrition** board, a part of the Institute of Medicine, declared choline an essential nutrient. Choline is found naturally in meats, egg yolks, dairy foods, and soy products. Lecithin is a source of choline.

A study published by the United States Department of Agriculture in 2001 found that the human body needs both folate and choline in order to continue to produce sufficient quantities of choline. A balanced diet rich in meats and vegetable products is recommended to help obtain sufficient amounts of choline.

General use

Choline has multiple important roles in the body. Choline is used to treat high **cholesterol**, improve memory, and safeguard the liver. It aids in the absorption and use of fats. Without choline, fat accumulates within the liver, damaging the organ. Choline also serves as an essential component in the making of acetylcholine. The latter is necessary for muscle control, storage of memory, and other neurological activities. Choline has gained popularity among body builders and athletes. According to a 2003 article in *Psychology Today*, choline reduced **fatigue** in long-distance runners and improved speed in a 20-mile run.

In 2003, scientists from the Massachusetts Institute of Technology released a study showing the positive effect of choline on boosting memory when laboratory rats took in a CDP-choline supplement. Choline is also important in the formation of DNA and other genetic compounds. A study released in 2006 found that a diet deficient in choline was linked with DNA damage. Choline is involved in the conversion of homocystine into **methionine**. This is an important physiological function because an accumulation of homocystine can increase risk for **heart disease** or **stroke**.

In 1999, the National Institutes for Health estimated that one percent of the United States population suffered from a genetic disorder that resulted in a fishy **body odor** due to a build-up of trimethylamine. A diet restricted in choline was suggested as a potential aide for these individuals.

Newborns require large amounts of choline to help their tiny organs undergo rapid growth and to achieve membrane biosynthesis. Choline and compounds containing choline are found in human breast milk and, in varying degrees, in infant formula.

A study released in 2007 found that supplements containing choline were beneficial for children with cystic fibrosis. A 2001 study involving rats found that pre- and postnatal supplementary choline prevented a loss of memory function associated with status epilepticus. As of 2008 more study in this area was needed.

Preparations

The recommended dose of choline, set by the Food and Nutrition Board of the National Academies of Science, is 425 mg per day for women and 550 mg

---

KEY TERMS

Biosynthesis—A process that produces chemical compounds from simpler components.

Folate—A vitamin used to treat a number of medical conditions.

Homocysteine—An amino acid found in the body. High levels raise the risk for heart disease and stroke.

Lecithin—A fatty substance found in plant and animal material, particularly egg yolk.

Methionine—An amino acid that provides benefits for the liver, as well as for conditions such as osteoarthritis, depression, fibromyalgia, and a host of other medical issues.

Trimethylamine—A product of decomposition associated with a fishy odor. Its build-up can result from excessive choline.

---

per day for men. Choline is available in capsules, tablets, and liquid form.

Precautions

Prior to taking choline, individuals should inform their physician if they are pregnant, breastfeeding, or if they have a chronic illness. A study released in 2007 found a potential link between ingestion of choline and increased risk of colon polyps in women. Its role in the formation of such polyps may be related to its ability to help form the outer shell of the polyps. However, researchers noted that other factors in the study, such as intake of red meat, may also be related to the rise in colon polyps. Scientists cautioned that more information is needed before conclusions can be drawn about choline intake and the development of colon polyps. A study involving men was planned.

Side Effects

In general, choline is considered to be a well tolerated supplement. Individuals who experience the following side effects should stop taking choline and report right away to their physician because they may be experiencing an allergic reaction:

- Problems breathing or tightness in the throat or chest
- Pain in the chest
- Rash, hives, itchiness, or swelling of the skin
  Other side effects include:
- Stomach pains or upset stomach
- Increased saliva

- Decreased appetite
- Sweating
- A fishy body odor

Interactions

As of 2008, there were no known negative interactions. Choline works in conjunction with other compounds, such as folate. Choline is a precursor to *betaine.*

Resources

BOOKS

Gaby, Alan R., (ed.) *The A-Z Guide to Vitamin-Drug-Herb Interactions: How to Improve Your Health and Avoid Problems When Using Common Medications and Natural Supplements Together* (2nd ed.). New York: Three Rivers Press, 2006.

PERIODICALS

Da Kosta, Kerry Ann, et al. "Choline Deficiency Increases Lymphocyte Apoptosis and DNA Damage in Humans." *American Journal of Clinical Nutrition* 84, no. 1 (July 2006): 88–94.

Innes, Sheila M., et al. "Choline-related Supplements Improve Abnormal Plasma Methionine-Homocysteine Metabolites and Glutathione Status in Children with Cystic Fibrosis." *American Journal of Clinical Nutrition* 85, no. 3 (March 2007): 702–708.

OTHER

Gangula, Ishani. "Choline May Increase Risk of Colon Polyps: Study." *Reuters* August 7, 2007. http://www.reuters.com.

PDRHealth. *Physicians' Desktop Reference.* http://www.pdrhealth.com.

ORGANIZATIONS

Institute of Medicine of the National Academies, 500 Fifth St. NW, Washington, DC, 20001, (202) 234-2352, http://www.iom.edu.

United States Department of Agriculture Research Service, Jamie L. Whitten Building. 1400 Independence Ave. SW, Washington, DC, 20250, http://www.ars.usda.gov.

Rhonda Cloos, RN

Chondroitin

Description

Chondroitin is a substance found in human and animal cartilage that is used to treat several physical disorders, most importantly arthritis, **psoriasis**, and **cancer**. It is the most plentiful type of glycosaminoglycan (GAG) found in cartilage. Glycosaminoglycans (GAGs) are complex carbohydrates that are found in the various types of connective tissue in the body. GAGs account for 5–20% of cartilage tissue. Chondroitin occurs in connective tissue as a sulfate composed of repeating disaccharide units; the first unit is either **glucosamine** or galactosamine; the other unit is glucuronic acid.

General use

Chondroitin has been studied in humans since about 1975 as a treatment for psoriasis, cancer, and arthritis. It is also used by veterinarians to treat animals for arthritis. These different applications are derived from different properties of chondroitin. In the early 2000s, chondroitin has been used in conjunction with another dietary supplement called glucosamine to help treat joint **pain** caused by **osteoarthritis** and to help stop cartilage loss in patients with the disease.

Psoriasis

Studies have been conducted in the United States since 1990 to determine whether chondroitin from shark cartilage can speed wound healing in psoriasis and related conditions. No conclusive findings had been reported as of early 2008.

Cancer

The use of cartilage products to treat cancer is based on the popular belief that cartilaginous fish (sharks, skates, and rays) do not get cancer. Samples of these fish indicate, however, that they do in fact develop a variety of tumors, mostly soft-tissue cancers.

There are several theories as to why chondroitin and cartilage products containing it may be useful in treating cancer. One theory is that they slow or stop the formation of blood vessels that supply the cancer with oxygen and nutrients. Another theory is that chondroitin blocks the formation of certain enzymes that tumors produce to invade surrounding tissue. The third theory suggests that cartilage products stimulate the immune system. As of late 1999 the National Cancer Institute was conducting a multicenter clinical trial of liquid cartilage extract.

Osteoarthritis

An estimated 20 million Americans suffer from joint-related disease and about 15 million of these people suffer from osteoarthritis. Chondroitin is best known to the general public as a remedy for osteoarthritis, which is a form of arthritis caused by wearing away or degeneration of the cartilage that cushions the ends of bones. In particular, it is thought that the drying of cartilage tissue in osteoarthritis is a major cause of tissue destruction. Chondroitin sulfate is given together with glucosamine, a building block of GAGs. The chondroitin helps to attract and hold fluid within cartilage tissue. Tissue fluid keeps cartilage healthy in two ways: it acts as a shock absorber within the joints of the body, thus protecting cartilage from being worn away by the bones; and it carries nutrients to the cartilage. The cartilage in the joints of the human body has no blood vessels, so it must receive its nutrients from tissue fluid.

In addition to drawing tissue fluid into cartilage, chondroitin is also thought to protect cartilage in the following ways:

- Acting as an anti-inflammatory activity.
- Inhibiting the activity of enzymes that break down cartilage.
- Counteracting enzymes that interfere with the transport of nutrients to the cartilage.
- Stimulating the production of proteoglycans, glycosaminoglycans, and collagen. These complex molecules are the building blocks of new cartilage.

Results of several European studies demonstrated that oral as well as injected chondroitin helps to increase joint mobility and reduce pain. A landmark 2001 study showed that combining glucosamine and chondroitin worked better than either worked alone in preventing cartilage damage and that both supplements worked well when taken orally. However, the Glucosamine/chondroitin Arthritis Intervention Trial reported in 2006 that glucosamine and chondroitin did not effectively reduce pain in people with osteoarthritis of the knee. Nearly 1,600 patients with osteoarthritis of the knee took part in the study conducted at 16 centers across the United States. Not all of the news from the study was discouraging, however. Among study participants who reported moderate to severe pain, as opposed to mild pain, 79% reported significant pain reduction when taking glucosamine and chondroitin supplementation. The study lasted for six months and a majority of the participants said they suffered from mild osteoarthritis of the knee. An ancillary study lasting an additional 18 months was conducted to see if glucosamine and chondroitin can reduce overall osteoarthritis pain if taken longer than six months. The results were expected in early 2008.

Preparations

The normal (non-vegetarian) adult diet already contains a certain amount of chondroitin; it is found in most animal tissues, particularly the gristle attached to bones.

Chondroitin sulfate can be taken orally as a pill, powder, or liquid. It can also be administered by injection. Oral preparations of chondroitin, alone or in combination with glucosamine, are available in the United States as over-the-counter (OTC) dietary supplements. They can be purchased over the Internet, at pharmacies, health food stores, and some grocery stores. Because they are marketed as dietary supplements, they do not require testing or approval by the Food and Drug Administration (FDA). As of 2008, there were no specific quality control requirements or clear manufacturing process (GMP) standards for these products.

There are, as of 2008, no standard patterns for administration of chondroitin as a treatment for psoriasis or cancer. When chondroitin is used together with glucosamine as a treatment for osteoarthritis, the daily dosage is based on the patient's weight. Suggested dosages are: 1,000 mg glucosamine + 800 mg chondroitin sulfate for 120 lbs or less; 1,500 mg glucosamine + 1,200 mg chondroitin sulfate for 120-200 lbs; and 2,000 mg glucosamine + 1,600 mg chondroitin sulfate for heavier than 200 lbs.

For maximum effectiveness, patients are advised to divide their daily dosage into 2 to 4 doses and take them throughout the day with food. They are also encouraged to take **vitamin C** and **manganese** supplements since these substances appear to increase the effectiveness of the chondroitin.

Precautions

There are two important precautions regarding chondroitin as a dietary supplement for osteoarthritis. The first is to avoid self-diagnosing and self-medicating. Persons with stiff or sore joints should consult a medical doctor (M.D.), osteopathic physician (D.O.), or naturopathic physician (N.D.) for an evaluation to determine if the problem is indeed osteoarthritis. **Gout**, **bursitis**, **rheumatoid arthritis**, **fibromyalgia**, and several other conditions can also cause pain and stiffness in the joints. These conditions are not helped by chondroitin. The supplement has not been studied in children or in pregnant or nursing women.

The second precaution is to purchase chondroitin made by a reliable manufacturer. The lack of government regulation of products sold as dietary supplements means that that there is no guarantee that claims made on the label are accurate. Thus a product that claims to contain chondroitin may not actually contain it, may not contain the amount that it claims

KEY TERMS

Cartilage—A firm, whitish elastic connective tissue found in humans and other animals. Chondroitin is an important component of cartilage.

Glucosamine—A complex carbohydrate composed of glucose and an amino acid called glutamine. It is an important building block of cartilage and is often taken together with chondroitin as a treatment for osteoarthritis.

Osteoarthritis—A degenerative disease of the joints, characterized by pain and stiffness related to loss or destruction of the cartilage in the joints.

Psoriasis—An inflammatory disorder of the skin characterized by scaly patches. Chondroitin may be a possible treatment for psoriasis.

to, or may not be free from contamination and safe to use. One helpful guideline is to look for the words *pharmaceutical grade* on the label. This standard ensures that the product is pure and that it contains the stated amount of chondroitin.

With regard to potential overdose problems, chondroitin sulfate appears to be nontoxic. One six-year study of people taking doses of 1.5-10 grams per day of chondroitin found no toxicity in the subjects.

Side effects

Chondroitin sulfate has no known significant side effects. Some people report having a bad taste in the mouth or mild **nausea** when taking large doses of oral chondroitin on an empty stomach. **Gas** or bloating has also been reported. A few people who have received chondroitin by injection report a mild soreness around the injection site.

Interactions

Chondroitin sulfate is not known to cause any significant interactions with other medications. A paper presented at the 1999 annual meeting of the American Academy of Orthopaedic Surgeons, however, stated that because the chondroitin sulfate molecule is similar to the heparin molecule, its use together with anticoagulant drugs is questionable.

Resources

BOOKS

Elkins, Rita. *Glucosamine and Chondroitin.* Orem, UT: Woodland, 2007.

Foltz-Gray, Dorothy. *The Arthritis Foundation's Guide to Good Living with Osteoarthritis,* 2nd ed. Atlanta, GA: Arthritis Foundation, 2006.

PERIODICALS

Band, Philip A. "Several Meta-Analyses Have Analyzed Its Safety and Effectiveness—Chondroitin Sulfate for Osteoarthritis: Interpreting Divergent Evidence." *Journal of Musculoskeletal Medicine* (October 1, 2007): 422.

Child, Rob. "Joint Pain and Supplements: The Recent GAIT Study on Glucosamine and Chondroitin for Chronic Joint Disease Sent Shock Waves Throughout the Industry, But What Did It Really Say about Their Effectiveness?" *Functional Foods and Neutraceuticals* (May 2006): 40.

Fox, Beth Anne, et al. "Glucosamine and Chondroitin for Osteoarthritis." *American Family Physician* (April 1, 2006): 1245.

Marshall, Peter D., and Elizabeth M. Tweed. "Do Glucosamine and Chondroitin Worsen Blood Sugar Control in Diabetes?" *Journal of Family Practice* (December 2006): 1091(3).

Schardt, David. "Arthritis Fighters: Do Glucosamine and Chondroitin Work?" *Nutrition Action Healthletter* (September 2006): 9(3).

Walsh, Nancy. "Chondroitin Reduces Joint Space Narrowing in OA." *Internal Medicine News* (January 1, 2007): 24.

ORGANIZATIONS

American Institute of Homeopathy, 801 N. Fairfax St., Suite 306, Alexandria, VA, 22314, (888) 445-9988, http://www.homeopathyusa.org.

Arthritis Foundation, PO Box 7669, Atlanta, GA, 30357, (800) 283-7800, http://www.arthritis.org.

Homeopathic Medical Council of Canada, 3910 Bathurst St., Suite 202, Toronto, ON, M3H 3N8, Canada, (416) 638-4622, http://www.hmcc.ca.

National Center for Alternative and Complementary Medicine, 9000 Rockville Pike, Bethesda, MD, 20892, (888) 644-6226, http://www.nccam.nih.gov.

Office of Dietary Supplements, National Institutes of Health, 6100 Executive Blvd., Room 3B01, MSC 7517, Bethesda, MD, 20892, (301) 435-2920, http://www.ods.od.nih.gov.

Rebecca Frey
Ken R. Wells

Christian Science healing

Definition

Christian Science healing is a method of spiritual healing based on the beliefs of the Christian Science, or Church of Christ, Scientist, church. The church's healing practices are based on the divine healing work of Jesus. Adherents hold that the material world is a false reality and that health is a condition of mind, God, and truth. Thus, Christian scientists believe that ill health can be cured by spiritual education, understanding of the truth, and **prayer**.

Origins

Mary Baker Eddy, the founder of Christian Science, was born Mary Baker in Bow, New Hampshire, on July 16, 1821, into a family of strict Christian practice and Puritan values. Baker was ill for much of her childhood and early adult life. She explored medical therapies popular in her time, including **homeopathy**, and found no relief for her chronic illness.

Between 1862 and 1865 Baker was a patient of a charismatic healer named Phineas Parkhurst Quimby. A former hypnotist, Quimby developed a philosophy of mental healing based on the belief that he had rediscovered the secret of Jesus' ability to heal the sick. It is thought that Quimby's ideas may have influenced Baker in the development of her philosophy of Christian Science healing, although she herself denied it.

In 1866, the same year that Phineas Quimby died, Baker suffered a spinal injury from a fall. This proved to be a critical turning point in her life. Seeking strength in the Bible to sustain her through the injury, Baker read a New Testament account of Jesus' healing. While she was reading, she experienced a sudden insight into how Jesus' healing was accomplished, and as she read, she found herself suddenly released from her injury and restored to health.

This transformation inspired Baker to spend the next three years studying the scriptures and codifying her discoveries about healing. She called her discoveries Christian Science, and believed that she had found the one and only "truth." She put her principles into action by healing others, including those who had illnesses declared by medical practitioners of the day to be incurable.

As Baker studied the Bible and practiced healing, she came to believe that she could teach others to heal following God's truth as she had discovered it. In 1870 in Lynn, Massachusetts, she taught her first class and began to develop a following that shared her belief in Christian Science healing.

In 1875, while still living in Lynn, Mary Baker published *Science and Health*, later renamed *Science and Health with Key to the Scriptures*. This book, revised by Baker Eddy over the next 35 years, is the fundamental document explaining the doctrine of Christian Science healing.

In 1877 Mary Baker married fellow Christian Scientist Asa Gilbert Eddy and by 1879 had established enough of a following to found the first Church of Christ, Scientist in Boston, Massachusetts. This church became her headquarters and is known as the Mother Church. The regulatory structure of the denomination was set forth in her book *The Manual of the Mother Church* published in 1895.

Throughout the late 1800s, Christian Science continued to attract converts. Most of these conversions were brought about by demonstrations of Christian Science healing. Eddy also established the Massachusetts Metaphysical College to teach Christian Science healing. It is estimated that by 1895 there were about 250 Christian Science congregations, mainly in New England.

Mary Baker Eddy died on December 3, 1910. At the time of her death, there were about 1,200 Christian Scientist congregations in the United States. By the 1930s the number had increased to about 2,400. The United States Bureau of the Census in 1936 estimated church membership in the United States at about 269,000. Meanwhile congregations were also being established overseas.

After World War II, the number of Christian Science congregations began to decline. Beginning in the 1980s the church had to deal with negative publicity from court cases alleging that the failure of Christian Science parents to seek conventional medical treatment for children who had illnesses considered treatable by mainstream medicine constituted child endangerment. Convictions, many of which were overturned on appeal, further hurt church membership. The number of Christian Scientist practitioners, as those people whom the Church of Christ, Scientist officially recognizes as spiritual healers are called, dropped from about 8,000 in 1960 to about 2,000 in 1998.

Today Mary Baker Eddy is recognized both as a mind-body healer and as a pioneer in the area of equality for women. In the Church of Christ, Scientist, men and women function equally as leaders and healers, an idea that was revolutionary in Eddy's lifetime. In 1995 she was elected to the National Women's Hall of Fame in recognition of being the only American woman to found an internationally established religion.

In addition to its practices of spiritual healing, Christian Science is best known today for its publishing activities, spearheaded by the international newspaper the *Christian Science Monitor* founded by Eddy in 1908. Each congregation also provides a public Christian Science Reading Room where the public may read Christian Science literature and ponder spiritual matters.

Benefits

For believers, Christian Science healing brings both spiritual and physical well being to those who are ill. Its healing practices make no distinction among different types of illnesses. It uses no material methods or laying on of hands to restore people to health and can be practiced in almost any setting.

Description

To understand Christian Science healing one must also understand Christian Science theology, because the two are inextricably linked. On the first page of *Science and Health with Key to the Scriptures* Eddy writes, "The prayer that reforms the sinner and heals the sick is an absolute faith that all things are possible to God...and a spiritual understanding of Him, an unselfed love... Prayer, watching, and working, combined with self-immolation, are God's gracious means for accomplishing whatever has been successfully done for the Christianization and health of mankind."

Christian Science teaches that the ordinary physical world that we perceive is a misconception. Matter is not created by God, but appears because of man's limited perception. Jesus, Eddy explains, was able to heal the sick, the blind, and the lame, because he saw beyond their material form and saw the spirit essence of the person.

In writing on the human body in *Science and Health with Key to the Scriptures*, Eddy states, "To measure intellectual capacity by the size of the brain and strength by the **exercise** of muscle, is to subjugate intelligence, to make the mind mortal, and to place this so-called mind at the mercy of material organization and non-intelligent matter. Obedience to the so-called physical laws of health has not checked sickness. Diseases have multiplied since man-made material theories took the place of spiritual truth. You say that **indigestion, fatigue**, sleeplessness, cause distressed

stomachs and aching heads. Then you consult your brain in order to remember what has hurt you, when your remedy lies in forgetting the whole thing; for matter has no sensation of its own and the human mind is all that can produce pain."

For believers, Christian Science healing is the triumph of mind over matter and the spiritual over the material world. Ill health is simply an illusion. Good health occurs when the mind achieves awareness of itself, which is synonymous with awareness of God. The goal of healing is not to remove physical suffering, but to lead the ill person to Christ and transform the consciousness into a more pure and spiritual state that knows God. Healing is seen as a measure of the depth of one's sincerity and belief.

Since health does not reside in the body, and is not controlled by physical laws, Christian Science healing cannot occur when a person is in a state of moral sinfulness or lack of belief. The basis of disease is fear, ignorance, or sin. Health is a spiritual fact to be demonstrated.

Christian Science teaches that all believers can be taught to heal. Those people officially sanctioned as healers by the Church of Christ, Scientist are called Christian Science practitioners. Practitioners may be either male or female. These people must pledge to devote themselves to the practice of healing full time. They may be paid by their patients for their work. In 2000 there were about 2,000 officially recognized Christian Science practitioners in the United States, and that number is declining.

Practitioners do not use any material props or even touch to heal their patients; only prayer is used. The practitioner approaches the patient with a clear conviction of the omnipotence of God and the firm belief that God is good and produces only good things. Practitioners who hold false beliefs, or error, even unwitting error, blended with the truth, have weak healing abilities and may be guilty of malpractice. If the healer realizes the truth, it will free his patient from symptoms of disease, discord, and disharmony and lead the patient to Christ. This is said to leave the patient feeling calm, refreshed, and healthy.

Many converts come to Christian Science through the demonstration of its power to heal. Traditionally, Wednesday night meetings are given over to healing testimony and witnessing of the healing power of God's truth.

Preparations

The purpose of Christian Science healing is not to free the body from disease, but to lead the patient to a higher spiritual understanding of God. Patients are best served if they are receptive to Christian Science beliefs and practices prior to the start of a healing session.

Precautions

There are no reasons other than disbelief or spiritual unreadiness not to participate in Christian Science healing. However, patients that do this must understand that they may be exacerbating their health problems by denying themselves access to traditional medical care.

Side effects

No side effects are reported from practicing Christian Science healing. There is, as noted above, danger posed by replacing traditional medical care with Christian Science practices in the case of serious illness.

Research and general acceptance

Christian Science healing is seen by the traditional medical community as quackery, since it denies any relationship between the physical universe and illness. It rejects the concepts of germs, contagion, and healing through the application of drugs.

All "proof" of the effectiveness of Christian Science healing is anecdotal. Many physicians believe that in certain cases of psychosomatic illness Christian Science healing may indeed bring about improvement in symptoms, but in diseases with a clear physical origin, it is ineffective.

Training and certification

The Church of Christ, Scientist recognizes some of its healers as official practitioners whose full-time job is healing. About 2,000 were in practice in the United States in 2000.

Resources

BOOKS

Eddy, Mary Baker. *Science and Health with Key to the Scriptures.* Boston: Christian Science Publishing Company, 1875 (reprinted 1994).

PERIODICALS

Sheler, Jeffrey L. "Mrs. Eddys House." *U.S. News Online* February 16, 1998. http://www.usnews.com/usnews/issue980216/16eddy.htm.

ORGANIZATIONS

Church of Christ, Scientist. http://www.ChristianScience.org.

OTHER

The Mary Baker Eddy Library for the Betterment of Humanity. *http://www.marybakereddy.org:86/.*
Virtual Christian Science Reading Room. http://www.mtn.org.

Tish Davidson

Chromium

Description

Chromium is a mineral that is essential to humans. It is found naturally in a variety of foods, and supplements are available in capsules or tablets. Supplements are prepared using a number of formulas, including chromium (III), chromium aspartate, chromium chloride, chromium citrate, chromium nicotinate, chromium picolinate, GTF chromium, and trivalent chromium.

General use

Chromium supports the normal function of insulin, which is a hormone secreted by the pancreas. Insulin helps transport glucose from the bloodstream into liver, muscle, and fat cells. Once it is inside these cells, the sugar is metabolized into a source of energy. Insulin is also involved in regulating protcin, fat, and catalytic enzyme processes. People with diabetes do not produce insulin (or produce very little) or their bodies cannot properly use the insulin that is produced. As a result, sugar builds up in the bloodstream, causing serious health effects. Numerous scientific studies have shown that chromium is useful in treating **insulin resistance** (metabolic syndrome) and diabetes. Diabetic **peripheral neuropathy**, a form of nerve damage that is a direct result of diabetes, is indirectly related to a lack of sufficient chromium.

Several studies have shown that chromium supplements may improve insulin sensitivity and lower blood glucose and elevated body fat. In February 2004, the University of Pennsylvania School of Medicine began a comprehensive study of chromium as a therapy for insulin resistance. This condition occurs when the body fails to respond properly to the insulin it already produces. People who are insulin resistant may have the ability to overcome this problem by producing more insulin. However, if the body cannot produce sufficient amounts of insulin, glucose levels in the bloodstream rise, and type 2 diabetes ultimately occurs. It is estimated that up to 80 million Americans have insulin resistance.

Adequate intake of chromium

Age	mcg/day
Children 0-6 mos.	0.2
Children 7-12 mos.	5.5
Children 1-3 yrs.	11
Children 4-8 yrs.	15
Boys 9-13 yrs.	25
Girls 9-13 yrs.	21
Boys 14-18 yrs.	35
Girls 14-18 yrs.	24
Men 19-50 yrs.	35
Women 19-50 yrs.	25
Men > 50 yrs.	30
Women > 50 yrs.	20
Pregnant women ≤ 18 yrs.	29
Breastfeeding women ≤ 18 yrs.	44
Pregnant women ≥ 19 yrs.	30
Breastfeeding women ≥ 19 yrs.	45

Foods that contain chromium	mcg
Broccoli, 1/2 cup	11
Grape juice, 1 cup	8
English muffin, whole wheat, 1	4
Garlic, dried, 1 tsp.	3
Potatoes, mashed, 1 cup	3
Basil, dried, 1 tbsp.	2
Beef cubes, 3 oz.	2
Orange juice, 1 cup	2
Turkey breast, 3 oz.	2
Whole wheat bread, 2 slices	2
Red wine, 5 oz.	1-13
Apple, unpeeled, 1 med.	1
Banana, 1 med.	1
Green beans, 1/2 cup	1

mcg = microgram

(Illustration by GGS Information Services. Cengage Learning, Gale)

A study conducted by Isala Clinics and University Hospital Groningen in the Netherlands, released in 2003, showed that a daily dose of 1,000 micrograms of chromium significantly reduced blood sugar levels in people with poorly controlled type 2 diabetes who use insulin. However, a subsequent study, conducted by Louisiana State University in Baton Rouge, indicated that the response to chromium supplementation by diabetics may be in part genetically mediated, so not all patients respond to chromium.

Chromium has also been used as an effective treatment for polycystic ovarian syndrome (PCOS), a hormonal condition affecting about two million American women. The condition can lead to **infertility** if untreated and is associated with insulin resistance and type 2 diabetes. A study released in 2003 by the State University of New York at Stony Brook showed that insulin sensitivity increased an average of 35 percent after two months of daily treatment with 1,000 micrograms (mcg) of chromium.

Through its involvement with insulin function, chromium plays an indirect role in lowering blood lipids. Studies suggest, but as of the early 2000s had not proven, that chromium supplementation can reduce the risk of cardiovascular (heart) disease in men and may decrease total **cholesterol** and triglyceride levels. However, several studies contradict these claims. Studies in animals suggest chromium supplementation may reduce **hypertension** (high blood pressure). Lipid reduction is secondary to insulin regulation and control; therefore, persons whose insulin is well regulated and controlled may not achieve reduced **heart disease** risk by taking chromium supplements.

Chromium supplements in high doses—1,000 mcg or more a day—are sometimes used in weight loss and muscle development. However, a number of scientific studies have found that chromium supplements are not effective in these areas. In fact, precautions warn against chromium doses exceeding 1,000 mcg per day. Weight loss and muscle development are secondary to insulin regulation and control. Therefore, when insulin is well regulated and controlled, chromium may not impact weight loss or muscle development. A controlled study by the United States Department of Agriculture in which 83 women were fed a controlled diet but received either chromium piccolinate, piccolinic acid, or placebo, failed to demonstrate any changes in body composition between the three groups.

Preparations

A complete lack of chromium is rare, and the United States Food and Drug Administration (FDA) has not established recommended dietary allowances (RDA) for the mineral. However, national statistics on the prevalence of diabetes, heart disease, and **obesity** suggest that chromium deficiencies may be common. Chromium occurs naturally in meat, seafood, dairy products, eggs, whole grains, black pepper, and almonds. According to *The PDR Family Guide to Natural Medicines and Healing Therapies*, the usual chromium supplement dose for children ages seven and older and adults is 50–200 mcg a day in tablets or capsules. For persons with type 2 diabetes who are not taking insulin, doses from 200–1,000 mcg daily may be taken. However, persons should only take doses at these levels after consulting with a physician. Chromium should not be taken in doses exceeding

KEY TERMS

Calcium carbonate—A salt that is used in many antacids.

Diabetes—Several metabolic disorders in which the body produces insufficient insulin.

Glucose—Sugar.

Hypertension—High blood pressure, which, if untreated, can lead to heart disease and stroke.

Insomnia—The inability to sleep.

Insulin—A hormone that helps liver, muscle, and fat cells take up sugars, starches, and other foods for conversion into energy the body needs.

Insulin resistance—Also called metabolic syndrome, a condition in which the body fails to properly respond to the insulin it produces.

Polycystic ovarian syndrome—PCOS, a hormonal condition in women that if untreated can lead to the inability to have children.

1,000 mcg a day. The cost of a bottle of 100 tablets or capsules (200 mcg) of chromium piccolinate ranges from \$5 to \$10 for a generic or house brand preparation.

Precautions

Doses of 200–1,000 mcg of chromium should be taken only after consultation with a physician. Pregnant or breastfeeding women are advised to consult a physician before taking chromium supplements. Chromium should not be taken in doses exceeding 1,000 mcg a day. Increased dietary sugar may be associated with higher urinary excretion of chromium.

Side effects

Several studies have noted occasional reports of irregular heartbeats with chromium use. Infrequently, chromium has been reported to cause such sleep pattern changes as **insomnia** and increased dream activity. Irritability has also been reported. In rare instances, persons may be allergic to a chromium formula. The symptoms of an allergic reaction include difficulty breathing, chest **pain**, **hives**, rash, and itchy or swollen skin. If any of these symptoms occur, the patient is advised to seek medical care immediately. High doses may also cause liver and kidney damage or gastric irritation, although these side effects are rare.

Interactions

Persons who are taking antacids are advised to talk with a physician before taking chromium supplements. Studies in animals suggest that antacids, especially those containing **calcium** carbonate, may reduce the body's ability to absorb chromium. Studies have shown that chromium may enhance the effectiveness of drugs taken by people who have type 2 diabetes or insulin resistance. These drugs include glimepiride, glipizide, glyburide, insulin, and metformin. Individuals taking these drugs should discuss chromium supplementation with a physician because improved insulin function may necessitate medication dosage changes.

Resources

PERIODICALS

Lukaski H. C., W. A. Siders, and J. G. Penland. "Chromium Picolinate Supplementation in Women: Effects On Body Weight, Composition, and Iron Status." *Nutrition* (March 23, 2007): 187–95.

Ken R. Wells
Sam Uretsky, PharmD

Chronic fatigue syndrome

Definition

Chronic **fatigue** syndrome (CFS) is a condition that causes extreme tiredness. People with CFS have debilitating fatigue that lasts for six months or longer. CFS does not have a known cause, but it appears to result from a combination of factors.

Description

CFS is the most common name for this disorder, but it also has been called chronic fatigue and immune disorder syndrome (CFIDS), myalgic encephalomyelitis, low natural killer cell disease, post-viral fatigue syndrome, Epstein-Barr disease, and yuppie flu. Reports of a CFS-like syndrome called neurasthenia date back to 1869. Subsequently, people with similar symptoms were said to have **fibromyalgia** because one of the main symptoms is myalgia, or muscle **pain**. Because of the similarity of symptoms, fibromyalgia and CFS are considered to be overlapping syndromes.

In the early to mid-1980s, there were outbreaks of CFS in some areas of the United States. Although many CFS patients had high levels of antibodies to

Symptoms of chronic fatigue syndrome

Unexplained fatigue

Unrefreshing sleep

Muscle aches and weakness

Insomnia or oversleeping

Swollen lymph nodes

Forgetfulness, confusion

Lack of concentration

Recurrent sore throat

Headaches (of a new type or severity)

Joint pain (without redness or swelling)

Long-lasting symptoms that continue for six months or longer

(Illustration by Corey Light. Cengage Learning, Gale)

the Epstein-Barr virus (EBV), which causes **mononucleosis**, many healthy people also had high levels of EBV antibodies. Scientists also found high levels of other viral antibodies in the blood of CFS patients. These findings led many scientists to believe that a virus or combination of viruses may trigger CFS.

Although CFS can affect people of any gender, age, race, or socioeconomic group, most patients diagnosed with CFS are 25 to 45 years old and female. Estimates of how many people are afflicted with CFS vary due to the similarity of CFS symptoms to other diseases and the difficulty in identifying it. The Centers for Disease Control and Prevention (CDC) has estimated that about one million people in the United States have CFS.

Causes and symptoms

There is no single known cause for CFS. Studies have pointed to several different conditions that might be responsible. These include:

• viral infections
• chemical toxins
• allergies
• immune abnormalities
• psychological disorders

Many doctors and researchers think that CFS may not be a single illness but a group of symptoms caused by several conditions. One theory is that a microorganism, such as a virus, or a chemical injures the body and damages the immune system, allowing dormant viruses to become active. When these viruses start growing again, the immune system may overreact and produce chemicals called cytokines that can cause flu-like symptoms. Immune abnormalities have been found in studies of people with CFS, although the same abnormalities are also found in people with **allergies**, autoimmune diseases, **cancer**, and other disorders.

In late 2001, a panel of experts concluded that a virus or bacteria acting on the immune system may indeed cause CFS; the experts agreed that the published evidence was substantial enough to prove that the immune system is involved in CFS. They stated that **infections** may also play a role in the condition, but they did not identify one single agent common to all patients with CFS. Further research was recommended. The panel also concluded that reproductive hormones may play a role in the condition, which might explain the higher prevalence among women. In spite of these findings, the CDC continued as of 2008 to report that the causes for CFS had yet to be identified.

The role of psychological problems in CFS is controversial. Because many people with CFS are diagnosed with **depression** and other psychiatric disorders, some experts concluded that the symptoms of CFS are psychological. However, many people with CFS do not have psychological disorders before getting the illness. Many doctors think that patients become depressed or anxious because of the effects of the symptoms of their CFS. One study concluded that depression was the result of CFS, not its cause.

People with CFS have severe fatigue that keeps them from performing their normal daily activities. They may have sleep disturbances that keep them from getting enough rest or they may sleep too much. When they **exercise** or try to be active in spite of their fatigue, people with CFS experience debilitating exhaustion that can confine them to bed for days.

Other symptoms of CFS include:

• muscle pain (myalgia)
• joint pain (arthralgia)
• sore throat
• headache
• fever and chills
• tender lymph nodes
• trouble concentrating
• memory loss

One study at Johns Hopkins University found an abnormality in blood pressure regulation in 22 of 23 patients with CFS. This abnormality, called neurally mediated hypotension, causes a sudden drop in blood pressure when a person has been standing, exercising, or exposed to heat for a while. When this response occurs, patients feel lightheaded and may faint. They often are exhausted for hours to days after one of these episodes. When treated with salt and medications to stabilize blood pressure, many patients in the study had marked improvements in their CFS symptoms. Follow-up research on this topic was limited as of 2008.

Diagnosis

CFS is diagnosed by evaluating symptoms and eliminating other causes of fatigue. Doctors carefully question patients about their symptoms, any other illnesses they have had, and medications they are taking. They also conduct a physical examination, neurological examination, and laboratory tests to identify any underlying disorders or other diseases that cause fatigue. In the United States, many doctors use the CDC case definition to determine if a patient has CFS.

To be diagnosed with CFS, patients must meet both of the following criteria:

- Unexplained continuing or recurring chronic fatigue for at least six months that is of new or definite onset, is not the result of ongoing exertion, and is not mainly relieved by rest, and causes occupational, educational, social, or personal activities to be greatly reduced.
- Four or more of the following symptoms: loss of short-term memory or ability to concentrate; sore throat; tender lymph nodes; muscle pain; multi-joint pain without swelling or redness; headaches of a new type, pattern, or severity; nonrefreshing sleep; and post-exertional malaise (a vague feeling of discomfort or tiredness following exercise or other physical or mental activity) lasting more than 24 hours. These symptoms must have continued or recurred during six or more consecutive months of illness and must not have started before the fatigue began.

Treatment

There is no specific cure for CFS, but many treatments are available to help relieve the symptoms. Treatments usually are individualized to each person's particular symptoms and needs. The first treatment recommended is a combination of rest, exercise, and a balanced diet. Prioritizing activities, avoiding overexertion, and resting when needed are key to maintaining existing energy reserves. Treatment of airborne allergies is an important facet in the treatment of CFS.

Diet

Drinking eight to 12 glasses of water daily helps fight fatigue. Food allergies can worsen CFS symptoms. Common food allergies include milk, wheat, eggs, citrus, alcohol, chocolate, and coffee. An extract from shiitake mushrooms (LEM) has been shown in Japanese studies to benefit CFS patients.

Ayurvedic medicine stresses that energy is derived from food. Energy-producing foods include: fresh fruits and vegetables, whole milk, wheat and wheat products, rice, barley, honey, olive oil, mung bean soup, raisins, dates, figs, almonds, clarified butter, and yogurt. Foods that deplete energy include: red meat, aged or fermented foods, onions, **garlic**, mushrooms, potatoes, sugar, alcohol, and coffee.

Ayurvedic medicine dictates that complete digestion of food is necessary to obtain the maximum amount of energy. The following measures can be taken to optimize digestion:

- eating in a quiet place
- following established mealtimes
- sitting while eating
- not eating while upset
- eating only until satiety (fullness)
- avoiding ice cold foods and drinks
- not talking while chewing
- eating at a moderate pace

Supplements

The following supplements have been used in treating CFS.

- Vitamin B_{12} deficiency causes fatigue, muscle aches, confusion, poor memory, and arm and leg numbness.
- Magnesium helps muscles to relax. Persons with kidney or heart disease should not take magnesium.
- Iron treats anemia, which can cause tiredness and improve mental clarity. This supplement should be taken only if a physician has diagnosed an iron deficiency.
- Manganese works with the supplements above to relieve CFS symptoms.
- Copper deficiency can cause inflammation. Maximum recommended daily dose for adults is 2 to 3

mg. Pregnant women should consult a physician before taking copper supplements.

- Zinc may boost the immune system.
- Coenzyme Q10 can increase immune health.
- NADH may lead to improvement in energy, cognitive ability, sleep patterns, headaches, and depression.
- Carnitine helps to better utilize fats for energy production. The recommended daily dose is 500 to 3,000 mg.
- Alpha lipoic acid enhances energy.
- 5-HTP helps to regulate sleep patterns.
- DHEA deficiency causes fatigue in females and low sex drive in males. It should be taken only under the direction of a physician.

Fluoride is a potentially toxic substance and should be avoided.

Other treatment options

Chinese medicine, including **acupuncture** and **cupping**, works to bring the body back into balance. Herbals that may help relieve symptoms of CFS include:

- astragalus (huang chi) to increase energy
- licorice (gan t'sao) for stomach and liver problems, adrenal exhaustion, and blood pressure warming
- ginger root for digestion
- turmeric for inflammation
- linden flowers for the heart
- echinacea for stimulating the immune system but taken for no more than 10 to 14 consecutive days
- Siberian ginseng (*Eleutherococcus senticosus*) to increase resistance to stress and boost the immune system
- ginkgo to increase blood flow through the brain but also thin the blood
- evening primrose (*Oenothera biennis*) oil to increase energy levels
- borage seed (*Borago officinales*) oil
- quercetin
- flaxseed oil

Some CFS patients use **fasting** only under the direction of a healthcare practitioner. **Probiotics** using *Lactobacillus acidophilus* can restore a normal balance to the intestinal bacterial.

Chiropractic adjustments may help relieve symptoms of CFS. **Osteopathy** helps some CFS patients. Osteopaths developed the craniosacral method that involves manipulation of the bones and membrane attachments of the head. Naturopathic physicians routinely treat CFS patients. Components of Ayurvedic treatment of CFS include **stress** reduction, daily oil massage, improving sleep, improving bowel function, and light to moderate exercise.

Psychological and spiritual counseling are important facets of CFS treatment. Cognitive behavior therapy helps patients manage activity levels to reduce fatigue. The type of **psychotherapy** employed is less important than having good rapport with the therapist.

For patients who are employed, modifications to the workplace are essential to maintaining good health. Vocational rehabilitation counseling allows the patient to maximize his or her work potential.

Exercise and physical therapy can have a dramatic impact on the health of CFS patients. Stretching exercises and moderate aerobic activity are beneficial. Too much exercise can worsen fatigue and other CFS symptoms. Exercise programs such as physical therapy, **t'ai chi**, **yoga**, chi kung, the **Alexander technique**, and muscle balance and function development (MBF) are all options.

There is a lengthy list of therapies used by CFS patients to find relief. These are not cures, and many have not been tested in clinical studies. CFS patients may find relief, if only temporarily, in the following:

- sessions with a spiritual healer
- yoga
- reflexology
- hydrotherapy
- sound therapy
- chocolate therapy
- magnet therapy
- meditation
- visualization
- spiritual cleansing rituals
- biofeedback

A 2002 report noted a study that showed some results from **homeopathy** for CFS patients. For the study, patients underwent six months of treatment chosen by one of four homeopaths and changed as needed. Sixty-five percent of patients reported some improvement, feeling fitter, more rested, and less tired. A 2002 review of research on the effectiveness of homeopathy in the treatment of CFS found mixed results, however. Authors of the review pointed out that the studies they examined were often poorly done, producing results that were difficult to interpret.

KEY TERMS

Alexander technique—A movement therapy that identifies and changes poor physical habits that may cause fatigue. The body is put into a state of relaxation and balance through the use of simple movements.

Arthralgia—Joint pain.

Depression—A psychological condition, with feelings of sadness, sleep disturbance, fatigue, and inability to concentrate.

Epstein-Barr virus (EBV)—A virus in the herpes family that causes mononucleosis.

Fibromyalgia—A disorder closely related to CFS. Symptoms include pain, tenderness, and muscle stiffness.

Lymphocytes—White blood cells that are involved in the immune system.

Mononucleosis—A flu-like illness caused by the Epstein-Barr virus.

Muscle balance and function development (MBF)—A movement therapy that strives to realign body posture through a series of exercises.

Myalgia—Muscle pain.

Natural killer (NK) cell—A lymphocyte that acts as a primary immune defense against infection.

Neurally mediated hypotension—A rapid fall in blood pressure that causes dizziness, blurred vision, and fainting, and is often followed by prolonged fatigue.

Neurasthenia—Nervous exhaustion. A disorder with symptoms of irritability and weakness, commonly diagnosed in the late 1800s.

Allopathic treatment

Drugs

Nonsteroidal anti-inflammatory drugs (NSAIDs), such as ibuprofen and naproxen, may be used to relieve pain and reduce **fever**. Another medication that is prescribed to relieve pain and **muscle spasms** is cyclobenzaprine (Flexeril).

Many doctors prescribe low dosages of antidepressants for their sedative effects and to relieve symptoms of depression. Antianxiety drugs, such as benzodiazepines or buspirone, may be prescribed for excessive **anxiety** that has lasted for at least six months.

Other medications that have been tested or were being tested as of 2008 for treatment of CFS are:

- Fludrocortisone (Florinef), a synthetic steroid, has helped some CFS patients who have neurally mediated hypotension.
- Beta-adrenergic blocking drugs, including atenolol (Tenoretic, Tenormin) and propranolol (Inderal), are sometimes prescribed for neurally mediated hypotension.
- Gamma globulin, which contains human antibodies, has been used experimentally to boost immune function in CFS patients.
- Ampligen, a drug which stimulates the immune system and has antiviral activity, improved mental function in some CFS patients.

Expected results

The course of CFS varies widely for different people. Some get progressively worse over time, while others gradually improve. Some persons have periods of illness that alternate with periods of good health. While some people with CFS do fully regain their health, those who do not find relief from symptoms and adapt to the demands of the disorder by carefully following a treatment plan combining adequate rest, **nutrition**, exercise, and other therapies.

Prevention

Because the cause of CFS is not known, there are no recommendations for preventing the disorder.

Resources

BOOKS

Bassman, Lynette. *The Feel-Good Guide to Fibromyalgia & Chronic Fatigue Syndrome: A Comprehensive Resource for Recovery*. Oakland, CA: New Harbinger Publications, 2007.

Bested, Alison C., and Alan C. Logan. *Hope and Help for Chronic Fatigue Syndrome and Fibromyalgia*. Nashville, TN: Cumberland House, 2006.

Bharadvaj, Daivati. *Natural Treatments for Chronic Fatigue Syndrome*. Westport, CT: Praeger Press, 2007.

Skelly, Mari, and Helen Walker. *Alternative Treatments for Fibromyalgia and Chronic Fatigue Syndrome*, 2nd ed. Alameda, CA: Hunter House, 2006.

PERIODICALS

Burley, Lucy, Diane L. Cox, and Leslie J. Findley. "Severe Chronic Fatigue Syndrome (CFS/ME): Recovery Is Possible." *British Journal of Occupational Therapy* (August 2007): 339–344.

Gray, Suzanne Elizabeth, and D. R. Rutter. "Illness Representations in Young People with Chronic Fatigue Syndrome Title." *Psychology and Health* (February 2007): 159–174.

Jason, Leonard A., Karine Corradi, and Susan Torres-Harding. "Toward an Empirical Case Definition of CFS." *Journal of Social Service Research* (December 2007): 43–54.

Matthews, Rosalind, and Anthony Komaroff. "Changes in Functional Status in Chronic Fatigue Syndrome Over a Decade: Do Age and Gender Matter?" *Journal of Chronic Fatigue Syndrome* (May 2007): 33–42.

Smith, Cath, and Leigh Hale. "The Effects of Non-pharmacological Interventions on Fatigue in Four Chronic Illness Conditions: A Critical Review." *Physical Therapy Review* (December 2007): 324–334.

Staud, Roland. "Treatment of Fibromyalgia and Its Symptoms." *Expert Opinion on Pharmacotherpy* (August 2007): 1629–1642.

OTHER

"Chronic Fatigue Syndrome." Centers for Disease Control and Prevention. [cited March 19, 2008]. http://www.cdc.gov/cfs/.

ORGANIZATIONS

CFIDS Association. Community Health Services, PO Box 220398, Charlotte, NC, 28222-0398, (704) 362-2343, http://www.cfids.org/.

National CFIDS Foundation, 103 Aletha Rd., Needham, MA, 02192, (781) 449-3535, http://www.ncf-net.org/index.html.

National Chronic Fatigue Syndrome and Fibromyalgia Association, PO Box 18426, Kansas City, MO, 64133, (913) 321-2278, http://www.ncfsfa.org/.

Belinda Rowland
Teresa G. Odle
David Edward Newton, Ed.D.

Chronic pain *see* **Pain**

Chrysanthemum flower

Description

The chrysanthemum, of which there are many varieties, has been known by a host of common names throughout history. Some of the chrysanthemum's common names include pellitory, **feverfew**, ox-eye daisy, and sunflower among others. It is a flower that has grown in gardens all around the world as far back as any records can tell, and seems to have been employed everywhere at some time or another as a cure for a host of complaints.

Chinese chrysanthemum flower

The Latin name for Chinese chrysanthemum flower is *Chrysanthemum indicum*, and it is known in China as Ju Jua. The plant grows profusely throughout China and is both an emblem to the Chinese and greatly prized for its medicinal properties, particularly as an anti-inflammatory.

The best flowers for medicinal purposes are considered to be the yellow fragrant ones. They are classified as being acrid, bitter, and slightly cold in the Chinese pharmacopoeia. Traditionally, they are harvested in the fall, when they are in full bloom.

The herb is taken internally for headaches, **dizziness**, and hearing disorders. It is also useful as a treatment for high blood pressure (**hypertension**). It is used as a compress or eye wash for inflammation of the eyes and for other eye problems such as dry-eye, blurred vision, and spots before the eyes. The herb can also be taken internally as an infusion and is combined with **honeysuckle** for the treatment of colds, the flu, and infected sores. It has a calming effect and can also be good for **stress**. Chrysanthemum is known to be a powerful antiseptic and antibiotic. However, people suffering from **diarrhea** should take it with caution.

Dalmatian pellitory

There are many plants that go by the name of pellitory, but this one is also a member of the chrysanthemum family. Its botanical name is *Chrysanthemum cinerariafolium*, and it originated in Dalmatia. It is cultivated in both Dalmatia and California. Previously, Persian pellitory was the most widely used, but it has been superceded by Dalmatian pellitory in practical use due to ease of cultivation.

Feverfew

The variety of chrysanthemum that is perhaps the most useful as far as herbal medicine is concerned, is feverfew, or *Chrysanthemum parthenium*. Most species of chrysanthemum are tall daisy-like flowers and feverfew is no exception. It is commonly found in England and the United States, and is similar to **chamomile** in appearance. Feverfew differs from chamomile in that it is larger and the white petals are arranged around a flat yellow center, as opposed to conical, which is the case with chamomile. The hairy stems of feverfew grow to about 2 ft (61 cm) tall, and the leaves are serrated and downy. Feverfew is also known by other common names, including featherfew, featherfoil, flirtwort, bachelor's buttons, and wild chamomile.

KEY TERMS

Decoction—These are made to be taken immediately (not for storage): simmer herbs for half an hour and strain, in the same way as for syrup, but sweetened to taste only.

Fluid extract—Made by simmering a plant and reducing the water until the mixture is thickened. This resulting liquid has a concentrated form of the active constituents of a plant. Alcohol, glycerin, or tincture of Benzoin may be added as a preservative.

Infusion—This is made in the same way that one would make tea, i.e., adding boiling water to the dried herb and allowing it to stand for a while.

Syrup—An herbal preparation that is made generally by boiling the herb with water, adding sugar as a preservative, and boiling until it thickens. The syrup may be stored.

Tincture—Herbs that are not soluble in water are bruised and steeped in alcohol. This liquid is placed in a bottle and may be filtered with coffee filters. The same procedure may be followed using vinegar instead of alcohol.

Ox-eye daisy

The botanical name for the ox-eye daisy is *Chrysanthemum leucanthemum*. It is a common sight in Britain, where it is known as dun daisy or maudlinwort. It is common throughout Europe, Russia, and Asia. Again, it is a yellow-centered flower with white petals. It grows to a height of 1-2 ft (30-61 cm) and has small leaves with serrated edges.

Sunflower

The sunflower is a native of Mexico and Peru, and is commonly grown in the United States and many other areas of the world. This is the largest of the chrysanthemum family, and there are several subspecies, varying slightly in size. Generally it grows to a height of 3-12 ft (91-366 cm), with flower heads that may measure more than 6 in (15 cm) across. The leaves are serrated and rough.

General use

The Flower Essence Society (FES) of California has a chrysanthemum essence that they recommend for those seeking spiritual growth.

According to many herbalists, species of chrysanthemum have many medicinal uses.

Dalmatian pellitory

This is commonly known as insect powder due to its insecticide properties. An advantage is that the powder is completely harmless to humans, and so does not have side effects (as is the case with all chemical insecticides), and can be used as a lotion and applied to the skin as an insect repellant. If the flowers are burned, the smoke that is given off can be valuable in exterminating insects.

Feverfew

Feverfew is chiefly regarded for its ability to treat fevers, reduce swelling, and for its analgesic properties; it is an excellent cure for a **headache** or any other **pain**. It is also used to promote menstrual flow, as an antidote to **depression** and nervous disorders, and as a general tonic. In addition, feverfew can be used to help in cases of difficult breathing, particularly associated with **asthma**, and chest **infections**. It has been used as a treatment for insect **bites** and even rat bites. In the past, feverfew was recommended for planting around dwellings because of its antiseptic properties. It wards off disease and prevents pests and diseases from attacking other plants. Similar to Dalmatian pellitory, it also has a repellant effect on insects. It can be used externally for flatulence and **colic**.

Ox-eye daisy

The herb has a soothing effect and is recommended for night sweats, especially those associated with **tuberculosis**. It is recommended for use in cases of **whooping cough**, asthma, and nervous tension. Generally its action can be compared to that of chamomile. It is useful for relieving chronic coughs and bronchial catarrh. Externally, it can be used as a lotion for **wounds**, **bruises**, and some skin conditions. In this regard, some herbalists recommend it as an ointment for treating swellings and it is also known for treating **gout**. Others recommend it for treating **jaundice** and also as a diuretic and tonic.

Sunflower

The sunflower is chiefly grown for its seeds which produce an oil, similar to olive oil, that is both cheap to produce and a valuable source of fatty acids. In many parts of the world, the sunflower provides much needed **nutrition** in poorer areas. The seeds can be used medicinally for treatment of bronchial complaints. A tincture of the seed has been used successfully in areas such as Russia, Turkey, and Persia for fevers (even **malaria**), where it has been found to be free of the complications sometimes associated with the use of quinine.

Preparations

Dalmatian pellitory

PARTS USED: FLOWERS. The chief use for Dalmatian pellitory is as an insecticide, or as an ointment to ward off insects. It is mainly dried and ground to a powder to this end.

Feverfew

PARTS USED: BARK, FLOWERS, AND LEAVES. For coughs it is generally made up into a syrup (decoction) with sugar or honey. The herb, when bruised and added to a little oil, can be used as an external application for flatulence and colic. For swellings and bites, it can be made up into a tincture, two teaspoonfuls of which should be mixed with half a pint of cold water and applied. As an infusion, made with boiling water and allowed to cool, feverfew will soothe pain of any kind, (muscular, nerve-related, rheumatic or intestinal). Chewing the leaves (one to four per day) can be effective in the case of migraine. It has also been used in this way to treat cases of **worms**.

Ox-eye daisy

PARTS USED: FLOWERS, ROOTS, AND LEAVES. This plant is mainly employed as an infusion. But in the case of tuberculosis, 15–60 drops of the fluid-extract should be taken in water. The flowers boiled with the leaves and stalks and sweetened with a little honey are a treatment for chest complaints.

Sunflower

PARTS USED: SEEDS AND LEAVES. Chest complaints: boil two ounces of the seeds in one quart of water until the water is reduced to 12 oz. Strain and add six ounces of Holland gin and six ounces of sugar. The dose is one to two teaspoonfuls of the mixture three times a day. Roasting the seeds and making an infusion is recommended for whooping **cough**.

Precautions

As with any herbal preparations, all of the above should be used with care and preferably under the supervision of an herbal practitioner.

Side effects

Feverfew should not be used for migraine that is a result of some kind of deficiency in the body (whether nutritional or otherwise). It is possible that feverfew may cause **dermatitis**, allergic reactions, or sores in the mouth in susceptible individuals. It should not be taken by pregnant women due to its ability to stimulate the uterus.

Interactions

Feverfew has been known to interfere with blood-clotting ability, and so a doctor should be consulted before it is used in conjunction with anticoagulants.

Resources

BOOKS

Buchman, Dian Dincin. *Herbal Medicine*. London: Tiger Books International, 1993.
Culpeper, Nicholas. *Culpeper's Complete Herbal*. London: Bloomsbury Books, 1992.
Grieve, Mrs. M. *A Modern Herbal*. London: Tiger Books International, 1992.

ORGANIZATIONS

Flower Essence Society. P.O. Box 459, Nevada City, CA 95959. (800) 736-9222. mail@flowersociety.org. http://www.flowersociety.org.

Patricia Skinner

Chymotrypsin

Description

Chymotrypsin is a digestive enzyme that breaks down proteins (i.e., it is a proteolytic enzyme; it can also be referred to as a protease). It is naturally produced by the pancreas in the human body. However, it can also be taken as an enzyme supplement to improve health and digestion and aid in the treatment of various diseases.

The pancreas, which produces chymotrypsin and other **digestive enzymes**, is a digestive organ in the abdomen that is located just below the stomach. Its primary job is to produce enzymes required for the digestion and absorption of food. Each day the pancreas secrets about 1.5 qt (1.4 L) of pancreatic juice, consisting of enzymes, water, and electrolytes (primarily bicarbonate) into the small intestine. The enzymes are secreted in an inactive form (as proenzymes) so that they will not digest the pancreas. The pancreas secretes an inhibitor to ensure that the enzymes are not activated too early. When the pancreatic juice reaches the small intestine, the enzymes become activated. The small intestine is not digested because it contains a protective mucous lining. However, self-digestion can occur if the pancreatic duct becomes blocked or if the pancreas is damaged. The proenzymes can overwhelm the inhibitor, causing the enzymes to become active while in the pancreas. This condition, called acute **pancreatitis**, can result in a lifetime of pancreatic insufficiency.

The enzymes secreted by the pancreas break down food by breaking the chemical bonds that hold food molecules together. Enzymes secreted include **lipase**, which, along with bile, digests fat; amylases, which break down starch molecules into smaller sugars; and protease, which breaks protein molecules into dipeptides and some single **amino acids**. In addition to chymotrypsin, other protease enzymes secreted by the pancreas include trypsin and carboxypeptidase.

Chymotrypsin, as a hydrolase type of enzyme (which means it adds a water molecule during the breakdown process) acts by catalyzing the hydrolysis of peptide bonds of proteins in the small intestine. It is selective for peptide bonds with aromatic or large hydrophobic side chains on the carboxyl side of this bond. Chymotrypsin also catalyzes the hydrolysis of ester bonds. Chymotrypsin does not digest blood proteins because of protective factors in the blood that block the enzyme.

General use

Generally, the primary uses of chymotrypsin are as a digestive aid and as an anti-inflammatory agent. The presence and amount of chymotrypsin in a person's stool is sometimes measured for diagnostic purposes as a test of pancreatic function. Testing for fecal chymotrypsin is noninvasive, unlike some other tests of pancreatic function.

Chymotrypsin, along with the other pancreatic enzymes, is most often used in the treatment of pancreatic insufficiency. Pancreatic insufficiency is characterized by impaired digestion, malabsorption and passing of undigested food into the stool, nutrient deficiencies, **gas**, and abdominal bloating and discomfort. Pancreatic deficiency also occurs in persons with cystic fibrosis, a rare inherited disorder. It may also occur in those with chronic pancreatitis, as well as in the elderly. Other conditions that could result in chymotrypsin deficiency include physical injuries, chemotherapy, and chronic **stress**.

Starch and fat digestion can be accomplished without the help of pancreatic enzymes; however, the protease enzymes (i.e., chymotrypsin, trypsin, and carboxypeptidase) are required for proper protein digestion. Incomplete digestion of proteins may result in the development of **allergies** and the formation of toxic

substances produced by putrefaction, the breakdown of protein materials by bacteria. Protease enzymes and other intestinal secretions are also required to keep the small intestine free from parasites such as bacteria, yeast, protozoa, and intestinal **worms**. A laboratory analysis of a stool sample along with physical symptoms are used to assess pancreatic function.

As an anti-inflammatory agent, the chymotrypsin and the other protease enzymes prevent tissue damage during inflammation and the formation of fibrin clots. Protease enzymes participate in the breakdown of fibrin in a process called fibrinolysis. Fibrin causes a wall to form around an area of inflammation, resulting in the blockage of blood and lymph vessels, which leads to swelling. Fibrin can also cause the development of **blood clots**. In autoimmune diseases, the protease enzymes aid in the breakdown of immune complexes, which are antibodies produced by the immune system associated with the compounds they bind to (antigens). High levels of immune complexes in the blood are associated with autoimmune diseases.

Specifically, chymotrypsin is used to:

- Aid in digestion.
- Treat inflammation and reduce swelling (i.e., soft tissue injuries, acute traumatic injuries, sprains, contusions, hematomas, ecchymoses, infections, edema

of the eyelids and genitalia, muscle cramps, and sports injuries).

- Treat arthritis and such other autoimmune diseases as lupus, scleroderma, and multiple sclerosis.
- Treat ulcerations and abscesses.
- Liquefy mucus secretions.
- Treat enterozoic worms and other parasites in the digestive tract.
- Treat cancer (a controversial use that requires much more scientific study, though chymotrypsin may be helpful in alleviating effects of radiation treatment or chemotherapy).
- Treat shingles and acne.
- Decrease effects of sun damage and age spots.

Preparations

Chymotrypsin is produced from fresh hog, beef, or oxen pancreas. It can be taken orally, topically, or by injection (by injection only by a physician in severe life-threatening situations), but is commonly taken orally in tablet form. As a tablet, it may be uncoated, microencapsulated, or enterically coated (to prevent digestion in the stomach so that the enzyme will be released in the small intestine). Other forms include coated granules, powder, capsules, and liquids. Creams and ointments are used to break down proteins and debride dead tissue resulting from **burns**, **wounds**, and abscesses. The enzyme preparation should be stored in a tight container with a moisture-proof liner in a dry, cool place. An opened container stored properly should maintain enzyme activity for about two to three months.

Usually chymotrypsin is included in a combination with other enzymes. A typical formulation may include: chymotrypsin (0.5–1 mg), **bromelain** (a plant protease) (25–45 mg), pancreatin (a mixture of many pancreatic enzymes) (100 mg), papain (a plant protease similar in action to chymotrypsin) (25–60 mg), and trypsin (a pancreatic protease) (24 mg). Formulations may also include vitamins, herbs, phytochemicals, and other nutrients to enhance the activity of the enzyme supplement.

Enzyme activity should be considered when a supplement is selected. Activity is usually indicated in units; however there is no one standard for enzyme activity level. Recognized guidelines for measuring enzyme activity include Food Chemicals Codex (FCC), United States Pharmacopoeia (USP), Federation Internationale du Pharmaceutiques (FIP), British Pharmacopoeia (BP), and Japanese Pharmacopoeia (JP). For example, the United States Pharmacopoeia

has set a strict definition for level of activity that must be reported in a enzyme supplement. A 1X chymotrypsin product must contain not less than 25 USP units for chymotrypsin activity. A preparation of higher potency is given a whole number multiple indicating its strength. For example, a full-strength undiluted extract that is 10 times stronger than the USP standard would be referred to as 10X USP. A consumer can compare enzyme activity levels among enzyme products within a single guideline system, but unfortunately the information is not interchangeable among guideline systems.

The dose required will vary on the quantity (amount in mg) and the quality (activity level) of the enzyme in the preparation, which is usually tablet form. The dose will also depend on the condition being treated. In most cases, for oral ingestion and for topical application, the directions on the bottle or tube label can be followed. Enterically coated tablets should be swallowed and not chewed or ground up. Tablets should also be taken with at least 8 oz of water to help activate the enzyme. Chymotrypsin taken to enhance digestion is usually taken just before, during, or just after meals, or before going to bed at night. With proper dosages, improvements in digestion should be noted within a few hours.

For inflammatory or chronic conditions, chymotrypsin should be taken on an empty stomach, either one hour before meals or at least two hours after meals. When chymotrypsin is taken for an inflammatory condition, some improvement may be noted within three to seven days. Those with chronic conditions such as arthritis may require one to three months or more to notice a change in conditions.

Precautions

Chymotrypsin is generally well tolerated and not associated with any significant side effects. However, since a safe dose has not been established, it should only be used when there is apparent need.

People who should not use **enzyme therapy** include those with hereditary clotting disorders such as hemophilia, those suffering from coagulation disturbances, those who are just about to or have undergone surgery, those on anticoagulant therapy, anyone suffering from protein allergies, and pregnant women or those breast-feeding. Since there is not much known about the effects of enzyme therapy on children, it would be prudent to avoid giving enzyme supplements to children.

When protective mechanisms against self-digestion in the body break down, chymotrypsin should not be used. For example, if a patient has stomach ulcers, chymotrypsin therapy should be discontinued.

Side effects

There do not appear to be any long-term side effects from chymotrypsin therapy if precautions for its use are followed. Studies have shown that at recommended doses, enzymes cannot be detected in blood analysis after 24–48 hours. Temporary side effects that may occur (but that should disappear when therapy is discontinued or dosage is reduced) include changes in the color, consistency, and odor of the stool. Some individuals may experience gastrointestinal disturbances, such as flatulence, a feeling of fullness, **diarrhea**, **constipation**, or **nausea**. With high doses, minor allergic reactions such as reddening of the skin may occur.

Interactions

Chymotrypsin is most often used in combination with other enzymes to enhance its treatment potential. In addition, a well-balanced diet or the use of vitamin and mineral supplements are recommended to stimulate chymotrypsin activity.

Some types of seeds, including jojoba and wild soja seeds, have been found to contain proteins that inhibit the activity of chymotrypsin. These proteins can be inactivated by boiling the seeds.

Chymotrypsin should not be used together with acetylcysteine, a drug used to thin mucus in the lungs. It should also not be used together with anticoagulant (blood thinning) drugs, as it increases their effects. Chloramphenicol, a medication used to treat eye **infections**, may counteract the effectiveness of chymotrypsin ophthalmic solutions.

Resources

BOOKS

Bland, Jeffrey. *Digestive Enzymes*. New Canaan, CT: Keats Publishing, Inc., 1993.

Cichoke, Anthony J. *The Complete Book of Enzyme Therapy*. Garden City Park, NY: Avery Publishing Group, 1999.

PERIODICALS

Deshimaru, M., R. Hanamoto, C. Kusano, et al. "Purification and Characterization of Proteinase Inhibitors from Wild Soja (Glycine Soja) Seeds." *Bioscience, Biotechnology, and Biochemistry* 66 (September 2002): 1897-1903.

Fujino, H., T. Aoki, and H. Watabe. "A Highly Sensitive Assay for Proteases Using Staphylococcal Protein Fused with Enhanced Green Fluorescent Protein." *Bioscience, Biotechnology, and Biochemistry* 66 (July 2002): 1601-1604.

Shrestha, M. K., I. Peri, P. Smirnoff, et al. "Jojoba Seed Meal Proteins Associated with Proteolytic and Protease Inhibitory Activities." *Journal of Agricultural and Food Chemistry* 50 (September 25, 2002): 5670-5675.

Zintl, A., C. Westbrook, H. E. Skerrett, et al. "Chymotrypsin and Neuraminidase Treatment Inhibits Host Cell Invasion by *Babesia divergens* (Phylum Apicomplexa)." *Parasitology* 125 (July 2002): 45-50.

ORGANIZATIONS

American Dietetic Association (ADA). 216 West Jackson Blvd., Suite 800, Chicago, IL 60606. (312) 899-0040. http://www.eatright.org.

Digestive Disease National Coalition (DDNC). 711 Second Street NE, Suite 200, Washington, DC 20002. (202) 544-7497. http://www.ddnc.org.

National Digestive Diseases Information Clearinghouse, National Institute of Diabetes and Digestive and Kidney Disease, and National Institutes of Health. 2 Information Way, Bethesda, MD 20892-3570. (310) 654-3810.

Judith Sims
Rebecca J. Frey, PhD

Cicada

Description

Cicada is an animal-derived substance used in **traditional Chinese medicine** (TCM). It is extracted from or prepared by grinding the empty shell shed every seven years by the cicada, (*Cryptotympana atrata* or *Cryptotympana pustulata*), which is a winged insect that makes a distinctive chirping sound and belongs to the Cicadidae family.

Cicadas are commonly found in mainland China, Taiwan, and Japan. They had religious significance in ancient China and symbolized reincarnation or immortality, as the Chinese compared the cicada's periodic molting of its shell with a person's leaving the physical body behind at the time of death. Bronze vessels as old as 1500 B.C. ornamented with cicadas have been found in Chinese tombs, along with white pottery and jewelry featuring cicada designs. During the Han dynasty (202 B.C. to A.D. 220), the Chinese carved small cicadas out of precious jade and placed them in the mouths of the dead.

The pharmaceutical name of the substance made from this insect is *Periostracum cicadae*, or *chan tui* in Chinese. It is prepared from the exuvium, or cast-off

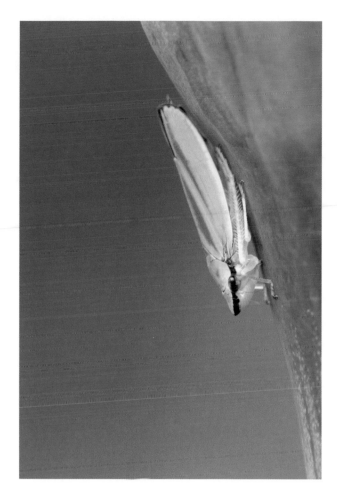

Cicada is an animal-derived substance used in traditional Chinese medicine extracted from or prepared by grinding the empty shell shed every seven years by the cicada, shown here. *(© Arco Images / Alamy)*

shell of the nymph form of the insect. The empty shell is shiny, translucent, and yellow-brown in color. As it would appear in a living cicada, the shell has three portions: head (with two eyes), chest (with wings and a crossed gap), and abdomen (with three pairs of feet).

General use

The medicinal uses of cicada include treatment of **fever** and associated seizures; skin **rashes**; and such eye disorders as **conjunctivitis, cataracts,** and blurred vision.

Due to its antipyretic effect, cicada-containing preparations are often used to treat high fevers, such as those associated with the **common cold** or **influenza**. Western news media reported in April 2003 that the Chinese were using combinations of cicada and silkworm droppings to treat the fever associated with SARS. In addition to reducing fever, cicada is also used in TCM to treat other symptoms of colds and flu, including **laryngitis, headache,** restless sleep, or nightmares.

Cicada is said to be effective in relieving itchy rashes and **eczema**. Its special use is for the treatment of rashes or skin eruptions that occur in the early stages of **measles** or chicken pox. According to traditional Chinese medicine, the sooner the rashes appear, the shorter and less severe these diseases will be. Therefore, a Chinese herbalist may suggest cicada preparations to hasten the eruption of the rash.

Cicada is said to prevent or reduce **muscle spasms** by reducing the tension of the striated muscles. It may also delay transmission of nerve signals at the neuromuscular junction, thereby reducing muscle spasms. Its actions may be similar to those of Western barbiturates, sedatives, and anticonvulsants (antiseizure medications).

Cicada has also been used in TCM to treat eye diseases associated with wind and heat, including blurred vision and conjunctivitis (inflammation of the membrane that lines the eyelids). It is usually mixed with chrysanthemum flowers (*Chrysanthemum morifolium*, or *ju hua* in Chinese) when used to treat cataracts.

Preparations

The usual dosage of cicada when taken alone is 3–9 grams per day. As of 2004, whole cicadas cost about 10 cents per gram when purchased in bulk from suppliers of Chinese medicinal herbs. Cicada may be prepared as a decoction, which means that the insect shells are boiled down to a concentrated broth or tea to be taken internally. Other forms of cicada preparations include ground powder and water and alcohol extracts.

Precautions

A general precaution when using herbs or other alternative medicines is to purchase them only from reputable sources. In the case of traditional Chinese remedies, this precaution is particularly important because many of them are imported from countries without strict production or labeling standards. In the case of cicada, the United States Food and Drug Administration (FDA) reported in June 2003 that a shipment described as "Cicada Molting Herbal Food Supplement" from Taiwan was refused entry into the United States and considered dangerous. In this instance, the FDA defined "dangerous" in these terms: "The article appears to be dangerous to health when used in the dosage or manner, or with the frequency or duration, prescribed, recommended, or suggested in the labeling thereof."

Practitioners of TCM state that pregnant women should not use cicada because of the risk of miscarriage.

Side effects

No side effects from cicada preparations have been reported in the United States as of early 2008.

Interactions

As of 2008, cicada decoctions have not been reported to interact with any Western prescription medications.

Resources

BOOKS

Bensky, Dan, and Andrew Gamble. *Chinese Herbal Medicine: Materia Medica.* rev. ed. Seattle: Eastland Press, 1993.

Kang-Ying, Wong, and Martha Dahlen. "Cicada." In *Streetwise Guide to Chinese Herbal Medicine.* San Francisco: China Bks. & Periodicals, Inc., 1996.

Molony, David. *The American Association of Oriental Medicine's Complete Guide to Chinese Herbal Medicine.* New York: The Philip Lief Group, 1998.

Reid, Daniel P. *Chinese Herbal Medicine.* Boston: Shambhala, 1993.

Williams, Tom. *The Complete Illustrated Guide to Chinese Medicine: A Comprehensive System for Health and Fitness.* Boston: Element Books, Inc., 1996.

PERIODICALS

Hsieh, M.T., W.H. Peng, F.T. Yeh, et al. "Studies of the Anticonvulsive, Sedative and Hypothermic effects of Periostracum Cicadae Extracts." *Journal of Ethnopharmacology* 35 (January 1991): 83–90.

Riegel, Garland. "Cicada in Chinese Folklore." *Cultural Entomology Digest* 3 (November 1994). http://www.insects.org/ced3/cicada_chfolk.html.

ORGANIZATIONS

American Foundation of Traditional Chinese Medicine. 505 Beach Street, San Francisco, CA 94133. (415) 776-0502.

American Herbal Products Association. 8484 Georgia Ave., Suite 370, Silver Spring, MD 20910. (301) 588-1174. http://www.ahpa.org.

Food and Drug Administration (FDA). 5600 Fishers Lane, Rockville, MD 20857. (888) 463-6332. http://www.fda.gov.

National Center for Complementary and Alternative Medicine. NCCAM Clearinghouse, National Institute of Health, P.O. Box 8218, Silver Spring, MD 20907-8218. (888) 644-6226. Fax: (301) 495-4957. http://nccam.nih.gov.

National Oriental Medicine Accreditation Agency (NOMAA). 3445 Pacific Coast Highway, Suite 300, Torrance, CA 90505. (213) 820-2045. http://www.nomaaa.org.

OTHER

Food and Drug Administration (FDA). "Refusal Actions by FDA as Recorded in OASIS (Organization for the Advancement of Structured Information Standards), Taiwan, Republic of China." Rockville, MD: FDA, June 2003. http://www.fda.gov/ora/oasis/6/ora_oasis_c_tw.html.

Rebecca Frey

Cimicifuga racemosa see **Black cohosh**

Cinnamon bark

Description

Cinnamon bark (*Cinnamomum verum, C. zeylanicum, C. cassica*) is harvested from a variety of evergreen tree that is native to Sri Lanka, China, and India. The tree has thick, reddish brown bark, small yellow flowers, and its leathery leaves have a spicy smell. It grows to a height of approximately 20–60 ft (8–18 m) and is found primarily in tropical forests. Cinnamon bark belongs to the Lauraceae family. Related species are *Cinnamomum cassia* and *Cinnamomum saigonicum* (Saigon Cinnamon).

Cinnamon bark is cultivated in such tropical regions as the Philippines and the West Indies. It is not grown in the United States. Every two years the trees are cut to just above ground level. The bark is harvested from the new shoots, then dried. The outer bark is stripped away, leaving the inner bark, which is the main medicinal part of the herb.

The use of cinnamon dates back thousands of years to at least 2700 B.C. Chinese herbals from that time mentioned it as a treatment for **fever**, **diarrhea**, and menstrual problems. Indian Ayurvedic healers used it in a similar manner. Cinnamon was introduced around 500 B.C. to the Egyptians, who then added it to their embalming mixtures. Hebrews, Greeks, and Romans used it as a spice, perfume, and for **indigestion**. Moses is said to have included cinnamon in an anointing oil that he used. By the seventeenth century, cinnamon was considered a culinary spice by Europeans. American nineteenth-century physicians prescribed cinnamon as a treatment for stomach cramps, **nausea**, **vomiting**, diarrhea, **colic**, and uterine problems.

General use

Cinnamon bark is a common ingredient in many products such as toothpaste, mouthwash, perfume, soap, lipstick, chewing gum, **cough** syrup, nasal sprays, and cola drinks. A popular food flavoring, it is valued as one of the world's most important spices. It is also valuable in the treatment of various ailments. Modern herbalists prescribe cinnamon bark as a remedy for nausea, vomiting, diarrhea, and indigestion. Chinese herbalists recommend it for **asthma** brought on by cold, some digestive problems, backache, and menstrual problems.

The medicinal value of the herb is attributed to the oil extracted from the inner bark and leaves. The cinnamon bark harvested from the young branches is primarily used for culinary purposes. In fact, the cinnamon sticks commonly used in cooking are actually pieces of rolled outer bark.

The active ingredients of the bark have antibacterial, antiseptic, antiviral, antispasmodic, and antifungal properties. A study published in 2002 indicated that oil from cinnamon bark inhibits the production of listeriolysin, a protein released by *Listeria* bacteria that destroys healthy cells. Japanese research has shown cinnamaldehyde, one of the constituents of cinnamon bark, to be a sedative and analgesic. Eugenol, another component, contains pain-relieving qualities.

Cinnamon bark is helpful in strengthening and supporting a weak digestive system. Research indicates that cinnamon bark breaks down fats in the digestive system, making it a valuable digestive aid. It is used to treat nausea, vomiting, diarrhea, stomach ulcers, acid indigestion, **heartburn**, lack of appetite, and abdominal disorders.

A traditional stimulant in Chinese medicine, cinnamon bark has a warming effect on the body and is used for conditions caused by coldness. The twigs of cinnamon enhance circulation, especially to the fingers and toes.

Cinnamon bark contains antiseptic properties that help to prevent infection by killing decay-causing bacteria, fungi, and viruses. One German study showed that the use of cinnamon bark suppressed the cause of most urinary tract **infections** and the fungus responsible for vaginal yeast infections. It is also helpful in relieving **athlete's foot**.

Cinnamon bark is a frequent ingredient in toothpaste, mouthwash, and other oral hygiene products because it helps kill the bacteria that causes tooth decay and **gum disease**. Inflammations of the throat and pharynx may be relieved through its use.

Cinnamon bark is also known to control blood sugar levels in diabetics. United States Department of Agriculture (USDA) researchers found that cinnamon bark may reduce the amount of insulin required for glucose metabolism. A dose of 1/8 to 1/4 tsp of ground cinnamon per meal for diabetic patients may help to regulate their blood sugar levels. Several studies in the early 2000s produced mixed results on the effectiveness of cinnamon in treating type 1 and type 2 diabetes. All of the studies were on small groups of participants.

Cinnamon is believed to have strong antioxidant properties and to enhance the activity of insulin in diabetics. A 2003 study in Pakistan, published in the December 2003 issue of *Diabetes Care*, reported that daily consumption of 1, 3, or 6 grams of cinnamon significantly reduced blood glucose, LDL (bad) **cholesterol**, total cholesterol, and triglycerides in people with type 2 diabetes. A study by the University of Connecticut School of Pharmacy, published in the January 2008 issue of *Diabetes Care*, analyzed five previous studies and concluded that cinnamon did not significantly improve A1C, **fasting** blood glucose, or cholesterol levels in patients with type 1 or type 2 diabetes. A1C is a test that measures a diabetic's average blood sugar (glucose) levels over two to three months. The Connecticut study is contrasted by a 2007 European study that reported 3 grams of cinnamon extract taken daily lowered fasting blood sugar levels by 10% among diabetics after four months.

The spice has also garnered quite a reputation as an aphrodisiac. A study at the Smell and Taste Research Foundation in Chicago tested medical students' reactions to various aromas by attaching measurement devices to the students' penises. The smell of hot cinnamon buns generated the most blood flow of all the scents.

Cinnamon bark promotes **menstruation**. It has been used to treat menstrual **pain** and **infertility**. Women in India take it as a contraceptive after **childbirth**.

Other conditions in which cinnamon bark may be helpful include fevers and colds, coughs and **bronchitis**, infection and wound healing, some forms of asthma, and blood pressure reduction.

Cinnamon bark has been shown to be an effective natural snake repellent that is safer to use than synthetic pest management chemicals.

Preparations

Cinnamon bark is available in several forms from Chinese pharmacists, Asian grocery stores, and health food stores: fresh or dried bulk, pill, tincture, and as an essential oil.

Dosage

In Chinese medicine, cinnamon is usually taken in combination with other herbs. Below are some typical dosages for cinnamon alone.

- Tincture: Take up to 4 ml with water three times daily.
- Tea: Take 1 cup 2–3 times daily at mealtimes.
- Crushed: Take 1/2 tsp (2–4 g) daily.

Precautions

- Cinnamon bark may cause an allergic reaction in some individuals.
- Cinnamon bark is not recommended for pregnant or nursing women.
- Essential oil of cinnamon bark ought not to be taken internally unless under professional supervision. Internal ingestion may cause nausea, vomiting, and possible kidney damage.
- Essential oil of cinnamon bark is one of the most hazardous essential oils and should not be used on the skin. External application of the oil may cause redness and burning of skin.
- Cinnamon bark should not be given to children under two years of age.

> ## KEY TERMS
>
> **A1C**—A test that measures a diabetic's average blood sugar (glucose) levels over two to three months.
>
> **Analgesic**—A pain-relieving substance.
>
> **Antispasmodic**—A substance that relieves muscle spasms or cramping.
>
> **Aphrodisiac**—A drug or other substance that arouses or is thought to arouse sexual desire.
>
> **Essential oil**—A concentrated oil that has been distilled from a plant.
>
> **Sedative**—A drug or herb that has a calming and relaxing effect. Sedatives are used to aid sleep and ease pain and are often given as mild tranquilizers.

- Cinnamon bark is considered toxic if taken in excess.
- Cinnamon bark should not be given to persons with inflammatory liver disease; in large quantities, it can irritate the liver.

Side effects

Mild side effects include stomach upset, sweating, and diarrhea. Large doses can cause changes in breathing, dilation of blood vessels, sleepiness, **depression**, or convulsions. Excessive use of cinnamon bark may cause red, tender gums; mouth ulcers; inflamed taste buds; and a severe burning sensation in the mouth.

Interactions

Some interactions with other medications have been reported. Cinnamon oil may cause skin irritation if applied to the skin together with **acne** medications that contain retinoic acid. Cinnamon bark has also been reported to intensify the effects of medications given to lower blood pressure. Persons taking cinnamon bark should discontinue its use two weeks before any surgery requiring general anesthesia because of the herb's tendency to lower blood pressure.

Resources

BOOKS

Teuscher, Eberhard. *Medicinal Spices*. Stuttgart, Germany: MedPharm Scientific Publishers, 2005.

PERIODICALS

Baker, William L., et al. "Effect of Cinnamon on Glucose Control and Lipid Parameters." *Diabetes Care* (January 2008): 41–43.

Blevins, Steve M., et al. "Effect of Cinnamon on Glucose and Lipid Levels in Non-Insulin-Dependent Type 2 Diabetes." *Diabetes Care* (September 2007): 2236–2237.

Chase, Celtina K., et al. "Cinnamon in Diabetes Mellitus." *American Journal of Health-System Pharmacy* (May 15, 2007): 1033(3).

Gray, Lisa Waterman. "Cinnamon: Common Spice, One-of-a-Kind Remedy: Can Cinnamon Ease Diabetic and Cardiovascular Symptoms as It Flavors Your Food? This Sweet Spice Has Been Used for Centuries for Its Health-Enhancing Powers." *Better Nutrition* (April 2007): 18.

Sego, Sherril. "Cinnamon." *Clinical Advisor* (May 2007): 152(2).

ORGANIZATIONS

American Association of Acupuncture and Oriental Medicine, PO Box 162340, Sacramento, CA, 95816, (866) 455-7999, http://www.aaaomonline.org.

American Institute of Homeopathy, 801 N. Fairfax St., Suite 306, Alexandria, VA, 22314, (888) 445-9988, http://www.homeopathyusa.org.

Homeopathic Medical Council of Canada, 3910 Bathurst St., Suite 202, Toronto, ON, M3H 3N8, Canada, (416) 638-4622, http://www.hmcc.ca.

National Center for Alternative and Complementary Medicine, 9000 Rockville Pike, Bethesda, MD, 20892, (888) 644-6226, http://www.nccam.nih.gov.

Jennifer Wurges
Ken R. Wells

Cirrhosis

Definition

Cirrhosis refers to various types of chronic degenerative disease of the liver in which normal liver cells are damaged and then replaced by scar tissue.

Description

Cirrhosis changes the structure of the liver and the blood vessels that nourish it. The disease reduces the liver's ability to manufacture proteins, complex carbohydrates, fats, **cholesterol**, and to process hormones, nutrients, medications, and poisons. Cirrhosis worsens over time and can be life-threatening.

Cirrhosis is the seventh leading cause of disease-related death in the United States. It is the third most common cause of death in adults between the ages of 45 and 65. It is twice as common in men as in women. The disease occurs in more than half of all malnourished chronic alcoholics. Some authorities estimate that cirrhosis and related complications are responsible for the deaths of more than 40,000 people a year in the United States with direct healthcare costs of more than $1 billion. In Asia and Africa, however, most deaths from cirrhosis are due to chronic **hepatitis** B.

Types of cirrhosis

There are several typs of cirrhosis:

- Portal, or nutritional cirrhosis, the most common form of the disease in the United States. About 30 to 50% of all cases of cirrhosis are this type. Nine out of every 10 people who have nutritional cirrhosis have a history of alcoholism. Portal cirrhosis is also called Laënnec's cirrhosis.
- Biliary cirrhosis, caused by liver bile-duct diseases that impede bile flow. Bile is formed in the liver and carried via ducts to the intestines. Bile then helps digest fats in the intestines. Biliary cirrhosis can result in the scarring or blockage of these ducts. It accounts for 15 to 20% of all cases of cirrhosis.
- Postnecrotic cirrhosis. Caused by chronic infections, this form of the disease affects up to 40% of all patients who have cirrhosis.
- Pigment cirrhosis (hemochromatosis). Disorders such as the inability to metabolize iron and similar disorders may cause pigment cirrhosis, which accounts for 5 to 10% of all instances of the disease.

Causes and symptoms

Causes and risk factors

Long-term **alcoholism** is the primary cause of cirrhosis in the United States. Men and women respond differently to alcohol. Although most men can safely consume two to five drinks a day, one to two drinks a day can cause liver damage in women. Individual tolerance to alcohol varies, but people who drink more and drink more often have a higher risk of developing cirrhosis. In some people, one drink a day can eventually cause liver scarring.

Chronic liver **infections**, such as hepatitis B and particularly hepatitis C, are commonly linked to cirrhosis. People at high risk of contracting hepatitis B include those exposed to the virus through contact with blood and body fluids. This group includes healthcare workers and intravenous (IV) drug users. In the past, people have contracted hepatitis C through blood transfusions. As of 2003, cirrhosis resulting from chronic hepatitis has emerged as a

leading cause of death among HIV positive patients; in Europe, about 30% of HIV-positive patients are coinfected with a hepatitis virus.

Liver injury, reactions to prescription medications, certain autoimmune disorders, exposure to toxic substances, and repeated episodes of heart failure with liver congestion can cause cirrhosis. A family history of diseases can genetically predispose a person to develop cirrhosis. These genetic problems include:

- a lack of a specific liver enzyme (alpha$_1$-antitrypsin deficiency)
- the absence of a milk-digesting enzyme (galactosemia)
- an inability to convert sugars to energy (glycogen storage disease)
- an absorption deficit in which excess iron is deposited in the liver, pancreas, heart, and other organs
- a disorder characterized by accumulations of copper in the liver, brain, kidneys, and corneas (Wilson's disease)

In the 2000s **obesity** was recognized as a risk factor in nonalcoholic hepatitis and cirrhosis. Some surgeons recommend that patients scheduled for weight-reduction surgery have a liver biopsy to evaluate the possibility of liver damage.

Symptoms

Symptoms of cirrhosis are usually caused by the loss of functioning liver cells or organ swelling due to scarring. The liver enlarges during the early stages of illness. Patients may experience one or more of the following symptoms:

- anemia
- bleeding gums
- constipation
- decreased interest in sex
- diarrhea
- dull abdominal pain
- extremely dry skin and intense itching
- fatigue
- fever
- fluid in the lungs
- hallucinations
- indigestion
- lethargy
- lightheadedness
- loss of appetite
- muscle weakness
- musty breath
- nausea

- painful nerve inflammation (neuritis)
- portal hypertension (This type of hypertension can be life threatening; it can cause veins to enlarge in the stomach and esophagus; the enlarged veins, called varices, can rupture and bleed massively.)
- redness of the palms of the hands
- slurred speech
- tremors
- dark yellow or brown urine and black or bloody stools
- vomiting
- weakness
- weight loss
- yellowish whites of the eyes and skin, indicating the development of jaundice

As the disease progresses, other symptoms usually appear:

- spleen enlarges and fluid collects in the abdomen (ascites) and legs (edema)
- spider-like blood vessels appear on the chest and shoulders and bruising becomes common
- men sometimes lose chest hair; their breasts may grow and their testicles may shrink
- women may have menstrual irregularities

If the liver loses its ability to remove toxins from the brain, the patient may have additional symptoms. The patient may become forgetful and unresponsive, neglect personal care, have trouble concentrating, and acquire new sleeping habits. These symptoms are related to ammonia intoxication and the failure of the liver to convert ammonia to urea. High protein intake in these patients can also lead to these symptoms.

Cirrhosis worsens over time and can become potentially life-threatening. This disease can cause:

- excessive bleeding (hemorrhage)
- impotence
- liver cancer
- coma due to accumulated ammonia and body wastes (liver failure)
- sepsis (blood poisoning)
- death

Diagnosis

A patient's medical history can reveal illnesses or a lifestyle likely to lead to cirrhosis. Liver changes can be seen during a physical examination. A doctor who suspects cirrhosis may order blood and urine tests to measure liver function. Because only a small number

of healthy cells are needed to carry out essential liver functions, test results may be normal even when cirrhosis is present.

In about 10% of all patients, the cause of cirrhosis cannot be determined. Many people who have cirrhosis do not have any symptoms (often called compensated cirrhosis). Their disease is detected during a routine physical examination or when tests for an unrelated medical problem are performed. This type of cirrhosis can also be detected when complications occur (decompensated cirrhosis).

Computed tomography scans (CT), ultrasound, and other imaging techniques can be used during diagnosis. They can help determine the size of the liver, indicate healthy and scarred areas of the organ, and detect **gallstones**. Cirrhosis is sometimes diagnosed during surgery or by examining the liver with a laparoscope. This viewing device is inserted into the patient's body through a tiny incision in the abdomen.

Liver biopsy is usually needed to confirm a diagnosis of cirrhosis. In this procedure, a tissue sample is removed from the liver and examined under a microscope in order to learn more about the organ's condition and to properly diagnose any liver disease.

A newer and less invasive test involves the measurement of hyaluronic acid in the patient's blood serum. As of 2008 the test was often used to monitor the progress of liver disease and to indicate when a liver biopsy may be necessary. The test for hyaluronic acid was not anticipated to completely replace liver biopsy in the diagnosis of cirrhosis.

Treatment

Before starting on any alternative treatment program, patients should consult their doctor regarding monitoring side effects and estimating effectiveness of treatment. Any nutritional changes should be discussed with the primary care provider. Alternative treatments that may be of help to cirrhotic patients include nutritional and juice therapy, Western herbal therapy, **traditional Chinese medicine**, and **homeopathy**.

Nutritional therapy

To support liver function and slow disease progression, a naturopath may recommend the following:

• Avoid liver toxins. Cirrhotic patients must completely avoid alcohol. Alcohol accelerates liver failure and hastens death in cirrhotic patients. In addition, even over-the-counter drugs, such as acetaminophen (Tylenol), should be avoided because they can be toxic in cirrhotic patients.

• Juice therapy helps the liver detoxify the body. Patients should mix one part of pure juice with one part of water before drinking.

• Eat smaller meals. To avoid overworking the liver, five or six smaller, lighter meals per day are recommended.

• Avoid fatty foods, especially those prepared with animal fats or hydrogenated oils and all processed foods. These types of foods put additional demands on the liver.

• Eat only meals containing lean proteins (containing no fats) and in limited amounts. Vegetable proteins, such as those found in legumes or tofu, and whole grains are preferred. High protein intake causes increases in ammonia levels in the blood, possibly resulting in mental confusion, and in severe cases, coma. However, individuals ought not to limit severely their protein intake, as this may cause protein deficiency and impair the healing process.

• Increase consumption of fruits and steamed vegetables. Fruits and vegetables are easy to digest, thus less work for the liver. In addition, they are good sources of vitamins, minerals, and antioxidants that help the liver detoxify and heal.

• Practice intermittent fasting.

• Take supplements that can improve digestion and help the liver heal and prevent further injury to the liver. These include pancreatic enzymes, milk thistle (*Silybum marianum*), lipotropic agents such as vitamin B_6, vitamin B_{12}, folic acid, choline, alpha lipoic acid, betaine, and methionine.

Many health practitioners have long recommended the use of **milk thistle** in treating cirrhosis and other liver diseases. The active component in milk thistle, silymarin, promotes liver protein synthesis. The National Center for Complementary and Alternative Medicine (NCCAM) selected milk thistle as one of the alternative treatments to study in more detail. As of 2008, the center had found mixed results from the studies it had reviewed and inconclusive evidence to support claims for milk thistle use. In 2008 NCCAM was supporting research on the possible health benefits of using milk thistle to treat liver diseases, **cancer**, and HIV disease.

Other therapies

Other types of therapies the patient may want to consider are naturopathic **hydrotherapy** and treatments that may improve immune function, including **stress** reduction, **guided imagery**, and massage.

Traditional Chinese medicine

Depending on a patient's specific condition, an expert Chinese herbalist may prescribe herbal remedies that may help improve liver function. Animal studies have shown that the following Chinese herbs may have protective effects on the liver:

- Propolis
- *Bupleurum chinense,* a frequently used herb for a variety of liver diseases
- *Phellodendron wilsonii*
- *Clementis chinensis*
- *Solanum incanum*
- *Ixeris chinensis*
- *Gardenia jasminoides*

Western herbal therapy

Patients should consult an experienced herbalist for specific herbal treatments.

Homeopathy

For homeopathic therapy, patients should consult a homeopathic physician who may prescribe specific remedies based on knowledge of the underlying cause.

Allopathic treatment

The goal of treatment is to cure or reduce the condition causing cirrhosis, prevent or delay disease progression, and prevent or treat complications.

Salt and fluid intake is often limited, and physical activity is encouraged. A diet high in calories and moderately high in protein can benefit some patients. Tube feedings or vitamin supplements may be prescribed if the liver continues to deteriorate. Patients must not consume alcohol.

Medication

Iron supplements, diuretics, and antibiotics may be used for **anemia,** fluid retention, and ammonia accumulation associated with cirrhosis. Vasoconstrictors are sometimes needed to stop internal bleeding and antiemetics may be prescribed to control **nausea.**

Laxatives help the body absorb toxins and accelerate their removal from the digestive tract. Beta-blockers may be prescribed to control cirrhosis-induced portal **hypertension.** Interferon medicines may be used by patients with chronic hepatitis B and hepatitis C to prevent post-hepatic cirrhosis.

Surgery

Medication that causes scarring can be injected directly into veins to control bleeding from varices in the stomach or esophagus. Varices may require a special surgical procedure called balloon tamponade ligation to stop the bleeding. Surgery may be required to repair disease-related throat damage. It is sometimes necessary to remove diseased portions of the spleen and other organs.

In the 2000s the incidence of liver cancer related to cirrhosis in the United States had increased 75% since the early 1990s. Partial surgical removal of the liver in patients with early-stage cancer of the liver appeared to be as successful as transplantation, in terms of the 5-year survival rate.

Liver transplants can benefit patients with advanced cirrhosis. However, the new liver will eventually become diseased unless the underlying cause of cirrhosis (such as alcoholism) is removed.

Supportive measures

A balanced diet promotes regeneration of healthy liver cells. Eating five or six small meals throughout the day should prevent the sick or bloated feeling patients with cirrhosis often have after eating. Alcohol and **caffeine,** which destroy liver cells, should be avoided, as should any other foods that upset the stomach. Patients with brain disease associated with cirrhosis should avoid excessive amounts of protein in the diet.

A patient can keep a food diary that describes what was eaten, when it was eaten, and how the patient felt afterwards. This diary can be useful in identifying foods that are hard to digest and in scheduling meals to coincide with the times the patient is most hungry.

Patients who have cirrhosis should weigh themselves every day and notify their doctor of a sudden gain of 5 lb (2 kg) or more within a one to two week period. A doctor should also be notified if symptoms of cirrhosis appear in anyone who has not been diagnosed with the disease. A doctor should be notified if a patient diagnosed with cirrhosis experiences the following:

- vomits blood
- passes black stools
- seems confused or unresponsive
- shows signs of infection (redness, swelling, tenderness, pain)

KEY TERMS

Compensated cirrhosis—Asymptomatic cirrhosis of the liver.

Edema—An excessive accumulation of fluid in body tissue.

Portal hypertension—A type of hypertension that can be life threatening; veins enlarge in the stomach and esophagus, and the enlarged veins, called varices, can rupture and bleed massively.

Sepsis—Blood poisoning.

Expected results

Cirrhosis-related liver damage cannot be reversed, but further damage can be prevented by patients who do the following:

- eat properly
- get enough rest
- do not consume alcohol
- remain free of infection

If the underlying cause of cirrhosis cannot be corrected or removed, scarring will continue. As scarring continues, the liver will fail, and the patient will probably die within five years. Patients who stop drinking after being diagnosed with cirrhosis can increase their likelihood of living more than a few years from 40% to 60-70%.

Prevention

Eliminating alcohol abuse could prevent 75 to 80% of all cases of cirrhosis.

Other preventive measures include:

- maintaining a healthy diet that includes whole foods and grains, vegetable, and fruits
- obtaining counseling or other treatment for alcoholism
- taking precautions (practicing safe sex, avoiding dirty needles) to prevent hepatitis
- getting immunizations against hepatitis if a person is in a high-risk group
- receiving appropriate medical treatment quickly when diagnosed with hepatitis B or hepatitis C
- having blood drawn at regular intervals to rid the body of excess iron from hemochromatosis
- using medicines (chelating agents) to rid the body of excess copper from Wilson's disease
- wearing protective clothing and following product directions when using toxic chemicals at work, at home, or in the garden

Resources

BOOKS

Chen, T. M., ed. *Liver Cirrhosis: New Research.* Hauppauge, NY: Nova Biomedical Books, 2005.

Dickerson, James L. *The First Year: Cirrhosis: An Essential Guide for the Newly Diagnosed.* New York: Marlowe & Company, 2006.

Dillon, Kevin H., ed. *Trends in Liver Cirrhosis Research.* Hauppauge, NY: Nova Biomedical Books, 2006.

The Official Patient's Sourcebook on Cirrhosis of the Liver: A Directory for the Internet Age. San Diego, CA: ICON Health Publications, 2005.

PERIODICALS

Fourcher, J., et al. "Diagnosis of Cirrhosis by Transient Elastography (FibroScan): A Prospective Study." *Gut* (March 2006): 403–408.

Klatsky, A. L., et al. "Coffee, Cirrhosis, and Transaminase Enzymes." *Archives of Internal Medicine* (May 2007): 980–982.

Méndez-Sánchez, Nahum, et al. "Treating Nonalcoholic Fatty Liver Disease." *Liver International* (November 2007): 1157–1165.

Villa, Erica. "Role of Estrogen in Liver Cancer." *Women's Health* (January 2008): 41–50.

ORGANIZATIONS

American Liver Foundation, 75 Maiden Lane, Suite 603, New York, NY, 10038-4810, (800) GO-LIVER (465-4837), http://www.liverfoundation.org.

United Network for Organ Sharing, PO Box 2484, Richmond, VA, 23218, (888) 894-6361, http://www.unos.org.

Mai Tran
Teresa Norris
Rebecca J. Frey, PhD
David Edward Newton, Ed.D.

Clap *see* **Gonorrhea**

Clinical ecology *see* **Environmental therapy**

Club moss

Definition

Club moss is the common name for the approximately 200 species of plants that make up the genus *Lycopodium*. This genus is a member of the order Lycopodiales, the only extant order of the class Lycopodiopsida in the plant kingdom. A second order, Drepanophycales, is now extinct, having flourished during the late Silurian to late Devonian periods (about 450 million to 350 million years ago). Members of the two orders are very different from each other,

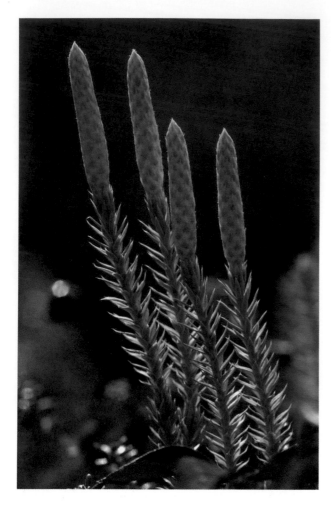

Club moss. (© tbkmedia.de / Alamy)

with the earlier plants growing to the size of trees with stems several millimeters to centimeters in diameter. Their decayed remains have become constituents of coal deposits found throughout the world.

Description

Modern club mosses look like true mosses, but are structurally very different in that they are vascular plants. They tend to be epiphytic (that is, subsisting on other plants without causing them harm) or terrestrial with extended, creeping stems. They are lacking in flowers and have abundant masses of tiny scale- or needle-like leaves. They produce sexually in two stages, one of which occurs beneath ground, by the production and distribution of spores.

Uses

Yellow spores collected from certain species of club moss, especially *Lycopodium clavatum*, are used

for a variety of purposes, including fingerprint identification, fireworks displays, and coatings for pills. Spore preparations are commonly known as **lycopodium** powder or vegetable **sulfur**. In **traditional Chinese medicine**, the spores have been dried and ground into a powder for use in the treatment of **fever** and inflammation. In this form the material is usually called Chinese club moss, or *qian ceng ta*.

Recent research has focused on one of the components of qian ceng ta, the alkaloid known as huperzine A. The substance has been found to be effective in treating the **dementia** associated with a number of neurological disorders, such as **Alzheimer's disease**. Huperzine A apparently interferes with the enzyme acetylcholinesterase, which breaks down the neurotransmitter acetylcholine in the central nervous system. Reduced levels of acetylcholine are thought to be related to the development of dementia. Other studies have suggested that huperzine A may be effective in treating the symptoms of myasthenia gravis and poisoning from a class of compounds known as the organophosphates. Results are preliminary, however, and experts point out that further studies are needed to confirm the therapeutic effects of huperzine A.

Some researchers suggest that the beneficial effects of club moss for the treatment of fever and **pain** may be the consequence of its dehydrative effects on cells. As cells lose water, they tend to contract, causing less pressure on nerves with which they may be associated. Definitive evidence for this hypothesis is, however, not yet available.

Side effects

The most serious side effect of using Chinese club moss is arrhythmia, irregular heart beat. With people who have a history of seizure, arrhythmia may increase the likelihood of additional, more serious seizures. Less serious side effects associated with use of the drug include:

- nausea
- diarrhea
- dizziness
- drooling
- excessive sweating
- blurred vision
- stomach cramps

Interactions

Chinese club moss and related drugs may interact with a variety of prescription drugs that inhibit the

KEY TERMS

Acetylcholine—A neurotransmitter that operates in the central nervous system.

Acetylcholinesterase—An enzyme that interferes with the function of acetylcholine.

Neurotransmitter—A chemical that carries a message between two neurons (nerve cells) in the body

Spore—A reproductive cell produced by simple organisms, such as fungi and ferns.

action of acetylcholine, so-called anticholinergic drugs, such as:

- atropine
- propantheline
- glycopyrrolate
- dicyclomine (Bentyl®)
- hyoscyamine sulfate (Levsin®)
- scopolamine (Transderm Scop®)

Resources

BOOKS

Fan, Warner J. W. *Manual of Chinese Herbal Medicine: Principles and Practice for Easy Reference*. Boston: Shambhala Publications, 2003.

PERIODICALS

Orhan, L., et al. "Appraisal of Anti–inflammatory Potential of the Clubmoss, Lycopodium Clavatum." *Journal of Ethnopharmacology* (July 2006): 146–150.

Fu, X. C., et al. "Preparation and in Vivo Evaluation of Huperzine A-loaded PLGA Microspheres." *Archives of Pharmaceutical Research* (September 2005): 1092–1096.

Gordon, R. K., et al. "Oral Administration of Pyridostigmine Bromide and Huperzine A Protects Human Whole Blood Cholinesterases from ex Vivo Exposure to Soman." *Chemico–Biological Interactions* (December 2005): 239–246.

Liu, W. H., et al. "Preparation and in Vitro and in Vivo Release Studies of Huperzine A Loaded Microspheres for the Treatment of Alzheimer's Disease." *Journal of Controlled Release* (October 2005): 417–427.

OTHER

Drug Digest. "Chinese Club Moss." ExpressScripts. http://www.drugdigest.org/DD/DVH/HerbsWho/0,3923,552633%7CChinese%2BClub%2BMoss,00.html (February 6, 2008).

Wikipedia. "Lycopodiopsida." http://en.wikipedia.org/wiki/Clubmoss (February 6, 2008).

David Edward Newton, Ed.D

Cnidium seeds

Description

A variety of carrot unknown to most Americans, *Cnidium monnieri* is a leafy annual with flowers that grow in clusters. The herb has been a popular remedy in Asian folk medicine for millennia, being first described about 2,000 years ago in the Chinese herbal classic *Shen Nong Ben Cao Jing*. Cnidium's reputation for treating itchy skin conditions persists to this day. Only the seeds and essential oil of *Cnidium monnieri*, which belongs to the Apiaceae family, are used as a drug.

The seeds, which are also referred as *she chuang zi* or *she chuang dze*, are somewhat yellow in color and have a sweet smell. They are believed to have several important therapeutic properties, including antibacterial, antifungal, and astringent effects. Some of these claims have been supported by animal and laboratory studies. In one test tube investigation, published in the Chinese journal *Chung Kuo Chung Yao Tsa Chih* in 1991, researchers demonstrated that *Cnidium monnieri* was effective against several **strains** of bacteria and fungi. *Cnidium monnieri* also appears to have antipruritic activity, meaning that the herb may help to alleviate **itching**. In a study of mice, published in the Japanese journal *Biological & Pharmaceutical Bulletin* in 2000, cnidium was shown to significantly reduce the itch-scratch response in rodents.

In the somewhat ethereal parlance of Chinese folk medicine—in which diseases are often believed to occur due to disruptions in the flow of bodily energy—cnidium seeds are considered warm, bitter, and acrid. The **essential oils** derived from the seeds include camphene, borneol, pinene, and terpineol.

General use

While not approved by the FDA, cnidium seeds have been reported to have several beneficial effects. Because the seeds have not been extensively studied in people, their effectiveness is based mainly on animal studies and their ancient reputation as a folk remedy in China. In modern times, the herb is primarily used to treat skin conditions such as **scabies**, **eczema**, ringworm, and itchy, oozing skin lesions. It is also thought to be helpful in the treatment of **vaginitis** and vaginal discharge. Cnidium is used externally for all the purposes mentioned above. The seeds may also be taken internally to treat **impotence** as well as **infertility** in both sexes.

KEY TERMS

Astringent—An agent that helps to contract tissue and prevent the secretion of internal body fluids such as blood or mucus. Astringents are typically used to treat external wounds or to prevent bleeding from the nose or throat.

Eczema—A condition characterized by inflamed, itchy skin. Eczema may also involve oozing, crusting, and scaling.

Essential oil—A term describing a wide variety of concentrated plant-derived oils. They are often used to make soaps and perfumes, as well as being used extensively in natural medical remedies.

Osteoporosis—An age-related disease in which bones become fragile and prone to debilitating fractures.

Ringworm—A fungal skin infection that predominantly affects children. The condition is characterized by reddish, scaly rings on the skin.

Scabies—A contagious rash caused by the *Sarcoptes scabiei* mite, which burrows into the upper layer of the skin in order to lay eggs. Scabies is characterized by intense itching.

Vaginitis—An inflammation of the mucous membrane that lines the interior of the vagina. It often results from a *Candida* or other fungal infection, and is accompanied by pain, itching, and discharge.

Cnidium has shown some intriguing activity against **asthma** and **osteoporosis** in animal studies, though the clinical implications of these findings are not yet known. In one investigation, published in the Chinese journal *Chung-kuo Chung Ya Yao Tsa Chih* in 1990, chemicals in *Cnidium monnieri* called coumarins appeared to protect guinea pigs from the effects of bronchial asthma, which the animals experienced after inhaling histamine. The researchers also demonstrated that the coumarins can relax the tracheal muscles of guinea pigs in test tube experiments. A possible link between cnidium and osteoporosis was examined in two rodent studies published in the Chinese journal *Chung-kuo Yao Li Hsueh Pao* in 1994 and 1997. Both studies suggest that cnidium can help to prevent osteoporosis induced by glucocorticoid drugs.

Preparations

The optimum dosage of cnidium seeds has not been established with any certainty. Dosage may range from 3-12 g. Because cnidium seeds have been recommended for a variety of purposes, and can be used internally and externally, consumers are advised to consult a doctor experienced in the use of alternative remedies or Chinese medicine to determine proper dosage.

To treat skin conditions, the herb is usually applied to the skin in the form of a solution or ointment. Vaginitis and vaginal discharge are treated with a douche prepared from the seeds.

In Chinese folk medicine, cnidium seeds are often combined with other herbs or minerals. When used externally, the seeds may be mixed with stemona and sophora for itchy, oozing skin lesions or with calomel for scabies and eczema (including genital eczema). Taken internally, cnidium seeds are often combined with **schisandra** or **cuscuta** to treat impotence or infertility.

Cnidium seeds are generally available in bulk or in combination products (such as powders or pills) that contain several different herbs.

Precautions

Cnidium seeds are not known to be harmful when taken in recommended dosages, though it is important to remember that the long-term effects of taking the seeds (in any amount) have not been investigated. Due to lack of sufficient medical study, cnidium seeds should be used with caution in children, women who are pregnant or breast-feeding, and people with liver or kidney disease.

Cnidium seeds should not be applied to skin that is hot, dry, and sore.

Do not confuse cnidium seeds with the essential oil derived from them. While the seeds may be taken internally, the essential oil should not be ingested except under the supervision of a doctor.

While cnidium has shown some activity against bronchial asthma and osteoporosis in animal studies, it is not yet recommended for either of these conditions. Both diseases are potentially serious and require a doctor's care.

Side effects

When taken in recommended dosages, cnidium seeds are not associated with any bothersome or significant side effects.

Interactions

Cnidium seeds should not be used at the same time as croton seeds, **fritillaria**, or peony root, according to practitioners of Chinese folk medicine. When used externally, cnidium seeds have been combined with stemona, sophora, and calomel without apparent harm. When used internally, the seeds have been safely mixed with schisandra and cuscuta.

Resources

BOOKS

Editors of Time-Life Books. *The Drug and Natural Medicine Advisor*. Alexandria, VA: Time-Life Books, 1997.

PERIODICALS

Cai, J., B. Yu, G. Xu, et al. "Studies on the quality of fructus Cnidii-comparison of antibacterial action." *Chung Kuo Chung Yao Tsa Chih* 16, no. 8 (1991): 451-453, 510.

Chen, Z. and X. Duan. "Mechanism of the antiasthmatic effect of total coumarins in the fruit of *Cnidium monnieri (L.) Cuss*." *Chung Kuo Chung Yao Tsa Chih* 15, no. 5 (1990): 304-305, 320.

Liao, J. M., Q. A. Zhu, H. J. Lu, et al. "Effects of total coumarins of Cnidium monnieri on bone density and biomechanics of glucocorticoids-induced osteoporosis in rats." *Chung Kuo Yao Li Hsueh Pao* 18, no. 6 (1997): 519-521.

Tohda, C., Y. Kakihara, K. Komatsu, et al. "Inhibitory effects of methanol extracts of herbal medicines on substance P-induced itch-scratch response." *Biol Pharm Bull* 23, no. 5 (2000): 599-601.

Xie, H., Q. N. Li, L. F. Huang, et al. "Effect of total coumarins from dried fruits of *Cnidium monnieri* on glucocorticoid-induced osteoporosis in rats." *Chung Kuo Yao Li Hsueh Pao* 15, no. 4 (1994): 341-344.

ORGANIZATIONS

American Botanical Council. P.O. Box 144345, Austin, TX 78714-4345.

OTHER

OnHealth. http://www.onhealth.com.
MEDLINE. http://igm.nlm.nih.gov.

Greg Annussek

Cobalain *see* **Vitamin B$_{12}$**
Cocklebur *see* **Burdock root**

Codonopsis root

Description

Codonopsis is the fresh or dried root of the plant *Codonopsis pilosula*. Codonopsis is a small perennial native to Asia. It is especially abundant in the Shanxi and Szechuan provinces of China. Codonopsis grows to a height of about 5 ft (1.5 m) in dense brushy thickets and at the edges of woods where the soil remains moist. Codonopsis is well known in Chinese herbalism. Its Chinese name is *tang shen*. The plant is also cultivated in many other parts of the world, including the United States, because of its distinctive bell-shaped greenish-purple flowers. Other names for codonopsis include bastard ginseng and bonnet bellflower.

General use

Codonopsis, or *tang shen*, has been used in China for more than 2,000 years. It is one of the best-known and most widely used herbs in Chinese medicine. In the Chinese system of health, the *yin* aspects of nature, which have to do with cold, moisture, dark, and passivity, must be kept in balance with the *yang* aspects, which have to do with heat, dryness, light, and activity. Ill health occurs when the energies and elements of the body are out of balance with nature or in interior disharmony. Health is restored by taking herbs and treatments that restore this balance. In **traditional Chinese medicine**, codonopsis is said to have a neutral nature and a sweet taste. It is used as a tonic for the lungs and spleen and to strengthen and nourish the blood and balance metabolic function.

Like ginseng, codonopsis is an adaptogen. Adaptogens are substances that non-specifically enhance and regulate the body's ability to withstand **stress**. They increase the body's general performance in ways that help the whole body resist disease. Codonopsis is thought to benefit the entire body by boosting strength, increasing stamina and alertness, rejuvenating the body, strengthening the immune system, aiding recovery from chronic illness, reducing stress, and stimulating the appetite. It belongs to a class of herbs called stomachics, which means that they tonify the stomach to improve digestive functions.

Codonopsis is sometimes called the "poor man's ginseng." It is often substituted in Chinese herbal formulas for ginseng, although it has a milder action that lasts for a shorter time. Scientists have shown that the actions of ginseng and codonopsis, although similar, are caused by very different chemical compounds. This type of substitution based on function rather than chemical structure, however, is considered acceptable in Chinese medicine.

In addition to the whole-body effects of codonopsis, the herb is used for a number of other specific conditions. It can be taken internally, in various combinations with other herbs, for **anemia**; **asthma**; **cancer**; **diarrhea**; headaches, especially tension

KEY TERMS

Adaptogen—A substance that regulates a body system, either stimulating or suppressing it to bring it back within its normal range.

Decoction—An extract of a plant made by boiling it, then straining the solid material out. The resulting liquid is the decoction.

Galactogogue—A substance or medication that increases the flow of breast milk in nursing mothers.

Stomachic—A substance or medication that tonifies the stomach to improve digestive functions.

Tincture—A plant extract prepared in a solution of alcohol and water.

Yang aspects—In traditional Chinese medicine, yang aspects are qualities of nature such as warmth, activity, light, and dryness.

Yin aspects—Yin aspects are the opposite of yang aspects and are represented by qualities such as cold, moisture, darkness, and passivity.

headaches; **hemorrhoids**; high blood pressure; mucus in the lungs and shortness of breath; **nausea** and **vomiting**; neck tension; and a prolapsed (collapsed) uterus. Codonopsis can also be taken internally as a galactogogue, which means that it increases the supply of breast milk in nursing mothers.

University and medical researchers only became interested in codonopsis in the 1980s. Most of the research work has been done in China. Overall research findings suggest that codonopsis is relatively effective and safe. Most of this work has been done in test tubes and on small laboratory animals. Large-scale controlled human studies have yet to be done.

In many studies, scientists have found that extract of codonopsis root helps mice withstand stress, whether that stress comes from swimming, high temperatures, or oxygen deprivation. Other studies show that codonopsis boosts the immune system. In research done in China in 1997, codonopsis was shown to protect laboratory animals against gastric ulcers.

Other research has shown that codonopsis can increase the number of red blood cells and hemoglobin in animals. It also improves the production of antibodies. Studies are being done to determine if codonopsis would be useful in treating HIV infection; such autoimmune diseases as **systemic lupus erythematosus** (SLE), or immune systems that have been weakened by chemotherapy. Although the results are promising, definitive answers cannot be obtained until controlled studies on humans are performed.

Preparations

Codonopsis root comes in different grades. Roots at least three years old are harvested in the autumn after the leaves of the plant have died back. The best quality roots are large, clean, and dry on the surface, but moist inside when chewed. Codonopsis has a pleasant taste when eaten raw. Poor quality codonopsis is almost tasteless and may be dry and dirty.

Although codonopsis is sometimes eaten raw, the dried root is usually made into a decoction, which is an extract of the plant made by boiling. Tinctures, which are solutions of alcohol and water containing plant matter, are used in the West but not in traditional Chinese medicine. Commercially produced tablets, capsules, and tinctures of codonopsis are available. Dosage varies with the condition being treated. Codonopsis is often used in Chinese preparations, and may replace ginseng in almost any formula.

Precautions

Years of use in China suggest that codonopsis is not toxic and can be used by almost everyone. In China, babies are sometimes given pieces of codonopsis root to teethe on. It is given to children to help them grow strong, and breast-feeding women use it as a tonic to increase the quantity of milk they produce.

Side effects

No unwanted side effects are reported with the use of codonopsis.

Interactions

There are few, if any, studies of how codonopsis interacts with traditional Western medicines. It has been used for many years in combination with other Chinese herbs without incident.

Resources

BOOKS

Chevallier, Andrew. *Encyclopedia of Medicinal Plants.* New York: DK Publishing, Inc., 1996.

Molony, David. *Complete Guide to Chinese Herbal Medicine.* New York: Berkeley Books, 1998.

Teegaurden, Ron. *The Ancient Wisdom of the Chinese Tonic Herbs.* New York: Warner Books, 1998.

ORGANIZATIONS

American Association of Oriental Medicine (AAOM). 433 Front Street, Catasauqua, PA 18032. (610) 266-2433. http://www.aaaomonline.org.

Tish Davidson

Coenzyme Q10

Description

Coenzyme Q_{10} is a fat-soluble nutrient also known as CoQ_{10}, vitamin Q_{10}, ubidecarenone, or ubiquinone. It is a natural product of the human body that is primarily found in the mitochondria, which are the cellular organelles that produce energy. It occurs in most tissues of the human body; however, the highest concentrations are found in the heart, liver, kidneys, and pancreas. Ubiquinone takes its name from a combination of the word ubiquitous, meaning something that is found everywhere, and quinone 10. Quinones are substances found in all plants and animals. The variety found in humans has a 10-unit side chain in its molecular structure. Apart from the important process that provides energy, CoQ_{10} also stabilizes cell membranes and acts as an antioxidant. In this capacity, it destroys free radicals, which are unstable molecules that can damage normal cells.

General use

CoQ_{10} is used extensively in Canada, Western Europe, Japan, and Russia to treat congestive heart failure. It is available as a prescription medication almost everywhere it is sold, although it is sold over-the-counter as a nutritional supplement in the United States. Some studies have shown it to be effective for as many as 70% of patients with congestive heart failure. It appears to improve patient health and well-being, and to increase cardiac efficiency. The dosage generally recommended for this condition is 100–300 mg a day, preferably in divided doses. According to Dr. Karl Folkers in *Prevention's Healing with Vitamins*, it takes one to three months to achieve desired results from supplementation, and as long as six months to attain maximum benefit.

CoQ_{10} may also help people with some forms of cardiomyopathy. Patients should consult their physician about the possible benefits of supplementation for this condition.

The usefulness of CoQ_{10} in lowering blood pressure is not well documented. One study suggests that the supplement is helpful for **hypertension**, but the results are in question as it was not a double-blind, controlled research project. The dose recommended is 200–250 mg a day, with results taking several months to appear. It is possible that some patients with essential hypertension who are initially low in CoQ_{10} may eventually be able to decrease the amount of their

KEY TERMS

Angina—Symptoms of pressure or burning in the chest that result from inadequate oxygen in the heart, generally due to coronary artery spasm or blockage.

Antioxidant—An enzyme or other substance that is capable of countering the damaging effects of oxidation in the body's tissues. Coenzyme Q_{10} performs antioxidant activity.

Cardiomyopathy—A condition of damaged, diseased, thickened, or stretched heart muscle, resulting in weakness of the heart. Cardiomyopathy often occurs following heart attacks due to scarring, but may also have an infectious or nutritional origin.

Friedreich's ataxia—An inherited disease that usually manifests in childhood or adolescence, characterized by loss of muscular coordination (ataxia), curvature of the spine, impaired speech, and cardiomyopathy.

Huntington's disease—A fatal inherited disorder characterized by progressive neurologic symptoms including loss of motor and cognitive function.

other blood pressure medications. This must be done under the care of a health care provider.

Oral supplementation of CoQ_{10} has been shown to improve periodontal disease, as it decreases the size of abnormally deep pockets in the gums, and also reduces the extent of bacterial contamination. Other possible benefits of CoQ_{10} are to decrease **angina** symptoms, improve immune function in patients with **AIDS** and other immune deficiencies, improve control of blood sugar, lower **cholesterol**, improve physical stamina, and help people with muscular dystrophy and Huntington's disease. A group of researchers at the University of California at San Diego reported in 2002 that coenzyme Q_{10} appears to slow the progress of **Parkinson's disease**, Friedreich's ataxia, and other conditions marked by degeneration of the central nervous system. The supplement can also reduce the toxicity of some types of chemotherapy. Doxorubicin, a chemotherapeutic agent, is known to sometimes damage the heart. Concomitant supplementation seems to reduce this toxic effect. The possible benefits of CoQ_{10} should be discussed with a nutritionally-oriented health care provider.

Since 1961, when it was first noticed that **cancer** patients in Sweden and the United States had low levels of the enzyme, coenzyme Q_{10} has been studied as a possible cancer treatment. Researchers believe that coenzyme Q$_{10}$ may protect against cancer by stimulating the immune system, and functioning as an antioxidant. Although animal studies have been conducted, as of 2008 no report of a randomized clinical trial involving human subjects whose survival times were lengthened by using coenzyme Q$_{10}$ in addition to a traditional cancer treatment has been reported in a peer-reviewed medical journal.

Deficiency

Patients with certain conditions tend to have lower levels of CoQ$_{10}$, and may benefit from supplements. Some diseases that are associated with decreased amounts of this nutrient are AIDS, chronic **fatigue**, congestive heart failure, cardiomyopathy, and inflammatory **gum disease**. Levels of CoQ$_{10}$ tend to decrease with age; tests for its presence in the body are not widely available. Adverse effects from this supplement are rare and mild, so anyone suffering from one of the listed conditions should consider discussing supplementation with a health care provider.

Preparations

Natural sources

Food products are a good source of CoQ$_{10}$, and provide approximately half of the body's requirement. Cold-water fish such as mackerel, salmon, sardines, and tuna are particularly high in CoQ$_{10}$. Vegetable oils and meats also provide good sources. The liver manufactures adequate amounts to fulfill the need not met in the diet. People who are deficient in B vitamins, **selenium**, **vitamin C**, and **vitamin E** may not be able to make as much CoQ$_{10}$ as they need because these nutrients are required for production. Consumption of foods rich in CoQ$_{10}$ and production of the nutrient in the liver will not provide the amounts needed to treat heart failure and other conditions that may contribute to a deficiency of this nutrient. In those cases, supplements are required.

Supplemental sources

Supplements of CoQ$_{10}$ are widely available; however, its cost varies considerably. In 2004, it was available in the United States, ranging in price from $7.79 for a bottle of 40 30-mg capsules to $38.95 for a bottle of 60 100-mg capsules. It is found in various forms including capsules, gelcaps, liquids, and tablets. The latter may be the best choice, as this form generally includes a source of fat that improves absorption. Vitamin E is a helpful stabilizing additive as well. Most of the CoQ$_{10}$ products currently available on the

market are manufactured in Japan. Like other supplements, Co$_{10}$ is best kept in a cool, dry place, out of direct light, and out of the reach of children.

Precautions

As of 2008, the safety of CoQ$_{10}$ for pregnant or breast-feeding women has not been established, and its use is not recommended under these conditions. It is also not recommended for young children. People diagnosed with heart failure, diabetes, kidney problems, or liver disease should use particular care with this supplement, as the dosage of other medications may require adjustment. These individuals should consult a physician before taking coenzyme Q$_{10}$.

Side effects

Reported adverse effects related to supplemental CoQ$_{10}$ use include **diarrhea**, irritation of the stomach, poor appetite, and **nausea**. These effects are rarely reported and are mild. CoQ$_{10}$ is considered extremely safe for most people. If doses over 300 mg per day are taken, liver enzyme levels may be affected, and may need monitoring.

Interactions

It is possible that CoQ$_{10}$ decreases the action of **sodium** warfarin (known by the brand name, Coumadin), which is prescribed to prevent the formation of **blood clots** in patients at risk of **heart attack** or **stroke**. Some oral diabetes medications may also interfere with the action of CoQ$_{10}$. Cholesterol-lowering drugs in the statin group may have this effect as well.

Resources

BOOKS

Bratman, Steven, and David Kroll. *Natural Health Bible.* Roseville, CA: Prima Publishing, 2000.

Griffith, H. Winter. *Vitamins, Herbs, Minerals & Supplements: The Complete Guide.* Tucson, AZ: Fisher Books, 2000.

Pressman, Alan H., and Sheila Buff. *The Complete Idiot's Guide to Vitamins and Minerals.*, 2nd ed. Indianapolis: Macmillan General Reference, 2000.

Therapeutic Research Faculty Staff. *Natural Medicines Comprehensive Database.* Stockton, CA: Therapeutic Research Faculty, 1999.

PERIODICALS

Baker, S. K., and M. A. Tarnopolsky. "Targeting Cellular Energy Production in Neurological Disorders." *Expert Opinion on Investigational Drugs* 12 (October 2003): 1655–79.

Naini, A., V., J. Lewis, M. Hirano, and S. DiMauro. "Primary Coenzyme Q$_{10}$ and the Brain." *Biofactors* 18 (2003): 145–52.

Shults, C. W. "Coenzyme Q$_{10}$ in Neurodegenerative Diseases." *Current Medical Chemistry* 10 (October 2003): 1917–21.

Shults, C. W., D. Oakes, K. Kieburtz, et al. "Effects of Coenzyme Q$_{10}$ in Early Parkinson's Disease: Evidence of Slowing of the Functional Decline." *Archives of Neurology* 59 (October 2002): 1541–50.

Vedanarayanan, V. V. "Mitochondrial Disorders and Ataxia." *Seminars in Pediatric Neurology* 10 (September 2003): 200–9.

ORGANIZATIONS

Food and Drug Administration (FDA). 5600 Fishers Lane, Rockville, MD 20857. (888) 463-6332. http://www.fda.gov.

National Cancer Institute (NCI). http://www.nci.nih.gov.

National Center for Complementary and Alternative Medicine (NCCAM) Clearinghouse. P. O. Box 7923, Gaithersburg, MD 20898-7923. (888) 644-6226. Fax: (866) 464-3615. http://nccam.nih.gov.

OTHER

National Cancer Institute (NCI). *Complementary and Alternative Medicine (CAM) Information Summary: Coenzyme Q$_{10}$.* Bethesda, MD: NCI, 2003. [cited June 3, 2004]. http://www.nci.nih.gov/cancerinfo/pdq/cam/coenzymeQ10.

National Institute of Neurological Disorders and Stroke (NINDS). "Study Suggests Coenzyme Q$_{10}$ Slows Functional Decline in Parkinson's Disease." NINDS press release, 14 October 2002. [cited June 3, 2004]. http://www.ninds.nih.gov/news_and_events/pressrelease_parkinsons_coenzymeq10_10140.

Rebecca Frey

Coix

Description

Coix is a grain plant whose botanical name is *Coix lacryma-jobi*. It belongs to the Gramineae (or Poaceae) family. Coix is used in **traditional Chinese medicine**, where it is called *yi yi ren*. In English it is also known as Job's tears. Coix is also a food. In addition, the seeds are used to make jewelry and items such as rosaries and **prayer** beads.

Coix is an annual plant that grows wild to a height of about 3 ft (1 m) in sunny but moist grasslands. It is also cultivated in many parts of Asia. Coix may have originated in East Asia, but it is now found throughout East India, China, Japan, the Philippines, northern Africa, the Caribbean, Central America, northern South America, and the United States. The plant has narrow, ribbon-like leaves. The seed with the husk removed is used medicinally. In some areas, coix is cultivated as a food grain. The seeds contain about 52% starch, 18% protein, and 7% fat, giving them a higher protein-to-carbohydrate ratio than other cereal grains.

General use

Coix is used as both a healing herb and a food. It was used in folk medicine to treat conditions ranging from arthritis and **halitosis** (bad breath) to rheumatism and **worms**. The seeds, with the husks removed, are important in traditional Chinese medicine. These are said to have a cool nature and a sweet, bland taste. In traditional Chinese medicine, coix seed is used to treat internal dampness and damp-heat conditions, especially disorders of the spleen, stomach, lungs, and large intestine.

Chinese herbalists use coix to improve water flow through the body. It is used to promote urination and as a diuretic to treat **edema**. It can be used to reduce **pain** and spasms in the legs when there is also swelling of the legs. Coix is also used to treat such conditions of the gastrointestinal system as **diarrhea**, poor digestion, and abdominal bloating.

Other claims are also made for coix seed. It is said that a tea made from the boiled seeds will help to cure **warts**. Coix is thought to be beneficial for the skin, helping to nourish and soften it so that skin looks smooth and healthy.

Coix is often used in formulas that treat arthritis and rheumatism, conditions believed to be caused by excess dampness according to traditional Chinese medicine. Chinese herbalists also use it to treat appendicitis, lung disease, lung abscesses, beriberi, and **cancer**.

The seeds of coix are said to have anti-inflammatory, antiseptic, and fever-reducing properties. It is claimed that they can prevent spasms, lower blood sugar, and act as a sedative. The coix root has been used to treat menstrual disorders.

There is no doubt that coix also has value as a food grain, although the seed coat is hard to remove, making it difficult to produce flour. Coix can be cooked like barley or rice, however, and the flour can be used to make bread. Parched coix seeds are used to make tea, and a coffee substitute can be made from the roasted seeds of some Chinese subspecies.

With so many claims made for coix, scientific interest in the plant was quite high in the 2000s.

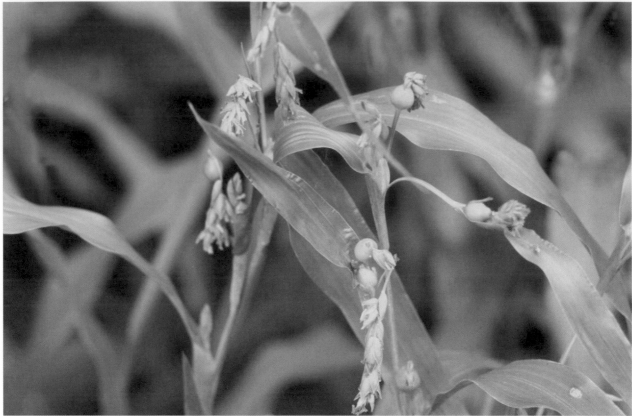

Coix (Coix lacryma-jobi). *(© blickwinkel / Alamy)*

Agricultural scientists were investigating the genetics of coix with an eye toward growing it as a food crop, and medical researchers were looking at its healing properties. Kanglaite, a compound obtained from the coix seed, had been studied in Asia as a treatment for conditions, including cancer. As of 2008, research included Phase II clinical trials studying people with non-small-cell **lung cancer**, according to the University of Texas M. D. Anderson Cancer Center.

Although coix may be proven effective in treating medical conditions, the American Cancer Society cautioned that many studies involving Chinese herbs were written in Chinese. Some journal articles about clinical trials did not include details such as how studies were conducted, information needed to compare the results with research performed in the United States.

The society's assessment paralleled the results of a February 2008 review of publications accessed through *PubMed* (http://www.ncbi.nlm.nih.gov/PubMed), an online service of the U.S. National Library of Medicine and the National Institutes of Health. A literature search for studies of kanglaite (KLT) produced five English-language abstracts (summaries) of articles originally written in Chinese or Russian.

The October 2005 issue of *Zhongguo Zhongyao Zazhi* (*China Journal of Chinese Materia Medica*) contained an article titled "Effect of Kanglaite Injection Oncyclooxygenase Activity in Lung Carcinoma A549 Cell." Few details were provided in the article, which was written in Chinese.

An article in the November 2004 issue of *Hepatobiliary and Pancreatic Diseases International* described a study involving 40 rats. Although KLT appeared to be effective in the treatment of liver tumors, researchers concluded that it was less effective than ethanol in terms of liver function, according to the article titled, "Efficacy of Intra-Tumor Injection of Kang-Lai-Te in Treating Transplanted Hepatoma in Rats."

Preparations

Coix seeds are harvested when the plant ripens in the autumn. The husks are removed and the seed is used fresh, boiled, roasted, or fermented. In traditional Chinese medicine, liquor fermented from coix seeds may be given for rheumatism. Coix is also used in combination with other herbs in rheumatism and arthritis formulas such as ginseng and **atractylodes** formula. When coix is used for medicinal purposes, the usual daily dose is 10–30 g.

Combination treatments include a remedy for arthritis. The combination consists of 30 g of coix combined with cinnamon twig tea. The mixture is cooked with rice and consumed.

Coix may be eaten as nourishment. That makes it different from other herbs, which are given in limited doses. Puffed coix, similar to puffed wheat or puffed rice cereals, is sold in health food stores and in markets that sell Asian food.

Precautions

Traditional Chinese herbalists suggest that pregnant women not use coix.

Furthermore, the United States Food and Drug Administration does not regulate herbal remedies such as coix, which means that the remedies have not proven to be safe or effective. The safety of coix has not been established for use by children, pregnant women, and nursing mothers. In addition, ingredients are not standardized to comply with federal regulations.

As of 2008, there was limited information about research claims into the effectiveness of coix as a remedy. The lack of information raises questions such as how coix would interact with other medications and herbs. In addition, the lack of detailed information about product ingredients drew cautions from organizations, including the American Cancer Society. After the California Department of Health tested Chinese herbal remedies, the tests revealed that close to 33% contained prescription drugs or were contaminated with toxic metals such as mercury, arsenic, and lead, according to the society.

Side effects

In traditional Chinese medicine, coix has been used without any undesirable side effects. Although there were no known side effects as of 2008, there were indications that people who eat large amounts of coix as a food may become dehydrated.

Interactions

Coix has been used for thousands of years in conjunction with other herbs with no reported interactions. Since coix is used almost exclusively in Chinese medicine, there were no studies of its interactions with Western pharmaceuticals as of 2008.

KEY TERMS

Beriberi—A serious disease caused by a deficiency in vitamin B1 and characterized by a slow degeneration of the nerves of the digestive system and heart.

Diuretic—Any substance that increases the production of urine.

Edema—Water retention in the body that often causes swelling of the hands and feet.

Resources

OTHER

"Chinese Herbal Medicine." American Cancer Society, June 26, 2007. http://www.cancer.org/docroot/ETO/content/ETO_5_3x_Chinese_Herbal_Medicine.asp (February 23, 2008).

"Coix lacryma-jobi." Plants for a Future. http://www.pfaf.org (February 23, 2008).

"Traditional Chinese Medicine: Overview of Herbal Medicines." University of Texas M. D. Anderson Cancer Center. http://www.mdanderson.org/departments/cimer/display.cfm?id=1b608136-f1c3-43b5-a3e14b864d2d14c6&method=displayfull&pn=6eb86a59-ebd9-11d4-810100508b603a14 (February 23, 2008).

ORGANIZATIONS

American Association of Acupuncture and Oriental Medicine, PO Box 162340, Sacramento, CA, 95816, (866) 455-7999, http://www.aaom.org.

American Botanical Council, 6200 Manor Rd., Austin, TX, 78723, (512) 926-4900, http://abc.herbalgram.org.

Herb Research Foundation, 4140 Fifteenth St., Boulder, CO, 80304, (303) 449-2265, http://www.herbs.org.

National Center for Complementary and Alternative Medicine, National Institute of Health (NCCAM), 9000 Rockville Pike, Bethesda, MD, 20892, (888) 644-6226, http://nccam.nih.gov.

Tish Davidson
Liz Swain

Cola nut *see* **Kola nut**

Colchicum

Definition

Colchicum is a genus of flowering plant consisting of about sixty species, perhaps the best known of which is *Colchicum autumnale*. *C. autumnale* is also known as "naked lady," "meadow saffron," or "autumn

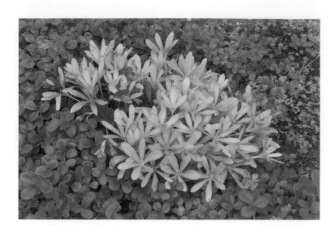

Colchicum (Colchicum autumnale). *(Nature's Images / Photo Researchers, Inc.)*

crocus." The first of these names derives from the fact that the plant develops beautiful pink, purple, or white flowers before leaves appear. The plant is "naked," therefore, in regard to its lack of leaves although flowers have already appeared. In 2008, Botanic Gardens Conservation International, a program dedicated to the conservation of threatened and endangered plant species, declared that the best known form of colchicum, *C. autumnale*, was at risk of extinction. The primary reason for this situation, as with other plants of medicinal value, was overharvesting by commercial operators.

Description

Colchicum is usually an annual (less commonly, perennial) plant that grows best in rich soils. It is found in western Asia, along the Mediterranean coast, in England, and throughout many parts of Europe and the United States. The plant's name derives from the region of Colchis, near present-day Georgia and Turkey. In addition to its colorful flower, the plant has somewhat broad (about an inch), longish (about a foot) dark green leaves.

The leaves, seeds, and corms of the plant contain the alkaloid colchicine, which is very toxic. It is the colchicine, taken in moderate doses, that provides the plant's medicinal value. Herbalists use the corm as the primary source of colchicine for their medical preparations.

The first mention of the use of colchicum for medical purposes appears to be a treatise by the Greek physician Pedanius Dioscorides (c. 40 A.D - c. 90 A.D) in his work *De Materia Medica*. Colchicine was first isolated from the colchicum plant by French chemists P. S. Pelletier and J. Caventon in 1820.

Medical Use

Historically, the primary use for colchicum has been in the treatment of **gout**, first mentioned by Dioscorides in the first century A.D. That application continues to be the most popular today. In addition, colchicum has been recommended for use with rheumatism, **gonorrhea**, **neuralgia**, enlarged prostate, pericarditis, dropsy (**edema**), **hepatitis**, **cirrhosis**, and inflammatory conditions. Research is currently being conducted on its possible use as an anti-cancer agent. In the United States, colchicine has been approved by the Food and Drug Administration (FDA) for use in the treatment of gout, familial Mediterranean **fever**, secondary amyloidosis, scleroderma, and Behçet's disease. Researchers have found that the basis of colchicine's action is its tendency to bind to tubulin, a chemical compound found in microtubules, basic components of cell structure. The presence of colchicine interferes with the process of mitosis (cell division), slowing down or interrupting the continued growth of cells. It is this property that makes colchicine a candidate as an anti–cancer agent since an essential characteristic of **cancer** cells is the rapid rate at which they reproduce.

Preparation

Medicinal extracts of colchicum are prepared from the plant's seeds or corm. If the later, the corm is harvested during and just following the plant's flowering. The bulb is dried whole or after first having been cut into thin slices. The dried product is then used to make an extract, tincture, or wine for medical use.

Side Effects

Colchicum has a relatively low therapeutic index. Therapeutic index is the ratio of a drug's potential benefits to its risks. Drugs with low therapeutic index must be carefully monitored since even a modest increase in the amount of drug ingested can cause serious side effects. Among the less serious side effects of colchicum are the following:

- nausea
- loss of appetite
- diarrhea
- hair loss

A number of more serious side effects may occur, requiring medical attention. These effects include:

- skin rash and/or itching
- stomach pain
- blood in the urine

- muscle weakness
- numbness or tingling in the hands or feet
- fever or chills
- swelling of the mouth or face
- pain or difficulty in urinating

Interactions

As of 2008, the International Programme on Chemical Safety has reported no interactions of colchicum with other herbal medications or drugs.

Resources

PERIODICALS

Brvar, Miran, et al. "Case Report: Fatal Poisoning with Colchicum Autumnale." *Critical Care* (January 2004): R56–R59.

Kumar, Andras, Saban Elitok, and Ralph Kettritz. "Colchicum ad Nauseum." *Nephrology Dialysis Transplantation* (October 2003): 2197–2198.

Morris, I., G. Varughese, and P. Mattingly. "Colchicine in Acute Gout." *BMJ* (November 2003): 1275–1276.

Ong, Michael, et al. "Safety of Colchicine Therapy during Pregnancy." *Canadian Family Physician* (August 2003): 967–969.

Ting, Joseph Yuk Sang. "Acute Pancreatitis Related to Therapeutic Dosing with Colchicine: A Case Report." *Journal of Medical Case Reports* (August 2007): 64.

OTHER

Dowd, Matthew J. "Colchicine." http://www.phc.vcu.edu/Feature/oldfeature/colchicine/colchicine.html (February 6, 2008).

Henriette's Herbal Homepage. "Colchicum." http://www.henriettesherbal.com/eclectic/kings/colchicum-autu.html (February 6, 2008).

"Pharmacology of Colchicine." http://biotech.icmb.utexas.edu/botany/colch.html (February 6, 2008).

David Edward Newton, Ed.D.

Cold, common *see* **Common cold**

Cold sore

Definition

A cold sore is a fluid-filled blister that usually appears at the edge of the lips. Cold sores are caused by a herpes simplex virus infection.

Description

A cold sore is a fluid-filled, painful blister that is usually on or around the lips. Other names for cold sores are **feverblisters**, oral herpes, labial herpes, herpes labialis, and herpes febrilis. Cold sores most often occur on the lips, distinguishing them from the common canker sore that is usually located inside the mouth. Cold sores do not usually occur inside the mouth except during the initial episode. **Canker sores** usually form either on the tongue or inside the cheeks.

Cold sores are caused by a herpes virus. There are eight different kinds of human herpes viruses. Only two of these, herpes simplex, types 1 and 2, can cause cold sores. It is commonly believed that herpes simplex virus type 1 infects above the waist and herpes simplex virus type 2 infects below the waist. This is not completely true. Both herpes virus type 1 and type 2 can cause herpes lesions on the lips or genitals but recurrent cold sores are almost always type 1.

Oral herpes is very common. More than 60% of Americans have had a cold sore and almost 25% of those infected experience recurrent outbreaks. Most of these persons became infected before age 10. Anyone can become infected by herpes virus and once infected, the virus remains latent for life. Herpes viruses are spread from person to person by direct skin-to-skin contact. The highest risk for spreading the virus is the time period beginning with the appearance of blisters and ending with scab formation. However, infected persons need not have visible blisters to spread the infection to others since the virus may be present in the saliva without obvious oral lesions.

Viruses are different from bacteria. While bacteria are independent and can reproduce on their own, viruses enter human cells and force them to make more virus. The infected human cell is usually killed and releases thousands of new viruses. The cell death and resulting tissue damage causes the actual cold sores. In addition, herpes virus can infect a cell and instead of making the cell produce new viruses, it hides inside the cell and waits. Herpes virus hides in the nervous system. This is called "latency." A latent virus can wait inside the nervous system for days, months, or even years. At some future time, the virus "awakens" and causes the cell to produce thousands of new viruses which causes an active infection.

This process of latency and active infection is best understood by considering the cold sore cycle. An active infection is obvious because cold sores are present. The first infection is called the "primary" infection. This active infection is then controlled by the body's immune system and the sores heal. In between active **infections** the virus is latent. At some point in the future, latent viruses become activated and once again cause sores. These are called "recurrent" infections. Although it is unknown what triggers a latent virus to activate, several conditions seem to bring on infections. These include **stress**, illness, **fatigue**, exposure to sunlight, **menstruation**, fever, and diet.

Causes and symptoms

While anyone can be infected by herpes virus, not everyone will show symptoms. The first symptoms of herpes occur within two to 20 days after contact with an infected person. Symptoms of the primary infection are usually more severe than those of recurrent infections. The primary infection can cause symptoms like other viral infections including fatigue, **headache**, fever, and swollen lymph nodes in the neck.

Typically, 50–80% of persons with oral herpes experience a prodrome (symptoms of oncoming disease) of **pain**, burning, **itching**, or tingling at the site where blisters will form. This prodrome stage may last anywhere from a few hours, to one or two days. The

herpes infection prodrome occurs in both the primary infection and recurrent infections.

In 95% of patients with cold sores, the blisters occur at the outer edge of the lips which is called the "vermilion border." Less often, blisters form on the nose, chin, or cheek. Following the prodrome, the disease process is rapid. First, small red bumps appear, which quickly form fluid-filled blisters. The painful blisters may either burst and form a scab or dry up and form a scab. Within two days of the first red bumps, all the blisters have formed scabs. The skin heals completely and without scarring within six to 10 days.

Some children have a very serious primary (first episode) herpes infection called gingivostomatitis. This causes fever, swollen lymph glands, and numerous blisters inside the mouth and on the lips and tongue, which may form large, open sores. These painful sores may last up to three weeks and can make eating and drinking difficult. Because of this, young children with gingivostomatitis are at risk for dehydration (excessive loss of water from the body).

Most people experience fewer than two recurrent outbreaks of cold sores each year. Some people never experience outbreaks while others have more frequent occurrences. In most people, the blisters form in the same area each time and are triggered by the same factors (such as stress, sun exposure, etc.).

Diagnosis

Because oral herpes is so common, it is diagnosed primarily by symptoms. It can be diagnosed and treated by the family doctor, dermatologists (doctors who specialize in skin diseases) and infectious disease specialists. Laboratory tests may be performed to look for the virus. Because healing sores do not shed much virus, a sample from an open sore is taken for viral culture. A sterile cotton swab is wiped over open sores and the sample used to infect human cells in culture. Cells that are killed by herpes virus have a certain appearance under microscopic examination. The results of this test are available within two to 10 days.

Oral herpes may resemble a bacterial infection called **impetigo**. This skin infection is most commonly seen in children and causes herpes-like blisters around the mouth and nose. Also, because oral herpes can occur inside the mouth, the blisters could be mistaken for common canker sores. Therefore, doctors need to determine whether the blisters are oral herpes, canker sores, or impetigo. The diagnosis and treatment of herpes infections should be covered by most insurance providers.

Treatment

There is no cure for cold sores but many alternative treatments can reduce outbreaks and shorten healing time. During an outbreak of cold sores, salty foods, citrus foods (oranges etc.), and other foods that irritate the sores should be avoided. Wash the sores once or twice a day with a warm, saline solution and pat gently to dry. Application of ice or a cold wet teabag for 10 minutes four or five times a day can relieve the itching and burning.

Supplements

Vitamin and mineral supplements and diet may have an effect on the recurrence and duration of cold sores. In general, cold sore sufferers should eat a healthy diet of unprocessed foods such as vegetables, fruits, and whole grains. Alcohol, **caffeine**, chocolate, nuts, and sugar should be avoided.

An imbalance in the **amino acids lysine** and **arginine** is thought to be a contributing factor in herpes virus outbreaks. A diet that is rich in the amino acid lysine may help prevent recurrences of cold sores. Foods that contain high levels of lysine include most vegetables, legumes, fish, turkey, and chicken. In one study, patients taking lysine supplements had milder symptoms during an outbreak, a shorter healing time, and had fewer outbreaks than patients who did not take lysine. Patients should take 1,000 mg of lysine three times a day during a cold sore outbreak and 500 mg daily on an ongoing basis to prevent recurrences. The effectiveness of lysine supplementation in treating herpes infections is controversial. Intake of the amino acid arginine should be reduced. Foods rich in arginine that should be avoided are chocolate, peanuts, almonds, and other nuts and seeds.

Vitamin C and **bioflavonoids** (a substance in fruits that helps the body to absorb and use vitamin C) have been shown to reduce the duration of a cold sore outbreak and reduce the number of sores. The **vitamin B complex** includes important vitamins that support the nervous system where herpes viruses are dormant. B complex vitamins also can help manage stress, an important contributing factor to the outbreak of herpes viruses. Some studies have shown that correcting **iron**, folate, vitamin C, or **vitamin B_{12}** deficiencies improves cold sores. **Vitamin E** speeds healing and reduces pain. Squeeze the oil from a vitamin E capsule onto a cotton ball and apply to the sore for 30 minutes to one hour.

Herbals

Mints are effective antivirals. **Lemon balm** or Melissa (*Melissa officinalis*) is comparable to the antiviral acyclovir in the treatment of cold sores. Apply lemon balm cream to the sore several times a day. Alternatively, prepare lemon balm tea, drink the tea and apply the dregs to the sore for one or two hours. The patient may also drink several strong cups of teas prepared from **hyssop**, oregano, **rosemary**, **thyme**, and **sage**. **Licorice** may be added to the tea.

Licorice (*Glycyrrhiza glabra*) is an antiviral and immune system stimulant. Licorice is available as a capsule or an ointment. Gradually take up to 300 mg a day. Apply ointment that contains glycyrrhetinic or glycyrrhizic acid directly to the sore as necessary. Ingestion of licorice may cause loose stools and high blood pressure.

Chinese medicine

Treatment with Qing Dai San (Natural Indigo Powder) mixed with cold boiled water and applied to the sore is generally all that is needed. For recurrent cold sores, the following oral preparations can be taken:

- Yin Huang Kou Fu Yi (Honeysuckle and Scutellaria Fluid): one ampule three times daily
- Yin Qiao Jie Du Pian (Honeysuckle and Forsythia Tablet to Resolve Toxin): two to four tablets three times daily
- Huang Lian Shang Qing Wan (Coptis Pill to Clear Heat of Upper Jiao): 5 g, two to three times daily

Other treatments for cold sores include:

- Pepto-Bismol Rub liquid into cold sore.
- Laser therapy. Ten daily treatments with low-intensity laser significantly lowered the incidence of oral herpes outbreaks as compared to placebo.
- Mild electric current. Preliminary studies of a small device that delivers a mild electric current to the cold sore site have shown shorter duration of pain and blisters.

Allopathic treatment

There is no cure for herpes virus infections. There are antiviral drugs available which have some effect in lessening the symptoms and decreasing the length of herpes outbreaks. There is evidence that some may also prevent future outbreaks. These antiviral drugs are most effective when taken as early in the infection process as possible. For the best results, drug treatment should begin during the prodrome stage before blisters are visible.

Acyclovir (Zovirax) has been the drug of choice for herpes infection and can be given intravenously or taken by mouth. It can be applied directly to sores as an ointment but is not very useful in this form. A liquid form for children is also available. Acyclovir is effective in treating both the primary infection and recurrent outbreaks. When taken by mouth to prevent an outbreak, acyclovir reduces the frequency of herpes outbreaks. In 2001, a report showed that use of high-dose acyclovir during primary infection will reduce the extent of latent infection. The use of penciclovir (Denavir) cream as soon as the prodrome symptoms appear speeds healing.

Over-the-counter lip products which contain the chemical phenol (such as Blistex Medicated Lip Ointment) and numbing ointments (Anbesol) help to relieve cold sores. Pharmacists also recommend the over-the-counter medicine Abreva, the only cold sore medicine approved by the U.S. Food and Drug Administration (FDA) to shorten healing time. Acetaminophen (Tylenol) or ibuprofen (Motrin, Advil) may be taken if necessary to reduce pain and fever.

Expected results

Oral herpes can be painful and embarrassing but it is not a serious infection. There is no cure for oral herpes but outbreaks usually occur less frequently after age 35. Alternative medicines can reduce the pain, prevent outbreaks, and shorten the course of cold sores. The spread of herpes virus to the eyes is very serious. Herpes virus can infect the cells in the cornea and cause scarring that may impair vision.

Prevention

The only way to prevent oral herpes is to avoid contact with infected persons. This is not an easy solution because many people are not aware that they are infected and can easily infect others. As of 2008 there were no known herpes vaccines available, although vaccines are being tested.

Several practices can reduce the occurrence of cold sores and the spread of virus to other body locations or people. These practices are:

- Avoidance of sun exposure to the face. Before getting prolonged exposure to the sun, apply sunscreen to the face and especially to the lips. Wearing a hat with a large brim is also helpful.
- Avoid touching cold sores. Squeezing, picking, or pinching blisters can allow the virus to spread to other parts of the lips or face and infect those sites.
- Wash hands frequently. Persons with oral herpes should wash their hands carefully before touching

others. An infected person can spread the virus to others even when he or she has no obvious blisters.

- Avoid contact with others during active infection. Infected persons should avoid kissing or sexual contact with others until after the cold sores have healed.
- Wear gloves when applying ointment to a child's sore.
- Be especially careful with infants. Never kiss the eyes or lips of a baby who is under six months old.
- Be watchful of infected children. Do not allow infected children to share toys that may be put into the mouth. Toys that have been mouthed should be disinfected before other children play with them.
- Maintain good general health. A healthy diet, plenty of sleep, and exercise help to minimize the chance of getting a cold or the flu, which are known to bring on cold sores. Also, good general health keeps the immune system strong which helps to keep the virus in check and prevent outbreaks.
- Participate in a stress reduction program. Yoga, massage, aromatherapy, meditation, hypnosis, or biofeedback can relieve stress which may reduce outbreaks.

Resources

BOOKS

Gorbach, Sherman, John Bartlett, and Neil Blacklow, eds. *Infectious Diseases.* Philadelphia: W. B. Saunders Co., 1998.

Ying, Zhou Zhong, and Jin Hui De. "Herpes Zoster and Herpes Simplex." In *Clinical Manual of Chinese Herbal Medicine and Acupuncture.* New York: Churchill Livingston, 1997.

PERIODICALS

"Abreva Recommended Most by Pharmacists for Cold Sores." *Virus Weekly* (November 13, 2001): 12.

Khalsa, Karta Purkh Singh. "Simple Solutions for Cold Sores." *Let's Live* 67 (May 1999): 66+.

Nash, Karen. "Cold Sore Treatment: Take Whatever Works, Including Placebos." *Dermatology Times* 19 (July 1998): 37+.

Sawtell, N. M. "Early Intervention with High-Dose Acyclovir Treatment During Primary Herpes Simplex Virus Infection Reduces Latency and Subsequent Reactivation in the Nervous System in Vivo." *The Journal of the American Medical Association* 286, no. 23 (December 19, 2001): 2922.

Schindl, Andreas, and Reinhard Neumann. "Low-Intensity Laser Therapy is an Effective Treatment for Recurrent Herpes Simplex Infection. Results from a Randomized Double-Blind Placebo-Controlled Study." *The Journal of Investigative Dermatology* 113 (1999): 221–223.

OTHER

MayoClinic.com. [cited October 2002]. http://www.mayo clinic.com.

Belinda Rowland
Teresa Norris

Coleus

Description

Coleus forskohlii is a perennial plant in the mint family with a strong, camphor-like odor. It is native to areas of India, Myanmar, Nepal, and Sri Lanka and grows well in warm temperate or subtropical areas. Coleus has long been used in traditional Indian (Ayurvedic) medicine, but it gained popularity when forskolin, a chemical extract of the root, demonstrated properties that make it a potential treatment for **asthma**, **bronchitis**, **glaucoma**, congestive heart failure, and other conditions. Forskolin was first identified by Western researchers in the 1970s, but as of 2008 the effects of the whole coleus plant and its extracts had not been as well studied.

Another species of coleus, *Coleus kilimandschari*, is found in parts of Africa and has been used in Rwandan folk medicine to treat **infections** and autoimmune diseases. Some studies of Rwandan coleus indicate that it is effective against a variety of disorders involving destruction of red blood cells. As of 2008, however, Rwandan coleus had not been studied as intensively as *Coleus forskohlii*, and its extracts awaited further analysis.

General use

Forskolin increases the levels of a cell-regulating compound called cyclic adenosine monophosphate (cAMP). This property allows it to stabilize mast cells that contain histamine and other inflammatory substances. Mast cells are one type of cell responsible for allergic response. Preventing the release of these compounds could make forskolin valuable in the treatment of diseases with an allergic component, such as asthma and **eczema**.

Another benefit of the increase of cAMP is forskolin's ability to relax smooth muscles. The bronchioles, uterus, arteries, gastrointestinal tract, and bladder all contain smooth muscle that is responsive to the antispasmodic effects of forskolin. As an antispasmodic, forskolin has potential, as yet unproven

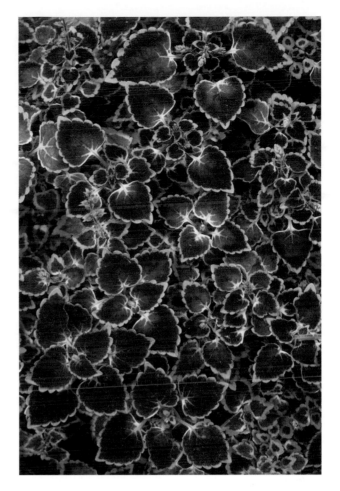

Coleus. *(© John Glover / Alamy)*

in humans, to treat conditions that involve cramping or smooth muscle contraction. These include asthma, painful menstrual periods, **angina**, **irritable bowel syndrome**, bladder infections, and high blood pressure.

People with asthma may benefit from the use of forskolin in its capacity as an antispasmodic. During an asthma attack, the smooth muscle within small passageways of the lungs (bronchioles) constricts and makes breathing difficult. The action of forskolin is similar to that of some standard inhalers containing such medications as albuterol, a beta agonist bronchodilator. Both substances relax the smooth muscle and improve the person's breathing ability. Studies of forskolin for the treatment of asthma have shown positive results in both oral and inhaled preparations. By 2008, several small studies had shown that coleus extract and forskolin effectively relax smooth muscle in human airways.

Other allergic conditions, including eczema, may also respond well to forskolin. Levels of cAMP are reduced in the bronchioles and skin of people suffering from asthma and eczema. The lack of cAMP causes histamine release and subsequent allergic symptoms, including bronchoconstriction and local reaction. Forskolin may be able to prevent the onset of symptoms in susceptible people by increasing cAMP levels. It can theoretically be helpful for any condition that is caused, wholly or partially, by an allergic reaction. Professional help should be sought regarding the use forskolin for this indication, particularly because of potential interactions with other medications used for asthma.

Psoriasis can be treated by taking forskolin supplements. In this condition, skin cells multiply at a rate much greater than normal. Itchy, silvery patches are formed on the skin. This condition may be due to an imbalance of cell regulating chemicals, including cAMP, that can be normalized by forskolin.

Cardiovascular diseases, such as congestive heart failure, angina, and high blood pressure, have the potential to be treated by forskolin. As of 2008, several small studies suggest that the extract appears to relax the smooth muscles in the walls of the arteries. The **relaxation** of the arteries decreases blood pressure, **pain** due to angina, and strain on the heart. Maximum benefit may be achieved in conjunction with other botanicals or medications, such as dobutamine. Cardiovascular effects of forskolin are an active area of research.

Blood vessels in the brain are dilated by forskolin, which could have clinical applications for patients who are at risk of, or recovering from, **stroke**. Forskolin also decreases the risk of abnormal blood clotting. This is another desirable effect for stroke patients and those with other cardiovascular conditions that cause, or result from, increased susceptibility to **blood clots**. However, as of 2008, these effects had not been well studied in humans.

The high pressure inside the eye that occurs with glaucoma has been reduced with forskolin in some small studies in humans. No safety data are available about this use, nor has the effectiveness of forskolin been compared to other products that are available to reduce pressure within the eye.

A 2007 study at Duke University found that forskolin extract injected into mice was effective in treating bladder infections. As of 2008, no research had been done to determine if this benefit carries over to humans taking oral supplements of forskolin.

An infusion of the leaves of *Coleus forskohlii* has traditionally been used in Indian medicine for the treatment of **gas**, bloating, abdominal pain, and menstrual cramps. Other unproven uses include treatment on melanoma (an aggressive **skin cancer**), **AIDS**, **hypothyroidism**, **insomnia**, irritable bowel disease, **schizophrenia**, diabetes, erectile dysfunction, **depression**, **cancer** metastasis, immune dysfunction, and parasites. As of 2008, there was no accepted scientific evidence to indicate coleus/forskolin is effective in treating any of these diseases.

As of 2008, dietary supplements containing forskolin were heavily promoted as an aid to weight loss and building lean body mass. There was no scientific evidence in humans, however, that forskolin is effective in this capacity.

Preparations

Crude preparations of *Coleus forskohlii* may not contain enough forskolin to exert a clinical effect. Forskolin extracts are available. One recommended dose is 50 mg two or three times daily of a preparation containing 18% forskolin. A healthcare provider knowledgeable in the clinical use of botanicals should be consulted before undertaking treatment with this extract.

Precautions

Forskolin can be a powerful medication and has effects on many systems of the body. It has been described as a central nervous system depressant that can cause sedation. It should not be taken without a person being aware of potential effects on other parts of the body. For this reason, professional supervision is recommended.

People with low blood pressure or gastric ulcers may wish to avoid forskolin due to potential exacerbation of these conditions. Children and women who are pregnant or breastfeeding should also avoid this substance. There is some evidence that use of forskolin by pregnant women delays fetal development. Those individuals who have chronic liver or kidney disease should use great caution in taking this medication, particularly if other herbs or medications are being used due to the current lack of data about potential risks.

Side effects

Forskolin does not appear to be toxic based on studies done on animals; however, it has been reported by veterinarians to lower the blood pressure of cats and dogs. As of 2008, the most common side effect reported for coleus leaves is **contact dermatitis** (skin rash) in people who are allergic to the plant. The overall safety and side effects of forskolin, however, had not yet received in-depth analysis as of 2008.

Interactions

Forskolin may intensify the effects of other medications taken concurrently. Caution should be used when taking any botanical or prescription medication. Forskolin should not be taken in conjunction with anti-asthmatic, anticoagulant, or antihypertensive medications without the supervision of a health care provider.

Resources

BOOKS

Chevallier, Andrew. *Herbal Remedies.* New York: DK Publishing, 2007.

Foster, Steven, and Rebecca Johnson. *National Geographic Desk Reference to Nature's Medicine.* Washington, DC: National Geographic Society, 2006.

Yarnell, Eric and Karen Abascal. *Clinical Botanical Medicine,* 2nd rev. ed. Larchmont, NY: Mary Ann Liebert, 2008.

OTHER

"Coleus (*Coleus forskohlii, Lamiaceae*) and Forsklin (Coleonol, IIL, 362)." *Intelihealth.com* May 3, 2005. http://www.intelihealth.com/. (April 12, 2008).

ORGANIZATIONS

Alternative Medicine Foundation, PO Box 60016, Potomac, MD, 20859, (301) 340-1960, http://www.amfoundation.org.

American Holistic Medical Association, PO Box 2016, Edmonds, WA, 98020, (425) 967-0737, http://www.holisticmedicine.org.

Centre for International Ethnomedicinal Education and Research (CIEER), http://www.cieer.org.

National Institute of Ayurvedic Medicine, 375 Fifth Ave., Fifth Floor, New York, NY, 10016, (212) 685-8600, http://niam.com/corp-web/index.htm.

Judith Turner
Tish Davidson, A. M.

Colic

Definition

Colic is persistent, unexplained crying and discomfort in an otherwise healthy baby between the ages of two weeks and about five months.

Description

Colic affects 10-20% of all infants. It is more common in boys than in girls and most common in a family's first child. Symptoms of colic usually appear when a baby is 14-21 days old, reach a peak at the age of three months, and disappear within the next eight weeks.

Causes and symptoms

Some babies who have colic are simply fussy. Others cry so hard that their faces turn red, then pale. Episodes may occur frequently but intermittently, usually beginning with prolonged periods of crying in the late afternoon or evening. Crying may intensify, taper off, and then get even louder. It can last for just a few minutes or continue for several hours. During a colicky episode, babies' bellies often look swollen, feel hard, and make a rumbling sound. Many babies grow rigid, clench their fists, curl their toes, and draw their legs toward their body. A burp or a bowel movement can end an attack. Most babies who have colic do not seem to be in **pain** between attacks.

One cause of colic may be the swallowing of large amounts of air, especially during feeding time. Air may then become trapped in the digestive tract and cause discomfort. Other possible causes include:

- immaturity of the digestive system
- food intolerances

- too little or too much food
- lack of sleep
- loneliness
- overheated formula
- overstimulation resulting from too much noise, light, or activity
- stress and tension on the part of the mother and other caregivers
- foods the mother eats, if breast-feeding, which are allergens or irritants for the baby

Diagnosis

Colic is suspected in an infant who:

- has cried loudly for at least three hours a day at least three times a week for three weeks or longer
- is not hungry but cries for several hours between dinnertime and midnight
- demonstrates the clenched fists, rigidity, and other physical traits associated with colic

The baby's medical history and a parent's description of eating, sleeping, and crying patterns are used to confirm the diagnosis of colic. Physical examination and laboratory tests are used to rule out infection, intestinal blockage, and other conditions that can cause abdominal pain and other colic symptoms.

Treatment

Parents should consult their healthcare practitioner before giving any herbal or allopathic medications to very young children. Teas made with **chamomile** (*Matricaria recutita*), **lemon balm** (*Melissa officinalis*), **peppermint** (*Mentha piperita*), **catnip** (*Nepeta cataria*), or dill (*Anethum graveolens*) can lessen bowel inflammation and reduce **gas**. **Slippery elm** powder (*Ulmus fulva*) is soothing and healing for the digestive system. Homeopathic remedies that may be effective for colic include *Bryonia* 30c every five minutes as needed, and *Chamomilla* 6c every five minutes for up to an hour. A homeopath can be further consulted for remedies to help strengthen the child's entire constitution. In addition, it is helpful to give the Bach flower essence called **Rescue Remedy** to the infant and to the caregivers. This will help to calm both baby and caregivers.

Hands-on treatments are often helpful in treating colic. Squeezing the **acupressure** point at the webbing between the thumb and index finger of either hand can calm a crying child. Gently massaging the abdomen with a circular motion can also be soothing. Applying warm compresses over the child's abdomen can also relieve cramping.

Soothing movements may help to calm the baby. Colicky babies cry less when they are soothed by the motion of a swing, a car ride, or being carried in a parent's arms. Taking the infant for a walk may also be soothing and encourage sleep. Rocking the baby in a quiet, darkened room can reduce overstimulation as well.

Giving small, frequent feedings rather than a few large feedings will be easier on digestion for a bottle-fed baby. For those who breastfeed, food allergens can be transmitted through the milk of the mother. Therefore, foods that cause problems in the infant should be removed from the mother's diet. These are most often likely to be coffee, tea, chocolate, citrus fruit, peanuts, wheat, and vegetables belonging to the cabbage family, including broccoli.

Allopathic treatment

Medications do not cure colic. Doctors sometimes recommend simethicone (Mylicon drops) to relieve gas pain. Generally, parents are advised to take a practical approach, using home remedies. However, a doctor should be notified if a baby with colic:

- develops a rectal fever higher than 101°F (38.3°C)
- cries for more than four hours without relief
- vomits
- has diarrhea or stools that are black or bloody
- continually loses weight
- continually eats less than normal

Expected results

Colic is distressing, but it is not dangerous. Symptoms almost always disappear before a child is six months old.

Prevention

To help prevent air from being swallowed during feedings, the infant's back can be gently massaged to release trapped gas bubbles. Keeping the infant in a sitting position while feeding is also helpful. Bottle-fed babies can swallow air if the nipple holes in the bottle are either too large or too small. This can be checked by filling the bottle with formula, turning it upside down, and counting the number of drops released as the bottle is being shaken or squeezed. The hole should allow the release of formula at the rate of one drop per second. Alternatively, a different style of nipple may improve nursing. A pharmacy should be consulted for additional guidance.

Cow's milk can often be disruptive to an infant's digestion. When cow's milk is the source of the symptoms, bottle-fed babies should be switched to a **soy protein** formula. (Regular soymilk should not be used, as it is not formulated for the nutritional needs of a nursing infant.) Goat's milk is easier to digest than cow's milk, and is also an acceptable substitute. Alternately, a tablespoon of **acidophilus** liquid or powder can be added to eight ounces of the infant's formula. A tablespoon of yogurt can also be used for this purpose. If an intolerance to cow's milk is suspected in a breastfed infant, the mother should eliminate dairy products from her diet, gradually reintroduce after seven days, and monitor the baby's symptoms. This should be done with any suspected allergen or irritating foods.

Resources

BOOKS

Editors of Time Life Books. *The Medical Advisor: The Complete Guide to Alternative & Conventional Treatments.* Alexandria, VA: Time-Life Books, 1996.

Taylor, Robert, ed. *Family Medicine Principles and Practice.* New York: Springer-Verlag, 1994.

Weed, Susun. *Wise Woman Herbal for the Childbearing Year.* New York: Ash Tree Publishing, 1986.

ORGANIZATIONS

American Academy of Family Physicians. 880 Ward Parkway, Kansas City, MO 64114. http://www.aafp.org.

Patience Paradox

Colitis

Definition

Colitis, also called ulcerative colitis, is an **inflammatory bowel disease** closely related to Crohn's disease. In individuals with colitis, the lining of the colon (large intestine) becomes inflamed, cells lining the wall die, and ulcers form on the colon wall.

General Description

Colitis is an inflammatory bowel disease of uncertain origin. In this disease, the lining of the colon and rectum become inflamed and develop sores (ulcers) that produce pus and mucus. In mild cases, only the lining of the intestine is affected, but in severe cases, these ulcers may penetrate deeper layers of the colon or even perforate (break through) the colon wall. In ulcerative colitis, the inflamed area is continuous and develops only in the rectum and colon. This condition contrasts with Crohn's disease in which the inflamed area develops in patches and can occur in multiple places in the digestive system from the mouth to the rectum.

About 2 million Americans have ulcerative colitis, which is a lifelong disease. The disease develops most often before the individual reaches age 30, although it can develop as late as age 60. People of European ancestry and those of Jewish ethnicity are more likely to develop ulcerative colitis. There is no cure, although treatment can bring symptoms under control or cause them to go into remission (disappear) for long periods.

Causes and symptoms

The cause of colitis is unclear. As of 2008, scientists believed that persons who develop colitis carry an inherited susceptibility to developing the disease. Research has shown that people who have a parent or sibling with colitis are more likely to develop the disease, and identical twins are both highly likely to be affected. However, inheritance does not completely predict who will develop colitis. Researchers believe that when a person with an inherited susceptibility to the disease is exposed to an outside agent, an inappropriate autoimmune reaction is triggered. As a result, the immune system attacks the body's own cells lining the intestine. No single outside trigger agent has been isolated. Suspect agents are bacteria, viruses, and environmental toxins. In the past, it was thought that food **allergies** could trigger colitis. Practitioners of conventional medicine subsequently suspected that this was not the cause, although some alternative medical practitioners continued to accept the food allergy theory.

Symptoms associated with colitis include abdominal **pain** and cramps; frequent, urgent bowel movements; **diarrhea** and blood, pus, and mucus in the stool; and **fever**. Other signs of colitis occur because the disease interferes with the ability of the digestive system to absorb nutrients. These symptoms include **fatigue**, loss of appetite, weight loss, dehydration, and in severe cases, electrolyte imbalance. Because the immune system responds inappropriately, other parts of the body may be affected. The individual may develop joint pain, liver, kidney, and eye problems, and skin **rashes**. Although colitis is not caused by **stress** or food allergies, stress and certain foods tend to worsen symptoms.

Diagnosis

Symptoms of colitis mimic those of several other bowel diseases. Colitis is often diagnosed after extensive testing has ruled out other causes. After a health history and physical examination, the physician will order additional tests, including blood tests and a stool sample. The stool sample is examined for blood and parasites. Imaging tests include a barium enema and x rays of the intestine. By cleansing the intestine and filling it with barium, a white, chalky, non-toxic substance, abnormalities of the bowel are more easily seen on the x-ray film. Ultrasound and computed tomography, two non-invasive imaging techniques, may also be done. A definitive diagnosis is usually obtained by a colonoscopy, an invasive procedure that allows the physician to examine the colon lining for the entire length of the colon.

Treatment

The goal of colitis treatment is to control symptoms. As of 2008, there was no cure for the disease. Treatment is individualized and depends on the severity of the disease, but usually conventional pharmaceuticals are needed. Nevertheless, complementary treatments listed below often help relieve symptoms and improve quality of life when used with conventional treatment. Patients should discuss the use of complementary treatments with their physician before beginning any treatment.

Diet

Certain foods seem to worsen symptoms of colitis in many people. Individuals must determine their own problem foods and learn to avoid them. General suggestions for dietary changes that help many people include the following:

- Drink 8–10 glasses of water or clear fluids daily to prevent dehydration, which is especially important for people who have frequent watery bowel movements.
- Avoid high fiber foods. If symptoms are under control, some high-fiber foods may gradually be added back into the diet.
- Experiment with whether dairy products worsen symptoms; many people find that milk and cheese seem to exacerbate their symptoms.
- Avoid caffeine because it stimulates the digestive tract.
- Avoid drinking alcohol.
- Eat a low-fat diet.
- Eat smaller, more frequent meals.

Herbs

Certain herbal remedies have been shown to improve symptoms for some people. These include the following:

- Psyllium. Recommended by both alternative and conventional physicians, psyllium absorbs water and adds bulk to the stool.
- Boswellia resin (*Boswellia sacra*.) is thought to have anti-inflammatory properties. In a small study, when taken with sulfasalazine (a pharmaceutical drug), it increased the number of patients whose symptoms went into remission.
- Aloe (*Aloe vera*) juice or oral gel is thought to improve the chance of remission.
- Turmeric *Curcuma longa* is thought to have useful anti-inflammatory properties.

Supplements

Many people with moderate to severe symptoms develop vitamin and mineral deficiencies that need to be corrected with supplements and/or a multivitamin. Alternative practitioners also recommend a wide range of supplements that have shown mixed results in small trials. Some of these are:

- Probiotics. Probiotics are beneficial living organisms, usually bacteria that supplement the beneficial bacteria normally found in the intestines. Some studies have found that a non-disease producing strain of *Escherichia coli* helps some people with ulcerative colitis remain in remission. Probiotics and their effects on digestive diseases were active areas of research in 2008. Several Food and Drug Administration approved clinical trials of probiotics were being conducted in the United States for people with colitis. Information on trials enrolling participants is available at the Clinical Trials Web site (http://www.clinicaltrials.gov). There is no cost to the patients who participate.
- Fish oil. Some studies have found that fish oil supplements increased weight gain and decreased the need for anti-inflammatory drugs, while others found fish oil was ineffective in patients with ulcerative colitis.
- Folic acid (Vitamin B-9). Sulfasalazine inhibits the absorption of folic acid, so people taking this drug may need supplementation. However, taking folic acid supplements can mask a vitamin B-12 deficiency, so people taking folic acid may also need to take B-12.
- Dehydroepiandrosterone (DHEA). This natural steroid hormone is produced in small amounts by the body. Improvement was seen only with large

supplement doses with a high likelihood of undesirable side effects.

- Iron. People who have a lot of blood in their stool are at risk of becoming iron deficient.

Stress reduction

Although stress does not cause colitis, it often worsens symptoms, so stress reduction techniques should be incorporated into the daily routine.

- Exercise. Mild to moderate exercise can help stabilize bowel function and improve mood.
- Yoga helps to relax the body and relieve tension.
- Meditation calms the body and mind.
- Biofeedback training helps individuals have more control over their body and allows individuals to consciously enter a relaxed state.
- Support groups allow people to share tips and frustrations in an atmosphere of mutual understanding.

Allopathic treatment

Conventional medicine treats the symptoms of ulcerative colitis primarily with pharmaceutical drugs, although many conventional practitioners also recommend some of the complementary therapies suggested above.

Medications used to treat diarrhea symptoms include diphenoxylate (Lomotil, Lofene), and loperamide (Imodium, Kaopectate). Anticholinergic drugs, which block the communication between nerves and muscles and thus reduce contraction of the intestine, include Anaspaz, Cystospaz, and Bentyl.

Anti-inflammatory drugs are at the heart of conventional medical treatment for ulcerative colitis. Sulfasalazine is the most common anti-inflammatory drug used because patients can take it for long maintenance periods, and it can be given with other drugs. Other anti-inflammatories include Asacol and Pentasa. If these drugs do not provide adequate symptom relief, patients may be given corticosteroids such as prednisone. Corticosteroid drugs have substantial side effects and can be taken only for a short time during symptom flare-ups.

People with severe symptoms and complications beyond the digestive system may be hospitalized and given intravenous (IV) steroid drugs or drugs that suppress the immune system. Since colitis is suspected of being caused by an inappropriate immune system response, suppressing the activity of the immune system should reduce symptoms. Once a flare-up is controlled, the patient continues on a maintenance dose

---

KEY TERMS

Colonoscopy—A procedure in which the colon is cleansed and the a lighted fiber optic instrument is inserted through the anus to allow the physician to view the entire length of the colon and detect abnormalities in the colon lining, including polyps and ulcers.

Electrolyte—Ions in the body that participate in metabolic reactions. The major human electrolytes are sodium (Na+), potassium (K+), calcium (Ca 2+), magnesium (Mg2+), chloride (Cl-), phosphate (HPO4 2-), bicarbonate (HCO3-), and sulfate (SO4 2-).

Rectum—The last few inches of the large intestine that store waste until it is eliminated from the body through the anus.

Steroid—A family of compounds that share a similar chemical structure. This family includes estrogen and testosterone, vitamin D, cholesterol, and the drugs cortisone and prednisone.

---

of some combination of diarrhea-control, anti-inflammatory, and immunosuppressant drugs.

Between 25% and 40% of people with ulcerative colitis develop symptoms so severe that they eventually need surgery to remove their colon. When the colon is removed, the final portion of the small intestine is connected to a hole (stoma) in the abdomen. The individual wears a bag outside the body to collect waste. The bag must be emptied at regular intervals. Alternately, if part of the rectum is left intact the small intestine may be connected directly to the rectum after the colon is removed. Waste leaves the body through the anus in the regular manner. Bowel movements are more frequent and watery, as fluid that would normally be absorbed in the colon now passes out of the body.

Expected results

Colitis cannot be cured. Most people go though periods of remission followed by periods of flare-ups when symptoms worsen. Remission can last from months to years depending on the individual.

Prevention

Ulcerative colitis cannot be prevented. About 5% of people who have ulcerative colitis later develop colon **cancer**. Regular yearly colonoscopies can detect colon cancer early when it can be easily treated.

Resources

BOOKS

Harper, Virginia. *Controlling Crohn's Disease: The Natural Way*. New York: Kensington, 2002.

OTHER

"Colitis." *eMedicineHealth.com* October 4, 2005. [cited April 6, 2008]. http://www.emedicinehealth.com/colitis/article_em.htm.

"Ulcerative Colitis." *Mayo Clinic* August 17, 2007 [cited April 6, 2008]. http://www.mayoclinic.com/health/ulcerative-colitis/DS00598.

"Ulcerative Colitis." *PeaceHealth.org* September 1, 2007 [cited April 6, 2008]. http://www.peacehealth.org/KBASE/cam/hn-1282001.htm.

ORGANIZATIONS

Alternative Medicine Foundation, PO Box 60016, Potomac, MD, 20859, (301) 340-1960, http://www.amfoundation.org.

American Holistic Medical Association, PO Box 2016, Edmonds, WA, 98020, (425) 967-0737, http://www.holisticmedicine.org.

Crohn's & Colitis Foundation of America, 386 Park Avenue South, New York, NY, 10016, (800) 932-2423, http://www.ccfa.org.

National Digestive Diseases Information Clearinghouse (NDDIC), 2 Information Way, Bethesda, MD, 20892-3570, (800) 891-5389, http://digestive.niddk.nih.gov.

Tish Davidson, A. M.

Colloidal silver

Description

A colloid is a suspension of submicroscopic particles in a medium of a different material. Colloidal silver is metallic silver suspended in water.

Some minerals are required in the diet for optimum health. These are known as essential minerals. Contrary to claims by some manufacturers of colloidal products, silver is not an essential mineral.

On the other hand, silver undoubtedly has antimicrobial properties, as do some other metals such as **copper**. Historically, coins or other items made of silver were used to help keep water from becoming contaminated and to keep milk fresh for longer periods when refrigeration was not available. This method may still be used today in some remote areas of the world. Silver is also impregnated into some water filtration systems used both for swimming pools and for drinking water.

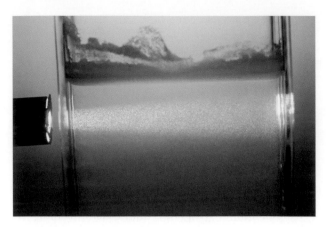

Light shines through a colloidal solution. *(Charles D. Winters / Photo Researchers, Inc.)*

Despite the proven antibacterial, antiviral, and antifungal properties of silver in vitro, it is unclear whether it can exert the same effects when taken into the body. It is unclear what concentration of silver reaches the area where the infection is occurring before being bound, disseminated, or excreted. Another question is whether the ingested silver would have an adequate time of contact with the target organisms to produce the desired effect. Silver has a greater chance of benefiting a patient with local and topical **infections**.

Colloidal silver products are often touted as the answer to the problem of microbial resistance to antibiotics. While it is certainly true that antibiotics are overused, leading to antibiotic-resistant bacteria, substantive evidence that colloidal silver is a safe and effective replacement for antibiotics does not yet exist.

General use

Silver is already used in some compounds that are commonly used against infections. Silvadine is a frequently used agent to prevent infection in burn patients. Silver nitrate was used in the eyes of newborns for years to prevent blindness caused by contracting **gonorrhea**, a sexually transmitted disease (STD), during the passage through the birth canal. The medication was not, however, effective against **chlamydia**, another STD that causes neonatal **conjunctivitis**. Silver nitrate can also be very irritating to the tissues of the eye. Erythromycin and tetracycline are now more frequently used in the United States for neonatal prophylaxis.

The claims made for colloidal silver are innumerable. Silver has been said to be effective against hundreds of **strains** of bacteria, and to be supportive in the treatment of colds and flu, **hepatitis**, Epstein-Barr

KEY TERMS

Antimicrobial—A substance that destroys or inhibits the growth of disease-causing organisms.

Epstein-Barr—A virus in the herpes family that causes mononucleosis and other diseases.

In vitro—An artificial environment; not in a living organism.

virus, **pneumonia**, **bronchitis**, and yeast infections. It has also been recommended for topical use in the mouth, eyes, ears, nose, sinuses, and for a wide variety of skin conditions. It is difficult to determine which of the claims, if any of them, have merit because substantive research data are lacking. Most of the reported effects are based on in vitro or anecdotal evidence. Extrapolations from such testimonials would be challenging due to the variability in particle size, concentration, quality of the preparation, and total dose.

Preparations

Silver colloid is created by grinding, wave method (such as ultrasonic), liquid, chemical, or electrical modes of manufacture. Methods vary according to how large the particles of silver are that are produced, and whether they carry an electrical charge. Particles that are very small and charged repel each other enough that they tend to remain in a suspended state for a longer time rather than settling. Currently, the electrocolloidal process is the most used, and considered to be the best at creating very small, charged particles.

Colloidal silver may be purchased ready for use, but products have been found to be inconsistent in content, varying from 15–120% of the silver concentration they are labeled to contain. Commercially produced products vary greatly in particle size, potency, stability, and contents. Some contain stabilizers or trace elements in addition to silver, which are considered undesirable. Others have been found to have bacterial contaminants.

The Food and Drug Administration (FDA) at one time considered it a medication that was exempted from the standard regulations as a result of being used and marketed prior to 1938. Since that time, the exemption has been revoked. In the United States, silver is now considered a dietary supplement as opposed to an over-the-counter medication. As such, specific claims to benefit or treat medical conditions cannot be made.

As an alternative to manufactured colloidal silver products, assorted kits are available to make colloidal silver for personal use. These kits generally use an electrical current to disperse particulate silver into the carrier. Important factors for producing colloidal silver at home are the purity of the silver, the purity of the water, and proper timing to form the desired concentration. Stability of the colloid is variable, and the silver will tend to gradually settle as the charge on the particles dissipates.

Precautions

The deposition of silver under the skin can cause a condition called argyria. This condition is not common, but the skin of those who are affected is permanently stained a blue or gray color. The type of silver compound, length of treatment, concentration, and total dose required to cause argyria is a matter of some debate. There seems to be a great individual variation in susceptibility. Proponents claim that the true colloidal form of silver cannot cause the condition, but for safety purposes, all silver consumed should be considered a potential contributor to argyria. Some colloidal silver products include this warning on the label.

Extremely large doses of silver, much beyond what is recommended by proponents for therapeutic use, may cause neurologic signs or organ damage. Most of the studies of toxicity have been performed using salts of silver, such as silver nitrate, which have a higher silver concentration and greater toxicity than colloidal forms. The latter are generally in the range of 5–10 parts per million (PPM), which is equal to a 0.0005–0.001% solution.

Side effects

There are no reported side effects.

Interactions

Interaction of colloidal silver with foods, medications, or herbs are not documented.

Resources

BOOKS

Baranowski, Zane. *Colloidal Silver: The Natural Antibiotic Alternative*. New York: Healing Wisdom Publications, 1995.

OTHER

Barrett, Stephen. *Colloidal Silver: Risk Without Benefit*. http://www.quackwatch.com/01QuackeryRelatedTopics/PhonyAds/silverad.html. 1999.

Hill, John. *A Brief History of Silver and Silver Colloids in Medicine.* http://www.clspress.com/history.html. 1998.

Weil, Andrew. *Charmed by Colloidal Minerals?* http://www.pathfinder.com/drweil/qa_answer/0,3189,252,00.html. 1997.

Weil, Andrew. *Colloidal Silver: Better than Antibiotics?* http://www.pathfinder.com/drweil/qa_answer/0,3189,1665,00.html. 1999.

Judith Turner

Colonic irrigation

Definition

Colonic irrigation is also known as **hydrotherapy** of the colon, high colonic, entero-lavage, or simply colonic. It is the process of cleansing the colon by

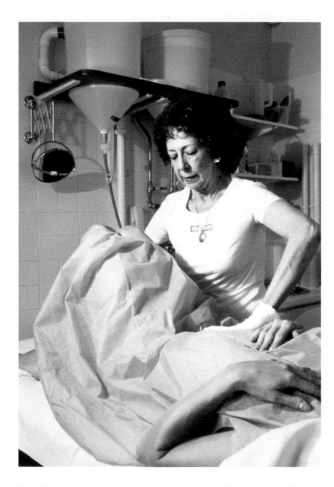

Practitioner massaging a patient's lower abdomen during colonic irrigation, a procedure in which the colon is flushed out with water or another liquid. *(Annabella Bluesky / Margie Finchell / Photo Researchers, Inc.)*

passing several gallons of water through it with the use of special equipment. It is similar to an enema but treats the whole colon, not just the lower bowel. This has the effect of flushing out impacted fecal matter, toxins, mucous, and even parasites, which often build up over the passage of time. It is a procedure that should only be undertaken by a qualified practitioner.

Origins

Cleansing the colon with the use of hydrotherapy is not a new concept. Forms of colonic irrigation have been used successfully for decades to relieve chronic toxicity and even acute cases of toxemia.

Benefits

Anyone suffering from **gas**, bloating, cramping pains, **acne** and other skin complaints, arthritis, and a list of bowel complaints such as **diverticulitis** and irritable bowel etc., may benefit from colonic irrigation. In particular, **cancer** patients are often advised to undertake a course of colonic irrigation sessions as an essential part of their treatment. When a biological cancer therapy begins to enable the body to breakdown a cancerous mass, it is essential that speedy and effective elimination of the resulting toxins is achieved.

Colon and bowel cancer remain among the leading causes of death in the United States, and alternative practitioners suggest that it can be prevented by efficient hygiene procedures. Providing that care is taken to replace the natural organisms that flourish in the bowel, many health benefits can be expected from colonic irrigation. In general, alternative practitioners maintain that an ill-functioning bowel is the source of all disease, and therefore keeping it clean will be an effective protection against disease.

Removing large amounts of toxic matter relieves the patient and can lead to the alleviation of symptoms such as arthritis, **chronic fatigue syndrome**, candidiasis, and a host of other illnesses. Properly executed, colonic irrigation can help restore normal peristaltic action to a sluggish bowel, thus reducing the need for more hydrotherapy treatments over time. In addition, removing the layer of fecal matter which coats the intestines in many individuals allows improved assimilation of the nutrients from foods and can alleviate symptoms of vitamin and other nutrient deficiencies. Many alternative health practitioners consider some form of hydrotherapy for the bowel to be essential in the treatment of degenerative diseases.

KEY TERMS

Dysbiosis—The condition that results when the natural flora of the gut are thrown out of balance, such as when antibiotics are taken.

Peristalsis—The natural wave-like action of a healthy bowel that transports matter from one end of the bowel to the other.

Probiotics—Supplements of beneficial microorganisms that normally colonize the gut.

Toxemia—Poisoning of the blood.

Description

Over time, many people develop a thick layer of fecal matter that coats their colon. It hardens and becomes impacted, reducing the efficiency of the bowel, and in some cases completely obstructs normal elimination of waste matter from the body. It is quite common for people to only have one bowel movement per day, some as few as one or two per week.

Alternative practitioners advise that we probably should have one bowel movement for every meal that we eat. If not, then we are not eliminating wastes completely, and if input exceeds output, then we will surely suffer the consequences at some point.

Incomplete elimination of body wastes may result in the following, depending on where the deposits end up:

- sluggish system
- joint pain and arthritis
- irritable bowel syndrome
- diverticulitis
- Crohn's disease
- leaky gut syndrome
- heart problem
- migraine
- allergies
- bad breath
- acne and other skin problems such as psoriasis
- asthma
- early senility and Alzheimer's disease
- chronic fatigue syndrome
- cancer, particularly of the bowel
- multiple sclerosis

During colonic irrigation, a small speculum is passed into the patient's bowel through the rectum.

This is attached to a tube, which leads to a machine that pumps temperature-controlled water into the colon at a controlled rate (to be controlled by either the practitioner or the patient). The temperature of the water should ideally be kept as close to body temperature as possible.

The patient will temporarily be filled with water up to the level of the entire colon. Patients say they can feel the water up under their ribs but that the process, although sometimes uncomfortable, is not painful. The amount of water will vary but will generally be in the region of between two and six liters (or quarts) at any one time. This triggers peristaltic action and the patient will begin to expel the water along with fecal matter back through the tube and into the machine.

The fecal matter is flushed out through a viewing tube, so that what is eliminated may be monitored. Quite often, unsuspected parasites are expelled, along with very old fecal material, very dark in color, which may have been in the colon for years. Some therapists comment that it looks like aging rubber.

During the treatment, the therapist will gently massage the patient's abdomen to help dislodge impacted fecal matter. In addition to massage, sometimes acupressure, reflexology, or lymphatic drainage techniques may be used to loosen deposits and stimulate the bowel. It is important that the right amount of water is used, as too much will cause discomfort and too little will be ineffective. If correctly done, colonic irrigation is not painful at all and some patients claim to sleep through their treatment.

Sanitation is vital to this process. The tubes and speculums used are generally disposable, but other parts of the machine, such as the viewing tube, must be sterilized after each patient.

Normally, a series of treatments will be required to achieve desired results regarding the elimination of impacted, decaying matter, and restoration of bowel regularity. Initially only gas and recent fecal matter may be expelled. The residue attached to the colon wall is usually the result of years of neglect, and therapists say that one cannot expect complete relief in only one session.

Impacted fecal matter can cause an imbalance of the natural organisms that normally populate the bowel, causing what is known as dysbiosis. Under ideal conditions, the bowel is populated by a variety of naturally occurring organisms. It seems that the enzymes occurring in fresh fruit and vegetables encourage these beneficial organisms. One of the results of eating processed denatured foods is that this natural balance is upset, and food may begin to rot in the bowel instead of being processed.

Decomposing matter can cause a toxic condition and may lead to many health problems, as **constipation** causes backed up pollution of the body cells. The process of repair and elimination of wastes enters a downward spiral which at best will cause **fatigue**, lack of energy and premature aging, and at worst can cause degenerative diseases, among them **allergies**, and even cancer and **Alzheimer's disease**.

The cost of colonic irrigation treatments varies, but is generally between $35-70 per session, which may last from 45 minutes to one hour. The cost of the machine itself ranges from $4,000-12,000, but again, it should be noted that only qualified therapists should conduct sessions.

Preparations

Most practitioners prefer that distilled or purified water is used for colonic irrigation, but others use sterilized tap water.

Precautions

It may be advisable to use a probiotic pessary after colonic irrigation, to ensure replacement of desirable natural flora. There are certain conditions that either partly or completely preclude the use of colonic irrigation, such as an active attack of **Crohn's disease**, bleeding ulcers, and hyperacidosis. If in doubt, a qualified practitioner should be consulted. Anyone suffering from these conditions should always notify the practitioner when receiving colonic irrigation treatments.

Side effects

Some allopathic practitioners claim that colonic irrigation flushes out essential electrolytes and friendly bacteria from the bowel and that it can be dangerous. Practitioners counter that this can easily be remedied with the use of **probiotics**, and that in any case, these possible disadvantages are easily offset by the benefits of having large amounts of putrefying matter, harmful organisms, and parasites removed from the system.

Research and general acceptance

Although many alternative health care practitioners swear by colonic irrigation, there is a large allopathic lobby that claims that there are no benefits to be had, and that there are dangers involved. However, there are many decades of records and research from the alternative health care community that

indicate that this therapy may have a valuable place in the treatment of degenerative diseases and toxic conditions.

Training and certification

Trained technicians should conduct colonic irrigation sessions.

Resources

BOOKS

Bonk, Melinda, ed. *Alternative Medicine Yellow Pages.* Tiburon, CA: Future Medicine Publishing, Inc., 1994.

ORGANIZATIONS

California Colon Hygienist Society. 333 Miller Ave., Suite 1, Mill Valley, CA 94941. (415) 383-7224.

Intestinal Health Institute. 4427 East Fifth St., Tucson, AZ 85711. (520) 325-9686. info@sheilas.com. http://www.sheilas.com.

Patricia Skinner
Teresa G. Odle

Color therapy

Definition

Color therapy, also known as chromatherapy, is based on the premise that certain colors are infused with healing energies. The therapy uses the seven colors of the rainbow to promote balance and healing in the mind and body.

Origins

Color therapy is rooted in Ayurveda, an ancient form of medicine practiced in India for thousands of years. Ayurveda is based on the idea that every individual contains the five basic elements of the universe: earth, water, air, fire, and ether (space). These elements are present in specific proportions unique to an individual's personality and constitution. When these elements are thrown out of balance through unhealthy living habits or outside forces, illness results. **Ayurvedic medicine** uses the energies inherent in the colors of the spectrum to restore this balance.

Color therapy was also used in ancient Egypt and China. In **traditional Chinese medicine** (TCM), each organ is associated with a color. In **qigong**, healing sounds are also associated with a color, which in turn corresponds to a specific organ and emotion.

Benefits

Each of the seven colors of the spectrum are associated with specific healing properties.

Violet

Violet promotes enlightenment, revelation, and spiritual awakening. Holistic healthcare providers use violet to soothe organs, relax muscles, and calm the nervous system.

Indigo

Indigo is also sedative and calming. It is said to promote intuition. Indigo may be useful in controlling bleeding and abscesses.

Blue

Blue promotes communication and knowledge. It eliminates toxins, and is used to treat liver disorders and **jaundice**.

Green

Because it is located in the middle of the color spectrum, green is associated with balance. Green is calming, and is used by Ayurvedic practitioners to promote healing of ulcers. It is said to have antiseptic, germicide, and antibacterial properties and is sometimes used by holistic color therapists to treat bacterial **infections**.

Yellow

Yellow is a sensory stimulant associated with wisdom and clarity. Yellow is thought to have decongestant and antibacterial properties, and is useful in stimulating both the digestive system and the lymphatic system.

Orange

Orange promotes pleasure, enthusiasm, and sexual stimulation. Ayurvedic practitioners believe it has antibacterial properties and may be useful in easing digestive system discomforts (e.g., flatulence, cramps).

Red

Red promotes energy, empowerment, and stimulation. Physically, it is thought to improve circulation and stimulate red blood cell production.

Description

The color spectrum is composed of different frequencies and wavelengths of light energy. Ayurvedic medicine uses the energy of colors to promote harmony and healing. The colors are said to be imbued with certain healing properties (i.e., red is energizing, blue is calming) and the vibrations generated by each color balance the individual.

Holistic healthcare providers who practice color therapy often relate the seven colors of the color spectrum to specific areas of the body known as the *chakras*. In **yoga**, the chakras are specific spiritual energy centers of the body. The therapeutic action of colors is related to the chakra they represent:

- first (root; or base of spine): red
- second (sacral; or pelvis/groin area): orange
- third (solar plexus) chakra: yellow
- fourth (heart) chakra: green
- fifth (throat) chakra: blue
- sixth (brow) chakra: indigo
- seventh (crown) chakra: violet

Therapeutic color can be administered in a number of ways. Practitioners of Ayurvedic medicine wrap their patients in colored cloth chosen for its therapeutic hue. Patients suffering from **depression** may be wrapped in reds and oranges chosen for their uplifting and energizing properties. Patients may also be bathed in light from a color-filtered light source to enhance the healing effects of the treatment.

Another method of color therapy treatment recommended in Ayurvedic medicine is to treat water with color and then drink the water for its purported healing properties. This is achieved by placing translucent colored paper or colored plastic wrap over and around a glass of water and placing the glass in direct sunlight so the water can soak up the healing properties and vibrations of the color.

Color may also be used environmentally to achieve certain calming or healing effects. Paint, wall and window treatments, furniture, and decorative accessories may all be selected in specific color families. Clothing may be chosen in specific colors for its healing properties.

Color therapy can be used in conjunction with both **hydrotherapy** and **aromatherapy** to heighten the therapeutic effect. Spas and holistic healthcare providers may recommend color baths or soaks, which combine the benefits of a warm or hot water soak with healing **essential oils** and the bright hues used in color therapy.

Because color is composed of different light frequencies, certain types of music and **sound therapy** are sometimes used as a companion to the treatment by holistic healthcare providers. One such method, known as the 49th Vibrational Technique, uses a mathematical formula to translate the inaudible vibrations produced in the color spectrum to their audible counterparts. Red is associated with the musical note G, orange is A, yellow is A#, green is C, blue is D, indigo is D#, and violet is E. By combining both visual colors and their audible frequency counterparts, the therapeutic value of the color frequency is thought to be enhanced.

Preparations

Before administering any treatment, practitioners of Ayurvedic medicine will perform a thorough examination of and interview with the patient to determine his *prakriti*, or constitution. In Ayurveda, an individual's prakriti is determined at conception and remains unchanged during his or her lifetime. Treatment colors will be chosen based on the prakriti and the individual's specific imbalance of *doshas*, or energies. There are three doshas—vata, pitta, and kapha—that correspond to a person's temperament and body type. Most are a combination of the three (tridosha) with one predominating.

In some cases, holistic providers may take a photographic image of the patient's aura, or individual energy field, using a special camera that reads electrical impulses from the patient's hands. The camera produces an image of the patient with bands of color(s) around the body. The colors are then analyzed to determine the patient's unique aura energy pattern, and to decide what type of color therapy would be complementary to that aura.

Precautions

While color therapy may be an effective treatment for promoting **relaxation** and overall well-being, and as an adjunct, or complementary therapy in treating some disorders and illnesses, individuals with serious chronic or acute health problems should not rely solely on the therapy for treatment. Anyone with a chronic or acute health concern should seek the advice of a qualified medical practitioner.

Side effects

There are no known side effects to common practices of color therapy.

Research and general acceptance

Ayurvedic medicine has been a firmly entrenched practice of medicine in India for thousands of years. However, it is largely regarded as a complementary practice in the United States, although its popularity has grown in recent years as Ayurvedic spas and medical practices have grown in number. The benefits of color therapy have not been researched extensively and it is still considered a fringe therapy by the allopathic medical community.

Training and certification

Individuals practicing as color therapists and/or practitioners of Ayurvedic medicine do not require special certification or licensing.

Resources

BOOKS

Klotsche, Charles. *Color Medicine: The secrets of color/vibrational healing*. Sedona, AZ: Light Technology Publishing.

Lad, Vasant. *The Complete Book of Ayurvedic Home Remedies*. New York: Three Rivers Press, 1998.

PERIODICALS

Sandroff, Ronni. "Color Me Healthy." *Vegetarian Times* (June 1999): 46-48.

Paula Ford-Martin

Colorectal cancer

Definition

Colorectal **cancer** is a malignancy of the colon (bowel) and/or rectum. Excluding skin cancers, colorectal cancer is the third most common cancer diagnosed in men and in women in the United States. The American Cancer Society reported that about 112,000 new cases of colon cancer (55,000 men and 57,000 women) and 41,500 new cases of rectal cancer

(24,000 men and 17,500 women) were diagnosed in 2007. Colorectal cancer is the second leading cause of cancer-related deaths in the United States and is expected to have caused about 52,000 deaths (26,000 men and 26,000 women) in 2008.

Description

Colorectal cancer occurs in either the last 6 ft (1.8 m) of intestine, known as the large bowel or colon, and/or in the rectum, where the colon terminates and waste (feces) leaves the body. The majority of malignancies that occur in colorectal cancers are called *adenocarcinomas*. When an individual develops colorectal adenocarcinomas, malignant cancer cells grow inside the colon and/or the rectum. Large clusters of these cells form structures known as tumors.

Causes and symptoms

Causes and risk factors

The exact cause of colorectal cancer is unknown. However, there are a number of known risk factors that increase the odds for developing the disease. They include:

- Family history. Individuals who have one or more close relatives who were diagnosed with colorectal cancer may be at increased risk for the disease. In 2003, research showed that about 5% of colorectal cancer patients had inherited syndromes.
- History of bowel disease and/or colon polyps. Certain types of colon polyps, which are tumor-like, benign outgrowths of tissue within the colon, may act as an early warning sign of or a precursor to colorectal cancer. They may develop into malignancies later in life. Colon diseases that cause inflammation and irritation of the bowel, such as Crohn's disease and inflammatory bowel disease, also can increase an individual's risk of developing a colorectal malignancy.
- Obesity. Overweight individuals, especially those with an apple-shaped body type (where fat is concentrated around the waist) as opposed to a pear-shaped body (where fat is stored in the hips and thighs), are at an increased risk for colorectal cancer. A high fat diet also increases an individual's chance of developing colorectal cancer.
- Age. Individuals over age 50 are at an increased risk for colorectal cancer.
- Sedentary lifestyle. A moderate exercise program is thought to have a preventive effect against cancer.
- Night work. A 2003 study showed that working the night shift actually may increase risk of colorectal

cancer in women. Exposure to light at night suppresses the body's natural production of melatonin, a hormone that helps keep certain intestinal cancers from proliferating.

Symptoms

Symptoms of colorectal cancer include:

- blood on the rectum or in the stool
- feelings of fecal urgency (feeling as if one has to have a bowel movement all the time)
- stomach and/or abdominal pain
- changes in bowel habits, including constipation, diarrhea, and/or pencil-thin stools
- extreme fatigue
- decreased appetite

Diagnosis

Early diagnosis is critical in successfully treating colorectal cancer. The simplest screening tests for colorectal cancer are a digital rectal exam and a fecal occult blood test (FOBT). In the digital rectal exam, a physician inserts a gloved finger into the rectum and feels for any irregularities. In the FOBT, stool samples are tested for traces of blood. The test can be done at home and sent to a lab for analysis. FOBT can reduce the death rate by about 33%. Unfortunately, in the United States, less than 35% of the population has received a FOBT.

A flexible sigmoidoscopy and/or a colonoscopy may be performed to view the interior of the colon. The former examines the rectum and lower colon for cancer, and the latter examines the full length of the colon. During these procedures, a doctor passes a flexible tube with a tiny, fiber-optic camera device (an endoscope) through the rectum and into the colon. The doctor can carefully examine the lining of the intestine for signs of cancer. Also, if a polyp is found during the examination, it is removed, usually by severing it with a sharp wire loop attached to the device. Since all polyps are removed, it prevents nonmalignant ones from developing into cancer. A tissue sample (a biopsy) of the colon is usually taken through the endoscope to examine under a microscope for evidence of malignancy. Both tests can cause discomfort and may be done under a local anesthetic if desired.

A lower GI (gastrointestinal) x-ray series can be helpful in determining how much of the intestine is involved in the disease. A chalky solution called barium, which acts as a contrast agent to illuminate the gastrointestinal tract on x-ray film, is administered in enema form to the patient. In some cases, air also is pumped into the rectum to provide a clearer view of the large intestine. This is called a double-contrast barium enema. The pressure in the patient's abdomen from the air and barium contrast likely will cause some discomfort.

As of 2007, researchers were developing alternative screening methods that caused less or no discomfort compared to an endoscope. An x-ray technique using computed tomographic scanning (a CT scan) called virtual colonoscopy was in limited use as of 2007. Other methods being developed would use feces or blood samples to screen for cancer.

Several reasons are given for the low percentage of people over the age of 50 who get screened for colorectal cancer. One is that the procedure is uncomfortable and time-consuming. Another disincentive is the laxative preparation usually required prior to a colonoscopy. It is hoped that newer, less invasive detection techniques will increase the percentage of people who get tested.

For most people, a colonoscopy or sigmoidoscopy is recommended starting at age 50 and then repeated every 10 years for a colonoscopy and every five years for a sigmoidoscopy. Colonoscopies were first used in 1969.

After colorectal cancer is diagnosed, further testing is required to determine how far the cancer has spread. This procedure is known as staging. There are five different stages of colorectal cancer:

- Stage 0 (carcinoma in situ). The earliest stage of colorectal cancer indicates that cancerous cells have not spread beyond the colon lining.
- Stage I. The cancer has spread to the second and third layers of the inside wall of the colon but is still contained within the colon.
- Stage II. The cancer has spread beyond the colon but has not spread to the lymph nodes.
- Stage III. The cancer has spread to a nearby lymph node but has not spread throughout the body.
- Stage IV. The cancer has spread throughout the body.

There is a sixth subtype of cancer, called recurrent, which is used to classify colorectal cancer that was treated, seemed to resolve, and later recurs either in the colon or in another part of the body.

Treatment

The best chance for successful treatment is to detect colorectal cancer early. Colorectal cancer is a life-threatening disease, and a correct diagnosis and appropriate treatment with surgery, chemotherapy, and/or radiation is critical to controlling the illness.

Acupuncture and **guided imagery** may be useful tools in treating **pain** symptoms and improving immune function associated with colorectal cancer. Acupuncture involves the placement of a series of thin needles into the skin at targeted locations on the body, known as acupoints, in order to harmonize the energy flow within the human body.

Guided imagery involves creating a visual mental image of pain as a means of **relaxation**. Once the pain can be visualized, patients can adjust the image to make it more pleasing, and thus more manageable to them.

Movement therapies, such as **yoga**, t'ai chi, and **qigong** can aid recovering patients. These therapies may lessen pain symptoms and help individuals to relax and reduce **stress**.

A number of herbal remedies also are available to lessen pain symptoms and promote relaxation and healing. However, cancer patients should consult with their healthcare professional before taking them. Depending on the preparation and the type of herb, these remedies may interact with or enhance the effects of other prescribed medications. Herbs that promote healing of the digestive tract include **slippery elm** bark (*Ulmus rubra*), **marsh mallow** root (*Althaea officinalis*), and **goldenseal** (*Hydrastis canadensis*).

An analysis of five previous studies of nearly 1,500 participants reported that getting the recommended daily dosage of **vitamin D** can greatly reduce the risk of getting colorectal cancer. The study projected a two-thirds reduction in the risk of getting colorectal cancer for people who took 2,000 IU of vitamin D daily. As of 2007, the U.S. Food and Drug Administration (FDA) recommended that adults ages 50–70 should have a daily intake of 400 IU of vitamin D. The maximum safe daily intake set by the FDA of vitamin D is 2,000 IU.

Allopathic treatment

Treatment options include surgery, chemotherapy, and radiation. Colorectal cancer is treated in two ways, locally to eliminate tumor cells from the colon by surgery and radiation, and to systemically destroy cancer cells that have traveled to other parts of the body. Systemic therapy includes the use of chemotherapy drugs.

Surgery

The extent of surgery depends on the type of colorectal cancer, whether the disease has spread, and the patient's age and health. A surgical procedure known as a bowel resection is performed for colon cancers, where the length of colon containing the cancerous cells is removed, along with nearby tissues and lymph nodes. The two ends of the remaining colon are then sewn back together.

For cancer affecting the rectum, several other surgical methods may be employed, including local excision of the cancer (where cancerous cells and nearby tissues are cut out of the rectum) and transanal resection, where invasive cancerous tissue is removed along with normal anal tissue.

Depending on the stage of the cancer and the degree of surgery required, some patients may need to have a colostomy. A colostomy involves surgically attaching the bowel to an opening in the abdominal wall where waste is eliminated into an attached bag.

The presence of cancer cells in the lymph nodes may require more extensive surgery. If the cancer has spread to the nodes, the patient will need either radiation, chemotherapy, hormone therapy, or a combination of all three after surgery. This is called "adjuvant therapy."

Radiation

Once the cancer has been removed, the doctor may recommend radiation treatment to destroy any remaining cancer cells. In cases where the cancer is located in hard to reach areas, radiation may be used to shrink the cancer growth or tumor. Radiation stops the cancer cells from dividing. It works especially well on fast-growing tumors. Unfortunately, it also stops some types of healthy cells from dividing. Healthy cells that divide quickly, like those of the skin and hair, are affected the most. For this reason, radiation can cause **fatigue**, skin problems, and **hair loss**.

Radiation therapy can be internal, where particles of radioactive materials are implanted into a tumor, or external, where energy rays (radiation) are directed at the cancer from outside the body. External radiation, the most common type of treatment for colorectal cancer, is usually administered five days a week for several weeks. Some studies indicate that radiation therapy decreases the likelihood of local recurrence of colorectal cancer by a significant margin. Some clinicians argue that the therapy is most effective when given before surgery rather than after. No definitive clinical trials proved the most effective timing as of late 2001.

Chemotherapy

Colorectal cancer surgery may be followed by chemotherapy in even the earliest stages. Chemotherapy is administered either orally or by injection into a blood vessel. It is usually given in cycles, followed by a period of time for recovery, followed by another course of drugs. Treatment time may range between four and nine months. In the fall of 2001, the Food and Drug Administration (FDA) approved trials for a new vaccine to help treat colorectal cancer. Investigators planned to give the vaccine in conjunction with chemotherapy to help prevent recurrence of the disease. In 2003, the FDA approved a new chemotherapy drug called Avastin to help fight metastatic spread of colorectal cancer.

Some types of chemotherapy produce significant side effects, including **nausea** and **vomiting**, temporary hair loss, mouth sores, skin **rashes**, fatigue, a weakened immune system, and **infertility**. However, most side effects are temporary and disappear once treatment has ended.

Expected results

The death rate for the disease has declined steadily over the last several decades of the 20th century, and since 1985, annual deaths due to colorectal cancer have declined at an average rate of 1.6% per year. Early detection is key to improved survival; patients with colorectal cancers detected early (at stage I) have a 96% survival rate. In comparison, patients who are diagnosed with stage IV colorectal cancer only have a 5% survival rate.

Prevention

Proper diet and **exercise** have been shown to help prevent many types of cancers, including colorectal cancer. Research published in 2003 confirmed the benefits of physical activity in reducing risk of colon and rectal cancers. A well-balanced diet consisting of a minimum of five servings of fruits and vegetables and six servings of food from other plant sources (i.e., cereals, grains, pastas) is recommended by the American Cancer Society. Additionally, patients may opt for a diet of whole foods. A number of fruits and vegetables have been shown to have antioxidant properties and may be useful in preventing cancer. These include **carotenoids**, which are found in fruit pigments; flavenoids found in vegetable pigments; and particularly **lycopene**, which is found in tomato juice.

Some clinical studies also have indicated that regular use of **green tea** (produced from the *Camellia sinensis* plant) may reduce the risk of certain types of cancer, including colorectal cancers. Green tea contains polyphenols, an antioxidant substance that also may inhibit the growth of existing cancer cells. In some

KEY TERMS

Adjuvant therapy—Treatment involving radiation, chemotherapy (drug treatment), hormone therapy, or a combination of all three.

Antioxidants—Enzymes that bind with free radicals to neutralize their harmful effects.

Free radicals—Reactive molecules created during cell metabolism that can cause tissue and cell damage like that which occurs in aging and with disease processes such as cancer.

Lymph nodes—Small, bean-shaped masses of tissue scattered along the lymphatic system that act as filters, removing fluids, bacteria, or cancer cells that travel through the lymph system. Cancer cells in the lymph nodes are a sign that the cancer has spread.

Malignant—Cancerous.

Polyp—A benign, tumor-like outgrowth.

animal studies, injections of tea extracts reduced the size of cancerous tumors. The antioxidant effects of green tea need to be studied further to more clearly define the role of the herb in cancer treatment and prevention.

Because early detection is so critical to recovery from colorectal cancer, patients considered at risk for the disease due to genetic, lifestyle, or environmental factors should undergo regular screening after age 50 (and possibly before, depending on the individual's personal and medical history). The American Cancer Society recommends the following screening tests:

- an annual FOBT plus a flexible sigmoidoscopy every five years; or
- a colonoscopy every 10 years; or
- a double contrast barium enema every five to 10 years.

A digital rectal exam also is recommended during each screening session.

Resources

BOOKS

Alschuler, Lise N., and Karolyn A. Gazella, eds. *Alternative Medicine Magazine's Definitive Guide to Cancer: An Integrative Approach to Prevention, Treatment, and Healing.* San Francisco: Celestial Arts, 2007.

American Cancer Society. *American Cancer Society's Complete Guide to Colorectal Cancer.* Atlanta, GA: American Cancer Society, 2007.

Lange, Vladimir. *Be A Survivor: Colorectal Cancer Treatment Guide.* Los Angeles: Lange Productions, 2006.

Tovey, Philip. *Complementary and Alternative Medicine in Cancer Care.* London: Routledge, 2007.

PERIODICALS

Beebe, Timothy J., et al. "Assessing Attitudes Toward Laxative Preparation in Colorectal Cancer Screening and Effects on Future Testing: Potential Receptivity to Computed Tomographic Colonography." *Mayo Clinic Proceedings* (June 2007): 666(6).

Harder, Ben. "The Screen Team: Less Unpleasant Colon Exams Might Catch More Cancers." *Science News* (August 19, 2006): 122(3).

Mahoney, Diana. "Exercise May Help Cut Colon Cancer Risk in Men." *Family Practice News* (January 1, 2007): 40.

McCarty, Mark. "Physicians Seek Better Tools to Diagnose, Treat Colon Cancer." *Diagnostic Update* (May 31, 2007): NA.

Meyerhardt, Jeffrey A. "Preventing and Treating Colon Cancer." *Harvard Special Health Report* (July 2006): 34(2).

"Vitamin D May Reduce Your Risk of Colorectal Cancer: Maintaining the Recommended Vitamin D Blood Level Could Cut Your Risk in Half." *Healthy Years* (April 2007): 4.

ORGANIZATIONS

American Cancer Society, 250 Williams St., Atlanta, GA, (800)227-2345, http://www.cancer.org.

British Association for Cancer Research. Institute of Cancer Research, McElwain Laboratories, Cotswold Road, Sutton, SM2 5NG, U.K., (44) 020-8722-4208, http://www.bacr.org.uk.

Canadian Cancer Society, 10 Alcorn Ave., Suite 200, Toronto, ON, M4V 3B1, Canada, (416) 961-7223, http://www.cancer.ca.

Colon Cancer Alliance, 5411 North University Dr., Suite 202, Coral Gables, FL, 33067, (877) 422-2030, http://www.ccalliance.org.

National Cancer Institute, 6116 Executive Blvd., Room 3036A, Bethesda, MD, 20892, (800) 422-6237, http://www.cancer.gov.

Paula Ford-Martin
Ken R. Wells

Colostrum

Description

Colostrum is a thick yellow fluid, rich in protein, growth factors, and immune factors. It is secreted by the mammary glands of all female mammals during the first few days of lactation. It also contains essential nutrients and protease inhibitors that keep it from being destroyed by the processes of digestion. Humans produce relatively small amounts of colostrum in the first two days after giving birth, but cows produce about 9 gallons (36 L) of colostrum. Bovine colostrum can be transferred to all other mammals, and is four times richer in immune factors than human colostrum.

Although colostrum has received widespread attention as a dietary supplement only since the late 1990s, it has a lengthy history of medicinal use. Ayurvedic physicians in India have used colostrum as a treatment for thousands of years. In the United States, mainstream medical practitioners recommended colostrum as a natural antibiotic before the discovery of penilcillin and sulfa drugs. In the 1950s, colostrum was used to treat **rheumatoid arthritis** (RA). Dr. Albert Sabin, the researcher who developed the first oral vaccine for poliomyelitis, found that colostrum contains antibodies against polio. He recommended colostrum as a dietary supplement for children who were vulnerable to polio.

The major components of colostrum include the following substances:

- Immunoglobulins. Immunoglobulins are globulin proteins that function as antibodies. They are the most plentiful immune factors found in colostrum. Immunoglobulin G (IgG) counteracts bacteria and toxins in the blood and lymphatic system; immunoglobulin M (IgM) seeks out and attaches itself to viruses in the circulatory system; immunoglobulins D and E (IgD and IdE) remove foreign substances from the bloodstream and activate allergic reactions. High-quality colostrum is certified to contain a minimum of 16% immunoglobulins.
- Lactoferrin. Lactoferrin is a protein that transports iron to red blood cells and helps to deprive viruses and harmful bacteria of iron.
- Proline-rich polypeptide (PRP). PRP is a hormone that regulates the thymus gland, helping to calm a hyperactive immune system or stimulate an underactive immune system.
- Growth factors. The growth factors in bovine colostrum include insulin-like growth factors (IgF-1 and IgF-2), an epithelial growth factor (EgF), transforming growth factors (TgF-A and TgF-B), and a platelet-derived growth factor (PDGF). Growth factors stimulate normal growth as well as the healing and repair of aged or injured skin, muscle, and other tissues. In addition, growth factors help the body to burn fat instead of muscle for fuel when a person is dieting or fasting.
- Growth hormone. Growth hormone slows some of the signs of aging.
- Leukocytes. Leukocytes are white cells that stimulate production of interferon, a protein that inhibits viruses from reproducing.
- Enzymes. Colostrum contains three enzymes that oxidize bacteria.
- Cytokines and lymphokines. These are substances that regulate the body's immune response, stimulate the production of immunoglobulins, and affect cell growth and repair.
- Vitamins. Colostrum contains small amounts of vitamins A, B$_{12}$, and E.
- Glycoproteins. Glycoproteins, or protease inhibitors, are complex proteins that protect immune factors and growth factors from being broken down by the acids in the digestive tract.
- Sulfur. Sulfur is a mineral that is an important building block of proteins.

General use

Colostrum is presently used to treat a variety of diseases and disorders. Applications that have been investigated in clinical trials include the following:

Bacterial and viral infections

A number of recent clinical studies have shown that colostrum is effective in reversing the inflammation of the digestive tract in HIV/AIDS patients caused by opportunistic **infections**. The antiviral, antifungal, and antibacterial properties of colostrum enable it to kill such pathogens as *E. coli*, *Candida albicans*, rotaviruses, and *Cryptosporidium*.

In 1980, a British researcher showed that a large proportion of the antibodies and immunoglobulins in colostrum are not absorbed by the body but remain in the digestive tract. There they attack food- and water-borne organisms that cause disease. More recent clinical studies have demonstrated that colostrum is effective in preventing intestinal infections by first keeping the bacteria from attaching themselves to the intestinal wall, and second by killing the bacteria themselves. Colostrum has proved to be capable of killing *Campylobacter*, *Helicobacter pylori*, *Listeria*, *Salmonella*, *Shigellosis*, and five types of streptococci.

Allergies and autoimmune diseases

The PRP in colostrum has been demonstrated to reduce or eliminate the **pain**, swelling, and inflammation associated with **allergies** and autoimmune diseases (**multiple sclerosis**, rheumatoid arthritis, lupus, myasthenia gravis). These effects are related to PRP's

KEY TERMS

Cytokines—Substances of low molecular weight that affect cell growth and repair, tissue inflammation, and immunity to diseases.

Glycoproteins—Complex proteins that protect immune factors and growth factors from being broken down by stomach acids. Glycoproteins are also called protease inhibitors.

Immunoglobulins—A group of globulin proteins that function as antibodies.

Lactoferrin—A protein found in colostrum that carries iron to red blood cells and appears to have anti-cancer activity.

Lymphocyte—A type of white blood cell that is important in the production of antibodies.

Opportunistic infection—A type of infection caused only under certain circumstances, as when a person's immune system is impaired.

Proline-rich polypeptide (PRP)—A hormone found in colostrum that regulates the thymus gland and the immune system. It helps to make colostrum an effective treatment for autoimmune disorders and possibly heart disease. Proline is an amino acid.

T cell—A type of lymphocyte that develops in the thymus gland, circulates in the blood and lymph, and regulates the body's immune response to infected or malignant cells.

ability to inhibit the overproduction of lymphocytes (white blood cells) and T-cells.

Heart disease

Recent research suggests that cardiovascular disease may be caused in part by alterations in the patient's immune system. One study indicated that 79% of patients with heart diseases had a certain type of *Chlamydia* (an intracellular parasite closely related to certain bacteria) associated with the formation of plaque in their arteries. The PRP in colostrum may be able to reverse **heart disease** in the same way it counteracts allergies and autoimmune diseases. In addition, the growth factors and growth hormone in colostrum appear to lower the blood levels of "bad" **cholesterol** while raising the blood levels of "good" cholesterol. These growth factors also repair damage to heart muscle and support the growth of new blood vessels in the part of the circulatory system that surrounds the heart.

Cancer

Since 1985, the cytokines contained in colostrum have been a major area of research in seeking a cure for **cancer**. Researchers have found that the lactoferrin in colostrum has some anti-cancer activity. In addition, the combination of immune factors and growth factors in colostrum appears to inhibit the growth of cancers.

Weight loss

The growth factor called IgF-1 that is contained in colostrum is needed by the body in order to metabolize fat. As humans grow older, their bodies produce less IgF-1. These lower levels of growth factor are associated with a higher rate of type 2 diabetes in older adults and with increased difficulty losing weight in spite of **exercise** and careful attention to diet. While colostrum by itself will not cause weight loss, it appears to be a useful part of a weight reduction program because of its IgF-1 content.

Sports medicine

The immune factors in colostrum appear to be helpful in protecting athletes from infections caused by the physical and emotional **stress** of competition. Using colostrum as a dietary supplement also increases the efficiency of the digestive tract for athletes in training. The intestines are able to make more nutrients available to the muscle cells and the body's vital organs. A 2002 report stated that cyclists taking 20 to 60 grams of bovine colostrums supplements per day showed significant performance improvements following a two-hour ride.

Open wounds

The growth factors in colostrum have been found to stimulate the growth of new skin and to repair tissues damaged by ulcers, injuries, **burns**, surgery, or inflammation. They are able to do this through their direct action on the cells' DNA and RNA. Powdered colostrum has been used in topical preparations for **gum disease**, sensitive teeth, mouth ulcers, **cuts**, and burns.

Other

Colostrum has been used outside clinical research to treat a variety of other conditions. Satisfied individuals have reported that colostrum has successfully treated skin disorders, **emphysema**, baldness in males, anger outbursts, **feverblisters**, **shingles**, **tendinitis**, thyroid disorders, **gout**, insect **bites**, vaginal yeast infections, and **anemia**.

Preparations

Colostrum is presently available in a variety of forms, including tablets, liquids, powders, and encapsulated powders. In general, the powdered forms are recommended as preferable to liquids or tablets, on the grounds that liquid colostrum has a short shelf life and the processing necessary to produce tablets destroys much of colostrum's biological activity. The recommended dose for adults with disease symptoms is 1,000–2,000 mg of powdered colostrum in capsules, taken twice daily with 8–12 oz of water. Preventive doses are left to the patient's choice. Children can be given colostrum but require less than adults.

In the United States, colostrum is taken from dairy cows within 24 hours after the birth of a calf. Only dairy cows that meet USDA health standards and have been raised on a feed supplemented with nutrients are used to supply colostrum. The calf needs four gallons of the nine that the cow produces. The remaining five gallons are collected by a USDA-certified dairy. The colostrum is frozen and kept at a temperature of 17°F (-8.3°C). After the frozen colostrum is taken to a processing plant, it is carefully thawed and evaluated for quality and immunoglobulin content. About 30% is rejected at this stage. The fat is then removed from the remaining colostrum, after which the colostrum is spray-dried at low heat. The colostrum is repeatedly tested during processing for freedom from bacterial contamination.

Precautions

Persons who are using colostrum as a dietary supplement in the United States should obtain it from a source licensed by the USDA.

Side effects

With the exception of allergic reactions in persons who are known to be allergic to cow's milk, colostrum does not produce any major side effects at any level of consumption. Mild flu-like symptoms that disappear with continued use of colostrum have been reported in children.

Interactions

No significant drug interactions between colostrum and standard pharmaceuticals have been reported.

Resources

PERIODICALS

Coombes, Jeff S., et al. "Dose Effects of Oral Bovine Colostrum on Physical Work Capacity in Cyclists." *Medicine and Science in Sports and Exercise* (July 2002): 1184.

ORGANIZATIONS

National Association of Alternative Medicines (NAAM). P. O. Box 35189, Chicago, IL 60707-0189. (708) 453-0080. Fax: (708) 453-0083.

OTHER

Health/Link: Alternative Health Directory. http://www.selene.com/healthlink/bovine.html.

Rebecca Frey, Ph.D.
Teresa G. Odle

Coltsfoot

Description

Coltsfoot is the plant *Tussilago farfara*, a member of the daisy family (Asteraceae). Coltsfoot is a perennial herb that grows to a height of 4-10 inches (10-25 cm). The stem is covered with white, downy fibers. Its leaves are hoof-shaped, and the flowers are yellow. The leaves, flowers, and occasionally the root are used medicinally.

Coltsfoot is a tough, invasive plant that lives in marginal soil, wasteland, roadsides, and sand dunes. In some areas coltsfoot is considered an undesirable weed. Although native to Europe, coltsfoot grows wild in North America and the temperate parts of China. Other names for coltsfoot are **cough** wort, horsefoot, horsehoof, bull's foot, ass's foot, foal's foot, British tobacco, butterbur, field hove, and flower velure. In Chinese it is called *kuan dong hua*.

General use

Coltsfoot has been used as a cough remedy in both **Western herbalism** and **traditional Chinese medicine** for at least 2,500 years. Coltsfoot was such a well-known and well-respected herb in eighteenth century France that apothecary shops advertised their presence by painting a picture of the herb on their signs. Chinese herbalists prefer to use the flower and flower buds, while Western herbalists most often choose to use the leaves.

Coltsfoot is recommended to treat:

- asthma
- bronchitis
- dry, hacking cough
- laryngitis and hoarseness

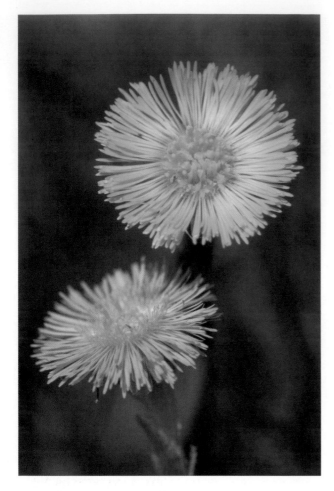

Coltsfoot has been used as a cough remedy in both Western herbalism and traditional Chinese medicine for at least 2,500 years. *(© Arco Images / Alamy)*

- lung cancer symptoms
- mouth and throat irritations
- sore throat
- wheezing

A decoction (boiling the herb down to a concentrated broth or tea to be taken internally) of coltsfoot root is sometimes used to induce sweating. Externally, a poultice of flowers is sometimes applied to the skin to treat **eczema**, **stings**, **bites**, and skin inflammations. Sometimes coltsfoot leaves are smoked to relieve cough.

Modern scientific investigation shows that coltsfoot contains a substance called mucilage (about 8%) that coats and soothes the throat. It is the presence of this substance that appears to make coltsfoot so effective in treating coughs and respiratory problems. Coltsfoot tea also appears to help clear the airways of mucus in some animal studies. **Smoking** coltsfoot will probably do more to irritate the throat than to soothe it.

Inhaling steam from a pot of boiling coltsfoot leaves is likely to produce little effect because so little of the medicinal material will reach the throat. The German Federal Health Agency's Commission E, established in 1978 to independently review and evaluate scientific literature and case studies pertaining to herb and plant medications, has approved the use of fresh or dried coltsfoot leaf in products to treat dry cough, hoarseness, and mild throat or mouth inflammations.

Despite evidence that coltsfoot does generally work, it is not without its problems. The leaves, and to a greater degree the buds and flowers, contain compounds called pyrrolizidine alkaloids. These compounds are known to damage the liver. They can cause liver **cancer** with extended exposure and may also cause the blood vessels of the liver to narrow dangerously. In one laboratory study, rats fed a diet of coltsfoot flower developed a high rate of cancerous liver tumors.

In the United States, the Food and Drug Administration (FDA) has labeled coltsfoot an herb of "undefined safety." Coltsfoot leaf also falls under some legal restrictions in Austria. German authorities, however, simply recommend that preparations containing coltsfoot leaf should not be taken for more than four to six weeks each year. There is, however, fairly unanimous agreement that the level of pyrrolizidine alkaloids in coltsfoot flowers is much higher than the level found in the leaves, and that medicinal preparations that use the flower or flower bud should be avoided. Some American herbalists are recommending that the internal use of coltsfoot be discontinued as a precaution until further research clarifies the risks involved.

Preparations

Coltsfoot leaves are harvested in early summer and can be used fresh or dried. In China, the flower heads are dug up in winter, before they emerge from the ground. When the root is used, it is harvested in the autumn.

Coltsfoot is most commonly prepared as a tea. It can also be made into a cough syrup when combined with **licorice**, **thyme**, or black cherry. Commercial preparations are also available.

Precautions

The safest course is to avoid the internal use of coltsfoot. Pregnant and nursing women and children under the age of six should not be given coltsfoot. People who choose to use coltsfoot should avoid ingesting more than 1 gram of pyrrolizidine alkaloids daily. However, accurate measurement of pyrrolizidine alkaloids is difficult and this information is not easily available to many consumers.

Side effects

Coltsfoot is believed to increase the incidence of liver damage and cancerous liver tumors in both laboratory animals and humans.

Interactions

There are no studies of the interactions of coltsfoot with conventional pharmaceuticals or other herbal remedies.

Resources

BOOKS

Chevallier, Andrew. *Encyclopedia of Medicinal Plants.* New York: DK Publishing, Inc., 1996.
PDR for Herbal Medicines. Montvale, NJ: Medical Economics Company, 1999.
Peirce, Andrea. *The American Pharmaceutical Association Practical Guide to Natural Medicines.* New York: William Morrow and Company, 1999.
Weiner, Michael and Janet Weiner. *Herbs that Heal.* Mill Valley, CA: Quantum Books, 1999.

OTHER

Plants for a Future "Tussilago farfara." http://www.pfaf.org.

Tish Davidson

Comfrey

Description

Comfrey (*Symphytum officinale*), or common comfrey, has been known by many names, including **boneset**, knitbone, bruisewort, black wort, salsify, ass ear, wall wort, slippery root, gum plant, healing herb, consound, or knit back. This distinctive herb, considered by the English herbalist Culpeper to be "under the dominion of the moon," is a member of the Boraginaceae family. The genus name *Symphytum* is from the Greek word *sympho* meaning to unite. The common name comfrey is from the Latin *confirmare* meaning to join together. The herb is named after its traditional folk use in compress and poultice preparations to speed the healing of **fractures**, broken bones, **bruises**, and **burns**. Comfrey is a perennial native of

Europe and Asia and has been naturalized throughout North America. There are about 25 species of the herb, including prickly comfrey (*S. asperum*) and Russian comfrey (*S. × uplandicum,* known as okopnik). In Russian medicine, the herb is considered poisonous when used excessively.

Comfrey grows well in rich, moist, low meadows, or along ponds and river banks, where it may reach a height of 4 ft (1.2 m). Comfrey root is large, branching, and black on the outside with a creamy white interior containing a slimy mucilage. Hollow, erect stems, also containing mucilage, are covered with bristly hairs that cause **itching** when in contact with the skin. The thick, somewhat succulent, veined leaves are covered with rough hairs. They are alternate and lance shaped, with lower leaves as large as 10 in (25 cm) in length, and dark green on top and light green on the underside. Small, bell-shaped flowers grow from the axils of the smaller, upper leaves on red stalks. Flowers are mauve to violet and form in dense, hanging clusters, blooming in summer. The cup-like fruits each contain four small, black seeds.

General use

Comfrey root and other parts of the herb have been valued medicinally for more than 2,000 years. The specific name *officinale* designates its inclusion in early lists of official medicinal herbs. Comfrey has been prepared as a poultice or compress with healing properties for blunt injuries, fractures, swollen bruises, **boils**, carbuncles, varicose ulcers, and burns. The external application of comfrey preparations may minimize the formation of scar tissue. Poultices were also applied to ease breast **pain** in breast-feeding women. Comfrey, taken internally as a tea or expressed juice, has been used to soothe ulcers, hernias, **colitis**, and to stop internal bleeding. As a gargle it has been used to treat mouth sores and bleeding gums. The herbal tea has also been used to treat nasal congestion and inflammation, **diarrhea**, and to quiet coughing. The hot, pulped root, applied externally, was used to treat **bronchitis**, **pleurisy**, and to reduce pain and inflammation of **sprains**.

The herb is thought to loosen congestion, soothe irritated membranes and skin, reduce bleeding, tighten tissues, and heal **wounds**. The allantoin in comfrey, found most abundantly in the flowering tops, has been identified as the source of much of the herb's healing actions. Comfrey, applied externally to superficial wounds, promotes the healing of connective tissue, bones, and cartilage. Other constituents found in comfrey include tannins, resin, essential oil, gum, carotene, rosmarinic acid, **choline**, glycosides, sugars, betea-sitosterol, and steroidal saponins.

KEY TERMS

Carbuncle—A skin infection creating deep, pus-filled boils.

Pleurisy—Inflammation of the pleura, the membranes enclosing the lungs and lining the chest cavity.

Comfrey contains vitamins A and B$_{12}$, and is high in **calcium**, **potassium**, and **phosphorus**. The herb has long been used as a cooked green vegetable in early spring, and the fresh, young leaves have been added to salads. The widespread suffering caused by the Irish potato famine of the 1840s motivated Henry Doubleday, an Englishman, to fund research into comfrey's potential as a nutritional food crop. Farmers have valued comfrey as a nutritious fodder for cattle. When the leaves are soaked in rainwater for a few weeks, they will produce a valuable fertilizer for the garden, especially beneficial to tomatoes and potatoes.

Modern herbalists, however, disagree strongly about comfrey's safety, particularly when herbal preparations are taken internally. A Japanese study in 1968 implicated comfrey constituents (known as pyrrolizidine alkaloids) as being toxic to the liver even when taken in small amounts. The study involved large amounts of comfrey extract rather than the whole herb. The most toxic of these pyrrolizidine alkaloids, according to Varro Tyler of the Purdue University School of Pharmacy, is echimidine. This alkaloid is found primarily in Russian comfrey and prickly comfrey rather than the common comfrey. However, Tyler cautions that other alkaloids toxic to the liver are present in common comfrey, and commercial preparations may not distinguish between the types of comfrey contained in the products offered for sale. Herbal products containing echimidine are prohibited for sale in Canada as medicines. In fact, all comfrey products made from the root, which contains a higher concentration of pyrrolizidine alkaloids, are restricted in Canada.

A 1978 Australian study reported that rats fed a large diet of comfrey leaf developed liver **cancer**. The research literature has reported some cases of liver toxicity attributed to long-term, internal use of comfrey. However, some Japanese doctors still continue to recommend a vinegar extract of comfrey to treat cases of **cirrhosis** of the liver, despite these previous research findings of the hazards associated with internal use. The research on the safety and effectiveness of comfrey as a medicine continues with some conflicting research results. In Germany, where standardized comfrey remedies are commercially available, the allowed dosage and duration of treatment is regulated. In the United States, however, commercial preparations may not be standardized to meet these dosage restrictions.

Preparations

Ointments, salves, and oil extracts of comfrey are available for external treatment. The crushed or powdered root and extracted juice of the herb are used to make poultices for external applications. Comfrey extract is an ingredient in commercially prepared medicines for chest congestion, coughs, and pain relief.

Precautions

Comfrey should not be used, either externally or internally, by pregnant or breast-feeding women. Many herbalists caution against internal use of comfrey. This caution is due to the dangers of the pyrrolizidine alkaloids that are toxic to the liver and may have cancer-causing effects, even in small amounts. Consumers should avoid external use of comfrey on deep wounds because the herb may promote premature healing of surface tissue before the deeper damage has been healed. Wounds must be thoroughly cleaned before application of comfrey remedies to avoid tissue forming over dirt particles. Comfrey preparations should not be used for more than four weeks. Gathering comfrey in the wild may be dangerous for the novice herbalist because the early spring leaves somewhat resemble the deadly ones of nightshade and, in some reported cases, ingesting comfrey in preparations contaminated with deadly nightshade has led to poisoning.

Side effects

No side effects are known with proper preparation and administration of *Symphytum officinale* in external, therapeutic applications. Internal use of herbal preparations should be avoided pending further research.

Interactions

None reported.

Resources

BOOKS

Hutchens, Alma R. *A Handbook of Native American Herbs.* Boston: Shambhala Publications, Inc., 1992.

McIntyre, Anne. *The Medicinal Garden.* New York: Henry Holt and Company, 1997.

Ody, Penelope. *The Complete Medicinal Herbal.* New York: Dorling Kindersley, 1993.

PDR for Herbal Medicines. Montvale, NJ: Medical Economics Company, 1998.

Polunin, Miriam, and Christopher Robbins. *The Natural Pharmacy.* New York: Macmillan Publishing Company, 1992.

Tyler, Varro E., Ph.D. *The Honest Herbal.* New York: Pharmaceutical Products Press, 1993.

Clare Hanrahan

Common cold

Definition

The common cold is a viral infection of the upper respiratory system, which includes the nose, throat, sinuses, eustachian tubes, trachea, larynx, and bronchial tubes. Although more than 200 different viruses can cause a cold, 30 to 50% are caused by a group known as rhinoviruses. Almost all colds clear up in less than two weeks without complications.

Description

Colds, sometimes called rhinovirus or coronavirus **infections**, are the most common illness to strike any part of the body. Repeated exposure to viruses causing colds creates partial immunity. Although most colds resolve on their own without complications, they are a leading cause of visits to the doctor and of time lost from work and school. Treating symptoms of the common cold has given rise to a multi-million dollar industry in over-the-counter medications, yet none of these medications is actually anti-viral to the rhinovirus.

Cold season in the United States begins in early autumn and extends through early spring. It is unclear why colds occur more frequently in winter. Although it is not true that getting wet or being in a draft causes a cold (a person has to come in contact with the virus to catch a cold), certain conditions may lead to increased susceptibility. These include:

- fatigue and overwork
- emotional stress
- poor nutrition
- smoking
- inadequate rest or sleep
- living or working in crowded conditions

Colds make the upper respiratory system less resistant to secondary bacterial infection. Secondary bacterial infection may lead to a number of other complications, including middle **ear infection, bronchitis, pneumonia, sinus infection,** or **strep throat**. People with chronic lung disease, **asthma,** diabetes, or a weakened immune system are more likely to develop these complications.

Demographics

It is estimated that the average person has more than 50 colds during a lifetime. Anyone can get a cold, although preschool and grade school children catch them more frequently than adolescents and adults (five to seven episodes per year in preschool children compared with two to three episodes per year in adulthood). Among employed adults, colds cause an estimated 40 percent of all time lost from jobs.

According to a telephone survey published in the *Archives of Internal Medicine* in 2003, about 500 million non-influenza viral respiratory infections occur annually, with direct costs of $17 billion and indirect costs of $22.5 billion.

Causes and symptoms

Colds are caused by more than 200 different viruses. The most common groups include rhinoviruses and coronaviruses. Different groups of viruses are more infectious at different seasons of the year, but knowing the exact virus causing the cold is not important in treatment.

People with colds are contagious during the first two to four days of the onset of symptoms. Colds pass from person to person in several ways. When an infected person coughs, sneezes, or speaks, tiny fluid droplets containing the virus are expelled. If these are breathed in by other people, the virus may establish itself in their noses and airways.

Colds may also be passed through direct contact. For example, if a person with a cold touches his runny nose or watery eyes, then shakes hands with another person, some of the virus is transferred to the uninfected person. If that person then touches his mouth, nose, or eyes, the virus is transferred to an environment where it can reproduce and cause a cold.

Finally, cold viruses can be spread through inanimate objects (door knobs, telephones, toys) that become contaminated with the virus, a common method of transmission in child care centers. Another vector of transmission is air travel, due to closed air circulation.

Once acquired, the cold virus attaches itself to the lining of the nasal passages and sinuses, which causes the infected cells to release a chemical called histamine. Histamine increases the blood flow to the infected cells, causing swelling, congestion, and increased mucus production. Within one to three days, the infected person begins to show cold symptoms.

The first cold symptoms are usually a tickle in the throat, runny nose, and **sneezing**. The initial discharge from the nose is clear and thin. Later, it may change to a thick yellow or greenish discharge. Most adults do not develop a **fever** when they catch a cold. Young children may develop a low fever of up to 102°F (38.9°C).

Other symptoms of a cold include coughing, sneezing, nasal congestion, **headache**, muscle ache, **chills**, **sore throat**, hoarseness, watery eyes, **fatigue**, dull hearing and blocked eustachian tube (a danger when flying), and lack of appetite. The **cough** that accompanies a cold is usually intermittent and dry.

Most people begin to feel better four to five days after their cold symptoms become noticeable. All symptoms are generally gone within 10 days, except for a dry cough that may linger for up to three weeks.

Colds make people more susceptible to secondary bacterial infections such as strep throat, middle ear infections, and sinus infections. A person should consult with a doctor if the cold does not begin to improve within a week. A doctor should also be consulted if the individual experiences chest **pain**, fever for more than a few days, difficulty breathing, bluish lips or fingernails, a cough that brings up greenish-yellow or grayish sputum, skin rash, swollen glands, or whitish spots on the tonsils or throat. These may be signs of a secondary bacterial infection that needs to be treated with an antibiotic.

People who have **emphysema**, chronic lung disease, diabetes, or a weakened immune system—either from diseases such as **AIDS** or **leukemia** or as the result of medications (corticosteroids, chemotherapy drugs)—should consult their doctor if they get a cold. People with these health problems are more likely to develop a secondary infection.

Diagnosis

Colds are diagnosed by observing a person's symptoms and symptom history. There are no laboratory tests as of 2008 for detecting the cold virus. However, a doctor may perform a throat or nasal culture or blood test to rule out a secondary infection.

Influenza is sometimes confused with a cold, but the flu causes much more severe symptoms and is generally accompanied by a fever. **Allergies** to molds or pollens also can cause a runny nose and eyes. Allergies are usually more persistent than the common cold. An allergist or a physician can perform tests to determine if the cold-like symptoms are being caused by an allergic reaction. Also, some people get a runny nose when they go outside in winter and breathe cold air. This type of runny nose, however, is not a symptom of a cold.

Treatment

Patients should drink plenty of fluids and eat nutritious foods. In fact, the old adage, "Feed a cold, starve a fever," was scientifically proven true in 2002. Dutch scientists found that cold-fighting immune responses rose after consuming a full meal, while **fasting** increased those that combat most fevers. Chicken soup with **ginger**, scallions, and rice noodles is nutritious and has properties that help people recover. Rest, to allow the body to fight infection, is very important. Gargling with salt water (half teaspoon salt in one cup of water) helps to soothe a sore throat. A vaporizer also will make sufferers feel more comfortable. Rubbing petroleum jelly or some other lubricant under the nose will prevent irritation from frequent nose blowing. For babies, nasal mucus should be suctioned gently with an infant nasal aspirator. It may be necessary to soften the mucus first with a few drops of salt water.

Herbals

Herbals can be taken to stimulate the immune system, for antiviral activity, and to relieve symptoms. The following herbs are used to treat colds:

- Ginger (*Zingiber officinale*) reduces fever and pain, has a sedative effect, settles the stomach, and suppresses cough.
- Forsythia (*Forsythia suspensa*) fruit can be taken as a tea for its anti-inflammatory, fever reducing, and antimicrobial properties.
- Honeysuckle (*Lonicera japonica*) flower can be taken as a tea for its anti-inflammatory, fever reducing, and antimicrobial properties.
- Aniseed (*Pimpinella anisum*) can be added to tea to expel phlegm, induce sweating, ease nausea, and ease stomach gas.
- Slippery elm powdered bark (*Ulmus fulva*) can be taken as a tea or slurry or capsules to soothe sore throat, to ease cough, and to thin mucous.

- Echinacea (*Echinacea purpurea, augustifolia*), or *pallida*) may relieve cold symptoms and reduce the severity of symptoms and duration of colds, but as of 2008 further clinical studies were needed to demonstrate its effects on the common cold. The usual dosage is 500 mg of crude powdered root or plant thrice on the first day, then 250 mg four times daily thereafter. Echinacea may also be taken as a tincture. (*Andrographis*, also known as Indian echinacea, is another form of echinacea that has been shown to reduce the symptoms of colds as well as increase resistance to colds. However, echinacea does not appear to be effective in children.)

- Garlic may reduce the severity of cold symptoms and the duration of colds. A 2007 study published in *Molecular Nutrition & Food Research* showed that participants who received garlic were almost two-thirds less likely to develop a cold than those receiving placebo, and those who did have a cold recovered about one day faster in the garlic group as compared to the placebo group.

- Goldenseal (*Hydrastis canadensis*) has fever reducing, antibacterial, anti-inflammatory, and antitussive properties. The usual dose is 125 mg three to four times daily. Goldenseal should not be taken for more than one week. Goldenseal may also be prepared as a tincture.

- Astragalus (*Astragalus membranaceus*) boosts the immune system and improves the body's response to stress. The common dose is 250 mg of extract four times daily.

- Cordyceps (*Cordyceps sinensis*) modulates and boosts the immune system and improves respiration. The usual dose is 500 mg two to three times daily.

- Elder (*Sambucus*) has antiviral activity, increases sweating, decreases inflammation, and decreases nasal discharge. The usual dose is 500 mg of extract thrice daily.

- American ginseng (*Panax quinquefolius*) can help prevent colds and reduce the severity and duration of cold symptoms. In seniors, American ginseng may help prevent flu-like illnesses. The usual dose is 400 mg once daily.

- Stinging nettle (*Urtica dioica*) has antihistamine and anti-inflammatory properties. The common dose is 300 mg four times daily.

- Schisandra (*Schisandra chinensis*) helps the body fight disease and increases endurance.

- Grape (*Vitis vinifera*) seed extract has antihistamine and anti-inflammatory properties. The usual dose is 50 mg three times daily.

- Eucalyptus (*Eucalyptus globulus*) or peppermint (*Mentha piperita*) essential oils added to a steam vaporizer may help clear chest and nasal congestion and disinfect room air.

- Boneset infusion (*Eupatroium perfoliatum*) relieves aches and fever.

- Yarrow (*Achillea millefolium*) is a diaphoretic.

- Supplemental larch from the inner bark of the western larch tree has been shown in some clinical trials to fight persistent colds and ear aches.

Chinese medicines

Chinese herbal treatments are based on the specific symptoms of colds and include a variety of *Radix*, *Rhizoma*, *Semen*, and *Herba* species. Chinese patent medicines for cold include:

- Wu Shi Cha (Noon tea): once or twice daily.

- Yin Qiao Jie Du Pian (Honeysuckle and Forsythia Tablet to Overcome Toxins): four to six, twice daily.

- Sang Ju Gan Mao (Mulberry Leaf and Chrysanthemum to Treat Common Cold): one packet of infusion or four to eight tablets, twice or thrice daily.

- Ling Yang Gan Mao Pian (Atelopis Tablet for Common Cold): four to six, twice daily.

- Ban Lan Gen Chong Ji (Isatidis Infusion): one packet twice or thrice daily.

- Huo Xiang Zheng Qi (Agastache to Rectify Qi): 6 g or four to six tablets.

Other remedies

Exercise of moderate intensity, over a period of one year, has been shown to decrease the incidence of self-reported colds. However, further research was needed as of 2008 to define the specific effects of exercise on the common cold.

Ayurvedic medicine practitioners recommend gargling with a mixture of water, salt, and **turmeric** powder or astringents such as alum, sumac, **sage**, and **bayberry** to ease a sore throat.

Homeopaths recommend microdoses of Viscue album, Natrum muriaticum, **Allium cepa**, or Nux vomica.

VITAMIN C. Vitamin C supplements, at a daily dose of 1,000 mg, can help to slightly reduce the symptoms and duration of colds when taken throughout the cold season. Vitamin C supplementation at the onset of cold symptoms is not effective in reducing the symptoms or duration of a cold, and it does not prevent colds.

VITAMIN E. Vitamin E supplements, at a daily dose of 200 IU, can help to slightly reduce the incidence of colds when taken throughout the cold season. Further studies were needed as of 2008 to evaluate the effects of vitamin E supplementation on the common cold.

ZINC. The effectiveness of zinc in nasal gels or throat lozenges for preventing or treating the common cold, as well as reducing the severity and duration of cold symptoms, continued to be investigated in the late 2000s. Numerous studies have generated inconsistent, although generally positive, results. For example, one study of over 100 employees of the Cleveland Clinic who used zinc lozenges immediately after the onset of cold symptoms showed the duration of colds decreased by one-half, although there were no differences in duration of fevers or level of muscle aches. It has been suggested that the effectiveness of the zinc lozenge is dependant on its formulation. For example, certain flavoring agents, including citric acid and tartaric acid, and the sweetener glycine in some lozenge formulations may bind zinc and reduce effectiveness. The recommended dosage is to suck on one lozenge every two hours while awake, beginning at the first cold symptoms. Side effects are bad taste, nausea, and vomiting. The results of studies using zinc nasal gel are more controversial because side effects such as nasal pain and loss of smell may override potential benefits. Further research was needed in the late 2000s to determine the effects of zinc compounds on the common cold.

Allopathic treatment

As of 2008, there were no known medicines proven to prevent or cure the common cold. Antibiotics are useless against a cold and can enhance bacterial resistance, if used carelessly. Nonprescription products to relieve cold symptoms include ipratropium bromide, cromolyn sodium, antihistamines, antitussives (cough suppressants), expectorants, decongestants, and/or pain relievers, but none has been found to shorten the duration of a cold. Over-the-counter cold remedies should not be given to infants without consulting a doctor first. Care should be taken not to exceed the recommended dosages, especially when combination medications or nasal sprays are taken. Aspirin should not be given to children with a cold because of its association with a risk of Reye's syndrome, a serious disease.

Ipratropium bromide, delivered via nasal spray, has been shown to improve symptoms of runny nose and sneezing, although side effects of nasal dryness and blood-tinged mucus can occur. Cromolyn sodium is a type of asthma medication—delivered via nasal spray, powder-filled inhalation capsules, or an aerosol via a metered dose inhaler—that has been shown to reduce the duration of cold symptoms.

Antihistamines are taken to relieve the symptoms of sneezing, runny nose, itchy eyes, and congestion. Side effects include dry mouth and drowsiness, especially with the first few doses. Some people have allergic reactions to antihistamines. Common over-the-counter antihistamines include Chlor-Trimeton, Dimetapp, Tavist, and Actifed. The generic name for two common antihistamines are chlorpheniramine and diphenhydramine.

Antitussives (cough suppressants), such as dextromethorphan and benzonatate, block the cough reflex and can be used to relieve symptoms of a non-productive cough. However, these medications are not recommended by the American College of Chest Physicians for treatment of cough associated with upper respiratory infections. Common brand names of over-the-counter dextromethorphan antitussives include Benylin, Delsym, Drixoral, Pertussin, and Robitussin. Tessalon is a common brand of benzonatate antitussive.

Expectorants, such as guaifenesin, help thin mucus so that coughing can remove secretions from the airway. Over-the-counter expectorant brands include Guiatuss, Robitussin, and Tusibron.

Decongestants reduce congestion and open inflamed nasal passages, making breathing easier. Decongestants can make people feel jittery or keep them from sleeping. They should not be used by people with heart disease, high blood pressure, or glaucoma. Some common decongestants are Neo-Synepherine, Novafed, and Sudafed. The generic names of common decongestants include pseudoephedrine and phenylephrine and in nasal sprays naphazoline, oxymetazoline, and xylometazoline. Nasal sprays and nose drop decongestants can act more quickly and effectively than decongestants found in pills or liquids because they are applied directly in the nose. Congestion returns after a few hours. Persons can become dependent on nasal sprays and nose drops, so they should not be used for more than a few days.

Many over-the-counter medications are combinations of both antihistamines and decongestants; an ache and pain reliever, such as acetaminophen (Datril, Tylenol, Panadol) or ibuprofen (Advil, Nuprin, Motrin, Medipren); and a cough suppressant (dextromethorphan). Common combination medications include Tylenol Cold and Flu, Triaminic, Sudafed Plus, and Tavist D.

Expected results

Given time, the body will make antibodies to cure itself of a cold. Most colds last seven to 10 days. Most people start feeling better within four or five days. Occasionally, a cold will lead to a secondary bacterial infection that causes strep throat, bronchitis, pneumonia, sinus infection, or a middle ear infection.

Prevention

Prevention focuses on strengthening the immune system by eating a healthy diet low in sugars and high in fresh fruits and vegetables, practicing **meditation** to reduce **stress**, getting adequate sleep, and getting regular moderate exercise. Some steps persons can take to prevent catching a cold and to reduce their spread include:

- washing hands well and frequently
- covering the mouth and nose when sneezing
- avoiding close contact with someone who has a cold during the first two to four days of their infection
- not sharing food, eating utensils, or cups
- avoiding crowded places where cold viruses can spread
- keeping hands away from the face
- avoiding cigarette smoke
- taking Echinacea; 250 mg up to four times daily for three weeks on, one week off
- taking astragalus; 250 mg to 500 mg daily
- taking a multivitamin with zinc

- taking vitamin C; 1,000 mg
- taking *Anas barbariae hepatis*; one dose weekly

Research has shown that transmission of the rhinovirus may be prevented through the use of antiseptic skin cleansers containing salicylic acid or pyroglutamic acid. The cleansers have properties that can kill the viruses and help prevent hand-to-hand transmission, but further research on their effectiveness remained to be done in the late 2000s.

Resources

BOOKS

Gruenwald, Joerg. *PDR for Herbal Medicines,* 4th ed. Montvale, NJ: Thomson Healthcare, 2007.

Judd, Sandra J., ed. *Complementary & Alternative Medicine Sourcebook (Health Reference Series).* Detroit, MI: Omnigraphics, 2006.

PERIODICALS

Pittler, Max H., and Edzard Ernst. "Clinical Effectiveness of Garlic *(Allium sativum)." Molecular Nutrition & Food Research* 51, no. 11 (November 2007): 1382–1385.

Simasek, Madeline, and David A. Blandino. "Treatment of the Common Cold." *American Family Physician* 75, no. 4 (February 15, 2007): 515

ORGANIZATIONS

Alternative Medicine Foundation, PO Box 60016, Potomac, MD, 20859, (301) 340-1960, http://www. amfoundation.org.

National Center for Complementary and Alternative Medicine, National Institutes of Health, 9000 Rockville Pike, Bethesda., MD, 20892, (888) 644-6226, http://www.nccam.nih.gov.

Office of Dietary Supplements, National Institutes of Health, 6100 Executive Blvd., Room 3B01, MSC 7517, Bethesda, MD, 20892-7517, (301) 435-2920, http://ods.od.nih.gov.

Belinda Rowland
Teresa G. Odle
Angela M. Costello

Coneflower *see* **Echinacea**

Conjunctivitis

Definition

Conjunctivitis is an inflammation of the transparent membrane lining of the conjunctiva, which covers the white part of the eye and the underside of the eyelid. Conjunctivitis can be caused by viral or bacterial infection, allergic reaction, or less commonly by physical agents such as chemicals splashed into the eye or exposure of the eye to infrared or ultraviolet light. Conjunctivitis is also known as pink eye.

Description

Conjunctivitis is a common eye problem because the conjunctivae are continually exposed to microorganisms and environmental agents that can cause **infections** or allergic reactions. Conjunctivitis can be acute (short term) or chronic (long term) depending upon how long the condition lasts, the severity of symptoms, and the type of organism or agent involved. It can affect one or both eyes. Viral and bacterial conjunctivitis is highly contagious; physical transfer can easily spread it to others. Bacterial conjunctivitis is particularly likely to spread among children in childcare centers or schools.

Causes and symptoms

Conjunctivitis may be caused by a viral infection, such as a cold, acute respiratory infection, **measles**, herpes simplex, or herpes zoster. Symptoms include mild to severe discomfort in one or both eyes, redness, swelling of the eyelids, and a watery, yellow, or greenish discharge. The symptoms may last several days to several weeks. Infection with an adenovirus may cause a significant amount of pus-like discharge and a scratchy sensation in the eye. These symptoms may be accompanied by swelling and tenderness of the lymph nodes near the ear.

Bacterial conjunctivitis occurs in adults or children but is more common in children. It is caused by such organisms as *Staphylococcus*, *Streptococcus pneumoniae*, and *Haemophilus influenzae*. Symptoms of bacterial conjunctivitis include a pus-like discharge and crusty eyelids upon awakening. Redness of the conjunctivae can be mild to severe and may be accompanied by swelling. In people who are sexually active, conjunctivitis may be caused by **chlamydia** or the bacteria that cause **gonorrhea**. In these cases, there may be large amounts of pus-like discharge. Other symptoms may include hypersensitivity to light (photophobia), a watery mucous discharge, and tenderness in the lymph nodes near the ear that may persist for up to three months.

Non-contagious conjunctivitis can be caused by such environmental hazards as wind, smoke, dust, and allergic reactions caused by pollen, dust, or grass. Symptoms range from **itching** and redness to a mucous discharge. Persons who wear contact lenses may develop allergic conjunctivitis caused by the various lens solutions and foreign proteins contained in them.

Other less common causes of conjunctivitis include looking at the sun, sun lamps, plant lamps, or the electrical arcs used during welding. Accidental chemical splashes in the eye can also cause non-contagious conjunctivitis, as can blocked tear ducts in newborns.

Diagnosis

Although inflammation of the eye is often obvious, accurate diagnosis of the cause of conjunctivitis requires taking the patient's history to learn when symptoms began, how long the condition has existed, and the specific symptoms experienced. Diagnostic tests may include an eye examination and culture of the eye discharge to determine the organism responsible for causing the condition. Obtaining samples for culturing is relatively painless.

Treatment

Conjunctivitis caused by bacteria and gonococcal or chlamydial infection usually requires prescription antibiotics. Immune system enhancement with dietary supplements can aid in the resolution of allergic and viral conjunctivitis. Removal of the allergic agent is an essential step in treating allergic conjunctivitis. If home care brings no improvement within 48 to 72 hours, a physician should be consulted.

Nutritional therapy

The following dietary changes may be helpful in managing conjunctivitis by supporting and strengthening the immune system:

- Taking 25,000 IU (international units) of beta-carotene twice daily for 7 days. However, taking megadoses of beta-carotene for an extended time has been shown to increase the risk of developing lung cancer in smokers but not in non-smokers.
- Taking 500–1000 mg of vitamin C three times daily for 7 days.
- Taking 25 mg of zinc with meals three times daily for 7 days.

Homeopathy

A number of homeopathic remedies are designed to treat acute conjunctivitis. These include *Argentum nitricum* (silver nitrate), **pulsatilla** (windflower), **belladonna**, *Arsenicum album* (arsenic trioxide), sulphur (elemental sulphur) and **eyebright** (*Euphrasia officinalis*). Eye drops prepared with homeopathic remedies may be a substitute for pharmaceutical eye drops.

Herbal therapy

Herbal eyewashes made with eyebright (1 tsp dried herb steeped in 1 cup of boiling water for 10 minutes, then strained and used at once) or **chamomile** (*Matricaria recutita*; 2–3 tsp in 1 pint of boiling water) may be helpful. Eyewashes should be strained and cooled before use. They should be discarded promptly after use, as old infusions may become contaminated (non-sterile).

Other home remedies may help relieve the discomfort associated with conjunctivitis. A boric acid eyewash (1 tsp boric acid in 1 cup of water) can be used to clean and soothe the eyes. A warm compress applied to the eyes for 5 to 10 minutes three times a day can help relieve the discomfort of bacterial and viral conjunctivitis and may help open a blocked tear duct. A clean washcloth soaked in warm water can be used as a warm compress. The patient should close both eyes and apply the compress to the affected eye. A cool compress or cool, damp tea bags placed on the eyes can ease the discomfort and itching of conjunctivitis.

Allopathic treatment

The treatment of conjunctivitis depends on what agent caused the condition. In all cases, warm compresses applied to the affected eye several times a day may help to reduce discomfort.

Conjunctivitis due to a viral infection is usually treated by applying warm compresses to the eye. Viral conjunctivitis is not treatable by antibiotic eye drops or ointment. Usually symptoms of viral conjunctivitis worsen for three to five days then begin to improve, and the disease clears on its own. If there is no improvement, a doctor should be consulted.

In cases of bacterial conjunctivitis, a physician usually prescribes an antibiotic eye ointment or eye drops containing **sodium** sulfacetamide (Sulamyd) to be applied daily for 7 to 14 days. As with all antibiotics, it is important to complete the entire course of treatment and not stop using the medicine simply because symptoms improve. Patients should contact their doctor if the eyes fail to improve after 72 hours.

Antibiotic eye drops are instilled (put in drop by drop) into the eye by having the patient tilt the head back and pulling down the lower eyelid. The patient is asked to look upward while the medication is instilled into the conjunctival sac. The dropper should not touch the skin to prevent discharge from the eye from contaminating the eye drop solution. After the drops have been instilled, the patient should gently close the eyes for one minute in order not to squeeze out any of the medication.

For cases of conjunctivitis caused by a gonococcus (the bacteria that causes gonorrhea), a physician may prescribe an injection of ceftriaxone (Rocephin) and a topical antibiotic ointment containing erythromycin or bactracin to be applied four times daily for two to three weeks. For chlamydial infections, a topical antibiotic ointment containing erythromycin (Ilotycin) may be prescribed to be applied one or two times daily.

To apply an antibiotic ointment, the eye should be gently wiped with a sterile cotton ball moistened with sterile water to remove any discharge. Then, the lower eyelid can be pulled down and a thin ribbon of ointment applied in the lower conjunctival sac. If possible, single-dose dispensers of ointment should be used as a protection against contamination of the medication. The eyelids can be closed and massaged gently to distribute the ointment. Patients may find that their vision is blurry for a few minutes after the ointment is applied, but this is a normal side effect. In addition to topical antibiotics, oral erythromycin or tetracycline therapy may be indicated for three to four weeks. Sexual partners should also be treated.

Allergic conjunctivitis is treated by removing the allergic substance from a person's environment, if possible, applying cool compresses to the eye, and by administering eye drops four to six times daily for four days. Also, the antihistamine diphenhydramine hydrochloride (Benadryl) may help to relieve itchy eyes. Some doctors may prescribe ophthalmic steroids, but they are often unnecessary and have the potential to cause complications in some patients.

Expected results

Conjunctivitis caused by an allergic reaction should clear up once the allergen is removed. Allergic conjunctivitis, however, is likely to recur if the individual again comes into contact with the particular allergen. Conjunctivitis caused by a bacterium or a virus, if treated properly, usually resolves in about ten days. If there is no relief of symptoms in 48 to 72 hours or if there is moderate to severe eye **pain** or changes in vision, a physician should be notified immediately. If untreated or treated inappropriately, conjunctivitis may cause vision impairment by spreading to other parts of the eye such as the cornea.

Prevention

Many states require that children with conjunctivitis remain at home until the eye redness is gone in order to prevent spreading this highly contagious disease. Conjunctivitis sometimes can be prevented or the course of the disease shortened by following some simple practices:

KEY TERMS

Adenovirus—A virus that affects the upper respiratory tract.

Chlamydia—A common sexually transmitted disease in the United States that often accompanies gonorrhea. It is caused by a rickettsia called *Chlamydia trachomatis*.

Gonococcus—The bacterium *Neisseria gonorrheae* , which causes gonorrhea, a sexually transmitted infection of the genitals and urinary tract that may occasionally affect the eye, causing blindness if not treated.

Herpes simplex virus—A virus that can cause fever and blistering on the skin, mucous membranes, or genitalia.

Herpes zoster virus—Acute inflammatory virus attacking the nerve cells on the root of each spinal nerve with skin eruptions along a sensory nerve ending.

Inflammation—The body's response to tissue damage, with symptoms of warmth, swelling, redness, and pain in the affected part.

Staphylococcus—A genus of bacteria, which resembles a cluster of grapes, that can infect various body systems.

- Washing hands frequently using antiseptic soap and using single-use towels during the disease to prevent spreading the infection
- Avoiding sharing towels and wash cloths
- Avoiding chemical irritants and known allergens
- In areas where welding occurs, using the proper protective eye wear and screens to prevent damaging the eyes
- Using a clean tissue to remove discharge from eyes and washing hands to prevent the spread of infection
- If medication is prescribed, finishing the course of antibiotics as directed to make sure that the infection is cleared up and does not recur
- Avoiding wearing eye makeup or contact lenses during the infection and do not share eye makeup with others

Resources

BOOKS

Chevallier, Andrew. *Herbal Remedies*. New York: DK Publishing, 2007.

Foster, Steven, and Rebecca Johnson. *National Geographic Desk Reference to Nature's Medicine*. Washington, DC: National Geographic Society, 2006.

Mayo Clinic Book of Alternative Medicine: The New Approach to Using the Best of Natural Therapies and Conventional Medicine. New York: Time Inc. Home Entertainment, 2007.

Weil, Andrew, *Natural Health, Natural Medicine*, rev. ed. New York: Houghton Mifflin, 2004.

OTHER

"Conjunctivitis." *American Optometric Association*. [cited April 20, 2008]. http://www.aoa.org/conjunctivitis.xml.

"Conjunctivitis (Pink Eye)." *MedicineNet.com* December 7, 2007 [cited April 20, 2008]. http://www.medicinenet.com/pink_eye/article.htm.

"Pink eye (Conjunctivitis)." *Mayo Clinic* May 25, 2006 [cited April 20, 2008]. http://www.mayoclinic.com/health/pink-eye/DS00258.

Silverman, Michael. "Conjunctivitis." *eMedicine.com* May 8, 2007 [cited April 20, 2008]. http://www.emedicine.com/emerg/topic110.htm.

ORGANIZATIONS

Alternative Medicine Foundation, PO Box 60016, Potomac, MD, 20859, (301) 340-1960, http://www.amfoundation.org.

American Academy of Family Physicians, PO Box 11210, Shawnee Mission, KS, 66207, (913) 906-6000, http://www.aafp.org.

American Holistic Medical Association, PO Box 2016, Edmonds, WA, 98020, (425) 967-0737, http://www.holisticmedicine.org.

American Institute of Homeopathy, 801 N. Fairfax St., Suite 306, Alexandria, VA, 22314, (888) 445-9988, http://homeopathyusa.org.

National Center for Homeopathy, 801 N. Fairfax St., Suite 306, Alexandria, VA, 22314, (703) 548-7790, http://www.homeopathic.org/contact.htm.

National Eye Institute, 2020 Vision Place, Bethesda, MD, 20892-3655, (301) 496-5248, http://www.nei.nih.gov.

Mai Tran
Teresa G. Odle
Tish Davidson, A. M.

Constipation

Definition

Constipation is an acute or chronic condition in which bowel movements occur less often than usual or consist of hard, dry stools that are painful or difficult to pass. Bowel habits vary, but an adult who has not had a bowel movement in three days or a child who has not had a bowel movement in four days is considered constipated.

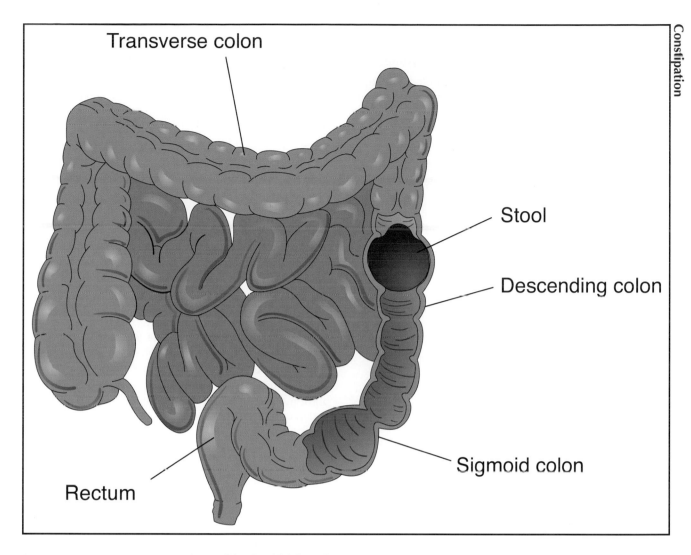

Transverse colon

Stool

Descending colon

Sigmoid colon

Rectum

Constipation is an acute or chronic condition in which bowel movements occur less often than usual or consist of hard, dry stools that are painful or difficult to pass. *(Iustration by Electronic Illustrators Group. Cengage Learning, Gale)*

Description

Constipation is one of the most common medical complaints in the United States. Estimates show that chronic constipation affects between 2% and 28% of adults. In the United States, constipation results in more than 2.5 million visits to physicians and 92,000 hospitalizations each year, according to an article in the October 1, 2007 issue of *Family Practice News*. Studies have shown chronic constipation is two to three times more common in women than men. The highest rates per age group are in people aged 65 years or older. However, it can occur at any age and is more common among individuals who resist the urge to move their bowels at the body's signal. This often happens when children start school or enter daycare and feel shy about asking permission to use the bathroom.

Although this condition is rarely serious, it can lead to the following:

- bowel obstruction
- chronic constipation
- hemorrhoids (a mass of dilated veins in swollen tissue around the anus)
- hernia (a protrusion of an organ through a tear in the muscle wall)
- spastic colitis (irritable bowel syndrome, a condition characterized by alternating periods of diarrhea and constipation)
- laxative dependency

Chronic constipation may be a symptom of **colorectal cancer**, **depression**, diabetes, diverticulosis (small pouches in the muscles of the large intestine), **lead** poisoning, or **Parkinson's disease**. An opioid overdose (as in excessive codeine from **cough** suppressants or heroin addiction) also may result in constipation.

In someone who is elderly or disabled, constipation may be a symptom of bowel impaction, a more serious condition in which feces are trapped in the lower part of the large intestine. A doctor should be called if an elderly or disabled person is constipated for more than a week or if a child seems to be constipated.

A doctor should be notified whenever constipation occurs after starting a new prescription, vitamin, or mineral supplement or is accompanied by blood in the stools, changes in bowel patterns, **fever**, or abdominal **pain**.

Causes and symptoms

Constipation usually results from not getting enough **exercise**, not drinking enough water or clear fluids, or from a diet that does not include an adequate amount of fiber-rich foods such as beans, bran cereals, fruits, raw vegetables, rice, and whole-grain breads.

Other causes of constipation include anal fissure (a tear or crack in the lining of the anus), chronic kidney failure, colon or rectal **cancer**, depression, hypercalcemia (abnormally high levels of **calcium** in the blood), **hypothyroidism** (underactive thyroid gland), illness requiring complete bed rest, **irritable bowel syndrome**, imbalanced bowel from food and flora **allergies**, and **stress**.

Constipation can also be a side effect of the following:

- aluminum salts in antacids
- antihistamines
- antipsychotic drugs
- aspirin
- belladonna (*Atopa belladonna,* source of atropine, a medication used to relieve spasms and dilate the pupils of the eye)
- beta blockers (medications used to stabilize irregular heartbeat, lower high blood pressure, reduce chest pain)
- blood pressure medications
- calcium channel blockers (medication prescribed to treat high blood pressure, chest pain, some types of irregular heartbeat and stroke, some non-cardiac diseases)
- codeine or opioids
- diuretics (drugs that promote the formation and secretion of urine)
- iron or calcium supplements

- narcotics (potentially addictive drugs that relieve pain and cause mood changes)
- tricyclic antidepressants (medications prescribed to treat chronic pain, depression, headaches, and other illnesses)

An adult who is constipated may feel bloated, have a **headache**, swollen abdomen, pass rock-like feces, or strain, bleed, or feel pain during bowel movements. A constipated baby may strain, cry, draw the legs toward the abdomen, or arch the back when having a bowel movement.

Diagnosis

Everyone becomes constipated once in a while, but a doctor should be notified if significant changes in bowel patterns last for more than a week or if symptoms continue more than three weeks after increasing activity and fiber and fluid intake.

The patient's observations and medical history help a primary care physician diagnose constipation. The doctor uses his fingers to see if there is a hardened mass in the abdomen and may perform a rectal examination. Other diagnostic procedures include a barium enema, which may reveal a blockage inside the intestine; laboratory analysis of blood and stool samples for internal bleeding or other symptoms of systemic disease; and a sigmoidoscopy (examination of the sigmoid area of the colon with a flexible tube equipped with a magnifying lens).

Physical and psychological assessments and a detailed history of bowel habits are especially important when an elderly person complains of constipation.

Treatment

Initially, alternative practitioners suggest that the patient drink an adequate amount of water each day (six to eight glasses), exercise on a regular basis, and eat a diet high in soluble and insoluble fibers. Soluble fibers include pectin, flax, and gums. Insoluble fibers include **psyllium** and bran from grains such as wheat and oats. Fresh fruits and vegetables contain both soluble and insoluble fibers, and since constipation is aggravated by folate, calcium, and **magnesium** deficiencies, sources of these nutrients, such as asparagus, spinach, **parsley**, and other dark green leafy vegetables, should be part of the daily diet. Various fruit juices can also help maintain normal bowel function: Sorbitol, the natural sugar found in apple juice, has known laxative properties. **Castor oil**, applied topically to the abdomen and covered by a heat source (a heating pad or hot water bottle), can help relieve constipation when used nightly for 20–30 minutes. For babies, about 1 tablespoon of corn syrup mixed with warm water might help relieve constipation.

Acupressure

This form of needleless **acupuncture** is said to relax the abdomen, ease discomfort, and stimulate regular bowel movements when diet and exercise fail to do so. After lying down, patients close their eyes and take deep breaths. For two minutes, the practitioner applies gentle fingertip pressure to a point about two inches below the navel. **Acupressure** can also be applied to the outer edges of one elbow crease and maintained for 30 seconds before pressing the crease of the other elbow. This should be done three times a day to relieve constipation.

Aromatherapy

Six drops of **rosemary** (*Rosmarinus officinalis*) and six drops of **thyme** (*Thymus spp.*) diluted by one ounce of almond oil, olive oil, or another carrier oil can relieve constipation when used to massage the abdomen. A circular motion for massage is recommended, beginning up the right side of the abdomen, coming across the top, and down the left side. Massaging the leg from knee to hip in the morning, at night, and before trying to move the bowels is said to relieve constipation.

Herbal therapy

A variety of herbal therapies can be useful in the treatment of constipation. Several herbs, including **chamomile** (*Matricaria recutita*), **dandelion** root (*Taraxacum officinale*), and burdock (*Arctium lappa*), act as **bitters** which stimulate the movement of the digestive and excretory systems. There are also laxative herbs that assist with bowel movement. Two of these are **senna** and **buckthorn**. These laxative herbs are stronger acting on elimination than bitters and can sometimes cause cramping (mixing them with a calming herb like **fennel** or caraway can help reduce cramping). Both senna and buckthorn are powerful herbs that are best used with direction from an experienced practitioner, since they can have adverse side effects and the patient may become dependent on them. In fact, practitioners caution that senna can cause severe cramping.

Yoga

The knee-chest position, said to relieve **gas** and stimulate abdominal organs, involves the following moves:

- standing straight with arms at the sides
- lifting the right knee toward the chest

- grasping the right ankle with the left hand
- pulling the leg as close to the chest as possible
- holding the position for about eight seconds
- repeating these steps with the left leg

The cobra position, which can be repeated as many as four times a day, involves the following moves:

- lying on the stomach with legs together
- placing the palms just below the shoulders, holding elbows close to the body
- inhaling, then lifting the head (face forward) and chest off the floor
- keeping the navel in contact with the floor
- looking as far upward as possible
- holding this position for three to six seconds
- exhaling and lowering the chest

The spinal twist is another pose that is recommended for daily use in relieving constipation. Practicing **relaxation** and **meditation** can also have a powerful effect on the digestive system. Slow, steady music can relieve tension that leads to constipation.

Allopathic treatment

If changes in diet and activity fail to relieve occasional constipation, an over-the-counter laxative may be used for a few days. Preparations that soften stools or add bulk (bran, psyllium, ducosate **sodium**) work more slowly but are safer than Epsom salts and other harsh laxatives or herbal laxatives containing senna (*Cassia senna*) or buckthorn (*Rhamnus purshianna*), which, if used long term, can harm the nerves and lining of the colon because they are stimulants that cause waves of involuntary muscle contractions in the intestines.

A woman who is pregnant should never use a laxative. She can use **flaxseed**, bran, ducosate sodium, prunes, or oatmeal. Anyone who is experiencing abdominal pain, **nausea**, or **vomiting** should also avoid laxatives. A warm-water or mineral oil enema can relieve constipation, and a non-digestible sugar (lactulose) or special electrolyte solution is recommended for adults and older children with stubborn symptoms. If a patient has an impacted bowel, the doctor may insert a gloved finger into the rectum and gently dislodge the hardened feces.

One study compared a non-toxic food ingredient called polyethylene glycol to lactulose for relieving constipation in children. It showed that it may work faster, prove easier to administer, and be just as safe and effective. However, more research was suggested before recommending the substance over lactulose. A small-scale study of children with chronic constipation reported in 2006 that an intake for four weeks of a cocoa husk supplement produced beneficial results.

In 2007, the anti-constipation prescription drug tegaserod (Zelnorm) was removed from the market after an analysis of previous studies (meta-analysis) of more than 18,000 people showed it increased the risk of cardiovascular events, including **heart attack**, **stroke**, and unstable **angina**. The risk was small but considered significant. The drug was used to treat people with irritable bowel syndrome who had constipation or chronic constipation. There was no proof the drug itself caused the cardiovascular events since all 13 people in the studies who reported cardiovascular events had pre-existing heart problems or had risk factors for **heart disease**.

Expected results

Changes in diet and exercise usually eliminate the problem of constipation.

Prevention

Most Americans consume between 11–18 grams of fiber a day. Consumption of 30 grams of fiber and between 6–8 glasses of water each day can generally prevent constipation, and 35 grams of fiber a day (an amount equal to five servings of fruits and vegetables, and a large bowl of high-fiber cereal) can relieve constipation. Fiber supplements containing psyllium (*Plantago psyllium*) usually become effective within about two days and can be used every day without causing dependency. Powdered flaxseed (*Linium usitatissimum*) works the same way. Insoluble fiber, such as wheat or oat bran, is as effective as psyllium but may give the patient gas at first.

Daily use of 500 mg **vitamin C** and 400 mg magnesium can prevent constipation. If symptoms do occur, each dosage can be increased by 100 mg a day, up to a maximum of 5,000 mg vitamin C and 1,000 mg magnesium. Use of preventive doses should be resumed after relief occurs. If the patient develops **diarrhea**, the vitamin C should be decreased. Calcium is also important. Children over five can take up to 1,300 mg and adults ages 19–50 can take up to 2,000 mg.

Sitting on the toilet for 10 minutes at the same time every day, preferably after a meal, can induce regular bowel movements. This may not become effective for a few months, and it is important to defecate whenever necessary.

Resources

BOOKS

Dhingra, Anand. *Constipation Causes & Cure*. Charleston, SC: BookSurge, 2006.

Gauss, Harry. *So You Feel Sluggish Today: The Causes and Treatment of Constipation*. Whitefish, MT: Kessinger, 2007.

PERIODICALS

Castillejo, Gemma, et al. "A Controlled, Randomized, Double-Blind Trial to Evaluate the Effect of a Supplement of Cocoa Husk that Is Rich in Dietary Fiber on Colonic Transit in Constipated Pediatric Patients." *Pediatrics* (September 2006): 1229–1230.

Drost, Jennifer, and Lucinda A. Harris. "Diagnosis and Management of Chronic Constipation: Diagnosis Is a Challenge Because Patients and Clinicians Often Define Constipation Differently. The History, Physical Examination, and Appropriate Diagnostic Procedures Are Key." *Journal of the American Academy of Physicians Assistants* (November 2006): 24(6).

Gaby, Alan R. "Food Allergy as a Cause of Chronic Constipation." *Townsend Letter: The Examiner of Alternative Medicine* (April 2007): 64.

Harrington, Kendra L., and Esther M. Haskvitz. "Managing a Patient's Constipation with Physical Therapy." *Physical Therapy* (November 2006): 1151(9).

Lembo, Anthony J. "Best Practices In: Chronic Constipation in the Elderly." *Family Practice News* (October 1, 2007): 10.

Wendling, Patrice. "Enemas Fail to Improve Intractable Constipation." *Pediatric News* (July 2007): 49.

OTHER

Jaeck, Brenda. "Constipation" (CD-ROM). *Seeds to Change*, 2007. http://seedstochange.com/ (February 25, 2008).

ORGANIZATIONS

Association of Gastrointestinal Motility Disorders, 12 Roberts Dr., Bedford, MA, 01730, (781) 275-1300, http://www.agmd-gimotility.org.

Irritable Bowel Syndrome Association, 1440 Whalley Ave., Suite 145, New Haven, CT, http://www.ibsassociation.org.

National Center for Alternative and Complementary Medicine, 9000 Rockville Pike, Bethesda, MD, 20892, (888) 644-6226, http://www.nccam.nih.gov.

National Digestive Disease Information Clearinghouse, 2 Information Way, Bethesda, MD, 20892-3570, (800) 891-5389, http://www.digestive.niddk.nih.gov.

Kathleen Wright
Ken R. Wells

Constitutional homeopathic remedies *see* **Homeopathy, constitutional prescribing**

Consumption *see* **Tuberculosis**

Contact dermatitis

Contact dermatitis

Definition

Contact **dermatitis** is the name given to any skin inflammation that results from surface contact. There are two kinds of contact dermatitis, irritant and allergic.

Description

Thousands of natural and synthetic substances can cause contact dermatitis, which is the most common skin condition requiring medical attention, and the foremost source of work-related disease. Florists, domestic workers, hairdressers, food preparers, and employees in heavy industry, construction, carpentry, dry cleaning, farming, health care, and the military are the people most at risk of contracting work-related contact dermatitis. Americans spend roughly $300 million a year in their quest for relief from contact dermatitis, not counting the considerable sums devoted by governments and businesses to regulating and policing the use of skin-threatening chemicals in the workplace. But exactly how many people suffer from contact dermatitis remains unclear; a 1997 article in the *Journal of the American Medical Association* notes that figures ranging from 1–15% have been put forward for Western industrial nations.

Causes and symptoms

Irritant contact dermatitis (ICD) is the more commonly reported of the two types of contact dermatitis, accounting for about 80% of cases. It can be caused by soaps, detergents, solvents, adhesives, fiberglass, and other substances that are able to directly injure the skin. Most attacks are mild and confined to the hands and forearms, but can affect any part of the body that comes in contact with the irritating substance. The symptoms can take many forms: redness, **itching**, crusting, swelling, blistering, oozing, dryness, scaliness, thickening of the skin, and a feeling of warmth at the site of contact. In extreme cases severe blistering can occur and open sores can form. Occupations that require frequent skin exposure to water, such as hairdressing and food preparation, can make the skin more susceptible to ICD.

Allergic contact dermatitis (ACD) results when repeated exposure to an allergen (an allergy-causing substance) triggers an immune response that inflames the skin. Tens of thousands of drugs, pesticides, cosmetics, food additives, commercial chemicals, and other substances have been identified as potential

allergens. Fewer than 30, however, are responsible the majority of ACD cases. Common culprits include poison ivy, poison **oak**, and poison sumac; fragrances and preservatives in cosmetics and personal care products; latex items, including gloves and condoms; and formaldehyde. Many people find that they are allergic to the nickel in inexpensive costume jewelry. ACD is usually confined to the area of skin that comes in contact with the allergen, typically the hands or face. Symptoms range from mild to severe and resemble those of ICD. A patch test may be needed to determine which kind of contact dermatitis a person is suffering from.

Diagnosis

Diagnosis begins with a physical examination and asking the patient questions about his or her health and daily activities. When contact dermatitis is suspected, the doctor attempts to learn as much as possible about the patient's hobbies, workplace duties, use of medications and cosmetics, etc.—anything that might shed light on the source of the disease. In some cases an examination of the home or workplace is undertaken. If the dermatitis is mild, responds well to treatment, and does not recur, ordinarily the investigation is at an end. More difficult cases require patch testing to identify the specific allergen.

Two methods of patch testing are currently used. The most widely used method, the Finn chamber method, employs a multiwell aluminum patch. Each well is filled with a small amount of the allergen being tested and the patch is taped to normal skin on the patient's upper back. After 48 hours the patch is removed and an initial reading is taken. A second reading is made a few days later. The second method of patch testing involves applying a small amount of the test substance directly to normal skin and covering it with a dressing that keeps air out and keeps the test substance in (occlusive dressing). After 48 hours the dressing is taken off to see if a reaction has occurred. Identifying the allergen may require repeated testing, can take weeks or months, and is not always successful. Moreover, patch testing works only with ACD, though it is considered an essential step in ruling out ICD.

Treatment

Herbal therapy

Herbal remedies have been used for centuries to treat skin disorders, including contact dermatitis. An experienced herbalist or naturopathic doctor can recommend the remedies that will be most effective for a person's condition. Among the herbs often recommended are:

- Burdock (*Arctium lappa*). Burdock is taken internally as a tea or tincture.
- Calendula (*Calendula officinalis*). Calendula is a natural antiseptic and anti-inflammatory agent. It is applied topically in a lotion, ointment, or oil to the affected area.
- Aloe (*Aloe barbadensis*). Aloes soothes skin irritations. Its gel is applied topically to the affected area.

Poison ivy, poison oak, and poison sumac are common culprits in cases of allergic contact dermatitis. Following exposure to these plants, the development of the characteristic rash may be prevented by washing the area with soap and water within 15 minutes of exposure. The leaves of jewelweed (*Impatiens* spp.), which often grows near poison ivy, may neutralize the poison ivy allergen if rubbed on the skin right after contact. Several topical herbal remedies may help relieve the itching associated with allergic contact dermatitis, including the juice of **plantain** leaves (*Plantago major*); a paste made of equal parts of green clay and **goldenseal** root (*Hydrastis canadensis*); a paste made of salt, water, clay, and **peppermint** (*Mentha piperita*) oil; and calamine lotion.

Homeopathy

A homeopath treating a patient with contact dermatitis will do a thorough investigation of the individual's history and exposures before prescribing a remedy. Common homeopathic remedies include:

- Rhus toxicodendron
- Croton tiglium
- ledum
- anacardium
- graphites
- sulfur

Allopathic treatment

The best treatment for contact dermatitis is to identify the allergen or irritating substance and avoid further contact with it. If the culprit is, for instance, a cosmetic, avoidance is a simple matter, but in some situations, such as an allergy to an essential workplace chemical for which no substitute can be found, avoidance may be impossible or force the sufferer to find new work or make other drastic changes in his or her life. Barrier creams and such protective clothing as gloves, masks, and long-sleeved shirts are ways of coping with contact dermatitis when avoidance is impossible, though they are not always effective.

For the symptoms themselves, treatments in mild cases include cool compresses and nonprescription lotions and ointments. When the symptoms are severe, corticosteroids applied to the skin or taken orally are used. Contact dermatitis that leads to a bacterial skin infection is treated with antibiotics.

Expected results

If the offending substance is promptly identified and avoided, the chances of a quick and complete recovery are excellent. Otherwise, symptom management— not cure—is the best that medical treatment can offer. For some people, contact dermatitis becomes a chronic and disabling condition that can have a profound effect on employability and quality of life.

Prevention

Avoidance of known or suspected allergens or irritating substances is the best prevention. If avoidance is difficult, barrier creams and protective clothing can be tried. Skin that comes in contact with an offending substance should be thoroughly washed, the sooner the better.

Resources

BOOKS

Swerlick, Robert A., and Thomas J. Lawley. "Eczema, Psoriasis, Cutaneous Infections, Acne, and Other Common Skin Disorders." In *Harrison's Principles of Internal Medicine*. Anthony S. Fauci, et al., eds. New York: McGraw-Hill, 1998.

Ullman, Dana. *The Consumer's Guide to Homeopathy: The Definitive Resources for Understanding Homeopathic Medicine and Making It Work for You*. New York: G.P. Putnam's Sons, 1995.

Wolf, John E., Jr. "Contact Dermatitis." In *Conn's Current Therapy*. Robert E. Rakel, ed. Philadelphia: W.B. Saunders, 1998.

PERIODICALS

Leung, Donald Y. M., et al. "Allergic and Immunologic Skin Disorders." *Journal of the American Medical Association* 278 (1997): 1914+.

Rietschel, Robert L. "Occupational Contact Dermatitis." *Lancet* 349 (1997): 1093+.

Mai Tran

Copper

Description

Copper is an essential mineral that plays an important role in **iron** absorption and transport. It is considered a trace mineral because it is needed in very small amounts. Only 70 to 80 mg of copper are found in the body of a normal healthy person. Even though the body needs very little copper, it is an important nutrient that has many vital physiological functions.

Copper is essential for normal development of the body because it functions in the following ways:

- Participates in a wide variety of important enzymatic reactions in the body.

- Is a component of or a cofactor for approximately 50 different enzymes. These enzymes need copper to function properly.

- Is essential for iron absorption and transport. Iron is needed to make hemoglobin, a main component of red blood cells. Therefore, copper deficiency is often linked to iron-deficiency anemia.

- Is required to build elastin and collagen, which are important components of bones and connective tissues. Therefore, copper is believed to protect the bones and joints against degeneration and osteoporosis.

- Is required for melanin production. People with copper deficiency may have pale skin and hair.

- Is a key mineral for the immune system. Copper promotes wound healing. Studies show that premature infants or children with genetic copper defects are at high risk of getting infections and significantly improve with copper supplementation.

- Attacks free radicals. A strong antioxidant, copper works by attaching itself to the enzyme superoxide dismutase (SOD). Copper also binds to a protein to form ceruloplasmin, which is an antioxidant.

- Helps the body produce energy. Copper participates in many oxidative reactions that break down fats in fat tissue to produce much needed energy. Copper

Adequate intake of copper	
Age	**mcg/day**
Children 0-6 mos.	200 (AI)
Children 7-12 mos.	220
Children 1-3 yrs.	340
Children 4-8 yrs.	440
Children 9-13 yrs.	700
Children 14-18 yrs.	890
Adults ≥ 19 yrs.	900
Pregnant women	1,000
Breastfeeding women	1,300

Foods that contain copper	mcg
Beef, liver, 3 oz.	1,240
Oysters, cooked, 6 med.	374
Chocolate, semisweet, 1 cup	176
Mushrooms, shiitake, cooked, 1 cup	130
Cashews, dry roasted, 1 oz.	70
Peas, black-eyed, cooked, 1/2 cup	70
Soybeans, boiled, 1 cup	70
Beans, white, canned, 1 cup	60
Sunflower seeds, 1/4 cup	59
Chickpeas, cooked, 1 cup	57
Baked beans, with pork, 1 cup	54
Lentils, cooked, 1 cup	50
V-8 juice, canned, 1 cup	48
Potato skin, baked, 1	47
Raisins, seedless, 1 cup	46
Salmon, baked, 3 oz.	30

AI = Adequate Intake
mcg = microgram

(Illustration by GGS Information Services. Cengage Learning, Gale)

deficiency has been associated with high cholesterol levels.

- Is necessary for normal functioning of insulin. Copper deficiency is also associated with poor blood glucose control.

- Is needed for normal functioning of the cardiovascular system.

- Protects the structure and function of the nervous system, including the brain. Copper protects nerve fiber by maintaining myelin, the insulating sheath that surrounds nerve cells. It also aids the transmission of nerve signals in the brains.

General use

Copper supplements may be beneficial in treating or preventing copper deficiency. Copper deficiency used to be relatively rare because the body requires so little of it, only about 2 mg per day. In addition, it is available naturally in a variety of foods such as whole grains, shellfish, nuts, beans, and leafy vegetables. Additional sources of copper are the copper water pipes that run through homes or the copper cookware in the kitchen. These sources leach copper into the water we drink and the food we eat. The level of copper in drinking water is sometimes so high that it becomes a public concern. However, scientists now realize that copper deficiency, especially borderline cases, is more common than once thought. Copper deficiency is currently on the rise due to a decrease of whole foods in the diet and high consumption of fatty and processed foods.

Studies have showed that vegetarian **diets** generally contain more copper than diets of omnivores but that the absorption efficiency is lower for lacto-ovo vegetarians than for nonvegetarians. Since vegetarians ingest more copper, however, the lower efficiency is not a problem in the diet of vegetarians.

Besides dietary causes, certain diseases or conditions may reduce copper absorption, transport, or increase its requirements, resulting in abnormally low copper blood levels. Increased copper intake through diet or supplementation may be necessary in the following conditions:

- premature infants fed only cow's milk
- pregnant women
- malnutrition
- celiac disease, sprue, cystic fibrosis, or short-bowel syndrome (these diseases cause poor absorption of dietary copper)
- kidney disease
- high consumption of zinc or iron (these minerals interfere with copper absorption)
- highly processed foods (copper is stripped away during food processing)
- Menkes syndrome (copper deficiency caused by genetic defects of copper transport). Menkes syndrome patients cannot efficiently use copper supplied by the diet.

Symptoms of copper deficiency include:

- anemia
- malnourished infants
- prominently dilated veins
- pale hair or skin
- poorly formed bones
- nervous system disorders
- high cholesterol levels

- heart disease
- loss of taste
- increased susceptibility to infections
- infertility
- birth defects

Exceeding the daily requirement of copper is dangerous, however, because copper toxicity tends to occur. Copper toxicity is a very serious medical problem. Acute toxicity due to ingestion of too much supplement, for example, may cause **nausea**, **vomiting**, abdominal **pain**, **diarrhea**, **dizziness**, **headache**, and a metallic taste in the mouth. Chronic toxicity is often caused by genetic defects of copper metabolism, such as Wilson's disease. In this disease, copper is not eliminated properly and accumulates to toxic levels. Copper is, therefore, present at high concentration where it should not be, such as in the liver, the lens of the eye, kidneys, and brain.

Disease prevention

Copper is a good antioxidant. It works together with an antioxidant enzyme, superoxide dismutase (SOD), to protect cell membranes from being destroyed by free radicals. Free radicals are any molecules that are missing one electron. Because this is an unbalanced and unstable state, a radical acts in such a way as to complete its electron pair. Therefore, it reacts with any nearby molecules to either steal an electron or give away the unpaired electron. In the process, free radicals initiate chain reactions that destroy cell structures. Like other **antioxidants**, copper scavenges or reacts with these highly reactive radicals and changes them into inactive, less harmful forms. Therefore, it can help prevent **cancer**. In 2001, a study reported that concentrations of copper sulfate and ascorbate may inhibit **breast cancer** growth. With further study, the combination may even prove useful as a chemotherapy agent for certain breast cancer patients.

Copper may also help prevent degenerative diseases or conditions such as premature **aging**, **heart disease**, autoimmune diseases, arthritis, **cataracts**, **Alzheimer's disease**, or diabetes.

Osteoporosis

Copper may play a role in preventing **osteoporosis**. **Calcium** and **vitamin D** have long been considered the mainstay of osteoporosis treatment and prevention. However, one study has shown that they can be even more effective in increasing bone density and preventing osteoporosis if they are used in combination with copper and two other trace minerals, **zinc** and **manganese**.

Rheumatoid arthritis

Copper has been a folklore remedy for **rheumatoid arthritis** since 1500 B.C. in ancient Egypt. Some people believe that wearing jewelry made of copper may relieve arthritic symptoms. Some researchers have attempted to verify the use of copper bracelets as a treatment for rheumatoid arthritis, but without success. Most studies show no effect at all, and the few that do were so poorly designed as to be of little use.

Preparations

Copper is contained in many multivitamin/mineral preparations. It is also available as a single ingredient in the form of tablets. These tablets should be swallowed whole with a cup of water, preferably with meals, to avoid stomach upset. A person may choose any of the following preparations: copper gluconate, copper sulfate, or copper citrate. However, copper gluconate may be the least irritating to the stomach.

Zinc and copper compete with each other for absorption in the gastrointestinal tract. As a result, excessive copper intake may cause zinc deficiency and vice versa. Therefore, a person should take zinc and copper supplements together in ratios of 10:1 or 15:1.

Precautions

Individuals who add copper supplements to their diets should consider the following precautions:

- Informing their doctors in order to gain proper instruction and monitoring of side effects. Copper toxicity due to excessive doses of copper supplements has been reported.
- Considering that recommended daily allowance (RDA) for copper varies with age and sex. It ranges from about 200 mcg/day for infants under the age of one year to 900 mcg/day for adult males and females. The RDA for pregnant and lactating women is 1,000 mcg/day and 1,300 mcg/day, respectively. Nausea and vomiting may occur in persons taking more than 20 mg of copper daily.
- It is not known if copper supplementation may harm a fetus. However, as with any drugs, pregnant or nursing women should not take copper or any other supplements or drugs without first consulting their doctors.
- In certain areas, drinking water may contain high levels of copper. Periodic checks of copper levels in drinking water may be necessary.

- Because individual antioxidants often work together to defend the body against free radicals, the balance among copper, zinc, and iron must be maintained. Excessive intake of one nutrient might result in a deficiency of other minerals and decreased resistance to infections and increased risk of heart disease, diabetes, arthritis, and other diseases.

Side effects

A person should stop taking copper supplements and seek medical help immediately if any of the following signs or symptoms occurs:

- anemia
- nausea
- vomiting
- abdominal pain

Interactions

Factors that increase copper concentrations

Certain disorders have been known to increase copper levels. Persons with these conditions should not take copper supplements as they may cause copper toxicity.

- recent heart attacks
- lupus erythematosus
- cirrhosis of the liver
- schizophrenia
- leukemia and some other forms of cancer
- viral infections
- ulcerative colitis (This inflammatory bowel disease may cause accumulation of copper in the body. Excessive amount of copper may worsen many

symptoms of this disease by increasing susceptibility to infections and inhibiting wound healing.)

- Wilson's disease (This disease causes accumulation of copper in the tissues. As a result, patients have liver disease, mental retardation, tremor, and poor muscle coordination. They also have copper deposits in the cornea of the eye. To manage this disease, patients are put on a low-copper diet and given penicillamine, a drug that attaches itself to copper and increases its excretion.)

Resources

BOOKS

Haas, Elson M., and Buck Levin. *Staying Healthy with Nutrition, 21st Century Edition: The Complete Guide to Diet & Nutritional Medicine.* Berkeley, CA: Celestial Arts, 2006.

Kirschmann, John D. *Nutrition Almanac.* New York: McGraw-Hill, 2006.

PERIODICALS

Ferrari, Carlos K. B. "Minerals: From Basic Aspects to Newly Discovered Physiological and Nutritional Actions." *Evidence-Based Integrative Medicine* 2, no. 3 (2005): 123–131.

Lamb, David J., et al. "Dietary Copper Supplements Modulate Aortic Superoxide Dismutase, Nitric Oxide, and Atherosclerosis." *International Journal of Experimental Pathology* (August 2005): 247–255.

Lynes, Michael A., et al. "Heavy Metal Ions in Normal Physiology, Toxic Stress, and Cytoprotection." *Annals of the New York Academy of Sciences* (October 2007): 159–172.

Qureshi, G. Ali, et al. "The Emerging Role of Iron, Zinc, Copper, Magnesium, and Selenium and Oxidative Stress in Health and Diseases." *Biogenic Amines* (September 2005): 147–169.

Stern, Bonnie Ransom, et al. "Copper and Human Health: Biochemistry, Genetics, and Strategies for Modeling Dose-response Relationships." *Journal of Toxicology and Environmental Health, Part B: Critical Reviews* (April 2007): 157–222.

Mai Tran
Teresa Norris
David Edward Newton, Ed.D.

Coptis

Description

Coptis is the underground stem (rhizome) or root of the plant *Coptis chinensis*. It is used in **traditional Chinese medicine** as a stomachic (a medication to

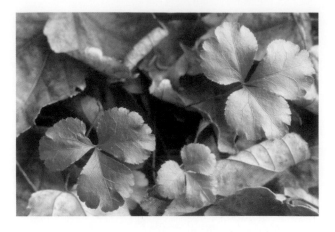

Coptis is used in traditional Chinese medicine as a stomachic (a medication to improve digestive functions) and an antiseptic. *(© Ross Frid / Alamy)*

improve digestive functions) and an antiseptic. Other related species are also called coptis and used in similar ways in other parts of the world. *Coptis anemonaefolia* is used in Japan. *Coptis trifolia* is used in North America, and *Coptis teeta* grows in India and is used in **Ayurvedic medicine**.

Coptis is a low, creeping perennial evergreen that grows in damp boggy spots in woods. The plant produces a mass of thread-like golden rhizomes that are used in healing. *C. chinensis* is native to the cooler parts of Asia and is extensively cultivated in Szechwan province in China. *C. trifolia* is native to eastern North America as far south as the mountains of Tennessee. Other names for the various species of coptis used in healing include goldthread, Chinese goldthread mouth root, cankerroot, yellowroot, coptidis, mishmi bitter, and chonlin. The Chinese name for *C. chinensis* is *huang lian*.

General use

Coptis, or *huang lian*, has a long history of use in China. In traditional Chinese medicine (TCM), coptis is used to treat conditions associated with excess dampness and excess heat, such as **insomnia** and irritability. Heat in TCM means excessive activity, not high temperature, although the diseased part of the body could be red or inflamed. Coptis is said to have a cold nature and a bitter taste. In TCM, coptis is considered one of the 50 fundamental herbs. It is associated with the heart, liver, stomach, and large intestine.

More specifically, coptis is used to treat such gastrointestinal problems as **diarrhea**, **vomiting**, and bacterial dysentery. It is also used to treat chronic gall bladder inflammations. Other gastrointestinal

KEY TERMS

Berberine—A white or yellow water-soluble alkaloid with antibacterial properties. Coptis, goldenseal, and barberry are all plants that contain berberine.

Hemostatic—A type of medication that is given to stop bleeding.

Rhizome—A rootlike underground plant stem that typically produces new shoots from its upper surface and new roots from the lower one. Coptis rhizomes are the parts of the plant most commonly used for medicinal purposes.

Stomachic—A type of medication that is given to tonify the stomach or improve digestive functions.

Tincture—An alcohol-based extract prepared by soaking plant parts.

conditions treated with coptis include abdominal cramps, acid reflux (**heartburn**), ineffective or painful bowel movements, and bloody stools. Coptis is effective as a hemostatic, which means that it can be used to stop bleeding.

Chinese herbalists also use preparations made from coptis to relieve high **fever** and delirium. These preparations can be used as a gargle to relieve sore throats. Externally coptis can be used as a mouthwash to treat all kinds of mouth sores, including **canker sores**, tongue ulcers, and swollen gums. As an eyewash it is used for **conjunctivitis** (pink eye). On the skin it is used topically to treat **acne**, **boils**, carbuncles, **burns**, and infected **cuts**.

C. triflora is used in North America in some similar ways. In an interesting parallel, some Native American tribes used their native species of coptis as a wash for eye and mouth problems in much the same way as the Chinese. It was also used as a gargle for sore throats. Although it is not as popular in North America as in China, modern North American herbalists use coptis to treat **indigestion**. It is also used externally as a douche to treat vaginal **infections**. The herb is used in similar ways in India.

Modern scientific research supports many of the traditional uses of coptis. All species of this herb contain the compound berberine, which is a white or yellow water-soluble alkaloid. Berberine is known to have strong antibiotic effects. In test tube studies, berberine was shown to inhibit the growth of streptococcal bacteria responsible for some forms of **pneumonia**. This antibacterial activity supports the use of coptis to treat skin, mouth, eye, and vaginal infections.

Berberine also is known to stimulate the production of saliva, gastric juice, pancreatic juice, and bile, suggesting that there is a chemical basis for the traditional use of coptis in treating gastrointestinal disorders. Berberine is also found in such other healing plants as **goldenseal**, **barberry**, and Oregon grape. Preliminary test tube studies of berberine suggest that it may also be effective against **fungal infections**, some viruses, and certain intestinal parasites. The high level of interest in berberine in the research community means that more studies of coptis may soon be available.

Preparations

The rhizomes and roots of coptis are harvested in the autumn and are used either dried or fresh. The herb is available powdered or as a tincture. The dosage varies according to the condition being treated. The actions of coptis are similar to the actions of goldenseal (*Hydrastis canadensis*), and it is sometimes substituted for goldenseal in herbal remedies.

In Chinese herbalism, coptis is rarely used alone, but can be found as an ingredient in many formulas. These include hoelen and polyphorus, leonoris and achyranthes, tang gui and **gardenia**, and at least half a dozen other formulas.

Precautions

Berberine is known to cause contractions of the uterus in laboratory animals. For this reason, it is recommended that pregnant women not take coptis or any other herb containing berberine.

Side effects

No unwanted side effects have been reported when coptis is used in the amounts recommended by herbalists.

Interactions

Coptis is has been used for thousands of years in China in conjunction with other herbs with no reported interactions. Since coptis is used most extensively in Asian medicine, there are no studies of its interactions with Western pharmaceuticals.

Resources

BOOKS

Chevallier, Andrew. *Encyclopedia of Medicinal Plants.* New York: DK Publishing, Inc., 1996.

Molony, David. *Complete Guide to Chinese Herbal Medicine*. New York: Berkeley Books, 1998.

PDR for Herbal Medicines. Montvale, NJ: Medical Economics Company, 1999.

ORGANIZATIONS

American Association of Oriental Medicine (AAOM). 433 Front Street, Catasauqua, PA 18032. (610) 266-2433.

OTHER

"Coptis chinensis." Plants for a Future. http://www.pfaf.org.

Tish Davidson

Cordyceps

Description

Cordyceps sinensis, also called Chinese caterpillar fungus, Cs-4, *Dong Chong Xia Caoor*, or *semitake*, is a fungus native to the Tibetan plateau in China. The fungus is parasitic and grows in the moth caterpillar. Spores enter the host, germinate, and ultimately kill the larva. Although species of cordyceps are seen in Europe and the Americas, only the Chinese form has been used medically.

General use

Cordyceps has a long history of use in Chinese medicine. Its traditional roles have been restorative; improving the quality of life, and increasing energy and longevity.

Traditional uses of the thousand year "rejuvenation" herb include the following:

- impotence treatment
- increase fertility
- stimulate immune system
- improve resistance to bacteria
- increase resistance to viruses
- relieve fatigue
- vitality tonic for mind and body, especially in aging men

While most of the cordyceps research has been conducted in China, published studies in Europe and elsewhere indicate that the fungus may have many potentially useful properties. A Korean study of a related species of cordyceps indicates that it has components that may inhibit coagulation, making it potentially beneficial in **stroke** and **heart attack** prevention. A hot water extract of the fungus appeared

to stimulate the immune system. This immune modulation effect is seen in other studies, which have reported that cordyceps may be useful in treating **Hepatitis** B. A study from Thailand reported that *Cordyceps nipponica* may have value in the treatment of **malaria**. Additional studies have indicated its possible benefit in preventing a recurrence of Lupus nephritis. However, another study that looked at herbs used as performance enhancers (to improve **exercise** and athletic performance), was unable to validate cordyceps' value for this purpose.

Another review concluded that cordyceps may be promising as a possible aid for **fatigue**, **stress**, heart health, lung function, and toxin exposure.

Cordyceps has physiological properties and benefits if used over time as a tonic, but taking it for a specific disease or problem remains an area needing further human studies and research. The traditional use of cordyceps was as an ongoing daily tonic, beginning in mid-life.

Preparations

Cordyceps capsules are available in varying strengths (400 mg, 450 mg, 615 mg, and 800 mg). The liquid preparation is sold in 1 gram per 1.5 ml strength.

Precautions

Cordyceps appears to be an exceptionally safe product with no established toxic dose. In 1996, there were two reports of cordyceps products contaminated with lead, but this does not appear to be an ongoing problem.

There is a risk of allergic reaction to either the fungus or other ingredients in the formulation.

Formulations of cordyceps are not standardized. Products are labeled in terms of the quantity of dried fungus contained, but there is no way to determine the amount of active components in any product. Because of this, activity may vary between brands and between individual samples from the same company.

Side effects

Side effects appear to be mild. Patients have reported stomach upset, **dry mouth**, and **nausea**.

Interactions

At this time, the only established interaction is due to the anticoagulant effects of the fungus, which may increase the risk of bleeding in patients taking warfarin (commonly known by the brand name Coumadin) or other anticoagulant drugs.

Because of the many different activities that have been attributed to cordyceps, it seems likely that other drug interactions will be reported in the future.

Resources

BOOKS

Jones, K. *Cordyceps: Tonic Food of Ancient China.* New Mexico: Sylvan, 1997.

PERIODICALS

Bucci, L. R. "Selected Herbals and Human Exercise Performance." *American Journal of Clinical Nutrition* (August 2000): 624S–36S.

Chen, Y. J., M. S. Shiao, S. S. Lee, and S. Y. Wang. "Effect of Cordyceps sinensis on the Proliferation and Differentiation of Human Leukemic U937 Cells." *Life Science* (1997): 2349–59.

Der Marderosian, A., Beutler, et al., editors. "Review of Natural Products." *Facts & Comparisons* (February 2004).

Isaka, M., M. Tanticharoen, P. Kongsaeree, and Y. Thebtaranonth. "Structures of Cordypyridones A-D, Antimalarial N-hydroxy- and N-methoxy-2-pyridones from the Insect Pathogenic Fungus Cordyceps nipponica." *Journal of Organic Chemistry* (July 13, 2001): 4803–8.

Pegler, D. N., Y. J. Yao, and Y. Li. "The Chinese Caterpillar Fungus." *Mycologist* (February 8, 1994).

Wu, T. N., K. Yang, C. M. Wang, J. S. Lai, K. N. Ko, P. Y. Chang, and S. H. Liou. "Lead Poisoning Caused by Contaminated Cordyceps, a Chinese Herbal Medicine: Two Case Reports." *Science of the Total Environment* (April 5, 1996): 193–5.

Yu, K. W., K. M. Kim, and H. J. Suh. "Pharmacological Activities of Stromata of Cordyceps Scarabaecola." *Phytother Res* (March 17, 2003): 244–9.

Samuel Uretsky, Pharm.D.

Corns and calluses

Definition

A corn is an overgrowth of skin on a bony prominence, usually occurring on the feet and toes. It manifests as a rough and painful bump. A callus is a rough, thickened lump of dead skin that is usually painless. It may be found on the feet, the hands, or anywhere else there is repeated friction and pressure.

Description

Corns and calluses affect about 5% of the population of the United States. Women have corns more often than men, probably due to wearing ill-fitted shoes more often. Although calluses may form anywhere on the body, they are generally found on the heels and balls of the feet, the knees, and the palms of the hands. Calluses are usually larger than corns—they may measure more than an inch (2.5 cm) wide. Calluses usually only hurt if pressure is applied to them.

Causes and symptoms

Corns and calluses form to prevent injury to skin that is repeatedly pinched, rubbed, or irritated. Hereditary calluses may develop where there is no apparent friction. This condition runs in families and occurs most often in children.

The most common causes of the formation of corns and calluses are:

- shoes that have very high heels and shoes that do not fit properly
- tight socks or stockings
- deformities of the toes
- walking or standing on a hard surface for an extended time
- jobs or hobbies that cause steady or recurring pressure on the same spot

Corns may be extremely sore and surrounded by inflamed, swollen skin. A sharp **pain** will probably occur whenever downward pressure is applied, and a dull ache may be felt at other times.

Diagnosis

Corns can be recognized on sight. They are sometimes mistaken for **warts**. However, if the lesion is a wart, it will bleed when scraped with a sharp implement. A callus will not bleed, but will shed a layer of dead skin. This can provide the basis of a general diagnosis.

Treatment

Standing and walking correctly can sometimes eliminate excess foot pressure and minimize the development and recurrence of corns and calluses. Bodywork systems such as **Aston-Patterning**, the **Feldenkrais** method, and **rolfing**, may help to correct body imbalances that lead to corns and calluses.

Two or three daily applications of **calendula** (*Calendula officinalis*) salve can soften skin and prevent inflammation. A mixture of one teaspoon of lemon juice, one teaspoon of dried **chamomile** (*Martricaria recutita*), and one crushed **garlic** clove (*Allium sativa*) can be applied directly to dissolve thickened skin.

A recommended Ayurvedic remedy is the nightly application of a paste made by combining one teaspoon of **aloe** vera gel with one half teaspoon of **turmeric** (*Curcuma longa*). The corn or callus should be covered with the paste and bandaged overnight. It should be soaked in warm water for 10 minutes every morning, and given a daily massage with mustard oil (*Brassica cruciferae*).

Allopathic treatment

The attention of a physician may be required if there is numbness, reduced feeling, or severe pain. Occasionally, an orthopedist may have to perform surgery to correct toe deformities or remove bits of bone that may be causing corns or calluses to develop. Medical attention is not usually required unless **diabetes mellitus**, poor circulation, or other problems make self-care difficult. The first step in home care of corns and calluses is to identify and eliminate sources of pressure and friction. Doughnut-shaped pads, wads of cotton, lamb's wool, or other kinds of inserts can be used to cushion affected areas. Soaking the feet in a solution of Epsom salts, or using hydrocortisone creams, petroleum jelly, or lanolin lotions can soften calluses. After which, they can be reduced or removed by rubbing the area with a pumice stone. This is not recommended for corns, however, as rubbing just makes them more painful.

It is important to consult with a healthcare provider if there is broken skin because it may become infected. In the case of an infection, affected layers of skin need to be removed, and pus may need to be drained. Oral antibiotics may be given to eliminate the infection. Cortisone may be injected into the affected area to decrease pain or inflammation.

Expected results

Most corns and calluses disappear within three weeks after the pressure that caused them is eliminated. However, if the causes of the condition are not remedied completely, or are allowed to recur, the corns and calluses may return. If there is continual pain associated with corns, it can change the way a person stands or walks. Such changes may eventually cause pain and dysfunction in the ankles, back, hips, or knees.

If a corn develops near a toe joint, **bursitis** may result, causing severe pain and inflammation. If cracks or other breaks in the skin develop, a staph infection may result. This is especially serious for people who have diabetes or poor circulation, as **gangrene** may develop from a resistant infection.

Prevention

Corns and calluses can usually be prevented by wearing shoes that fit properly. Feet should be measured, while standing, whenever buying new shoes. It is best to shop for shoes late in the day, when feet are likely to be swollen. It is also important to buy shoes with toe-wiggling room and to try new shoes on both feet. Pointy-toed shoes and high heels should be avoided. Worn down or uneven shoe soles and heels should be replaced or repaired. Corrective footwear or special insoles may be necessary. Socks and stockings should also be fitted appropriately at the feet. Gloves, kneepads, and other protective gear should be worn as needed to prevent rubbing and friction, especially when engaging in heavy work or sports activities. Cutting or paring dead skin should be avoided, as it may lead to further injury or infection.

Resources

BOOKS

Editors of Time-Life Books. *The Medical Advisor: The Complete Guide to Alternative and Conventional Treatments*. Alexandria, VA: Time-Life, 1996.

Gottlieb, Bill, ed. *New Choices in Natural Healing*. Emmaus, PA: Rodale Press, 1995.

ORGANIZATIONS

American Podiatric Medical Association. 9312 Old Georgetown Road, Bethesda, MD 20814-1698. http://www.apma.org.

Patience Paradox

Cornsilk

Description

Cornsilk (*Zea mays*) is an herbal remedy made from stigmas, the yellowish thread-like strands found inside the husks of corn. The stigmas are found on the female flower of corn, a grain that is also known as maize and is a member of the grass family (Gramineae or Poaceae). The stigmas measure 4–8 in (10–20 cm) long and are collected for medicinal use before the plant is pollinated. Cornsilk can also be removed from corn cobs for use as a remedy.

If fertilized, the stigmas dry and become brown. Then yellow corn kernels develop. Corn is native to North America and now grows around the world in warm climates.

Cornsilk is also known as mother's hair, Indian corn, maize jagnog, Turkish corn, yu mi xu, and stigmata maydis.

General use

Some historians believe that corn has grown for more than 7,000 years in North America. About the time that Christopher Columbus brought the first corn to Europe, the grain grew throughout North and South America. The venerable plant's stigmas have long been used in folk medicine to treat urinary conditions including inflammation of the bladder and painful urination.

Cornsilk also served as a remedy for heart trouble, **jaundice**, **malaria**, and **obesity**. Cornsilk is rich in

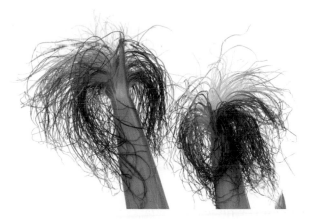

Cornsilk. *(Emilio Ereza / Alamy)*

vitamin K, making it useful in controlling bleeding during **childbirth**. It has also been used to treat **gonorrhea**.

For more than a century, cornsilk has been a remedy for urinary conditions such as acute and inflamed bladders and painful urination. It was also used to treat the prostate. Some of those uses have continued into modern times; cornsilk is a contemporary remedy for all conditions of the urinary passage.

Drinking cornsilk tea is a remedy to help children stop wetting their beds, a condition known as enuresis. It is also a remedy for urinary conditions experienced by the elderly.

Cornsilk is used to treat urinary tract **infections** and **kidney stones** in adults. Cornsilk is regarded as a soothing diuretic and useful for irritation in the urinary system. This gives it added importance, since today, physicians are more concerned about the increased use of antibiotics to treat infections, especially in children. Eventually, overuse can lead to drug-resistant bacteria. Also, these drugs can cause complications in children.

Furthermore, cornsilk is used in combination with other herbs to treat conditions such as cystitis (inflammation of the urinary bladder), urethritis (inflammation of the urethra), and parostitis (**mumps**).

Cornsilk is said to prevent and remedy infections of the bladder and kidney. The tea is also believed to diminish prostate inflammation and the accompanying **pain** when urinating.

Since cornsilk is used as a kidney remedy and in the regulation of fluids, the herb is believed to be helpful in treating high blood pressure and water retention. Cornsilk is also used as a remedy for **edema** (the abnormal accumulation of fluids).

Cornsilk is used to treat urinary conditions in countries including the United Sates, China, Haiti, Turkey, and Trinidad. Furthermore, in China, cornsilk as a component in an herbal formula is used to treat diabetes.

In addition, cornsilk has some nonmedical uses. Cornsilk is an ingredient in cosmetic face powder. The herb used for centuries to treat urinary conditions acquired another modern-day use. Cornsilk is among the ingredients in a product advertised to help people pass their drug tests.

Preparations

Some herbalists say that cornsilk is best used when fresh, but it is also available in dried form. Cornsilk can be collected from the female flower or from corn cobs. In addition, cornsilk is available commercially in powdered and capsule form and as an extract. Cornsilk is usually brewed as a tea, a beverage that is said to be soothing.

Cornsilk tea or infusion can be made by pouring 1 cup (240 ml) of boiling water over 2 tsp (2.5 g) of dried cornsilk. The mixture is covered and steeped for 10–15 minutes. The tea should be consumed three times daily.

In addition, a tincture of 1 tsp (3-6 ml) of cornsilk can be taken three times daily. Tincture can be purchased over the counter, or made at home by mixing the herb with water or alcohol at a ratio of 1:5 or 1:10.

Cornsilk is also available in capsule form. The usual dosage for 400-mg capsules is two capsules. These are taken with meals three times daily.

A remedy for bedwetting

Herbal remedies can be part of the treatment when children wet their beds. Methods of stopping this behavior include having the child **exercise** during the day, drink fewer beverages in the evening, and drink a cup of cornsilk tea one hour before bedtime. Cornsilk could be the only ingredient in the tea. However, cornsilk can be part of an herbal combination if **bedwetting** is caused by lack of nervous control of the bladder.

Cornsilk combinations

Cornsilk combines well with other herbs to remedy a range of urinary conditions. One remedy for a bed-wetting tea is to combine one part of cornsilk, **St. John's wort**, **horsetail**, **wild oat**, and **lemon balm**.

An herbal practitioner can recommend other combination remedies to treat more complicated conditions. For example, when a person has cystitis, cornsilk can be combined with **yarrow**, **buchu**, couchgrass, or bearberry.

Furthermore, cornsilk may be an ingredient in a commercial remedy taken to maintain the urinary tract system. Other ingredients could include yarrow and **marsh mallow**.

Precautions

Cornsilk is safe when taken in proper dosages, according to sources including *PDR (Physician's Desk Reference) for Herbal Medicines*, the 1998 book based on the findings of Germany's Commission E. The commission published its findings about herbal remedies in a 1997 monograph.

Before beginning herbal treatment, people should consult a physician, practitioner, or herbalist. Herbs like cornsilk are not regulated by the U.S. Food and Drug Administration (FDA), a process that involves research and testing.

If a person decides to collect fresh cornsilk, attention should be paid to whether the plants were sprayed with pesticides.

Side effects

There are no known side effects when cornsilk is taken in designated therapeutic dosages.

Interactions

Information is not available about whether there is an interaction when cornsilk is taken with medication. People taking medications should first check with their doctor or health practitioner before using cornsilk.

Resources

BOOKS

Duke, James A. *The Green Pharmacy*. Emmaus, PA: Rodale Press, Inc., 1997.

Keville, Kathi. *Herbs for Health and Healing*. Emmaus, PA: Rodale Press, Inc., 1996.

Medical Economics Staff. *PDR for Herbal Medicines*. Montvale, NJ: Medical Economics Company, 1998.

Ritchason, Jack. *The Little Herb Encyclopedia*. Pleasant Grove, UT: Woodland Health Books, 1995.

Squier, Thomas Broken Bear with Lauren David Peden. *Herbal Folk Medicine*. New York: Henry Holt and Company, 1997.

PERIODICALS

Edney, Mark T, et al. "Putting Antimicrobials to Best Use in Pediatric Urology." *Contemporary Urology* (July 2002): 35–39.

ORGANIZATIONS

American Botanical Council. P.O. Box 201660, Austin, TX 78720. (512) 331-8868. http://www.herbalgram.org/.

Herb Research Foundation. 1007 Pearl St., Suite 200, Boulder, CO 80302. (303) 449-2265. http://www.herbs.org.

OTHER

HealthWorld Online. http://www.healthy.net (January 17, 2001).

Holistic Online. http://www.holisticonline.com (January 17, 2001).

Liz Swain
Teresa G. Odle

Cornus

Description

Cornus (*Cornus officinalis*) is a tree of the dogwood family used in Chinese medicine. Its Chinese name is *shan zhu yu*. Cornus grows to a height of 30 ft (10 m) in the woodland regions of East Asia from China to Korea. The fruit is used in healing. It is harvested when ripe, then dried for future use. The small fruits can also be eaten as food, either raw or cooked. They contain about 8.6% sugar and have a slightly astringent taste. The bark from the stem is also used as an anti-malarial tonic.

Chinese cornus should not be confused with the North American tree *Cornus florida*, better known as dogwood or American boxwood. Dogwood and Chinese cornus are in the same plant family but have somewhat different healing properties. The bark of *Cornus florida* is used in Western herbal healing.

General use

Cornus has been used in China for more than 2,000 years. In the Chinese system of health, yin aspects must be kept in balance with yang aspects. Ill health occurs when the energies and elements of the body are out of balance or in disharmony. Health is restored by taking herbs and treatments that restore this balance.

Cornus is strongly associated with the kidneys, the reproductive system, and, to a lesser extent, the liver. It is made into a slightly warm yin tonic and classified as having a sour taste. In Chinese medicine sour herbs are believed to help control body fluids and conditions such as bed-wetting, excessive sweating, heavy or prolonged **menstruation**, and premature ejaculation.

Cornus is rarely used alone. It is an ingredient in many herbal formulas where it is used to stabilize and bind. It has astringent properties that are thought to boost the power of other herbs. Cornus can be combined with both yin and yang herbs to remedy deficiencies in either area because it conserves *jing*, the essence of life. In Chinese medicine jing, when referring to a man, means sperm. The ability to conserve jing is a result of the stabilizing and binding properties and the ability to control body fluids.

Although the results are not completely clear, some studies have shown that the fruit of cornus has antibacterial and antifungal properties. In some studies extracts of the fruit inhibited the growth of some **strains** of *Staphylococcus* bacteria. It may also be effective against *Salmonella* and *Shigella*, both bacteria that cause gastrointestinal disturbances. Chinese researchers also claim that cornus reduces the blood sugar level in animals, enhances immune system response, and increases sperm motility. Few scientific studies have been done on this herb outside of China.

Cornus fruit is also used in formulas that strengthen the back and knees, both areas associated with kidney jing. It is also used in formulas that control body fluids and treat excessive sweating, urine leakage, sperm leakage (spermatorrhea), and heavy, prolonged menstruation. Cornus is also an ingredient in formulas that treat ringing of the ears (**tinnitus**), poor hearing, **dizziness**, extreme shock, and a wide range of other conditions. The bark is boiled, and the resulting astringent decoction is used in formulas that treat fevers and as an anti-malarial. Interestingly, in **Western herbalism** the bark of dogwood, cornus's cousin, is also used against **malaria**. Cornus is also used to treat diabetes, arthritis, and **impotence**.

Preparations

Both cornus fruit and bark usually are prepared as a decoction that can be added to other tonics and healing formulas. They can also be prepared as a tincture. The dosage varies depending on the formula.

Some formulas that contain cornus include:

- eight immortal long life pill
- phellodendron
- supreme creation
- Buddha's yang
- dragon jing
- endocrine health
- essence restorative

Precautions

People experiencing painful or difficult urination should not use cornus.

Side effects

Since cornus is rarely used alone, it is difficult to separate any side effects it may cause from those caused by other herbs in the formula. No side effects specifically attributable to cornus have been reported.

Interactions

Cornus is has been used for thousands of years in conjunction with other herbs with no reported interactions. Since cornus is used almost exclusively in Chinese medicine, there are no studies of its interactions with Western pharmaceuticals, although it should not be used while taking a diuretic since cornus is an antidiuretic.

Resources

BOOKS

Bensky, Dan, et al.*Chinese Herbal Medicine: Materia Medica,* 3rd ed. Seattle, WA: Eastland Press, 2004.

PERIODICALS

Zhang YaJun and YunYan Goa. "Chemical Constituents of Asiatic Cornelian Cherry (*Cornus officinalis*) and Its Pharmaceutical Functions." *Chinese Journal of Information on Traditional Chinese Medicine* 9 no. 10 (2000): 81-82. http://www.cababstractsplus.org/google/abstract.asp?AcNo=20053161779.

ORGANIZATIONS

Alternative Medicine Foundation. P. O. Box 60016, Potomac, MD 20859. (301) 340-1960. http://www.amfoundation.org.

American Association of Oriental Medicine. PO Box 162340, Sacramento, CA 95816. (866) 455-7999 or (914) 443-4770 http://www.aaaomonline.org.

Centre for International Ethnomedicinal Education and Research (CIEER). http://www.cieer.org.

OTHER

"Cornus officinalis." *Plants for a Future.* [cited February 17, 2008]. http://www.pfaf.org/database/plants.php?Cornus+officinalis.

Tish Davidson, A. M.

Coronary artery disease *see* **Heart disease**

Coronary thrombosis *see* **Heart attack**

Corydalis

Description

Corydalis is the name of a group of herbs used in different parts of the world to relieve **pain**. *Corydalis yanhusuo* is a species used primarily in Chinese herbal medicine. *C. gariana*, native to the Himalayas, is used medicinally in India. A related species, *Corydalis cava*, is used in European herbalism. Another closely related species, is *Corydalis canadensis* (also called *Dicentra canadensis*) and known by the common name corydalis or turkey corn, is found in North America. There are other species of *Corydalis* found throughout the world. Although the names are somewhat confusing, many are used by herbal therapists in similar ways and are included under the umbrella label corydalis.

C. yanhusuo is a small herb that grows in mixed sun and shade at the edge of woodlands. It is native to Siberia, northern China, and Japan, but is cultivated in other cool parts of China. *C. yanhusuo* grows to about 8 in (20 cm) in height and has narrow leaves and pink flowers. The rhizome (underground stem) is used in healing. *C. yanhusuo* is called *yan hu suo* in Chinese. Some sources suggest that *C. yanhusuo* is used interchangeably with the related species *C. solida*, which is called by the same Chinese name.

C. cava is a perennial that grows in shady forests. It is native to southern Europe and has spread throughout the continent. *C. cava* grows to a height of about 11 in (30 cm). Its flowers range in color from red to yellowish to white, with occasional lilac, brownish-red, or dark blue flowers. The tubers (knobby, fleshy underground stems) are used medicinally. Alternative names for the North American species of corydalis include turkey corn, squirrel corn, and early fumitory.

KEY TERMS

Corydaline—An alkaloid derived from corydalis that has some effectiveness as a pain reliever.

Decoction—A liquid made by simmering an herb in water and then straining it.

Diuretic—A substance or medication that increases the production of urine.

Qi—In traditional Chinese medicine, the vital life force or energy that permeates the body.

Tincture—An alcohol-based extract prepared by soaking plant parts.

General use

In **traditional Chinese medicine** (TCM), *C. yanhusuo* is said to have a warm nature and a pungent, bitter taste. It is associated with the heart, liver, and spleen. *C. yanhusuo* is used to relieve pain resulting from almost any cause. It is especially used to treat menstrual cramps, chest pains, and abdominal pain. Corydalis is also the preferred herb in treating pain from traumatic injuries. Some herbalists report that frying corydalis in vinegar enhances its ability to ease pain.

Along with its ability to relieve pain, *C. yanhusuo* is used as a general aid to blood circulation and to promote the circulation of *qi*, or vital energy. Some Chinese herbalists also report using corydalis as a sedative and to lower blood pressure. The herb is frequently found in combination with other plants in Chinese formulas that treat stabbing pain sensations, painful periods, and the like.

In Western medicine, the various corydalis species are used to treat shaking and involuntary tremors. They can be used to treat people with **Parkinson's disease**. Corydalis is also used as a painkiller; a diuretic; a sedative that slows the pulse and depresses the central nervous system; and a tonic that invigorates the circulation. Occasionally it is used to treat mild forms of **depression**. In fact, the uses of the various corydalis species are surprisingly similar around the world.

Research scientists have isolated several potent alkaloid compounds from corydalis. The strongest of these is corydaline. It has the ability to block certain receptors in the brain associated with the sensation of pain. There is good evidence from Chinese studies that corydalis is effective in relieving pain and menstrual cramps. Evidence for the other uses of corydalis is limited to test tube and animal studies. One 1999 study at the University of Maryland Dental School found that an extract of *C. yanhusuo* was successful in reducing artificially induced inflammation in the paws of rats, although it was less successful than some other TCM herbs that were tested.

Preparations

Corydalis tubers and rhizomes are dug either in the spring or fall, before or after the leaves are actively growing. They are dried and kept in a cool place before use. Corydalis can be made into a tea, a tincture, or a decoction. Commercial extracts are also available.

Corydalis is usually combined with other herbs. One popular treatment for menstrual pain is a decoction of corydalis and cinnamon. In traditional Chinese medicine, corydalis is found in almost all formulas to treat menstrual pain, other pain formulas, and formulas to improve the circulation.

Precautions

Chinese herbalists report that pregnant women should not take corydalis. Since corydalis contains a compound that depresses the central nervous system, it should be used cautiously when using other central nervous system depressant drugs or alcohol. This herb should be taken under the supervision of a trained herbalist.

Side effects

Although no poisonings from corydalis have been reported, overdose is likely to produce shaking and tremors.

Interactions

Some Western herbalists report that corydalis is incompatible with tannic acid and vegetable astringents. Corydalis has been used in many Asian formulas without any reported interactions. Few, if any, scientific studies have been done on its interactions with Western pharmaceuticals.

Resources

BOOKS

Chevallier, Andrew. *Encyclopedia of Medicinal Plants*. New York: DK Publishing, Inc., 1996.

PDR for Herbal Medicines. Montvale, NJ: Medical Economics Company, 1999.

ORGANIZATIONS

American Association of Oriental Medicine (AAOM). 433 Front Street, Catasauqua, PA 18032. (610) 266-2433.

OTHER

"Corydalis." *Plants for a Future*. http://www.pfaf.org.

Tish Davidson

Cotton root bark

Description

Cotton root and the cotton plant are known as *Gossypium herbaceum*. Cotton is a member of the mallow or Malvaceae family. The cotton plant is an evergreen shrub that is native to Asia and Africa. It is also grown in the southern United States, Egypt, and countries along the Mediterranean Sea. The plant was cultivated to produce cotton fiber for clothing. Cotton root bark, the inner bark, and cotton seeds are all used as herbal remedies. While the seeds also served as a food, cotton root bark has been known for centuries as a "female medicine."

The herbal remedy is known as cotton root bark, *Gossypium herbaceum*, and cotton.

General use

Gossypium is the Latin word for cotton-producing plant, and this evergreen shrub has been cultivated for thousands of years in India. That form of cultivation was brought to China and Egypt in approximately 500 B.C. Europeans brought cotton cultivation to the New World in 1774.

Traditional uses

While *Gossypium herbaceum* was grown to produce cotton fiber, other parts of the plant served as medical remedies and food products. Cotton root bark was used as a folk remedy for numerous female conditions ranging from nonmenstrual bleeding from the uterus to inducing labor contractions. While it was used to make **childbirth** easier, cotton root bark was also taken as an abortifacient (to induce miscarriages).

Cotton root bark was not just a woman's remedy. Chewing on the roots was said to stimulate the sexual organs, giving cotton root the reputation of being an aphrodisiac. The root also had uses not related to reproduction. Cotton was also a remedy for conditions including snake bite, dysentery, and **fever**. Furthermore, cotton seed was once a food product and a remedy. A seed oil emulsion was given as an intravenous treatment for people with nutritional deficiencies.

Some of cotton root bark's remedial uses came to North America with the Africans enslaved by Europeans. Women used cotton bark root to stimulate menstrual flow and for help with difficulties during childbirth. Cotton had a different use when slave owners raped women; they drank cotton root tea to induce abortions.

Contemporary uses

Contemporary uses of cotton root bark cover nearly every aspect of the female reproductive system. Generally, a tea made from this herb is consumed to produce a normal menstrual cycle. Numerous other uses are listed in such sources as the *PDR (Physician's Desk Reference) for Herbal Medicines*, the 1998 book based on the findings of Germany's Commission E. The European group's findings about herbal remedies were published in a 1997 monograph.

Cotton root bark is used as an aid during childbirth and as a remedy for the absence of **menstruation**, irregular menstruation, and painful menstruation. Pregnant women take cotton root bark to increase uterine contractions, to expel the afterbirth, and to help with the secretion of milk. Cotton root bark is also taken for difficulties experienced during **menopause**.

Furthermore, cotton root bark is currently used as a male contraceptive in China because it is said to immobilize the sperm. Cotton root bark supposedly blocks production of sperm without affecting a man's potency. In June 2000, clinical trials were underway regarding this use of cotton root bark.

In addition, cotton root bark still has a reputation as an aphrodisiac. Evidence of this property of the herb, however, is anecdotal. No clinical research or studies have proven that cotton root bark stimulates or increases sexual desire.

In addition to the medicinal uses of cotton root, oil from cotton seed is currently used in soap and in the production of margarine, shortening, cooking oil, and salad oil.

Preparations

While cotton root bark was taken as a tea in folk medicine, other forms of the herb are used in contemporary alternative medicine. Cotton root bark is currently used as a liquid extract or a tincture. The dosage for both the tincture and liquid extract is 0.5–1 tsp (2–4 ml) of either solution. This amount can be divided into two daily doses; a single dose consists of 20–40 drops (0.25–0.5 tsp). The extract or tincture can be added to a small amount of water.

Cotton root bark can be combined with **goldenseal** (*Hydrastis canadensis*) in herbal preparations.

Precautions

Cotton root bark has varied uses, and opinions are varied about whether this remedy is safe to use. According to the *PDR for Herbal Medicines*, cotton root bark is safe when taken in therapeutic doses. Other herbalists state that no part of *Gossypium herbaceum* should be taken internally without first consulting with a doctor or health practitioner. This precaution is particularly important for pregnant women. Although cotton root bark is a remedy for conditions related to childbirth, manufacturers of herbal products advise women to seek medical advice before using it.

Although health risks have not been reported, poisonings have occurred when animals ate cottonseed cakes over a long period of time. Some of those cases were fatal.

In addition, gossypol is a chemical found in cottonseed oil that is believed to immobilize sperm. Men who cook with this oil may find themselves temporarily infertile.

Side effects

Cotton root bark has not been identified as producing side effects.

Interactions

There are no identified interactions associated with taking cotton root bark.

Resources

BOOKS

PDR for Herbal Medicines. Montvale, NJ: Medical Economics Co., 1998.

Ritchason, Jack. *The Little Herb Encyclopedia*. Pleasant Grove, UT: Woodland Health Books, 1995.

Squier, Thomas Broken Bear, with Lauren David Peden. *Herbal Folk Medicine*. New York: Henry Holt and Company, 1997.

ORGANIZATIONS

American Botanical Council. P.O. Box 201660, Austin TX, 78720. (512) 331-8868. http://www.herbalgram.org/.

Herb Research Foundation. 1007 Pearl St., Suite 200. Boulder, CO 80302. (303) 449-2265. http://www.herbs.org.

OTHER

Health Mall Online. http://www.healthmall.com.

Liz Swain

Cough

Definition

A cough is a forceful release of air from the lungs that can be heard. Coughing protects the respiratory system by clearing it of irritants and secretions.

Description

While people can generally cough at will, a cough is usually a reflex triggered when an irritant stimulates one or more of the cough receptors found at different points in the respiratory system. These receptors then send a message to the cough center in the brain, which in turn tells the body to cough. A cough begins with a deep breath in, at which point the opening between the vocal cords at the upper part of the larynx (glottis) shuts, trapping the air in the lungs. As the diaphragm and other muscles involved in breathing press against the lungs, the glottis suddenly opens, producing an explosive outflow of air at speeds greater than 100 mi (160 km) per hour.

In normal situations, most people cough once or twice an hour during the day to clear the airway of irritants. However, when the level of irritants in the air is high or when the respiratory system becomes infected, coughing may become frequent and prolonged. It may interfere with **exercise** or sleep, and it may also cause distress if accompanied by **dizziness**, chest **pain**, or breathlessness. In the majority of cases, frequent coughing lasts one to two weeks and tapers off as the irritant or infection subsides. If a cough lasts more than three weeks, it is considered a chronic cough, and physicians will try to determine a cause beyond an acute infection or irritant.

Coughs are generally described as either dry or productive. A dry cough does not bring up a mixture of mucus, irritants, and other substances from the lungs (sputum), while a productive cough does. In the case of a bacterial infection, the sputum brought up in a productive cough may be greenish, gray, or brown. In the case of an allergy or viral infection it

KEY TERMS

Antitussives—Drugs used to suppress coughing.

Expectorant—Drug used to thin mucus.

Gastroesophageal reflux—Condition in which stomach acid backs up into the esophagus.

Glottis—The opening between the vocal cords at the upper part of the larynx.

Larynx—A part of the respiratory tract between the pharynx and the trachea, having walls of cartilage and muscle, and containing the vocal cords.

Sputum—The mixture of mucus, irritants, and other substances expelled from the lungs by coughing.

may be clear or white. In the most serious conditions, the sputum may contain blood.

Causes and symptoms

In the majority of cases, coughs are caused by respiratory **infections**, including:

- colds or influenza, the most common causes of coughs
- bronchitis, an inflammation of the mucous membranes of the bronchial tubes
- croup, a viral inflammation of the larynx, windpipe, and bronchial passages that produces a bark-like cough in children
- whooping cough, a bacterial infection accompanied by the high-pitched cough for which it is named
- pneumonia, a potentially serious bacterial infection that produces discolored or bloody mucus
- tuberculosis, another serious bacterial infection that produces bloody sputum
- fungal infections, such as aspergillosis, histoplasmosis, and cryptococcoses

Environmental pollutants, such as cigarette smoke, dust, or smog, can also cause a cough. In the case of cigarette smokers, the nicotine present in the smoke paralyzes the hairs (cilia) that regularly flush mucus from the respiratory system. The mucus then builds up, forcing the body to removed it by coughing. Post-nasal drip, the irritating trickle of mucus from the nasal passages into the throat caused by **allergies** or sinusitis, can also result in a cough. Some chronic conditions, such as **asthma**, chronic **bronchitis**, **emphysema**, and cystic fibrosis, are characterized in part by a cough. A condition in which stomach acid backs up into the esophagus (gastroesophageal reflux) can cause coughing, especially when a person is lying down. A cough can also be a side effect of medications that are administered via an inhaler. It can also be a side effect of beta-blockers and ACE inhibitors, which are drugs used for treating high blood pressure.

Diagnosis

To determine the cause of a cough, a physician should take an exact medical history and perform an exam. Information regarding the duration of the cough, what other symptoms may accompany it, and what environmental factors may influence it aid the doctor in his or her diagnosis. The appearance of the sputum will also help determine what type of infection, if any, may be involved. The doctor may even observe the sputum microscopically for the presence of bacteria and white blood cells. Chest x rays may help indicate the presence and extent of such infections as **pneumonia** or **tuberculosis**. If these actions are not enough to determine the cause of the cough, a bronchoscopy or laryngoscopy may be ordered. These tests use slender tubular instruments to inspect the interior of the bronchi and larynx.

Treatment

Coughs due to bacterial or viral upper respiratory infections may be effectively treated with complementary therapies. The choice of remedy will vary and be specific to the type of cough the patient has. Lingering coughs or coughing up blood should be treated by a trained practitioner.

Nutrition & diet

Many health practitioners advise increasing fluid intake and breathing in warm, humidified air as ways of loosening chest congestion. Avoiding mucous-producing foods can be effective in healing a cough condition. These mucous-producing foods can vary, based on individual intolerance, but dairy products are a major mucous-producing food for most people. Other foods to avoid are sugar and foods high in **sodium**. Others recommend hot tea flavored with honey as a temporary home remedy for coughs caused by colds or flu.

Various vitamins may be helpful in preventing or treating conditions (including colds and flu) that lead to coughs. They include **vitamin C**, **vitamin E**, **zinc**, **vitamin A**, and **folic acid**.

Herbal medicine

There are many Western herbs, as well as herbs used in **traditional Chinese medicine** (TCM), that soothe the throat, quiet coughs, and act as expectorants. Some include:

- marsh mallow
- licorice
- aniseed
- fritillaria
- loquat

Homeopathic remedies

Depending on the type of cough and its duration, several homeopathic remedies include:

- Aconite for dry coughs with fever
- Antimonium tartaricum for productive coughs
- Bryonia for intense, dry coughs accompanied by thirst
- Drosera for violent coughing
- Rumex crispus for tickling coughs

Allopathic treatment

Treatment of a cough generally involves addressing the condition causing it. An acute infection such as pneumonia may require antibiotics, an asthma-induced cough may be treated with the use of bronchodialators, or an antihistamine may be administered in the case of an allergy. Cough medicines may be given if the patient cannot rest because of the cough or if the cough is not productive, as is the case with most coughs associated with colds or flu. The two types of drugs used to treat coughs are antitussives and expectorants.

Expected results

Because the majority of coughs are related to the **common cold** or **influenza**, most will end in 7-21 days. The outcome of coughs due to a more serious underlying disease depends on the pathology of that disease.

Prevention

It is important to identify and treat the underlying disease and origin of the cough. Avoid **smoking** and coming in direct contact with people experiencing cold or flu symptoms. Wash hands frequently during episodes of upper-respiratory illnesses.

Resources

BOOKS

The Burton Goldberg Group. *Alternative Medicine: The Definitive Guide.* Tiburon, CA: Future Medicine Publishing Inc., 1995.

Chandrasoma, Parakrama, and Clive R. Taylor. *Concise Pathology.* East Norwalk, CT: Appleton and Lange, 1991.

Schumann, Lorna. "Alterations in Respiratory Function." In *Perspectives on Pathophysiology.* Lee-Ellen Copstead, ed. Philadelphia: W.B. Saunders, 1994.

Time-Life Books Editors. *The Alternative Advisor.* Alexandria, VA: Time-Life Books, 1997.

PERIODICALS

Philp, Elizabeth B. "Chronic Cough." *American Family Physician* 56 (October 1, 1997).

ORGANIZATIONS

National Heart, Lung, and Blood Institute Information Center. P.O. Box 30105, Bethesda, MD 20824. (301)251-1222.

Coughwort *see* **Coltsfoot**

Crab lice *see* **Lice infestation**

Cradle cap

Definition

Cradle cap is a form of seborrheic **dermatitis**, a minor inflammatory disease of the scalp, face, and occasionally other areas of the body. It is a common scalp problem in infants and younger children.

Description

Cradle cap appears as thick, oily yellowish or brownish patches on the skin, particularly the scalp. It is also often found around the eyebrows, around the nose, behind the ears, and in the genital area. The skin itself often appears to be red, flaky, and irritated underneath the oily patches. It most often affects children who are between two weeks and two years old. Although cradle cap may be unsightly, it is usually not harmful to the child.

Causes and symptoms

During infancy and early childhood, the glands that produce sweat and oil are in a highly reactive state. Cradle cap is most likely due to a buildup of sweat and oil produced by these overactive glands. This buildup may also cause an irritation of the skin. Sometimes an overgrowth of the yeast called *Pityrosporum ovale* may also contribute to the condition. Occasionally, cradle cap is a symptom of more serious problems.

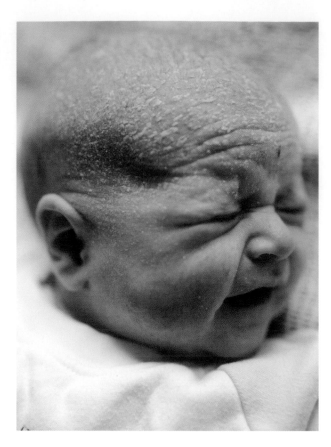

Newborn infant suffering from cradle cap, a form of seborrheic dermatitis, an itchy, flaky rash. *(Ian Boddy / Photo Researchers, Inc.)*

Diagnosis

Cradle cap is easily recognizable, and usually it requires no further diagnosis. However, if the rash seems to be very itchy or irritating, it may be necessary to rule out **eczema**. If there are additional symptoms, a healthcare provider should be consulted for a physical exam and possible testing.

Treatment

Most remedies for cradle cap can be applied directly to the oily patches on the skin. Tannins, for example, can help to slow down oil production, as well as clear away the cradle cap. Warm caffeinated tea, German **chamomile** tea (*Matricaria recutita*), burdock tea (*Arctium lappa*), or diluted **witch hazel** extract (*Hamamelis virginiana,*) can be rubbed into the skin with a cloth several times per day.

A **comfrey** rinse can also be used. It should be rubbed onto the affected area with a washcloth. The rinse can be used after shampooing or bathing, or it can be applied to dry skin. This treatment can be given

nightly for up to ten days until the symptoms are gone. The comfrey rinse can be made by boiling two ounces (about 57 grams) of comfrey root, *Symphytum officinale,* in one quart (or one liter) of water. The tea should be simmered for 20 minutes and then allowed to cool. A batch of the comfrey rinse can be used and stored in the refrigerator for up to four days.

A rule of thumb in science is that like dissolves like; therefore, any type of food grade oil can be used to dissolve the oily buildup found in cradle cap. Olive oil, **wheat germ** oil, and **sesame oil** are particularly favored. **Aromatherapy** may be used by adding in 1-2 drops of the essential oil of **lavender**, *Lavandula angustifolia*. The oil should be applied to the skin and left overnight. It can then be removed gently and slowly with a baby brush or a fine-tooth comb. The area should be washed or shampooed afterwards with a very mild soap.

Slippery elm (*Ulmus fulva*) is useful in soothing a variety of skin problems, and can be applied to affected areas several times per day. The herb can also be misted liberally with water or used as a tea. Ointments containing *Calendula officinalis* or **plantain** (*Plantago major*) are also appropriate to use on areas of cradle cap. These herbs can often clear up an outbreak in as little as four days.

Internal remedies for cradle cap can be quite effective. These include tincture of **burdock root**, which can help to balance oil and sweat production. Burdock is also a good general tonic to take to keep the skin healthy. Burdock should be given for at least three weeks for full effect. A tincture of the wild pansy flower, *Viola tricolor,* can also be given. **Biotin**, a B vitamin, works well for cradle cap and can be given at dosages of 10 micrograms (mcg) for age 0-6 months; 15 mcg for age 6-12 months, and 20 mcg for age one to three years.

Allopathic treatment

Generally, cradle cap does not need to be treated medically. If the condition is resistant to treatment or it starts spreading, however, an over-the-counter **dandruff** shampoo may be used once per day until the cradle cap has improved. Shampoos containing coal tar derivatives may be highly irritating and are not recommended for use on children under two.

A 0.5% or 1% hydrocortisone cream is available over-the-counter and can be applied two or three times per day to stubborn cases of cradle cap. If a *Pityrosporum ovale* infection is suspected, a dermatologist may prescribe ketoconazole (Nizoral) cream or shampoo.

These medications are strong and should be used for as short a time as possible.

If crusting, pus, redness, or **pain** are present, a physician should be consulted. There may be an underlying infection caused by the infant's scratching, which can introduce bacteria into the skin. Antibiotics may have to be prescribed. Other symptoms, such as poor growth or **diarrhea** may point to immune system problems requiring medical assessment and treatment.

Expected results

Usually cradle cap will eventually resolve with no aftereffects, even without treatment. However, it can take quite some time to clear. Most home remedies should clear up cradle cap in a few weeks or months.

Prevention

Washing the hair more often than two or three times per week may dry the skin out, making it more vulnerable to cradle cap, so limited hair washing is recommended.

Resources

BOOKS

Foley, Denise, et al. *The Doctors Book of Home Remedies for Children: From Allergies and Animal Bites to Toothache and TV Addiction, Hundreds of Doctor-Proven Techniques and Tips to Care for Your Kid.* Emmaus, PA: Rodale Press, 1999.

Kemper, Kathi J., M.D. *The Holistic Pediatrician.* New York: HarperPerennial, 1996.

OTHER

DermaMed Pharmaceutical Incorporated. http://www.dermamed.com/aboutscalp.htm (January 17, 2001).

Health World Online. http://www.healthy.net/asp/templates/book.asp?PageType = Book&ID = 787 (January 17, 2001).

Patience Paradox

Cramp bark

Description

Cramp bark (*Viburnum opulus*) is a deciduous tree or shrub that is native to Europe and the eastern United States. It is a member of the Caprifoliaceae family. It is also cultivated for use as an ornamental tree or shrub. Other names for cramp bark include guelder rose, snowball tree, king's crown, high **cranberry**, rose **elder**, water elder, Whitsun rose, May rose,

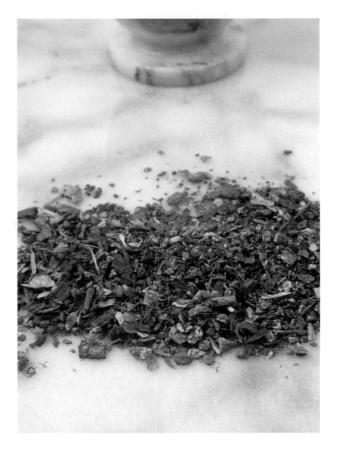

Dried cramp bark of the Viburnum opulus plant can be used to relieve menstrual, muscle and stomach cramps. *(Geoff Kidd / Photo Researchers, Inc.)*

dog rowan tree, Whitsun bosses, silver bells, and gaiter berries.

Cramp bark grows in low grounds, woodlands, thickets, and hedges. This large shrub grows 5-10 ft (1.5-3 m) tall. The flowers, which appear in spring and summer, are large (3-5 in [8-13 cm] across), flat-topped clusters of snow-white florets. The inner florets are very small, complete flowers while the florets along the outer edge of the cluster are large and showy but cannot produce fruit. The fruits, which appear in August, are drooping clusters of bright red oval shiny, translucent berries. Cramp bark berries are edible, but have a very bitter taste. The leaves of cramp bark are lobed and turn a rich purple color in the fall. The bark is grayish-brown, faintly cracked lengthwise, and has scattered brown-colored **warts**. The bark has a strong odor and a bitter, astringent taste.

Constituents and bioactivities

Cramp bark contains a wide variety of biologically active compounds. The constituents of cramp bark are very similar to those of a close relative called **black haw** (*Viburnum prunifolium*). Cramp bark and black haw may be used interchangeably under certain conditions but should not be considered interchangeable in the strict sense. The constituents of cramp bark include:

- acid compounds (acetic, baldrianic, capric, chlorogenic, cinnamic, citric, malic, ursolic, and valerianic)
- amyrins (alpha-amyrin and beta-amyrin)
- astragalin
- beta-sitosterol
- coumarins (scopoletin and scopoline)
- elements (aluminum, calcium, chromium, cobalt, iron, magnesium, manganese, phosphorus, potassium, selenium, silicon, sodium, tin, and zinc)
- esculetin
- glucosides (viburnine)
- glycosides (quercetin)
- hydroquinones (arbutin, methylarbutin, and free hydroquinone)
- myricyl alcohol
- paeoniside
- pectin
- protein
- resin
- tannins (catechin and epicatechin)
- viopudial

Cramp bark has antispasmodic (relieves **muscle spasms**), anti-inflammatory (relieves inflammation), nervine (calms and soothes the nerves), hypotensive (lowers blood pressure), astringent (causes local contraction), emmenagogic (induces **menstruation**), and sedative (reduces activity and excitement) properties. The berries of cramp bark have antiscorbutic (effective against scurvy) properties due to their **vitamin C** content.

General use

Historically, the Native American Meskwaki people used cramp bark to treat cramps and pains located anywhere in the body, whereas the Penobscot people used cramp bark to treat **mumps** and swollen glands. Cramp bark was named for its primary medicinal use—to relieve **muscle cramps** and other conditions caused by muscle overcontraction.

Cramp bark is presently used to relieve any overly tense muscle or muscle spasm of the body. This includes the muscles of the uterus, air passages, intestines, arms, legs, and back. In addition, it can be used to prevent muscle tension and **pain**. Cramp bark is

---

KEY TERMS

Antiscorbutic—An agent that is effective against scurvy, like the vitamin C found in cramp bark.

Astringent—A substance that constricts or binds skin cells.

Emmenagogue—A substance or medication given to bring on a woman's menstrual period.

Prophylactic—Use of a treatment to prevent a disease or condition before symptoms appear.

Sedative—A substance or medication used to soothe or reduce nervous irritation or overstimulation.

Tincture—An alcoholic solution prepared from herbal medicinal agents.

---

also used to treat symptoms that are associated with excess muscle tension, including menstrual pain (**dysmenorrhea**) caused by uterine muscle contractions, and breathing difficulties associated with **asthma**. **Colic**, spastic **constipation**, **irritable bowel syndrome**, and the physical indications of nervous tension are also treated with cramp bark.

Cramp bark has also been used to treat hysteria, nervous complaints, debility, convulsions, fits, lockjaw, heart palpitation, tension headaches, spasmodic stricture (narrowing of a passage), bladder muscle spasms, high blood pressure, rheumatism, circulatory problems, and **heart disease**. It is effective in treating cases of arthritis in which joint pain and weakness have led to severe muscle contractions. Cramp bark relaxes the muscles, allowing improvement in blood circulation that can return normal function to the arthritic joints.

Cramp bark is used to treat excessive blood loss during menstruation and **menopause**, and to induce menstruation in women with light or delayed periods. A woman may treat dysmenorrhea prophylactically (before symptoms appear) by taking cramp bark the day before painful menstruation is expected. Cramp bark is also used to treat **endometriosis** and threatened miscarriage.

In addition to its medicinal uses, cramp bark has a few culinary applications. Cramp bark berries have been used to make jelly and alcoholic beverages, and they are used in certain food dishes.

Preparations

The bark of cramp bark is peeled off the tree during the spring and summer months. The bark

---

should be peeled off in strips carefully in order not to kill the tree. The bark is chopped up and dried. Cramp bark can be made into a decoction (a water extract), a tincture (an alcoholic extract), or a lotion. Liquid preparations of cramp bark have a reddish-brown color, a slight odor, and an astringent taste.

The decoction is prepared by adding 2 tsp of the dried bark to 1 cup water. The mixture is brought to a boil, the heat is reduced, and the decoction is simmered gently for 10–15 minutes.

Although the recommended doses of the decoction are variable, it is safe to drink up to three cups daily. The dose of decoction for menstrual pain is 0.5 cup every three hours.

Tinctures are more concentrated and act faster (within 30 minutes) than teas or decoctions. The tincture may be taken for long-term conditions caused by muscular tension such as irritable bowel syndrome. Again, the recommended doses vary somewhat, but up to 8 ml may be taken three times a day. The suggested dose of tincture for irritable bowel syndrome is 0.5 tsp in hot water twice a day. The suggested dose of tincture for menstrual cramps is 1 tsp in water three times a day.

A lotion prepared from cramp bark may be rubbed into the skin to relieve painful muscles.

To relieve cramping and back pain at night, cramp bark may be mixed with **lobelia** (*Lobelia inflata*). Cramp bark may also be used with **Mexican yam** (*Dioscorea villosa*) for ailments of the gastrointestinal and genitourinary systems.

Precautions

Some sources state that the berries of cramp bark are toxic and should not be eaten.

Side effects

Cramp bark is safe for both short- and long-term use. In 2008, there were no indications that cramp bark causes any side effects. Pregnant women and women who are lactating (breast-feeding), however, should not use any herbal medicines without first consulting a physician.

Interactions

As of 2008, there were no indications of any interactions between cramp bark and any other drug or herbal medicine.

Resources

BOOKS

Chevallier, Andrew. *The Encyclopedia of Medicinal Plants.* New York: DK Publishing, Inc., 1996.

ORGANIZATIONS

American Botanical Council. P.O. Box 201660, Austin TX, 78720. (512) 331-8868. http://www.herbalgram.org/.
Herb Research Foundation. 1007 Pearl St., Suite 200, Boulder, CO 80302. (303) 449-2265. http://www.herbs.org.

OTHER

Alternative Medicine Foundation. *HerbMed.* http://www.am foundation.org/herbmed.htm.
"Cramp bark." Planet Botanic. http://www.planetbotanic.com/cramp.htm.

Belinda Rowland

Cranberry

Description

The cranberry plant, a familiar source of berries used in juices and relishes in the United States, has been in existence since the Iron Age. The Romans were the first to recognize its medicinal uses by the local inhabitants of what is now England. Herbalist Henry Lyte documented its healing effects in 1578. Since then, the cranberry plant has been a popular folk remedy for a variety of illnesses, including **gout**, rheumatism, **diarrhea**, **constipation**, scurvy, fevers, skin **infections** and other skin problems such as **eczema**. Cranberries are well known as a treatment for such women's health problems as cystitis, and urinary and genital infections.

Currently, there are approximately 150 species of cranberry. The best known and most popular is the American cranberry (*Vaccinium macrocarpon*), because of the size and juiciness of its fruit. It is a member of the Heath (*Ericaceae*) family. *Vaccinium macrocarpon* is a low-lying fruit plant grown commercially in North America. The shrub bears beautiful pink flowers that grow into rounded reddish-black berries. The berries are harvested early in the fall, and made into juices, jellies, or relishes. Juice made from cranberries is a popular, tart fruit drink. The United States presently produces about 98% of the world's cranberries.

Scientists have learned that the chemical composition of cranberries includes many substances that promote healing, such as:

- Proanthocyanidins and anthocyanins. These bioflavenoids make up the pigment of the leaves, and produce the color of the berries. More importantly, proanthocyanidins are responsible for cranberry's best-known medicinal effect, preventing bladder and urinary tract infections by inhibiting bacterial colonization. They may also help relieve diarrheal symptoms.

- Organic acids, including quinic, malic, and citric acids. Quinic acid is considered the most important among these organic acids. These compounds, which are responsible for the sour taste of cranberries, acidify the urine and prevent kidney stones.

- Vitamins and minerals. Cranberries are rich sources of vitamins including vitamin A, carotene, thiamine, riboflavin, niacin, and vitamin C. They also contain many essential minerals such as sodium, potassium, calcium, magnesium, phosphorus, copper, sulfur, iron, and iodide. These vitamins and minerals are strong antioxidants that enable cranberries to help protect the body against such infections as colds or influenza. Because of their high vitamin C content, cranberries were used in the past to prevent a vitamin C deficiency known as scurvy.

- Fiber. Like many other fruits, cranberries are a good source of fiber.

General use

Prevention and treatment of urinary tract infections

Urinary tract infections (UTIs) are extremely common in women, affecting one of every two females during their lifetime. Men have urinary infections as well, but less frequently than women. A woman contracts a urinary tract infection when bacteria gets into the relatively short female urethra and moves up to the bladder. Once in the bladder, the bacteria grow and spread to other parts of the urinary tract. If left untreated, UTIs can cause serious **kidney infections** that may require hospitalization. The disease is relatively easy to treat, but tends to recur.

In the United States, urinary tract infections result in more than five million medical treatment visits each year. The most frequently prescribed treatment for urinary tract infections is antibiotics. There are also simple self-protective measures that women can take against UTIs. These include:

- Drinking a lot of fluid, which increases the amount of urine produced and helps to flush out infectious microorganisms.

- Emptying the bladder immediately after having intercourse.

- Using oral contraceptives rather than a diaphragm, which tends to put pressure on or irritate the urethra.

- Drinking cranberry juice as a preventive measure for women. As early as the 1840s, German physicians observed that cranberry juice prevented urinary tract infections. This effect was attributed to the cranberry's high acidity.

Recent research has confirmed the effectiveness of cranberries in preventing UTIs. Two studies in the mid-1990s, one involving women 65 years or older and the other with younger women between the ages of 18 and 45, showed that cranberries are effective in preventing bladder infections. Regardless of age, women can significantly reduce their risk of urinary tract infections by consuming 10 ounces of cranberry juice daily. Scientists, however, have learned that the effectiveness of cranberry juice is not related to its acidity, as was previously believed. Researchers found that the cranberry's antibacterial properties come from its proanthocyanidins (or condensed tannins). Proanthocyanidins inhibit *chia coli* bacteria from attaching to the inside walls of the bladder, allowing them to be easily flushed out with urine before they multiply and cause infections.

A careful review of all studies involving the cranberry's role in preventing UTIs concluded that cranberry juice or concentrate is beneficial in preventing infections in women, but its benefits have not been proven in children or males. The reviewers also noted that many women did not complete the full one-year study period.

Prevention of kidney stones

Kidney stones are most often caused by high levels of ionized **calcium** (as in calcium salts) in the urine. Cranberries can help prevent this condition because they are rich in quinic acid, which increases the acidity of the urine. As a result, the levels of ionized calcium in the urine are lowered.

A person needs to drink 16 ounces of unsweetened cranberry juice (two glasses) daily to effectively prevent kidney stones. Cranberry capsules or powdered concentrates are also available. It is important not to consume too much cranberry, because very high acidity in the urine actually increases the risk of kidney stones. A person would need to drink at least one liter of cranberry juice per day for a prolonged period of time for this to occur.

Prevention of colds and influenza

A daily glass of cranberry juice is a good source of **vitamin C** and **antioxidants**. These nutrients help support the body's immune function and prevent **cancer** as well as such common infections as colds or **influenza**.

Other uses

Cranberries may serve as a digestive aid. Because of their high acidity, they help to digest fatty foods and to increase the appetite.

Some early laboratory studies suggest that cranberries may help to prevent gingivitis (**gum disease**) and coronary (heart) disease. These studies have not yet been confirmed by clinical research in humans.

Cranberry has been a folk remedy for diarrhea. Proponents of this use suggest that the proanthocyanidins in cranberries, in addition to having antibacterial activity, also act as astringents. They cause proteins to clump together to form rigid cakes that prevent bacteria from using the proteins for food. However, the effectiveness of cranberries in the treatment of diarrhea remains unproven.

Various cranberry preparations have also been used to treat skin disorders such as **acne**, **dermatitis**, and **psoriasis**; bed-wetting; **burns** and **wounds**; and **stress** and **depression**. There is currently insufficient scientific evidence to support these uses.

A recent study suggests that cranberry juice may inhibit the formation of dental plaque by preventing bacteria from collecting (coaggregating) on the tooth film formed by proteins in the saliva. These preliminary findings await further testing.

Preparations

There are many types of cranberry preparations available, partly because cranberry products are among the top 10 best sellers in the health food market. They include:

- Cranberry juice. For prevention of urinary tract infections and kidney stones, recommended products include those containing pure cranberry juice rather than mixtures that are only 25–27% cranberry juice. Four to six ounces of unadulterated cranberry juice daily is recommended for the prevention of UTIs. Some herbalists advocate the use of cranberry for treatment of mild urinary tract infections; dosages of 10–32 oz (0.3–1 kg) daily have been used. Cranberry juice may not be effective, however, for established infections. It should be taken only as a complementary measure rather than as an alternative to antibiotics in the treatment of active UTIs. If a woman experiences such symptoms of cystitis as chills, fever, fatigue, and burning pain during urination, she should contact her doctor immediately for antibiotic treatment.
- Dried cranberry powder capsules (475–500 mg). Because most commercial cranberry juice contains high levels of sugar, these capsules may be a better alternative for diabetic patients or dieters. Each capsule equals 0.5 ounces of cranberry juice. Nine to 15 capsules daily is the recommended dosage for the prevention of urinary tract infections.
- Powdered concentrates. These forms of cranberry are available in different strengths. Women should follow the dosages recommended by manufacturers.
- Fresh or dried cranberries. Dried untreated cranberries can be found in health food stores. They can be stored up to a year. Cranberries are also available fresh or frozen in most grocery stores or supermarkets. Because of their tartness, most people may find it difficult to consume them in sufficient quantity to obtain their therapeutic benefits.
- Cranberry herbal teas. These products can be obtained from health food stores or via the Internet.

Precautions

Cranberries should be used with care or modification in patients with certain diseases, including:

- Active urinary tract infections. Cranberries should not be substituted for antibiotic treatment, but used only as a supplementary therapy.

- Irritable bowel syndrome (IBS). Large quantities of cranberry juice or capsules may cause diarrhea in IBS patients.
- Diabetes. Patients with diabetes should use sugar-free cranberry juice, or take capsules or powdered concentrates.

Side effects

The most common side effects associated with excessive cranberry consumption are diarrhea and an increased risk of developing kidney stones.

Regular cranberry consumption by women trying to prevent UTIs may result in *vulvovaginal candidiasis*. Alterations in the normal vaginal bacteria may lead to increased fungal growth.

Interactions

There are no identified drug interactions associated with cranberry consumption.

Resources

BOOKS

Davies, Jill Rosemary. *Healing Herbs—In a Nutshell: CRANBERRY*. Boston: Element Books, Inc., 2000.

Fetrow, Charles W., and Juan R. Avila. *The Complete Guide to Herbal Medicines*. Springhouse, PA: Springhouse Corporation, 2000.

McCaleb, Robert, Evelyn Leigh, and Krista Morien. *The Encyclopedia of Popular Herbs: Your Complete Guide to the Leading Medicinal Plants*. Rocklin, CA: Prima Health, 2000.

Murray, Michael, and Joseph Pizzorno. *Encyclopedia of Natural Medicine*. Rocklin, CA: Prima Health, 1998.

PERIODICALS

Avorn J., M. Monane, J.H. Gurwitz, et al. "Reduction of Bacteriuria and Pyuria after Ingestion of Cranberry Juice." *Journal of the American Medical Association (JAMA)* 271 (1994): 751-4.

Jepson R., L. Mihaljevic, and J. Craig. "Cranberries for preventing urinary tract infection." *Cochrane Database Syst Rev* (2004).

Patel, D.A., B. Gillespie, J.D. Sobel, et al. "Risk factors for recurrent vulvovaginal candidiasis in women receiving maintenance antifungal therapy: Results of a prospective cohort study." *American Journal of Obstetrics and Gynecology* March (2004): 644–53.

Weiss, E.I., A. Kozlovsky, D. Steinberg, R., et al. "A high molecular mass cranberry constituent reduces mutans streptococci level in saliva and inhibits in vitro adhesion to hydroxyapatite." *FEMS Microbiol Lett* (March 2004): 89–92.

ORGANIZATIONS

American Association of Naturopathic Physicians. 601 Valley St., Suite 105, Seattle, WA 98109. (206) 298-0126. Fax: (206) 298-0129. http://www.naturopathic.org.

American Herbal Products Association. 8484 Georgia Ave., Suite 370, Silver Spring, MD 20910. (301) 588-1174. http://www.ahpa.org.

National Center for Complementary and Alternative Medicine (NCCAM). NCCAM Clearinghouse, PO Box 8218, Silver Spring, MD 20907-8218. (888) 644-6226. Fax: (301) 495-4957. http://nccam.nih.gov.

Samuel Uretsky, Pharm.D.

Cranial manipulation *see* **Craniosacral therapy**

Craniosacral therapy

Definition

Craniosacral therapy is a holistic healing practice that uses very light touching to balance the craniosacral system in the body, which includes the bones, nerves, fluids, and connective tissues of the cranium and spinal area.

Origins

The first written reference to the movement of the spinal nerves and its importance in life, clarity, and "bringing quiet to the heart" is found in a 4,000-year-old text from China. Craniosacral work was referred to as "the art of listening." Bone setters in the Middle Ages also sensed the subtle movements of the body. They used these movements to help reset **fractures** and dislocations and to treat headaches.

In the early 1900s, the research of Dr. William Sutherland, an American osteopathic physician, detailed the movement of the cranium and pelvis. Before his research it was believed that the cranium was a solid immovable mass. Sutherland reported that the skull is actually made up of 22 separate and movable bones that are connected by layers of tissue. He called his work cranial **osteopathy**. Nephi Cotton, an American chiropractor and contemporary of Sutherland, called this approach craniology. The graduates of these two disciplines have refined and enhanced these original approaches and renamed their work as sacro-occipital technique, cranial **movement therapy**, or craniosacral therapy.

Dr. John Upledger, an osteopathic physician, and others at the Department of Biomechanics at Michigan State University, College of Osteopathic Medicine learned of Sutherland's research and developed it further. He researched the clinical observations of various osteopathic physicians. This research provided the basis for Upledger's work which he named craniosacral therapy.

Benefits

According to Upledger, craniosacral therapy is ideally suited for **attention-deficit hyperactivity disorder**, headaches, chronic middle **ear infection**, **pain**, and general health maintenance. It is recommended for **autism**, **fibromyalgia**, **heart disease**, **osteoarthritis**, **pneumonia**, **rheumatoid arthritis**, chronic sinus **infections**, and **gastroenteritis** (inflammation of the lining of the stomach or small intestine). It is also used with other therapies to treat **chronic fatigue syndrome**, back pain, and menstrual irregularity. In addition, other craniosacral practitioners have reported benefits for eye dysfunction, **dyslexia**, **depression**, motor coordination difficulties, temporomandibular joint dysfunction (TMD), hyperactivity, **colic**, **asthma** in babies, floppy baby syndrome, whiplash, **cerebral palsy**, certain birth defects, and other central nervous system disorders.

Description

Craniosacral therapy addresses the craniosacral system. This system includes the cranium, spine, and sacrum which are connected by a continuous membrane of connective tissue deep inside the body, called the dura mater. The dura mater also encloses the brain and the central nervous system. Sutherland noticed that cerebral spinal fluid rises and falls within the compartment of the dura mata. He called this movement the primary respiratory impulse; today it is known as the craniosacral rhythm (CSR) or the cranial wave.

Craniosacral therapists can most easily feel the CSR in the body by lightly touching the base of the skull or the sacrum. During a session they feel for disturbances in the rate, amplitude, symmetry, and quality of flow of the CSR. A therapist uses very gentle touch to balance the flow of the CSR. Once the cerebrospinal fluid moves freely, the body's natural healing responses can function.

A craniosacral session generally lasts 30–90 minutes. The client remains fully clothed and lays down on a massage table while the therapist gently assesses the flow of the CSR. Upledger describes several techniques which may be used in a craniosacral therapy session. The first is energy cyst release. "This technique is a hands-on method of releasing foreign or disruptive energies from the patient's body. Energy cysts may cause the disruption of the tissues and organs were they are located." The therapist feels these cysts in the client's body and gently releases the blockage of energy.

Sutherland first wrote about a second practice called direction of energy. In this technique the therapist intends energy to pass from one of his hands, through the patient, into the other hand.

The third technique is called myofascial release. This is a manipulative form of bodywork that releases tension in the fascia or connective tissue of the body. This form of bodywork uses stronger touch.

Upledger's fourth technique is position of release. This involves following the client's body into the positions in which an injury occurred and holding it there. When the rhythm of the CSR suddenly stops the therapist knows that the trauma has been released.

The last technique is somatoemotional release. This technique was developed by Upledger and is an offshoot of craniosacral therapy. It is used to release the mind and body of the residual effects of trauma and injury that are "locked in the tissues."

The cost of a session varies due to the length of time needed and the qualifications of the therapist. The cost may be covered by insurance when the therapy is performed or prescribed by a licensed health care provider.

Precautions

This gentle approach is extremely safe in most cases. However, craniosacral therapy is not recommended in cases of acute systemic infections, recent skull fracture, intracranial hemorrhage or aneurysm, or herniation of the medulla oblongata (brain stem). Craniosacral therapy does not preclude the use of other medical approaches.

Side effects

Some people may experience mild discomfort after a treatment. This may be due to re-experiencing a trauma or injury or a previously numb area may come back to life and be more sensitive. These side effects are temporary.

Research and general acceptance

More than 40 scientific papers have been published that document the various effects of craniosacral

WILLIAM SUTHERLAND (1873–1954)

William Garner Sutherland studied osteopathy under its founder, Andrew Taylor Still. Dr. Sutherland made his own important discovery while examining the sutures of cranial bones the skull bones that protect the brain. What he noticed is that the sutures were designed for motion. Sutherland termed this motion the *Breath of Life*. Through his experiments and research he determined that primary respiration was essential to all other physiological functions.

When Sutherland developed his techniques for craniosacral therapy, he wanted it to serve as a vehicle for listening to the body's rhythmic motions, and treat the patterns of inertia, when those motions become congested.

He believed that the stresses—any physical or emotional trauma—created an imbalance in the body that needed correction to restore it to full health. The therapy is a hands-on method so that the therapist can feel the subtleties of the patterns of movement and inertia. Sutherland felt that this was the way to encourage self-healing and restoration of the body's own mechanisms, taking a holistic approach to creating optimal health.

The Craniosacral Therapy Educational Trust, based on Sutherland's pioneering work is located at 10 Normington Close, Leigham Court Road, London SW16 2QS, United Kingdom. The phone number is 07000 785778.

---

therapy. There are also 10 authoritative textbooks on this therapy. The most notable scientific papers include Viola M. Fryman's work documenting the successful treatment of 1,250 newborn children with birth defects. Edna Lay and Stephen Blood showed the effects on TMD, and John Wood documented results with psychiatric disorders. The American Dental Association has found craniosacral therapy to be an effective adjunct to orthodontic work. However, the conventional medical community has not endorsed these techniques.

Training and certification

Craniosacral therapy is offered as part of the standard training in osteopathy, **chiropractic**, and **rolfing**. Massage therapists, nurses, dentists, physical therapists, and other health care practitioners can receive training through a series of workshops and seminars. The Upledger Institute offers two levels of national certification, involving a rigorous three part exam process of written, oral, and hands-on testing. The Milne Institute certifies practitioners through a two year training program that covers anatomy, physiology, symptomatology, psychology, **meditation** practice, and training in sensitivity, perception and intuition. Today there are around 40,000 practitioners certified to practice crainiosacral therapy.

Resources

BOOKS

Knaster, Mirka. *Discovering the Body's Wisdom*. New York: Bantam Books, 1996.
Milne, Hugh. *Heart of Listening: A Visionary Approach to Craniosacral Work: Anatomy. Technique, Transcendence*. 2nd ed. Berkeley, CA: North Atlantic Books, 1998.
Upledger, John E. "CranioSacral Therapy." In *Clinician's Complete Reference to Complementary and Alternative Medicine*. Donald Novey, ed. St. Louis, MO: 2000.

Upledger, John E. *Your Inner Physician and You: Cranio-Sacral Therapy Somatoemotional Release*. Berkeley, CA: North Atlantic Books, 1991.
Upledger, John E., and John Vredevoogd. *Craniosacral Therapy*. Seattle: Eastland Press, 1983.

ORGANIZATIONS

Milne Institute Inc. P.O. Box 2716, Monterey, CA 93942-2716. (831) 649-1825. Fax: (831) 649-1826. http://www.milneinstitute.com. milneinst@aol.com.
Upledger Institute. 11211 Prosperity Farms Road, Palm Beach Gardens, FL 33410. (800) 233-5880. Fax: (561) 622-4771. http://www.upledger.com.

OTHER

Milne, Hugh. *A Client's Introduction to Craniosacral Work*. Pamphlet. Milne Institute.

Linda Chrisman

Creatine

Definition

Creatine is a nitrogenous organic acid that occurs in vertebrates. Its molecular formula is $C_4H_9N_3O_2$.

Description

With its promises of bigger muscles and improved athletic performance, creatine has generated more interest and controversy than almost any other dietary supplement in the 2000s. It is widely used by body builders and athletes at all levels, from famous baseball sluggers to high school jocks. Even without taking supplements, all people have a small amount of this compound in their bodies. Some of it comes from food, especially meat and fish, while the rest is made by the body from **amino acids**. No one disputes the fact that creatine plays an important role in converting food into energy. The real question is whether taking extra amounts of creatine can make muscles bigger, boost athletic performance, or improve the health of people with muscle or nerve disease.

Creatine is considered important because it can increase the amount of energy available to working muscles. The compound is used by the body to make a chemical compound called adenosine triphosphate (ATP), the immediate fuel source used by muscles during short but intense bursts of activity. Through its conversion into phosphocreatine, a related substance, creatine appears to delay muscle **fatigue** by re-supplying muscles with ATP. Because creatine can be stored for later use by cells, consuming extra amounts of the substance may create a deeper energy reserve for muscles and other tissues. Excess creatine is eliminated by the kidneys, which means that creatine supplements may be of little value to people who have sufficient levels of the compound, since the kidneys automatically remove extra amounts.

A significant amount of research was required as of 2008 to determine the long-term effects of taking creatine, proper dosage, and whether age, gender, or the presence of existing diseases can affect use of the supplements. As of 2008, a review of research on 12 proposed uses of the drug reported by the National Institutes of Health found, in all cases, inconclusive scientific evidence for the suggested application. The 12 uses were as follows:

- Congestive heart failure
- Enhanced athletic performance and endurance
- Enhanced muscle mass/strength
- GAMT (guanidinoacetate methyltransferase) deficiency
- Heart muscle protection during heart surgery
- High cholesterol
- Huntington's disease
- Hyperornithinemia
- McArdle's disease
- Muscular dystrophy
- Myocardial infarction
- Neuromuscular disorders

General use

Creatine supplements are generally used by weight lifters and athletes who wish to optimize their workouts or enhance athletic performance. It is important to distinguish fact from myth regarding the possible benefits of creatine. The scientific evidence suggests that creatine may not have much usefulness as a muscle-enhancing agent, although it does appear to moderately improve performance in exercises or sports that require short, repeated bursts of high-energy activity. For example, creatine may provide a slight energy boost to the muscles of a weight lifter during extended repetitions or a basketball player who makes yet another drive to the hoop. However, creatine does not appear to increase aerobic capacity or improve performance in endurance-type activities such as marathon running. Apart from its uses in body building and athletics, creatine may prove beneficial in the treatment of certain diseases involving the muscles or nerves.

As of 2008, more than 3,200 research studies on creatine had been conducted in the preceding three decades. Many of those studies investigated the effects of creatine on athletic performance in a wide variety of sports, including short- and long-distance running, rugby, weight-lifting, swimming, hockey, and tennis. In September 2007, the National Library for Health (NLH) conducted a study of research on the use of creatine for enhancing athletic performance. It focused first on two research reviews carried out in 2005. One study of all the research conducted since 1999 found activities involving jumping, sprinting, or cycling generally benefited from the ingestion of creatine. For other types of athletic activity, the results were contradictory. The second report covered more than 500 studies on the use of creatine for the enhancement of athletic performance. The report found that 70% of the studies reviewed reported statistically significant improvement in at least some types of athletic performance.

The NLH also reviewed four studies that had been completed in the two preceding years. It found that three of the four placebo-controlled studies found no relationship between the use of creatine supplements and improved athletic performance among ice hockey players, tennis players, sprinters, and other types of runners.

In addition to its possible use in sports, creatine has been recommended for the treatment of a number of other diseases affecting the muscles or nerves, including Huntington's disease, **Lou Gehrig's disease** (ALS, amyotrophic lateral sclerosis), and congestive heart failure. Creatine is not considered a cure for these diseases but may help to alleviate symptoms (such as muscle weakness and fatigue) or possibly extend survival. Most research reported as of 2008 suggested that patients with neuromuscular disorders tolerate creatine therapy satisfactorily, but they do not appear to benefit significantly from the therapy.

Preparations

Dosage of creatine usually consists of a loading dose of 10 to 30 g a day (divided into several doses) for four to six days, followed by a maintenance dose of 2 to 5 g a day. It is not clear if the high loading dosage is actually necessary. Smaller dosages (3 g a day) may achieve the same effects if taken for several weeks.

Even without taking supplements, most people get about 1 g of creatine from food. Some authorities believe it is safer for people to avoid creatine supplements altogether in favor of eating foods that contain creatine. The best sources of creatine are meat, poultry, and fish. Getting too much dietary creatine is not considered a significant risk because only small amounts of the substance are present in food.

Precautions

Creatine supplements are not known to be harmful when taken in recommended dosages, although some precautions should be observed. People with kidney disease should not use creatine without medical supervision. Due to lack of sufficient medical study, creatine should be used with caution in children under age 16, women who are pregnant or breast-feeding, and people with liver disease.

The long-term health risks associated with taking creatine were unknown as of 2008. Surprisingly, though, use of the supplement was increasing in the late 2000s, even among children and adolescents. Some adults have used the drug on a long-term basis without knowing the effects of long-term use.

Side effects

A slight weight gain due to water retention is probably the most common side effect. **Nausea**, cramping, dehydration, **diarrhea**, and increased blood pressure have also been reported.

To avoid possible side effects, individuals ought not to take creatine immediately before or during **exercise**.

Individuals ought to drink plenty of fluids (six to eight glasses a day) while using creatine in order to prevent dehydration.

Interactions

Taking creatine with large amounts of carbohydrates may increase its effectiveness. **Caffeine** may decrease the effects of the supplement.

The international review group Natural Standard suggests that interactions are possible between

---

KEY TERMS

Amino acids—The building blocks of protein.

Meta-analysis—An analysis of previous medical studies.

---

creatine and a number of drugs and herbs, including diuretics such as hydrochlorothiazide and furosemide; drugs that may damage the kidneys, such as trimethoprim and cimetidine; anti-inflammatory drugs, such as ibuprofen, cyclosporine, amikacin, gentamicin, and tobramycin; cholesterol-lowering medications, such as lovastatin; and two herbal preparations, **bitter melon** (*Momordica charantia*) and red yeast (*Monascus purpureus*).

Resources

BOOKS

Appleton, Jeremy. *Creatine*. Chapmanville, WV: Woodland Press, 2008.

Paterson, Ellen R., compiler. *Anabolic Steroids and Sports, Testing, Creatine, Androstenedione, and Other Ergogenic Aids: Spring 1998—spring 2005: An Annotated Bibliography*. Albany, NY: Whitston, 2006.

Stout, Jeffrey R., Jose Antonio, and Douglas Kalman, eds. *Essentials of Creatine in Sports and Health*. Totowa, NJ: Humana Press, 2007.

PERIODICALS

Bemben, Michael G., and Hugh S. Lamont. "Creatine Supplementation and Exercise Performance: Recent Findings." *Sports Medicine* (February 2005): 107–125.

Buford, Thomas W. "International Society of Sports Nutrition Position Stand: Creatine Supplementation and Exercise." *Journal of the International Society of Sports Nutrition* (August 2007): 4–9.

Glaister, M., et al. "Creatine Supplementation and Multiple Sprint Running Performance." *Journal of Strength and Conditioning Research* (May 2006): 273–277.

Matich, Andrea Jensen. "Performance-enhancing Drugs and Supplements in Women and Girls." *Current Sports Medicine Reports* (December 2007): 387–391.

ORGANIZATIONS

American College of Sports Medicine, 401 W. Michigan St., Indianapolis, IN, 46202-3233, (317) 637-9200, http://www.acsm.org.

Grand Forks Human Nutrition Research Center, 2420 Second Ave. N, Grand Forks, ND, 58202, http://www. gfhnrc.ars.usda.gov.

Greg Annussek
Teresa G. Odle
David Edward Newton, Ed.D.

Crohn's disease

Definition

Crohn's disease is a type of **inflammatory bowel disease** (IBD), resulting in swelling and dysfunction of the intestinal tract.

Description

Crohn's disease involves swelling, redness, and loss of function of the intestine, especially the small intestine. Research suggests that this inflammation is caused by an error in the immune system, which attacks the body itself instead of attacking foreign invaders, such as viruses or bacteria. The inflammation of Crohn's disease most commonly occurs in the last part of the ileum (a section of the small intestine), and often includes the large intestine (the colon). However, inflammation may also occur in other areas of the gastrointestinal tract, including the mouth, esophagus, or stomach. Crohn's disease differs from ulcerative **colitis**, the other major type of IBD, in two important ways:

- The inflammation of Crohn's disease may be discontinuous, meaning that areas of involvement in the intestine may be separated by normal, unaffected segments of intestine. The affected areas are called regional enteritis, whereas the normal areas are called skip areas.
- The inflammation of Crohn's disease affects all the layers of the intestinal wall, while ulcerative colitis affects only the lining of the intestine.

Also, ulcerative colitis does not usually involve the small intestine; in rare cases it involves the terminal ileum (so-called backwash ileitis).

In addition to inflammation, Crohn's disease causes ulcerations, or irritated pits, in the intestinal wall. These pits occur because the inflammation has made areas of tissue shed away.

While Crohn's disease and ulcerative colitis are similar, they are also very different. Although it can be difficult to determine whether a patient has Crohn's disease or ulcerative colitis, it is important to make every effort to distinguish between these two diseases. Because the long-term complications of the diseases are different, treatment depends on careful diagnosis of the specific IBD present.

Crohn's disease may be diagnosed at any age, although most diagnoses are made between the ages of 15 to 35. About 20 to 40 people out of 10,000 suffer from this disorder, with men and women having an

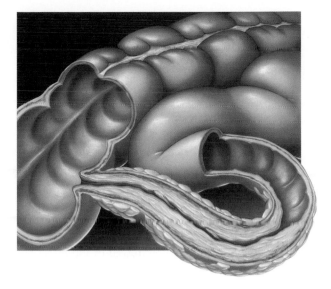

Crohn's disease, inflammation of the ileum, the terminal portion of the small intestine, and characterized by abdominal pain and deep ulceration. *(Brian Evans / Photo Researchers, Inc.)*

equal chance of being stricken. Caucasians are more frequently affected than other racial groups, and people of Jewish origin appear three to six times as likely to suffer from IBD. IBD runs in families; an IBD patient has a 20% chance of having relatives who are fellow sufferers.

Crohn's disease is a chronic disorder. While the symptoms can be improved, there is no known cure for the underlying disease as of the late 2000s.

Causes and symptoms

The cause of Crohn's disease is unknown. No infectious agent (virus, bacteria, or fungi) has been identified as the etiologic agent. Still, some researchers have theorized that some type of infection may have originally been responsible for triggering the immune system, resulting in the continuing and out-of-control cycle of inflammation that occurs in Crohn's disease. Other evidence for a disorder of the immune system includes the high incidence of other immune disorders that may occur along with Crohn's disease.

The first symptoms of Crohn's disease may include **diarrhea**, **fever**, abdominal **pain**, inability to eat, weight loss, and **fatigue**. Some patients experience severe pain that mimics appendicitis. It is rare, however, for patients to notice blood in their bowel movements. Because Crohn's disease severely limits the ability of the affected intestine to absorb the nutrients from food, a patient with Crohn's disease can have signs of malnutrition, depending on the amount of intestine affected and the duration of the disease.

The combination of severe inflammation, ulceration, and scarring that occurs in Crohn's disease can result in serious complications, including obstruction, **abscess** formation, and fistula formation.

An obstruction is a blockage in the intestine. This obstruction prevents the intestinal contents from passing beyond the point of the blockage. The intestinal contents back up, resulting in **constipation**, **vomiting**, and intense pain. Although rare in Crohn's disease (because of the increased thickness of the intestinal wall due to swelling and scarring), a severe bowel obstruction can result in an intestinal wall perforation (a hole in the intestine). Such a hole in the intestinal wall allows the intestinal contents, usually containing bacteria, to enter the abdomen. This complication can result in a severe, life-threatening infection.

Abscess formation is the development of a walled-off pocket of infection. A patient with an abscess has bouts of fever, increased abdominal pain, and, in some cases, a lump or mass that can be felt through the wall of the abdomen.

Fistula formation is the formation of abnormal channels between tissues. These channels may connect one area of the intestine to another neighboring section of intestine. Fistulas may join an area of the intestine to the vagina or bladder, or they may drain an area of the intestine through the skin. Abscesses and fistulas commonly affect the area around the anus and rectum (the very last portions of the colon where waste leaves the body). These abnormal connections allow bacteria that normally live in the intestine to enter other areas of the body, causing potentially serious **infections**.

Patients suffering from Crohn's disease also have a significant chance of experiencing other disorders. Some of these may relate specifically to the intestinal disease, and others appear to have some relationship to the imbalanced immune system. The faulty absorption state of the bowel can result in **gallstones** and **kidney stones**. Inflamed areas in the abdomen may press on the tube that drains urine from the kidney to the bladder (the urethra). Urethra compression can cause urine to back up into the kidney, enlarge the urethra and kidney, and can potentially lead to kidney damage. Patients with Crohn's disease also frequently suffer from the following:

- arthritis (inflammation of the joints)
- spondylitis (inflammation of the vertebrae, the bones of the spine)
- ulcers of the mouth and skin
- painful, red bumps on the skin
- inflammation of several eye areas
- inflammation of the liver, gallbladder, and/or the channels (ducts) that carry bile between and within the liver, gallbladder, and intestine

The chance of developing **cancer** of the intestine is greater than normal among patients with Crohn's disease, although this chance is not as high as among those patients with ulcerative colitis.

Diagnosis

Diagnosis is first based upon a patient's symptoms. Blood tests may reveal an increase in certain types of white blood cells, an indication that some type of inflammation or infection is occurring in the body. Blood tests may also reveal **anemia** and other signs of malnutrition due to malabsorption (low blood protein; variations in the amount of **calcium**, **potassium**, and **magnesium** present in the blood; and changes in certain markers of liver function). Stool samples may be examined to make sure that no infectious agent is causing the diarrhea, and to see if the waste contains blood.

A colonoscopy may be performed to view the interior of the colon. During colonoscopy, a doctor passes a flexible tube with a tiny, fiber-optic camera device (an endoscope) through the rectum and into the colon. The doctor can then carefully examine the lining of the intestine for signs of inflammation and ulceration that might suggest Crohn's disease. A tissue sample (biopsy) of the intestine can also be taken through the endoscope to examine under a microscope for evidence of Crohn's disease.

Both an upper and lower GI (gastrointestinal) x-ray series can be helpful in determining how much of the intestine is involved in the disease. In the upper GI (also called a small bowel series), the patient drinks a chalky solution consisting of a salt of barium, which acts as a contrast agent to illuminate the gastrointestinal tract on x-ray film. After the barium is ingested, x rays are taken at specific time intervals as the barium passes through the stomach and into and through the small intestine. The lower GI series provides an x-ray study of the large intestine. The patient is given an enema containing a barium salt, and in some cases, air is also pumped into the rectum to provide a clearer view of the large intestine. This procedure is called a double-contrast barium enema.

Treatment

Crohn's disease is a chronic, often progressive, illness. A correct diagnosis and appropriate treatment with anti-inflammatory medications is critical to controlling the disease.

Some Crohn's patients find that certain foods are hard to digest, including milk, large quantities of fiber, and spicy foods. Dietary adjustments are usually necessary to minimize pain, diarrhea, and other symptoms.

Acupuncture and **guided imagery** may be useful tools in treating pain associated with Crohn's disease. Acupuncture involves the placement of thin needles into the skin at targeted locations on the body known as acupoints in order to harmonize the energy flow within the human body. To treat chronic pain, such as that involved with Crohn's disease, an acupuncturist frequently places the acupuncture needles along what is known as the large intestine meridian.

Guided imagery involves creating a visual mental image of one's pain in one's mind. Once the pain can be visualized, the patient can adjust the image to make it more pleasing and, thus, more manageable.

Several herbal remedies are also available to lessen pain symptoms and promote **relaxation** and healing. These include **peppermint** oil, **slippery elm** (*Ulmus rubra*), **marsh mallow** (*Althaea officinalis*), and Chinese herbs. However, Crohn's patients should consult with their healthcare professional before taking them. Depending on the preparation and the type of herb, these remedies may aggravate the digestive tract or interact with prescription drugs that are being taken to control the inflammation of Crohn's disease.

Allopathic treatment

Allopathic treatments for Crohn's disease try to reduce the underlying inflammation, the resulting malabsorption/malnutrition, the uncomfortable symptoms of cramping abdominal pain and diarrhea, and any possible complications (obstruction, abscesses, and fistulas).

Inflammation can be treated with a drug called sulfasalazine. Sulfasalazine is made up of two parts. One part is related to the sulfa antibiotics; the other part is a form of the anti-inflammatory chemical, salicylic acid. Sulfasalazine is not well-absorbed from the intestine, so it stays mostly within the intestine, where it is broken down into its components. It is believed that the salicylic acid component actively treats Crohn's disease by reducing inflammation. Some patients do not respond to sulfasalazine, particularly those with more severe disease. These patients require steroid medications (such as prednisone). Steroids, however, must be used carefully to avoid the complications of these drugs, including increased risk of infection and weakening of bones (**osteoporosis**).

In 2001, the Food and Drug Administration (FDA) approved use of budesonide capsules for mild and moderate cases of Crohn's disease involving the small and large intestines. Although a steroid, budesonide allows the drug to release into the intestines, where it can be mostly metabolized. As a result, less of the drug enters the patient's system, meaning fewer undesirable side effects may occur. Some potent immunosuppressive drugs that interfere with the products of the immune system and hopefully decrease inflammation may be used for those patients who do not improve on steroids. One addition to the various drugs used to treat Crohn's disease is natalizumab (Tysabri), originally developed and approved for the treatment of **multiple sclerosis**. The U.S. Food and Drug Administration (FDA) approved natalizumab in January 2008 for use with moderate to severe cases of Crohn's disease.

Serious cases of malabsorption/malnutrition may need to be treated by providing nutritional supplements. These supplements must be in a form that can be absorbed from the damaged, inflamed intestine. When patients are suffering from an obstruction, or during periods of time when symptoms of the disease are most acute, they may need to drink specially formulated, high-calorie liquid supplements. Those patients who are severely ill may need to receive their **nutrition** through a needle inserted intravenously.

A number of medications are available to help decrease the cramping and pain associated with Crohn's disease: loperamide, tincture of opium, and codeine. Some fiber preparations (methylcellulose or **psyllium**) may be helpful, although some patients do not tolerate them well.

The first step in treating an obstruction involves general attempts to decrease inflammation with sulfasalazine, steroids, or immunosuppressive drugs. A patient with a severe obstruction must stop taking all food and drink by mouth, allowing the bowel to rest. Abscesses and other infections require antibiotics. Surgery may be required to repair an obstruction that does not resolve on its own, to remove an abscess, or to repair a fistula. Such surgery may involve the removal of a section of the small intestine. In extremely severe cases of Crohn's disease of the colon that do not respond to treatment, a patient may need to have the entire large intestine removed (an operation called a

KEY TERMS

Abscess—A walled-off pocket of pus caused by infection.

Endoscope—A medical instrument that can be passed into an area of the body (e.g., the bladder or intestine) to allow examination of that area. The endoscope usually has a fiber-optic camera, which allows a greatly magnified image to be shown on a television screen viewed by the operator. Many endoscopes also allow the operator to retrieve a small sample (biopsy) of the area being examined.

Fistula—An abnormal channel that creates an open passageway between two structures that do not normally connect.

Gastrointestinal tract—The entire length of the digestive system, including the mouth, pharynx, esophagus, stomach, small intestine, large intestine, rectum, and anus.

Immune system—The body system responsible for producing various cells and chemicals that fight infection by viruses, bacteria, fungi, and other foreign invaders. In autoimmune disease, these cells and chemicals turn against the body itself.

Inflammation—The result of the body's attempts to fight off and wall off an area that is infected. Inflammation results in the classic signs of redness, heat, swelling, and loss of function.

Obstruction—A blockage.

Ulceration—A pitted area or break in the continuity of a surface, such as the skin or mucous membrane.

colectomy). In this case, a piece of the remaining small intestine is pulled through an opening in the abdomen. This bit of intestine is fashioned surgically to allow a special bag to be placed over it. This bag catches the body's waste, which no longer can be passed through the large intestine and out through the anus. This opening, which remains in place for life, is called an ileostomy. However, as an alternative to ileostomy, small intestines are often shaped into substitute rectal pouches, and the patient may not always need the ileostomy.

Expected results

Crohn's disease is a lifelong illness. The severity of the disease can vary, and patients can experience periods when the disease is not active and they are symptom free. However, the complications and risks of Crohn's disease tend to increase over time. Well over 60% of all patients with Crohn's disease require surgery, and about half of these patients require more than one operation over time. About 5 to 10% of all Crohn's patients die of their disease, primarily due to massive infection.

Prevention

Crohn's disease is a chronic, lifelong disorder for which there is no prevention as of 2008. Some drugs, including azathioprine (Imuran, Azasan), 6-mercaptopurine (Purinethol), and methotrexate may help keep the disease in remission, although each drug has some potentially serious side effects also.

Resources

BOOKS

Dahlman, David. *Why Doesn't My Doctor Know This? Conquering Irritable Bowel Syndrome, Inflammatory Bowel Disease, Crohn's Disease, and Colitis.* Garden City, NY: Morgan James, 2008.

Parker, Philip M. *Crohn's Disease: A Bibliography and Dictionary for Physicians, Patients, and Genome Researchers.* San Diego, CA: ICON Group International, 2007.

Warner, Andrew S., and Amy E. Barto. *100 Questions & Answers About Crohn's Disease and Ulcerative Colitis: A Lahey Clinic Guide.* Sudbury, MA: Jones & Bartlett, 2007.

PERIODICALS

Bernard, André. "A Systematic Review of Patient Inflammatory Bowel Disease Information Resources on the World Wide Web." *American Journal of Gastroenterology* (September 2007): 2070–2077.

Clark, M., et al. "American Gastroenterological Association Consensus Development Conference on the Use of Biologics in the Treatment of Inflammatory Bowel Disease." *Gastroenterology* (July 2007): 312–339.

Feagan, Brian G., et al. "Health-Related Quality of Life During Natalizumab Maintenance Therapy for Crohn's Disease." *American Journal of Gastroenterology* (December 2007): 2737–2746.

Van Kruiningen, Herbert J., et al. "Search for Evidence of Recurring or Persistent Viruses in Crohn's Disease." *Apmis* (August 2007): 962–968.

Van Limbergen, Johan, et al. "The Genetics of Inflammatory Bowel Disease." *American Journal of Gastroenterology* (December 2007): 2820–2831.

ORGANIZATIONS

Crohn's & Colitis Foundation of America, 386 Park Ave. S., 17th Floor, New York, NY, 10016-8804, (800) 932-2423, http://www.ccfa.org/.

Paula Ford-Martin
Teresa G. Norris
David Edward Newton, Ed.D.

Croup

Definition

Croup is a common ailment of early childhood involving inflammation of the larynx, trachea, bronchial tubes, and lungs. The condition is characterized by a harsh, barking **cough, wheezing**, and difficulty in breathing.

Description

Croup is most likely to be found in children between the ages of three months to six years. Most incidences occur during the cold weather seasons.

Spasmodic croup is usually mild and may be due to bacterial infection or **allergies**. For the most part, the child will not have a **fever**. Viral croup, also called laryngotracheobronchitis, is more severe and is often accompanied by fever. Both types follow a very similar course, which depends on the severity of the illness.

In many instances, a child may have had a cold or the flu just before the onset of croup symptoms. These symptoms tend to come on very suddenly. It is not uncommon for a child with croup to waken in the middle of the night coughing violently and gasping for breath. In fact, the croup symptoms will usually be worse at night and get better during the day.

Causes and symptoms

During the immune system response to an infection or an allergic reaction, the respiratory passages become swollen, and they are congested with mucus and fluid. They also become more and more irritated. There is a great deal of coughing, and the child may become hoarse. The airways are narrowed, and the breathing is difficult and noisy. This leads to the characteristic symptom of stridor, or noisy aspiration, as the child attempts to draw in air through narrowed passages. The constriction of these airways is usually accompanied by a high-pitched cough, often described as sounding like the bark of a seal.

Diagnosis

Diagnosis of croup is primarily based on a good history taken by the health care provider, including the physical symptoms of the illness, the presentation of the illness, and its progression. If a physical exam is performed, it will probably include listening with a stethoscope for the breathing sounds which are characteristic of croup. When the symptoms appear to be severe, or the history suggests it, x rays may be taken

---

KEY TERMS

Aspiration—Accidental inhaling of an object such as food into the airway passages. This is dangerous, in that it may cause obstruction and difficulty breathing.

Corticosteroid—A hormonal drug that acts on the immune system to control inflammation and swelling.

Epiglottitis—A serious bacterial infection that can develop rapidly and lead to airway obstruction.

Epinephrine—A hormonal drug used chiefly to stimulate to the heart

Inflammation—Reaction by body tissues to infection or injury. Usually the area will be hot, red, painful, and swollen due to the immune response.

Intravenous fluids—In cases of immediate need for hydration, nourishment, or medicine, a needle with tubing is inserted directly into the vein.

Intubation—A procedure in which a flexible tube is carefully passed down the throat to keep the breathing passage open.

Stridor—A noisy wheezing sound during breathing that may indicate an airway obstruction.

---

to rule out epiglottitis (infection of the epiglottis) or aspiration of a foreign body, which are emergency situations.

Treatment

Supportive measures

Most treatment can be done at home, using relaxing and supportive measures to relieve symptoms. Steam inhalation is quite helpful in this respect. A cool-mist humidifier is recommended, as a hot vaporizer is often hazardous, especially around young children.

One of the best ways to produce a lot of moist air in a short time is to make use of the bathroom shower. The procedure is to close the bathroom door and turn on the cool water shower faucet full blast. Then the child can be a held while seated on a chair or the closed commode, breathing in steam as it fills the room. This can be done for up to 15 minutes, and often brings instant relief from congestion.

Cool air seems to relax and soothe the respiratory system. Therefore, taking a car ride with the window down will sometimes effect good results in reducing the coughing associated with croup.

There is a strong possibility of dehydration due to the illness. Increasing fluid intake as much as possible and insuring plenty of rest will enhance immune functioning, helping the body to help itself. In addition, **smoking** should be prohibited within the house.

Herbs

Respiratory herbs can be used to soothe swollen and irritated tissues, reduce inflammation, and gently loosen and expel mucus. The following herbs should be given three times per day diluted in water or other liquids until symptoms are gone:

- *Grindelia* spp., gum weed, 1-2 ml
- *Sambucus nigra,* elder flowers, 2-4 ml
- *Glycyrrhiza glabra,* licorice root, 1-3 ml
- *Verbascum thapsus,* mullein, 2-4ml
- *Astragalus senticocosus,* 2-4 ml (This herb is an immune system stimulant and should be given as a preventative for those who have chronic bouts of croup.)

Slippery elm bark can also be taken, as it is soothing to the throat.

Homeopathy

Aconite is the most favored remedy to use for croup. If it does not work, Spongia can be tried, especially if the breathing sounds as if wood were being sawed. Alternately, try Hepar sulphuris, indicated by a mucus-filled cough. Give a dosage of 12X or 30C every 30 minutes until the child is able to fall asleep.

Allopathic treatment

In most cases, croup can be easily and successfully treated at home. However, if the symptoms become severe, the child will need to be seen by a physician. Prompt medical attention is needed if:

- The child's fever goes up to 104°F (39.9°C).
- The child seems pale or bluish around the mouth or fingernails.
- The child refuses all liquids or can't swallow.
- The child is drooling a great deal.
- The child's breathing becomes increasingly rapid or difficult.

Severe cases may warrant the use of inhalants, such as epinephrine, to reduce swelling and ease the child's breathing. Inhalants have limited effectiveness over time, and care must be taken to avoid undesirable side effects. Oxygen may also be administered in more severe cases. Corticosteroids are given to decrease **pain** and swelling.

If a child is hospitalized for further observation or treatment, intravenous (IV) fluids may be given to reduce dehydration. In a few very severe cases, a tube has to be inserted through the nose or mouth (intubation) to keep the airway passage open for breathing. There is a slight risk of injury to the respiratory system during the introduction and the removal of the tube.

Expected results

Croup ordinarily lasts three to seven days. Most cases are mild and gradually improve with care. Some children have recurring bouts with croup, but they usually outgrow this by seven years of age.

It is important to monitor a child with croup throughout the night. An adult should probably consider sleeping or resting nearby. If the child is having a serious struggle with breathing, emergency services should be contacted immediately. This means either calling 911 or making a trip to the nearest emergency room. Hospital visits are necessary in about one to 15% of the reported cases of croup.

Prevention

Croup is generally the result of an infectious disease. Avoiding exposure to others with respiratory **infections** is the best way to avoid getting croup. Children should be taught to maintain good hygiene practices such as not eating food from the silverware or dishes of others and washing their hands. Care should be taken with colds and the flu so that there is no progression to symptoms of croup.

In general, an adequate intake of vitamins A and C, **bioflavonoids**, and **zinc** can help to prevent the respiratory infections and allergic reactions that lead to croup.

Resources

BOOKS

Bunch, Bryan, ed. *The Family Encyclopedia of Diseases: a Complete and Concise Guide to Illnesses and Symptoms.* New York: Scientific Publishing, Inc., 1999.

The Editors of Time-Life Books. *The Medical Advisor: The Complete Guide to Alternative and Conventional Treatments.* Alexandria, VA: Time-Life, Inc., 1997.

OTHER

"Childhood Infections" The Nemours Foundation. http://kidshealth.org. (1999).

"The Common Cold" Natural Medicine Online. http://www.nat-med.com. (2000).

"Croup" Merck & Co., Inc. http://www.merck.com.

"Croup and Your Young Child" American Academy of Pediatrics. http://www.aap.org. (2000).

Patience Paradox

Crystal healing

Definition

A crystal is a mineral that is nearly transparent and colorless or has a slight color. Practitioners of crystal healing believe that crystals, particularly quartz crystals such as amethyst or clear quartz, contain energy that enhances healing of both body and mind. They believe that crystals can be "charged" with this healing energy, in a manner similar to the charging of a flashlight battery. The charged crystal can then be used to alter the energy patterns in the person receiving treatment. Some crystal healers also say that arrowheads and other stones can be used to diagnose illness.

Origins

Aboriginal, shamanistic cultures throughout the world, including Native Americans and the Inuit of northern Canada, have long believed in the healing properties of semiprecious and precious stones. These views were further developed and widely popularized during the late twentieth century by New Age healers.

Benefits

Crystal healing is used to enhance healing of a wide range of physical and mental ailments. For example, amethyst is said to be useful against **acne**, atacamite against venereal diseases, agate against ulcers, and lapis lazuli against **stroke** symptoms. Crystals may also be used to counter environmental hazards such as electromagnetic radiation, food additives, and polluted air and water. They are thought by some to minimize the detrimental effects of **caffeine**, tobacco, and alcohol. In addition, some practitioners use crystals before and after surgery to minimize trauma.

Description

Although its effectiveness is disputed, crystal healing is generally safe and inexpensive. Crystals are used in a wide variety of ways. The best results are said to occur when both the patient and the healer are holding crystals. The healer may hold a stone in one hand while using the other to touch the body part in need of healing. Crystals may also be worn as pendants (this is said to be particularly effective in treating thymus gland problems). Appropriate stones can be selected, healers say, by simply picking up various crystals and determining which ones seem to harmonize with the frequencies of the patient's body. This may be indicated by a feeling of warmth or tingling. Some healers work solely with crystals while others combine them with aura or chakra work.

Preparations

Numerous techniques are used to prepare crystals before therapeutic use. One such technique is clearing, which involves using an invocation to remove negative emotional energy from the stone. Another method is cleansing, which is said to maintain the crystal's existing energy level but converts negative energy to positive. This may be accomplished by immersing the stone for a minimum of 24 hours in dry salt or saline solution. Crystals can also be charged, like a battery, by exposing them to running water, magnets, sunlight, moonlight, pyramids, fire, laser light, or living animals, birds, fish, or plants.

Some practitioners attempt to charge stones by putting them near a mother who is giving birth, or someone who is dying. Crystals have been wrapped in a newborn's placenta, then given to the child seven years later. Gem stones that have been near meteorite fragments, earthquakes, volcanoes, or trees struck by lightening are also highly valued for healing properties.

Some healers believe that healing crystals can be programmed with human thoughts. This may be done by placing a crystal against the forehead, then visualizing a desired outcome.

Precautions

Crystal healing is largely viewed as an enhancement to other therapies. It should not be used exclusively in cases of serious illness.

Side effects

There are few, if any, proven side effects to crystal healing.

Research and general acceptance

Medical professionals place little credence in crystal therapy, attributing any observed benefits to **placebo effect**. Their skepticism stems from a lack of scientific evidence for the healing effects of crystals, and from differences of opinion among practitioners about how the therapy actually works.

Training and certification

Practitioners of crystal healing tend to be New Age spiritual healers. A number of schools in Europe and North America offer courses in crystal therapy, but the field is largely unregulated. Many individuals use crystals for self-healing.

Resources

BOOKS

Elsbeth, Marguerite. *Crystal Medicine*. St. Paul: Llewellyn Publications, 1997.

ORGANIZATIONS

The International Association of Crystal Healing Therapists. P.O. Box 344, Manchester, M60 2EZ, United Kingdom. Telephone: (UK) 01200-426061. Fax: (UK) 01200-444776. info@iacht.co.uk. http://www.iacht. co.uk/.

David Helwig

Cupping

Definition

Cupping is a technique used in **traditional Chinese medicine** (TCM) for certain health conditions. Glass or bamboo cups are placed on the skin with suction, which is believed to influence the flow of energy and blood in the body. Cupping should not be confused with the percussive technique in **Swedish massage** called "cupping" or "clapping."

Origins

Cupping was originally called "horn therapy" in ancient China, but variations of it have been used in Turkey, Greece, France, Italy, and Eastern Europe. Cupping has a long history of use in **acupuncture** practice and has been combined with bloodletting, but it is a therapy in its own right. There are specialist cupping practitioners in Japan.

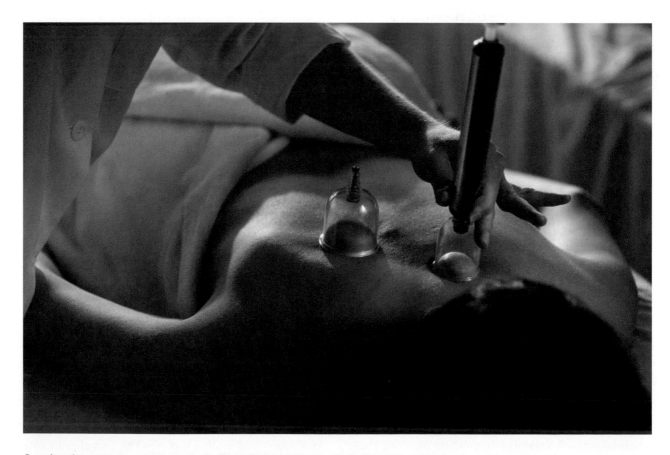

Cupping therapy on woman's back. *(© Photo Researchers, Inc. Reproduced by permission.)*

Benefits

Cupping is a safe, non-invasive, and inexpensive technique. It is used by practitioners of Chinese medicine to treat colds, lung **infections**, and problems in the internal organs. It is also used to treat muscle and joint **pain** and spasms, particularly in the back. Cupping can be used on people for whom the injection of acupuncture needles poses a problem or risk. Cupping therapy is thought to stimulate blood circulation.

Description

Practitioners of traditional Chinese medicine begin treatment by diagnosing a patient through interviews, close examinations of the pulse, tongue and other parts of the body, and other methods. TCM strives to balance and improve the flow of *qi*, or life energy, which travels throughout the body in channels called meridians. According to traditional Chinese medicine, illness is caused when qi does not move properly in the body. Acupuncturists are trained to determine where qi is stagnated, weak, or out of balance.

Acupuncturists use cupping for specific problems in the flow of qi. Cupping disperses and moves qi by exerting suction and pressure. Cupping is used when the qi is blocked at certain points, or when qi needs to be drawn to the surface of the body from deep within. For instance, cupping is used to treat lung infections and colds, because it is believed that the suction disperses and energizes the qi that has become blocked and stagnated in the lungs. Cups can also pull out "wind-cold" that in Chinese medicine is believed to cause lung infections.

Patients usually lie down for a cupping treatment. Cups are made of bamboo or strong glass. To create a vacuum, a flame from a lighter or a burning cotton ball is placed in an upside-down cup. When the oxygen in the cup is burned off, the cup is placed directly on the skin, where it is held in place by a surprisingly strong suction. Often, the skin inside the cup visibly rises. There are also cups available that use pumps instead of burning to create the proper suction. Cupping is generally a painless procedure.

Multiple cups may be used at a time to cover an area thoroughly. Cups may be left in the same place for several minutes, or removed quickly and placed elsewhere. Cups are sometimes placed over acupuncture needles that have been inserted. Moving cupping may also be performed, by first rubbing the skin with a small amount of oil to allow the cups to slide around. After cupping, patients may remain lying down for several minutes. When cups are used to treat colds and lung infections, patients are advised to wrap up in blankets to stay warm after treatment. Acupuncturists may also prescribe herbal remedies, dietary changes, and other health recommendations.

Precautions

Cupping should be performed by experienced professionals. Although it is a simple treatment, people should not attempt it on themselves. Improper glass vessels can shatter and cause injury, and cupping may cause bruising.

Side effects

Cupping causes blood to be drawn to the surface of the skin, which can cause red marks, swelling, and bruising.

Resources

BOOKS

Fleischman, Dr. Gary F. *Acupuncture: Everything You Ever Wanted to Know.* Barrytown, NY: Station Hill, 1998.

Williams, Tom, Ph.D. *The Complete Illustrated Guide to Chinese Medicine.* Rockport, MA: Element, 1996.

ORGANIZATIONS

American Association of Acupuncture and Oriental Medicine. 433 Front St., Catasaugua, PA 18032. (610) 266-1433.

Douglas Dupler

Curanderismo

Definition

Curanderismo is a holistic system of Latin American folk medicine. This type of folk medicine has characteristics specific to the area where it is practiced (Guatemala, Nicaragua, Honduras, Argentina, Mexico, the southwestern region of the United States, etc.).

Curanderismo blends religious beliefs, faith, and **prayer** with the use of herbs, massage, and other traditional methods of healing. Curanderismo can be defined as a set of traditional beliefs, rituals, and practices that address the physical, spiritual, psychological, and social needs of the people who use it.

The Spanish verb *curar* means to heal. Therefore, curanderismo is translated as a system of healing. The goal of curanderismo is to create a balance between the patient and his or her environment, thereby sustaining health.

The healer who practices curanderismo is referred to as a *curandero* (male healer) or *curandera* (female healer). Healing terms vary with the language and culture of the area in which the system is practiced. For example, a female healer in Argentina is called a *remedieras*.

Origins

Curanderismo in Mexico is based on Aztec, Mayan, and Spanish influences. The ancient native cultures believed that a delicate balance existed between health, nature, and religion. Illness occurred when one of these areas was out of balance.

The use of nature's resources was very important to the native cultures. In the fifteenth century, the Huaxtepec garden was developed by the Aztec leader Montezuma I. This garden was a collection of several thousand medicinal plants. The Aztec priests used this garden to perform research on the medicinal properties of the plants.

When the Spanish conquistadors came to Mexico in the sixteenth century, they destroyed the garden and all of the priests' research because the Catholic Church considered these "sciences" to be blasphemous. Although the written knowledge was destroyed, the plant wisdom was remembered, passed down by the native peoples, and became an integral part of curanderismo.

The Spanish missionaries who were sent to the New World introduced the native peoples to the Catholic religion and European healing philosophies. Prayers to Catholic saints were soon integrated into healing rituals. Another doctrine that was passed on to the native peoples by the Europeans was their belief in witchcraft, sorcery, and other superstitions, and the philosophy that illness is often caused by supernatural forces.

As the native and Spanish cultures intermingled over the centuries, a new culture was formed, as was the folk medicine of curanderismo.

Benefits

Curanderismo is used to treat ailments arising from physical, psychological, spiritual, or social conditions. Illness is said to be caused by either natural or supernatural forces.

Naturally caused illness is treated with herbal medicine, massage, and prayer. Much of this illness is thought to be brought about by intense emotions caused by trauma or a specific event. Susto, for example, is an illness that is caused by fright. A startling event such as a fire, earthquake, dog attack, car accident, or death may cause the patient to become ill. Symptoms of susto are **insomnia**, **diarrhea**, extreme nervousness, sadness, **depression**, loss of appetite, loss of brilliance in the eyes, and lack of dreams. The events are thought to dislodge a person's spirit from the body.

Bilis is an ailment that is the result of excessive emotional **stress**. Bilis is caused by prolonged anger and fear. The ailment is thought to occur when excessive bile is trapped in the system and causes tension, irritability, and loss of appetite.

Empacho and **colic** are ailments treated by massage and herbs. Empacho is a blocked intestine disease where the intestines are plugged by something indigestible such as chewing gum or unbaked dough. To treat this condition, the curandera performs a massage in which she pulls on the skin of the back just above the coccyx (tailbone). When the skin makes a snapping noise the food has been loosened. Herbal tea is also given to complement the massage.

Colic is caused by excessive coldness of the stomach, and mint is used for such digestive problems.

Supernaturally caused illnesses or conditions are initiated by witchcraft, sorcery, or hexes. Physical symptoms might manifest as nervous breakdowns, paranoia, **schizophrenia**, depression, or excessive worrying. Supernatural forces can also create social problems. A person who has a streak of continued bad luck, or who suffers from marital problems, the loss of a job, or car troubles will deem the problem to be caused by a supernatural force. To heal these ailments and remove the hex or problem, the curandera uses rituals, spiritual cleansings, herbs, and prayer.

Description

Prayer is the foundation of curanderismo. Curanderas have strong religious faith and believe that they were given the ability to heal as a gift from God. Curanderas pray to spirits and/or Catholic saints for help in healing their patients, often praying to specific saints for particular conditions.

A traditional healing session may include one or more of the following: spiritual cleansing (*limpia*), ritual, massage, and/or herbal therapy. Curanderas use a variety of objects in their healing sessions, including herbs and spices, eggs, lemons, flowers, fruits, holy water, pictures of saints, crucifixes, candles, incense, and oils. Each object has a specific purpose.

Holy water is used for protection from negativity or evil spirits. Eggs and lemons are patted on the patient's body to absorb negative energies. **Rosemary**, basil, and rue branches are brushed on the body to remove negativity.

Candles are burned to absorb negative energy and create a healing environment. Different colored candles are burned for different reasons: red for strength, blue for harmony, pink for good will. Incense is used to purify the room, while **garlic** and oils are used as protection from negativity and bad spirits.

Research and general acceptance

Although much of the Hispanic community is currently devoted to the practice of curanderismo, many people fear that it will be lost from lack of interest on the part of the younger generation or reliance on mainstream medical procedures. There is a great deal of research on curanderismo in the field of anthropology.

Training and certification

Curanderas are generally trained informally. The information is passed from generation to generation (i.e., mother to daughter). Often the curandera starts out as an apprentice to a more experienced curandera.

Resources

BOOKS

Perrone, Bobette, Henrietta H. Stockel, and Victoria Kruger. *Medicine Women, Curanderas, and Women Doctors.* Norman, OK: University of Oklahoma Press, 1989.

Sandoval, Annette. *Homegrown Healing: Traditional Remedies From Mexico.* New York: Berkley Books, 1998.

Trotter, Robert T., II, and Juan Antonio Chavira. *Curanderismo: Mexican American Folk Healing.* 2nd ed. Athens, GA: The University of Georgia Press, 1997.

Jennifer Wurges

Curcumin

Definition

Curcumin is a biologically active phytochemical compound found in the root and rhizome of **turmeric** (*Curcuma longa L.*). Turmeric is native to India and cultivated throughout China, Southeast Asia, and in other tropical climates. It is a perennial species in the **ginger** (Zingaberaceae) family of flowering plants. Curcumin (diferuloyl methane), Demethoxycurcumin and Bisdemethoxycurcumin, collectively called curcuminoids, are polyphenolic pigments extracted from the orange-gold colored root of turmeric. Curcumin is the most abundant curcuminoid found in the turmeric root, providing about 75 percent of the total curcuminoids, which together comprise less than 10 percent of turmeric.

General use

The aromatic, pungent, and spicy-flavored turmeric root is one of the key ingredients in many Indian curries, imparting its distinctive color. This tropical herb is a staple dietary spice throughout Asia and India. It has been used for centuries as a food preservative, fabric dye, cosmetic, and ritual herb. More recently turmeric was used as a non-toxic food coloring agent in mustards and other foods. In scientific laboratories, turmeric paper, made by soaking paper in a tincture of turmeric, is used to detect alkaloids and boric acid.

Chinese and Ayurveda medicine

The wide range of therapeutic benefits of curcumin-rich turmeric root have long been recognized in Chinese herbal medicine, where the herb is known as *jianghuang*. In Ayurveda, India's ancient system of medicine, turmeric is called *haldi* and is valued as the internal healer. Turmeric has proven effective in the extensive clinical practice of eastern medicine for treatment of inflammation, **pain**, gastrointestinal, pulmonary and liver disorders, and numerous other conditions.

Curcumin acts to promote digestion, stimulate the gall bladder and the flow of bile, aid in nutrient absorption, check **diarrhea**, prevent **blood clots**, lower **cholesterol**, regulate menses, and treat **premenstrual syndrome** (PMS). Curcumin's pain relieving qualities are helpful with arthritis, **toothache**, **colic** and chest and abdominal pain, among other traditional uses.

For external treatments, the antibiotic, astringent, and antiseptic turmeric root is prepared as an ointment or poultice to treat **bruises**, **cuts** and abrasions, **scabies** (combined with **neem**(*Azadirachta indical*), **boils** and other infected areas of the skin, and as a remedy for ailments of the eyes, including **conjunctivitis**. The volatile oils of turmeric root also act as a mosquito repellant and prevent bacterial infection in **wounds**. In India a common folk tonic for new mothers is a beverage made of turmeric and ginger root powder added to warm milk and honey. A paste of turmeric is sometimes applied to the skin to protect against sun damage.

Western medicine

Extensive scientific research was underway in the late 2000s to validate in western terms the traditional uses in Eastern medicine for the remarkably diverse turmeric root and its constituent curcumin. Many studies of curcumin have been in laboratory or animal research. Animal studies, however, do not always prove as successful in human clinical trials. Curcumin extract has been investigated with both *in vivo* and *in vitro* research. Numerous studies have demonstrated curcumin to be an effective treatment for a wide range of medical conditions, including the following:

- Alzheimer's disease
- Cardiovascular risks
- Crohn's disease
- Digestive disorders
- Herpes simplex
- Melanoma and other cancers
- Rheumatoid arthritis
- Gallbladder disease
- Type II diabetes

Research

Laboratory and animal research has demonstrated the anti-inflammatory, antioxidant, and anti-cancer properties of turmeric and its constituent curcumin. Scientists have demonstrated curcumin's action to induce apoptosis, a naturally occurring form of cell death that eliminates damaged or diseased cells in cases of lymphoma and melanoma. Additional research is needed with humans to further verify the health benefits of a turmeric-rich diet and dietary supplements of curcumin extract.

In laboratory tests in the 1990s, researchers at Harvard Medical School and elsewhere reported curcumin as active against both acutely and chronically infected HIV cells. However, later clinical trials called into question the efficacy of curcumin extract in treatment of HIV.

A study published in 2006 in the *Journal of Alzheimer's Disease* reported that curcumin extract may protect against progression of Alzheimer's because of its action to inhibit the build-up of amyloid plaques in the brain. Curcumin can cross the blood-brain barrier and bind to the amyloid plaques that cause Alzheimer's, aiding in their removal from the system. In a 2006 study of non-demented elderly Asians who consumed a regular diet of turmeric-rich curry, cognitive function was found to be higher than in individuals who did not consume dietary turmeric.

Toronto scientists, reporting in the *Journal of Clinical Investigation* in 2008, found that curcumin could prevent and reverse hypertrophy, restore heart function, and reduce scar formation in mice with enlarged hearts. Additional studies have demonstrated the heart-healthy action of curcumin and its ability to protect against **heart disease** by lowering high blood cholesterol levels and preventing blood clotting.

One clinical trial in patients with **rheumatoid arthritis** compared curcumin to phenylbutazone, a nonsteroidal anti-inflammatory drug (NSAID) prescribed to alleviate arthritic pain. Patients receiving the curcumin extract showed significant improvement with therapeutic effects comparable to those obtained with phenylbutazone, though without the risk of possible serious side effects of the prescription drug.

A 2008 study at Michigan State University demonstrated that curcumin in low concentrations acted to interfere with replication of *Herpes simplex* virus. Scientists began testing curcumin as a possible treatment for skin, breast, and colon **cancer**.

Curcumin extract helps to stimulate the production of bile and break down fats and has been shown in animals to reduce secretion of stomach acid. Curcumin, taken orally, has been shown to have activity against Crohn's disease. Curcumin's use as a digestive aid has been approved by the German Commission E, formed by the German government to evaluate the safety and efficacy of herbs and herb combinations. The official monographs of the Commission, available through the American Botanical Council, provide "approved uses, contraindications, side effects, dosage, drug interactions and other therapeutic information essential for the responsible use of herbs and phyto-medicines," according to the council.

Preparations

Turmeric root

Turmeric root is traditionally collected in winter when the aerial part is dying off. The root is washed, boiled or steamed thoroughly, dried and then ground into a powder just prior to use.

Curcumin extract

Curcumin is commercially available as a fluid extract, capsule, or tincture. For maximum effectiveness, curcumin must be taken with a meal. Researchers have discovered that curcumin undergoes a chemical transformation during absorption from the intestine. Although the phytochemical is almost totally insoluble in water, it is completely soluble in fat. In India, raw turmeric juice is mixed with warm milk and taken as a morning drink to purify blood, relieve bronchial **asthma**, or as a general tonic. The digestive enzyme **bromelain**, extracted from the stem and the fruit of the pineapple plant *(Ananas comosus)*, is sometimes taken in combination with curcumin. The medical benefit depends upon the chemical content and biological activity of the curcumin supplements.

Recommended doses for adults range from 250 to 500 mg of turmeric extract capsules standardized at 90 to 95%; curcumin, three times daily, with a meal. The root, sliced or ground, can be taken in amounts up to 3,000 mg per day. The tincture can be taken in dosages up to 30 drops, four times daily. If taken on an empty stomach, curcumin may cause gastric irritation and ulceration.

Precautions

Turmeric root has been demonstrated in numerous human trials to be safe in amounts up to 2,500 mg per day. It is traditionally used freely as a food spice with no significant adverse effects. Curcumin has been shown to stimulate the production of bile and to facilitate the emptying of the gallbladder, so persons with gastrointestinal disorders, ulcer, **gallstones**, or bile duct obstructions should not take curcumin. The safety of curcumin extract for use by very young children or pregnant or nursing women has not been established.

Drug interactions

People should not take curcumin while taking certain blood thinning medicines. **Breast cancer** patients undergoing chemotherapy are advised to limit intake of dietary turmeric and avoid use of the

---

KEY TERMS

Amyloid plaques—Protein fragments produced normally in the body that accumulate and form hard, insoluble plaques between the nerve cells in the brain and interfere with neural activity.

Apoptosis—Structural changes within cells of a multi-cell organism leading to controlled and regulated cell death, also called programmed cell death (PCD); a natural means to eliminate unnecessary and unhealthy cells.

Crohn's disease—A chronic, recurrent inflammation of the intestine and digestive tract; an inflammatory bowel disease (IBD) that most commonly affects the small intestine.

in vivo—A Latin term meaning living. In science, the term denotes those experiments conducted on or within living organisms.

in vitro—A Latin term meaning glass. In science the term denotes those experiments conducted in a laboratory, but not with living organisms.

Phytochemicals—Beneficial chemical substances found in plants and fruits and thought to work synergistically in whole foods to provide disease protection and promote health.

Polyphenols—A group of phytonutrient compounds present in various foods, including onions, apples, grapes, berries, certain nuts, green tea and red wine. Polyphenolic compounds include tannins, lignins, and flavonoids and are an abundant source of dietary antioxidants.

---

curcumin extract as it may inhibit the anti-tumor action of cyclophosphamide, a chemical used in treating breast cancer.

Side effects

No side effects have been reported other than risk of stomach upset in very high dosages and if taken on an empty stomach.

Resources

BOOKS

Mateljan, George. *The World's Healthiest Foods: Essential Guide to the Healthiest Way of Eating.* Seattle, WA: George Mateljan Foundation, 2006.

Advances in Experimental Medicine and Biology, Vol. 595: The Molecular Targets and Therapeutic Uses of Curcumin in Health and Disease. New York: Springer US, 2007.

PERIODICALS

Brown, Donald. "Curcumin Helps Maintain Remission in Patient with Ulcerative Colitis." *Original Internist* (June 1, 2007).

Funk, J. L., et al. "Turmeric Extracts Containing Curcuminoids Prevent Experimental Rheumatoid Arthritis." *Journal of Natural Products* 69, no.3 (2006): 351–355.

Ng, T. P., C. P. Chiam, T. Lee, et al. "Curry Consumption and Cognitive Function in the Elderly." *American Journal of Epidemiology* 164, n. 9 (2006).

Siwak, D., et al. "Curcumin-induced Antiproliferative and Proapoptotic Effects in Melanoma Cells Are Associated with Suppression of 1kB Kinase and Nuclear Factor kB Activity and Are Independent of the B-Raf/Mitogen Activated/Extracellular Signal-regulated Protein Kinase Pathway and the Akt Pathway." *Cancer* 104, no. 4 (2005): 879–890.

"Spicing Up Your Life: Can Turmeric, the Spice that Adds Color and Flavor to Asian Foods, Play a Role in Preventing Alzheimer's Disease? Scientists Are Trying to Find Out." *Saturday Evening Post* 277, no. 3 (May 1, 2005): 70.

Uddin, S., et al. "Curcumin Suppresses Growth and Induces Apoptosis in Primary Effusion Lymphoma." *Oncogene* (2005): 1–9.

OTHER

"Chemical Found in Curry May Help Immune System Clear Amyloid Plaques Found in Alzheimer's Disease." *Science Daily,* October 3, 2006. http://www.sciencedaily.com/releases/2006/10/061003143643.htm. (March 2, 2008).

Dharmananda, Subhuti. "Turmeric: What's in an Herb Name? How Turmeric (Jianghuang) and Curcuma (Yujin) Became Confused." Institute for Traditional Medicine. http://www.itmonline.org. (March 1, 2008).

Higdon, Jane. "Curcumin." Linus Pauling Institute, Micronutrient Information Center, Oregon State University. http://lpi.oregonstate.edu/infocenter/phytochemicals/curcumin/. (February 28, 2008).

Li, Hong-Liang. "Curcumin Prevents and Reverses Murine Cardiac Hypertrophy." *Journal of Clinical Investigation,* 2008. http://www.pubmedcentral.nih.gov/articlerender.fcgi?artid=2248327. (March 1, 2008).

Pandeya, N. K. "Old Wives' Tales: Modern Miracles—Turmeric as Traditional Medicine in India." *Trees for Life Journal* 1 (2005): 3. http://www.tfljournal.org/article.php/20051201122521970. (March 5, 2008).

"Turmeric Prevents Experimental Rheumatoid Arthritis and Bone Loss." *UA News,* University of Arizona, October 23, 2006. http://uanews.org/node/12838. (March 2, 2008).

ORGANIZATIONS

American Botanical Council, PO Box 144345, Austin, TX, 78714-4345, (512) 926-4900, http://abc.herbalgram.org.

Clare Hanrahan

Cuscuta

Description

Cuscuta is the name of a group of plants in the morning glory family, of which the species *Cuscuta epithymum* is most commonly used in healing. A member of the Cuscutaceae family, species of cuscuta are found almost everywhere in the world, although cuscuta is more often called Chinese dodder in English-speaking countries. Other names are hellweed, devil's gut, beggarweed, strangle tare, scaldweed, dodder of **thyme**, greater dodder, and lesser dodder. In Chinese, cuscuta seeds are called *tu si zi*.

Cuscuta is a parasitic plant. It has no chlorophyll and cannot make its own food by photosynthesis. Instead, it grows on other plants, using their nutrients for its growth and weakening the host plant. Agriculturalists consider cuscuta a destructive weed and attempt to eradicate it. It parasitizes wild and cultivated plants and is especially destructive to such commercially valuable

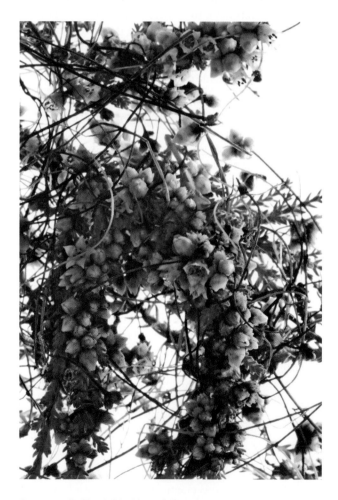

Cuscuta. *(© Frank Blackburn / Alamy)*

crops as flax, **alfalfa**, beans, and potatoes. It also grows on such common ornamentals as English ivy, petunias, dahlias, and chrysanthemums. For medicinal purposes, herbalists prefer *C. epithymum* that grows on thyme.

Cuscuta is a leafless plant with branching stems ranging in thickness from thread-like filaments to heavy cords. The seeds germinate like other seeds. The stems begin to grow and attach themselves to nearby host plants. Once they are firmly attached to a host, the cuscuta root withers away. The mature plant lives its entire life without attachment to the ground. The stems of cuscuta are used in **Western herbalism**, and the seeds are used in **traditional Chinese medicine** (TCM). Cuscuta is used as an individual remedy and in combination with other herbs.

General use

Despite the fact that cuscuta is unpopular with farmers, it has a long history of folk use. In Western herbalism, cuscuta was traditionally used to treat liver, spleen, and gallbladder disorders such as **jaundice**. It was also used to support liver function. It is still used, although rarely, in that way by modern herbalists. It is also a mild laxative. Other traditional Western claims for cuscuta are that it is a mild diuretic and that it can be used to treat **sciatica** and scurvy. Externally, it can be gathered fresh and applied to the skin to treat scrofuladerma. Extracts of the herb have a very bitter taste.

In traditional Chinese medicine, the seeds of cuscuta, called *tu si zi*, have been used for thousands of years. In the Chinese understanding of health, *yin* aspects inside the person and outside in the environment must be kept in balance with *yang* aspects. Ill health occurs when the energies and elements of the body are out of balance or in disharmony with nature. Health is restored by taking herbs and treatments that restore internal and external balance.

According to traditional Chinese healers, cuscuta seeds have a neutral nature and a pungent, sweet taste. They are associated with the liver and kidneys and are used in formulas that help both yin and yang deficiencies, depending on the patient's condition and the other herbs in the formula. Cuscuta was considered both an aphrodisiac and a longevity herb because it slowed down the loss of fluids from the body.

Contemporary Chinese herbalists use cuscuta in formulas to treat a range of conditions, including the following:

- impotence
- premature ejaculation
- sperm leakage
- frequent urination
- ringing in the ears
- lower back pain
- sore knees
- white discharge from the vagina (leucorrhea)
- dry eyes
- blurred vision
- tired eyes

Cuscuta is also used in the Indian system of Ayurvedic healing to treat jaundice, muscle **pain**, coughs, and problems with urination.

Cuscuta in combinations

Cuscuta is one of nine herbs included in the manufacture of two Chinese herbal remedies, Astra Essence and Equiguard. Each contains eight other similar ingredients according to package ingredients listed in 2008.

Astra Essence, a product of Health Concerns, contains the following herbs:

- Herba Epimedii (stem and leaves)
- Fructus Rosae Laevigatae (fruit)
- Fructus Rubi (fruit)
- Fructus Psoraleae (fruit)
- Radix Morindae Officinalis (root)
- Fructus Schisandrae (fruit)
- Fructus Ligustri Lucidi (fruit)
- Semen Cuscutae (seed)
- Radix Astragali (root)

The uses of Astra Essence include a tonic for **infertility**, **impotence**, balanced kidney tonfication, and to reduce the frequency of urination. Other uses are a preventative for **hair loss** and to balance blood glucose in diabetes. The formula is said to help slow **aging** and prevent adverse effects caused by premature aging and the kidney deficiency caused by a fast-paced lifestyle. These include the loss of memory and hearing. Furthermore, Astra Essence is said to help with the side effects of chemotherapy and radiation.

Equiguard, a product of Integrated Chinese Herbal Nutraceuticals, contains the following herbs:

- Herba Epimedii, Fructus
- Rosae Laevigatae
- Fructus Rubi, Fructus
- Psoraleae, Radix
- Morindae Officinalis
- Fructus Schisandrae

- Fructus Schisandrae
- Fructus Ligustri Lucidi
- Semen Cuscutae, Radix
- Astragali, Hydroxypropyl Methylcellulose

Equiguard is marketed as a natural blend of Chinese herbs that helps kidney and prostate disorders. Men age 50 and older may experience prostrate-related difficulties such as difficulty urinating, frequent urination, and discomfort when urinating. Equiguard is said to promote healthy kidney function, support prostate health, and normalize urination, according to the Web site maintained by Equiguard.

Cuscuta research

As of 2008, little scientific research had been performed in the West on cuscuta. A purgative compound had been isolated from the herb, however, that supports its traditional use as a liver and gallbladder tonic. Other research done at Asian universities indicated that cuscuta seeds contain a complex carbohydrate that stimulates the immune system and that it has some antioxidant properties as well. Research into the antioxidant properties of cuscuta included a study described in the April 2007 issue of the *Journal of Ethnopharmacology*. Researchers at Kaohsiung University in Taiwan studied the effect of cuscuta on rats and concluded that data suggested that cuscuta could prevent hepatic (affecting the liver) injuries and that this was probably done through cuscuta's **antioxidant** activities.

Equiguard research

Research performed at New York Medical College indicates that the combination of ingredients in Equiguard may be effective in the treatment of **prostate cancer**. The preparation inhibited the growth of **cancer** cells, increased the rate of self-destruction (apoptosis) of cancer cells, and prevented the surviving cells from forming colonies.

Preparations

In Western herbalism, the entire thread-like stems of cuscuta are used. They are boiled in water along with such herbs as **ginger** and allspice to make a decoction. In Chinese herbalism, only the seeds are used. They are almost always used in combination with other herbs, as in concha marguerita and ligastrum formulas.

Cuscuta is available in capsule and tablet form. Herbal combinations containing cuscuta are also available in tablet and capsule forms. The dosage

KEY TERMS

Antioxidant—An enzyme or other organic substance that is able to counteract the damaging effects of oxidation in living tissue.

Diuretic—Any substance that increases the production of urine.

Sciatica—Pain in the lower back, buttocks, hips, and thigh caused pressure on the sciatic nerve.

Scrofuloderma—Abscesses on the skin associated with tuberculosis and caused by mycobacteria.

Scurvy—A disease caused by the absence of vitamin C in the diet.

Yang aspects—Yang aspects, in nature and in the human body, include such qualities as warmth, activity, light, and forcefulness.

Yin aspects—Yin aspects are the opposite of yang aspects and are represented by such qualities as cold, stillness, darkness, and passivity.

depends on the strength of the remedy and the condition being treated.

Precautions

The United States Food and Drug Administration does not regulate herbal remedies such as cuscuta, which means that the remedies have not proven to be safe or effective. In addition, ingredients are not standardized to comply with federal regulations.

Women who are pregnant, nursing mothers, and children should not take cuscuta as a single herb or in combination products. No special precautions are necessary when cuscuta is used in the doses normally prescribed by herbalists.

Side effects

As of 2008, no side effects had been reported when cuscuta is used in doses prescribed by herbalists.

Interactions

Cuscuta has been used for centuries with other Chinese herbs without any reported interactions. There were no known interactions between cuscuta and Western pharmaceuticals, as of 2008.

Resources

PERIODICALS

Yen, F.L., T. H. Wu, L. T. Lin, C. C. Lin. "Hepatoprotective and Antioxidant Effects of Cuscuta Chinensis Against Acetaminophen-Induced Hepatotoxicity in Rats." *Journal of Ethnopharmacology* (April 2007): 123–128.

OTHER

"Cuscuta epithymum." *Plants for a Future.* http://www.pfaf.org. (February 27, 2008).
Equiguard Online. http://equiguardonline.com. (February 27, 2008).
"Learn About Prostate Cancer." American Cancer Society. http://www.cancer.org/docroot/LRN/LRN_0.asp?dt=36. (February 27, 2008).
"Study Finds Many Prostate Cancer Patients Use Complementary and Alternative Methods." American Cancer Society. http://www.cancer.org/docroot/NWS/content/NWS_1_1x_Many_Prostate_Cancer_Patients_Use_Complementary_and_Alternative_Methods.asp. (February 27, 2008).

ORGANIZATIONS

American Association of Acupuncture and Oriental Medicine, PO Box 162340, Sacramento, CA, 95816, (866) 455-7999, http://www.aaom.org.
American Botanical Council, 6200 Manor Rd., Austin, TX, 78723, (512) 926-4900, http://abc.herbalgram.org.
Herb Research Foundation, 4140 Fifteenth St., Boulder, CO, 80304, (303) 449-2265, http://www.herbs.org.
National Center for Complementary and Alternative Medicine, National Institute of Health (NCCAM), 9000 Rockville Pike, Bethesda, MD, 20892, (888) 644-6226, http://nccam.nih.gov.

Tish Davidson
Rebecca J. Frey, PhD
Liz Swain

Cuts and scratches

Definition

Cuts are **wounds** that break through the skin and sometimes reach the underlying tissue. Scratches are usually superficial wounds where the skin is scraped by a sharp object.

Description

The skin is a barrier between the environment and the rest of the body. Usually it offers protection from the invasion of infective organisms. If the skin is broken by cutting or scratching, there is an increased possibility of infection, along with **pain** and blood

---

KEY TERMS

Ghee—Butter heated to remove the fat, used in Ayurvedic foods and remedies.

Keloids—An excessive overgrowth of collagen scar tissue, often found in young women and African Americans.

Lymph nodes—Structures that form white blood cells and help fight infection in the body.

Poultice—Fresh chopped herbs applied to an injured part of the body, and often covered with a cloth, for healing pains, diseases, and infections.

---

loss. Most cuts and scratches are relatively minor and respond well to home remedies. Deep cuts may require medical help and repairing the skin with stitches to heal properly.

Causes and symptoms

A cut or scratch is often due to an accidental injury or intentional violence. Age-related changes may be a contributing factor, because the skin becomes more thin and fragile with age, and thus, more susceptible to cuts and scratches. Infection is a primary concern in dealing with cuts and scratches. Signs of infection include redness, pain or tenderness, local swelling, warmth, a discharge from the wound site, **fever**, swollen lymph nodes, and red streaks spreading out from the wound site.

Diagnosis

Minor cuts and scratches do not usually require diagnosis. However, if an infection sets in, the wound may need to be assessed by a healthcare provider taking a history of the injury and performing a physical exam.

Treatment

Homeopathic topical preparations can be useful in treating cuts and scratches. Calendula and *Hypericum perforatum* are herbs that can be applied topically as a cream, gel, or ointment. Hypericum 30c can be taken internally, as well. It is particularly indicated if the cut is very painful. Staphysagria 30c is indicated for deep cuts and stab wounds. **Aconite** 30c may be given every 30 minutes for up to three to five doses if a person is very anxious as well as injured.

Ayurvedic medicine recommends several simple applications for minor cuts and scratches. These include fresh **aloe** vera gel, plain ghee, and coconut oil. **Licorice** (*Glycirrhiza glabra*) and **turmeric** (*Curcuma longa*) can be added to any of these to make a paste that will help the skin heal.

Western herbal remedies that promote the healing of cuts and scratches include a strong tea made from *Calendula officinale* flowers, which can be used as a soak or a wash for wounds; distilled **witch hazel** (*Hamamelis virginiana*) which may also stop bleeding; **goldenseal** (*Hydrastis canadesis*) powder or salve, a specific for skin healing; a poultice of crushed **plantain** leaves (*Plantago* spp.); and **comfrey** root salve (*Symphytum officinale*). Raw honey can also be directly applied to help disinfect superficial wounds and to promote healing. *Echinacea* spp. tincture can also be used as a disinfectant or antimicrobial to the affected site. The alcohol in the tincture may cause the wound to sting. Topical applications should not be used on a deep wound until some initial healing has occurred.

According to **aromatherapy**, a spray of diluted **essential oils** can be used as an antiseptic. They may also repair skin damage and encourage new cell growth. Tea tree, **lavender**, **myrrh**, benzoin, bergamot, **chamomile**, tea tree, **eucalyptus**, **juniper**, **rosemary**, helichrysum, eucalyptus, rose geranium, and sandalwood are all appropriate to use on cuts and scratches. About 10 drops of the full-strength oil should be added, singularly or blended, to two ounces of distilled water and one half ounce of goldenseal tincture or alcohol. The essential oil mixture should be shaken well before each use, and it can then be sprayed on two or three times per day.

Vitamins E and A are necessary for the skin to heal well and quickly. These vitamin oils can be squeezed directly from their capsules onto the affected areas several times per day. They can be taken orally, as well, along with a multivitamin containing vitamins A, C, E, and B complex. Healing following an injury is also speeded up by supplementation with the **amino acidsarginine** and glycine. **Bromelain**, the digestive enzyme from pineapple, can be taken between meals as needed to reduce inflammation.

Allopathic treatment

Most cuts and scratches are minor and can be handled at home. A physician should be consulted if:

- The cut is very large or deep.
- There is uncontrolled bleeding.
- There is damage to muscles, nerves, or other deep tissues.

- The wound edges are very jagged or do not seem to join together for healing.
- The wound site is very dirty or contains difficult-to-remove foreign material, such as gravel.
- There is weakness or numbness below the injury.
- The cut is on the face, chest, fingers, genitals, back, stomach, palm of the hand, or over a joint.
- There are signs of infection.
- The lymph nodes become swollen.
- The injured person has a history of diabetes, poor circulation, mitral valve prolapse, an artificial heart valve, or an artificial hip.

A cut or scratch should be washed with a mild soap and water. Tweezers that have been disinfected by washing in hot, soapy water and soaking in rubbing alcohol can be used to remove any dirt, glass, or gravel remaining in the wound. Pressure can be applied directly to wound with clean gauze pad until bleeding has stopped. The wound can be protected while it heals by covering it with an adhesive bandage. The use of an antibiotic or antiseptic ointment is optional. The use of rubbing alcohol and hydrogen peroxide are not recommended for minor cuts and scratches, as they can cause irritation of the wound.

Aspirin, acetaminophen, or nonsteroidal anti-inflammatory drugs (NSAIDs), such as ibuprofen, naproxen, or ketoprofen can be taken to reduce pain. If there is a lot of bleeding, however, aspirin and NSAIDs should be avoided because they may interfere with blood clotting. Keeping the edges of the wound together can help keep dirt out, speeds healing, and decreases scarring. Stitches are helpful in this regard, but they, too, can cause scarring. Butterfly bandages or steri-strips may also be used to keep the wound closed. If a cut is more than 0.5 in (1.25 cm) deep, stitches will usually be needed.

Expected results

Most cuts and scratches are superficial, and heal within a few days. Sometimes keloids form, and these painless scars become gradually less prominent and visible over a period of months to years. Deep cuts may result in permanent decrease in function. Serious damage may also result if an infected wound is left untreated.

Prevention

It is especially easy to get cuts and scratches while working outdoors. Protective clothing and gloves are therefore recommended for any kind of manual labor outside the house. Using a moisturizer on the skin ensures that it will not become dried out. Dry skin is much more susceptible to cuts, scratches, and cracking than moist skin. Care should be taken to avoid accidents in the home. The safety of problem areas should be addressed. For example, hardwood floors and stairs are often slippery, as are loose rugs and broken steps or floorboards. Also, the shower can be a major site of home injuries. Furniture may have to be moved if there are repeated accidents. Overexposure to the sun's rays should be avoided, as it is a major cause of fragile skin leading to injury. In addition, a **tetanus** booster shot is recommended every 10 years.

Resources

BOOKS

Dollemore, Doug and Prevention Health Books for Seniors Staff. *The Doctors Book of Home Remedies for Seniors.* Emmaus, PA: Rodale Press, Inc., 2000.

Kirchheimer, Sid and Prevention Magazine Health Book Editors. *The Doctors Book of Home Remedies II: Over 1,200 New Doctor-Tested Tips and Techniques Anyone Can Use to Heal Hundreds of Everyday Health Problems.* Emmaus, PA: Rodale Press, Inc., 1993.

OTHER

Alternative Medicine.com. http://www.alternativemedicine.com

MotherNature.com. http://www.mothernature.com.

Patience Paradox

Cyanocobalamin *see* **Vitamin B₁₂**

Cymatic therapy

Definition

Cymatic therapy is a form of **sound therapy** that is not applied through hearing, but by instruments that send audible sound waves directly into the body through the skin. This process is said to promote a healing environment in the body. The process may be known as Cymatherapy, which is a trademarked name for an organization that sells instruments and provides cymatic training.

Origins

Sound, particularly in the form of music, drumbeats, or chanting, was used for healing purposes in numerous ancient traditions. The physiological effects of different types of music on blood pressure and other bodily indicators were first noticed during the late 1800s. Eighteenth-century German scientist Ernst Chladni demonstrated the relationship between sound and matter. Chladni, who came to be known as the "Father of Accoustics," discovered that when he moved a violin bow around a plate containing sand that the action caused the grains of sand to form geometric patterns. During the twentieth century, Hans Jenny, a Swiss scientist elaborated on that research.

Jenny studied the effect of sound on metal plates containing material such as sand, liquid, and powder. He discovered that the sound caused the formation of elaborate patterns in the materials. He coined the word "cymatics," deriving it from the Greek word *kyma* (a great wave). Jenny published his findings in a 1967 book titled *Cymatics: A Study of Wave Phenomena & Vibration,* which discussed the structure, dynamics, and effects of sound vibrations and featured photographs of his research on sound patterns. Jenny's book was republished in 2001.

Cymatic therapy was largely developed during the 1960s by Sir Peter Guy Manners, an English medical doctor and osteopath. He believed that everything vibrated to its own frequency and that when a frequency changed, so did its form. Manners maintained that conditions such as illness represented an imbalance in the sound or harmonic frequency of cells. If **cancer** waves affected a kidney, the person could be treated by exposure to the frequency of a healthy kidney. The application of the healthy frequency to the skin over time would restore a healthy balance to the kidney, according to Manners. He created a therapeutic cymatic instrument that was said to emit more than 800 controlled audible frequencies.

Benefits

Practitioners of cymatic therapy believe that sound is capable of rearranging the structure of molecules and, therefore, has unlimited potential as a tool for healing. They claim to have successfully treated otherwise incurable and terminal diseases. At the same time, they acknowledge that some patients seem to be unaffected by sound therapy. The treatment has been used on patients with tumors, internal **bruises**, calcified joints, bacterial or viral **infections**, blood diseases, and other problems.

Description

Sound consists of mechanical vibrations that travel through a medium such as air, water, or in the case of cymatic therapy, the body. Sound healers believe that all parts of the body vibrate and thus produce sound, either at a healthy, harmonious frequency, or at an inharmonious, unhealthy frequency. Using a computerized instrument, cymatic therapists direct healing frequencies into the body to restore resonance and harmony. The healing frequencies are related to those emitted by a healthy organ or body part. In this way, cymatic healers say, the immune system and other natural regulatory functions are stimulated. Frequencies may be applied directly or transmitted along **acupuncture** meridians.

Cymatic therapy does not directly heal, practitioners say. Rather, it creates a near-optimal environment for organs or cells. In such an environment, they say, the body can heal itself without drugs or surgical intervention. The therapy may also be delivered without such equipment, with the use of instruments such as tuning forks.

Products marketed by Cymatherapy in February 2008 included the Cyma 1000, an instrument registered with the United States Food and Drug Administration (FDA) as a therapeutic massager. The instrument was described as "an electrically powered device intended for medical purposes, such as to relieve minor muscle aches and pains," according to the registration that was revised on April 1, 2006. The registration as a Class 1 Device did not mean that the product was approved by the FDA, only that the registration was filed with the federal agency.

The Cyma 1000 is marketed on the Cymatherapy Web site as "simply an acoustic massager that emits relaxing tones" and not a product "intended to diagnose, treat, cure, or prevent any disease." The machine provided more than 500 "commuations (harmonious combinations of five frequencies)." It sold for $9,950 in 2008.

Precautions

Patients with cardiac pacemakers are advised to avoid this therapy. Because of the controversial nature of cymatic treatment, people with pre-existing medical conditions should consult a physician before beginning cymatic therapy treatment.

The FDA does not approve Class 1 devices such as cymatic therapy instruments, which means the instruments have not been rigorously tested for safety and effectiveness. In addition, the American Cancer Society cautioned that claims that sound waves could promote a healing environment were not scientifically proven. The society warned people not to rely solely on cymatic therapy or delay seeking conventional treatment for cancer.

Side effects

Cymatic therapy was thought to be generally free of adverse side effects, as of February 2008.

Research and general acceptance

The variability with which different body tissues absorb and reflect sound is universally acknowledged. It is this variability that makes ultrasound scanning a useful form of medical imaging. However, few physicians are convinced that healing can be facilitated by tuning a sound device to a patient's cellular vibrations. Hence, medical doctors tend to be highly skeptical about cymatic therapy. There were no large studies of the effectiveness of cymatic therapy as of February 2008.

Training and certification

Cymatic devices are used by a variety of alternative practitioners, including osteopaths, acupuncturists, and chiropractors. Specific training is needed to operate the machines. This can be obtained through books, tapes, seminars, and correspondence courses. In most jurisdictions, the field is unregulated and patients must, therefore, take care to ensure the competence of their healer.

Cymatherapy offered a certification course that consisted of 200 credit hours and cost $2,000 in February 2008, according to the Web site. Training as a certified cymatherapist included 182 hours of course credit and a three-day workshop. The topics studied included anatomy, psychology, and technology of sound (cymatics).

Resources

OTHER

"Cymatic Therapy." American Cancer Society, March 26, 2007. http://www.cancer.org/docroot/ETO/content/ETO_5_3X_Cymatic_Therapy.asp?sitearea=ETO. (February 26, 2008).

Manners, Peter Guy. "Vibrational Therapy." http://www.soundhealersassociation.org/sha/peter_guy_manners.html. (February 28, 2008).

ORGANIZATIONS

Cymatherapy International, (866) 909-0099, http://cymatherapy.com.

Sound Healers Association, PO Box 2240, Boulder, CO, (800) 246-9764, http://www.soundhealersassociation.org.

David Helwig
Liz Swain

Cyperus

Description

Cyperus refers to a family of marsh-dwelling grass-like plants known as sedges. Perhaps the best-known member of this family is the reed, which ancient Egyptians used to make papyrus. However, many other members of this family have proven useful as food and medicine. *Cyperus articulatus* and *Cyperus rotundus* are the two species most often associated with healing.

C. articulatus, also called adrue or Guinea rush, is a tall sedge that mainly grows in Jamaica, Turkey, and along the Nile River in Egypt. The medicinal part of the plant is its root or tuber. This part is blackish in color and shaped like a top. Tubers are usually about 0.7–1 in (1.1–2.5 cm) long and about 0.5–0.7 in (1.3–1.7 cm) in diameter. The tubers may be connected in groups of two or three by underground stems. They are harvested and dried for healing. The herb is bitter in taste and aromatic, similar to **lavender**.

C. rotundus is used primarily in Asia and Africa, but it also grows in Australia, Europe, and North America. It is an invasive plant that grows in low, damp places near water. Like *C. articulatus*, the tuber is the part of the plant used in healing. Its Chinese name is *xiang fu*, and it has been used in **traditional Chinese medicine** for thousands of years. *C. rotundus* is also called tiririca, nutsedge, nutgrass, musta, mutha, and a host of other local names.

General use

C. articulatus is used mainly for digestive disorders. It is an antiemetic, meaning that it suppresses **vomiting**. This is useful in reducing the symptoms of **morning sickness** during **pregnancy**. Because it gives the body a general feeling of warmth, *C. articulatus* is sometimes used as a sedative, generally in connection with suppressing **nausea**. Cyperus is also used to relieve **gas** in the stomach and intestines. In the Peruvian Amazon, native people use the herb to treat infection, and in Africa it is used to treat **epilepsy**.

There are few scientific studies of *C. articulatus*. An Argentinean study conducted in 1995 looked at the bacteria-killing properties of the herb. It concluded that decoctions of *C. articulatus* completely inhibited the growth of one species of *Staphylococcus* bacteria and partially inhibited the growth in one species of *Pseudominas* bacteria. Both of these bacteria **strains** are capable of causing severe, and sometimes fatal, **infections**. It was ineffective in tests against five other infection-causing organisms.

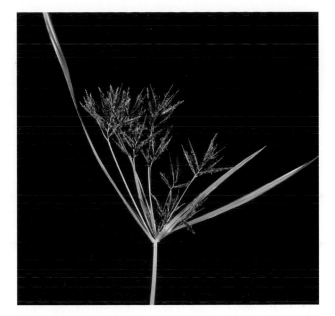

Cyperus rotundis flower spike. *(Nigel Cattlin / Photo Researchers, Inc.)*

Another study published in the *Journal of Ethnopharmacology* in 1996 by Swiss investigators found that extracts of *C. articulatus* reduced certain types of spontaneous neuron firings in the brains of rats. These scientists suggested that this suppression might be the basis for the effectiveness of *C. articulatus* in treating **headache** and epilepsy. In the early 2000s, no studies on *C. articulatus* were published in scholarly, peer-reviewed journals.

C. rotundus is used in Chinese medicine and Japanese Kampo formulations. It is rarely used alone and can be found in formulas that relieve **pain**, especially pain associated with **menstruation**. It is also used in formulas for stomachache and **diarrhea**, to improve menstrual function, to treat **impotence** or heighten sexual potency, to treat bacterial infections, dry or tired eyes, and in tonics for general wellness. In other Asian and African countries, *C. rotundus* is also used as a diuretic and to treat high blood pressure. It is also spread on the skin as a bactericide and a fungicide to prevent infection of **wounds**. A study published in 2007 supported the idea that *C. rotundus* has antibacterial properties. Researchers found that an extract of *C. rotundus* substantially reduced the growth of *Streptococcus mutans*, a bacteria responsible for the formation of dental plaque and tooth decay (dental caries).

Preparations

C. articulatus is usually prepared as a decoction or liquid extract to be taken internally. *C. rotundus* may

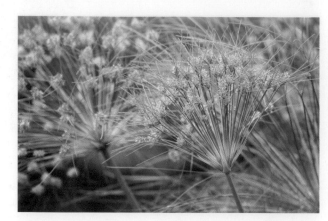

Cyperus. *(© blickwinkel / Alamy)*

be prepared two different ways. It can be boiled to make a liquid to be mixed with other herbs. The tubers can also be ground into a paste with or without other herbs. The paste can either be formed into pills to be taken internally or applied externally to wounds or skin **rashes**. This paste is also sometimes applied directly to the temples to treat headaches.

Precautions

As of early 2008, no particular precautions had been reported as being necessary in using cyperus.

Side effects

As of the early 2000s, no side effects had been reported in using cyperus. This herb has a long tradition of folk use, but its effects on humans had not been studied in any structured way.

Interactions

Cyperus is often used in conjunction with other herbs in Chinese formulations with no reported interactions. Cyperus is, however, reported to be mixed with hallucinogenic plants by certain tribes living in the Brazilian rain forest, in order to prolong the action of the hallucinogens. As of 2008, there were no studies of interactions between cyperus and standard Western pharmaceuticals. One Korean report on several compounds isolated from cyperus, however, indicated that it inhibits the action of benzodiazepine tranquilizers and modifies the effectiveness of several neurotransmitters in the central nervous system.

Resources

BOOKS

Chevallier, Andrew. *Herbal Remedies.* New York: DK Publishing, 2007.

Foster, Steven, and Rebecca Johnson. *National Geographic Desk Reference to Nature's Medicine.* Washington, DC: National Geographic Society, 2006.

PDR for Herbal Medicines, 4th ed. Montvale, NJ: Thomson Healthcare, 2007.

PERIODICALS

Yu, H. H., D. H. Lee, S. J. Seo, and Y. O. You. "Anticariogenic Properties of the Extract of *Cyperus rotundus.*" *American Journal of Chinese Medicine.* 35 no. 3 (2007): 497–505.

OTHER

Dharmananda, Subhuti. "Cyperus: Primary Qi Regulating Herb of Chinese Medicine." Institute for Traditional Medicine, March 2005. http://www.itmonline.org/arts/cyperus.htm (February 10, 2008).

ORGANIZATIONS

Alternative Medicine Foundation, PO Box 60016, Potomac, MD, 20859, (301) 340-1960, http://www.amfoundation.org.

American Association of Oriental Medicine, PO Box 162340, Sacramento, CA, 95816, (866) 455-7999 or (914) 443-4770, http://www.aaaomonline.org.

Centre for International Ethnomedicinal Education and Research (CIEER), http://www.cieer.org.

Tish Davidson, A. M.
Rebecca J. Frey